PENGUIN BOOKS

MEDICAL TREATMENTS: THE BENEFITS AND RISKS

Peter Parish is a Professor Emeritus of the University of Wales. He has had a distinguished career as a professor and physician and is recognized nationally and internationally for his valuable contributions to our knowledge and understanding of the prescribing and use of drugs.

MEDICAL TREATMENTS

THE BENEFITS AND RISKS

PETER PARISH, MD

PENGUIN BOOKS

PENGUIN BOOKS

Published by the Penguin Group
Penguin Books Ltd, 27 Wrights Lane, London W8 5TZ, England
Viking Penguin, a division of Penguin Books USA Inc.
375 Hudson Street, New York, New York 10014, USA
Penguin Books Australia Ltd, Ringwood, Victoria, Australia
Penguin Books Canada Ltd, 2801 John Street, Markham, Ontario, Canada L3R 1B4
Penguin Books (NZ) Ltd, 182–190 Wairau Road, Auckland 10, New Zealand

Penguin Books Ltd, Registered Offices: Harmondsworth, Middlesex, England

First published 1991
1 3 5 7 9 10 8 6 4 2

Printed in England by Clays Ltd, St Ives plc
Filmset in Monophoto Photina

This book is dedicated to Dr Jim Struthers who, as a Principal Medical Officer at the Ministry of Health in the sixties, was instrumental in my obtaining a major research grant from government to study the prescribing of drugs by general practitioners. That support set me off on a twenty-year research career studying the prescibing and use of drugs. Throughout those years Jim Struthers acted as my mentor and friend.

Contents

Introduction xi

1 The benefits and risks of drug treatments 1
2 The autonomic nervous system 9
3 Colds 32
4 Coughs 45
5 Throat infections and laryngitis 54
6 Disorders of the ears 61
7 Disorders of the nose 67
8 Sinusitis and catarrh 72
9 The immune system 75
10 Allergies 88
11 Immunizations 108
12 Asthma 143
13 Disorders of the mouth 169
14 Nausea, vomiting, motion sickness and vertigo 175
15 Indigestion and peptic ulcers 187
16 Diarrhoea 214
17 Constipation 232
18 Haemorrhoids (piles) and other disorders of the anus 245
19 Disorders of the gall bladder 250
20 Angina 253
21 Raised blood pressure (hypertension) 281
22 Heart failure 315
23 Disorders of heart rhythm and rate 337
24 Disorders of the circulation 352
25 Deposits of cholesterol and fats in arteries (atherosclerosis) 366
26 Bleeding disorders and thrombosis 379
27 Pain 400
28 Local anaesthetics 423
29 Migraine 428
30 Rheumatoid arthritis 439
31 Osteoarthritis, chronic back pain and Paget's disease 464
32 Gout 472
33 Disorders of the urinary tract 484
34 Sexually transmitted diseases 503

35 Eye diseases 521
36 Parkinson's disease and parkinsonism 543
37 Epilepsy 558
38 Sleep disorders 572
39 Depression 584
40 Anxiety 604
41 Schizophrenia and other serious mental illnesses 626
42 Stimulants 638
43 Slimming 646
44 Tonics 654
45 Vitamins 659
46 Minerals 686
47 Anaemias 704
48 Anti-bacterial drugs – antibiotics 726
49 Penicillins 735
50 Cephalosporins 746
51 Tetracyclines 750
52 Aminoglycosides 754
53 Other anti-bacterial drugs 758
54 Sulphonamides and trimethoprim 766
55 Tuberculosis 772
56 Fungal infections 779
57 Viral infections 788
58 Malaria 796
59 Some parasitic infections (including worms) 804
60 The pituitary gland 819
61 The adrenal glands 827
62 Corticosteroids 832
63 Thyroid disorders 846
64 Disorders of the parathyroid glands 859
65 Diabetes 861
66 Female sex hormones 887
67 Oral contraceptive drugs 902
68 Menstrual problems, menopause, osteoporosis and hormone replacement therapy 919
69 Infertility 942
70 Vaginal and vulval conditions 946
71 Abortion, labour and childbirth 951
72 Male sex hormones 955
73 Anabolic steroids 961
74 Drugs and sex 967
75 Skin diseases 976
76 Cancer 1052

77 How to use drug treatments effectively and safely 1068
78 Some harmful drug effects and what to do if you develop them 1078
79 Pregnancy and the risks of drug treatments 1116
80 Breast feeding and the risks of drug treatments 1129
81 Babies, infants and children, and the risks of drug treatments 1134
82 Elderly people and the risks of drug treatments 1136
83 Liver disease and the risks of drug treatments 1141
84 Kidney disease and the risks of drug treatments 1159
85 Inherited abnormalities and the risks of drug treatments 1178
86 Stomas and the risks of drug treatments 1180
87 Risks of drug treatments in people who drink alcohol 1183
88 Risks of drug treatments in people who drive 1186
89 Risks of one drug reacting with another drug (drug–drug interaction) 1188
Appendix 1 Generic prescription drugs and their brand names 1243
Appendix 2 Update 1263
Index 1275

Introduction

Thanks to research-based drug companies we have a wide range of safe and effective drugs of quality to treat and to prevent disease. If used responsibly, the benefits of these drugs far outweigh any possible risks. Nevertheless, different people may react differently to any one drug and therefore no drug is 100 per cent safe in all of us. Because of this potential for risk in some of us, any drug treatment should always be tailored to our individual needs and responses, particularly in those of us who may be more vulnerable to the effects of a drug than others; for example, unborn babies, babies and infants, elderly people, and people who suffer from liver or kidney disease.

Drug treatments may produce unwanted and sometimes harmful effects as well as beneficial effects. Fortunately, most harmful effects produced by drugs are mild and merely unpleasant and can easily be avoided by reducing the dose of the drug, by stopping drug treatment or by changing to another drug. Very occasionally, some drugs may produce serious harmful effects but even the frequency of these can be reduced if those drugs that are known to produce such harmful effects are used with caution, particularly in vulnerable people.

In general, the safety of drug treatments depends upon how safely drugs are used, and this demands knowledge of the disorder being treated, knowledge of the drugs that are available for treating that particular disorder and, above all, knowledge of the individual who is being treated. I have therefore written this book in order to share some of this knowledge with you, the reader, because I believe that if we have knowledge of ourselves and our disorder and of available drug treatments we should be able to ensure that we get maximum benefits from any drug treatment that we may take. I hope it will also be of value to doctors, nurses and other health care workers.

In medical books mild harmful effects from drugs are usually referred to as *side effects* to differentiate them from more rare and serious harmful effects, which are referred to as *adverse effects*. However, in this book I refer to all unwanted effects as *harmful effects*, whether they are very mild and occur commonly or are serious and occur very rarely. This is in order to avoid any confusion and to warn you that although the benefits of drug treatments generally outweigh the risks, they none the less have a potential for harm.

To make the book as up to date as possible, Appendix 2 has been added at proof stage. It contains additional information that became available before going to press. Wherever you see the symbol (U) in the book, please refer also to Appendix 2 – Update.

Peter Parish MD
Swansea, 1990

1

The benefits and risks of drug treatments

Drugs are used for many purposes; for example, to cure disease (e.g. the use of antibiotics to treat bacterial infections), to relieve symptoms (e.g. pain, nausea, vomiting), to change the natural progression of a disease (e.g. the drug treatment of raised blood pressure), to suppress symptoms and change the progression of a disease (e.g. asthma, epilepsy), to provide replacement for an underlying deficiency (e.g. hormone replacement treatment in thyroid disease, insulin in diabetes), to suppress symptoms without altering the progression of the underlying disease (e.g. the use of anti-inflammatory drugs to relieve the pain, swelling and stiffness of joints in rheumatoid arthritis), to produce an altered state of mind (e.g. anti-anxiety drugs, anti-depressant drugs), and to produce an altered state of consciousness (e.g. sleeping drugs, general anaesthetics). Drugs are also used to prevent disease (e.g. vaccinations), to diagnose disease, to prevent conception, to procure an abortion and to assist childbirth.

The many uses of drugs provide substantial benefits in terms of relief of suffering and the prevention of illness and death. However, these benefits have to be balanced against the risks of producing harmful effects, because no drug is totally safe in all people. When it comes down to treating individuals, the expected benefits have to be balanced against the risks of using a particular drug to treat a particular disorder in that person. This is because different individuals and different disorders may respond differently to the same drug (see later). Therefore, it is important to remember that no drug is without the potential for producing harmful effects in some individuals and the potential risks of using a drug must always be recognized. We must not expect drugs to be totally safe, and we must be aware that drugs may *produce* suffering and deaths as well as *relieving* suffering and preventing deaths.

There are two main factors that balance the benefits and risks of drug use in each individual. The first is the quality, safety and effectiveness of the *drug* to be used, and the second is the appropriate and safe *use* of that drug in the person being treated.

The quality, safety and efficacy of a drug are principally in the hands of the manufacturer of that drug who has to meet stringent government regulations. The appropriate and safe use of a drug are in the hands of those who prescribe (doctors), dispense (pharmacists) and administer it. The last (the administration of a drug) is usually in the hands of the individual who self-administers the drug; however, in hospital it is the nursing staff who are responsible.

Suffering and deaths caused by drugs (and other treatments) are referred to as iatrogenic diseases (diseases caused by doctors). Those caused by drugs obviously make a contribution to our overall suffering but to what extent we will never know because of the problems involved in recognizing, reporting and confirming that a particular disorder or death was caused by a particular drug. However, iatrogenic disease is a well recognized hazard of drug treatment – just think how many people are addicted to benzodiazepine sleeping drugs and tranquillizers and how many elderly people develop serious harmful effects from anti-rheumatic drugs.

Studying the benefits and risks of drug treatments

Because drug treatments are always a balance of benefits to risks, drugs are carefully tested in animals and then in humans before they become available for general use. However, the testing of drugs in animals is of limited value in predicting the benefits and risks in humans, let alone in individual people suffering from disease. In the end the benefits and risks of a drug must always be assessed in the person suffering from the disorder which the drug is supposed to benefit.

The testing of a drug in humans is usually carried out in four phases. In phase 1, tests are carried out on a small number of healthy human volunteers in order to assess how the body deals with the drug in terms of its absorption from the intestine, its distribution around the body, its breakdown and its excretion from the body. In phase 2, the drug is tested in a few hundred patients suffering from the disease to be treated and then if these results are promising in terms of benefits against risks the drug is tested in several hundred patients (phase 3) in order to further evaluate its benefits and risks. If these results are satisfactory it is then approved for general marketing to doctors, which is followed by a period of surveillance of the benefits and risks in several thousand patients (phase 4).

The need for a scientific approach

To study the benefits and risks of using a particular drug to treat a particular disorder it is necessary to be as scientific as possible. This is because there are many factors other than the drug treatment which may influence a person's response to treatment. People may feel better for many reasons other than the fact that they took the drug. Much improvement is often 'in the mind' because the individual believes the drug will do some good and because he/she believes in the doctor. Also doctors may influence a patient's 'improvement' by their enthusiasm and their own belief in the drug and their wish to try something new. Therefore, if we are to assess the benefits and risks of a drug we need more than the subjective opinions of the patients and the doctors. We need to eliminate this bias and to make the study as objective as possible. In other words, we need to eliminate (or control) as many of those factors as possible that may influence the response of the patients and doctors, because we need to know whether or not it is the drug itself that produces benefits.

Factors that may affect a patient's response to drug treatment other than those produced by the actions of the drug in the body are often referred to as *non-drug* factors. We therefore design studies that attempt to control these non-drug factors, and there are several ways of doing this. One of the most effective ways is to study a number of patients who receive the drug treatment and to compare their responses with the responses of an equal number of patients who do not receive the drug treatment or who receive an alternative treatment. To eliminate bias we also need to make sure that patients are selected randomly 'for treatment' or 'no treatment', that is without the doctor or anyone else making a choice. It is also important that the patients are drawn from equivalent groups of patients so that the two groups do not differ in terms of their age, sex, race, duration and severity of the disease, etc. The two groups should also be treated during the same period of time and in the same type of facility in order to control for any factors in time (e.g. seasons) or place (e.g. hospital or general practice). The results of the studies are collected and subjected to statistical analysis in order to determine whether the benefits in the treated group were significantly better than those experienced by the untreated group. These studies are referred to as *randomized controlled trials* because the patients are selected randomly for treatment or non-treatment and they are designed to control for non-drug factors.

Another method of studying the benefits and risks of a drug is to test the 'active' drug against a 'dummy' drug (placebo) that has the same shape, colour and taste. If the patient does not know whether he is receiving the active drug or the dummy drug we call it a 'single-blind' trial, and if neither the patient nor the doctor knows we call it a 'double-blind' trial. The latter is an important way of studying a drug because it eliminates the bias of both the patient and the doctor. The active drug and the dummy drug are secretly coded (usually known only to the pharmacist) so that the doctor and patient do not know which is which. Patients are then randomly allocated to treatments with the dummy or the active drug. Sometimes the patient may have a course of the dummy drug followed by a course of the active drug and vice versa. The patients' responses are recorded by the doctor and the results from each doctor are then collected and subjected to statistical analysis to test whether there was any difference in response between those patients treated with the active drug and those treated with the dummy drug and to assess whether any improvement on the active drug was actually due to the drug or whether it could have occurred purely by chance.

When there is already an effective drug on the market for treating a disorder, it may be quite unethical to test a new drug against a dummy. In these cases the new active drug is compared with the known effective drug and the results are analysed; this avoids the patients having to be given dummy tablets.

The need for a personal approach

The above has been a very sketchy description of some of the techniques used to study the benefits and risks of a drug. They are very valuable and ensure that doctors have access to effective drugs of quality. However, having obtained access to quality drugs that have been shown to be effective, doctors and patients must then use them appropriately and safely. To ensure the appropriate and safe use of a drug, the treatment of an individual should be tailored to his particular needs, having taken into consideration the various physical, mental, social and environmental factors that may influence him, his disease and his response to treatment. In other words, if drug treatments are to be *effective* in practice, not only must they be based on scientific studies of their benefits and risks, they must also be based upon what is appropriate for each individual being treated and upon how each individual responds to treatment.

Risks of drug treatments

The testing of a new drug in animals before it is tried in humans will not completely predict its potential harmful effects in humans. Equally, the testing of a drug in healthy human volunteers and then in groups of patients (clinical trials) will not completely predict its potential harmful effects in other individuals. Nor will any of these tests be able to predict completely what harmful effects may develop when a patient uses a drug over a prolonged period of time. *The hard fact of life is that we must learn about most of the risks of drugs through using them in everyday practice.* In the end we learn about the harmful effects of drugs through using them and because some individuals develop harmful effects and some die. This is a painful way to learn but, as I keep repeating, any drug treatment is always a balance of benefits to risks in the individual being treated.

Lack of information

Unfortunately, and despite the sacrifice made by those who experience harmful effects from drugs, our knowledge of the extent and nature of harmful effects caused by drugs is inadequate because of difficulties in recognizing, reporting and confirming such events. It is often very difficult to prove that a certain drug caused a certain harmful effect. This is because patients are often taking several drugs at the same time and often have several things wrong with them. This is particularly true in elderly people who may be taking three, four or more different drug treatments at any one time. In addition, a patient taking prescribed drugs may also be taking other drugs that have been purchased without a prescription.

With drugs that have been on the market for years we have accumulated useful information over time, and doctors are informed about their harmful effects by the drug companies and by government. However, with new drugs we have to learn about their harmful effects day by day, and their benefits and risks need careful monitoring.

Since we learn about the benefits and risks of drugs through use, every medical 'event' we experience while on a new drug should be reported to our doctor; it does not matter whether it is a headache and dizziness or a skin rash – any *new* symptom or problem should be reported. Your doctor should then report the event to the Medicines Control Agency (MCA) because it will only be by collecting such information on a sufficient number of patients over time that we will get an early warning that a new drug is beginning to cause problems. This process is called post-market surveillance.

NOTE Doctors are advised on which new drugs to watch out for – they are marked with a ▲ in the British National Formulary and publications provided by drug companies (MIMS and ABPI Data Sheet Compendium). Doctors are asked to report any harmful or any unexpected event, however minor, which could possibly be caused by the drug. They are asked to make reports to the MCA even if they are uncertain whether the new drug caused the problem, whether or not the 'event' is well recognized, and also if other drugs have been given to the patient at the same time.

The need to monitor patients taking drug treatments

Because any drug treatment is always a balance of benefits to risks, each patient should always be assessed before treatment starts and at regular intervals during treatment. This is because any disorder in a particular individual is always in a state of change and what may seem appropriate treatment today may not be appropriate in a few weeks' time.

If you are on any long-term drug treatment you should consult your doctor at regular intervals and not just pick up a repeat prescription month after month. By seeing the doctor each time it will make it easier for your doctor to look out for any developing harmful effects from the drug and to decide whether you really need to continue taking the drug, whether the dose should be changed or whether an alternative drug may be of more benefit to you. He or she will also be able to carry out any special tests that may be necessary; for example, blood tests and tests of kidney and liver function.

We shall learn about the harmful effects of drugs only if we report any new symptom to our doctor and if doctors regularly check their patients for harmful effects and report them to the MCA when appropriate. An important step in helping to determine the extent and nature of harmful effects from drugs is for all patients who develop a new symptom to ask themselves 'could this be caused by any drug I am taking?' and for all doctors who see a patient with a new symptom to ask themselves 'could this be due to any drug treatment I am prescribing?'

Variations between individuals

In any individual, the development of harmful effects from drugs will depend upon many factors such as age, sex, nutritional state, diet, general physical and mental health, the disease or diseases being treated, genetic characteristics and the presence or absence of other diseases.

When considering the risks of taking drugs it is therefore important to remember that different people react differently – one man's meat is another man's poison! The same dose of a drug may produce differing responses in different individuals, and different doses of a drug may be needed to produce a similar response in different people. This is another argument against the use of standard doses and standard treatments – it is an argument for the individualization of treatments.

Inappropriate use increases risks

The responsible use of drugs should ensure that a patient is treated with a drug only when it is expected to produce more benefits than risks. The drug should then be used in the right dose, at the right intervals of time and for the right duration of time. Unfortunately, some harmful effects occur because drug treatments are used when they should not be used – sometimes no treatment is better and safer for the patient. In addition, drug treatments may not be used properly; for example, the dose may be inappropriate (too large for that patient with that disorder; e.g. elderly patients) or the drug may be prescribed at too frequent intervals throughout the day which may cause the drug to accumulate in the body to reach toxic levels and produce harmful effects. The long-term use of certain drugs may also cause harmful effects; e.g., addiction to sleeping drugs and benzodiazepine tranquillizers.

Dose-related harmful effects

Most of the commonly occurring harmful effects caused by drugs are due to an exaggerated response. They are usually related to the doses used and are easily controlled by reducing the dose. They are referred to as dose-related harmful effects and account for most of the harmful effects listed in this book.

Some of us are more sensitive to drugs than others

Some of us may be very sensitive (over-sensitive) to the effects of certain drugs. We develop an exaggerated response; for example, most anti-histamines produce some drowsiness in most of us but some people can become very drowsy and sleepy. You may also get opposite effects in some people; for example, if most of us take a tranquillizer we will feel calm but some people may become over-excited and restless – this is called a *paradoxical effect*.

Not only may some people be more sensitive to some drugs than others but also, within an individual, some organs and tissues in the body may be more sensitive than others to the effects of a drug. It may therefore be helpful to remind you that a drug acts like shot from a shotgun – some shot lands on target but the rest does not. Likewise a drug not only acts on the target tissues or organs (e.g. the heart) but it also acts on many other tissues and organs in the body, some of which may be very sensitive; for example, we may get blurred vision from a drug taken to relieve stomach pains or wheezing from a drug taken to relieve angina.

Harmful drug effects may be caused by how the body deals with drugs

Harmful effects from drugs are determined by how the body deals with a drug once it has entered the body; for example, harmful effects from certain drugs may be more frequent and severe if you have liver or kidney disease, heart disease or a disorder of the circulation. The liver and kidneys are particularly important because the liver plays a principal role in breaking down drugs and the kidneys play a principal role in eliminating drugs from the body.

The effectiveness of the liver in breaking down drugs varies between individuals and between drugs. Some individuals break down drugs more slowly than other people, and the level of a drug in the bloodstream may increase to reach toxic levels and produce harmful effects. These people run a greater risk of developing harmful effects on standard doses than those who break the drug down at a 'normal' rate – they need to be given smaller daily dosages. Likewise, any impairment of kidney function will cause the concentration of a drug which is normally excreted by the kidney to rise in the bloodstream to reach toxic levels and produce harmful effects. This is a particular risk in elderly people whose kidney function may be impaired – they too will need smaller dosages.

Liver disease and harmful drug effects are discussed in Chapter 83.

Kidney disease and harmful drug effects are discussed in Chapter 84.

Serious and unexpected harmful effects

Some harmful effects of drugs are not simply an exaggeration of their normal effects which can be reduced or stopped by reducing the dose of the drug. These harmful effects are *unexpected* and often cannot be predicted although we learn about them over time. They include allergic reactions, blood disorders, bleeding disorders, kidney damage, liver damage, effects on the brain and nervous system, effects on the eyes, skin rashes and effects on fertility. These serious and unexpected harmful effects are very rare but some of them may be fatal.

The most common causes of serious and unexpected harmful effects from drugs are due to factors in the individual. These may be genetic or they may be due to extremes of age, for example old age or infancy. They may be due to impaired liver or kidney function, heart disease and chest disease or to a predisposition to allergic reactions. An unborn baby may be damaged by a drug its mother takes during pregnancy and a breast-fed baby may develop harmful effects from drugs taken by his breast-feeding mother and excreted into the milk.

2

The autonomic nervous system

The nervous system (the brain, spinal cord and nerves supplying all tissues and organs) can roughly be divided into voluntary and involuntary systems. The voluntary part of our nervous system (the somatic nervous system) is largely under our control and maintains our communications with the external environment – it has a sensory division that responds to sensations (e.g. pain, temperature, touch, sight, hearing, smell, etc.) and a motor division that controls movements.

The involuntary nervous system is self-governing (autonomous) and is therefore known as the autonomic nervous system. It serves mainly to regulate the functions of internal organs, to adjust their response to changing needs and therefore to maintain the status quo of the internal environment of the body. Most of these activities cannot be voluntarily controlled.

The autonomic nervous system is responsible for controlling the functions of many organs; for example, the heart and circulation; stomach and intestines, lungs and breathing tubes, sweat glands, bladder, eyes and sexual organs. The system is principally involved in what are called reflex arcs – automatic responses.

These automatic (reflex) responses occur because nerve receptors in the autonomic nervous system are programmed to respond reflexly to all kinds of stimulations – pain, stretching, chemicals, pressure, etc. Any such stimulation will immediately fire off a local or general response, causing contraction of the muscles in the different organs (blood vessels, eyes, lungs, stomach, intestine, bladder, genitals, etc.) and in addition produce changes in the functioning of the heart and changes in various glands in the body. A good example of these automatic reflexes which you can easily see for yourself is obtained by shining a light in someone's eyes: the muscles in the iris of each eye contract immediately to constrict the pupils. Simple reflexes occur within the organ itself, whereas complex ones are referred automatically to the brain.

The control centre in the brain (the hypothalamus)

In the brain there is a centre that is responsible for controlling the whole of the autonomic nervous system; it is called the hypothalamus. This centre also controls certain other divisions of the nervous system and the glandular system (endocrine system) of the body.

The hypothalamus is the most important organ for controlling the internal environment of the body. It controls the body's temperature, water and salt balance and hormone production (it controls the master gland, the pituitary). It also prepares the body for 'fight or flight' in response to stress or fear (the alarm reaction or defensive reaction), exercises control over nutrition by controlling the blood supply to the stomach and intestine, and controls sexual behaviour and activities, including regulation of pregnancy.

Overall control and integration of the autonomic nervous system with other systems take place at a higher level in the cortex of the brain.

Divisions of the autonomic nervous system in the body

The autonomic nervous system outside of the brain is organized into two divisions which are structurally and functionally different. These two parts are known as the *sympathetic* and the *parasympathetic* divisions.

The sympathetic division

As the nerves of the sympathetic division leave the spinal cord they enter small 'switchboxes' (ganglia) which are located along side the spine in the neck and abdomen. The nerves leading into these ganglia are called pre-ganglionic nerves and the ones that leave them to supply the organs of the body are called post-ganglionic nerves. About 20 post-ganglionic nerve fibres leave each ganglion (switchbox) for every one pre-ganglionic nerve fibre that enters it.

The chemical messenger (neurotransmitter) that transmits nervous impulses within the ganglia is acetylcholine – it transmits messages from the pre-ganglionic nerves coming out of the spinal cord to the post-ganglionic nerves that supply the organs. The neurotransmitter in the sympathetic division that transmits messages from the post-ganglionic nerve fibres to the nerve receptors in organs is noradrenaline (known as norepinephrine in the USA).

noradrenaline at their nerve endings) and parasympathetic nerve fibres (that use acetylcholine at their nerve endings). The results will therefore be mixed. These effects will be in addition to the stimulating effects of acetylcholine at the nerve/muscle junction in skeletal muscles, its direct effects on arteries in skeletal muscles, and its effects on the brain and adrenal medulla.

Physostigmine is an example of an anticholinesterase drug. It is used to cause constriction of the pupil in the treatment of glaucoma and to treat the harmful effects on the brain of drugs that block the effects of acetylcholine (see below).

Neostigmine is an anticholinesterase drug which also stimulates acetylcholine receptors. It is used to stimulate the bowels and bladder after surgery. It is also used to treat myasthenia gravis, which is a disease that affects the muscles and is due to an impaired conduction of nervous impulses from the nerves to the muscles, producing excessive muscle weakness and fatigue. The disease is due to an abnormal immune response in the body (auto-immune disease) in which are formed antibodies that block acetylcholine receptors. The abnormal production of antibodies is caused by a disorder of the thymus gland.

Pyridostigmine, distigmine and ambenonium produce effects similar to those produced by neostigmine but they are longer acting. Edrophonium is related to neostigmine but its effects wear off rapidly; it is used to diagnose myasthenia gravis.

Drugs that aggravate myasthenia gravis

Drugs that may make myasthenia gravis worse or cause symptoms like myasthenia gravis include aminoglycoside antibiotics (e.g. gentamicin, kanamycin, neomycin, streptomycin), some beta blockers (e.g. propranolol); phenytoin and lithium. Penicillamine, used to treat rheumatoid arthritis, may actually stimulate the production of antibodies to block acetylcholine receptors and produce a syndrome just like myasthenia gravis; most patients recover when the drug is stopped.

Drugs that block the actions of acetylcholine

Drugs that block the effects of acetylcholine may be divided into three groups:

1. Anticholinergic drugs
2. Ganglion blocking drugs
3. Neuromuscular blocking drugs

Anticholinergic drugs

Anticholinergic drugs block the action of acetylcholine on acetylcholine receptors in the tissues and organs of the body. In addition some of them have a weak effect in blocking acetylcholine in the main switchboxes (ganglia) of the autonomic nervous system (affecting both sympathetic and parasympathetic divisions). No anticholinergic drug blocks the action of acetylcholine at nerve endings in voluntary muscles, except propantheline in very high doses.

There are several groups of anticholinergic drugs which produce differing degrees of effects in the body. For example, some produce more effects on the brain and/or the eyes than the others, some produce more effects on the stomach or intestine, and some are much more selective in their actions than others.

Anticholinergic drugs obtained from plants include atropine, belladonna, hyoscine and hyoscyamine. They produce similar effects and their uses are listed later.

Synthetic anticholinergic drugs may be divided into three groups according to whether their principal actions are drying up secretions and reducing movements of the intestines (anti-secretory and anti-spasmodic); whether they reduce the shaking and excessive salivation in patients with parkinsonism (anti-parkinsonism effects); or whether their main effects are upon the eyes (mydriatic and cycloplegic effects).

Those used mainly for their *anti-secretory/anti-spasmodic* effects include dicyclomine, emepronium, glycopyrronium, poldine and propantheline.

Those used mainly to treat *parkinsonism* include benzhexol, benztropine, biperiden, chlorphenoxamine, methixene, orphenadrine, procyclidine.

Those used mainly to treat *eye disorders* include cyclopentolate and tropicamide.

Effects produced by atropine

Atropine is usually taken as the main example of the anticholinergic drugs. It blocks acetylcholine receptors and stops acetylcholine from stimulating them – it is an acetylcholine blocker. Its overall effect, therefore, is to depress these receptors; however, initially it may produce some transient stimulation of them.

The results of the acetylcholine blocking effects of atropine are:

- To dry up all secretions in the body except milk – sweating stops, the eyes dry up, the nose and breathing passages dry up and the mouth becomes dry; the secretion of stomach juices (including acid) and intestinal secretions are also reduced by atropine

- To relax the muscles in the stomach and intestine and reduce movements, producing constipation
- To relax muscles in the bronchial tubes and relieve wheezing
- To relax the muscles in the bladder, making it difficult to empty the bladder and pass urine (this may cause particular problems in elderly men with enlarged prostate glands who may develop retention of urine)
- To relax the muscles in the walls of the ureters and ducts of the gall bladder
- To dilate the pupils and increase the pressure inside the front chamber of the eyes – this may trigger an attack of glaucoma
- To paralyse the muscles involved in focusing, which makes focusing difficult and also makes the eyes sensitive to light
- To increase the heart rate by blocking the effects of the main nerve to the heart (the vagus nerve) which normally exercises a slowing effect. In overdose, atropine relaxes the muscles in arteries causing dilatation (e.g. flushing)
- To stimulate the brain, producing restlessness and excitement, mania, confusion, delirium and hallucinations
- To stimulate the temperature control centre in the brain, to raise the body temperature which is made higher by the reduced sweating
- To block the effects of acetylcholine on the movement co-ordinating centre in the brain and relieve some of the symptoms of Parkinson's disease and parkinsonism
- To block the effects of acetylcholine on the vomiting centre and the organ of balance and reduce the symptoms of motion sickness

Disorders treated with anticholinergic drugs

The varied effects produced by atropine are shared to a greater or lesser extent by other anticholinergic drugs, and according to their principal effects they are used to treat different disorders.

Asthma Ipratropium is used to relieve wheezing in asthma; it is given by inhaler.

Dilating the pupils Anticholinergic drugs used mainly on the eyes to dilate the pupils for detailed eye examination include atropine, cyclopentolate, homatropine and tropicamide.

Disorders of heart rhythm Atropine and certain other anticholinergic drugs are used to treat disorders of heart rhythm and heart block.

Intestinal colic Anticholinergic drugs used mainly to slow down movement

Table 2.1 Some examples of the uses of anticholinergic drugs

Drugs	*Uses*
atropine	The use of atropine is now limited to dilating the pupils, relieving painful spasms (colic) of the intestine, treating slow heart rate and as a pre-medication before surgery to dry up the mouth and bronchial tubes and to control the heart rate
belladonna	Various preparations of belladonna have been used in the past to treat colic (painful spasms) of the intestine, gall bladder, kidney and bladder, to treat asthma and bedwetting and to reduce acid production in the stomach in the treatment of peptic ulcers
benzhexol	Its main use is in the treatment of parkinsonism
benztropine	Its main use is in the treatment of parkinsonism
biperiden	Its main use is in the treatment of parkinsonism
cyclopentolate	Used to dilate the pupils
dicyclomine	Used to treat colic (painful spasms) of the intestine, gall bladder, kidneys and bladder, and to reduce acid production in the stomach in the treatment of peptic ulcers
emepronium	Previously used to treat incontinence and frequency of urine in elderly people
glycopyrronium	As tablets to relieve colic (painful spasms) of the intestine, to reduce acid production in the treatment of peptic ulcers; injections used as a pre-medication for surgery to dry up the mouth and bronchial tubes and to control the heart rate; as a local powder to relieve sweating of the hands and feet
homatropine	Used principally to dilate the pupils
hyoscine (scopolamine)	Used principally as a pre-medication for surgery to dry up the mouth and bronchial tubes, control the heart rate and to calm the patient (also used for this purpose combined with papaveretum: Omnopon-Scopolamine). It is used to treat motion sickness. Was previously used in childbirth along with morphine or pethidine to produce the so-called 'twilight sleep'
hyoscyamine	To reduce acid production in the treatment of peptic ulcers, to relieve painful spasms (colic) of the intestine and to treat excessive sweating
ipratropium	Used by inhalation to treat asthma and other wheezing disorders
lachesine	Used to dilate the pupils
mepenzolate	To slow down or to relieve painful spasms (colic) of the intestine
methixene	Used mainly to treat parkinsonism
orphenadrine	Used mainly to treat parkinsonism. Also used to relieve spasms of voluntary muscles
pipenzolate	Used to reduce acid production in the treatment of peptic ulcers
pirenzepine	This is a selective-acting anticholinergic drug used to reduce acid production in the treatment of peptic ulcers. It is the best anticholinergic drug to use for this purpose

Table 2.1 Some examples of the uses of anticholinergic drugs (*cont.*)

Drugs	*Uses*
poldine	Used to relieve colic (painful spasms) of the intestine, gall bladder, kidneys or bladder; to reduce acid production in the treatment of peptic ulcers; to treat bedwetting and sweating
procyclidine	Used mainly to treat parkinsonism
propantheline	Used to reduce acid production in the treatment of peptic ulcers, to treat bedwetting, sweating, and to treat colic (painful spasms) of the intestine
stramonium	Should no longer be used to relieve wheezing in asthma
tropicamide	Used to dilate the pupils

and/or to relieve painful spasm (colic) in the stomach and intestine include dicyclomine, glycopyrronium, mepenzolate, pipenzolate, poldine and propantheline.

Kidney colic Anticholinergic drugs used to relieve painful spasm (colic) in the urinary tract (e.g. ureteric colic) include emepronium and flavoxate.

Motion sickness Hyoscine is the main anticholinergic drug used to relieve motion sickness; it is also used as pre-medication before surgery (see below).

Parkinsonism Those anticholinergic drugs whose main actions are on the movement control centre in the brain are used to treat parkinsonism. They include benzhexol, benztropine, biperiden, methixene, orphenadrine and procyclidine. They are also given to relieve the symptoms of parkinsonism caused by anti-psychotic drugs given in the treatment of schizophrenia and other serious mental disorders.

Peptic ulcer Belladonna, dicyclomine, glycopyrronium, pirenzepine, poldine and propantheline are examples of anticholinergic drugs used to reduce acid production in the treatment of peptic ulcers.

Pre-medication before surgery Anticholinergic drugs are used before a general anaesthetic to reduce secretions in the bronchial tubes, to control the heart rate and to calm the patient. They include atropine, glycopyrronium and hyoscine.

Table 2.2 Anticholinergic drugs – harmful effects and warnings

Harmful effects of anticholinergic drugs vary between different drugs and between different individuals. They vary in frequency, severity and type. Most harmful effects produced by anticholinergic drugs are mild and are usually related to the doses used. They can easily be controlled by reducing the dose. More serious harmful effects are usually caused by high doses and/or by how a particular individual reacts. The following harmful effects have been reported and should be borne in mind whenever an anticholinergic drug is used.

Harmful effects produced by anticholinergic drugs include dryness of the mouth and difficulty in swallowing, dryness of the nose and throat, blurred vision, flushing and dryness of the skin, slowing followed by quickening of the heart rate, palpitations, disorders of heart rhythm, desire to pass urine but with an inability to do so, constipation, giddiness, confusion, vomiting, unsteadiness, and pain in the chest due to acid reflux from the stomach up into the oesophagus. High doses cause rapid beating of the heart, high temperature, restlessness, confusion, excitement, mania, delirium, hallucinations and a rash on the face and chest.

Warnings Anticholinergic drugs should not be used in people with enlarged prostate glands, paralysis of the intestine, narrowing of the outlet from the stomach (pyloric stenosis), acid reflux up the oesophagus or closed-angle glaucoma. Do not use when the environmental temperature is high, particularly in children. They should be used with caution in elderly men and in anyone with a fever, a rapid pulse rate (e.g. due to overworking of the thyroid gland) or heart failure or during heart surgery. Reduced bronchial secretions caused by anticholinergic drugs may make it difficult for people with bronchitis to cough up phlegm, which may accumulate and cause a blockage. People with Down's syndrome are sensitive to the effects of anticholinergic drugs, whereas albinos appear to be resistant.

Risks in elderly people Harmful effects may be more frequent and severe in the elderly; therefore use with caution. The risk of producing confusion in elderly people is greater than in younger people. Difficulty in passing urine leading to retention of urine may be a problem in elderly men, particularly those with enlarged prostate glands. Glaucoma may be triggered by anticholinergic drugs.

Ganglion blocking drugs

These drugs block acetylcholine in the main switchboxes (the ganglia) of the whole of the autonomic nervous system. They therefore block both the sympathetic and the parasympathetic divisions of the system. They were originally used to treat raised blood pressure but caused so many harmful effects that they are no longer used. They include hexamethonium, mecamylamine, pempidine and pentolinium.

Neuromuscular blocking drugs (myoneural blocking drugs)

When an impulse passes down a motor nerve to a voluntary muscle (skeletal muscle) it causes the release of acetylcholine at the nerve ending which acts on special areas in the muscle fibres called 'motor end-plates'. This action triggers a contraction of the muscle. Drugs that block this action of acetylcholine to produce a nerve/muscle block are referred to as neuromuscular blocking drugs or myoneural blocking drugs and sometimes as muscle relaxants. There are two main groups: competitive and depolarizing neuromuscular blocking drugs.

Competitive neuromuscular blocking drugs (or non-depolarizing muscle relaxants)

These drugs compete with acetylcholine at the acetylcholine receptors in neuromuscular junctions. They block its action, causing the muscles to go floppy and paralysed. These actions are usually reversed by giving neostigmine, an anticholinesterase drug (i.e. a drug that stops the breakdown of acetylcholine; see earlier). They include alcuronium, atracurium, gallamine, pancuronium, tubocurarine and vecuronium.

Competitive neuromuscular blocking drugs produce prolonged paralysis of muscles and are used during surgical operations to relax abdominal muscles, diaphragm and vocal cords (so that a breathing tube can be passed into the windpipe).

Table 2.3 Competitive neuromuscular blocking drugs – harmful effects and warnings

NOTE Patients who have received a neuromuscular blocking drug should always have their breathing assisted until the drug has been inactivated by giving the anticholinesterase drug neostigmine. Atropine or glycopyrronium should be given before or with the neostigmine to prevent excessive production of saliva and slowing of the pulse rate.

Harmful effects These drugs are used to provide muscle paralysis, along with general anaesthetics during surgery, but it is important to remember that consciousness may not be impaired although the patient cannot move. If the general anaesthetic (e.g. nitrous oxide) is not given in concentrations sufficient to cause unconsciousness the patient may be totally paralysed and unable to communicate and yet be able to hear and feel everything that is going on. There are very rare reports of this happening. Harmful effects to bear in mind when using some of these drugs include a transient fall in blood pressure and a slight increase in pulse rate. Occasionally, breathing difficulty may occur after the operation. Rarely, there may develop allergic reactions which include wheezing and skin rashes due to the release of histamine.

Warnings They should not be used in anyone with myasthenia gravis or severe lung disease. Some of them should be used with caution in people who suffer from allergies (e.g. asthma, eczema, hayfever), or impaired kidney function. Their effects are increased by inhalational anaesthetics.

alcuronium (Alloferin)
The dose should be reduced in anyone suffering from impaired kidney function.

atracurium (Tracrium)
May cause allergic reactions due to release of histamine. It does not affect the heart

Table 2.3 Competitive neuromuscular blocking drugs – harmful effects and warnings (*cont.*)

rate or blood pressure. It may be used in people with impaired kidney or liver function. Low body temperatures (hypothermia) may prolong its effects. It does not accumulate in the body on repeated dosing.

gallamine (Flaxedil)
May cause rapid pulse rate and it should not be used in anyone with severe impairment of their kidney function.

pancuronium (Pavulon)
Does not cause allergy or changes in blood pressure. The dose should be reduced in obese individuals and in anyone with impaired kidney function. It should be used with caution in people whose condition could be made worse by an increase in heart rate (e.g. angina) and in patients with impaired liver function.

tubocurarine (Jexin, Tubarine)
May cause allergic reactions due to release of histamine and an instant fall in blood pressure. The dose should be reduced in anyone with impaired kidney function.

vecuronium (Norcuron)
Does not cause allergic reactions or changes in heart rate or blood pressure. Large doses may accumulate in the body and so increase its effects.

Depolarizing neuromuscular blocking drugs

These drugs imitate the action of acetylcholine on the nerve/muscle receptors and cause contraction of the muscles, but they are not destroyed immediately like acetylcholine. However, the contraction does not last and the muscles rapidly become floppy and paralysed. This is because they cannot be stimulated again while the drugs are acting. The effects of these drugs cannot be reversed by neostigmine (an anticholinesterase drug); it may in fact make the paralysis worse.

Suxamethonium, (Anectine, Scoline) is the only one of these drugs that is used. Its duration of action is only about 5 minutes and it is therefore used to provide muscle relaxation for procedures such as passing a tube into the lungs.

Table 2.4 Suxamethonium – harmful effects and warnings

Harmful effects The enzyme acetylcholinesterase is usually referred to as 'cholinesterase'. It is present in the blood and the tissues, at the end of parasympathetic nerves and in the muscles at the end of motor nerves. Another cholinesterase enzyme (pseudocholinesterase) is also present in the blood. It splits choline esters other than acetylcholine. It is responsible for destroying suxamethonium. The local anaesthetics procaine and amethocaine are also destroyed by pseudocholinesterase and may therefore prolong the action of suxamethonium by competing with it for pseudocholinesterase. About 1 person in 2,500 is deficient in pseudocholinesterase and cannot destroy suxamethonium as rapidly as normal people. In these people the paralysis produced by suxamethonium

Table 2.4 Suxamethonium – harmful effects and warnings (*cont.*)

will last for hours rather than 4–5 minutes. Treatment consists of using a respirator until the paralysis has cleared up. Suxamethonium may cause a slowing of the heart rate and occasionally disorders of heart rhythm. A serious and often fatal rise in body temperature (malignant hyperpyrexia) may occur very rarely in patients given suxamethonium with a general anaesthetic. It occurs in apparently healthy individuals who appear to have some genetic abnormality that makes them prone to develop this complication. The symptoms include an increased temperature, rigid muscles and the appearance of muscle protein in the urine. Very rarely, the patient may go on to develop heart failure, destruction of red blood cells (haemolysis) and brain damage. Suxamethonium may occasionally cause allergic reactions, including wheezing in some patients, and muscle pains may occur for a short period after the operation. It may sometimes increase the frequency of bowel movements, raise the pressure inside the eyes (see 'glaucoma' in Chapter 35), cause the salivary glands in the cheeks (parotid glands) to increase in size, increase the production of saliva and increase the production of gastric juices.

Warnings Suxamethonium should not be used in individuals with severe burns, disorders of muscle tone or an abnormality of cholinesterase (see earlier), serious eye injuries or extensive body injuries, liver disease, malnutrition or severe anaemia, or who have been exposed to organophosphate weedkillers or insecticides, which may cause a low level of pseudocholinesterase in the blood. Nor should they be used in anyone with myasthenia gravis, nerve or brain damage, phaeochromocytoma, or kidney failure (particularly those with high blood potassium levels). It should be used with caution in people with heart disease. In order to prevent too much slowing of the heart or an increase in secretions in the bronchial tubes, atropine should be given *before* suxamethonium.

Risks in elderly people Harmful effects, particularly on the heart and circulation, may be more frequent and severe; therefore suxamethonium must be used with caution.

Noradrenaline

Noradrenaline is the neurotransmitter at most *sympathetic* post-ganglionic nerve endings and at some nerve junctions in the brain, especially in the hypothalamus. From the adrenal glands both adrenaline and noradrenaline are released into the bloodstream to be carried to their sites of action where they reinforce the stimulation produced by the sympathetic nerves. They also stimulate tissues not reached by these nerves.

Nerve fibres that use noradrenaline as a neurotransmitter are called adrenergic nerves, and we talk about the adrenergic transmission of impulses (i.e. using noradrenaline).

Noradrenaline in the sympathetic nervous system is manufactured at adrenergic nerve endings where it is also stored. The release of noradrenaline is triggered by impulses travelling along the nerves. It may also be released by stimulant drugs such as the amphetamines and ephedrine and by drugs that lower blood pressure, such as guanethidine and reserpine.

Intravenous infusion of noradrenaline will replenish the stores at nerve endings.

Noradrenaline receptors (adrenoceptors) are divided into two main groups – alpha receptors and beta receptors – according to how they respond to stimulation by adrenaline and noradrenaline. These two groups are further subdivided into alpha-1 and alpha-2 receptors and beta-1 and beta-2 receptors.

Alpha-1 receptors are in most organs and tissues supplied by sympathetic nerves. One of their principal actions when stimulated is to cause constriction of small arteries (vasoconstriction). Alpha-2 receptors are at nerve endings and control the amounts of noradrenaline released – if noradrenaline release falls, they stimulate further release of noradrenaline in order to keep the level up; if it rises too high, they reduce its release.

Stimulation of alpha receptors produces dilatation of the pupils; constriction of small arteries, particularly in the skin and intestine; and sweating of the skin. It also makes the hairs stand on end. Stimulation of alpha receptors is also involved in ejaculation, and in contraction of the bladder to pass urine.

Stimulation of beta receptors increases the heart rate and produces other effects on the heart (mainly a beta-1 effect); dilatation of small arteries, particularly the ones supplying skeletal muscles (a beta-2 effect); relaxation of the muscles in the bronchial tubes (a beta-2 effect); relaxation of the womb (a beta-2 effect); tremor of skeletal muscles (a beta-2 effect); and relaxation of the bladder.

Relaxation of the muscles in the intestine is a combined alpha and beta effect. Alpha stimulation causes a rise in levels of potassium in the blood while beta-2 stimulation causes a fall in blood potassium levels. Beta-2 stimulation also causes a rise in the level of glucose in the blood as a result of glucose being made by the liver, and it causes the splitting up of fats.

Sympathomimetic drugs

Drugs that mimic the actions produced by stimulating the sympathetic nerves are called sympathomimetic drugs. They produce 'adrenaline-like' effects on the body. They may produce these effects by acting directly on adrenoreceptors, indirectly by causing a release of noradrenaline from nerve endings or by a mixture of both. They may work on both alpha and beta receptors or they may be selective and stimulate only alpha or beta receptors. They may even be more selective and stimulate predominantly beta-2 receptors. However, it is important to remember that when given in high enough doses their selectivity goes and they start stimulating other adrenoreceptors.

Sympathomimetic drugs that act directly on adrenoreceptors include adrenaline, isoprenaline, metaraminol, methoxamine, noradrenaline and xylometazoline. Those that act indirectly by causing a release of noradrenaline from its stores at nerve endings include amphetamines and tyramine. Those that produce both actions include dopamine and ephedrine.

A diminishing response to frequent and continuous use of sympathomimetic drugs may occur, particularly to the indirect acting ones (e.g. amphetamines: 'speed'). This diminishing response to frequent and continuous use is referred to as tachyphylaxis.

Other drugs that affect adrenergic nerve activity

Other drugs may affect adrenergic nerves in several ways:

- By blocking adrenoreceptors directly – e.g. betablockers
- By preventing the re-uptake of noradrenaline back into storage at the nerve endings – e.g. cocaine, tricyclic anti-depressants
- By preventing the breakdown of noradrenaline at nerve endings – e.g. monoamine oxidase inhibitor (MAOI) anti-depressants
- By using up the stores of noradrenaline at nerve endings – e.g. reserpine
- By preventing the release of noradrenaline from nerve endings – e.g. guanethidine
- By producing a false nerve transmitter at nerve endings – e.g. methyldopa

These actions help to explain the effects and uses of these drugs – for example, the stimulation produced by amphetamines and cocaine; the lift of mood produced by anti-depressant drugs (tricyclic, cyclic and MAOIs); the blood pressure lowering effects of reserpine, guanethidine and methyldopa; the 'protection' of the heart against stimulation offered by the beta blockers; and the constriction of arteries produced by drugs with sympathomimetic actions.

Uses of sympathomimetic drugs

Asthma Sympathomimetic drugs used to treat asthma are discussed in Chapter 12.

Heart failure Sympathomimetic drugs used to treat heart failure are discussed in Chapter 22.

Nasal decongestants Sympathomimetic drugs used to treat blocked and runny noses are discussed in Chapter 3.

Premature labour Sympathomimetic drugs cause relaxation of the womb and may be used to stop premature labour. The ones most commonly used include isoxsuprine, orciprenaline, ritodrine, salbutamol, terbutaline.

Shock due to a serious fall in blood pressure Those sympathomimetic drugs which principally cause constriction of arteries were previously used to treat a sudden and serious fall in blood pressure. They included metaraminol, methoxamine, noradrenaline and phenylephrine. The danger in using these drugs to raise blood pressure is that the blood supply may be diverted away from vital organs such as the kidneys, which may cause serious damage. These drugs should no longer be used for this purpose.

The best treatment for shock is to raise the blood volume by giving blood or plasma. However, those sympathomimetic drugs that work principally on the heart may be given by intravenous injection or infusion to treat severe shock. They include dobutamine and dopamine.

Table 2.5 Sympathomimetic drugs – harmful effects and warnings

Harmful effects of sympathomimetic drugs vary between different drugs and between different individuals. They vary in frequency, severity and type. Most harmful effects produced by sympathomimetic drugs are mild and are usually related to the doses used. They can easily be controlled by reducing the dose. More serious harmful effects are usually caused by high doses and/or by how a particular individual reacts. The following harmful effects should be borne in mind whenever a sympathomimetic drug is used.

Harmful effects These include anxiety, restlessness, palpitations, rapid beating of heart, tremors, weakness, dizziness, headache, coldness of the hands and feet, breathlessness. These harmful effects may occur in people particularly sensitive to adrenaline (e.g. anxious and tense or with an over-active thyroid gland). Overdosing may produce disorders of heart rhythm, fluid on the lungs (pulmonary oedema) and brain haemorrhage. Local constriction of blood vessels may be so severe following an injection as to cause damage and death to the surrounding tissue. In people with arteriosclerosis (hardening of the arteries) or raised blood pressure these drugs may occasionally trigger a brain haemorrhage. In anyone with coronary artery disease (e.g. angina) they may trigger an attack of angina and/or a heart attack. Injections of local anaesthetic preparations that contain adrenaline may cause gangrene in tissues supplied by end-arteries (e.g. the fingers or the penis). Adrenaline eye drops may cause redness and swelling of the eyes, a brown pigmentation (melanin) of the cornea and conjunctiva, and blockage to the tear ducts. Inhalations of adrenaline and related drugs may be swallowed and cause stomach pains, therefore rinse the mouth out with water after each inhalation.

Warnings Sympathomimetic drugs should not be used in anyone with narrow-angle glaucoma. They should be used with caution in people with raised blood pressure, arteriosclerosis (hardening of the arteries), or coronary artery disease (e.g. angina) and in diabetics because the blood glucose may be increased. They should also be used with caution when taking other drugs (see under drug interactions, Chapter 89).

Risks in elderly people Harmful effects may be more frequent and severe in the elderly. Note the risks associated with hardening of the arteries (above).

Table 2.6 Some examples of the use of sympathomimetic drugs

Drugs	*Uses*
adrenaline	Used to treat acute attacks of asthma; to treat and prevent severe allergic reactions (anaphylaxis); given with a local anaesthetic to make it last longer; to stop bleeding from superficial wounds (e.g. nose bleeding); to treat glaucoma; and to stimulate the heart to start beating if it has stopped
dobutamine	Used to treat sudden heart failure associated with a sudden severe fall in blood pressure
dopamine	Used to treat sudden heart failure following a heart attack or heart surgery
ephedrine	Used to treat asthma, and in nasal decongestants and in cough medicines; and to treat bedwetting
etafedrine	Used to treat asthma and in cough medicines
fenoterol	Used to treat asthma
isoetharine	Used to treat asthma
isometheptene	Used to treat migraine
isoprenaline	Used to treat asthma; to treat slow heart rate; to treat serious allergic reactions (e.g. bee stings)
isoxsuprine	Used to treat uncomplicated premature labour
metaraminol	Used to treat a sudden fall in blood pressure
methoxamine	Used to treat a sudden fall in blood pressure during general anaesthesia
naphazoline	Used in nasal decongestants and in decongestant eye drops
noradrenaline	Used to treat a sudden fall in blood pressure or sudden stopping of the heart
orciprenaline	Used to treat asthma and uncomplicated premature labour
oxymetazoline	Used in nasal decongestants
phenylephrine	Used to treat asthma; in cough medicines; in nasal decongestants; to treat irritation of the eyes; and to treat bedwetting
phenylpropanol-amine	Used in cough and cold remedies as a decongestant and to treat hayfever
reproterol	Used to treat asthma
rimiterol	Used to treat asthma
ritodrine	Used to treat uncomplicated premature labour
salbutamol	Used to treat asthma and uncomplicated premature labour
terbutaline	Used to treat asthma and in cough medicines. Also used to treat uncomplicated premature labour
xylometazoline	Used in nasal decongestants

Table 2.7 Sympathomimetic drug preparations: injections

See the appropriate chapter for sympathomimetic drug preparations used to treat the following: allergic emergencies (Chapter 10), asthma (Chapter 12), bedwetting (Chapter 33), glaucoma and congestion of the eyes (Chapter 35), nasal allergy and congestion (Chapters 10 and 3), uncomplicated premature labour (Chapter 71), coughs (Chapter 4) and colds (Chapter 3).

Preparation	*Drug*	*Preparation*	*Drug*
adrenaline	adrenaline	Min-I-Jet Adrenaline	adrenaline
Aramine	metaraminol	Min-I-Jet Isoprenaline	isoprenaline
Dobutrex	dobutamine	phenylephrine	phenylephrine
dopamine	dopamine	Saventrine IV	isoprenaline
Intropin	dopamine	Select-A-Jet Dopamine	dopamine
Isuprel	isoprenaline	Sympatol	oxedrine
Levophed	noradrenaline	Vasoxine	methoxamine

Drugs that block adrenoreceptors

Drugs are available that block adrenoreceptors – some principally block alpha receptors (*alpha blockers*), others block beta receptors (*beta blockers*) and some block both alpha and beta receptors.

Alpha blockers

Most alpha blockers block both alpha-1 and alpha-2 receptors. The result is that the arteries dilate and cause a fall in the resistance to the flow of blood through them, which results in a fall in blood pressure, particularly on standing up after lying down and on exercise. This is an alpha-1 effect.

Normally when the blood pressure falls, pressure receptors in certain blood vessels send messages to the blood pressure control centre in the brain which then activates the sympathetic nerves to release noradrenaline, which causes constriction of arteries and also sends up the heart rate to compensate. When these effects are blocked by alpha blocking drugs this compensatory rise in heart rate does not occur. This aggravates the fall in blood pressure caused by the alpha blocking in these patients and they may experience dizziness, light-headedness and faintness on standing up after sitting or lying down (postural hypotension) or on exercise. This can be dangerous in elderly people, who may fall. Other harmful effects of alpha blockers include stuffy nose and failure to ejaculate.

Alpha blockers are used to treat raised blood pressure, heart failure and disorders of the circulation.

Beta blockers

Beta blockers are discussed in detail in Chapter 20.

Alpha and beta blockers

Labetalol is a non-selective beta blocker which also blocks alpha receptors. The alpha blocking effects reduce the constriction of arteries (e.g. cold fingers and toes) produced by beta blocking. Because of its alpha and beta blocking effects labetalol is suitable for controlling a raised blood pressure in patients who suffer from angina.

Drugs that block nerve endings

Drugs that block the nerve endings of sympathetic nerves (adrenergic neuron blocking drugs) cause less noradrenaline to be released and block it from being taken back into store. This causes the noradrenaline stores at the nerve endings to become used up. Drugs that produce these effects include guanethidine, bethanidine and debrisoquine. Their use to treat raised blood pressure is discussed in Chapter 21.

Reserpine is another drug that is used to treat raised blood pressure. In addition to its effects in the brain, it blocks the storage of noradrenaline at nerve endings so that less is available for release to stimulate the adrenoreceptors.

False transmitters

Methyldopa, used to treat raised blood pressure, is broken down in the body to methylnoradrenaline which acts as a false neurotransmitter and stimulates the blood pressure control centre in the brain to react as if there were too much noradrenaline in the blood. The centre responds by triggering mechanisms to reduce the activity of sympathetic nerves, which causes a fall in blood pressure.

Clonidine stimulates alpha receptors in the brain, causing the blood pressure control centre to reduce the activity of sympathetic nerves which causes a fall in blood pressure. In high doses it also works on sympathetic nerve endings to control the production of noradrenaline (see earlier). It is used to treat raised blood pressure and migraine.

Ganglion blockers

These drugs block the switchboxes (the ganglia) of the autonomic nervous system and produce effects on both the parasympathetic and the sympathetic systems. They were used to treat raised blood pressure but are now obsolete.

The adrenal medulla

The functions of the adrenal glands are discussed in Chapter 61. Stimulation of the inner parts (the medulla) of the adrenal glands by sympathetic (preganglionic) nerve fibres causes the release of adrenaline and noradrenaline. These are called catecholamines.

The manufacture and storage of these catecholamines in the adrenal glands are similar to those described at the adrenergic nerve endings (above), but, due to the presence of an additional enzyme, most of the noradrenaline is converted to adrenaline and dopamine (the precursor for noradrenaline) and stored. Some of the noradrenaline leaks away into surrounding tissues where an enzyme (monoamine oxidase) partly breaks it down and partly converts it to adrenaline. ACTH (adrenocorticotrophic hormone) and cortisol are also involved in the stimulation of the adrenal medulla (see below).

Normally, the adrenal medulla functions at a low basic level of activity, releasing only small quantities of adrenaline and noradrenaline into the bloodstream. However, through the effects of the hypothalamus, increased amounts of adrenaline and noradrenaline are released by the adrenal glands in response to physical work, cold, heat, low blood sugar, pain, oxygen deficiency, a drop in blood pressure, fear and anger. This amount of adrenaline and noradrenaline is sufficient to stimulate most cells in the body and put the body on full alert.

The essential role of adrenaline and noradrenaline in these 'stress' situations is to mobilize chemical energy (fats and glucose) and increase the supply of glucose to cells. This provides the extra fuel for muscle cells to burn up as energy ready for fight or flight. They also increase the heart rate, the output from the heart and the blood pressure. At the same time they cause the blood vessels supplying the intestine to close down so that more blood can be supplied to the muscles.

Phaeochromocytoma

This is a tumour which may occur anywhere in the sympathetic division of the autonomic nervous system, but 90 per cent are found in the adrenal glands. It is rare and results in the over-production of catecholamines (e.g. adrenaline and noradrenaline) which cause severe hypertension (raised blood pressure), which may be sustained or come on in episodes producing apprehension, paleness, sweating, palpitations, headache, pain in the stomach and tightness in the chest. Treatment is usually by surgical removal of the tumour; failing this, combined treatment with an alpha blocker (phenoxybenzamine) and a beta blocker is used. A sudden dangerous rise in blood pressure is treated with an injection of phentolamine. Metirosine (Demser) blocks the enzyme involved in the production of catecholamines and it is used to prepare for surgery patients suffering from a phaeochromocytoma. It is also used in the long-term treatment of patients who are not suitable for surgery. It may be necessary to add an alpha blocker (phenoxybenzamine) to the treatment if the patient does not improve on metirosine alone.

Other nerve transmitters

Dopamine

Dopamine is a nerve transmitter that stimulates dopamine receptors in the brain and nervous system, and also alpha and beta adrenoceptors. It can also stimulate the release of noradrenaline from nerve endings. It is used to treat shock due to acute heart failure.

Dopamine stimulants

Bromocriptine stimulates dopamine receptors in the brain. It is used to suppress milk production after childbirth because it stimulates nerves that block the release of the milk-producing hormone prolactin by the pituitary gland. It is also used to treat serious breast disorders associated with milk production, and to treat tumours that produce excessive amounts of prolactin. It also stimulates nerves that block the release of growth hormone by the pituitary gland, and may be used to treat over-production of this hormone (e.g. acromegaly). Another main use of bromocriptine is to treat parkinsonism in which there is a breakdown of dopaminergic nerve cells in the brain (see Chapter 36).

Amantadine stimulates an increase in concentration of dopamine in the brain. It is used to treat parkinsonism.

Levodopa is taken up by dopaminergic neurones and converted into dopamine. It is also used to treat parkinsonism.

Lysuride is a selective dopamine receptor stimulant used to treat parkinsonism.

Selegeline is a selective blocker of the enzyme that breaks down dopamine and is used to treat parkinsonism.

Dopamine blockers

Anti-psychotic drugs used to treat serious mental disorders block dopamine receptors. They may produce adverse effects similar to parkinsonism which is caused by a deficiency of dopamine in the brain (see Chapter 36).

Metoclopramide and domperidone are dopamine blockers used to treat nausea and vomiting due to disorders of the stomach and intestine or due to drugs (e.g. anti-cancer drugs). They block dopamine receptors in the chemoreceptor trigger zone in the brain (see Chapter 14).

Tetrabenazine reduces the concentration of dopamine in the brain and nervous system and is used to treat disorders of movement such as Huntington's chorea.

5-Hydroxytryptamine (5HT, serotonin)

This chemical is present in many cells in both plants and animals. It has a wide spectrum of activity by stimulating and blocking nerves in smooth muscles, particularly in the breathing tubes, producing wheezing, and in blood vessels, producing constriction in some (e.g. in the intestine and kidneys) or dilatation in others (e.g. in muscles). It produces a slowing of heart rate, a fall in blood pressure and affects the movements of the stomach and intestine. It also acts as a nerve transmitter in the brain.

Most of the 5HT in food is destroyed in the walls of the intestine and, if it is absorbed, in the liver and the lungs. It is therefore manufactured in the body from tryptophan (an essential amino acid in the diet).

5HT stimulants

Drugs that increase the amount of 5HT available in the brain are used to treat depression (see Chapter 39). They include:

5HT re-uptake inhibitors	–	fluoxetine and fluvoxamine
5HT precursors	–	tryptophan
Monoamine oxidase inhibitors	–	These block the breakdown of 5HT as well as other nerve stimulants in the brain
Tricyclic and related anti-depressants	–	These block the uptake of 5HT and other nerve stimulants in the brain

NOTE Reserpine, which is used to treat raised blood pressure (Chapter 21), depletes the store of 5HT in the brain and can cause depression.

5HT blockers

Methysergide blocks 5HT at its receptor sites and is used to prevent migraine (see Chapter 29). Pizotifen is a 5HT blocker that is also used to prevent migraine.

Anti-psychotic drugs block the activity of dopamine in the brain and they may also block the activity of 5HT (see Chapter 41).

Cyproheptadine is an antihistamine that also blocks the effects of 5HT. It is used to stimulate the appetite and as an antihistamine (see Chapter 10).

Fenfluramine and dexfenfluramine increase 5HT levels in the brain and are used as slimming drugs (see Chapter 43).

Odansetron is a selective 5HT blocker used to treat nausea and vomiting caused by anti-cancer drugs and radiation treatment (see Chapter 14).

3

Colds

The nose, sinuses, throat and air passages are lined by a membrane of mucus-producing cells (a mucous membrane) which is very richly supplied with blood vessels which ensure that the air we breathe is warm and moist. The blood supply increases when the air is cold and decreases when the air is warm. In addition, the surfaces are covered with tiny hair-like structures (cilia) and by a moist coat of mucus. The cilia and mucus have a very important function because they clean the air that we breathe by trapping dust and other particles, including bacteria, and propel them out to the surface so that they can be coughed up and spat out or blown out of the nose. The mucus contains chemicals that kill bacteria and viruses. It also contains antibodies and white blood cells which move out from the bloodstream to engulf and destroy micro-organisms. An increase in mucus production occurs if the surfaces become inflamed as a result of an infection (e.g. a cold), by allergy (e.g. hayfever) or by irritation (e.g. inhaling irritant vapours or dust). Mucus production may be interfered with by some cold and cough remedies that dry up the surfaces (see later) and of course by dry atmospheres and smoking. Therefore, an important part of treating coughs and colds is to keep the surfaces moist by drinking more fluids than usual, stopping smoking if you smoke, and avoiding dry atmospheres if possible. In addition, the inhalation of steam may help (see later).

Colds

A common cold (coryza, infectious rhinitis, acute rhinitis) is caused by one of many different types of cold viruses. They are principally spread by droplet infection, as a result of infected people coughing and sneezing. They produce inflammation of the nose (rhinitis), sore throat (pharyngitis), a hoarse voice (laryngitis), inflammation of the windpipe (tracheitis) and, occasionally, bronchitis.

The onset of a common cold is sudden, with sneezing, running nose, sore throat, smarting eyes and sometimes headache and mild feverishness.

Colds are is expensive to society because more time is lost from school and work due to colds than to all other disorders added together; yet we do not know how to prevent colds or what makes some people get more colds than others. We do not have a cure and we do not know how to shorten the duration of a cold. Whether we fill ourselves up with drugs or not, it will take 5–7 days for our body defences to get rid of the infection.

Colds are costly

Clearly we feel very sorry for ourselves when we have a cold, which probably explains why we spend millions of pounds each year on cough and cold remedies. It is very big business: manufacturers of cold remedies spend millions of pounds every year on advertising in order to persuade us to take some expensive product to relieve our aches and pains, dry up or unblock our noses, relieve our sore throats and/or stop our tickling coughs. We are very vulnerable to these pressures and feel better for taking some remedy, particularly if it smells, looks and/or tastes as if it could do us some good.

To treat or not to treat

In making a decision whether or not to take a cold remedy, it is important for you to understand that any cold remedy relies on the use of only a small number of active drugs which are used in varying doses and combinations. These are aimed at four groups of symptoms – reducing aches, pains and feverishness; relieving blocked and/or runny noses; relieving sore throats; and relieving coughs.

Relief of aches, pains and feverishness

Aches and pains are good warning signs that you may have an infection and that you should rest. The fever that you get with a cold is usually very mild and there is no evidence that such a mild fever is harmful but, on the other hand, there is no evidence that it is beneficial, although there is a probability that fever may help the body's defence system against infection. Nevertheless, aches, pains and feverishness are unpleasant and can easily be relieved. However, remember that if you relieve these symptoms with drugs you have done nothing to affect the underlying infection and although you may feel better, you should still take it easy for a few days and not do heavy physical work.

To relieve aches and pains and feverishness, aspirin, ibuprofen or paracetamol are very effective if used singly and in an appropriate dose. Despite this fact they are often mixed with other drugs in numerous cold remedies, which is quite unnecessary.

Some cold remedies contain salicylamide which is related to aspirin but it is rapidly broken down in the body and offers no advantage over aspirin. Preparations that contain pain relievers such as codeine, dextropropoxyphene or dihydrocodeine are not necessary because these drugs are not as effective as aspirin or paracetamol in relieving the aches, pains and feverishness of a cold.

For treating aches, pains and feverishness, it is better to stick to a *single* preparation of aspirin or paracetamol. Do not take mixtures. Tablets of soluble aspirin BP or tablets of paracetamol BP are the cheapest preparations to buy.

Paracetamol is the drug of choice, especially if aspirin upsets your stomach, if you have asthma or chronic bronchitis, haemophilia, if you are taking anticoagulants (anti-blood-clotting drugs), if you are allergic to aspirin or if you suffer from or have suffered in the past from stomach ulcers, duodenal ulcers, heartburn or chronic indigestion. It is the drug of choice in children under the age of 12 years.

Harmful effects and warnings on the use of aspirin and paracetamol are described in Chapter 27.

Warning *Do not give aspirin to children under the age of 12 years; use paracetamol instead. Do not take aspirin along with alcohol.*

For a common cold you will need to take no more than three standard doses of paracetamol or aspirin during the first 24 hours of your cold at intervals of no less than 4 hours.

NOTE Sponging the body with tepid water is the safest way of cooling a feverish child.

Relieving a blocked and runny nose

It will help you to understand this section better if you first read the chapter on the autonomic nervous system (Chapter 2). When you have a cold, the lining of the nose becomes inflamed, resulting in increased production of mucus, and it may also become swollen. This produces a runny nose followed by a blocked nose (congestion). Drugs that reduce the swelling of the mucous membrane and suppress mucus production are called decongestants. When taken by mouth in appropriate dosage these drugs act on nerves that supply the heart and blood vessels. They constrict small arteries and reduce the blood flow to many tissues in the body, including the nose where they shrink its lining and dry it up. They may also increase the heart rate and send up the blood pressure. They produce 'adrenaline-like' effects on the body. They are related to the amphetamines ('speed') and are usually referred to as sympathomimetic drugs because they mimic stimulation of the sympathetic nervous system which uses noradrenaline as a nerve messenger (see Chapter 2).

Decongestant drugs by mouth affect the whole body and may be harmful in some people

Drugs that produce adrenaline-like effects on the body (sympathomimetic drugs) to be taken by mouth to relieve congestion of the nose include phenylephrine, phenylpropanolamine, and pseudoephedrine. In addition to relieving congestion of the nose they may also produce general effects throughout the body which include an increase in the pulse rate and a rise in the blood pressure. In high doses they may cause restlessness, anxiety, insomnia, trembling, rapid beating of the heart, disorders of heart rhythm, dry mouth and cold hands and feet. They may be harmful to people who have a raised blood pressure or heart disease. They may also be harmful to anyone with diabetes, because they send the blood sugar up. In someone with an over-active thyroid gland (thyrotoxicosis) they may trigger an irregular heart beat. In somebody with coronary artery disease, the rise in pulse rate and blood pressure may trigger an attack of angina.

The message is clear – decongestant drugs by mouth may be harmful to some people because they constrict small arteries throughout the whole body as well as those in the nose.

Warning *Dangerous levels of phenylephrine, phenylpropanolamine and pseudo-ephedrine may occur in the body if you take a decongestant that contains one or more of these drugs by mouth and also use a decongestant nasal spray or nasal drops that also contain one or more of these drugs. They may be particularly dangerous in patients taking an MAOI anti-depressant drug or within 2 weeks of stopping such a drug.*

Decongestant drugs applied to the nose may also cause problems

Decongestant preparations that contain sympathomimetic drugs are available to be applied directly up the nose in the form of nose sprays and drops.

When applied in this way they cause the blood vessels to constrict and the lining of the nose to shrink. This dries up the nose if it is running and unblocks it if it is blocked. However, if used too frequently these nasal sprays and drops may cause a rebound swelling of the lining of the nose. In other words, when their effects have worn off, the congestion may become worse than it was before it was treated. This may lead you to use the decongestant nose spray or drops again, which will cause a further rebound effect. As a consequence, regular use may cause a chronic blocked nose which may be associated with overgrowth of the lining of the nose (see page 69).

The commonly used sympathomimetic drugs in decongestant preparations to be applied up the nose are ephedrine, naphazoline, oxymetazoline, phenylephrine, phenylpropanolamine, pseudoephedrine and xylometazoline. They provide relief from a blocked nose for about 2–6 hours but remember that these drugs may be absorbed into the bloodstream, and produce harmful effects in some people.

Nasal decongestants may cause irritation and dryness of the nose, throat and mouth. If over-used they may produce general harmful effects. Naphazoline and xylometazoline may, if over-used, be absorbed sufficiently into the bloodstream to depress the brain, causing coma and a marked reduction in body temperature, especially in infants.

Warning *Use nasal decongestant sprays or drops to relieve a runny or blocked nose only when it is really necessary; for example, if you have to go to a meeting and cannot get out of it. If you do have to use one, use it only two or three times daily for no more than a few days. Remember, steam inhalations may provide transient relief and salt solution nose drops may also produce relief, but buy only from a pharmacist who will make up a fresh solution.*

*Drops of oil from oily nasal solutions may be inhaled and cause pneumonia; they should **never** be used.*

Cold remedies containing antihistamine drugs

Antihistamines used in cold (and cough) remedies include brompheniramine, chlorpheniramine, diphenhydramine, doxylamine, pheniramine and promethazine.

Antihistamines are used to treat allergies such as hayfever because they block the effects of histamine which is released from injured cells following the breathing in of a foreign protein, for example pollen. The release of histamine produces 'inflammation' of the lining of the nose and throat, and causes symptoms like that of a bad cold.

In treating a common cold, the use of antihistamine drugs might be a

Table 3.1 Nasal decongestants taken by mouth

Preparation	*Drug*	*Drug group*	*Dosage form*
Actifed	pseudoephedrine triprolidine	sympathomimetic antihistamine	Tablets, syrup
Benylin Decongestant	pseudoephedrine diphenhydramine	sympathomimetic antihistamine	Syrup
Congesteze	pseudoephedrine azatadine	sympathomimetic antihistamine	Tablets, syrup, paediatric syrup
Dimotane Plus	pseudoephedrine brompheniramine	sympathomimetic antihistamine	Paediatric liquid, sugar-free
Dimotane Plus LA	pseudoephedrine brompheniramine	sympathomimetic antihistamine	Sustained-release tablets
Dimotapp	phenylephrine phenylpropanolamine brompheniramine	sympathomimetic sympathomimetic antihistamine	Sugar-free elixir and paediatric elixir
Dimotapp LA	phenylephrine phenylpropanolamine brompheniramine	sympathomimetic sympathomimetic antihistamine	Sustained-release tablets
Eskornade	phenylpropanolamine diphenylpyraline	sympathomimetic antihistamine	Sustained-release capsules, sugar-free syrup
Expurhin	ephedrine chlorpheniramine	sympathomimetic antihistamine	Paediatric linctus (sugar-free)
Galpseud	pseudoephedrine	sympathomimetic	Tablets, sugar-free linctus
Haymine	ephedrine chlorpheniramine	sympathomimetic antihistamine	Sustained-release tablets
Sudafed	pseudoephedrine	sympathomimetic	Tablets, elixir
Sudafed-Co	paracetamol pseudoephedrine	pain reliever sympathomimetic	Tablets
Sudafed Plus	pseudoephedrine triprolidine	sympathomimetic antihistamine	Tablets, syrup
Sudafed SA	pseudoephedrine	sympathomimetic	Sustained-release capsules
Triogesic	paracetamol phenylpropanolamine	pain reliever sympathomimetic	Tablets, sugar-free elixir
Triominic	phenylpropanolamine pheniramine	sympathomimetic antihistamine	Tablets, syrup
Uniflu with Gregovite C	phenylephrine diphenhydramine caffeine codeine paracetamol	sympathomimetic antihistamine stimulant pain reliever pain reliever	Tablets plus chewable tablets of vitamin C

Nasal decongestant preparations applied up the nose are listed in Table 7.1.

good idea if the symptoms were actually caused by an allergic reaction and the release of histamine; but inflammation in a cold is caused by a virus infection and there is no evidence that antihistamine drugs are of benefit in relieving this type of inflammation. However, in addition to their antihistamine effects, they affect the brain, producing drowsiness which may dampen down the cough control centre in the brain. They may also produce slight drying up of the linings of the nose and air passages. It is these usually unwanted harmful effects of antihistamines that are exploited when they are included in cold remedies.

The drying effect on the nose and air passages produced by antihistamines is a result of weak anticholinergic effects which these drugs produce. This drying effect is usually slight, but even so it may interfere with the natural protection which the mucus covering of the air passages provides and may possibly do more harm than good. Also, the drowsiness caused by antihistamine drugs may be dangerous because it may affect your ability to drive and operate moving machinery. Furthermore, antihistamines may be particularly dangerous when taken with alcohol because they increase its effects. They also increase the effects of sleeping drugs, tranquillizers and narcotic pain relievers.

Cold remedies that contain antihistamines known to produce marked drowsiness are usually recommended to be taken at bedtime; nevertheless, they may still produce hangover effects the next day in some people.

Warning *In the treatment of common cold symptoms there is no convincing evidence from adequate and well controlled studies that the benefits of taking a cold remedy containing an antihistamine outweigh the risks.*

Avoid cold remedies that contain anticholinergic drugs (e.g. atropine, belladonna, isopropamide)

It will help you to understand this section better if you first read the chapter on the autonomic nervous system (Chapter 2). Part of our nervous system is self-governing (autonomous). We have no voluntary control over it; for example, it controls our heart rate which increases automatically when we exercise and slows down when we rest. The self-governing nervous system has two parts, which work against each other to produce a balance. One part is called the sympathetic system and stimulation of this produces many adrenaline-like effects such as increasing the heart rate. The other system works alongside the sympathetic and is called the parasympathetic system. Stimulation of this system produces opposite effects to adrenaline. It makes you sweat, produce more saliva and tears, tightens up your bronchial tubes, slows your heart rate, increases the movements of your gut, contracts your bladder (to make you pass urine) and constricts your pupils. Stimulation also excites the brain.

These effects are produced by the release of a chemical messenger at nerve endings. This messenger is called acetylcholine and the effects produced are called cholinergic effects (acetylcholine effects). There are drugs that can produce these effects and they are called cholinergic drugs. There is also a group of drugs that block these effects; they are called anticholinergic drugs. Belladonna is an example of such a drug; it is found in the poisonous plant deadly nightshade. These chemicals (of which atropine is the best example) can affect all organs and tissues supplied by the parasympathetic nervous system. The ones included in some cold remedies include belladonna and isopropamide.

In the treatment of cold symptoms, anticholinergic drugs dry up the linings of the nose and air passages and act as decongestants. This may interfere with the natural protection against infection which the mucus on these linings offer (see earlier). What is more, if given by mouth in effective doses, they produce more harmful effects than benefits; for example, blurred vision, dry mouth, constipation, difficulty in passing urine and confusion. They should not be used. They are present in some herbal remedies but usually in doses so low as to produce no effect.

Warning *Cold mixtures that contain an anticholinergic drug and an antihistamine drug expose the user to both the drowsiness produced by the antihistamine and the drying up of the nose and air passages produced by both drugs. Such mixtures are not recommended.*

Vapour rubs and inhalants used to treat colds

Steam inhalations may help to provide transient relief from a blocked nose and may soothe an irritating cough. This treatment is safe and cheap but it obviously has no 'magic' in it; therefore it helps some individuals to add a substance whose vapour at least smells as if it might do some good. These are usually aromatic essential oils such as eucalyptus oil, peppermint oil or pine oil, or aromatic substances such as camphor or menthol. These aromatic substances are also included in vapour rubs and in preparations to be applied to handkerchiefs and clothing. Because it is not always convenient to use steam inhalations, these preparations offer an alternative way of breathing in the vapours for those individuals who believe in them.

Harmful effects of essential oil vapours

Essential oils (e.g. peppermint, pine, eucalyptus) may irritate the skin and produce dermatitis. Highly concentrated vapours of essential oils can kill mice and may produce sleepiness, coughs, headaches, and liver and kidney damage in workers exposed to such vapours. Highly concentrated vapours or the prolonged use of such vapours should therefore be avoided, especially in babies and infants.

Dangers of camphor

There have been reports of instant collapse of infants who have had a local application of camphor up their nostrils.

Camphorated oil is toxic if swallowed accidentally and should not be used.

Dangers of menthol

Menthol can cause allergic reactions in some patients, producing nettle rash (urticaria), flushing and headache. It may also cause dermatitis when applied to the skin. There are reports of immediate collapse following the application of menthol to the nose of infants. Also, menthol nose drops may cause spasm of the throat and make it difficult for young children to breathe.

Does inhaling vapours help?

There is no doubt that some people find the smell of menthol and eucalyptus (and other essential oils) attractive and that they believe that they provide some relief from cold symptoms. Certainly, the use of such vapours is an essential part of our folk medicine and they are very symbolic of caring and being cared for. It would be difficult to design a study to determine whether their principal effects are in the mind or whether they produce direct beneficial effects on the air passages. However, there is no convincing evidence from adequate and well controlled studies that they work, nor is there any convincing evidence that they do not work: and of course the same observation could be made about steam inhalations. Nevertheless, inhaled vapours from applications applied to a handkerchief, applied to clothing or a pillow, rubbed into the chest or inhaled from an inhaler appear to provide transient relief of symptoms in some people, and if used only occasionally appear to be harmless. However, they may be harmful if over-used. They should be used with *utmost caution* in babies under 1 month of age because strong applications may affect their breathing.

Wright's Vaporizing Fluid contains liquid chlorocresol (a disinfectant) which vaporizes when heated, using the small candles provided (night lights). Its antiseptic and rather 'clinical' smell may help some people to believe that they are being cared for or are providing care. Chlorocresol is irritant to the skin and, because it is corrosive, it is very dangerous if accidentally swallowed.

Vitamin C in the treatment of colds

The usefulness of high doses of vitamin C in the treatment of colds is a subject of controversy. Those in favour of its use produce evidence that when you have a cold your body's level of vitamin C is reduced and that you need to take additional vitamin C. Some researchers have shown that vitamin C kills viruses and bacteria; others have shown that it has anti-inflammatory and antihistamine properties and that it is involved in the body's immune system (defence against infections) and also involved in repair when cells have been damaged by infection. However, none of these observations has been definitely proved to be relevant to the treatment of colds, so there is still much controversy about whether or not vitamin C is beneficial. Evidence that vitamin C and aspirin taken together is beneficial in treating colds is also contradictory.

Risks of high doses of vitamin C

There are dangers to the daily use of high doses of vitamin C. It has been shown that we can become used to large daily doses so that when the daily dose is dropped back to normal daily requirements we may develop signs of deficiency (scurvy). High daily doses of vitamin C may also cause kidney stones.

In order to make large doses of vitamin C palatable, some preparations are made to dissolve in water as a fizzy drink. To produce the fizziness, the preparations usually contain high doses of sodium bicarbonate (bicarbonate of soda). This high amount of sodium may be harmful to patients with a raised blood pressure, kidney disease or heart disease.

Conclusion on the use of vitamin C

There is no convincing evidence from adequate and well controlled studies that taking any dose of vitamin C daily helps to prevent colds, reduces the severity of cold symptoms or shortens the duration of a cold.

Soothing throat lozenges and pastilles

We spend millions of pounds each year on what chemists and druggists call medicated confectionery – preparations used to soothe sore throats.

Apart from the release of vapours (e.g. menthol) which may produce some transient clearing of the nose in some people, throat lozenges and pastilles act as demulcents – which means that they coat the surface of the throat to soothe any soreness and protect it from irritation. However, this coating may easily be washed away by the saliva which is produced by sucking the lozenges or pastilles. Fortunately, saliva is the body's natural product for soothing the throat and preventing it from being irritated and this is what probably produces most of the relief. Ordinary toffees or even chewing gum may therefore work just as well as throat lozenges and pastilles, and they are much cheaper. Certainly it would be very difficult to disprove this. Nevertheless, there is a large psychological element involved, and those people who believe in them will feel better if they suck throat lozenges and pastilles, even though they are probably only very expensive sweets.

Warning *Some throat lozenges and pastilles are very high in sugar content and may be harmful to teeth (particularly in children) because they are sucked slowly between meals. They should not be used by diabetic patients.*

Anti-bacterial and/or antiseptic throat lozenges and pastilles

Some throat lozenges and pastilles contain an anti-bacterial drug and/or an antiseptic. Because most sore throats are caused by a virus infection and because anti-bacterial drugs have no effect on viruses, there is no point in taking these drugs to treat a sore throat. If your sore throat is caused by a bacterial infection, you need to take the most suitable antibiotic in a proper effective dosage. Furthermore, anti-bacterial or antiseptic drugs in throat preparations are usually present in a small dose and any of the drug which makes contact with the surface of the throat is quickly diluted and washed away by the saliva and swallowed.

Throat lozenges and pastilles that contain a local anaesthetic

Local anaesthetic drugs are included in some throat lozenges and pastilles in order to relieve pain. There is much controversy about the effectiveness of available preparations and the effectiveness of the various anaesthetics used in throat lozenges and pastilles. Their effectiveness will depend directly upon the concentration of the local anaesthetic. In an effective concentration they will provide transient relief from a sore throat caused by a cold virus but at this dose they may also mask symptoms and delay the individual from seeking effective treatment for a more serious disorder (e.g. a bacterial tonsillitis).

Gargles used to treat sore throats

Most sore throats are caused by viruses that are not affected by the concentrations of antiseptics used in gargles; therefore there is no point at all in using them. A sore throat caused by a bacterial infection needs appropriate treatment with an antibiotic.

Table 3.2 Drugs used to treat colds – harmful effects and warnings

Drugs used to relieve aches, pains and feverishness

Aspirin
For harmful effects and warnings, see Chapter 27; for preparations of aspirin, see Chapter 27.

Paracetamol
For harmful effects and warnings, see Chapter 27; for preparations of paracetamol, see Chapter 27.

Warning Cold remedies that contain aspirin or paracetamol combined with other drugs expose you to the risk of harmful effects from several drugs. For the relief of aches, pains and fever it is best to use single effective doses of aspirin or paracetamol rather than using a mixture.

Drugs used to relieve a blocked and/or runny nose

Decongestant drugs by mouth
Usually contain a sympathomimetic drug, which produces adrenaline-like effects on the body. The ones most commonly used are ephedrine, phenylephrine, phenylpropanolamine and pseudoephedrine.

Harmful effects Phenylephrine may produce a rise in blood pressure, nervousness, insomnia, headache, vomiting, light-headedness and, rarely, palpitations. *Ephedrine, phenylpropanolamine* and *pseudoephedrine* in high doses (normal doses in some people) may produce giddiness, headache, nausea, vomiting, palpitations, tremor, thirst, difficulty in passing urine, muscle weakness, anxiety, restlessness, chest pain, shortness of breath and insomnia. Raised blood pressure may occur. Overdose may cause serious mental symptoms, including delusions and hallucinations.

Warnings Ephedrine, phenylephrine, phenylpropanolamine and *pseudoephedrine* should not be used or used only with utmost caution by people who are over-excitable and may be sensitive to the effects of adrenaline-like drugs, or by people with over-active thyroid glands

Table 3.2 Drugs used to treat colds – harmful effects and warnings (*cont.*)

diabetes, raised blood pressure, hardening of the arteries (arteriosclerosis), disorders of the heart or circulation, or fast pulse rate. They should be used with caution by anyone with closed-angle glaucoma. They are related to amphetamines and frequent regular use may cause addiction. Avoid drinking too much tea, coffee or cola because the caffeine may add to the nervous symptoms in some individuals.

Risks in elderly people Harmful effects may be more frequent and severe; therefore, use with utmost caution.

Nasal decongestant sprays and drops
Usually contain a sympathomimetic drug which produces adrenaline-like effects on the body. The ones most commonly used include ephedrine, naphazoline, oxymetazoline, phenylephrine, phenylpropanolamine, pseudoephedrine and xylometazoline.

Harmful effects Nasal decongestants may all cause irritation and dryness of the nose. Prolonged use for more than 10 days may damage the lining of the nose. Some of the drug may be absorbed into the bloodstream to produce general effects (see under 'Decongestant drugs by mouth'). Harmful effects include light-headedness, palpitations and tremor. In addition, *naphazoline* and *xylometazoline* may cause nausea and headache, and their over-use may cause a fall in body temperature, sweating, slowing of the pulse, drowsiness and coma, particularly in children. A rise in blood pressure may be followed by a fall in blood pressure. *Oxymetazoline* may cause stinging or burning, sneezing and dryness of the mouth and throat.

Warnings They should not be used by people who are allergic to them, nor by anyone who suffers from closed-angle glaucoma. They should be used with caution by those who suffer from disorders of the heart or circulation, raised blood pressure, over-active thyroid gland or diabetes.

Infants and children may be very susceptible to the harmful effects of nasal decongestants; they should therefore be used with utmost caution by children under the age of 7 years; they should not be used by infants under 3 months of age. Drops of oil from oily nasal solutions may be inhaled and cause pneumonia; they should never be used.

Antihistamines used in cold remedies
May produce drowsiness and dry up the breathing passages. For harmful effects and warnings on the use of antihistamines, see Chapter 10.

Anticholinergic drugs used in cold remedies
May produce blurred vision, dry mouth, constipation, difficulty in passing urine and confusion. For other harmful effects produced by anticholinergic drugs, see Chapter 2.

Vapour rubs and inhalants
For harmful effects of essential oils (e.g. peppermint, pine, eucalyptus), camphor and menthol, see earlier.

Vitamin C
For harmful effects of high doses of vitamin C, see Chapter 45.

Soothing throat lozenges, pastilles and syrups
May damage the teeth because they are often high in sugar content and are sucked between meals. Diabetic patients should use sugar-free products.

Anti-bacterial throat preparations
May produce soreness, encourage the growth of fungus in the mouth, cause bacterial resistance to the particular antibiotic and produce allergic reactions.

Antiseptic throat preparations
May cause local irritation and soreness.

Warning Chrolaseptic throat spray should be used with utmost caution.

Anaesthetic throat preparations
May cause local irritation (U).

Gargles
May cause local irritation in the mouth and throat.

4

Coughs

Some coughs serve a useful purpose, for example to get rid of something that has 'gone down the wrong way' or to cough up phlegm. Common causes of coughing include infection of the bronchial tubes (bronchitis), inflammation of the air passages that occurs in asthma and breathing in irritants (e.g. smoking). Coughs, like the ones you get with colds, are caused by a virus infection and are often just dry and irritating, serving no useful purpose. Most acute coughs clear up on their own and are usually associated with a cold. Most long-standing coughs occur in smokers and in people the bronchitis and other chronic chest disorders.

When the chest is congested (e.g. acute bronchitis) we develop a rattly cough on the chest (a *congestive* cough) and may cough up phlegm (a mixture of mucus and pus). We describe this as a *productive* cough (i.e. a cough that produces phlegm when we cough). A dry cough not associated with congestion of the chest and producing no phlegm is called a *non-productive* cough. Congestion of the chest may produce a rattly cough which is also non-productive.

A congestive cough on the chest is helped by anything that 'loosens' the phlegm and makes it easier to cough up. Avoiding dry atmospheres, stopping smoking, drinking more fluids than normal and using steam inhalations are all beneficial, provided of course that any underlying infection, inflammation and wheezing are treated effectively. If these actions are taken, there is seldom need to take a cough medicine that is supposed to 'loosen' the phlegm and/or increase its production.

A dry, irritating, non-productive cough will also benefit from avoiding dry atmospheres, stopping smoking, drinking more fluids than normal and using steam inhalations. It may also benefit from the use of a cough suppressant (see later).

Cough medicines

There are three main types of cough medicine: soothing cough medicines for throaty coughs; ones that stop you coughing (cough suppressants or antitussives); and ones that are supposed to enable you to cough up phlegm more easily, called cough expectorants.

Soothing cough medicines

We spend millions of pounds every year on cough lozenges, pastilles and syrups to relieve dry coughs produced by irritation in the throat (often referred to as 'throaty' coughs). These are nearly always associated with a cold and last for only a short period of time – usually no more than a day or two.

Soothing cough medicines (lozenges, pastilles and syrups) contain sweet substances such as sorbitol, glycerol and syrup, and in addition they contain mixtures of chemicals such as peppermint, eucalyptus, lemon, clove, aniseed, menthol and camphor.

Soothing cough medicines coat the surface of the throat and protect it from irritation. They also make you produce more saliva which is the body's natural protection against irritation of the throat. It is probably this increase in the production of saliva that really helps to soothe your throat, and therefore sucking ordinary sweets or chewing gum probably works just as well. However, soothing cough medicines are part of our folk medicine and they are subjected to extravagant sales promotion. Some people believe that they work and it would be almost impossible to design a scientific study to unravel the problem. There is little harm in believing, but it is important for you to understand that they are often expensive and much of the money that you pay for these preparations has gone on television and newspaper advertising and sales discounts to pharmacists and druggists.

Warning *Because of the high sugar content of some soothing cough medicines and the fact that you take them between meals, they may be harmful to teeth, particularly in children. They should not be taken by diabetic patients.*

Cough suppressants

The throat and air passages are very sensitive to irritation, which triggers messages up to the brain where they are picked up in a special nerve centre called the 'cough centre'. The cough centre responds by sending messages back down to the nerves supplying the muscles of the chest wall, abdomen and diaphragm to tell them to contract; this produces a cough. This reflex may be very useful if you have inhaled something (note how you cough if something has 'gone down the wrong way'). However, it may be very annoying if you have a cold or some other disorder that makes you keep coughing all the time.

There are several effective drugs available which reduce the sensitivity of the cough centre and stop it sending messages out to cough. In other words, they suppress your cough. There are two groups of cough suppressants – those that may produce addiction and those that do not. They are used to relieve coughs that do not produce phlegm (non-productive coughs).

Cough suppressant drugs that may produce addiction (narcotic cough suppressants)

Diamorphine (heroin), methadone and morphine are narcotics which are very effective in suppressing coughs. Their use should be restricted to treating severe coughs; for example, in patients dying from cancer of the lung. In the doses used to treat coughs they affect the brain and may produce drowsiness, they may also cause constipation, depression of breathing and difficulty in passing urine. They are discussed in Chapter 27, under 'Narcotic pain relievers'.

Codeine is obtained from opium or made from morphine. Two salts of codeine (codeine sulphate and codeine phosphate) are used as cough suppressants. One or other appears in numerous cough medicines.

Codeine is a moderately effective cough suppressant. It may produce drowsiness, dizziness, nausea and constipation (which may be a particular problem in the elderly). Large doses may produce excitement, and in children convulsions may occur. Some patients may be allergic to codeine and develop nettle rash (urticaria) and itching skin (pruritus). If high, regular, daily doses of codeine cough medicine are used there is a risk that some individuals may come to 'rely' on the medicine and start having to increase the dose because not only are they becoming tolerant to the effects of the codeine but they are also becoming addicted to it. Babies have been born addicted to codeine because their mothers took codeine cough medicine daily during pregnancy. Codeine and other narcotic cough suppressants should not be given to children under one year of age

Cough suppressant drugs that do not produce addiction but that are weaker than codeine

Pholcodine is related to morphine. It may produce nausea and drowsiness. In high doses it may produce restlessness, excitement and lack of control over voluntary movement, producing, for example, difficulty in walking.

Dextromethorphan is nearly as potent as codeine but produces fewer harmful effects. It may cause drowsiness, dizziness, excitation, mental confusion, and stomach upsets. Very high doses may depress the rate and depth of breathing.

Noscapine is obtained from opium. It has no pain relieving properties and is not a drug of addiction, but is as effective as pholcodine. It may produce slight drowsiness, dizziness, headache and nausea, and it may cause allergic symptoms affecting the nose, eyes and skin.

Isoaminile is as effective as pholcodine. It may produce dizziness, nausea, constipation and diarrhoea.

Choosing a cough suppressant

For a dry, irritating, throaty cough associated with a cold there is seldom any need to take a cough suppressant. Sucking a sweet, whether medicated or not, will help because it will increase the production of saliva which will soothe the throat. If this does not work or the irritation is below the voicebox (where soothing cough lozenges, pastilles and syrups can have no effect because they are swallowed into the stomach), avoiding dry atmospheres, stopping smoking, drinking more fluids than normal and using steam inhalation will normally help. If this does not work or is inconvenient, it may be worth trying a cough suppressant, particularly if a dry, irritating cough is disturbing your sleep. Choose a cough medicine that contains *only one cough suppressant in an effective dose*; for example, codeine or one of the following – dextromethorphan, isoaminile, noscapine or pholcodine. There is little to choose between the latter provided they are taken in effective cough-suppressant doses. One dose should provide relief for up to 4 hours. With most acute coughs there is no need to take more than three or four doses daily for more than 2 to 3 days.

Cough expectorants

Our traditional liking for cough medicines goes back to the days when there were no antibiotics and tuberculosis (consumption), bronchitis and other chest diseases were rife. Doctors were able to do very little but prescribe bottles of brightly coloured medicines, which if they tasted awful were supposed to do you good! Paradoxically, despite the availability today of specific and effective treatments for these disorders the use of cough medicines continues, principally due to heavy advertising by drug companies and our faith in them.

Cough expectorant drugs are supposed to help you cough up phlegm by increasing its production but there is little evidence of such beneficial effects. There is evidence that they irritate the lining of the stomach and that in high doses this irritation will stimulate the vomiting centre in the brain to make you vomit. However, there is doubtful evidence that if they are taken in a dose not big enough to make you vomit that they stimulate, by a reflex mechanism, the cells in the bronchial tubes to produce more secretions that will soften the phlegm and make it easier to cough up. Yet this is the belief, even though it has never been convincingly proved that any of these drugs can help you to cough up phlegm. Despite this there are several drugs marketed for this purpose. They include acetic acid, ammonium salts, bromhexine, camphor, cocillana, creosote, guaiacol, guaiacol carbonate, guaiphenesin, iodides, ipecacuanha, liquorice, senega, squill and terpin.

These various chemicals used as expectorants may irritate the lining of the stomach and in high doses produce nausea and vomiting. They should be used with caution by people who suffer from peptic ulcers.

Harmful effects of cough expectorants

Ammonium chloride and other ammonium salts in large doses may produce vomiting, nausea, thirst, headache, rapid breathing, progressive drowsiness, make the blood acid (acidosis) and cause a fall in blood potassium.

Guaiacol may cause drowsiness.

Liquorice may cause salt and water to be retained from the urine and a loss of potassium in the urine. These effects may cause fluid retention in the body, raised blood pressure and disturbances in the chemistry of the blood.

Iodine as potassium iodide or sodium iodide is present in some cough medicines as an expectorant. The risks of regular daily use of cough medicines containing iodides include mental depression, nervousness, insomnia, sexual impotence, and under-activity of the thyroid gland. Goitres may occur in infants born to mothers who took cough medicines containing iodides regularly every day during pregnancy. Allergy may occur to iodides (iodism) and cause symptoms like a common cold – headache, pain and swelling of the salivary glands, watery eyes, weakness, conjunctivitis, fever, laryngitis and bronchitis. Skin rashes may occur such as a mild redness of face or acne of the face.

Ipecacuanha is of interest because it is used as a drug to make you vomit if you have taken an overdose of certain drugs (e.g. alcohol). It contains two drugs – emetine and cephaeline. It is irritant to the lining of the stomach and intestine, and in high doses it may produce vomiting, bloody diarrhoea and ulceration of the stomach and/or intestine. Such high doses may also damage the kidneys, producing proteins in the urine, and may be toxic to the heart.

Squill irritates the lining of the stomach, and in high doses it may produce nausea, vomiting and severe diarrhoea; it may also affect the heart, producing effects like those produced by digoxin. Cough medicines containing squill should not be taken by patients with kidney or heart disorders.

Other drugs used in cough medicines

Numerous other drugs are included in cough medicines despite the fact that there is no convincing evidence that they are of any benefit other than improving the colour, taste or smell – they include benzoic preparations, camphor, eucalyptus oil, menthol, peppermint oil, pine tar, sodium citrate, tolu and turpentine oil.

The use of antihistamine drugs in cough medicines

Antihistamine drugs used in cough medicines include chlorpheniramine, diphenhydramine, pheniramine, promethazine and triprolidine. They produce two effects that are exploited in cough medicines – they act on the brain, producing drowsiness and a damping down of the cough centre, and they dry up the lining of the nose and breathing passages.

Warnings *The drowsiness produced by antihistamines included in cough medicines may affect your ability to drive motor vehicles and operate moving machinery. Antihistamines may also increase the effects of alcohol, sleeping drugs, tranquillizers and narcotic pain relievers. Furthermore, their effects on drying up the lining of the breathing passages may actually make it harder for you to cough up phlegm if you have congestion on your chest.*

The drowsiness produced by antihistamines may interfere with breathing in people who suffer from chronic bronchitis and other serious chest disorders because it may cause a build-up of carbon dioxide in the blood.

The use of bronchodilator drugs in cough medicines

Irritation of the lining of bronchial tubes may cause them to constrict, which may cause coughing. For example, a cough may be an early symptom of asthma or allergy. In a cough of this kind it is important to take an effective dose of a drug that dilates the bronchial tubes, a bronchodilator, and to treat any associated infection and/or inflammation or allergy. The bronchodilators used in cough medicines (e.g. bufylline, ephedrine, theophylline) are usually present in such small doses as to be of little benefit if you suffer from asthma or some other wheezing disorder. Furthermore, if you do not suffer from a wheezing disorder they are of doubtful value.

The use of decongestant drugs in cough medicines

Decongestant drugs are discussed in detail in Chapter 3. They are included in some cough medicines. The three most commonly used are pseudoephedrine, phenylephrine and phenylpropanolamine. They are usually present in very small doses but if you overdose or use a nasal decongestant that contains one or more of these drugs at the same time, you may develop toxic symptoms, which include headache, nausea, vomiting, sweating, rapid beating of the heart, palpitations, muscle weakness, restlessness, anxiety, insomnia and difficulty in passing urine.

The use of anticholinergic drugs in cough medicines

Anticholinergic drugs (e.g. belladonna) dry up the lining of the air passages and dilate the bronchial tubes. The benefits and risks of using these drugs to treat the common cold are discussed in Chapter 3, and to treat asthma in Chapter 12. Because they dry the air passages, they may make it more difficult to cough up phlegm.

Warning *Any cough medicine that contains a decongestant, antihistamine and/or an anticholinergic drug may make it more difficult to cough up phlegm.*

Drugs that reduce the stickiness of phlegm and make it easier to cough up

Drugs that reduce the stickiness of phlegm are called mucolytics. They reduce the stickiness of sputum and help to liquefy the phlegm.

Mucolytic drugs may be taken by inhalation or by mouth.

Inhalational mucolytics Acetylcysteine is the one used most frequently but there is doubt about its effectiveness by inhalation, which may cause wheezing in some individuals particularly those who suffer from asthma.

Mucolytics that may be taken by mouth include acetylcysteine (Fabrol), carbocisteine (Mucodyne) and methylcysteine (Visclair). However, there is controversy over how much people benefit from their use even though they do liquefy the sputum.

Cough mixtures (compound cough medicine)

Cough mixtures contain small doses of several drugs aimed at reducing coughs. They are very popular and expensive. Some mixtures are quite irrational – combining a cough suppressant to stop you coughing with a cough expectorant to help you cough, or mixing small doses of a large number of drugs that produce the same effects.

Advice on treating coughs

For a dry irritating cough caused by a cold that is interfering with your sleep or disrupting your day it is best to use a cough medicine that contains a *single drug* (e.g. codeine linctus).

For a chesty rattly cough (congestive cough) where it is difficult to cough up phlegm, cough medicines are of little use even though they are supposed to 'loosen' the phlegm and make it easier to cough up. It is far more important to drink more fluids than usual and to use water or steam inhalations; to avoid dry, smoky atmospheres; to stop smoking if you smoke; to check whether any drug you are taking may dry up your bronchial tubes; and to seek medical advice and have specific treatment for any wheezing that may be due to infection and/or inflammation of the bronchial tubes.

Always seek medical advice for any cough that persists for more than 2 or 3 days, if your phlegm is yellowish-green or if it is bloodstained and/or if you have a fever associated with your cough.

Reducing the risks of cold and cough mixtures

If you still wish to take a cold and/or cough mixture be guided by the following warnings.

If you are on a low salt diet, a low sugar diet (e.g. if you are a diabetic), if you are allergic to any preservative or dyes in medicines or if you are allergic to any of the drugs included in cough and cold medicines, check with your pharmacist before purchasing a cold or cough mixture.

Cold and cough mixtures contain more than one active drug and many liquid cough mixtures contain alcohol; therefore check with your pharmacist if you wish to avoid using a cough mixture that contains alcohol or a drug that may cause a problem for you.

If you are pregnant or breast feeding it is safest to avoid the use of drugs if possible. It is certainly safer to avoid the use of mixtures of drugs. For harmful effects and warnings on the use of drugs in pregnancy, see Chapter 79 and when breast feeding, see Chapter 80.

Be most cautious about using cold and cough mixtures if you suffer from diabetes, asthma or other chronic chest disorders, enlarged prostate gland or any difficulty in passing urine, any disorder of the heart or circulation, raised blood pressure, kidney or liver disease or over-active thyroid gland. Consult your pharmacist before purchasing a preparation.

Always check with your pharmacist whether it is safe to take a cough or cold remedy along with alcohol or any other drug treatment you may be taking, whether prescribed by your doctor or purchased by you 'over-the-counter' (see Chapter 89).

Always ask your pharmacist for clear instructions on how to take a cold or cough remedy. Always take the stated dose; do not overdose because you will increase the risk of harmful effects.

Never take more than one cough or cold remedy or pain reliever without checking that it is safe to do so.

Remember that some cold and cough remedies may contain a drug that could irritate the stomach (e.g. aspirin). Such preparations should be taken *with* or *after* food and not on an empty stomach. Check with your pharmacist.

Sustained-release capsules or tablets should be swallowed whole and not chewed before swallowing.

It is not important if you miss out a dose of a cough or cold remedy. Take it as soon as possible; but if it is nearly time for your next dose, skip a dose. Never take a double dose in order to catch up.

Always keep cough and cold remedies out of reach of children and away from heat and direct light but not in the bathroom where heat and moisture may cause the drugs to break down.

Do not keep out-of-date cough and cold remedies; flush them down the toilet or, preferably, return them to your pharmacist for disposal.

5

Throat infections and laryngitis

An infection of the surface of the throat is called pharyngitis. If the infection focuses on to the tonsils it is called tonsillitis.

Virus infections are most common and you do not need antibiotics

The most common cause of a sore throat is a virus infection, for which there is no specific treatment apart from sucking a sweet or a throat lozenge and taking a pain reliever such as aspirin or paracetamol. Unfortunately, millions of tablets, capsules and bottles of antibiotics are taken every year by people suffering from virus infections of the throat. Not only is this unnecessary and very expensive, it may also be harmful because it exposes these people to the risks of allergic and other reactions for no benefit and it may encourage the development of antibiotic-resistant bacteria.

Bacterial sore throats

The commonest bacterial infection of the throat is caused by a streptococcal infection (a 'strep. sore throat'). This infection can cause tonsillitis and complications such as rheumatic fever and kidney disease. It needs treating quickly and effectively with the right antibiotic in the right dose for the right duration of time. Treatment should not be a hit and miss thing and it should preferably be based on laboratory identification of the infecting organism and tests of its sensitivity to selected antibiotics. In other words, a throat swab from the throat should, if possible, be taken before starting any treatment. Phenoxymethylpenicillin (penicillin V) is the drug of choice and it should be taken for a full 10 days. If the infection is severe an initial injection of benzylpenicillin (penicillin G) should be given into a muscle. If the patient is allergic to penicillin, erythromycin should be used.

Chronic sore throat

Chronic inflammation of the throat (chronic pharyngitis) is always due to some continuing irritant – e.g. shouting, over-singing, smoking, alcohol drinking and/or coughing. It may also be caused by chronic mouth breathing due to a blocked nose or a chronic sinus infection. Treatment is obvious and does not involve the use of drugs – stop smoking, stop drinking alcohol, stop shouting, etc.

Treatment of laryngitis

Laryngitis is an inflammation of the voicebox which affects the vocal cords, producing a hoarse voice. Acute laryngitis is often due to a virus infection (e.g. cold virus). It may also occur from shouting, over-singing, allergy and inhaling irritant fumes. Chronic laryngitis is often due to shouting or over-singing, what the specialists politely call 'vocal abuse'. It occurs particularly by straining the voice during an acute attack of laryngitis. It is made worse by coughing and smoking.

The best treatment for acute laryngitis is to rest the voice, inhale steam and avoid irritants (e.g. smoking). Cough or cold remedies will not be beneficial except for their psychological effects (i.e. their effects on the mind). If hoarseness persists for more than a week or so, you should ask your doctor to send you to see an ear, nose and throat (ENT) specialist for a check-up.

Summary of recommendations on the drug treatment of colds, sore throats and coughs

Relieving aches, pains and feverishness caused by a cold

There is no convincing evidence to show that any of the many cold remedies on the market are better than paracetamol or aspirin used alone in standard doses.

Paracetamol is the drug of choice for treatment. Soluble aspirin is equally effective but it should not be given to children under the age of 12 years, and there are several warnings and precautions to its safe use.

Relieving a runny and/or blocked nose caused by a cold

Decongestants by mouth

Taking any decongestant by mouth to relieve a runny and/or blocked nose produced by a cold is like taking a sledge hammer to crack a nut. They are of doubtful benefit and the risks of using them in some people may easily outweigh such benefit, particularly in those who suffer from raised blood pressure, over-active thyroid gland, coronary heart disease (e.g. angina) or diabetes. They may be especially dangerous to someone taking monoamine oxidase inhibitor (MAOI) anti-depressant drugs.

In addition to a decongestant, some cold remedies to be taken by mouth also contain an antihistamine; this produces an additional risk of drowsiness, which may affect ability to drive and is made very much worse by taking alcohol. These preparations may dry up the air passages and make it difficult to cough up phlegm.

Decongestant nasal sprays and drops

These preparations provide relief from a runny and/or blocked nose for 2–6 hours but remember that the risks from over-use may easily outweigh any benefits, because you may become trapped into a cycle of using them to relieve the rebound blockage of the nose which they cause. Regular and prolonged use may permanently damage the lining of the nose. The stronger drugs used in nasal drops (oxymetazoline, phenylephrine, xylometazoline) are more likely to cause rebound effects than the others.

Decongestant nasal sprays and drops should be used *only* when really necessary, only for two or three times in a day and for no longer than 7–10 days. Ephedrine Nasal Drop solution is an effective and cheap preparation to use.

Salt (sodium chloride 0.9%) nasal drop solution, if freshly made up by a pharmacist, may provide some transient relief, and so too will steam inhalations.

Vapour rubs and inhalants

There is no convincing evidence from adequate and well controlled studies of the benefits of using vapour rubs and inhalants. They may produce transient relief of a blocked nose in some people but there are dangers if they are over-used, particularly in infants. Steam inhalations are cheap and effective and the addition of an aromatic substance such as eucalyptus may encourage their use. Vapour rubs and inhalants should not be used in babies and infants under 1 month of age.

Cold remedies containing a mixture of drugs

Cold remedies to be taken by mouth which contain a mixture of drugs aimed at relieving aches, pains and fever and also at relieving a runny and/or blocked nose and other symptoms are examples of blunderbuss treatment. A blunderbuss is a short gun with a large bore, which fires many balls. These remedies are like these guns: they fire many drugs that land all over the body, from the brain to the heart; yet there is no evidence that they are any more effective than taking two paracetamol tablets and occasionally using a suitable decongestant up the nose.

The drowsiness produced by an antihistamine may well be helpful during the night but could be harmful in the daytime, particularly if you drive and/or drink alcohol. In effective doses, anticholinergic drugs are too harmful. Other drugs used in such remedies are either not effective or are present in too small a dose to be effective. Both antihistamines and anticholinergic drugs may dry up the air passages and make it difficult to cough up phlegm.

The use of vitamin C

There is no convincing evidence from adequate and well controlled studies that taking vitamin C in whatever dose helps to prevent colds, reduce their severity or shorten their duration.

Relieving a sore throat caused by a cold

Medicated confectionery (*throat lozenges, pastilles and syrups*)

These are very expensive sweets that contain, for example, menthol, eucalyptus oil or other essential oils. The vapours given off by these sweets may produce a transient clearing of the nose in some people but there is no convincing evidence from adequate and well controlled studies that they are any more effective than sucking ordinary toffees or chewing gum in soothing a sore throat, because it is your own saliva that soothes the throat and protects it from irritation. Some contain a high amount of sugar which may be harmful to the teeth, particularly in children, because they are sucked slowly between meals. Diabetic people should not use them.

Anti-bacterial and/or antiseptic throat lozenges and pastilles

These are of no benefit because most sore throats are caused by virus infections which are not affected by anti-bacterial drugs nor by the concentration of antiseptics used in throat lozenges. If a throat infection is caused by a bacterial infection, it is important to take a full course of treatment with an appropriate antibiotic.

Anaesthetic throat lozenges and pastilles

There is much controversy about the effectiveness of the various local anaesthetic throat lozenges and pastilles that are available. An effective concentration of an anaesthetic in a throat lozenge or pastille will produce transient relief of pain in the throat but preparations that may be bought over the counter (without a prescription) contain less than effective doses. Regular use of these preparations may cause irritation of the throat.

Gargles used to treat sore throats

Most sore throats are caused by viruses which are not affected by the antiseptics used in gargles. A sore throat caused by a bacterial infection needs appropriate treatment with an antibiotic.

Soothing cough medicines

Soothing cough medicines are of no use for treating a cough coming from below the voicebox, and for throaty coughs above the voicebox they are probably no more effective than sucking ordinary sweets or chewing gum. It is your own saliva that helps to reduce the irritation. Many cough medicines contain sugars which may damage the teeth, particularly in children since they are usually taken between meals. Diabetic people should not use these preparations.

Cough suppressants

Most acute, dry, irritating coughs are caused by a cold and seldom need treating. You should stop smoking if you smoke, avoid dry atmospheres and drink more fluids than normal. Steam inhalations may help if the cough is painful. Only if the cough is disturbing your sleep or your work should you take a dose of a cough suppressant. Take one that contains a *single drug*; for example, codeine linctus.

To treat a dry, irritating cough associated with a cold, a cough suppressant linctus should be taken not more than three or four times daily and for not more than 2–3 days. Cough suppressants may cause constipation and other harmful effects.

Cough suppressants containing codeine or other narcotics should preferably not be used in children, and certainly not if they are under 1 year of age.

You should not use a cough suppressant if you suffer from asthma, chronic bronchitis or other chronic chest disorder because it may make it harder for you to cough up phlegm. Steam inhalations and antibiotics will be more beneficial, combined with treatment to relieve any wheezing and/or inflammation that is present; and of course you should stop smoking if you smoke, drink more fluids than you do normally and avoid dry atmospheres.

For a painful, irritating cough in a person dying from, for example, lung cancer, diamorphine linctus, methadone linctus or a solution of morphine may be useful if given by mouth at regular intervals. However, they may make it difficult to cough up phlegm, so a form of steam inhalation should be used as well. They may cause constipation and this will need treating.

Cough expectorants

Millions of bottles of medicines to help you cough up phlegm are prescribed and bought every year, yet there is no convincing evidence from adequate and well controlled studies that these preparations are of benefit other than psychological; i.e. their beneficial effect is principally in the mind!

Cough mixtures

Cough mixtures may contain a cough suppressant, cough expectorant, antihistamine, bronchodilator, and/or decongestant drug. They often contain an irrational mixture of drugs and are expensive. The doses of drugs in cough mixtures are usually too low to be effective if used alone and without any evidence of their effectiveness when combined in a mixture. Some of the drugs used in cough mixtures actually oppose each other in their effects, which will not do your cough much good; for example, some contain a cough suppressant to stop you coughing and a cough expectorant to help you cough up your phlegm! Despite these warnings many people swear by them, but of course about 4 out of 10 of us would benefit from a dummy medicine if we believed it was going to help us!

Despite what the adverts say, there is little point in taking cough mixtures; but if you really believe in cough mixtures then use the simplest and cheapest – e.g. simple linctus.

Warning *Apart from patients who are dying from cancer of the lung or some other serious disorder that produces a persistent and distressing cough, you should not use a cough medicine for more than a few days at a time. You should not get into the habit of taking cough medicines regularly; it is costly, potentially harmful and does you no good, particularly if you continue to smoke.*

Drugs used to reduce the stickiness of phlegm and make it easier to cough up (mucolytics)

There is no convincing evidence from adequate and well controlled studies to show that the inhalation of these drugs is more beneficial than inhaling steam alone. They are of doubtful benefit when taken by mouth. Steam inhalations and physiotherapy (postural drainage) are probably the most effective treatments to help coughing in chronic chest disorders such as bronchiectasis.

Inhalations

Steam inhalations are beneficial for treating productive coughs associated with disorders such as bronchitis. The addition of menthol or eucalyptus, etc., to the inhalant gives an aroma which at least smells beneficial and may encourage the use of steam inhalations.

6

Disorders of the ears

There are four commonly occurring disorders of the ears for which drugs are used:

- Removal of wax from the ears
- Inflammation of the outer ear (otitis externa)
- Inflammation of the middle ear (otitis media)
- Disorders of the organ of balance (see Chapter 14)

Removal of ear wax

Wax (cerumen) in the ear is normal and it helps to protect the lining of the outer ear. It needs removing only if there is so much that it is causing deafness or if the doctor cannot examine the ear drum properly in a patient with some other ear complaint. To clean the wax out, the ear should be syringed with warm water by a doctor or nurse. If the wax is very hard, it can be softened before syringing by applying sodium bicarbonate ear drops, warm olive oil or almond oil. Preparations that contain a wetting agent (e.g. docusate sodium) or urea hydrogen peroxide may be equally effective. The latter releases oxygen bubbles when it comes into contact with ear wax and this helps to break up the wax.

Preparations that contain turpentine oil may irritate the lining of the ear, and some ingredients may cause a local allergic reaction; for example paradichlorobenzene (also used in insect sprays) and chloroxylenol (an antiseptic).

To apply ear drops you should lie down with the affected ear uppermost, apply the drops into the ear and lie still for 10 minutes; before you get up, apply a cotton wool plug into the ear, which you should keep in for an hour or two.

Warning *Preparations used to treat wax in the ear only soften the wax, they do not remove it. It still has to be cleaned out or syringed out by a doctor or nurse.*

Table 6.1 Applications used to remove wax from the ears

Preparation	*Ingredients*	*Preparation*	*Ingredients*
Cerumol ear drops	chlorbutol, paradichloro-benzene, arachis oil	sodium bicarbonate ear drops	sodium bicarbonate in glycerol
Dioctyl ear drops	docusate sodium in polythene glycol	Wax-Aid Ear Drops	paradichloro-benzene, chlorbutol, turpentine oil, arachis oil
Exterol ear drops	Urea–hydrogen peroxide complex in glycerin	Waxsol ear drops	docusate sodium
Molcer ear drops	docusate sodium		

Inflammation of the outer ear (otitis externa)

Otitis externa is inflammation of the skin lining the outer ear canal caused by eczema or an infection. It is dark and warm in the canal; if it becomes moist the lining may become softened (macerated) and this increases the risk of infection. It may produce pain and itching which may be made worse by attempting to clean it out with a match, hairpin or cotton wool swab. Such procedures are likely to damage the lining of the ear and increase the risk of infection with bacteria or fungi. Excessive moisture (e.g. from swimming – 'swimmer's ear') may also cause maceration of the skin and infection. This may be made worse by attempts to get the water out; for example, using the corner of a dirty towel. Once an infection develops in the outer ear, a discharge is likely to occur.

Eczema of the external ear may occur in people who suffer from seborrhoea.

Treatment of otitis externa

Acute attacks of otitis externa are often best treated by the doctor or nurse cleaning and drying the ear. If this fails, an application of a ribbon gauze (gauze wick) soaked in a drying solution (aluminium acetate) may help. Alternatively, a ribbon gauze soaked in a weak solution of a corticosteroid can be very beneficial provided no infection is present. A ribbon gauze helps the drug to stay in the ear; however, if it is not possible to apply such a gauze wick the ear should be cleaned and you should lie down with the affected ear uppermost, the ear should then be filled with the solution and left for at least 10 minutes. After this, a pad of cotton wool should be applied to the outside of the ear and the head turned so that the ear is now downwards – this will allow the solution to drain out. Do *not* poke anything into the ear to clean out the solution.

If pain is severe, aspirin or paracetamol tablets by mouth will help, along with a hot pad applied to the ear. There is no place for the use of local anaesthetic ear drops to relieve pain in otitis externa, and preparations that contain pain relievers such as choline salicylate or phenazone are of doubtful value.

If the ear is infected, an anti-infective preparation should be used (see later).

Chronic otitis externa is often accompanied by eczema of the lining, a discharge, itching and irritation. The best initial treatment is to get the ear cleaned and dried out by a doctor or nurse and then to apply drying drops (astringent drops) such as aluminium acetate. Corticosteroid applications are very effective at relieving chronic inflammation. If infection is present and causing a yellowish-green discharge, an *anti-bacterial application* such as the antiseptic clioquinol or the antibiotics framycetin or neomycin will help but the treatment should not be used daily for more than a week. Prolonged use may cause you to become allergic to the anti-bacterial drug, which may result in further irritation inside the ear. It may also lead to a fungus infection inside the ear, which may be very difficult to clear up. Sometimes the base of an anti-bacterial preparation may cause irritation (e.g. propylene glycol in chloramphenicol ear drops). If the ear is inflamed *and* infected then a combined corticosteroid and anti-bacterial preparation may be used.

It is very important that any person suffering from otitis externa be taught how to clean out the ear effectively and to apply an ointment or drops; if this is not possible, treatment should be carried out by a trained person – doctor, nurse, carer.

Some people with otitis externa may develop a discharge, and there is not a lot of point in trying to apply ointment or drops when all that will happen is that the discharge will wash them straight out. In such people the application should be applied on ribbon gauze and pushed into the ear after it has had a good cleaning out.

Warnings *With chronic* otitis externa *it is important not to neglect simple, regular cleaning of the ear and to remember that over-use of anti-bacterial applications may cause local allergic reactions, the development of resistant bacteria and the emergence of a fungal infection. The corticosteroid in corticosteroid/anti-bacterial preparations may mask some of these developments* *and cause further problems. Therefore, they should be used only under strict medical supervision and for as short a period of time as possible.*

People suffering from otitis externa should have their ear drums examined carefully to see if there is a perforation, because sometimes a discharge may come from the ***middle ear*** *through a perforation in the ear drum. In these cases, it is important to be careful and not to apply anti-bacterial drugs to the outer ear which, if they were to enter the middle ear, could cause deafness; for example, the antibiotics framycetin, gentamicin, neomycin or polymyxins, or the antiseptic chlorhexidine.*

Ear drops should be disposed of once a course of treatment has been completed.

Infection of the middle ear (otitis media)

Infection of the middle ear (otitis media) causes a deep-seated pain in the ear, often with fever and some deafness. It is the commonest cause of severe pain in infants and young children.

The infection spreads from the throat up the tubes that link the back of the throat with the middle ears (the eustachian, or pharyngotympanic, tubes). It may cause the tubes to swell and become blocked with pus. This may create a build-up of pressure in the middle ear, causing the drum to become red and swollen and then to perforate. Once the drum has perforated the pain goes.

If the otitis media is caused by a virus infection the child will be snuffly, may have a mild temperature and earache. No specific treatment is necessary except for fluids, plenty of nursing and something to relieve the pain (e.g. paracetamol by mouth). By the next day the earache should have gone, the temperature should be down and the child should look better. However, if it is caused by a bacterial infection the child is more severely ill, the drum may perforate and the fever persist. It should be treated quickly and effectively with an antibiotic,* which may have to be given by injection if the child is vomiting or keeps spitting the medicine out. If there is a discharge from the ear, a swab should be taken, if possible, and sent to the laboratory to identify the infecting organism and to carry out antibiotic sensitivity tests on it. This will help in the selection of the most effective antibiotic. Treatment should continue for 5–10 days. The ear drum should be re-examined after 2–3 days, and if there is no improvement a different antibiotic should be used.

Failure to treat otitis media effectively may lead to a chronic sticky discharge from the ear (glue ear) with some deafness and a proneness to

* Because of the risk of complications from bacterial infections and the difficulty of deciding whether an infection is bacterial or viral it is safer to treat all cases with antibiotics.

keep on developing attacks of otitis media. Children should be examined 2 months after an attack of otitis media to check for glue ear and any residual deafness.

If a child regularly gets middle ear infections, it is worth giving him or her an antibiotic daily throughout the winter in order to prevent attacks developing, but of course any benefits from such treatment should be balanced against the risks produced by the regular daily use of an antibiotic drug such as erythromycin or an anti-bacterial drug such as co-trimoxazole.

The use of a pain reliever (e.g. paracetamol) plus a decongestant to reduce the swelling of the eustachian (pharyngotympanic) tubes in order to allow the pus to drain out of the middle ear has been suggested as an alternative to antibiotic treatment but much more evidence of the benefits and risks of such treatment is needed before it can be recommended.

A chronic discharging middle ear requires regular cleansing, and antibiotics when necessary according to laboratory tests on the discharge to identify the infecting organism.

Table 6.2 Applications used to treat disorders of the outer ear (otitis externa)

Product	*Corticosteroid*	*Anti-infective*	*Pain reliever*	*Other*
Achromycin ointment		tetracycline		
aluminium acetate solution				aluminium acetate (astringent)
Audax ear drops			choline salicylate	glycerol
Audicort ear drops	triamcinolone	neomycin/ undecenoic acid		
Betnesol drops	betamethasone			
Betnesol-N drops	betamethasone	neomycin		
Canesten solution		clotrimazole (anti-fungal)		
chloramphenicol ear drops		chloramphenicol		propylene glycol
Cidomycin drops		gentamicin		
Framycort drops	hydrocortisone	framycetin		
Framygen drops		framycetin		
Garamycin drops		gentamicin		

Table 6.2 Applications used to treat disorders of the outer ear (otitis externa) (*cont.*)

Product	*Corticosteroid*	*Anti-infective*	*Pain reliever*	*Other*
gentamicin ear drops		gentamicin		
Genticin drops		gentamicin		
Gentisone HC ear drops	hydrocortisone	gentamicin		
Locorten-Vioform ear drops	flumethasone	clioquinol (anti-bacterial/ anti-fungal)		
Neo-Cortef drops	hydrocortisone	neomycin		
Otomize spray	dexamethasone	neomycin		
Otosporin ear drops	hydrocortisone	neomycin, polymyxin B		
Predsol drops	prednisolone			
Predsol-N drops	prednisolone	neomycin		
Sofradex drops and ointment	dexamethasone	framycetin, gramicidin		
Soframycin cream		framycetin, gramicidin		
Soframycin ointment		framycetin, gramicidin		
Terra-Cortril drops	hydrocortisone	oxytetracycline, polymyxin B		
Tri-Adcortyl Otic (ear) ointment	triamcinolone	gramicidin, neomycin, nystatin (anti-fungal)		propylene glycol
Vista-Methasone drops	betamethasone			
Vista-Methasone N drops	betamethasone	neomycin		

7

Disorders of the nose

There are three main disorders of the nose for which drugs are used:

- Allergies (e.g. hayfever) (see Chapter 10)
- Blockage of the nose
- Infections

Blockage of the nose

Acute blocked nose

The commonest causes of acute short-lasting obstruction to the nose are the common cold and allergies (e.g. hayfever). The treatment of the common cold is discussed in Chapter 3. Your special attention should be given to the dangers of using decongestants to relieve a blocked nose. The drug treatment of nasal allergies (e.g. hayfever) is discussed in Chapter 10.

Chronic blocked nose: vasomotor rhinitis

A common cause of chronic blockage in the nose is vasomotor rhinitis. In this disorder the normal ability of the lining of the nose to shrink or swell in response to the temperature (i.e. its air-conditioning function) is defective. The nose becomes blocked and it may be associated with sneezing and a runny nose. Attacks come and go but eventually long-lasting irritation of the lining of the nose causes it to swell and stay swollen, and it may hang in folds – these folds are called polyps and they block various parts of the nose.

Vasomotor rhinitis may be caused by working in a dry, warm atmosphere, by irritants in the air (e.g. tobacco smoke) and by emotional factors.

There are two types of vasomotor rhinitis according to whether the affected nasal tissue contains or does not contain special white cells (eosinophils) whose function is not fully understood but which is known to be associated with allergic reactions.

Non-eosinophilic vasomotor rhinitis causes profuse running of the nose but only moderate blockage. It seems to be caused by a malfunction of the nerves that supply the lining of the nose. Under-activity of the sympathetic nerves allows the lining to swell, and over-activity of the parasympathetic nerves stimulates the glands in the lining to produce a watery discharge (rhinorrhoea).

Eosinophilic vasomotor rhinitis causes marked blockage, moderate running of the nose and loss of the sense of smell. The condition may be due to some disorder of the lining of the nose, causing a deficiency of a chemical (a prostaglandin) that is involved naturally in causing the lining to shrink and dry up. The use of aspirin (which blocks the production of prostaglandins) is associated with this type of vasomotor rhinitis and is also often associated with nasal polyps and asthma.

The treatment of non-eosinophilic vasomotor rhinitis is difficult. Nasal decongestants applied up the nose are best avoided because they can produce rebound swelling of the lining of the nose and they are of limited use when taken by mouth. Antihistamines by mouth may help a few people, and some may be helped by corticosteroid applications.

The anticholinergic drug ipratropium applied in a metered dose spray (Rinatec) reduces the amount and duration of the discharge from the nose. It has a rapid onset of action and its effects last for about 6 hours. Some is absorbed into the bloodstream, so continuous use of high doses may cause a fall in pulse rate and blood pressure. It may produce dryness of the nose and should be used with caution in people with glaucoma and difficulty passing urine (e.g. men with enlarged prostate glands). Contact with the eyes should be avoided because of the risks of triggering glaucoma.

Eosinophilic rhinitis is helped by the use of corticosteroid applications. Treatment should be used daily for about 1 month and not repeated more than six times a year.

Nasal polyps

Long-lasting swelling of the lining of the nose caused by infection, irritation or allergy may result in rubbery swellings which hang down in lumps or folds – these are called polyps. They can block parts of the nose. They may recur unless the cause is removed (e.g. allergy to aspirin, smoking, etc.).

The local application of nasal decongestants may worsen the obstruction caused by polyps, due to a rebound swelling. Decongestants by mouth may help some people but see the risks discussed in Chapter 3. Combined treatment with an antihistamine and a decongestant by mouth may also benefit some people, as may the use of corticosteroid applications. It is important to stop any provoking factors (e.g. the use of aspirin, smoking, exposure to allergens); quite often the polyps will need to be removed surgically.

For *harmful effects* and *warnings* on the use of decongestants see Chapter 3, and for corticosteroids see Chapter 62.

Over-use of nasal decongestants

A common cause of nose blockage is the over-use of decongestant nasal sprays and drops. This is called rhinitis medicamentosa (inflammation of the nose caused by medicaments). ENT specialists often refer to it as iatrogenic obstruction – obstruction caused by doctors' treatment. Any decongestant nasal spray or drops will damage the lining of the nose if used daily for more than about 10 days. They cause the blood vessels to constrict and the lining of the nose to shrink; this may reduce the oxygen supply to the delicate lining of the nose, which may be damaged by repeated use. When the drug's effects have worn off the lining swells right up to block the nose again, often worse than before the decongestant was applied. The patient then takes more decongestant and a vicious circle is set up which leads to permanent damage to the lining of the nose, which stays swollen and becomes red, rubbery and no longer responds to decongestants. The treatment is to stop the drug and use a corticosteroid application.

Infections of the nose

The commonest infection of the nose is caused by the common cold virus and its treatment is discussed in Chapter 3. In many of us (up to 40 per cent) the lining of the nose may act as a reservoir for bacteria that cause boils (staphylococci). If you suffer from boils, this reservoir of bacteria may be knocked out by applying an anti-bacterial cream up each nostril four times daily for 10 days. An anti-bacterial cream applied daily up the nose will also prevent an individual who is in contact with a staphylococcal infection (e.g. a nurse) from spreading the infection to other patients. Fashionable applications at the present time are Naseptin cream, which contains an antiseptic (chlorhexidine) and an antibiotic (neomycin), and Bactroban ointment, which contains the antibiotic mupirocin. Unfortunately, re-colonization of the nose by the bacteria after such treatment is fairly frequent.

Naseptin should be kept out of the eyes and ears. It contains neomycin which, on prolonged use, may cause allergic skin rashes. Neomycin may also be absorbed from the nose into the bloodstream, and regular daily use for a prolonged time may, very rarely, damage hearing and balance – and also damage the kidneys. The chlorhexidine antiseptic may also cause a generalized allergic reaction.

Apart from the above use, there is seldom if any necessity for anti-bacterial drugs to treat disorders of the nose.

Warning *Preparations that contain an anti-bacterial drug should not be used to treat hayfever or the common cold because neither disorder is due to a bacterial infection; hayfever is due to allergy and a cold is caused by a virus infection.*

Table 7.1 Nasal decongestant preparations

Preparation	*Drug*	*Drug group*
Afrazine nasal drops and spray	oxymetazoline	sympathomimetic
Afrazine paediatric nasal drops	oxymetazoline	sympathomimetic
ephedrine nasal drops (0.5% and 1.0%)	ephedrine	sympathomimetic
Otrivine nasal drops and spray	xylometazoline	sympathomimetic
xylometazoline nasal drops	xylometazoline	sympathomimetic
xylometazoline paediatric nasal drops	xylometazoline	sympathomimetic

Table 7.2 Preparations used to treat allergic disorders of the nose

Preparation	*Drug*	*Drug group*
Beconase nasal aerosol (powder) and aqueous suspension atomizer	beclomethasone	corticosteroid
Betnesol drops	betamethasone	corticosteroid
Dexa-Rhinaspray nasal aerosol	dexamethasone neomycin tramazoline	corticosteroid antibiotic sympathomimetic
Rhinocort aerosol	budesonide	corticosteroid
Rinatec	ipratropium	anticholinergic
Rynacrom nasal drops, spray and insufflation	sodium cromoglycate	anti-allergic
Rynacrom Compound nasal spray	sodium cromoglycate xylometazoline	anti-allergic sympathomimetic
Syntaris nasal spray	flunisolide	corticosteroid
Vibrocil nasal drops, spray and gel	dimethindene phenylephrine neomycin	antihistamine sympathomimetic antibiotic
Vista-Methasone nasal drops	betamethasone	corticosteroid

Table 7.3 Applications used to treat infections of the nose

Preparation	*Drug*	*Drug group*
Bactroban nasal ointment*	mupirocin	antibiotic
Betnesol-N nasal drops †	betamethasone	corticosteroid
	neomycin	antibiotic
Locabiotal nasal aerosol	fusafungine	antibiotic
Naseptin nasal cream*	chlorhexidine	antiseptic
	neomycin	antibiotic
Vista-Methasone N†	betamethasone	corticosteroid
	neomycin	antibiotic

* To treat nasal carriers
† To treat inflammatory conditions with infection

8

Sinusitis and catarrh

The sinuses open into the back of the nose (the nasopharynx) and their surfaces have an effective self-cleaning mechanism. This mechanism involves the production of mucus which is swept into the back of the nose by the tiny hair-like structures, called cilia, which line all the surfaces of the air passages. Any foreign particles including bacteria are swept on a continuous blanket of mucus out through the sinus openings and into the nose. For this process to work effectively you require normal mucus, normal functioning cilia and clear openings from the sinuses into the back of the nose.

The self-cleaning mechanism of the sinuses and nose may be impaired when you have a cold or some other virus infection. The lining swells up, the cilia do not work as effectively and outlets from the sinuses may get blocked by the swollen linings. There is then a risk that the mucus stagnates in the sinuses and becomes secondarily infected by bacteria which are attacked by white blood cells. This produces what is called mucopus – the yellow–green discharge you get when you blow your nose. The cilia find it more difficult to sweep mucopus away because it is very sticky and the outlets from the sinuses may easily become blocked – you then have sinusitis. This explains why when you have a cold you should not sniff, you should blow your nose gently instead!

A common cold is the commonest cause of an acute blockage of the sinuses leading to the development of sinusitis.

Acute sinusitis

After a cold your symptoms do not clear up; you develop a yellow–green discharge from the nose, you may have a raised temperature and you develop pain in the face and/or forehead which is worse on straining or bending down. You have acute sinusitis.

Treatment of acute sinusitis

Without treatment sinusitis may clear up on its own within a few days to a few weeks. Antibiotics should be used if the sinusitis lasts for more than 2–3 days or if the symptoms are severe. Ampicillin or amoxycillin should be taken for a full course of treatment of 5–10 days. A 10-day course of doxycycline is also effective but should not be given to children. In addition, steam inhalations and a pain reliever (e.g. paracetamol) will help. Nasal decongestants by mouth are usually ineffective but decongestant nasal drops or sprays may be of limited benefit. They may, however, be harmful if used regularly every day for more than 10 days.

Chronic sinusitis

Chronic sinusitis may be infective or hyperplastic (meaning overgrowth).

Chronic infective sinusitis follows an acute attack of sinusitis that has not responded to treatment. The sinuses and nose become blocked; the affected sinuses contain a mixture of mucus and pus which causes a yellow–green discharge from the nose. Chronic infective sinusitis may also occur in an individual who is immune deficient due to drug treatment or to disease (e.g. AIDS). It may sometimes occur in people with long-standing chest disorders.

In *chronic hyperplastic sinusitis* the lining of the sinuses and nose overgrows and becomes swollen. It is associated with allergy (both seasonal and perennial) and may occur in people who are allergic to aspirin. The person develops catarrh at the back of the throat and a foul taste in the mouth, the nose may be blocked and there may be pain over the nose.

Treatment of chronic infective sinusitis

In order to get rid of the pus, the sinuses have to be washed out with saline by inserting a narrow tube (cannula) up the nose and into the infected sinus. This procedure is called a simple antrostomy.

Treatment of chronic hyperplastic sinusitis

A corticosteroid nasal spray may help if used two or three times daily for about 1 month – but not more than six times a year. Any polyps in the nose will need to be removed surgically, and if necessary the sinuses should be washed.

Catarrh

Catarrh is an inflammation of the lining membranes of the air passages. It may affect the nose (nasal catarrh), the space at the back of the nose (post-nasal catarrh) or any part of the air passages. It may be acute and caused by a cold or it may be chronic and be aggravated by smoking and a dry atmosphere. It may also be caused by many other factors; for example, allergy (e.g. hayfever), a dusty dry atmosphere or fungal spores in the air. Acute catarrh may produce a soreness of the affected area or it may produce a mucous discharge; for example, runny nose, mucus at the back of the throat, phlegm on the chest, or snuffles in a baby. The mucus may become sticky and hard to clear and it may become yellowish-green due to secondary bacterial infection.

Treatment of catarrh

In treating acute catarrh it is important to treat the cause, for example hayfever, and to stop smoking if you smoke and avoid dry, dusty and/or smoky atmospheres if possible. Parents of snuffly babies should not smoke in the home. This general advice also applies to the treatment of chronic catarrh.

Steam inhalation may help to clear catarrh; so may the use of a decongestant nasal spray but see (Chapter 3) the dangers of regular daily use and dangers in infants. Vapours and inhalations may help some people but see the dangers in infants (Chapter 3).

There is no convincing evidence from adquate and well controlled studies that mucolytics (drugs that dissolve phlegm) are beneficial in treating chronic catarrh despite their being heavily advertised. Preparations containing more than one drug are best avoided because the dose of one drug cannot be changed without changing the dose of the other drug or drugs. Furthermore, such preparations expose you to risk of harmful effects from more than one drug.

9

The immune system

Immunity

Immunity is a state of resistance to disease; it is our defence system against attack. It is influenced by many factors, and the mechanisms in the body that create immunity are very complex and not fully understood. What is more, the ability of the body to develop resistance (immunity) to a specific infection is only part of the story. The body also has the ability to recognize a whole range of foreign substances (other than infecting micro-organisms) that enter the body and react to them (see later).

Any substance that produces an immune response in the body is called an *antigen*, and an important function of the body's immune response is to produce *antibodies* specifically against invading antigens (e.g. infectious bacteria and viruses) in order to destroy them. Antibodies are proteins, and another name for them is *immunoglobulins*. Antibodies can also recognize unfamiliar cells (e.g. cancer cells) and cells of transplanted tissues. They are produced by certain white cells in the blood (see later).

Sometimes antibodies are produced that treat certain tissues of the body as if they were foreign antigens; this is called *autoimmunity* and it can produce serious diseases (see later).

Lymphocytes

The attachment of an antibody to an antigen is called an antigen/antibody reaction. The production of antibodies is under the control of white cells in the blood called lymphocytes, of which there are two types – 'T' lymphocytes and 'B' lymphocytes.

B lymphocytes produce antibodies

Antibodies are proteins made up of sub-units of amino acids in various arrangements. Different arrangements represent different antibodies, and these different arrangements are stored in the memories of the B lymphocytes by what is called genetic coding. They are activated by unfamiliar proteins (antigens) on the surfaces of invading micro-organisms. The lymphocytes are able to test various antibody combinations on their surfaces against specific antigens until one fits and the antigens are then locked into the activated B lymphocytes' surfaces at what are called binding sites. Once this has happened the lymphocytes divide rapidly into more simple cells called plasma cells, each carrying the special code in order to produce sufficient specific antibodies to react against that specific antigen.

T lymphocytes attack invading cells

T lymphocytes also 'recognize' antigens on abnormal or invading cells by using antibody-like receptors on their surfaces. Once they recognize an antigen, they multiply rapidly, each new cell being programmed to carry a specific antibody on its surface for that particular antigen. The contact with the antigens also makes each lymphocyte release special substances, called lymphokines, which bring about various immune responses in the body, including allergic responses. Interferons are lymphokines, which block the reproduction of viruses. The lymphocytes also release an 'arming' factor which enables the big white cells in the blood to kill cells which have the particular antigen that has been recognized. The big white cells engulf invaders (phagocytosis) and are attracted to an area of infection by chemicals released by the inflammatory response.

T lymphocytes may be divided into effector cells and regulatory cells. Effector cells are involved in delayed allergy, and regulator cells include suppressor cells which stop antibody production by B lymphocytes and helper cells (or inducers) which help B lymphocytes to produce antibodies. There are also T lymphocytes to destroy cells that contain viruses; these are called cytotoxic (cell-damaging) T lymphocytes.

The suppressor cells control the production of antibodies by blocking the production of antibodies by B lymphocytes. Relaxation of this control over antibody production may be a factor in autoimmune disease where the body produces antibodies to its own tissues.

About 75 per cent of lymphocytes in the blood are T lymphocytes, a third of which are helper cells. The activities of T lymphocytes are restricted by the HLA system (see later).

The coding programmes for the various antibodies are stored inside long-living T and B lymphocytes – these programmes are referred to as the cells' immunological memories.

Killer cells

Certain white cells in the blood and lymphoid tissue can become killer cells (or K cells) for specific antigens once they have been sensitized by contact with a specific antigen/antibody complex. They can kill and dissolve 'foreign' cells. Also in the blood are natural killer cells which keep an eye out for foreign cells produced by the body (e.g. cancer cells), cells infected with viruses and other foreign cells. They thus play a part in preventing cancers developing and in resistance to infections, and they may also contribute to red cell destruction.

Antibodies (immunoglobulins)

Antibodies are proteins, called globulins, which are made up of specially arranged amino acids that can be put together on demand in a special way in order to respond to a specific antigen. There are several classes of these 'immunoglobulins' and they have different properties. For short, immunoglobulin is referred to as Ig.

Immunoglobulin G (IgG) is the most abundant in healthy adults. It accounts for 73 per cent of the total serum immunoglobulins (or antibodies). It is active against bacteria and viruses, and passes from the mother into the unborn baby to provide protection for the baby during the first few months of its life.

Immunoglobulin M (IgM) is a big molecule which forms about 7 per cent of immunoglobulins (or antibodies). It is made up of five immunoglobulin units and is specifically adapted to deal with cell debris and bacteria in the blood. It is the first immunoglobulin to appear in an immune response but does not persist for long.

Immunoglobulin A (IgA) accounts for 19 per cent of immunoglobulins (or antibodies) and is especially secreted in colostrum (the first milk to be produced by a breast-feeding mother), saliva, intestinal juice and secretions in the respiratory system (nose, throat, bronchial tubes, etc.). These immunoglobulins produce a very important 'antiseptic' function on all of these mucous surfaces.

Immunoglobulin D (IgD) resembles IgG and may be active against food antigens.

Immunoglobulin E (IgE) is present on all cell surfaces and is responsible for producing allergic reactions. It may provide some defence against worm infection.

The complement system

This part of the immune system is very complex and is triggered by an antigen/antibody reaction. It activates all the various cells and processes involved in fighting infections.

Types of immune reactions

There are six main types of immune reaction.

Type I immune reaction (allergic reactions)

These are called anaphylaxic reactions or immediate hypersensitivity reactions. Anaphylaxis means a high degree of sensitivity to certain foreign proteins (antigens). It is called hypersensitivity, or *allergy*, and it occurs in some individuals and not in others; in certain individuals it occurs to some antigens (e.g. pollen) and not others (e.g. house dust). The first exposure to the antigen sensitizes the person and then any subsequent exposure to that particular antigen will produce an allergic reaction. This allergic reaction depends upon the route of entry of the antigen into the body, whether by mouth, breathed in, injected or by contact with the skin. These reactions occur most commonly to pollen and house dust, and they characteristically produce the symptoms of hayfever. If they are inhaled, they may produce wheezing (bronchospasm) in some patients.

Allergic symptoms may be very sudden and severe if an antigen (e.g. a bee sting) is injected into someone who is allergic to that antigen (i.e. someone who has been made allergic by a previous bee sting). People so affected develop severe wheezing (bronchospasm), swelling of the throat (so much so that they may suffocate) and a rapid fall in blood pressure. They may also suffer nausea, vomiting and diarrhoea. Reaction may even be such that the individual develops severe shock (anaphylactic shock) and may collapse and die.

An allergic reaction in the skin produces nettle rash (urticaria) with characteristic weals (raised white areas) and flares (bright red areas). It may develop from an antigen taken in by mouth and absorbed into the bloodstream – common food allergies include strawberries and shellfish. The nettle rash may be the only sign of allergy or it may be associated with other symptoms.

These allergic reactions are produced by IgE antibodies which stick to the surfaces of cells in most tissues in the body, particularly on what are called mast cells. The allergic reaction is triggered when the antigen/

antibody reaction occurs on the surfaces of these mast cells. This sets off a series of reactions in the cells which results in the release of histamine and other chemicals that cause the allergic reactions – they cause blood vessels to dilate, the bronchial tubes to constrict, the blood pressure to drop and produce a local reaction just like inflammation.

Type II immune reaction (e.g. autoimmune reaction)

In this reaction the antigen/antibody reaction on the cell surfaces destroys the cells. An example is autoimmune disease in which the body produces antibodies to its own cells (see later). Both IgG and IgM may be involved. Another example is blood transfusion reactions in which 'foreign' red blood cells are destroyed. These reactions are called antibody-mediated cytotoxic (cell killing) or blocking reactions.

Type III immune reaction

This is called an immune complex reaction, and may occur in response to infection with micro-organisms, to drugs or to the body's own tissues. It is the result of antigen/antibody complexes being deposited in various tissues and triggering an inflammatory response, producing damage to local tissues. These complexes may block small blood vessels in the kidneys and produce kidney damage. The antigen must be 'foreign' or from the body (autogenous). Examples are the kidney damage that can follow streptococcal throat infections and a drug-induced syndrome which includes a skin rash and fever associated with inflammation of joints, blood vessels, kidneys and the nervous system. Rheumatoid arthritis and virus hepatitis are other examples of tissue damage that may occur with this type of reaction.

Serum sickness is an example of a general upset produced by this reaction. It usually involves fever, skin rashes, joint pains and swollen glands. It may be an allergic reaction to an antiserum or to a drug such as penicillin.

Type IV immune reaction

This reaction is set off by T lymphocytes in which free antibody plays no part. The antigens stimulate the T lymphocytes to release lymphokines which trigger a number of reactions, including hypersensitivity (allergy). This occurs in autoimmune disease.

Type V immune reaction

Certain IgG antibodies have the ability to stimulate their target cells rather than killing them. An example of this type of effect is Graves disease, which causes over-activity of the thyroid gland. The antibodies latch on to thyroid-stimulating hormone (TSH) receptors in the thyroid gland, making it increase its production of thyroid hormones.

Type VI immune reaction

Killer cells (see earlier) can move in and kill certain cells that have developed an antigen/antibody reaction on their surfaces. These reactions are referred to as antibody-dependent cell-mediated cytotoxicity (cell killing) (ADCC). It may be involved in autoimmune disease (see later) and in defence against worm and protozoal infections.

Autoimmune disease

Autoimmune diseases are caused by the production of antibodies that react to some of the body's own tissues. Normally this does not happen and there are complex mechanisms to ensure that it does not. Sometimes, however, a defect may occur spontaneously or be caused by some outside factor. The defect may be very specific and affect the cells in just one organ (e.g. Hashimoto's disease of the thyroid gland) or it may be non-specific and produce a general reaction throughout the body (e.g. lupus erythematosus). There is a suggestion that there may be a loss of control by suppressor T lymphocytes over the function of B lymphocytes.

The HLA system and disease

The antigens in human tissues that trigger an immune response that results in the rejection of a transplanted organ are known as homologous (human) leucocytic antigens (HLA). They are genetically determined and are inherited in a specific chromosome (number 6) where they constitute what is called the major histocompatibility complex (MHC). 'Histocompatibility' refers to the compatibility of tissues (antigens) between donor and recipient of transplanted organs.

HLA antigens in body tissues can be detected and identified, and are divided into four series. Their identification forms the basis for tissue matching in organ transplant patients. The better the match the less is the chance of the body reacting to the transplanted organ and rejecting it. There are also strong associations between HLA and susceptibility to certain diseases, especially autoimmune diseases.

Drugs that suppress the immune system

In certain medical conditions it is necessary to dampen down (suppress) the activities of the immune system by using drugs. The drugs used for this purpose are referred to as immunosuppressive drugs. Immunosuppression is needed in treating autoimmune diseases in which the immune system attacks normal body tissues. This attack may be local as in Hashimoto's disease of the thyroid gland or it may be general and affect many organs and tissues (e.g. lupus erythematosus). Suppression of the immune system is also necessary in treating patients who have had an organ transplant, otherwise the immune system would cause rejection of the transplanted organ.

The production of antibodies and the cells involved in the immune system are dependent upon the production and multiplication of lymphocytes. Therefore any drug that interferes with the production or multiplication of lymphocytes will suppress the immune system. Low doses of certain anti-cancer drugs (which slow the production of all cells in the bone marrow) will produce these effects (see below). Cyclosporin is more selective than these anti-cancer drugs. It blocks multiplication (replication) of lymphocytes and affects T lymphocyte growth factor but not the activity of B lymphocytes.

The risk of immunosuppressive drugs is that by suppressing immunity (the body's resistance to infection) they throw the patient open to the risk of infection from various bacteria, fungi and viruses. Also, because lymphocytes prevent the multiplication of abnormal cells there is an increased risk of developing certain types of cancer.

Immunosuppressive drugs

Azathioprine, chlorambucil and cyclophosphamide are used to treat certain cancers. They are also used to stop lymphoid cells from dividing in order to reduce the immune response in diseases such as rheumatoid arthritis and ulcerative colitis. Azathioprine is also used to reduce the immune response in patients who have had a transplant, in order to reduce the risk of rejection of the transplanted organ.

Cyclosporin is a powerful immunosuppressive drug and is the main drug used to reduce the risk of rejection of transplanted organs.

Corticosteroids suppress the immune reaction by reducing the activity of B and T lymphocytes. They reduce the production of antibodies and are used to prevent transplant rejection.

Harmful effects and warnings on the use of immunosuppressive drugs

Azathioprine (Azamune, Imuran) prevents the multiplication of lymphocytes that occurs in response to foreign proteins (antigens); for example, transplanted organs. It helps the survival and functions of transplanted organs. It is also of benefit to some people suffering from rheumatoid arthritis and other autoimmune disorders, usually when corticosteroids have failed to control the symptoms.

Harmful effects include damage to the bone marrow, producing a reduction in the white blood cells (leucopenia) and a reduction in platelets (thrombocytopenia) – for early warning signs, see Chapter 78. It may also damage the production and development of red blood cells, causing a megalobastic anaemia. Other harmful effects include nausea, vomiting and loss of appetite. Very rarely, damage to the lining of the stomach and intestine may occur and be associated with bleeding and perforation. This appears to occur only in transplant patients who are also being treated with corticosteroids. Allergic reactions may, rarely, occur and include drug fever, skin rash and painful muscles and joints. Liver damage may occur very rarely, as may damage to the pancreas, causing abdominal pain and vomiting. Injected solutions may cause pain and soreness at the site of injection.

Warnings *Azathioprine should not be used by anyone who is allergic to it. It should be used only if the individual can be carefully monitored for harmful drug effects throughout the duration of the treatment. During the first 8 weeks of treatment, complete blood counts must be carried out at least every week and more frequently if high doses are used or if kidney or liver function is impaired. After the first 8 weeks of treatment, blood counts should be carried out twice monthly. Careful monitoring is essential, and reduction of dose may be necessary in anyone whose kidney or liver function is severely impaired. With certain disorders, suddenly stopping the drug may cause a serious flare-up of the disorder; therefore it is best to reduce the dose slowly over several days to weeks.*

Serious infections are a constant hazard of treatment with immunosuppressives. These include fungal, viral or bacterial infections and they should be treated vigorously. In transplant patients treated with azathioprine there is a very rare risk of developing skin cancer or cancer of the lymphoid tissue. Patients should avoid over-exposure to the sun and the skin should be examined at regular intervals.

Risks in elderly people Harmful effects may be more frequent and severe, therefore use with caution.

Risks in pregnancy Azathioprine and its breakdown products cross from the mother's blood into the baby's blood. There is therefore a potential for damage to the baby during the first 3 months of pregnancy and damage to the baby's immune system later in pregnancy. Azathioprine should be used only if the expected benefits outweigh the risks. Because of the risk of chromosomal damage it should be used with caution in patients (males and females) who may want children. It should not be used to treat rheumatoid arthritis in pregnant women.

Risks with other drugs Azathioprine is broken down in the body to mercaptopurine, therefore the effects of azathioprine are increased by allopurinol which is used to treat gout. The dose of azathioprine should be reduced to one-quarter of the dose when given along with allopurinol. It should be used with caution in people receiving or who have recently received any drug which may damage the bone marrow. It may block the effects of muscle relaxants such as tubocurarine and pancuronium. Do not use along with penicillamine. Any drug that affects the breakdown of azathioprine in the liver may affect its blood level and, therefore, its benefits and risks – these include such drugs as phenytoin, phenobarbitone and rifampicin.

Chlorambucil (Leukeran) is an effective anti-cancer drug which is used occasionally as an immunosuppressant to treat patients suffering from rheumatoid arthritis or related disorders.

Harmful effects include damage to the bone marrow, affecting the production of red and white blood cells. Nausea, vomiting, diarrhoea and ulceration of the mouth may occur infrequently. Other rare harmful effects include liver damage with jaundice, fever, allergic skin rashes, nerve damage (numbness and pins and needles in the hands and feet), pneumonia, inflammation of the bladder, seizures, loss of periods and reduced sperm count (with high doses) and damage to chromosomes.

Warnings *Bone marrow damage is usually reversible if the drug is stopped; however, it may be irreversible. (See early warning of bone marrow damage in Chapter 78.) Blood tests should be carried out before and at regular intervals during treatment.*

Chlorambucil should not be used in people who have recently had radiotherapy and/or treatment with other anti-cancer drugs. It should be used with caution in anyone with impaired kidney function. Such individuals should have regular blood counts because of the increased risk of bone marrow damage, and reduced doses may have to be used. It should be used with similar caution in patients whose liver function is severely impaired.

There are rare reports of chlorambucil being associated with the development of acute leukaemia in patients treated for chronic lymphatic leukaemia, but whether this was due to the drug or the disease or both is not certain. People treated for cancer of the ovaries also run a very rare risk of developing acute leukaemia, as do those who receive long-term treatment for breast cancer.

Risks in elderly people Kidney and liver function should be checked and, if impaired, the drug should be used with caution and be carefully monitored (see above).

Risks with other drugs Allopurinol may increase the blood levels of chlorambucil, producing an increase of harmful effects.

Cyclophosphamide (Endoxana) is an effective anti-cancer drug which is used occasionally as an immunosuppressant to treat patients suffering from rheumatoid arthritis or related disorders.

Harmful effects include nausea, vomiting and loss of hair (alopecia) in about 20 per cent of patients receiving over 100 mg daily. Loss of hair starts after the first 3 weeks of treatment and regrowth starts after about 3 months even though treatment may be continued. Other harmful effects include bone marrow damage causing reduction in red and white blood cell production (for early warning signs, see Chapter 78), bladder damage and blood in the urine, loss of periods, swelling of the breasts and reduced sperm count. High doses may cause heart damage. Pigmentation of the skin, fluid retention (e.g. ankle swelling), changes in blood sugar levels and disorders of the lungs may, rarely, occur.

Warnings *Cyclophosphamide should be used only when there are adequate facilities for carrying out regular tests of the blood and full medical examinations under the direction of a specialist in cancer treatment. Its use to treat disorders other than cancer should be taken only after the serious risks of using this drug have been balanced with any expected benefits; for example, to treat a life-threatening disorder. It should not be used in anyone who is allergic to it, nor in people with an acute infection, bone marrow disorder or acute urinary tract infections. Male and female patients should avoid sexual intercourse or use a mechanical form of contraceptive (e.g. a condom) during treatment with cyclophosphamide. It should be used with caution in debilitated patients, and in people with diabetes or with evidence of bone marrow damage, or who have recently received radiotherapy and/or anti-cancer drug treatment. It should not be used in patients with laboratory evidence of impaired kidney or liver function. To reduce damage to the kidneys and bladder, patients should drink plenty of fluids and pass urine frequently. Sometimes it may be necessary to give water tablets (diuretics) to achieve this. However, mesna (Uromitexan) may reduce the damage to the lining of the urinary tract and if this is used, frequent emptying of the bladder should be avoided.*

Cyclosporin (Sandimmun) blocks the multiplication of lymphocytes and blocks the production of a factor that makes T lymphocytes grow. It is a powerful immunosuppressant and is used to prevent rejection of transplanted organs and tissues. It does not damage the bone marrow.

Harmful effects are usually mild to moderate, and clear up if the dose is reduced. Reported harmful effects include overgrowth of hair on the body, tremor, impaired kidney function, impaired liver function, swelling of the gums, loss of appetite, nausea, vomiting, raised blood potassium, raised blood pressure in most heart transplant patients; rarely, a combination of raised blood pressure, fluid retention and convulsions may occur, mainly in children. Swelling of the face, burning sensation in the hands and feet in the first week of treatment, and allergic reactions (may be severe with infusions) may occur.

Warnings *Cyclosporin must not be used in people allergic to it. Some preparations for intravenous use (e.g. Sandimmun) contain polyethoxylated castor oil, to which some individuals may be severely allergic, so any such preparations should not be used in people allergic to it. It should not be used along with other immunosuppressive drugs except corticosteroids. Over-suppression of the immune system may, rarely, cause a risk of infections and cancer of the lymphoid tissue (lymphoma). Kidney and liver function tests should be carried out before and at regular intervals during treatment. Cyclosporin by mouth may produce an erratic response, therefore measurement of the level of the drug in the blood should be carried out at intervals.*

Risks in elderly people Harmful effects may be more frequent and more severe; therefore reduced doses may be necessary.

Risks in breast feeding Do not breast feed when taking this drug.

Risks with other drugs Any drug that may damage the kidney should be used with utmost caution in patients taking cyclosporin – e.g. aminoglycosides or amphotericin B. Trimethoprim (also in co-trimoxazole) may cause an irreversible deterioration in kidney function in patients taking cyclosporin. Ketoconazole increases the blood level of cyclosporin and may therefore increase its toxic effects. Phenytoin, rifampicin, isoniazid and intravenous sulphadimidine and trimethoprim decrease the blood levels of cyclosporin and therefore reduce its effectiveness. Their use should be avoided where possible. When they have to be used, the blood levels of cyclosporin should be measured and the dose adjusted accordingly.

Immune deficiency disorders

Immune deficiency occurs when the immune system fails to protect the body against infection or cancer. It may be present from birth because the body's immune system has not developed normally or it may be 'acquired' as a result of infection (e.g. AIDS), cancer drug treatment (e.g. anti-cancer drugs, corticosteroids) or radiotherapy for cancer.

Immune deficiency reduces the patient's resistance to bacterial, fungal, viral and other infections and certain types of cancer.

Types of immune deficiency

Immune deficiency may occur because of a deficiency of antibodies or of a deficiency of the cells (lymphocytes) involved in immunity. These deficiencies may occur separately or together.

A deficiency of the parent cells (stem cells) of both T and B lymphocytes will cause a deficiency of the cells involved in both immunity and antibody production (see earlier). This is called a combined deficiency state. It is very rare and occurs in infants.

Deficiency of antibodies

A deficiency of antibodies (immunoglobulins) produced by a selective deficiency of lymphocytes (see earlier) may be inherited or acquired. Most cases are acquired and are associated with autoimmune diseases such as pernicious anaemia or haemolytic anaemia.

Deficiency of different antibodies will produce different disorders. IgM deficiency is associated with meningococcal meningitis, whereas deficiency of IgA is associated with infections of the respiratory tract, the stomach and intestine. Such patients are treated with frequent injections of immunoglobulins.

In the last 3 months of pregnancy, IgG antibodies from the mother pass into the unborn baby so that if the baby is born at term it will have some protection against infections. Premature babies miss out on this and are prone to infections. They have to have injections of IgG immunoglobulin.

The ability of babies and infants to produce antibodies is not as effective as adults and therefore they are less resistant to coughs, colds and diarrhoea because they do not produce enough IgA antibody. However, IgA is present in colostrum (the first lot of breast milk produced after childbirth) and this provides some protection for the baby against diarrhoeal infections.

Drugs that depress the immune system include phenytoin and penicillamine. They induce an IgA deficiency.

Deficiency of lymphocytes

A deficiency of T lymphocytes may occur on its own or be secondary to some disease such as:

- *Hodgkin's disease* – anaemia plus enlargement of the lymph glands and overgrowth of lymphoid tissue in the spleen, liver and other organs
- *Sarcoidosis* – a generalized disease producing swelling (granuloma) of the lymph glands and lymphatic system; it may affect the tonsils, bone marrow, lungs, liver and spleen, sometimes the skin and occasionally other organs
- An attack of *measles* or *leprosy* or treatment with *anti-cancer drugs* may result in a deficiency of T lymphocytes
- *AIDS* (*acquired immune deficiency syndrome*) is a disorder caused by infection with the HIV virus; the virus invades certain cells, particularly T-helper lymphocytes and may interferes with the production of antibodies which normally fight infections and control the development of abnormal cells (see AIDS, chapter 34).

Immunostimulants

Agents used to stimulate the immune system include the bacterium *Corynebacterium parvum* (Coparvax), which has the ability to stimulate the immune system. The bacteria are inactivated and freeze dried. When reconstituted in saline the preparation is used to inject into the cavity of the chest or abdomen to treat fluid in the chest (pleural effusion) or in the abdomen (ascites), caused by cancer cells.

Harmful effects include fever, nausea and vomiting. Injection into the abdomen may cause discomfort and pain. Leakage into the tissue may cause tenderness. It may cause local scaring (fibrosis) in the chest or abdominal cavities.

Warnings *The incidence and severity of harmful effects following injection into the chest may be reduced if it is not used within about 10 days of surgical removal of the affected lung.*

10

Allergies

The preceding chapter on the immune system should be read before reading this chapter. It should help you to understand allergy more easily.

Allergy

In defence against infecting micro-organisms, the body produces antibodies that combine with protein in the micro-organisms to neutralize any effects which they may have upon the body. By means of this defence mechanism, the body develops resistance or immunity. This often gives protection against re-infection by the same micro-organism (e.g. you never get measles twice). A specific antibody reacts *only* with the protein (referred to as an antigen) of the infecting micro-organism responsible for its formation. There is no shared antibody formation with other micro-organisms; for example, there is no cross-immunity between measles and polio – getting measles does not protect you against polio. Antibodies are very specific to particular antigens.

Sometimes renewed exposure to an infection produces an excessive or altered response (see Chapter 9, under 'Immunity') – this is called allergy. Allergy to micro-organisms is rare and most allergic reactions are to proteins not naturally known to your body (foreign proteins). These act as allergens and may trigger an allergic reaction. Common ones include drugs, house dust, pollens and certain foods. The immune system tries to protect the body from a foreign protein by trying to eliminate it. On first exposure certain blood cells (lymphocytes) produce antibodies against the foreign protein (antigen). These antibodies then attach themselves to certain cells, called mast cells, which circulate all over the body. If the same allergen comes into contact with the surfaces of these cells, they bind to the antibodies, causing the cells to release chemicals, the most important of which is histamine (see Type I immune reaction, page 78).

It is not understood why some people become allergic to certain allergens and others do not – we are all, for example, exposed to pollen grains and yet some of us will develop hayfever and others will not. Nor is the nature of allergic reactions fully understood; it may be a fault in the immunity mechanisms, resulting in faulty production of antibody, or it may be due to an inherited defect in the tissues concerned.

Features of the allergic reaction

The features of the allergic reaction are largely due to the release locally into the tissue and/or into the bloodstream of histamine and several other chemicals. A single allergen may cause reactions at several sites; thus a patient allergic to a certain food may develop stomach symptoms, a rash and wheezing. Allergens may affect the body through the skin (e.g. contact allergy due to a cosmetic), in food (e.g. allergy to strawberries), by inhalation (e.g. hayfever due to grass pollens; farmer's lung) and by injection (e.g. insect bites and allergy to antisera).

Allergic reactions may appear as skin rashes (e.g. nettle rash, hives); as swollen patches of skin, swellings of the eyelids, face, lips or throat (angioedema or angioneurotic oedema); as abdominal symptoms (vomiting, diarrhoea and colic); or commonly as hayfever (itching eyes, running nose and sore throat) or as wheezing (asthma). Allergic reactions may be sudden and transient (e.g. sneezing) or last for years (e.g. eczema). They may be trivial, or so serious as to cause sudden death from what is called anaphylactic shock – collapse of the circulation, fall in blood pressure, swelling of the throat and acute wheezing. This usually occurs in patients given an injection that contains a protein to which they have already been made allergic by a previous injection (e.g. bee stings, penicillin).

Histamine

One of the chemicals mainly responsible for allergic reactions is histamine; it is present in most tissues of the body and is released when cells are injured. It causes small blood vessels (capillaries) to dilate, particularly those in the skin, making it hot and red. It also makes the vessels more permeable, so plasma flows from inside the blood vessels out into the surrounding tissues to produce swelling (oedema).

When histamine is injected into the human skin it produces what is called a triple response: (1) a localized red spot which extends within a few seconds, reaches a maximum in about a minute and then becomes bluish; (2) a bright red 'flame' spreads out from this spot; and (3) local swelling occurs, forming a weal. This reaction is often associated with itching and pain. Histamine also causes the blood vessels in the brain to dilate, which produces a headache.

Histamine causes a fall in blood pressure and may increase the heart rate. Large doses may produce a severe fall in blood pressure and collapse. It stimulates the muscles of the small bronchial tubes to constrict, resulting in wheezing, and it stimulates the production of acid in the stomach. It is released in anaphylactic shock, allergy and injury. Its concentration is particularly high in the skin, in the stomach lining and in the lungs.

The release of histamine does not account for all allergic reactions and it is obvious that what was thought to be a straightforward reaction is not so. There is a whole spectrum of allergic responses, both direct and indirect.

Tissue damage will cause the release of histamine. In the skin this may be caused by a physical process, such as sunburn, cold, sunlight, pressure, friction. The juice of the stinging nettle contains histamine which produces a skin rash called urticaria (nettle rash). This sort of rash may also appear in drug allergies.

Histamine released in response to an antigen/antibody reaction or to injury acts on histamine receptors in the skin, blood vessels, nasal passages and airways. These are referred as H_1 receptors. Histamine also acts on histamine receptors in the stomach lining, salivary glands and tear glands in the eyes. They are referred to as H_2 receptors.

The drug treatment of allergies

There are four main drug treatments of allergies:

- *Antihistamine drugs* block histamine receptors in the body and therefore stop the development of allergic reactions
- *Sodium cromoglycate* and related drugs (mast cell stabilizers) prevent the release of histamine by mast cells
- *Corticosteroid drugs* suppress the 'inflammatory' response produced by an allergic reaction
- *Adrenaline* relieves the symptoms of acute allergic reactions by opposing the actions of histamine

Antihistamines

Antihistamine drugs used to treat allergic reactions block H_1 histamine receptors throughout the body. They stop to varying degrees most, but not all, of the effects produced by histamine. They reduce its constricting actions on the muscles of the gut and the bronchial tubes, they reduce the weal in the skin produced by an injection of histamine (see earlier) and they reduce hayfever symptoms, itchy skin rashes and allergic swellings.

Antihistamines that block H_2 receptors are used to treat peptic ulcers and are discussed in Chapter 15.

Antihistamines (H_1 blockers) have many actions in the body other than blocking histamine receptors. For example, some of them block chemical messengers in the nervous system such as acetylocholine, producing anticholinergic-like effects, an action which accounts for some of their harmful effects such as blurred vision, dry mouth and constipation. They may also block the effects of adrenaline on some tissues; and they may produce some effects on dopamine receptors in the brain, affecting control of voluntary movements.

In the brain, antihistamines have both stimulating and depressing effects. Some people may become restless and nervous if they take an antihistamine, and quite small doses of an antihistamine may trigger an epileptic seizure in patients who suffer from focal epilepsy (see Chapter 37). Over-dose with an antihistamine may cause excitation and convulsions, particularly in infants. However, in most patients antihistamines cause depression of brain function, producing reduced alertness, slowed reaction times and drowsiness. They also produce a depressant effect on the cough centre and the vomiting centre, and some of them are used in cough and cold medicines and as anti-vomiting drugs. The newer antihistamines cause less drowsiness and other effects on the brain because they do not enter the brain from the bloodstream as easily as other antihistamines.

Conditions treated with antihistamines

Allergic conjunctivitis

Antihistamine eye drops are effective in relieving the redness and irritation caused by allergic conjunctivitis.

Allergic drug reactions

Many drug reactions respond well to antihistamines, particularly those that cause itching of the skin and nettle rash (urticaria) – but do not forget to stop taking the drug that caused the reaction.

Allergic emergencies

Antihistamines are of no benefit on their own in an acute allergic emergency (see later).

Allergic stomach upsets

Antihistamines are of no value in treating nausea, vomiting or diarrhoea caused by allergic reactions affecting the stomach or intestine.

Angioedema

This is an allergic, patchy swelling of the skin and/or mucous membranes (e.g. the lips and mouth). Antihistamines may relieve allergic swelling of the skin and mucous membranes but are of little value on their own if the swelling affects the throat and threatens life (see treatment of allergic emergencies, later).

Asthma

Antihistamines are of no benefit in treating allergic asthma because chemicals other than histamine appear to be involved; but see the use of ketotifen and oxatomide (Chapter 12).

Blood tranfusion reactions

Antihistamines are of benefit in treating blood transfusion reactions.

Coughs and colds

Harmful effects such as drowsiness and drying of the air passages may outweigh any benefit.

Hayfever

Antihistamines are useful for relieving the symptoms of seasonal hayfever but they have no effect upon the cause. Only about half the patients who suffer from perennial 'hayfever' respond to antihistamines. They are more effective when the course of treatment is started before an attack.

Insect stings and bites

When given by mouth or injection, an antihistamine will relieve the itching and swelling produced by an insect bite or sting. A local application of an antihistamine may also be effective but a corticosteroid preparation is more so (see Chapter 75).

Itching

Antihistamines by mouth may be used to relieve generalized itching but when applied to the skin there is a danger of producing allergic dermatitis. By mouth, antihistamines relieve itching caused by allergic reactions and certain other disorders. The new antihistamines that do not produce drowsiness do not relieve itching caused by non-allergic disorders, probably because they do not easily cross from the bloodstream into the brain. A corticosteroid application is more effective for relieving local itching and discomfort (see Chapter 75).

Motion sickness

Some antihistamines are effective in preventing motion sickness (see Chapter 14).

Pregnancy sickness

The use of antihistamines to treat pregnancy sickness is discussed in Chapter 14.

Serum sickness

Antihistamines are of use in relieving the rash in serum sickness (an allergic reaction following the injection of an antiserum), but they do not help the fever and joint pains very much.

Skin rashes

Some skin rashes, for example acute nettle rash (urticaria) caused by drug allergy, respond well to antihistamines by mouth. Long-standing rashes (e.g. eczema) are little affected.

Sleep

Some antihistamines produce drowsiness and are used to promote sleep, particularly if it is disturbed by an itching skin.

Vertigo and Ménière's disease

Some antihistamines are of benefit in some people with these conditions (see Chapter 14).

Choice of antihistamine

There are numerous antihistamine preparations to choose from, and different people may react differently to any one of them. Antihistamines differ mainly in the degree of drowsiness and in the degree of anticholinergic effects (see Chapter 2) that they produce. Diphenhydramine, promethazine (Phenergan) and trimeprazine (Vallergan) produce the most drowsiness and may be used at bed-time to relieve allergic symptoms during the night.

For day-time use there are now several antihistamines available which do not easily enter the brain from the bloodstream and therefore produce much less drowsiness than previous antihistamines. They include acrivastine (Semprex), astemizole (Hismanal), cetirizine (Zirtek), loratadine (Clarityn) and terfenadine (Triludan). Except for acrivastine, these need only be taken once daily. Acrivastine has to be taken three times a day.

With regard to the anticholinergic effects of antihistamines (dry mouth, constipation, difficulty passing urine, etc.), these are more marked with diphenhydramine (Benadryl), cyproheptadine (Periactin) and promethazine (Phenergan). The newer antihistamines (see above) produce fewer anticholinergic effects (if at all) and for this reason they remain the drugs of choice.

NOTE Some antihistamines may produce an increase in weight; for example, cyproheptadine (Periactin), astemizole (Hismanal) and oxatomide (Tinset).

For dangers of direct application of an antihistamine to the skin, see Chapter 75.

Antihistamines (H_1 blockers) used to treat allergies

acrivastine* (Semprex)
astemizole* (Hismanal)
azatadine (Optimine)
brompheniramine (Dimotane, Dimotane LA)
cetirizine* (Zirtec)
chlorpheniramine (Alunex, Piriton)
clemastine (Tavegil)
cyproheptadine (Periactin)
dimethindene (Fenostil Retard)
diphenhydramine
diphenylpyraline (Histryl, Lergoban)
loratadine* (Clarityn)
mequitazine (Primalan)
oxatomide (Tinset)
phenindamine (Thephorin)
pheniramine (Daneral SA)
promethazine† (Phenergan)
terfenadine* (Triludan)
trimeprazine† (Vallergan)
triprolidine (Actidil, Pro-Actidil)

* These antihistamines do not easily enter the brain from the bloodstream and therefore they produce less drowsiness than the other antihistamines. They are useful for day-time treatment. They are referred to as non-sedative antihistamines.

† These antihistamines produce drowsiness and are useful for night-time use.

Table 10.1 Antihistamine preparations*

Preparation	*Drug*	*Dosage form*
Actidil	triprolidine	Tablets, elixir
Alunex	chlorpheniramine	Tablets
Claritin	loratadine	Tablets
Daneral SA	pheniramine	Sustained-release tablets
Dimotane LA	brompheniramine	Sustained-release tablets
Fabahistin	mebhydrolin	Tablets, suspension
Fenostil-Retard	dimethindene	Sustained-release tablets
Hismanal	astemizole	Tablets, sugar-free suspension
Histryl	diphenylpyraline	Sustained-release capsules
Lergoban	diphenylpyraline	Sustained-release tablets
Optimine	azatadine	Tablets, syrup
Periactin	cyproheptadine	Tablets, syrup
Phenergan	promethazine	Tablets, elixir, injection
Piriton	chlorpheniramine	Tablets, sustained-release tablets (spandets), syrup, injection
Primalan	mequitazine	Tablets
Pro-Actidil	triprolidine	Sustained-release tablets
Semprex	acrivastine	Capsules
Tavegil	clemastine	Tablets, sugar-free elixir
Thephorin	phenindamine	Tablets
Tinset	oxatomide	Tablets
Triludan	terfenadine	Tablets, suspension
Triludan Forte	terfenadine	Tablets
Vallergan	trimeprazine	Tablets, syrup
Vallergan Forte	trimeprazine	Syrup
Zirtek	cetirizine	Tablets

* For nasal preparations containing an antihistamine combined with a decongestant see pages 70–71.

The following antihistamines are available without a doctor's prescription: To treat hayfever: Aller-eze (cemastine), Pollon-eze (astemizole) and Seldane (terfenadine). To treat occasional insomnia: Sominex (promethazine).

Table 10.2 Antihistamines – harmful effects and warnings

Harmful effects of antihistamine drugs vary between different drugs and between different individuals. They vary in frequency, severity and type. Most harmful effects produced by antihistamine drugs are mild and are usually related to the doses used. They can easily be controlled by reducing the dose. More serious harmful effects are rare and are usually caused by high doses and/or by how a particular individual reacts. Not all of the following harmful effects have been reported with every antihistamine drug but they have been reported with one or more of them and should be borne in mind whenever an antihistamine drug is used.

Harmful effects include sweating, chills; dry mouth, nose and throat; allergic skin rashes, severe allergic reactions, sensitivity of the skin to sunlight; fall in blood pressure, headaches, palpitations, rapid beating of the heart, extra heart beats; blood disorders, including damage to circulating red blood cells (haemolytic anaemia) and a reduction in white blood cells; sedation, sleepiness, dizziness, disturbed co-ordination leading to clumsiness; fatigue, confusion, restlessness, excitement, nervousness, tremors, irritability, insomnia, feeling of extreme well-being (euphoria), heaviness and weakness of the hands and feet, numbness and pins and needles in the hands and feet, blurred vision, double vision, vertigo, noises in the ears, convulsions; stomach upset, nausea, vomiting, diarrhoea, constipation; frequency of passing urine, difficulty in passing urine, retention of urine; early menstrual periods; thickening of the phlegm, tightness of the chest, wheezing. Children and elderly people are usually more sensitive to the harmful effects of antihistamines.

Warnings Antihistamines should not be used in patients who are allergic to them. Because of their anticholinergic effects they should be used with utmost caution in patients with glaucoma, narrowing of the outlet from the stomach (pyloric stenosis), enlarged prostate gland, or any obstruction to the outflow of urine from the bladder. They should be used with caution in patients who suffer from asthma, over-active thyroid gland, or raised blood pressure. Remember that antihistamines may produce excitement instead of drowsiness, particularly in young children, and that overdose in children may, very rarely, cause hallucinations, convulsions and death. Because antihistamines reduce allergic reactions they will interfere with skin tests for allergies. They should therefore be stopped at least 1 week before such a test.

Risks in elderly people Harmful effects may be more frequent and severe, particularly dizziness, feeling faint, drowsiness, difficulty in passing urine; dry mouth, nose and throat; nightmares, excitement, nervousness, restlessness; constipation. They should be used with caution.

Risks in driving Antihistamines may cause drowsiness and affect your ability to drive a motor vehicle or operate moving machinery. In this respect, antihistamines affect different patients differently but some antihistamines (e.g. diphenhydramine) produce more drowsiness than others. Do not drive until you know how the drug is going to affect you.

Risks with alcohol Antihistamines increase the effects of alcohol. This may be particularly dangerous to drivers. Do not drink alcohol when you are taking antihistamines.

Table 10.3 Non-sedative antihistamines – harmful effects and warnings (U)

Until recently the great problem of using antihistamines was the risk of producing drowsiness. However, new antihistamines rarely produce drowsiness, probably because they do not enter the brain from the blood stream as easily as the other antihistamines. They are therefore the antihistamines of first choice for treating allergic disorders during th daytime.

astemizole (Hismanal)
Is long acting and remains in the body for 1–4 weeks. It need only be taken once daily. It is therefore useful for long-term treatment of allergic disorders. High daily doses are required in the first week of treatment.

Harmful effects include weight gain. In very high doses it may cause a serious disorder of heart rhythm.

Warnings It should not be used in children under 6 years of age.

terfenadine (Triludan)
Is not as long acting as astemizole (Hismanal) and has to be taken twice daily. No increased dosage is necessary at the start of treatment, so it is suitable for intermittent treatment of allergic disorders.

Harmful effects include headache, sweating, stomach upsets and skin rashes. Harmful effects that have been reported *but not proved* include allergic reactions, alopecia, wheezing, disorders of heart rhythm, confusion, depression, convulsions, dizziness, breathlessness, fatigue, insomnia, jaundice, menstrual disorders (including painful periods), muscle and joint pains, nightmares, palpitations, pins and needles in the hands and feet, sensitivity of the skin to sunlight, fainting and visual disturbances.

Warnings Use with caution if liver function is impaired. It should not be used in children under 3 years of age or in anyone who is allergic to it.

Risks in driving Reports of drowsiness are extremely rare but some people may be sensitive to it; therefore do not drive until you know how the drug is going to affect you.

Table 10.4 Other anti-allergic drugs – harmful effects and warnings

ketotifen (Zaditen)
Possesses both antihistamine and mast cell stabilizing properties (see below, under 'Sodium cromoglycate').

Harmful effects include drowsiness, dry mouth and dizziness for a few days at the start of treatment.

Warnings Flare-up of asthma may occur but this is probably due to stopping other treatments too quickly.

Risks in driving May affect ability to drive during first few days of treatment; therefore do not drive until you know how it is affecting you.

Risks with alcohol It may increase the effects of alcohol; therefore do not drink alcohol when you are taking this drug.

oxatomide (Tinset)
Has both antihistamine and mast cell stabilizing properties (see later, under 'Sodium cromoglycate').

Harmful effects include drowsiness, dry mouth increase appetite and weight gain.

Warnings

Risks in driving It may cause drowsiness; therefore do not drive until you know how the drug will affect you.

Risks with alcohol It increases the effects of alcohol; therefore do not drink alcohol if you are taking this drug.

Sodium cromoglycate

Sodium cromoglycate (Intal, Nalcrom, Opticrom, Rynacrom) has a protective effect on the surfaces of special cells (mast cells) in the linings of the air passages and elsewhere, and prevents the cells from releasing histamine and other chemicals in response to an antibody/antigen reaction on their surfaces. It is called a mast cell stabilizer. It does not stop the antibody/antigen reaction but stops the consequences of that reaction on the surface of the affected cells. Because it is not effective after the reaction, it is used to *prevent* the allergic response (e.g. asthma due to constriction of the bronchial muscles) but is of no use once the reaction has occurred – it is *not* used to treat an acute attack of asthma.

Sodium cromoglycate is poorly absorbed from the intestine when taken by mouth and has to be inhaled in the treatment of allergic asthma and hayfever. Because it is poorly absorbed, it may be taken by mouth to treat food allergies, provided the particular item of food is reduced or eliminated from the diet.

Use of sodium cromoglycate (Intal) to treat asthma

Sodium cromoglycate to treat asthma is available in capsules (spincaps) that contain the finely powdered drug mixed with lactose. The contents of the capsule are inhaled by means of a special inhaler. Alternatively, a respiratory solution of the drug is available for use with a power-operated nebulizer, and it is also available in aerosol inhalers. Because it is used to prevent the consequences of an allergic reaction, it must be used regularly every day, even when you have no symptoms. It is usually used four times a day but this can be reduced.

Sodium cromoglycate is used for the prevention of bronchial asthma due to allergy and also in asthma that is brought on by exercise, cold air, a chemical or occupational dust. In these disorders, by preventing the consequences of an allergic reaction it prevents the constriction of the bronchial tubes (wheezing). Regular use may allow the doses of other drugs (e.g. corticosteroids or bronchodilators) to be reduced. Children seem to respond better to sodium cromoglycate than adults. Because it is difficult to predict which patient will respond to treatment, it is worth trying it in all patients whose asthma is not well controlled with bronchodilators. It should be tried for at least 4 weeks before deciding that it is of no use.

Because sodium cromoglycate prevents attacks of allergic asthma, if it is stopped suddenly a severe attack of asthma may develop. It is sensible, therefore, to reduce the daily dose gradually over about a week before stopping it. For further comments on the use of sodium cromoglycate to treat asthma, and harmful effects and warnings on the use of sodium cromoglycate, see Chapter 12.

The onset of action of sodium cromoglycate varies with the dose, dosage form and the condition being treated. Allergic conjunctivitis and seasonal hayfever may respond after several days whereas asthma and perennial hayfever may take 2–6 weeks to show an improvement. The drug usually works for about 4–6 hours.

Use of sodium cromoglycate (Rynacrom) to treat hayfever

Sodium cromoglycate is available for application into the nose in the treatment of both seasonal and perennial hayfever. A compound preparation of sodium cromoglycate with xylometazoline (Rynacrom Compound) is also available but you should be aware of the harmful effects produced by the regular use of nasal sprays containing xylometazoline and related drugs (Chapter 7).

Other uses

For the use of sodium cromoglycate to treat allergic conjunctivitis see Chapter 35, and to treat ulcerative colitis see Chapter 16.

Table 10.5 Sodium cromoglycate – harmful effects and warnings

Harmful effects include coughing, hoarseness, local irritation, very rarely nausea, vomiting, headache, joint pains, dizziness, wheezing, itching, skin rash, difficulty sleeping.	*Warnings* Do not take sodium cromoglycate if you are allergic to it. Do not use in children under 5 years of age, except in eye drops.

Ketotifen and oxatomide

These drugs produce actions and effects similar to those of sodium cromoglycate, but also possess some antihistamine properties (see Table 10.4). They are used to treat hayfever and other allergic reactions.

Corticosteroids

Corticosteroids are discussed in detail in Chapter 62. They reduce the symptoms of inflammation and allergy, and in the long term they reduce resistance to infections. They suppress the symptoms of hayfever, serum sickness, allergic drug reactions, bee stings and allergic swellings of the skin, mouth and throat (angioedema).

Corticosteroids by mouth or by intramuscular injection are very effective in relieving the symptoms of allergic asthma, but, because of the risk of harmful effects, they are safer if given by inhaler which allows the dose to be significantly reduced and also delivers the drug right to the target. (See Chapter 12 for discussion on the use of corticosteriods in asthma.)

Corticosteroids by mouth or by intramuscular injection are effective in relieving and/or preventing the symptoms of hayfever but any expected benefits must be balanced against the risks. They are safer if given by inhaler because a much smaller dose may be used. For a discussion of the treatment of hayfever, see later.

Sympathomimetic nasal decongestants

Sympathomimetic drugs applied locally to the nose constrict the arteries in the lining of the nose. This reduces the swelling and dries up any discharge. Repeated use causes damage to the lining of the nose and gives less and less benefit the more you use a nasal decongestant. When the effects of these drugs have worn off, the lining can swell right up and produce a blockage worse than before the treatment was started. This rebound swelling may cause permanent blockage to the nose. Any nasal application containing one of these drugs (see Tables 7.1 and 7.2) should be used with caution.

If taken by mouth to relieve nasal congestion these drugs may produce harmful effects particularly in people suffering from heart disease, raised blood pressure, over-active thyroid glands or diabetes. They should not be used to treat hayfever.

Adrenaline injections used to treat acute allergic reactions

Adrenaline is the drug of choice for treating acute allergic reactions. An injection of adrenaline under the skin quickly relieves itching of the skin, nettle rash (urticaria) and swelling of the skin, lips, eyelids, mouth, throat and tongue. The drug may be life saving if swelling of the lining of the voicebox (laryngeal oedema) is suffocating the patient. Adrenaline is the first drug that should be given to someone who develops allergic shock (see later).

Hyposensitization

NOTE Hyposensitization used to be called desensitization, but hyposensitization was a better term because treatment reduces but does not stop sensitization (allergic) reactions. However, it is now often referred to as immunotherapy.

Hyposensitization is a procedure aimed at reducing the frequency and/or severity of allergic reactions in people known to be allergic to specific allergens. The individual is given a graded series of doses of the specific antigen injected under the skin weekly for 9–10 weeks in order to stimulate antibody formation, with the hope that when the person is subsequently exposed to the antigen it may somehow prevent the reaction that occurs between that antigen and the specific antibody on the surface of mast cells. This reaction is responsible for the manifestation of the allergic reaction.

Hyposensitization – benefits

Hyposensitization may be beneficial in people who have suffered a severe allergic reaction to wasp or bee stings. It may occasionally be beneficial to someone who suffers from seasonal hayfever due to grass pollens or from perennial hayfever due to house dust mites. A decision to use hyposensitization treatment in such a person should be made only if, from skin tests and other special tests (e.g. radio-allergosorbent test, RAST), the patient has been shown to be allergic to a specific antigen (e.g. house dust mites) and provided other treatments have failed to relieve symptoms (e.g. antihistamines plus the use of local corticosteroids or sodium cromoglycate) for 2–3 months during exposure to the allergen. Hyposensitization may reduce symptoms such as runny nose and eyes but the duration of such improvement is not fully known. The use of hyposensitization to other allergens (e.g. animal dander) may be of benefit in some people who suffer from perennial hayfever. There is controversy about the potential benefits of hyposensitization in people who suffer from allergic asthma. However, some asthmatic children who are allergic to house dust mites may occasionally benefit and some people allergic to cats may benefit. Hyposensitization to several antigens is less effective than for a single antigen.

The benefits of hyposensitization in patients who suffer from eczema are doubtful.

Hyposensitization – risks

Local reactions at the site of injection include redness, swelling and itching. However, with hyposensitization injections there is always a risk of the patient developing a severe allergic reaction (anaphylaxis). Several patients die every year due to sudden collapse; in most cases adequate facilities to provide resuscitation were not available. The frequency of anaphylactic attacks is not known but it is evident that people with asthma are vulnerable.

Reducing the risks of hyposensitization

Some people are allergic to a wide range of antigens and therefore hyposensitization with a specific antigen will be of little benefit. Furthermore, skin tests of allergens may be unreliable and must only be used along with RAST (see earlier) and a very careful study of the patient's allergy history.

Hyposensitization with a mixture of several allergens contained in a single preparation is not recommended because there is no evidence that they are effective and the risk of producing a serious allergic reaction is increased.

Because of the risks, hyposensitization should be given only in well equipped clinics by specialists in allergic diseases. Full facilities for resuscitation must be immediately available and patients must be kept under careful observation before, during and for up to 2 hours after the injection. Patients with asthma are at special risk of developing a severe allergic reaction.

An antihistamine by mouth an hour before hyposensitization may help to reduce redness and swelling at the site of the injection and a bronchodilator (e.g. salbutamol) by inhaler or by injection under the skin may help to lessen any wheezing (see Chapter 12), which may occur about half an hour after the injection or be delayed for about 6 hours. If mild reactions occur, the next injection should be reduced to a level that causes no reaction and then built up again. If the reactions are moderate or severe, hyposensitization should be stopped.

The duration of benefit from hyposensitization is often uncertain, and with allergy to bee or wasp stings it may help to test the individual by stinging and then taking blood to assess the degree of antibody response. If this is high, a further course may be necessary.

Recent research into preparations of allergens to use for desensitization include the use of allergen polymers in the hope that polymerized allergens will reduce the risk of harmful effects. Polymerization is the combination of two or more molecules to form a compound (polymer). Another approach is to modify the allergen in such a way that it triggers an immune response but produces less risk of an allergic reaction.

Acute allergic shock

In acute allergic shock (anaphylactic shock), nettle rash (urticaria) may develop and there is a sudden and dramatic fall in blood pressure, producing collapse, the bronchial tubes constrict (bronchospasm) and their linings swell up, producing wheezing and difficulty in breathing. Sometimes there is swelling of the throat and lining of the voicebox (laryngeal oedema), which may cause suffocation and sudden death. Early signs include malaise, tiredness and smarting eyes.

Warning *Anaphylactic shock is very rare and is usually triggered by antisera, insect stings, antibiotics, iron injections, aspirin or other anti-inflammatory drugs (see Chapter 30), blood products, heparin or hyposensitization products. It is more likely to occur following an injection and in susceptible individuals who have a history of eczema, asthma and hayfever.*

Treatment of an acute allergic emergency

Treatment is urgent – the patient must be lain flat with the legs raised in order to try to raise the blood pressure. Then the following treatment is given.

- *Adrenaline* by injection under the skin or into a muscle in a dose of 0.5–1.0 mg (0.5–1 ml of 1 in 1000 adrenaline solution), repeated every 10 minutes up to a total of 2 ml
- If wheezing is severe, the patient may require, in addition to the adrenaline, another *bronchodilator* (e.g. salbutamol by nebulizer inhalation and/or by infusion into a vein 3–20 microgram/minute) or by slow intravenous injection (250 microgram, repeated if necessary), or aminophylline slowly into a vein (250–500 mg slowly over 20 minutes)*
- *Chlorpheniramine* (an antihistamine) by slow infusion into a vein: 10–20 mg when necessary up to a maximum dose of 40 mg in 24 hours
- *A transfusion of salt solution* (0.9% sodium chloride) into a vein will help to restore the volume of the blood and raise the blood pressure
- *Oxygen* by a face mask may be necessary
- *Hydrocortisone* by injection into a vein in a dose of 100–300 mg. This takes several hours to work but should be used in order to prevent deterioration.

Warnings *If an injection has caused the collapse, a tourniquet should be applied above the injection site to prevent the substance from being further absorbed into the bloodstream.*

* Individuals taking a beta-blocker may not respond to adrenaline and will need salbutamol by infusion into a vein.

If the patient develops swelling in the voicebox (laryngeal oedema) and cannot breathe, a breathing tube must be put down into the lungs (intubation) or a hole (tracheostomy) must be cut in the main windpipe below the voicebox (Adam's apple).

Patients allergic to insect bites should carry an adrenaline aerosol inhaler (e.g. Medihaler-Epi) or preferably a prefilled syringe of adrenaline.

Hayfever

Hayfever (allergic rhinitis) is either *seasonal* caused by an allergic reaction to, for example, grass pollens or *perennial* (all the year round) and caused by an allergic reaction to, for example, house dust mites or animal fur.

Exposure to grass pollens, house dust mites and other antigens trigger the production of antibodies. These antibodies concentrate on the surfaces of mast cells in the lining of the nose, air passages and elsewhere in the body. Once this development has occurred the individual is now allergic to that particular antigen. If he breathes it in again, there will be an immediate antibody/antigen reaction on the surface of these cells which will cause them to burst and release histamine and other chemicals which will produce a local allergic reaction just like acute inflammation. In hayfever, the lining of the nose becames inflamed and swollen, causing it to be blocked, runny and itchy. A similar reaction may occur in the eyes, producing watering, swelling and redness of the conjunctiva (allergic conjunctivitis).

Treatment of hayfever

Avoidance of allergens

The best treatment of hayfever is to try to avoid contact with the allergen, but this is obviously very difficult. With seasonal hayfever try to avoid going out into the garden or the country during the pollen season. Keep windows closed, use air filters in the home, and try wearing a face mask if you go out. With perennial hayfever, try an air filter in the home, particularly in the bedroom; clean the house regularly to reduce the dust, and cover mattresses and pillows with sealed plastic covers.

Drug treatment of hayfever

Antihistamine drugs by mouth

Antihistamine drugs are discussed earlier. They may be of benefit in both seasonal and perennial hayfever but different people react differently to antihistamines and it is often a matter of trying various ones until you find one that suits you. However, one of the principal harmful effects of antihistamines is drowsiness because of their effects on the brain.

This is why for day-time use it helps to use one of the newer antihistamines that produce less drowsiness. They include acrivastine (Semprex), astemizole (Hismanal), cetirizine (Zirtek), loratadine (Clarityn) and terfenadine (Triludan). Except for acrivastine, they need only be taken once daily. Acrivastine has to be taken three times daily.

Acrivastine (Semprex), cetirizine (Zirtek) and loratadine (Clarityn) are not recommended for children. Astemizole (Hismanal) and terfenadine (Triludan) are not recommended for children under 6 years, and half doses should be used in children aged 6–12 years.

Antihistamines by mouth are useful for relieving sneezing, runny nose and sore eyes but they do not produce much effect on blockage of the nose. Therefore it is usually necessary to use a local application up the nose (e.g. a corticosteroid, discussed below).

Antihistamine nose drops and sprays (see Table 7.2)

These preparations usually contain a decongestant drug as well as an antihistamine, and although they may provide relief of symptoms in some people there are dangers in using a nasal decongestant regularly every day. Preparations that also contain an antibiotic (e.g. neomycin) should not be used.

Decongestant nose drops and sprays (see Table 7.1)

These are discussed in detail in Chapter 3. There are dangers in using these preparations regularly every day, so they should be used only occasionally to treat hayfever.*

* Patients with perennial hayfever develop an over-reaction to irritants which stimulates parasympathetic nerve endings (see Chapter 2) to produce a running nose. This effect can be blocked by an anticholinergic drug e.g. ipratropium (Rinatec nasal spray). For details on ipratropium see page 146.

Nasal decongestants by mouth

These preparations are of doubtful value and may be harmful in some people (Chapter 3).

Corticosteroid nasal applications

beclomethazone (Beconase nasal aerosol and aqueous nasal spray)
betamethasone (Betnesol drops; Vista-Methasone nasal drops)
budesonide (Rhinocort nasal aerosol)
flunisolide (Syntaris nasal spray)

Corticosteroids are discussed in detail in Chapter 62. They suppress inflammation, and nasal preparations of corticosteroids are very beneficial in relieving the symptoms of hayfever in some people. Depending upon the type of application, they sometimes cause stinging and sneezing. The use of a saline nasal spray in between corticosteroid applications may help to reduce these harmful effects.

It takes several days of regular daily use of corticosteroid nasal applications to produce any beneficial effect, and it therefore helps if you also take an antihistamine drug by mouth, particularly if you also have eye symptoms. Compared with the dose of a corticosteroid that has to be taken by mouth, the dose in nasal applications is very small; nevertheless some of the drug is absorbed into the bloodstream and you should read Chapter 62 on the benefits and risks of using corticosteroids.

Sodium cromoglycate (Rynacrom spray, nasal drops and insufflator)

Sodium cromoglycate is not as effective in preventing nasal allergic reactions as it is in preventing allergic asthma but it is still worth trying if you suffer from hayfever. It must be used *regularly every day* even though you may have no symptoms, because it prevents the allergic reaction from developing; however, it has no effect once an allergic reaction has occurred and you have developed symptoms. It may occasionally irritate the nose in the first 4 days of treatment. Rarely, it may cause wheezing and tightness of the chest through inhaling the drug into the lungs. Rynacrom Compound contains sodium cromoglycate and a decongestant, xylometazoline. It is recommended for use where hayfever is associated with a blocked nose, but see Chapter 7 for the dangers of using a decongestant regularly every day. The dose of xylometazoline is low but, even so, some of the drug is absorbed into the bloodstream and there is a risk of harmful effects, which include headache, insomnia, drowsiness and palpitations. Locally in the nose it may cause irritation, dryness and sneezing. Regular daily use may cause a rebound swelling of the lining, resulting in blockage.

Eye applications

Corticosteroid eye applications should not be used to treat eye symptoms in hayfever because of the dangers (see Chapter 35).

Combined eye preparations containing an antihistamine and a decongestant may be helpful in some people. They include Otrivine-Antistin (antazoline and xylometazoline) and Vasocon-A (antazoline and naphazoline). These drugs may be absorbed into the bloodstream and you should read about the harmful effects and warnings on the use of antihistamines (Table 10.3) and decongestants (Chapter 3). They should not be used if you wear soft contact lenses or if you suffer from closed-angle glaucoma. They should be used with caution if you suffer from raised blood pressure, overactive thyroid gland, diabetes or coronary artery disease. They should not be used by patients taking an MAOI anti-depressant or within 2 weeks of stopping such drugs. They should only be used for a short period of time.

Opticrom eye drops and ointment contain sodium cromoglycate. They may be beneficial in some patients in *preventing* allergic reactions in the eyes, so they need applying *before* the allergic reaction develops (e.g. just before the hayfever season begins) and they should be applied regularly every day when the pollen count is high, even though you may have no eye symptoms. The applications may produce transient stinging of the eyes, and the ointment, like any eye ointment, may produce transient blurring of vision. It may help to use Opticrom drops in the day-time and Optricrom ointment at night. Soft contact lenses should not be worn while using Opticrom eye drops.

Corticosteroids by mouth or injection

For seasonal hayfever, when symptoms are severe and disabling it may be worth trying a short course of a corticosteroid by mouth or a long-acting injection of a corticosteroid such as methylprednisolone (Depo-Medrone). Corticosteroids work only when symptoms are present, so they should not be used to prevent hayfever. It is important that the benefits of relieving the symptoms of the hayfever are balanced against the risks of using a corticosteroid; these are discussed in detail in Chapter 62.

Sometimes in hayfever the inflammation of the lining of the nose produces swelling and blockage so that nose drops are difficult to apply. If this happens, it may help to take a corticosteroid by mouth for a few days in order to relieve the inflammation and to shrink the lining. Treatment may then be switched to a corticosteroid nasal application which will be able to penetrate the lining and produce beneficial effects.

11

Immunizations

Immunity is a state of resistance to disease, especially to a specific disease (see Chapter 9).

Active immunity to an infectious disease may come from having had a fully blown attack of the disease (e.g. an attack of measles protects you from getting another attack of measles for the rest of your life) or from having suffered only a mild attack of a disease (e.g. a mild attack of polio may cause just a slight headache and feeling off-colour but it protects you none the less against polio for the rest of your life). Such a mild attack is not sufficient to 'cause' the disease but is sufficient to trigger the body's immune system to produce antibodies against that disease. These antibodies will provide protection against the disease in the future. These 'mild' attacks are often referred to by doctors as 'sub-clinical' attacks of the disease, because the individual does not develop symptoms and signs of the fully blown disease, but only develops, for example, mild aches and pains and a slight fever.

Passive immunity is a short-term immunity to a disease which is transferred to an individual; for example, a newborn baby gets antibodies from his mother's milk which will protect him temporarily from certain diseases (see Chapter 9).

Knowledge of how the body can provide its own active immunity and passive immunity is used in immunizations which may provide an individual with either active or passive immunity to several diseases.

Immunization means the production of immunity by either active or passive means. Active immunization involves the production of active immunity by the injection (or by other means) of an antigen to which the body responds by producing its own specific antibodies. Passive immunization involves the injection of antibodies that have been produced in another human (human antibodies, or human immunoglobulins) or in an animal (referred to as antiserum).

Active immunity

This involves the injection or taking by mouth of a substance that can trigger an immune response and the production of antibodies specific to that substance. A substance that produces such effects is known as an antigen, but when we are talking about immunization we usually refer to this antigen as a vaccine.

The term 'vaccine' was originally applied only to the fluid from cowpox (vaccinia) which was used to vaccinate humans against smallpox. However, it has come to be used as a general term for any substance (antigen) used to produce active immunity. Vaccines may be bacterial or viral. They may consist of weakened (attenuated) live bacteria (e.g. BCG vaccine used to protect against tuberculosis) or killed bacteria (e.g. typhoid vaccination), or they may contain a toxic substance (or toxin) produced by a certain group of bacteria (e.g. tetanus vaccine). Virus vaccines may contain live but weakened viruses (e.g. polio vaccine), killed viruses (e.g. influenza vaccine), certain parts of the protein structure of the virus – viral antigens (e.g. some influenza vaccines), or harmless live viruses that trigger the same antibody reaction as the virus that causes a particular disease (e.g. smallpox vaccine).

Vaccination is the process of immunizing; the term may be used to cover any active immunization but often is reserved just for smallpox vaccination using vaccinia virus.

Vaccines stimulate the body's immune system and trigger the production of antibodies against that disease. They do not provide immediate protection against infection and it may take up to 4 weeks before full immunity develops. When immediate protection is needed, it may be necessary to provide passive immunity (see below) using immunoglobulins. With *live vaccines*, one dose will usually provide adequate protection for many years but not usually as long as if the individual developed the disease. The lasting protection provided by live vaccine is helped by the fact that the live organisms included in the vaccine multiply in the body to produce a powerful stimulation to antibody production. With the weakened viruses used in polio immunization, three doses have to be used at monthly intervals.

Dead vaccines and *inactivated vaccines* require a series of injections to make sure that the immune system is sufficiently stimulated to produce an adequate antibody response. These are usually given in three doses at monthly intervals, with a booster injection at some future date because the immunity will last only a few months to years (see each individual immunization schedule, later).

Passive immunity

Passive immunity is used for individuals who have recently been or may soon be exposed to a specific disease. Immunization consists of giving an injection of a preparation obtained from the plasma of individuals who have adequate levels of antibodies against the disease for which protection is sought. These antibodies are proteins (immunoglobulins) from the plasma of humans; they are therefore known as human immunoglobulins.

In the past, antibodies were also obtained from animals by giving them the disease – for example, the old anti-tetanus serum (ATS) was obtained from the plasma of horses that had been given tetanus. This is why it caused so much trouble – it contained horse protein to which many people became allergic. They developed severe reactions such as serum sickness (fever, rash, aching joints and swollen glands) or anaphylactoid shock (a serious allergic emergency, see Chapter 10). A preparation from an animal used to provide passive immunity is called an antiserum. Such antisera are seldom used these days.

Immunization vaccines

Anthrax vaccine

Anthrax is a bacterial disease transmitted as spores to humans through direct contact with animals or their carcasses, hides, furs or wools and also foodstuffs (e.g. bone meal, fish meat). It may produce severe ulcers and blisters of the skin, stomach and intestine and inflammation of the lungs and brain (meningitis).

An anthrax vaccine is available, made from inactivated bacteria, and given by injection into a muscle or deep under the skin. A dose is given every 3 weeks for three doses and then a fourth dose is given after 6 months. A booster dose is given every year. Prevention should also focus on good education, protective clothing and equipment in industry and good husbandry in farming.

Harmful effects and warnings

See the general statement on harmful effects and warnings on the use of vaccines in Table 11.1.

BCG vaccine (tuberculosis)

BCG stands for Bacillus Calmette–Guérin. It is a live weakened strain of tuberculosis bacteria from infected cattle. It stimulates an increased immune response in humans – a hypersensitive response. Calmette and Guérin were two French scientists who introduced the test. The vaccine protects against the consequences of a primary attack of tuberculosis. It reduces the incidence of tuberculosis of the lungs by up to 80 per cent and minimizes the risks of complications. It protects the individual but it does not reduce the spread of the disease within a community. Its effectiveness depends upon the increased immune response it produces; this enables the body to attack and kill any infecting tuberculosis bacteria before they can attack the tissues of the body.

The effectiveness of BCG vaccination programmes still remains controversial. They have been used extensively in the UK whilst in the USA they have not been used to the same extent. This is because vaccination interferes with any future use of the tuberculin test (see Chapter 55) in recognizing whether an individual is infected with tuberculosis, and because the major source of tuberculosis comes from already infected people.

In the UK, BCG vaccination is still carried out in most areas on children aged 10–14 years who have negative tuberculin tests. In some areas it is not now used if the infection rate of the population in that region is less than 1 per cent, but this decision often appears to be on the grounds of cost rather than on the benefits and risks to the individual and to the community.

Individuals who have contact with someone suffering from active tuberculosis of the lungs should be tuberculin tested and all those who are negative (i.e. have never had the disease) should be given BCG vaccine. This applies to children and adults. Babies should be vaccinated without first having a tuberculin test. College students, trainee teachers and nurses should be tuberculin tested and vaccinated if their tests are negative.

About 1 week after vaccination a small swelling appears at the injection site which turns into a small lump (papule) or ulcer over about 3 weeks and then clears up after about 6–12 weeks. It helps the ulcer to heal if it is exposed to the air. Prolonged ulceration or the development of an abscess are due to faulty methods of injecting the vaccine.

In the UK, all immigrants from countries where there is a high incidence of tuberculosis are tuberculin tested, and all those who are negative are given BCG vaccine – adults and children. All newborn babies coming from these countries are vaccinated against tuberculosis, without first being tuberculin tested.

Harmful effects of BCG vaccine

Harmful effects are rare. They include not only those harmful effects that are general to any vaccine (see Table 11.1) but also ulceration and abscess formation at the injection site, sometimes with tender swollen glands and inflammation of the underlying bone. Healing of a BCG ulcer may be slow and involve the growth of 'proud' flesh (keloid). Very rarely, a condition known as lupus vulgaris may develop at the site. This is tuberculosis of the skin, which forms soft nodules (apple jelly nodules), ulcers and red patches. Rarely, a generalized allergic reaction may occur and also a generalized BCG infection.

Warnings on the use of BCG vaccine

See general warnings on the use of vaccines (Table 11.1).

BCG vaccine should not be given to people who have leukaemia, cancer, acute illness (including tuberculosis), or to patients being treated with corticosteroids or drugs that suppress the immune system or to any patient with an immune deficiency (e.g. AIDS).

Administration

BCG is given by injection *into* the skin. It should no longer be given by multiple punctures through the skin (percutaneous). In babies, great care must be taken not to give the vaccine under the skin; this may cause a local abscess.

Botulism antitoxin

Botulism is a severe paralysing disease caused by toxins from the micro-organism *Clostridium botulinum*, which forms spores and is widely distributed in soil, agricultural products and marine life. Three types of toxin-producing micro-organisms have been recognized, and are referred to as types A, B and E.

The commonest form of the disease is food-borne botulism, which comes from eating food contaminated with toxins from the micro-organisms; it is one of the most dangerous toxins known in man. Food sources of the infection include home-canned foods in the USA, meat and meat products in Europe and fish products in Japan, Scandinavia and Russia. Types A, B and E (from fish) are found in food poisoning.

Passive immunization

Botulism antitoxin contains concentrated antibodies (immunoglobulins) obtained from the blood of healthy horses that have been immunized against the toxins produced by types A, B and E. It is used to treat botulism caused by eating infected food. It should be given as early as possible.

Harmful effects of botulism antitoxin

Because botulism antitoxin is prepared from horse protein there is always a serious risk that it will cause severe allergic reactions in susceptible individuals. At least 20 per cent of patients develop an allergic reaction and about 3–5 per cent develop a severe reaction (anaphylaxis) in which they start to wheeze, their throat swells up, their blood pressure falls, and they may collapse and die. Allergy may also take the form of serum sickness coming on some 7–12 days after treatment (see harmful effects of antisera, Table 11.2.)

Warnings on the use of botulism antitoxin

See the general warnings on the use of antitoxins, Table 11.2.

Harmful allergic reactions are more likely to occur in people who suffer from eczema, asthma, hayfever or other allergies and in patients who have previously received any antitoxins. All patients should be tested for allergy to the antitoxin by giving them a test dose one hour before treatment. If there is a history of allergy the antitoxin should be diluted.

Administration

Botulism antitoxin against toxins from types A, B and E organisms is given by intramuscular injection as soon after exposure as possible to prevent an attack. If an attack has already begun, the antitoxin is given by repeated slow intravenous infusions, followed by injections.

Infant botulism

Infant botulism results from the production of toxin (type A) in the bowel of an infant by an infecting micro-organism, which may come from honey. About 10 per cent of honey supplies have been found to contain spores of botulism and honey accounts for about one-third of the 30–80 cases that occur in the USA every year. The toxins cause paralysis and produce what is called a 'floppy' baby. The death rate is about 2 per cent. Passive immunization with botulism antitoxins is of no value.

Cholera vaccine

Cholera is a serious infectious disease that causes severe diarrhoea, vomiting and collapse. It is caused by bacteria and an epidemic usually starts with infection of the water supplies. It is present in the rivers of the Ganges, the rivers of the Far East and also in parts of the Near East and Africa. The organism is passed in stools and vomit from infected persons and it can survive in fresh water for up to 2 weeks and for up to 8 weeks in salt water. Transmission is normally through drinking infected water or through eating infected shellfish or food contaminated by flies or by the fingers of infected people who handled it.

Cholera vaccine contains dead cholera organisms. It provides protection for up to about 6 months but obviously does not control the spread of the disease. Because the vaccine is dead, it does not give lasting immunity and it is necessary to have booster injections every 6 months for those living in areas where cholera is prevalent. Even after vaccination, special hygienic precautions should always be taken, particularly with food and drinking water.

Harmful effects and warnings

See the general statement on harmful effects and warnings regarding vaccines in Table 11.1.

Slight tenderness, redness and swelling may occur at the injection site along with fever and malaise. Sometimes allergic reactions can occur which may be serious, and nerve damage and mental symptoms have occurred very occasionally.

Administration

It is given by two injections into a muscle or under the skin. The second dose should be given 4 weeks after the first dose but it may be given as close as 1 week after. To reduce the risk of harmful effects it helps if the second and subsequent doses are given *into* the skin (intradermally), but some countries insist that all injections should be given under the skin or into a muscle.

Diphtheria vaccines

Diphtheria is an infectious bacterial disease which usually attacks the throat to produce local inflammation with the production of an exudate that looks just like a 'wash-leather'. The neck may swell and the lymph glands become swollen. The bacteria produce a toxin that is highly dangerous and can cause collapse and death within 10 days of first becoming infected.

Diphtheria vaccines contain a toxin produced by diphtheria organisms.

Actually it is a *toxoid*, which is the material produced by treating a toxin in such a way that its toxic properties are inactivated whilst its ability to stimulate antibody production remains intact.

The toxin is inactivated by formaldehyde and it is therefore known as formol toxoid. The formol toxoid is then precipitated on to a mineral (e.g. aluminium hydroxide) which ensures that it is released slowly into the bloodstream after injection. 'APT' is alum-precipitated diphtheria toxoid (i.e. toxoid precipitated on to aluminium oxide). The initial course of vaccine for a child consists of three injections at monthly intervals, starting at 2 months of age, and then a booster dose 3 years later (at entry to play group or school). Protective antibodies persist for at least 10 years after the initial course of injections and after a booster dose.

Diphtheria immunization decreases the spread of the disease and the severity of the disease. Before 1950 it was a common and often fatal disease in the UK but, thanks to immunization, it is now so rare that most doctors have never seen a case. However, it is still around in other parts of the world and there is no cause for complacency with regard to diphtheria immunization.

Harmful effects and warnings

See the general statement on the harmful effects of vaccines in Table 11.1. Local redness and swelling at the site of injection may occur but these are usually slight.

Administration

A single diphtheria vaccine (monovalent vaccine) is available as 'diphtheria vaccine adsorbed' (Dip/Vac/Ads) for primary immunization of children who do not require immunizing against tetanus or whooping cough. It may also be used in adults who are susceptible to diphtheria as indicated by a positive Schick test (a local reaction caused by injection of a diluted diphtheria toxin into the skin). It may also be used in children over 10 years of age who are at particular risk and are Schick positive.

The dose is given by intramuscular or deep injection under the skin. Starting at 2–3 months of age, three doses are given at monthly intervals and a booster dose 3 years later at play group or school entry. Children over the age of 10 years or adults who have never been immunized against diphtheria and are Schick positive (i.e. susceptible) should receive two doses of adsorbed diphtheria vaccine at an interval of 4 weeks.

A dilute vaccine is available to boost immunity in adults who are at risk; for example, those who work in infectious disease units.

Diphtheria vaccine is usually combined with tetanus vaccine and whooping cough (pertussis) vaccine.

Adsorbed diphtheria, tetanus and pertussis vaccine (DTPer/Vac/Ads) – triple vaccine This is prepared from diphtheria formol toxoid, tetanus formol toxoid and pertussis vaccine precipitated (adsorbed) on to aluminium hydroxide to allow slow release after injection. It is the standard triple vaccine used to immunize children. Three injections (intramuscular or deep under the skin) are given at monthly intervals, with a booster dose usually 3 years later.

NOTE The adsorbed vaccine is preferred to non-adsorbed preparations.

Adsorbed diphtheria and tetanus vaccine (DT/Vac/Ads) This is prepared from diphtheria formol toxoid and tetanus formol toxoid precipitated (adsorbed) on to aluminium hydroxide to allow slow release after injection (see earlier). It is used for immunizing children when the use of whooping cough (pertussis) vaccine is not indicated or not wanted by the parents. The dose of this double vaccine is given by intramuscular or deep injection under the skin. Three doses are given at monthly intervals, with a booster dose usually 3 years later.

NOTE The adsorbed vaccine is preferred to the non-adsorbed vaccine.

Passive immunization against diphtheria

Diphtheria antitoxin contains mainly immunoglobulins (antibodies) from the serum of healthy horses that have been immunized against diphtheria toxin or toxoid. It neutralizes diphtheria toxin at the site of infection (e.g. the throat) with the diphtheria organism but it cannot affect any damage that the toxin has already caused. The passive immunity provided by the antitoxin lasts about 2 weeks. Diphtheria antitoxin should be given immediately the diagnosis is made, before the toxin causes too much damage on the tissues.

Harmful effects Because diphtheria antitoxin is prepared from horse protein there is always a serious risk that it will cause severe allergic reactions in susceptible individuals. This may take the form of an acute anaphylactic reaction in which the individual starts to wheeze, his throat swells up, his blood pressure falls and he collapses and may die. It may take the form of serum sickness, which develops in about 7–12 days and causes fever, nettle rash (urticaria), swollen glands and painful joints. This serum sickness comes on quicker (within 3–4 days) in people who have previously had an injection of horse serum (e.g. anti-tetanus serum). A test dose of antitoxin should always be given half an hour before the full dose.

German measles vaccine

German measles (rubella) is caused by a virus that spreads by droplet infection (coughs and sneezes). One attack of the disease gives a high degree of lasting immunity. The disease is usually trivial in children, but in pregnant women it may cause serious abnormalities in the unborn baby. The baby may be born with heart damage, mental impairment, cataracts and deafness. The danger is greatest in the first 4 months of pregnancy, and may be very serious in the first four weeks when the risk of damaging the baby may be as high as 70 per cent.

The time from first contact to the development of the disease (the incubation period) is 18 days.

Vaccination of all children

It is now the general policy to vaccinate all children (boys and girls) against measles, mumps and rubella in the hope of eliminating the spread of these diseases among children.

Vaccination of girls

In order to prevent damage to unborn babies, *all girls should be vaccinated against german measles before puberty* (usually between 10 and 14 years of age). Only those who have documented records that they have been previously vaccinated against german measles should be excluded. Reliance should *not* be based on a history that a girl has had a previous attack of german measles. The illness may have been misdiagnosed and this risk should never be taken. Obviously tests for antibodies to german measles could be carried out to see if the girl has had the disease, but it is quicker, cheaper and safer to vaccinate *all* girls who have not previously been vaccinated against german measles, or if there is any doubt.

Women of child-bearing age

In the UK it is recommended that all women of child-bearing age be vaccinated against german measles if they produce a negative test for antibodies (this shows that they have never had the disease and are at risk). In the USA they have gone further by attempting to vaccinate all women of child-bearing age who have not been previously vaccinated. This seems much more sensible.

Advice Any woman of child-bearing age who has no documented evidence that she has been vaccinated against german measles should be vaccinated.

She should *never* rely on evidence of a past attack of german measles, no matter how well documented.

The risk of german measles vaccination in pregnancy The inadvertent vaccination of women who are pregnant has shown that the weakened virus used in german measles vaccines enters the baby's tissues; but there has been no report of damage to babies caused by the german measles vaccine. Nevertheless, vaccination should be avoided in early pregnancy, and it makes sense to vaccinate only those women who are known *not* to be pregnant and to advise them to take contraceptive precautions for at least 1 month after vaccination.

A long-lasting depot injection of a progestogen is often used for contraception but its routine use in women who have been vaccinated against german measles should not be encouraged, particularly the practice of giving it without the women's knowledge. Such practices should only be with the written consent of the woman after she has had the benefits and risks explained to her in detail.

Warnings on german measles vaccination

German measles vaccination can fail;* therefore a woman should have an antibody test at the beginning of *every* pregnancy. If she does not have antibodies, there is a risk that the baby will be damaged if she contracts german measles.

The same advice applies to women who have just had a baby but whose blood tests show that they have never had german measles. These women should be vaccinated as soon as possible after the birth of their child and they should practise contraception for at least 1 month after the vaccination. This is an important group of women to protect because 60 per cent of all abnormalities in babies caused by german measles in pregnancy occurs in those born to women who have had more than one child. This shocking finding reflects just how bad screening for german measles used to be in pregnant women.

Additional protection for pregnant women is obtained by ensuring that all nurses and doctors working in obstetric units are (or have been) vaccinated against german measles.

Harmful effects of german measles vaccination

For general harmful effects of vaccines, see Table 11.1. Harmful effects of german measles vaccine include skin rashes, painful joints, cold-like symp-

* Re-infection with german measles may also occur occasionally.

toms, sore throats, fever, swollen glands and, very rarely, nerve damage (numbness and pins and needles in the arms and legs).

German measles vaccine should not be given to anyone with leukaemia, cancer or fever. It should not be given to those who may have immune deficiency due to drugs (e.g. corticosteroids, immunosuppressants) or disease (e.g. AIDS). It should be used with caution in people who suffer from allergic disorders (eczema, asthma, hayfever). It should not be given within 4 weeks of another live vaccine and it should not be given in pregnancy, particularly within the first 4 months of getting pregnant.

Administration

Rubella vaccine, live (Rub/Vac/Live) is a weakened, live german measle virus. A single dose is given by injection under the skin.

Passive immunization against german measles

Human normal immunoglobulins (antibodies also referred to as 'gamma-globulins') may lessen the likelihood of german measles developing in a pregnant woman who has not been vaccinated and/or who has no antibodies against the disease, and who has been in contact with someone with the active disease. However, if she has caught the infection, passive immunization may just mask the symptoms and provide no protection for the baby. Human normal immunoglobulin is given by injection into a muscle; it is repeated in 2 or 3 days.

Hepatitis B vaccine

Hepatitis is discussed in Chapter 83. Hepatitis B is due to a virus which cannot be grown in the laboratory. However, the virus and material from its surface circulate in the blood of infected individuals. This allows hepatitis B vaccine to be made from the blood of people who carry the virus. The blood is purified to remove whole virus, treated with formalin (to inactivate any remaining live virus) and then adsorbed on to alum. It is part of the capsule of the virus (the surface antigen) which stimulates the immune system and leads to the production of specific antibodies in the vaccinated person. It is also manufactured using biotechnology.

Hepatitis B vaccination is recommended for people who run a high risk of getting infected – for example, surgeons, dentists, dialysis workers and lab. technicians who work with blood. Susceptible patients include those on dialysis, those who receive multiple blood transfusions or blood products (e.g. haemophiliacs), sexually active and promiscuous male homosexuals, intravenous drug users who share syringes and equipment, male and female prostitutes and certain close family contacts.

Babies born to mothers who suffer from hepatitis B (i.e. they have evidence of the virus in their blood) should be vaccinated with hepatitis B vaccine and also given passive immunization using hepatitis B antibody (hepatitis B immunoglobulin) immediately after delivery.

Passive immunization

Passive immunization against hepatitis A and hepatitis B is available, see page 139.

Harmful effects and warnings on the use of hepatitis B vaccine

See the general statement on harmful effects and warnings of vaccines (Table 11.1).

Administration

H-B-Vax (a suspension of hepatitis B surface proteins [antigens] adsorbed onto alum) is given by intramuscular injections. Three doses are given; the second dose should be given 1 month after the first dose and the third dose should be given 5 months later.

Engerix B (a suspension of hepatitis B surface proteins [antigens]) is prepared from yeast cells by biotechnology; it is adsorbed on to aluminium hydroxide. It is given in the same way as H-B-Vax, except that for travellers the third dose may be given 2 months after the first dose, with a booster at 12 months.

Influenza vaccines

Three types of influenza virus have been described – A, B and C. Type A causes the major epidemics of influenza that spread throughout the world (pandemics). Several strains of influenza A virus have been identified (e.g. Asian flu, Hong Kong flu). Influenza B usually causes smaller and less serious outbreaks, and influenza C is very rare.

The immunity that we develop after an attack of flu is specific to a particular type of influenza virus and is short lasting. Immunity to influenza is made difficult by the fact that influenza viruses keep altering the protein structure on their surfaces and it is these protein structures that act as the antigens which trigger antibody production against them.

To be effective, an influenza vaccine has to keep pace with any changes in surface proteins on the influenza virus, the important ones being labelled H and N. Every year the World Health Organization publishes the latest position with regard to these protein changes, and the manufacturers of influenza vaccines prepare their vaccines accordingly.

Influenza vaccines do not control the spread of influenza; they merely offer protection to the individual. They are therefore recommended only for people at risk; for example, patients with diabetes, immune deficiency disorders, chronic heart or chest or kidney disorders, and elderly people, particularly those living in institutions and residential homes.

Inactivated influenza vaccine produces protection against influenza in about 2–3 weeks in about 70 per cent of those immunized but it lasts only for a few months.

Harmful effects of influenza vaccines

See the statement on harmful effects of vaccines (Table 11.1). The injection may produce redness and swelling at the site of injection, and there may be mild generalized reactions such as fever and malaise. Very occasionally, a severe fever may develop.

Warnings on the use of influenza vaccines

Influenza vaccine is grown in chick embryos, so the vaccine should never be used to treat people who are allergic to eggs or feathers: it may cause severe allergic reactions in them. It should be used with caution in people who suffer from allergies (e.g. hayfever, eczema, asthma). See also warnings on vaccines (Table 11.1).

Administration

Vaccines prepared from the surface proteins (antigens) of the influenza virus are called surface antigen vaccines. They are also known as split product vaccines (SPV). They are tolerated better than vaccines made from the whole virus. Surface antigen vaccines should be used in children in preference to whole virus vaccines; in the most vulnerable age groups (4–13 years) a purified form of surface antigen vaccine should be used. The dose of vaccine is given by intramuscular injection or injection under the skin.

Warning *The method of giving influenza vaccine using a jet gun should no longer be used because of the risk of transmitting AIDS.*

Measles vaccine

Measles is caused by a virus that is spread by droplet infection (coughs and sneezes). One attack gives a high level of lasting immunity. Most people develop measles in childhood. Babies up to the age of 6 months have immunity passed on to them by their mothers – i.e. they are given passive immunity by their mother's antibodies.

The time from first contact to the development of the disease (incubation period) is 10 days.

Measles can be a serious illness in some children and may cause convulsions. Secondary infection with bacteria may cause an abscess in the middle ear (otitis media) and pneumonia. The disease may be complicated by inflammation and soreness of the mouth (stomatitis), gastro-enteritis, appendicitis and inflammation of the brain (encephalitis). Measles causes many deaths in tropical countries.

Active immunization against measles

Measles vaccine contains a live, weakened virus. Because it contains a live virus, it has only to be given once.

In children over 1 year of age it produces a good antibody response in 90–97 per cent, although a gradual fall will occur if the child does not come into contact with the disease; nevertheless, antibodies are present for up to 15 years after a single injection of the vaccine. Failure of a live measles vaccine to protect a child is usually due to its use before the age of 1 year, when the child's antibodies from its mother may stop the virus multiplying. This multiplication of the virus in the body following vaccination is what stimulates an effective and lasting immunity.

NOTE A combined vaccine of measles, mumps and german measles is now given at 15 months of age.

Controlling an outbreak of measles

The incubation period of measles is 10 days and it is spread by droplet infection from those who have the disease. Vaccination programmes can therefore stop the spread of the disease if all contacts are vaccinated within about 2–3 days of the first case of measles developing in a group.

Harmful effects of measles vaccine

The vaccine may produce a mild measles-like illness with a rash and fever about 1 week after the injection.

Very rarely, convulsions have been reported following measles vaccination. It is difficult (from the evidence available) to decide whether these would have happened anyway, because there is always a risk of convulsions occurring in certain children who develop a fever; nevertheless, convulsions occur much less frequently with measles vaccination than in other conditions that cause a fever.

Very rarely, inflammation of the brain (encephalitis) has been reported following measles vaccination; but the number of children affected compared with the number vaccinated is very much less than the number of unvaccinated children who develop encephalitis from an attack of measles.

A serious type of encephalitis (subacute sclerosing panencephalitis) that may follow an attack of measles and which produces mental impairment occurs very rarely in unvaccinated children (5–10 cases in every million). In vaccinated children this risk is even less – 0.5–1.0 case per million doses of vaccine.

Warnings on the use of measles vaccine

Measles vaccine contains virtually no egg protein but, nevertheless, it should not be used in patients who are severely allergic to egg protein.

Children who suffer or who have suffered in the past from convulsions or whose parents or brothers or sisters have a history of idiopathic epilepsy (see Chapter 37) should be given measles vaccine but parents should be warned about the risk of fever and how to treat it with cooling (e.g. tepid sponging) and paracetamol at the earliest sign of a fever.

Children and adults who have immune deficiency because of drug treatment (corticosteroids, certain anti-cancer drugs) or disease (e.g. AIDS, leukaemia) should not be vaccinated against measles. If they are in contact with measles they should be given passive immunization using normal immunoglobulin.

NOTE Measles vaccine (which is live) should *never* be given to pregnant women.

Administration

Measles vaccine live is given by a single intramuscular injection or injection under the skin.

Comments

The benefits of measles vaccination far outweigh any risks, particularly if the warnings listed above are followed carefully. In the USA, because of vaccination the number of reported cases of measles has dropped dramatically in recent years. Unfortunately, in the UK the take-up of measles vaccination has been disappointing. This appears to be due to two main factors – ignorance of doctors about the benefits and risks of measles vaccination and their failure to adequately advise parents; and ignorance of parents based on their often-unfounded fears of vaccination because of the massive media coverage about the risks of whooping cough vaccine (see later). Hopefully the introduction of MMR (combined mumps, measles and rubella vaccine) and its accompanying publicity will reverse these trends (see later).

All children (except those listed on p. 127) *should be vaccinated against mumps, measles and rubella* (*MMR*) *in their second year of life. A child who has not received MMR vaccine in his second year of life should be MMR vaccinated before going to nursery or primary school or a play group, irrespective of whether he/she has had a measles 'jab' or an attack of mumps, measles or german measles.*

Passive immunization

Passive immunization against measles using human normal immunoglobulin may be used to modify an attack of measles in children in whom measles vaccine should not be used.

Meningitis vaccine

Meningitis is an inflammation of the membranes covering the brain and spinal cord. It may be caused by a viral, bacterial, fungal or protozoal infection. It may also be caused by irritation of the membranes, for example by blood from a haemorrhage between the two layers of the membrane.

Viral infection is the commonest cause of meningitis, and most patients recover. Bacterial infection is less common but much more serious, and much publicity has been given to a type of bacterial meningitis, called meningococcal meningitis, caused by *Neisseria meningitidis*, which can be fatal. It is the commonest cause of bacterial meningitis in Western countries and causes serious epidemics in some parts of Africa, particularly where the climate is hot and dry and living conditions are poor and overcrowded. It spreads from person to person through the air and enters the body through the linings of the nose and throat.

The disease starts with snuffles and symptoms like a cold for 1–2 days and then a fever develops with vomiting, headache and a rash (tiny red spots which spread from the buttocks over the legs and trunk). The patient may become very ill and have fits. Sometimes the infection can present as a sudden severe illness with collapse and widespread rash, and the patient can die within a few hours of the first symptoms despite treatment. Rarely, the disease can be chronic and cause fever, sweating, rash and joint pains which go on for weeks.

The diagnosis of meningococcal meningitis is confirmed by examining the spinal fluid and culturing the infecting bacteria – *Neisseria meningitidis*. Benzylpenicillin is the antibiotic of choice for treating meningococcal meningitis, and close contacts with an infected person should be given rifampicin.*

There are three types of the bacteria (*N. meningitidis*) that cause meningococcal meningitis: type A causes outbreaks throughout the world and accounts for about 3 per cent of attacks in Great Britain; type B accounts for about 57 per cent of attacks; and type C for about 20 per cent of attacks.

A vaccine is available against types A and C (AC Vax and Mengivac A+C). It produces protection in about 5–10 days in 85–95 per cent of individuals vaccinated. Immunity lasts about 3–5 years.

A and C vaccine is useful for people travelling abroad to countries such as Ethiopia, Sudan, Kenya, Middle East, India and parts of South America where meningitis A and C are prevalent.

Warnings on the use of meningitis vaccine

It may cause redness, tenderness and hardness at the site of injection, and occasionally fever, irritability and chills for about 24–72 hours. It should not be used in people who have an acute infection (e.g. a cold), fever or allergy to the vaccine. It should be used with utmost caution in women who are pregnant or breast feeding and in people who are immune deficient (e.g. due to AIDS).

Administration

A and C vaccine is given by injection deep under the skin or into a muscle.

Mumps vaccine

Mumps, or epidemic parotitis, is an acute infectious disease caused by a virus and spread by direct contact (kissing) and by droplet infection (e.g. coughing and sneezing). The time between first contact and the appearance of the disease (the incubation period) is 17–18 days. It causes a painful enlargement of one or other or both of the parotid salivary glands in the

* Sulphadimide is an alternative (if strain is known to be sensitive).

cheeks and/or other salivary glands. Complications include inflammation of the testicles (orchitis) in males after puberty, inflammation of the pancreas, and meningitis.

Active immunization

Mumps vaccine contains live, weakened mumps virus. Because it is a live vaccine only one dose needs to be given to produce a good immune response in 95–100 per cent of people. Vaccinated people do not spread the virus. The antibody levels produced are not as good as those produced by the natural disease but they last for 14–16 years. There is only one strain of mumps virus and therefore a single infection with the natural virus or the mumps vaccine virus will produce immunity.

Harmful effects and warnings

See Table 11.1 for a statement on harmful effects and warnings on live vaccines.

Administration

Mumps vaccine is given by injection under the skin to adults and to children over 1 year of age.

Passive immunization

Passive immunization against mumps using normal immunoglobulin seems to be of very doubtful value.

Measles, mumps and rubella vaccine (MMR)

MMR vaccine (measles, mumps and rubella [german measles] vaccine) is now available and should replace measles vaccine in the *second year of life*, and later if measles vaccine has not been given.

At the age of 4–5 *years* (before starting play group, or nursery or primary school) MMR vaccine should be given to children irrespective of whether they have previously had a measles jab or have had measles, mumps or rubella. Children who *should not* need MMR vaccine at this age include those with documented records of their having been vaccinated with MMR previously and/or laboratory evidence that they have immunity (i.e. possess antibodies) against measles, mumps and rubella.

Other people who may receive MMR vaccine include children of any age on the request of their parents and adults who have been shown not to have immunity to measles, mumps and rubella.

Measles vaccine or MMR vaccine can be given to prevent measles following exposure to measles. The vaccine should be given within 72 hours of exposure. The response to MMR is too slow to be of any value in preventing mumps or rubella.

Children who should *not* receive MMR vaccine include:

- Children with an acute feverish illness (e.g. tonsillitis) when they present for vaccination; MMR vaccine should be postponed until they are well again
- Children with allergies to neomycin or kanamycin or a history of severe allergic reactions (anaphylaxis) due to any cause
- Children who have received another live vaccine by injection within 3 weeks
- Children with untreated cancer or immune deficiency due to disease (e.g. AIDS) or drugs (e.g. immunosuppressant drugs or high doses of corticosteroids) or children receiving radiation treatment (radiotherapy)

MMR vaccine should not be given to children who are severely allergic to eggs – in other words, those who have a record of developing a generalized nettle rash (urticaria), swelling of the mouth and throat, difficulty with breathing, a fall in blood pressure and shock after eating eggs or foods containing eggs.

Harmful effects of MMR vaccine

Most commonly occurring harmful effects include malaise, fever and/or a measles-like rash which lasts for 2–3 days and comes on about 1 week after injection. Occasionally, some children may get a mumps-like swelling of the glands in the cheeks (parotid glands) which appears about the third week after vaccination.

Children who develop symptoms after being vaccinated with MMR are not infectious.

Warnings on the use of MMR vaccine

Children who suffer – or have suffered – from convulsions or whose brothers or sisters have a history of idiopathic epilepsy should be given MMR vaccine but parents should be warned about the risk of fever and how to treat it with cooling (e.g. tepid sponging) and paracetamol by mouth.

All girls aged 10–14 years of age should still receive rubella vaccine until such time that there is evidence of a high uptake of the MMR vaccine.

MMR vaccine should not be given within 3 months of an injection of immunoglobulin.

MMR vaccine should not be given to a woman who is, or might be pregnant. Pregnancy should be avoided for 1 month after MMR vaccination.

Immunoglobulin should not be given at the same time as MMR vaccine because it may block the immune response to mumps and rubella.

Whooping cough (pertussis) vaccine

Whooping cough (pertussis) is a very infectious disease caused by a bacterium (*Bordetella pertussis*). It is spread by droplet infection (e.g. coughs and sneezes), and the period from first contact to the appearance of the disease (the incubation period) is 7–14 days. It can affect all ages but about 90 per cent of cases are in children under the age of 5 years. It causes sore eyes, runny nose and severe bouts of coughing which may be so severe that children vomit.

The main complications of whooping cough are pneumonia and collapse of part of a lung. Rarely, this may cause permanent damage to the affected lung, leading to bronchiectasis in which the bronchial tubes are scarred, distorted and inflamed producing a chronic cough with yellow–green phlegm. A secondary bacterial infection of the middle ear may occur (otitis media) and, very rarely, meningitis and brain damage.

During paroxysms of coughing the blood supply to the brain may be reduced, producing convulsions, and the coughing may be so severe that blood vessels in eyes burst and the rectum is pushed out through the anus (prolapsed rectum).

Newborn babies are very susceptible to whooping cough, and most deaths occur in the first year of life.

The diagnosis of whooping cough is difficult until the paroxysms of coughing start, and yet it is in the early snuffly stage that it is highly infectious. This makes it difficult to control the spread of the infection.

Active immunization

There is now convincing evidence from adequate and well controlled studies that any fall in illness and deaths from whooping cough in the very young in a particular area can be directly related to the extent of whooping cough immunization in that area.

As stated earlier, the highest risk of illness and deaths from whooping cough is in infants under 1 year of age, and unfortunately newborn babies do not appear to have any protective antibodies passed on to them by their mothers. Therefore, active immunization should start as soon as the baby is capable of making its own antibodies; this is at about 2–3 months of age. The baby should receive three injections at 8-week intervals (the third injection may be at 4–6 weeks after the second injection).

Active immunization does not confer lasting immunity against whooping cough. About 80 per cent of those vaccinated will be protected against whooping cough for about 4 years. In other words, about 20 per cent will run a risk of developing the disease. This should be compared with the fact that 90 per cent of unvaccinated babies will develop whooping cough if exposed to the infection.

There is now little doubt that the number of illnesses and deaths from whooping cough can be directly related to failure to have babies vaccinated.

Harmful effects of whooping cough vaccine

See Table 11.1 for a general statement on the harmful effects of vaccines. Whooping cough vaccination may cause redness and swelling at the site of injection, a mild fever and irritability. In the 1960s some of the vaccines that were then available resulted in persistent screaming and collapse but these episodes are now very rare with the vaccines that have been introduced since then.

The real fear of using whooping cough vaccine is that it may very rarely produce convulsions and brain damage in some babies: but this risk must be put in perspective. The risk of vaccination causing permanent brain damage is about 1 in every 100,000 vaccinations. This risk is far less than leaving these children unvaccinated. Furthermore, major developments in the production of whooping cough vaccines are making them safer every year.

Warnings on the use of whooping cough vaccine (including DPT vaccine)

See Table 11.1 general statement on warnings on the use of vaccines.

A baby should not be vaccinated if he/she has a fever and/or a cough and cold or other disorder, until fully recovered.

The course of injections must be discontinued if the baby develops *any* severe local or general reaction or sign of nerve or brain irritation to the preceeding injection. Severe *local* reactions include the development of a large red, hard area in the skin, spreading out from the site of injection. Severe *general* reactions include a high fever within 2 days of the injection; a severe allergic reaction (collapse, wheezing and difficulty in breathing), convulsion, prolonged unresponsiveness and prolonged uncontrollable screaming coming on within 72 hours of the injection.

Take a child specialist's advice on whether to vaccinate:

- A baby who suffers from or has had fits or convulsions or who has suffered from any sort of brain damage or brain infection at or just after childbirth
- A baby whose parents, brothers or sisters suffer from idiopathic epilepsy (Chapter 37) because there is a risk of the baby's developing epilepsy regardless of whether he has been vaccinated or not
- A baby whose physical or mental development is delayed, which appears to be due to some abnormality in the brain

NOTE In the babies mentioned above the risk of the disease may be greater than risks associated with vaccination; the medical advisers and parents must take a joint decision based on the individual baby's needs.

Spina bifida, cerebral palsy or other stable nerve disorder is *not* a reason for not having a child vaccinated against whooping cough. Nor is a history of allergy in the child or his family (e.g. hayfever, eczema, asthma).

Administration

Pertussis vaccine (killed bacteria) is given by three injections into a muscle or deep under the skin, at monthly intervals.

Combined vaccine The common practice is to use a combined vaccine of *adsorbed diphtheria, tetanus and whooping cough* (*pertussis*). DTPer/Vac/Ads (see earlier).

Pneumococcal vaccine

Pneumococcal pneumonia is an infection of the lungs caused by bacteria (*Streptococcus pneumoniae*). The disease occurs at all ages but people at particular risk include those who have had their spleen removed or whose spleen is damaged through a disorder such as sickle-cell anaemia (Chapter 47) and elderly debilitated people who suffer from heart, lung, liver or kidney disease or diabetes.

A pneumococcal vaccine which contains products from the surface of the bacteria (capsular antigens) is available and this provides protection from infection for up to 5 years. It should be given to anyone at particular risk and anyone over 65 years of age.

Harmful effects of pneumococcal vaccine

See Table 11.1 statement and harmful effects of vaccines. Redness, soreness and hardness may develop at the site of injection. Fever, rash, painful joints and, rarely, nerve damage and severe allergic reactions may occur.

Warnings on the use of pneumococcal vaccine

Pneumococcal vaccine should not be given to people who have an active infection and/or fever, or to individuals on immunosuppressive drugs, who have Hodgkin's disease or who have had treatment with anti-cancer drugs and/or radiotherapy.

It should be used with great caution in people with severe heart or lung disease or in anyone who has had pneumonia in the previous 3 years, or with an active and/or feverish chest infection.

No patient should be re-vaccinated, because of the risk of allergic reactions.

It should not be used in pregnant women or in children under 2 years of age.

Administration

Pneumovax contains polysaccharides from the capsules of 23 types of pneumococcus which causes 90 per cent of all pneumococcal infections. It is given by intramuscular injection or injection under the skin.

Poliomyelitis vaccine

There are three types of poliovirus, and they occur throughout the world. Poliomyelitis is a virus infection that causes fever, meningitis (inflammation in the spinal cord and brain) and paralysis. Paralysis from an attack of poliomyelitis is more frequent with advancing age. Adults and adolescents are ten times more likely to develop paralysis than are children.

Humans carry the virus, and it is principally spread from person to person by hand-to-mouth contact. It may also be spread by droplet infection (coughs and sneezes) and possibly by insects. It enters the blood from the nose, throat and intestine and then invades the nervous system.

There are two types of poliomyelitis vaccine (against types 1, 2 and 3) – live vaccine to be given by mouth, and inactivated vaccine to be given by injection. The former is the most frequently used.

Harmful effects of poliomyelitis vaccine

See Table 11.1 for a general statement on the harmful effects of vaccine.

Harmful effects are rare with the live polio vaccine by mouth. Very rarely, diarrhoea, skin rashes and allergic reactions may develop. Poliomyelitis caused by the vaccine has been reported but it is estimated to occur only in 1 out of every 5 million persons vaccinated. The risk of a contact picking up polio from a vaccinated person is about the same.

The inactivated virus vaccine by injection may rarely cause redness and swelling at the site of injection, and has been suspected of, very occasionally, causing convulsions and brain damage.

Warnings on the use of poliomyelitis vaccine

See Table 11.1 for general warnings on the use of vaccines.

Live polio vaccine by mouth: should *not* be used:

- For infants or adults with a fever and/or acute illness
- For infants or adults who have diarrhoea or a disorder of the stomach or intestine which may affect absorption of the vaccine
- For infants or adults who have an immune deficiency because of drug treatment (e.g. corticosteroids, anti-cancer drugs, radiation) or because of disease (e.g. AIDS, leukaemia)
- In the first 3 months of pregnancy
- Within 1 month of any other live vaccine

The faeces from a vaccinated baby contain polioviruses so those who change the nappies should be hygienic and wash their hands afterwards.*

Administration

Poliomyelitis live vaccine by mouth is given in three separate doses, usually at the same time as routine vaccination against diphtheria, tetanus and whooping cough. A booster dose should be given at the same time as a booster diphtheria and tetanus vaccination at school entry, and a booster polio by mouth and a booster tetanus injection should be given on leaving school at 16–18 years of age.

Travellers who are visiting regions other than Europe, North America, Australia or New Zealand should be given a full course of vaccine if they have never been vaccinated against polio. Those who have been previously vaccinated should be given a booster dose if it is 10 years or more since their last dose of polio vaccine.

The inactivated vaccine is given by deep injection made under the skin or by intramuscular injection. A course of three injections is given at monthly intervals with a booster when required. This should be given to people in whom the live oral vaccine should not be used – for example, in pregnancy and people who are immune deficient.

* The virus may become more virulent as it passes through the intestine and may, very rarely, cause paralysis in a household contact, e.g. grandparents who have never been vaccinated. Any contact without a history of immunization against polio should be immunized.

Rabies vaccine

Rabies is an acute viral disease of warm-blooded animals (particularly foxes, wolves and bats) which may incidentally affect humans, almost always as a result of a bite by a rabid animal. Dogs are also infected through contact with other infected animals. The virus spreads through the saliva of the infected animal. The time from the bite to the appearance of the disease may be 2–6 weeks or longer. Only a small proportion of people who are bitten by a rabid animal develop the disease, but once it develops they will invariably die. The patient develops fever, anxiety, fear of water (hydrophobia), spasms, delusions, hallucinations and paralysis.

Prevention

People at high risk of catching rabies should be vaccinated – for example, those working in quarantine stations.

Merieux Inactivated Rabies Vaccine produces a good immune response and is given as an initial course of two injections (1 month apart) and then a booster dose 6–12 months later. To maintain a good antibody level, a booster dose should then be given every 3 years if the risk of infection continues.

Treatment following exposure

The first injection of vaccine should be given as soon as possible after the exposure (an animal bite) and followed by five further doses on days 3, 7, 14 and 30 and 90. The treatment schedule can be stopped if the animal is subsequently found not to be infected with rabies.

Protection of staff in contact with a patient suffering from rabies may be provided by four injections under the skin of Merieux Inactivated Rabies Vaccine. The injections are given on the same day at different sites on the body.

Harmful effects of rabies vaccine

See Table 11.1 for general statements on harmful effects of vaccines. Redness, swelling and tenderness may occur at the injection site during the first 48 hours. Fever may develop, and there is a risk of allergic reactions in people who suffer from allergies.

Passive immunization against rabies

Anti-rabies serum is obtained from the blood of healthy animals (usually a horse) that have been immunized against rabies. See Table 11.1 for the dangers of antisera. It should no longer be used and has been replaced by anti-rabies immunoglobulin injection. It is given at the same time as the first injection of rabies vaccine.

Rubella

See 'German measles'.

Smallpox vaccine

Smallpox vaccination is no longer required in the UK and other countries because the disease has been eradicated world wide. Travellers no longer need certificates to prove that they have been vaccinated.

Tetanus vaccine

Tetanus is caused by the bacterium *Clostridium tetani*, which lives in the intestines of humans and animals and in the soil. Spores from the micro-organism infect the ground and can enter the body through a wound. This happens most often in farmers and gardeners. It can occur in newborn babies if they are delivered in dirty surroundings and the stump of the umbilical cord gets infected.

If the spores enter a deep wound where there is a poor supply of oxygen, they germinate and the bacteria start to multiply, to produce a dangerous toxin which enters the nervous system and causes muscle spasms, rigidity, convulsions and death.

Preventing tetanus

The safest treatment for tetanus is to prevent it, and this is achieved by using tetanus vaccine. All children should have a course of tetanus vaccination, and this is usually included along with diphtheria and whooping cough vaccine (triple vaccine). This provides protection for 5–10 years.

Active immunization is also important in adolescents and adults who have never had, or who have failed to complete, a full course of tetanus vaccine. Very rarely, tetanus has occurred in patients following surgery on the bowel. Patients awaiting abdominal surgery should therefore check whether they have been immunized against tetanus; if not, they should have a course of tetanus immunization before the operation.

Administration

Tetanus vaccine and tetanus toxoid are prepared from tetanus toxin produced by bacteria grown on a culture medium. The toxin is converted to formol toxoid by adding formaldehyde (see earlier).

Adsorbed tetanus vaccine is formol toxoid precipitated on to a mineral (e.g. aluminium hydroxide, aluminium phosphate or calcium phosphate). It is the vaccine of choice because it is more effective at stimulating antibody production. A high degree of protection is provided for up to 5 years after an initial course of three injections (see later).

In children the triple vaccine (DTP: diphtheria, tetanus and pertussis [whooping cough]) gives protection against tetanus in childhood and provides a basic immunity that can be reinforced (boosted) at school entry, on leaving school, in adulthood and if there is a risk of tetanus following an injury.

Adults should be given a tetanus booster every 10 years (e.g. every decade birthday, 30, 40, 50, etc.). This should be continued into old age because half the deaths from tetanus (about 30–50 a year in the UK) occur in those over 65 years (who usually have injured themselves while gardening).

A full course of vaccine should be given to anyone who has never had a complete course of vaccine and then boosted every 10 years. When an individual is injured and has not had a booster for more than 5 years he should be re-vaccinated, particularly if the wound is dirty.

The adsorbed tetanus vaccine (Tet/Vac/Ads) is given by intramuscular injection or deep injection under the skin. For a full course, three doses should be given, with about 6–8 weeks between the first and second doses and 16–28 weeks between the second and third doses.

NOTE It is best not to have a tetanus vaccine booster too frequently (not less than every 5 years) in order to avoid the risk of allergic reactions occurring.

Passive immunization

Wounds that might be contaminated with tetanus-producing bacteria are carefully cleared of dead tissue and debris and the patient is given passive immunization using anti-tetanus immunoglobulin by intramuscular injection.

Passive immunization is usually routine in people who have not been vaccinated against tetanus. In addition, they should be started off on a course of tetanus vaccination, which will not help them at the time but it will in the future.

Until recently, human immunoglobulin was not available and patients were given anti-tetanus serum (ATS or tetanus antitoxin). This was obtained from healthy horses that had been immunized against tetanus toxin or toxoid. Because it contained horse protein it caused many serious allergic reactions and, sometimes, deaths. In fact, in the UK there were often more sickness and deaths from the use of the antitoxin than from tetanus. The risks of antisera are discussed in Table 11.1. Tetanus antiserum should no longer be used.

Typhoid vaccine

Salmonella infections

A group of bacteria called salmonella cause a number of different disorders in humans (e.g. typhoid and paratyphoid fevers, and gastro-enteritis). There are more than 1,500 different types of salmonella and most of them come from animals, especially poultry. They are transmitted directly to humans from the animals or in food prepared from the animals. There is one exception and that is *Salmonella typhi*, which is usually transmitted from human to human.

Typhoid and paratyphoid fever

The bacteria that cause typhoid and paratyphoid fever are transmitted from human faeces by infected persons who do not wash their hands properly after going to the lavatory and then handle food, and through human faeces contaminating drinking water, food or milk. Occasionally, shellfish can be infected from sewage-infected waters.

In some people the bacteria may live in the gall bladder for months or even years after an attack and keep infecting the faeces. These people are called 'carriers' because, although they have no symptoms of the disease, they still spread it in their faeces.

Prevention

The best prevention against typhoid and paratyphoid fever is good hygiene. If you go to a country where typhoid or paratyphoid is prevalent, do not drink the tap water (use bottled water or water that has been boiled or that has been treated with sterilizing tablets), do not eat salads and uncooked vegetables, eat fruits that can be peeled, avoid under-cooked or uncooked meats and fish, and be cautious about creams and ice creams.

Typhoid vaccine containing killed typhoid bacteria provides adequate protection in about 70 per cent of those vaccinated. The immunity lasts for about 2 years. For primary immunization of adults two doses are given by intramuscular injection or injection under the skin at an interval of 4–6 weeks. The second dose may be smaller, and given into the skin (intradermally). Booster doses may be given every 3 years.

Harmful effects of typhoid vaccine

See Table 11.1 for statements on the harmful effects of vaccines. Harmful effects are worse in people over about 35 years of age and are less marked if the vaccine is given into the skin (intradermally). Tenderness, pain and swelling at the injection site may develop in 2–3 hours, and fever, malaise and headache may occur and last for about 2 days. If severe reactions are experienced after the first injection, subsequent injections are given into the skin (intradermally) and not under the skin (subcutaneously).

Warnings on the use of typhoid vaccine

See Table 11.1 for warnings on the use of vaccines. Typhoid vaccine should not be used in patients with acute or chronic illness or in children under 1 year of age.

Typhus vaccine

Epidemics of typhus fever may be louse-borne, flea-borne, tick-borne or mite-borne. Typhus vaccine contains killed organisms (*rickettsiae*) and is used against louse-borne typhus. It does not provide complete resistance but lessens the severity of the disease. Two doses of vaccine should be given at an interval of 7–10 days, with a booster several months later and then every year. It does not protect against scrub typhus (mite-borne typhus). This vaccine is no longer available in the UK or the USA but can be obtained in Australia.

Yellow fever vaccine

The virus that causes yellow fever is transmitted to monkeys and to humans by the bite of a mosquito infected from biting an infected monkey or human. The virus infection causes fever and vomiting, affects the brain and kidneys, and causes liver damage, producing jaundice (yellowness of the skin and eyes) and bleeding from the gums, nose, stomach, intestine and bladder.

Yellow fever vaccine containing a live, weakened strain of the virus stimulates immunity within 10 days and provides protection for 10 years. A booster injection (after 10 years) provides further protection for another 10 years.

An international certificate of vaccination against yellow fever is valid only if the vaccine used is approved by the World Health Organization (WHO) and administered by designated vaccination centres.

Vaccination should be repeated every 10 years.

Harmful effects on yellow fever vaccines

See Table 11.1 for harmful effects of vaccines. Allergic reactions may occur in people allergic to egg protein because it is grown on chick embryo. Inflammation of the brain (encephalitis) may very rarely occur, especially in children under 9 months of age.

Warnings on the use of yellow fever vaccines

See Table 11.1 for warnings on the use of vaccines. Yellow fever vaccine should not be used in people allergic to egg protein, in infants under the age of 9 months (unless there is a serious risk of infection), in pregnancy, or in people who are immune deficient whether due to drugs or to disease (e.g. AIDS).

Passive immunization products

Passive immunity involves the injection of antibodies (immunoglobulins) that have been produced in another human being or in an animal. Immunoglobulins from animals (antisera) may cause serious allergic reactions to animal protein (see Table 11.2) and are now seldom used. Their place has been taken by human immunoglobulins.

Human immunoglobulins

Human immunoglobulins are proteins in the blood which function as antibodies against infections. The group also includes gammaglobulins, which are structurally related to immunoglobulins and also function as antibodies. Six distinct types of immunoglobulins (antibodies) are known (see Chapter 9).

Two types of human immunoglobulins are used – normal immunoglobulins and specific immunoglobulins.

Normal immunoglobulin

Normal immunoglobulin contains the antibodies *normally* present in adult humans. It is obtained from plasma and serum of healthy humans or from the blood from the placentas of healthy women just after childbirth. It is prepared from 'pooled' material from no fewer than 1,000 donors and treated in such a way as not to be capable of transmitting any infection. It is concentrated to give an antibody effect of ten times the original pooled material. No antibiotics are used to prevent contamination but preservatives may be added to the final product. It is available in a liquid form or a freeze-dried form for reconstitution. It is given by intramuscular injection to provide passive immunity against hepatitis, measles and german measles.

Special preparations of normal immunoglobulin are available for intravenous use as replacement treatment for patients who are not able to make their own.

Harmful effects Allergic reactions may, rarely, develop to human immunoglobulin. Pain and tenderness at the site of injection may occur.

Warnings *Live virus vaccines should not be given within 3 months of a normal immunoglobulin injection. If a live vaccine has been given, an injection of normal immunoglobulin should not be given within a 3-week period.*

Hepatitis A (See Chapter 83) Normal immunoglobulin* provides protection for 3 months for travellers into areas where hepatitis A is prevalent and for contacts of the disease in closed communities (e.g. boarding schools). Good hygiene is the best method of control. The immunoglobulin should be given every 4–6 months to visitors in highly infected areas.

Anti-hepatitis B virus immunoglobulin (HBIG) is available to provide immediate protection to people who have accidently become contaminated with the hepatitis B virus (e.g. laboratory staff handling infected blood who prick themselves) and newborn babies whose mothers become infected during pregnancy.

Measles Normal immunoglobulin may be used to modify or prevent an attack of measles in special-risk babies and/or in whom measles vaccination could be harmful.

Rubella (german measles) Normal immunoglobulin may decrease the risk of developing german measles in a pregnant woman who has been exposed to it. It is given in two doses separated by 2 or 3 days.

Specific immunoglobulins

Specific immunoglobulins (antibodies) are prepared by pooling blood from

* Normal immunoglobulin may be used to prevent Hepatitis A in immune deficient individuals and in people who have suffered severe burns.

patients who have just recovered from a particular disease or by collecting and pooling blood from blood donors who have recently had a booster injection against the disease.

Anti-rabies immunoglobulin should be injected immediately around the site of a bite from a rabid animal and also intramuscularly; at the same time a course of rabies vaccine should be started.

Anti-tetanus immunoglobulin should be used in people never previously immunized against tetanus and who have developed a wound that is dirty; is due to a puncture or penetrating injury; has much dead tissue in it; and/ or if more than 6 hours has passed since the wound was caused and no cleaning has been carried out. At the same time, the first injection of a course of adsorbed tetanus vaccine should be given as well as an antibiotic.

Other specific immunoglobulins include *anti-varicella-zoster immunoglobulin* (ZIG) against chickenpox and shingles and an *anti-herpes simplex immunoglobulin.*

Anti-D (rhesus) immunoglobulin is used to prevent a rhesus-negative mother forming antibodies to rhesus-positive red blood cells from her baby. This may happen when red blood cells from the baby enters the mother's bloodstream during childbirth or during an abortion. The anti-D immunoglobulin should be injected within 72 hours of delivery or abortion. The injected antibodies will destroy the baby's red blood cells in the mother's blood and make it unnecessary for her own immune system to start producing its own antibodies against the baby's red blood cells, which would then be stored in the 'memories' of certain of her white blood cells to cause problems if she were to become pregnant again with a baby who was rhesus positive. Her antibodies would then enter the baby's bloodstream and start destroying its red blood cells (see Chapter 26).

Table 11.1 Vaccines – harmful effects and warnings

Harmful effects Some vaccines may cause pain, swelling and inflammation at the site of injection. Local lymph glands may swell up (e.g. an injection in the forearm may produce swollen glands in the armpit). Very rarely, the site of injection of a vaccine may become hardened and an abscess may develop, particularly with vaccines containing alum and injected *under* the skin.

The injection of some vaccines may be followed by fever, headache and malaise starting a few hours after the injection and lasting for about 1 or 2 days.

Vaccines made from viruses grown on eggs may cause allergic reactions in people allergic to eggs.

Some vaccines may cause a very mild form of the disease (e.g. measles, german measles).

Very rarely, a serious infection has followed the use of a vaccine that

Table 11.1 Vaccines – harmful effects and warnings (*cont.*)

contained an inadequately weakened organism. Neuritis near the site of injection may, rarely, develop about 7–10 days after an injection of vaccine.

For other harmful effects, see the entry on each type of vaccine.

Warnings No one should be given a vaccine until careful enquiries have been made as to any previous allergic or other reactions to that or other vaccines and of other allergies such as hayfever, eczema and asthma.

Adequate resuscitation equipment should always be available in case an acute allergic emergency develops (anaphylactic shock).

Some vaccines contain small amounts of antibiotics and these should not be given to people allergic to those antibiotics.

Live vaccine should not be given to people with any immune deficiency, whether due to drug (e.g. corticosteroids, anti-cancer drugs, immunosuppressive drugs), radiotherapy or disease (e.g. AIDS or leukaemia). Live vaccine should not be used in people with a fever and/or an acute illness.

AIDS and vaccination

People with AIDS suffer from *immune deficiency* and are prone to infection from bacteria, viruses and fungi. Therefore vaccinations must be used with utmost caution.

HIV-positive people, whether they have AIDS or not, may receive the following vaccines.

Live vaccines

Measles vaccine If they are exposed to measles, they should receive normal immunoglobulin to protect them
Mumps vaccine
German measles vaccine (rubella)
MMR vaccine (mumps, measles and rubella)
Polio vaccine

NOTE The virus may be excreted in the faeces for longer periods than normal and therefore contacts should be most careful about washing their hands after contact with soiled nappies and linen. HIV-positive contacts are at a greater risk of infection from the polio vaccine than are non-HIV-positive contacts.

Inactivated vaccines

Cholera
Diphtheria

Hepatitis B
Whooping cough (pertussis)
Polio – see warnings, above, for live vaccine
Tetanus
Typhoid

HIV-positive individuals should *not* receive BCG or yellow fever vaccine.

Table 11.2 Antisera – harmful effects and warnings

Harmful effects Allergic reactions are liable to occur after the injection of any antiserum obtained from an animal. Severe allergic reactions (anaphylaxis) may occur, and full facilities for resuscitation should be immediately available. *Serum sickness* may occur 7–10 days after an injection of serum from an animal. It includes fever, vomiting, diarrhoea, wheezing, nettle rash, painful joints and muscles, and (rarely) inflammation of the kidneys, heart, nerves and/or eyes.

Warnings Before the injection of any antiserum from an animal, a careful history must be taken of any previous injections of antisera and any history of allergies (e.g. hayfever, eczema, asthma). If there is no history of allergies and/or the patient has never had an antiserum injection before, the injection may be given into a muscle. However, if there is any history of allergies and/or a previous reaction to an antiserum and/or history of a previous injection of an antiserum, or if there is any doubt at all, a *test dose* of the antiserum should be given. This consists of an injection of the antiserum under the skin. If no general reaction develops within 30 minutes the main dose can be given into a muscle.

After any antiserum injection the person should be kept under close observation for 30 minutes and an injection of adrenaline kept at the ready.

In all urgent cases, injection into a vein will be necessary but this should never be given unless an intramuscular injection has been given and no reaction has occurred over the subsequent 30 minutes.

For intravenous use, the antiserum should be at room temperature, the injection should be given slowly, and the person must remain lying down and under observation for at least 1 hour after the injection.

12

Asthma

Attacks of reversible wheezing caused by a narrowing of the bronchial tubes in the lungs are called asthma. It is usually associated with bouts of coughing, shortness of breath and tightness in the chest. The narrowing, which affects both large and small bronchial tubes (bronchi and bronchioles) is triggered by allergy, emotion or an infection, or by inhaling some irritant such as dust or a chemical. It can also be triggered by exercise or cold air.

In an asthmatic attack the linings of the airways are inflamed and over-react. This produces a release of chemicals which cause the muscles of the bronchi to contract so that it is difficult for the person to breathe, and he starts to wheeze. These chemicals also cause the lining of the airways to swell and produce sticky secretions. These secretions make the airways more narrow and they can actually block some of the smaller airways, making it even more difficult for the person to breathe.

The contraction of the muscles in the bronchial tubes (the bronchi) is referred to as 'bronchospasm'. It produces wheezing on breathing out, which is so characteristic of asthma.

Asthma in most people starts either in childhood or in middle age. *Early-onset asthma* is usually an allergic asthma and is often associated with eczema and hayfever and a family history of allergies. Common allergens are house mites in house dust, pollens, animal danders, feathers, moulds and wool. *Late-onset asthma* generally occurs in people who for some reason have a predisposition to develop asthma. They may or may not have a history of allergy (e.g. hayfever) but they may develop asthma following a bronchial infection after, for example, an attack of influenza. Attacks usually start between 35 and 45 years of age and about 10–15 per cent of patients are sensitive to aspirin.

Early-onset asthma (allergic asthma) is sometimes called 'extrinsic' asthma (caused by some 'factor' that is taken into the body), and late-onset asthma may be called 'intrinsic' asthma (caused by some predisposing factor within the body). However, it is probable that allergy is an important factor in both types.

Exercise-induced asthma usually occurs in children and young adults; it may or may not be associated with other types of asthma.

Bronchitis, bronchiectasis and emphysema

Narrowing of the bronchial tubes producing wheezing may also occur in long-standing chest disorders such as *bronchitis* which is an inflammation of the lining of the bronchial tubes. Bronchitis may be acute due to an acute chest infection or it may be chronic due to repeated attacks of acute bronchitis. Chronic bronchitis may be associated with scarring of the bronchial tubes (*fibrosis*) or with *bronchiectasis* in which the bronchial tubes become scarred, distorted and narrowed by repeated infections which make the glands in their linings overwork. They may increase in size and produce excess amounts of secretion which causes the patient to cough up large amounts of phlegm.

Bronchitis may also be associated with *emphysema* in which the lung tissue loses its natural elasticity. The bronchial tubes become stiffened and there is no natural 'give' when the patient breathes out. This makes it additionally difficult for the patient to breathe.

Chronic obstructive airways disease

Chronic bronchitis and emphysema frequently coexist, and each produces obstruction to the flow of air through the air passages. In chronic bronchitis this obstruction is caused mainly by swelling of the linings of the bronchial tubes and by thick, sticky phlegm blocking the tubes. In emphysema the obstruction to the flow of air is not inside the bronchial tubes but is caused by pressure on the bronchial tubes from outside. This pressure is caused by the lung tissue being over-distended with air which becomes trapped when the patient breathes out. Any chest infection will make these conditions worse. Chronic bronchitis and emphysema are often grouped together under the heading 'chronic obstructive airways disease' (COAD).

Peak flow meters

Peak flow meters measure the peak flow of air breathed out by an individual and are used to indicate the degree of obstruction to the airways. These machines are very useful in assessing the effectiveness of treatment and for monitoring the progress of the disease. All patients receiving treatment for asthma or other wheezing disorders should possess one and monitor their own progress. If there is any deterioration to their peak flow they should seek medical advice.

Drugs may trigger an attack of asthma

Examples of drugs that may trigger an attack of asthma in someone prone to develop asthma include:

Some anti-rheumatic drugs
Anti-psychotic drugs
Aspirin and related drugs
Beta blocker drugs
MAOI anti-depressant drugs
Nitrofurantoin
Oral contraceptives
Some antibiotics (e.g. erythromycin, penicillin)
Some anti-blood-pressure drugs (e.g. hydralazine, reserpine)
Some pain relievers (e.g. paracetamol, dextropropoxyphene, pentazocine)

Drugs used to treat asthma

Drugs that relieve wheezing – bronchodilators

It will help you to understand bronchodilators if you read the chapter on the autonomic nervous system (Chapter 2) before reading this section.

In Chapter 2 I explain that the autonomic nervous system (self-governing nervous system) controls all kinds of involuntary activities in the body from breathing to sexual responses and from sweating to digestion. It consists of two divisions – the sympathetic and the parasympathetic divisions. These divisions actually oppose each other but a careful balance is maintained by special centres in the brain. Noradrenaline is the chemical messenger used in the sympathetic system and acetylcholine is the chemical messenger used in the parasympathetic system.

Anticholinergic drugs

With regard to breathing, stimulation of the parasympathetic nerves produces constriction of the bronchial tubes and an increase in secretions by the glands in the lining surfaces. A group of drugs are available which block these effects – they are called anticholinergic drugs because they block the effects of the nerve transmitter, acetylcholine, of the parasympathetic nervous system. They all resemble belladonna which is a chemical from the plant deadly nightshade. By blocking the parasympathetic nerves, anticholinergic drugs relieve the constriction of the bronchial tubes and dry up the airways.

Dangers of taking anticholinergic drugs by mouth

Although widely used in the past and still available in herbal remedies, anticholinergic drugs by mouth are not recommended in the treatment of asthma and other wheezing disorders, because in the dose required to relieve wheezing they produce unacceptable harmful effects on other parts of the body – dry mouth, flushing, dry skin, palpitations, difficulty in passing urine, constipation and confusion. They also dry up the surfaces of the bronchial tubes and make the phlegm more sticky, which makes it much more difficult for the patient to cough it up.

Ipratropium – an anticholinergic drug taken by inhalation

When taken by inhalation a drug can be targeted straight to the site of action in the bronchial tubes and therefore a much smaller and safer dose can be used. Given in this way, an anticholinergic drug such as ipratropium is of use in relieving bronchospasm without drying up the bronchial secretions too much. It is also safer because it is more selective in its actions than other anticholinergics.

Ipratropium is the fashionable anticholinergic drug for inhalation at present. It is used in an inhaler or in a special inhalation solution (nebulizer solution), particularly to treat bronchospasm associated with chronic bronchitis.

Harmful effects and warnings on the use of ipratropium by inhalation Accidental release of the drug into the eyes will cause the pupils to dilate and the pressure in the front chamber of the eye to increase. This may trigger an attack of glaucoma in a susceptible person (see Chapter 35). Ipratropium inhalers should therefore be used with caution in people who suffer from glaucoma and in anyone likely to develop it. In elderly people, because some of the drug is always absorbed into the bloodstream, over-use of these inhalers may produce harmful effects; for example, constipation and dry mouth, and in elderly men with enlarged prostate glands it may cause difficulty in passing urine. Harmful effects and warnings on the use of anticholinergic drugs are listed in Table 2.2.

Warnings *You should always consult your doctor if you find that you are getting a reduced response to the drug. You should understand the dangers of accidental release into the eyes (see above), and if this happens consult your doctor straight away. Make sure that you are absolutely sure how to use the inhaler properly (ask your pharmacist to explain and to provide you with an instruction leaflet).*

Ipratropium should not be used in people known to be allergic to an anticholinergic drug such as atropine. It should be used with caution in patients who suffer from glaucoma or an enlarged prostate gland.

Preparations of ipratropium Ipratropium inhalation works in about 30–60 minutes and the effects last long enough to allow a dose of one to four puffs to be taken three to four times daily. Inhalers that deliver a fixed dose with each puff are available. They are referred to as metered dose inhalers, and include Atrovent and Atrovent Forte. An Atrovent nebulizer solution is also available for use in a nebulizer (see later). (U)

Adrenoreceptor stimulants (beta stimulants)

Stimulation of the sympathetic nervous system produces the release of noradrenaline at nerve endings, which acts on adrenaline receptors (adrenoreceptors) throughout the body. The effect of this stimulation of adrenoreceptors in the bronchial tubes is to dilate them and reduce the release of inflammation-producing chemicals by certain of the bronchial cells (mast cells). These actions are very beneficial to patients suffering from wheezing due to asthma, bronchitis or other wheezing disorders.

Drugs that stimulate adrenoreceptors (adrenoreceptor stimulants) to produce adrenaline-like effects on the body may act directly on adrenaline receptors at nerve endings (e.g. isoprenaline); indirectly, by stimulating the release of noradrenaline from its stores at nerve endings (e.g. amphetamines); or by both actions (e.g. ephedrine).

Improving the benefits and reducing the risks of adrenoreceptor stimulants

Briefly, adrenaline receptors are classified into alpha and beta-1 and beta-2 receptors. Stimulation of alpha receptors causes constriction of arteries in the skin and intestines, a rise in blood pressure and dilatation of the pupils. Beta-1 receptors are located principally in the heart, and stimulation produces an increase in heart rate and an increase in the output of blood from the heart. Stimulation of beta-2 receptors produces relaxation of bronchial muscles, relaxation of the womb and dilatation of arteries in muscles.

From this description, it is evident that unless an adrenoreceptor-stimulant drug is very selective in its actions on the airways (i.e. selective for beta-2 receptors) it will produce unwanted effects on the heart and circulation, causing a rise in blood pressure and heart rate. Non-selective adrenoreceptor stimulants which were widely used in the past and which are still available include adrenaline, ephedrine and isoprenaline. *Except for the use of adrenaline in emergencies, these drugs should no longer be used to treat asthma and other wheezing disorders whether by mouth or inhaler.*

You should use only a selective adrenoreceptor stimulant (beta-2 selective agonists). These preparations are listed in Table 12.2.

The safest way of taking adrenoreceptor stimulants is by inhalation. This allows a very much smaller dose of the drug to be targeted on to the bronchial tubes to produce its beneficial effects and reduces the amount of drug absorbed into the bloodstream to produce harmful effects elsewhere. Even so there are still dangers, particularly with the non-selective adrenoreceptor stimulants such as adrenaline, ephedrine and isoprenaline. Because selective adrenoreceptor stimulants by inhaler have reduced harmful effects on the heart and circulation they are safer to use in people suffering from heart disease or raised blood pressure.

Harmful effects of adrenoreceptor stimulants The harmful effects of non-selective adrenoreceptor stimulants affect principally the heart and circulation, producing rapid beating of the heart, disorders of heart rate and rhythm, and coldness of the hands and feet. These effects may be harmful to patients suffering from heart disease and/or raised blood pressure and they may cause problems in elderly people. They may also produce tremor, anxiety and nervousness. These harmful effects are less when a beta-2 selective adrenoreceptor stimulant such as salbutamol is used.

Warning *Adrenoreceptor stimulants (whether selective or not) may stimulate the heart, produce a fall in blood potassium levels and cause a heart attack. Fenoterol is particularly dangerous in these respects.*

Dangers of over-using inhalers containing adrenoreceptor stimulants One risk of using these inhalers is that if no relief is obtained from one inhalation, the individual may keep repeating the dose. This may result in overdosing and the risk of harmful effects on the heart and circulation.

An additional risk is that the individual may delay seeking medical advice. It is important to remember that relief of wheezing is not the whole treatment, and people who develop a flare-up will need an anti-inflammatory drug (e.g. a corticosteroid) as a matter of *urgency* (see later).

Use of selective adrenoreceptor stimulants to treat asthma Selective adrenoreceptor stimulants by inhalation (see Table 12.2) are the safest drug preparations to use. There is little difference between the various preparations that are available. The dose and frequency of dosage may be reduced if these inhalers are used along with other drug treatments (e.g. corticosteroid inhalations and sodium cromoglycate inhalations and/or theophylline by mouth).

They relieve wheezing but do not affect the underlying inflammation which needs suppressing by using anti-inflammatory drugs (e.g. corticosteroids), see later. If you are using a stimulant to relieve your wheezing, then you should measure your peak flow before and after using your inhaler in order to check whether it is working. It will also check whether you are using your inhaler effectively.

Selective adrenoreceptor stimulants by inhalation work quickly and provide relief for up to 6 hours. Slow-release preparations by mouth may be helpful at night in some patients (see later). Salbutamol or terbutaline may be given by injection into a vein, or occasionally under the skin, to treat an acute, severe attack of asthma (see later). Selective adrenoreceptor stimulants by inhalation are also beneficial in relieving and preventing wheezing that comes on with exercise.

Harmful effects of selective adrenoreceptor stimulants Selective adrenoreceptor stimulants by mouth or by injection may cause muscle tremor, particularly affecting the hands, and (rarely) tension. In high doses they may cause flushing, rapid beating of the heart and headache. They may lower blood potassium (see dangers, page 690).

Warnings *They should not be used by patients allergic to particular preparations. They should be used with caution in patients with over-active thyroid glands, coronary artery disease (e.g. angina), raised blood pressure and diabetes (blood sugar level should be measured because it may be increased by these drugs).*

Harmful effects of selective adrenoreceptor stimulants by inhaler are less frequent and less severe than if taken by mouth or injection, unless they are over-used (see Table 12.1).

Theophylline

Theophylline belongs to a group of drugs called xanthines. They are obtained from plants and include three main drugs – caffeine, theophylline and theobromine. They are similar in their actions and effects but vary in their potency. Caffeine and theophylline are present in tea; coffee contains caffeine and cocoa contains caffeine and theobromine. Cola drinks also contain caffeine (see Chapter 42).

Theobromine was widely used in the past, often combined with phenobarbitone to treat symptoms produced by disorders of the heart and circulation. It is now no longer used. Theophylline is still used to treat asthma because it is very effective at relieving wheezing if it is used properly.

Theophylline relaxes the bronchial muscles and relieves wheezing by blocking the actions of an enzyme that breaks down a chemical (cyclic-AMP) responsible for causing relaxation of the circular muscles in the bronchial tubes; its dilating effect on the bronchi is thus prolonged.

Preparations of theophylline

There were many problems with theophylline in the past – they irritated the lining of the stomach, produced nausea and vomiting and they were rapidly absorbed from the intestine into the bloodstream and then excreted. Although theophylline preparations provided prompt relief from an attack it was always difficult to get a steady effect from the drug throughout the day and night. Fortunately, preparations now available produce less irritation of the stomach, less nausea and vomiting, and slowly release the drug in the intestine over several hours. These are called sustained-release preparations. These sustained-release preparations of theophylline have greatly improved the effectiveness of theophylline treatment because they can provide a steady effective level of the drug in the blood for up to 12 hours and, taken every 12 hours, they provide relief throughout the day and night.

Aminophylline is a compound of theophylline and ethylenediamine that splits in the body to release theophyline. It is 20 times more soluble than ordinary theophylline. This is an advantage in preparations for injection, which may be used to treat asthmatic emergencies (see later).

Choline theophyllinate contains about 50 per cent of theophylline but there is no evidence that it produces less irritation of the stomach than sustained-release preparations of theophylline if given in equally effective doses.

Harmful effects and warnings on the use of theophylline are listed in Table 12.1.

The effective use of theophylline The key to the effective use of theophylline is to adjust the dose in order to keep the level of the drug in the blood steady within a certain range. At this level (usually between 10 and 20 micrograms/litre) the benefits will outweigh the risks. Below this optimal range the effectiveness will decrease and above this range harmful effects will increase because there is a narrow margin between effective levels and toxic levels of theophylline in the blood.

People vary widely in their response to theophylline, and adjustment of the daily dose of theophylline in an individual should therefore be guided by any improvement in breathing, by the appearance of any harmful effects (e.g. nausea, vomiting, headaches) and by measuring the blood level of the drug. Working out the timing of a dose can be difficult because different people break down and excrete the drug at different rates. Moreover, its excretion is increased by smoking and alcohol, and reduced by virus infections, heart failure, liver disease and some drugs. Because of this, treatment should always start with a small dose which is then gradually increased until the patient improves. Absorption of the drug when taken by mouth varies between available preparations and between individuals. Therefore working out the right treatment for an individual needs time and patience. It also highlights the risks of changing preparations in someone who is well controlled. Any change may cause excessive fluctuations in the blood levels and therefore changes in the balance between desired effects and unwanted harmful effects. This warning applies particularly to sustained-release preparations.

NOTE Monitoring the level of theophylline in the blood – a blood sample should be taken 1–2 hours after an immediate-release preparation and 5 hours after a sustained-release preparation. The patient should not have missed a dose in the previous 48 hours and not taken an extra dose. No one should be maintained on a dose that is producing harmful effects.

Misuse of theophylline The above observations raise questions about the effectiveness of theophylline treatments when standard doses are used at fixed intervals of time (e.g. three times daily) without varying the dose to the individual's needs and response. Of particular concern is the use of theophylline combined with another drug (e.g. phenobarbitone) into one fixed-dose tablet. Some of these preparations may be used without regard for the age and weight of the patient, whether he smokes or not or whether he drinks alcohol and/or drinks large amounts of tea or coffee. Such use of theophylline may not do the patient much good but those preparations that contain phenobarbitone may ensure that the patient becomes dependent on the drug preparation and keeps going back for more!

The main use of theophylline is to prevent night attacks of asthma. It is not a drug of first choice but may be used if other treatments have failed to control night-time symptoms. It may also be added to other treatments to try to improve day-time control.

A *sustained-release tablet* of theophylline at bed-time may be effective in preventing attacks of asthma that come on in the night and also in preventing early morning attacks of asthma. Ultra-slow release preparations of theophylline (e.g. Uniphyllin Continus) may be taken mid-evening and provide prolonged relief throughout the night.

Drugs that relieve inflammation

Corticosteroids

Corticosteroids are discussed in detail in Chapter 62. Since the discovery in the 1950s that cortisone dramatically reduces the symptoms of allergy and inflammation, corticosteroids have been widely used, and sometimes misused, to treat patients suffering from asthma. If used properly they can be very effective and are a mainstay of asthma treatment. However these drugs do not specifically suppress inflammation; they have many other effects on the body. If used in high doses and for prolonged periods of time they produce harmful effects to many tissues and organs in the body.

Harmful effects of corticosteroids

Harmful effects and warnings on the use of corticosteroids by mouth or by injection are discussed in detail in Chapter 62. Harmful effects increase if the daily dose is high (over 10 mg of prednisolone per day or an equivalent dose of any other corticosteroid) and if such daily treatment is continued for more than a few weeks. Briefly, *prolonged use of high doses* may cause an increase in salt and fluid volume in the body, producing a rise in blood pressure and weight gain; a loss of potassium which can lead to apathy, weakness and mental confusion; a rise in blood sugar; a loss of protein from the body, producing muscle wasting and weakness; softening of bones (osteoporosis), producing collapse of vertebrae and bending of the spine (kyphosis); and a redistribution of fat around the body so the individual develops a moon face and 'buffalo hump' around the neck. They suppress inflammation and may mask an underlying infectious disease such as tuberculosis. They may cause mood changes and, rarely, they may cause cataracts in the eyes. They retard the growth of children.

Regular daily use of high doses causes the adrenal glands to shrink, which means that the individual cannot produce an increased amount of corticosteroids in times of stress due to an accident, surgery or an infection. This can have disastrous consequences (see Chapter 62).

Because long-term daily use knocks out the adrenal glands, the sudden stopping of these drugs can cause serious problems. The daily dose must therefore be reduced very slowly over a matter of months before the drug is finally stopped.

Aerosol inhalations reduce the risks of corticosteroids Aerosol inhalations of corticosteroids offer an opportunity to significantly reduce the daily dose used and therefore the harmful effects. These preparations have revolutionized the treatment of asthma. However, it is important to remember that only a small proportion of the dose actually reaches the bronchial tubes – the rest is swallowed and absorbed into the bloodstream – and you should realize that the long-term use of more than six puffs a day from an inhaler may produce harmful effects on the body, particularly if a high-dose preparation is used.

Corticosteroid aerosol inhalations must be used at regular intervals throughout each day in order to work effectively and it may take up to a week before the individual feels any benefit. In people who find it difficult to use aerosol inhalers, insufflation cartridges of dry powder are available; these are worked by the individual breathing in. However, higher doses of the drug are required in these preparations than in aerosol inhalers.

The use of a *nebulizer* (a powered machine that produces a spray) is another method which is very helpful to people who cannot work aerosols and dry inhalers *but note that the dose inhaled is higher and the risks of overdosage are higher*.

If you are taking a corticosteroid by inhalation you should always carry a 'steroid warning' card with you, particularly if you are taking a high-dose preparation. In acute attacks you will require a corticosteroid by mouth for a few days, in reducing daily dosages.

Various inhaler devices (e.g. Nebuhaler, Volumatic) may help to prevent complications in the mouth (e.g. thrush) by reducing the amount of drug deposited in the mouth and throat during an inhalation. After using an inhaler, it helps to rinse the mouth out with water and then to spit the water out.

To ensure that the corticosteroid reaches the parts it is supposed to reach, it helps to inhale a selective adrenoreceptor stimulant drug about 10 minutes beforehand. This relieves any bronchospasm and opens up the airways so that the corticosteroid reaches further down the air passage.

Harmful effects of corticosteroids by mouth are discussed in Chapter 62. When used by inhaler, the dose is much smaller and so general harmful effects are less frequent; nevertheless, they may still occur because some of the inhaled drug is absorbed into the bloodstream, particularly with higher dose preparations. Local harmful effects include hoarseness and thrush of the mouth.

Warnings *Corticosteroid inhalers should not be used by people who are allergic to such preparations, and they should be used with caution in people suffering from quiet or active tuberculosis of the lungs.*

Dangers of changing from corticosteroids by mouth to corticosteroid inhalers Because the dose of corticosteroid by inhaler is very much smaller than the dose by mouth, people who have been taking corticosteroids by mouth should have the dose of their corticosteroid by mouth slowly reduced over several weeks while *at the same time* using an inhaler. Serious problems, including deaths, have occurred when a corticosteroid by mouth was stopped suddenly and a corticosteroid inhaler substituted.

Use of corticosteroids by mouth *Acute attacks* may need to be treated with short courses of a corticosteroid by mouth for a few days and then reducing the daily dose slowly according to response.

Some individuals with *chronic continuing* asthma may not respond to other treatments and may still require the regular daily use of a corticosteroid by mouth. In these people the smallest dose for the greatest benefit should be worked out. To try to avoid knocking out the adrenal glands, it is better to use no more than 7.5 mg daily of prednisolone (or an equivalent dosage of another corticosteroid), and it may help to give the dose just once a day in the mornings. A higher dose every other day is an alternative but it seldom works well on the second day.

NOTE It helps to keep on high doses of inhaled corticosteroids in the hope of reducing the dose by mouth to a minimum.

The dangers of long-term use of corticosteroids are discussed in Chapter 62.

If it is necessary for you to be kept on long-term treatment with corticosteroids by mouth, you should see your doctor regularly to check for any harmful effects from this treatment, and to check your breathing in order to assess whether the drugs are actually doing you any good. You should discuss reducing the dose slowly over time, and you should *never* stop the drugs suddenly.

Warning *If you are taking a corticosteroid, whether by mouth, injection or inhaler, you should always carry a* ***steroid warning card*** *with you wherever you go. You should also read Chapter 62 on corticosteroids.*

Sodium cromoglycate (Intal)

One of the main factors that trigger an allergic asthma attack is the release of chemicals by certain cells in the linings of the bronchial tubes. These cells are called mast cells, and if their surfaces are irritated (e.g. by an allergic reaction), they release chemicals that cause the bronchial muscles to contract (bronchospasm) and the linings of the bronchial tubes to become 'inflamed'. Sodium cromoglycate acts on the surface of the mast cells and prevents this action. It belongs to a group of drugs known as mast cell stabilizers. To be effective it must be on the surface of the mast cells before the allergic reaction occurs. It is therefore of use in *preventing* attacks of allergic asthma but of no use in treating an attack once it has started. It is of more benefit to children and young patients than to older patients, but it may also provide relief in older patients who develop late-onset asthma.

Sodium cromoglycate is also effective in relieving wheezing triggered by exercise, wood dusts, aspirin, industrial dusts, chemicals and cold air. A single inhalation before exposure to these will often *prevent* an attack of wheezing. Sodium cromoglycate is poorly absorbed by mouth and has to be given as a powder by inhaler (aerosol inhalation), by insufflator or by inhalation of a solution through a nebulizer.

Sodium cromoglycate prevents attacks of allergic asthma; therefore if it is suddenly stopped a severe attack of asthma may develop. It is sensible to reduce the daily dose gradually over about 1 week before stopping it.

Problems with compound preparations

Dry powder inhalation of sodium cromoglycate may cause irritation, producing wheezing and coughing in some people sensitive to the inhalation of the dry powder. In such individuals a bronchodilator drug (e.g. salbutamol) or a related drug should be inhaled a few minutes before inhaling sodium cromoglycate. Although the manufacturers of Intal produce Intal Compound (a combination of sodium cromoglycate with a bronchodilator drug – isoprenaline) it should be used with caution because isoprenaline does not have a selective effect on the bronchial tubes and may cause rapid beating of the heart and other harmful effects. Also, because isoprenaline relieves wheezing, the patient may use Intal Compound to produce relief rather than to prevent an attack.

Preventing attacks of asthma

Sodium cromoglycate should be used for the prevention of asthma that may be due to allergy, exercise, cold air or inhaled chemicals or occupational dusts. In people with chronic asthma who respond to sodium cromoglycate, regular use may allow the doses of other drugs (e.g. bronchodilators, corticosteroids) to be reduced. Because sodium cromoglycate may take 4–6 weeks to reach its maximum benefits, any other drug should be continued for at least 2 weeks and the daily dose then slowly reduced. Note the particular dangers of stopping corticosteroids suddenly (see Chapter 62).

Because it is difficult to predict which people will respond to treatment with sodium cromoglycate, it is worth trying it on all individuals whose asthma is not well controlled with bronchodilators and/or corticosteroids. The most important part of treatment is knowing how to use the inhaler properly. *Regular use throughout each day is also important, even when there are no symptoms.* It is usually used four times a day but this may be reduced. The drug should be tried for at least 4 weeks before deciding whether it is of no use.

NOTE Sodium cromoglycate administered with a nebulizer is useful for people who cannot manage dry powder inhalers or pressurized aerosols. When used to prevent asthma that occurs with exercise, it should be taken by inhaler half an hour before the exercise, in a single dose.

Harmful effects and warnings on the use of sodium cromoglycate
Harmful effects of inhaling sodium cromoglycate include irritation and coughing. These symptoms may be relieved by using a selective adrenoreceptor stimulant inhaler (e.g. salbutamol) a few minutes before inhaling the sodium cromoglycate. Rarely, the drug may cause severe wheezing at the beginning of treatment and have to be stopped.

Warning *The drug should be withdrawn slowly over a period of about 1 week by gradually reducing the daily doses.*

Nedocromil sodium

Nedocromil sodium (Tilade) acts principally by relieving inflammation in the bronchial tubes. When it is inhaled it blocks the release of chemicals that cause inflammation and constriction of the bronchial tubes. It is used as regular preventive treatment in people suffering from reversible obstructive airways diseases such as asthma, asthmatic bronchitis and wheezing triggered by cold air, allergy, dust, chemicals and other pollutants in the air. If used regularly it improves breathing and reduces wheezing, cough and the production of phlegm. Other treatments should not be stopped suddenly but should overlap with the use of nedocromil until there is evidence of benefit. They should then be slowly reduced or stopped. Note the dangers of stopping corticosteroids suddenly (see Chapter 62).

Harmful effects of nedocromil include nausea, headache and a bitter taste in the mouth. These are usually mild and transient.

Antihistamines

Antihistamines are of no use in treating asthma and Ketotifen (Zaditen) which is a mast cell stabilizer with some antihistamine properties is of doubtful value.

Harmful effects include drowsiness and, occasionally, dry mouth and slight dizziness for a few days at the start of treatment.

Warnings *Ketotifen should not be used by people who are taking anti-diabetic drugs by mouth because there is a risk of reversible thrombocytopenia (a reduced number of platelets in the blood). Rarely, asthma may get worse but this is probably due to stopping other treatment; therefore treatment should always overlap for at least 2 weeks.*

Risks with alcohol Ketotifen may increase the effects of alcohol, sleeping drugs, sedatives, tranquillizers and antihistamines.

Risks with driving During the first few days it may cause drowsiness and interfere with ability to drive and operate moving machinery.

Combined drug preparations for asthma

There are well founded objections to the use of more than one drug combined into a single preparation. One is that the dose of each drug cannot be changed, and so you are exposed to fixed doses of the drugs day in and day out whether you need to be taking all the drugs in those doses or not. Other objections are that if you develop harmful effects from such a preparation, it is difficult to know which drug is causing the problem. Also, if you take an overdose – whether accidentally or intentionally – treatment may be more difficult with fixed-dose combinations of drugs than with drugs used separately. Another major objection is that you may know only the preparation by its brand name and not know the drugs it contains, or their doses.

The main benefit of combined preparations is that it is easier for the patient to remember to take the preparation but this convenience may easily be outweighed by the risks of using such combined preparations. Furthermore, they are usually more expensive than the drugs used separately. Combined asthma preparations are listed in Table 12.3.

Inhaled preparations to treat asthma

Aerosol inhalers

Pressurized aerosol inhalers* are very effective at targeting a drug to the site of action in the bronchial tubes. If used properly they prevent attacks and they also provide quick relief of mild to moderate attacks of bronchospasm. Their beneficial effects can last for 3–5 hours. Only a small proportion of the drug actually gets to the site of action but this is sufficient to produce relief – the rest of the dose is swallowed and absorbed into the bloodstream; but, because of the low doses used in inhalers, the risk of developing harmful effects is much less than if the drug is taken by mouth as a tablet or capsule. For example, an average dose of salbutamol by mouth is 4 mg, whereas the dose of salbutamol in an inhaler is 0.01 mg – i.e. the dose by mouth is 400 times greater than by inhaler.

It is important that inhalers are used correctly; many failures of treatment occur because the patient uses the inhaler incorrectly. Most patients can manage, but obviously small children and some elderly people have difficulty. A *serious danger* with inhalers is excessive use. Patients may take a puff and then another puff almost straight away, whereas they would not dream of taking one tablet and then another tablet if the first one does not produce immediate relief. One puff or two puffs of an inhaler is the required dose, and to take another puff is to take an overdose and run the risk of developing harmful effects.

You should know the most appropriate number of inhalations that you should use at any one time, the optimal interval of time between puffs and the maximum number of puffs that you should take in any 24-hour period. Failure to follow these instructions may lead to underuse or overuse of your inhaler, either of which may be harmful.

Warning *Failure to obtain relief may be due to faulty technique but it may also be due to a worsening of your disorder. If you find treatment that was effective is no longer giving relief, you should consult your doctor straight away. It is far better to prevent a severe asthmatic attack than to have to treat it once it has developed.*

Powder inhalers

For people who have difficulty with pressurized aerosol inhalers (e.g. young children and the elderly) some drugs are available in cartridges for dry

* Aerosol containers are not ozone friendly because they contain CFCs.

powder inhalation. These devices deliver the powder when the patient breathes in. However, not so much drug actually reaches the target area as with pressurized aerosols and therefore higher doses of the drug are included in these preparations. They may be useful but the dry powder may make the patient cough. Devices include spinhalers, diskhalers and turbohalers.

Products designed to improve the efficiency of inhalers

Various devices are now available to improve the efficiency of inhalers. They provide a space between the inhaler and the mouth (they are referred to as spacers). This spacer reduces the speed of the drug particles and allows more time for the propellant to evaporate before the active drug enters the breathing tubes. In addition, the patient does not have to breathe in at exactly the same time as he presses the inhaler. They are therefore useful for people who find difficulty using inhalers. They are also useful if high doses have to be taken, for children and for preventing thrush in people using a corticosteroid inhaler.

Available devices include Bricanyl Spacer Inhaler for use with a Bricanyl Inhaler (terbutaline), Nebuhaler Spacer for use with Bricanyl (terbutaline) and Pulmicort (budesonide) Inhalers, Volumatic Spacer for use with Ventolin (salbutamol), Becotide (beclomethasone) Inhalers and a Rondo device for use with Salbuvent preparations.

Aerosol (nebulizer) solutions

A water-based aerosol (respiratory solution) given by a power-operated nebulizer (a machine that produces a spray) is a very effective way of taking a drug into the bronchial tubes. The aqueous aerosol is inhaled slowly over about 15 minutes. Small portable nebulizing machines are suitable for home use. In hospital the drugs are usually given through a mask connected to a ventilating machine. Very careful instructions should be given to the patient and it must be remembered that the doses of drugs in aqueous solutions are much higher than those used in inhalers. They should be used with the utmost caution.

How to use an inhaler

It is very important that you are supervised when you first try an inhaler and that you are allowed to test the various ones that are available in order to select the one that is the most efficient for you. This takes time and patience. It is also important that you should test your breathing before and after using the inhaler in order to see whether the drug is actually producing any beneficial effect and to determine whether you are using the inhaler efficiently. These tests should be repeated at regular intervals. Young children will need special help to select the most appropriate way of taking a drug to prevent or relieve their asthmatic attacks.

Warnings *Many patients use their inhalers inefficiently – this may be costly, ineffective and potentially harmful.*

Some nebulizer solutions may trigger a wheezing attack, which can be serious. If your wheezing gets worse while on treatment, consult your doctor; do not take additional doses, this could have serious consequences. This paradoxical effect is probably due to an allergic reaction to some chemical in the nebulizer solution, for example a preservative (e.g. benzalkonium). Preservative-free preparations of some products are now available – check with your pharmacist.

Summary of the use of available drugs to treat asthma

Drug treatment of asthma is aimed at relieving acute attacks and preventing recurrent attacks; obtaining maximum benefit in terms of lung function and freedom from asthmatic attacks for the minimum use of drugs; and preventing late chest and heart complications such as bronchiectasis, emphysema and congestive heart failure.

Selective adrenoreceptor stimulants (beta stimulants)

Inhalants containing a selective acting adrenoreceptor stimulant are very beneficial in relieving the wheezing in mild to moderate attacks of asthma if used as directed. Regular daily use also helps to prevent attacks.

There is little to choose between the various drugs that are available for inhalation. It is much more important that the inhaler is used properly and that breathing tests are carried out before and after initial use and at regular intervals during treatment in order to assess whether the inhaler is being used efficiently and the drug actually works. The selection of an inhaler device to suit a particular individual is very important, as is the use of special spacing devices.

Preparations of a selective adrenoreceptor stimulant for use *by mouth* are occasionally useful in children (use sugar-free preparations) and in people who cannot use an inhaler. A slow release preparation by mouth at bed-time may be effective in preventing early morning asthma attacks in some individuals. *Intravenous* and, occasionally, *subcutaneous injections* may be given in emergencies (see later).

Non-selective adrenoreceptor stimulants should *not* be used because of their potential harmful effects on the heart and circulation.

Anticholinergic drugs

The only anticholinergic drug that should be used is a preparation of ipratropium by inhalation. This may provide additional benefit when given with a selective adrenoreceptor stimulant to people who suffer from chronic bronchitis and who have not improved on an adrenoreceptor stimulant. Unlike other anticholinergic drugs, ipratropium does not increase the stickiness of phlegm and make it hard to cough up. It is slow to work (30–60 minutes) but needs to be taken only three times daily. Its benefits should be carefully assessed by using a peak flow meter.

Theophylline

Slow-release preparations of theophylline to be taken by mouth offer the advantage of less frequent dosages throughout the day, less fluctuation in blood levels of the drug and therefore less risk of harmful effects and more effective control of wheezing. However, variations in individual response and a narrow margin between the benefits and risks still remain a problem. Slow release preparations of theophylline are of benefit in preventing attacks of asthma in the night or early morning in patients who have not benefited from high doses of inhaled corticosteroids and standard doses of beta stimulants.

Theophylline by mouth may increase the effects of inhaled adrenoreceptor stimulants without causing a tremor, but it may increase the risk of disorders of heart rhythm in some people.

Sodium cromoglycate

A sodium cromoglycate preparation is of great benefit in preventing attacks of allergic asthma, and in treating exercise-induced asthma (used half an hour before exercise as a single dose). It is of more benefit in children and young adults than in older people, but it may also provide relief in older individuals who develop late-onset asthma. It is effective in preventing wheezing triggered not only by exercise but also by wood dust, aspirin, industrial dusts, chemicals and cold air. It should be tried for 1 month by all people who do not respond well to bronchodilators.

Nedocromil (Tilade)

Nedocromil relieves inflammation, and is possibly of more benefit than sodium cromoglycate in adults suffering from late-onset asthma and asthmatic bronchitis.

Ketotifen (Zaditen)

Ketotifen acts like sodium cromoglycate but can be taken by mouth to prevent asthma. However, it is less effective than sodium cromoglycate.

Corticosteroids

The availability of inhalations of corticosteroids has significantly reduced the risks and improved the benefits of corticosteroids. They must be used regularly every day to obtain maximum relief, and from first starting treatment they may take 3–7 days to produce their maximum benefit. They should be used in patients who need to use a beta stimulant inhaler more than once a day and/or who develop symptoms during the night. Treatment should start with high, frequent doses and then be slowly reduced according to breathing tests. Despite the availability of corticosteroid preparations for inhalation, some people still require to take them by mouth.

Suggestions for the treatment of asthma

It is very important to take your treatment as directed, to measure your progress regularly using a peak flow meter and to consult your doctor as soon as possible if your treatment seems to be failing and/or your asthma is getting worse.

Drug treatment of chronic, persistent asthma should be introduced in steps: for example, a beta stimulant by inhalation when necessary. If the inhaler has to be used more than once a day to relieve attacks and/or if you get asthma at night then an anti-inflammatory inhaler (i.e., a corticosteroid inhaler) should be added. You should monitor your peak flow regularly and if there is no improvement on high doses of corticosteroids plus standard doses of beta stimulants then it may be necessary to add ipratropium inhalations to the treatment or to try theopylline at night. Finally, it may be necessary to add corticosteroids by mouth to the treatment.

The above suggestion is only one example of step-by-step treatment. Each individual will need to have the treatment tapered to his/her particular needs: for example, children and some adults may do very well on sodium cromoglycate and will not need corticosteroids; others may respond well to nedocromil. Remember that failed treatment is often due to failure to take treatment as directed.

Emergency treatment of asthma

Emergency treatment of asthma involves the use of oxygen and high doses of salbutamol or terbutaline by nebulizer and an intravenous injection of hydrocortisone or prednisolone by mouth. If there is no improvement, ipratropium by nebulizer may be added to the treatment and aminophylline should be given by slow injection into a vein provided that the individual is not already taking theophylline by mouth; otherwise, salbutamol or terbutaline should be given by injection into a vein.

Table 12.1 Drugs used to treat asthma – harmful effects and warnings

Selective adrenoreceptor stimulants
Harmful effects By mouth: tenseness and tremor of skeletal muscles, affecting mostly the hands. The higher the dose, the greater the effect. These drugs may occasionally cause flushing, rapid beating of the heart and headache. High doses by *inhalation* may cause similar harmful effects, as may *injections*. The latter may also cause pain and stinging at the site of injection.

Warnings Do not use a particular preparation if you have had a previous allergic reaction to that preparation. Selective adrenoreceptor stimulants should be used with caution in anyone suffering from an over-active thyroid gland, angina, heart disease, raised blood pressure or diabetes. Blood sugar levels should be repeatedly checked in diabetic patients receiving intravenous injections, and the dose of insulin increased accordingly. Concurrent use of a corticosteroid may increase the dangers of a raised blood sugar in diabetic patients.

Non-selective adrenoreceptor stimulants
Harmful effects According to how they are used, these drugs may cause anxiety, restlessness, rapid beating of the heart, tremor, weakness, dizziness, headache, coldness of the hands and feet, dry mouth and a rise in blood pressure.

Warnings They should be used with utmost caution by anyone with angina, heart disease, raised blood pressure, over-active thyroid gland or diabetes. Tolerance to their bronchodilator effects may develop. Non-selective adrenoreceptor stimulants should be replaced by selective ones.

Risks in elderly people Harmful effects may be more frequent and severe. Because they may cause difficulty in passing urine, they must be used with caution in men with enlarged prostate glands.

Ipratropium by inhalation
Harmful effects include dry mouth, difficulty passing urine and constipation.

Warnings Do not use if you are allergic

Table 12.1 Drugs used to treat asthma – harmful effects and warnings (*cont.*)

to atropine or a related drug. Use it with caution if you have glaucoma or an enlarged prostate gland. Seek medical advice if you start getting a reduced response to the inhaler.

corticosteroids
For harmful effects and warnings on the use of corticosteroids by *mouth* and by *injection*, read Chapter 62.

Harmful effects by *inhalation* include thrush infection of the mouth and throat, hoarseness and cough. Some drug is absorbed into the bloodstream and regular use of high doses may cause problems (see Chapter 62).

Warnings Do not use a particular preparation if you have developed an allergy to that preparation. Deaths have occurred due to lack of adrenal gland function when patients have been transferred from corticosteroids by mouth to corticosteroids by inhalation. The inhalation should be started while the individual is still taking corticosteroids by mouth and then the dose of the latter should be reduced very slowly over several weeks to months, while the individual uses the full recommended daily dosage of a corticosteroid inhaler. Corticosteroid inhalers take several days to produce any benefit; they should not be used to treat acute attacks of wheezing.

Risks in elderly people As in adults, but with the additional risk of oesteoporosis.

theophylline
Harmful effects The following harmful effects are usually related to dose; they may be transient at the start of treatment but if they come on later it usually means the concentration in the blood has reached toxic levels and the dose should be reduced. They include rapid heart rate, irregular heart beats, palpitation, flushing, nettle rash (urticaria), nausea, vomiting, diarrhoea, dizziness, vertigo, light-headedness, nervousness, headaches, irritability, restlessness, over-excitability and, rarely, muscle twitching and convulsions.

Warnings Do not use a particular preparation that has produced an allergic reaction previously. In an individual taking regular daily treatment, the dose should not be increased for an acute attack without checking the concentration of theophylline in the blood. Defective excretion of the drug and therefore increased risk of toxic effects may occur in people with impaired kidney or liver function, those over 55 years (particularly males) or with chronic lung disease or heart failure from whatever cause; newborn babies, people taking certain drugs (see Chapter 89) and in anyone suffering from influenza or after influenza immunization. *Serious harmful effects (disorders of heart rhythm and convulsions) may come on without warning and are not necessarily preceded by less severe harmful effects* (e.g. nausea and restlessness, which occur in about 50 per cent of people). Smokers break the drug down faster than non-smokers and will require higher doses. Theophylline should be used with caution by people with severe heart disease, severe low blood oxygen levels, raised blood pressure, overactive thyroid gland, alcoholism, liver disease, congestive heart failure or peptic ulcers.

Risks with driving Harmful symptoms may affect your ability to drive, therefore do not drive until you know that it is safe to do so.

Warnings Adrenoreceptor stimulants (whether selective or not) may stimulate the heart, produce a fall in blood potassium levels and cause a heart attack. Fenoterol is particularly dangerous in these respects. Theophylline may also cause a fall in blood potassium therefore potassium levels should be checked at regular intervals.

Table 12.2 Preparations used to treat asthma

Preparation	*Drug*	*Drug group*	*Dosage form*
adrenaline	adrenaline	Sympathomimetic	Injection
Aerolin Autohaler	Salbutamol	Selective beta-2 stimulant	Aerosol
Alupent	orciprenaline	Partially selective beta-2 stimulant	Tablets, sugar-free syrup, aerosol
aminophylline	aminophylline	Xanthine	Tablets, injection, suppositories
Atrovent	ipratropium	Anticholinergic	Aerosol, nebulizer solution (preservative-free)
Atrovent Forte	ipratropium	Anticholinergic	Aerosol
Becloforte	beclomethasone	Corticosteroid	Aerosol (high dose)
Becodisks	beclomethasone	Corticosteroid	Disks containing powder for inhalation
Becotide 50 and 100	beclomethasone	Corticosteroid	Aerosol, rotacaps (powder for inhalation), nebulizer suspension
Berotec	fenoterol	Selective beta-2 stimulant	Aerosol, nebulizer solution
Biophylline	theophylline	Xanthine	Sugar-free syrup tablets
Bricanyl	terbutaline	Selective beta-2 stimulant	Tablets, sugar-free syrup, injection, aerosol (and Bricanyl Spacer Inhaler) respirator solution, powderinhaler(Bricanyl Turbohaler)
Bricanyl Respules	terbutaline	Selective beta-2 stimulant	Single dose units for nebulization
Bricanyl SA	terbutaline	Selective beta-2 stimulant	Sustained-release tablets
Bronchodil	reproterol	Selective beta-2 stimulant	Tablets, aerosol, respirator solution
Choledyl	choline theophyllinate	Xanthine	Tablets, syrup
Cobutalin	salbutamol	Selective beta-2 stimulant	Tablets
ephedrine	ephedrine	Adrenoreceptor stimulant	Tablets, elixir
Exirel	pirbuterol	Selective beta-2 stimulant	Capsules, syrup, aerosol

Table 12.2 Preparations used to treat asthma (*cont.*)

Preparation	*Drug*	*Drug group*	*Dosage form*
Intal	sodium cromoglycate	Mast cell stabilizer	Aerosol (breath activated), nebulizer solution, spincaps (inhalation cartridges)
Iso-Autohaler	isoprenaline	Non-selective beta stimulant	Aerosol
Lasma	theophylline	Xanthine	Sustained-release tablets
Medihaler-Epi	adrenaline	Sympathomimetic	Aerosol
Medihaler-Iso	isoprenaline	Non-selective beta stimulant	Aerosol
Medihaler-Iso Forte	isoprenaline	Non-selective beta stimulant	Aerosol
Monovent	terbutaline	Selective beta-2 stimulant	Tablets, syrup
Monovent SA	terbutaline	Selective beta-2 stimulant	Sustained-release tablets
Nuelin	theophylline	Xanthine	Tablets, liquid
Nuelin SA, Nuelin SA 250	theophylline	Xanthine	Sustained-release tablets
Numotac	isoetharine	Non-selective beta stimulant	Sustained-release tablets
Pecram	aminophylline	Xanthine	Sustained-release tablets
Phyllocontin Continus, Phyllocontin Paediatric, Phyllocontin Forte	aminophylline	Xanthine	Sustained-release tablets
Pro-Vent	theophylline	Xanthine	Sustained-release capsules
Pulmadil	rimiterol	Selective beta-2 stimulant	Aerosol
Pulmadil Auto	rimiterol	Selective beta-2 stimulant	Aerosol (breath activated)
Pulmicort	budesonide	Corticosteroid	Aerosol (high dose) powder inhaler (Turbohaler)
Pulmicort LS	budesonide	Corticosteroid	Aerosol (inhaler, Nebuhaler)
Sabidal SR	choline theophyllinate	Xanthine	Sustained-release tablets
Salbulin	salbutamol	Selective beta-2 stimulant	Tablets, aerosol
Salbuvent	salbutamol	Selective beta-2 stimulant	Tablets, syrup, aerosol, injection, respiratory solution

Table 12.2 Preparations used to treat asthma (*cont.*)

Preparation	*Drug*	*Drug group*	*Dosage form*
Slo-Phyllin	theophylline	Xanthine	Sustained-release capsules
Theo-Dur	theophylline	Xanthine	Sustained-release tablets
Tilade	nedocromil sodium	Bronchial anti-inflammatory	Aerosol
Uniphyllin Continus, Uniphyllin Paediatric Continus	theophylline	Xanthine	Sustained-release tablets
Ventodisks	salbutamol	Selective beta-2 stimulant	Rotating disks for inhalation
Ventolin	salbutamol	Selective beta-2 stimulant	Tablets, sustained-release tablets, sugar-free syrup, injection, solution for intravenous infusion, aerosol, nebules, rotacaps, respirator solution
Volmax	salbutamol	Selective beta-2 stimulant	Sustained-release tablets
Zaditen	ketotifen	Mast cell stabilizer	Capsules, tablets, elixir

Table 12.3 Combined preparations used to treat asthma

Preparation	*Drug*	*Drug group*	*Dosage form*
Bronchilator	isoetharine	Non-selective beta stimulant	Aerosol
	phenylephrine	Sympathomimetic	
CAM	ephedrine butethamate	Sympathomimetic Bronchodilator	Syrup (sucrose-free)
Duo-Autohaler	isoprenaline	Non-selective beta stimulant	Aerosol
	phenylephrine	Sympathomimetic	
Duovent	fenoterol	Selective beta-2 stimulant	Aerosol
	ipratropium	Anticholinergic	
Franol, Franol Plus	ephedrine theophylline	Sympathomimetic Xanthine	Tablets

Table 12.3 Combined preparations used to treat asthma (*cont.*)

Preparation	*Drug*	*Drug group*	*Dosage form*
Intal Compound	sodium cromoglycate	Mast cell stabilizer	Spincaps
	isoprenaline	Non-selective beta stimulant	
Labophylline	theophylline	Xanthine	Injection
	lysine	Amino acid	
Medihaler-duo	isoprenaline	Non-selective beta stimulant	Aerosol
	phenylephrine	Sympathomimetic	
Theodrox	aminophylline	Xanthine	Tablets
	aluminium hydroxide gel	Antacid	
Ventide	salbutamol	Selective beta-2 stimulant	Aerosol, rotacaps and paediatric rotacaps (powder for inhalation)
	beclomethasone	Corticosteroid	

13

Disorders of the mouth

All kinds of bacteria, fungi and other micro-organisms live in the mouth. They are kept under control in healthy people by an adequate diet, by the physical effects of eating and drinking and by cleaning the teeth. A poor diet lacking in vitamins, poor health and poor oral hygiene allow some of these micro-organisms to over-multiply and spread to produce inflammation of the mouth (stomatitis) and/or inflammation of the gum (gingivitis). These are particularly likely to happen when your resistance to infection is reduced. This immune deficiency may be caused by drugs used to suppress the immune system or by disease (e.g. AIDS).

Inflammation of the mouth caused by vitamin deficiency

A deficiency of vitamins due either to a lack of vitamins in the diet or to an inability to absorb them from food because of some disorder of the stomach or intestine can cause inflammation of the mouth and tongue. The vitamins especially involved are vitamin B_2 (riboflavine) and nicotinamide (niacin). In these deficiencies the mouth is sore, the tongue becomes red and painful (glossitis) and the lips and corners of the mouth may become sore (angular stomatitis). People who develop stomatitis due to vitamin deficiency usually suffer from multiple vitamin B deficiencies rather than a deficiency of just one particular B vitamin.

Folic acid deficiency causes anaemia and may cause a sore tongue, and Vitamin B_{12} deficiency causes anaemia in which patients often develop a smooth red tongue. Vitamin C deficiency (scurvy) may cause the gums to become swollen and fragile and to bleed easily.

Treatment of these disorders is to take the appropriate vitamin or vitamins (see Chapter 45).

Thrush infections of the mouth

Thrush (candidiasis) usually causes white patches like milk curd in the mouth, with very little surrounding inflammation, but it may cause inflammation and soreness without white patches in people who have had long courses of antibiotics by mouth (antibiotic tongue). It is caused by a yeast (*Candida albicans*) that normally lives in the mouth. It may multiply to cause thrush in debilitated people, particularly the elderly with poor fitting dentures and poor oral hygiene. It may also occur in patients who have an immune deficiency (e.g. AIDS). In addition to being caused by long courses of antibiotics, it may also be caused by anti-cancer drugs, immunosuppressive drugs, corticosteroids and radiotherapy, all of which may cause an immune deficiency. Thrush may occur in babies, spreading from the mother and possibly from poorly washed infected bottles and teats or soothers (dummies). It may occur in diabetes, malnutrition and severe anaemias. Drugs that dry the mouth may predispose to the development of thrush; for example, anticholinergics, anti-depressants, antihistamines and some drugs used to treat blood pressure.

The *most effective treatment* for thrush of the mouth is a preparation that contains an anti-fungal drug such as nystatin, amphotericin or miconazole (see below). Dequalinium and polynoxylin are less effective. Crystal violet is an old-fashioned treatment which stains the skin and clothes and may burn the surface of the mouth.

Drugs used to treat thrush infections of the mouth

amphotericin (Fungilin)
dequalinium (Dequadin, Labosept)
miconazole (Daktarin)
nystatin (Nystan, Nystatin-Dome)
polynoxylin (Anaflex)

Harmful effects of anti-fungal drugs are listed in Table 56.1.

Common mouth ulcers (aphthous ulcers, canker sores)

These are painful, superficial ulcers that occur in groups and keep recurring. They are most commonly called aphthous ulcers. We do not know what causes them and there is no cure. They appear to run in families and they may be caused by some type of 'allergic' reaction, possibly to a certain type of bacteria that live in the mouth.

A difficult problem with treatment is that whatever you apply to the ulcers is soon washed away in the saliva and swallowed, so it does not have much time to work, and the result is generally disappointing. All kinds of treatments have been tried but the most fashionable at present are the following.

Antibiotic mouth-washes may be useful in recurrent, severe ulceration of the mouth but they may trigger a thrush infection. The one in fashion at present is tetracycline mouth-bath, which contains a tetracycline mixture.

Antiseptics Any ulcer in the mouth may become secondarily infected with bacteria which will then delay healing. An antiseptic mouth-wash containing chlorhexidine may therefore help to reduce the infection and encourage healing. Harmful effects of antiseptic applications are discussed in Chapter 75.

Astringents to dry up the ulcer include sticks of toughened silver nitrate and alum. These are applied right on to the ulcer but they are too strong and may damage the ulcer and actually delay healing.

Carbenoxolone gel (e.g. Bioplex, Bioral) may be beneficial to some people. Carbenoxolone is also used to heal peptic ulcers (see Chapter 15).

Corticosteroid pellets or pastes are the most effective. They include hydrocortisone in Corlan pellets, and triamcinolone in Adcortyl in Orabase paste. They relieve inflammation and pain.

Local anaesthetics to relieve the pain are included in some preparations. Their effects are transient and they may cause local irritation and soreness of the mouth and lips. Also, if the local anaesthetic application is swallowed there is a risk of anaesthetizing the surface of the throat – if applied before meals this may produce choking when trying to swallow.

NOTE Compound benzocaine lozenges contain ten times more benzocaine than benzocaine lozenges combined with menthol.

Mouth rinses and sprays may be used to relieve pain and inflammation. An example is Difflam oral rinse and spray which contain benzydamine, a pain reliever.

Pain relievers such as a salicylate applied directly to an ulcer may relieve the pain of minor ulcers. Available preparations include choline salicylate dental gel; Bonjela oral gel, which contains choline salicylate; Pyralvex oral paint, which contains salicylic acid; and anthraquinone glycosides and Teejel oral gel, which contains choline salicylate and cetalkonium. Any of these preparations may cause stinging when applied to the ulcer, and excessive use or use under a denture may cause ulceration. Chlorbutol is also included as a pain reliever in some preparations but is of doubtful value. **Protective pastes or powders** to coat the surface of the ulcers (e.g. Orabase paste or Orahesive powder) contain carmellose and provide a physical protection over the ulcer and may help it to heal but they are easily washed away in the saliva.

Comment Over all, available treatments for aphthous ulcers are disappointing although some of them may provide transient relief of pain. Corticosteroid applications (e.g. Corlan pellets and Adcortyl in Orabase) appear to be the most effective, perhaps because they relieve inflammation. They should be used at the very first sign of an ulcer developing.

Vincent's infection (Vincent's stomatitis, Vincent's gingivitis)

This is a nasty infection that produces pain, bad breath and severe ulcers of the gums. It is rare but may occur in patients who have an immune deficiency (e.g. AIDS). The infection is treated by improving oral hygiene and the use of the antibiotic drug metronidazole or nimorazole by mouth.

Cold sores

'Cold sores' or 'fever blisters' are caused by the herpes simplex virus. They keep recurring, often in the same place. Herpes infections are discussed in Chapter 57. If the ulcers are severe, it is worth trying a tetracycline mouth bath, or an antiviral drug; for example, acyclovir in a cream (e.g. Zovirax cream). If the ulcers are severe and recur frequently, acyclovir may have to be given by injection. Otherwise, there is no specific treatment for cold sores and most treatments are based on 'old wives' tales'. Caustic applications should be avoided (e.g. phenol and silver nitrate), so should counter-irritants such as camphor. Corticosteroid applications (e.g. hydrocortisone) are best avoided because of the risks of spreading the infection (see Chapter 57). Drying applications should also be avoided because if the ulcers dry and crack there is an added risk of secondary infection. It is probably best to use a protective application (e.g. Orabase) or Vaseline petroleum jelly.

Special preparations used to treat disorders of the mouth

Mouth-washes and gargles

Despite what the adverts say, these are only of any value to certain people; for example, those who have mouth infections, those whose gums are inflamed and too sore for the teeth to be brushed, and those who are physically unable to brush their teeth and/or are severely debilitated. In 'healthy' people with normal oral hygiene the saliva and the mucus that covers the mouth and throat are the best protection against irritation. Most available mouth-washes and gargles contain an antiseptic, but there is no convincing evidence from adequate studies that their use is beneficial. A chlorhexidine mouth-wash helps to prevent plaque on teeth and may be useful additional treatment in people with a mouth infection when it is not possible to brush the teeth.

Antiseptic lozenges and sprays

These are best avoided. They are of little benefit and may cause a sore tongue and lips. Those that contain a local anaesthetic may cause an allergic reaction.

Artificial saliva products

These are designed to mimic saliva both chemically and physically. They are used to treat dry mouth but they do not stimulate the production of saliva; they only act as 'artificial saliva'. Dry mouth may be caused by shrinking of the salivary glands due to disease, radiation treatment to the neck, or advanced old age. Temporary dry mouth is often caused by drugs (e.g. anticholinergic drugs, anti-depressant drugs and antihistamine drugs). Persistent dry mouth causes a sore mouth and tongue, difficulty in swallowing and speaking, and tooth decay. Treatment should be directed at preventing dental decay and soreness of the mouth. Artificial saliva preparations relieve this soreness and are more effective than mouth-washes and lozenges. They do not affect the damage to the teeth and some may make it worse because they contain sugar alcohols. Some patients may be allergic to preservatives in these preparations. Preparations include Glandosane aerosol (carboxymethylcellulose sodium with sorbitol, potassium chloride, sodium chloride, magnesium chloride, calcium chloride, dipotassium hydrogen phosphate).

Table 13.1 Preparations used to treat thrush and other fungal infections of the mouth

Preparation	*Drug*	*Dosage form*
Anaflex	polynoxylin	Lozenges
Daktarin	miconazole	Oral gel
Diflucan	fluconazole	Capsules
Fungilin	amphotericin	Lozenges
Labosept	dequalinium	Pastilles
Nystan	nystatin	Pastilles, suspension, powder for suspension; sugar-, lactose-, gluten-free
nystatin mixture	nystatin	Mixture

14

Nausea, vomiting, motion sickness and vertigo

Nausea and vomiting are symptoms. These symptoms may occur with all kinds of physical disorders, some of which are quite simple and short-lived, such as food poisoning, and some very serious and long-lasting, such as cancer of the stomach or a brain tumour. Drugs often cause nausea and vomiting (e.g. morphine, digoxin, oestrogens) and so may motion, pregnancy and emotion (e.g. the sight of a severely injured road-accident victim). Nausea and vomiting may serve a useful purpose – as in food poisoning – but usually they are distressing symptoms which need relieving.

Mechanisms that cause vomiting

There is a vomiting centre in the brain which, if stimulated, activates the nerves that supply the muscles in the stomach and chest to make you vomit. It responds to stimulations from the stomach and intestine (e.g. irritation), from the brain (e.g. raised pressure in the brain), from the organ of balance, from other centres in the brain which are stimulated by sight, smell or emotion and from the chemoreceptor trigger zone. The last seems to respond to chemical stimulation. It triggers vomiting if it is stimulated by certain drugs (e.g. morphine) or by chemicals produced in the body in disorders such as diabetes or kidney failure. It is called the chemoreceptor trigger zone because the receptors pick up the chemicals and trigger messages to the vomiting centre to make you vomit.

Movement affects the organ of balance, which has link-ups with the vomiting centre. For example, motion produced by travelling in a car, on a boat or on a roundabout stimulates the organ of balance, which sends messages to the vomiting centre that may result in a feeling of nausea (sweating, salivation, rapid beating of the heart and a feeling you are going to vomit) and vomiting. Motion sickness is more common in children.

Certain movements (e.g. swinging) will make some people sick, whilst others who are not made sick by swinging may become sick at sea. Fear and anxiety can make things worse but, fortunately, over a period of a few days, our bodies can become tolerant to the motion and we stop being sick.

Anti-vomiting drugs

Drugs used to treat nausea and vomiting (anti-emetics) should be used only when you know what the cause is – for example, seasickness. Otherwise, their use may delay the diagnosis of an underlying disorder that may be causing the nausea and vomiting, or mask the harmful effects produced by some drug treatment that you are taking.

NOTE There are many drugs that produce nausea and vomiting and these symptoms usually clear up if the dose of the drug is reduced.

Drugs used to treat nausea and vomiting include anticholinergics, antihistamines, dopamine blockers and 5 HT (serotonin) blockers.

How do anti-vomiting drugs work?

Anticholinergics

The vomiting centre in the brain and the organ of balance appear to be stimulated by the nerve messenger, acetylcholine, and this explains why hyoscine and drugs that block the effects of acetylcholine (i.e. anticholinergic drugs) in the brain help to reduce nausea and vomiting as well as motion sickness. They also produce some anticholinergic effects on the nerves of the stomach and reduce its movements. They may also cause dry mouth, blurred vision and constipation.

Antihistamines

In addition to affecting the vomiting centre, antihistamines also affect receptors in the organ of balance and other receptors in the brain, including those in the chemoreceptor trigger zone. This may help to explain why antihistamines relieve nausea and vomiting due to different causes, including motion sickness. They appear to block not only histamine receptors but also acetylcholine and dopamine receptors.

Dopamine blockers

A nerve messenger that stimulates the chemoreceptor trigger zone is dopamine; this is why drugs that block dopamine (dopamine blockers or dopamine antagonists) produce their beneficial effects in relieving nausea and vomiting caused by drugs and diseases. Dopamine blockers include the phenothiazine drugs and the drugs metoclopramide and domperidone.

5 HT (Serotonin) blockers

Ondansetron is a drug that blocks 5 HT receptors in the intestine and chemoreceptor trigger zone. Unlike metoclopramide it has no effects on dopamine receptors and therefore it does not cause movement disorders.

Drugs used to prevent motion sickness

Motion sickness may be produced by all kinds of motion, including travelling in cars, trains, aeroplanes and boats. It develops when the brain is confused by the various messages coming from the organ of balance, the eyes and the body. These confused messages stimulate the vomiting centre. Anyone may develop motion sickness but children are particularly prone.

There is no drug which effectively prevents motion sickness that does not produce harmful effects in some people.

Once motion sickness has started, taking drugs by mouth may have no effect at all because the drug may be vomited straight up and/or the exit from the stomach into the intestine may be closed as a result of the vomiting. This closure of the exit from the stomach holds the drug back from entering the intestine from where it is normally absorbed into the bloodstream to produce its beneficial effects. In these circumstances (i.e. when someone is vomiting repeatedly) an anti-vomiting drug should be given by injection or by suppository into the rectum. Some preparations may be sucked and the drug absorbed directly into the bloodstream from the lining of the mouth (e.g. cinnarizine). Hyoscine (see later) is available in the form of a patch to be applied to the skin.

The aim of drug treatment should be to try to *prevent* an attack of motion sickness developing. A short-acting drug (e.g. hyoscine) should be taken for a short journey and a long-acting one (e.g. an antihistamine) for a long journey.

Available drugs

Hyoscine

Hyoscine (an anticholinergic drug) is the drug of choice. It acts principally on the organ of balance and the vomiting centre. It is very effective for treating motion sickness but is short acting and therefore useful only for short journeys. It should be taken by mouth half an hour before a journey. In high dosage and on repeated use it may produce drowsiness, blurred vision, dry mouth, constipation, difficulty in passing urine and rapid beating of the heart. It increases the effects of alcohol and interferes with the ability to drive or operate moving machinery

A preparation of hyoscine that can be applied to the skin is available (Scopoderm). The hyoscine is absorbed directly into the bloodstream and therefore a small dose can be used which results in less severe harmful effects. It also has a prolonged effect – up to 36 hours.

Antihistamines

Antihistamines are useful for treating motion sickness because they act on the organ of balance in addition to acting on the vomiting centre in the brain. They are discussed in detail in Chapter 10.

In using antihistamines to prevent motion sickness the greatest problem is drowsiness. It is the most common harmful effect and it may affect the ability to drive and operate moving machinery. If you wish to take an antihistamine for a journey, it is worth trying a dose a few weeks before, just to see how it affects you; then you will know what to expect. Paradoxically, in infants and young children antihistamines may produce stimulation rather than drowsiness. This may cause them to become restless and unable to sleep.

The antihistamines that are used to prevent motion sickness are less effective than hyoscine but produce less dry mouth and constipation. However, most of them produce drowsiness. There is no evidence that one antihistamine is better than all the others at relieving motion sickness. Some produce less drowsiness than others and some produce less dry mouth and constipation than others. However, over all it is a matter of trial and error because different people react differently to antihistamines. The newer antihistamines that do not produce drowsiness do not enter the brain and are therefore of little use in relieving motion sickness.

If sleep is needed (e.g. an overnight journey by boat) it is better to use an antihistamine that is known to produce drowsiness (e.g. promethazine or dimenhydrinate). In the day-time it is better to try cyclizine or cinnarizine because they produce less drowsiness than the others. The first dose of an antihistamine should be taken about half an hour before the journey (2 hours before for cinnarizine).

Dangers of antihistamines with alcohol and other drugs It is important always to remember that antihistamines increase the effect of alcohol and other drugs that depress the consciousness of the brain; for example, sleeping drugs, anti-anxiety drugs (tranquillizers) and anti-depressant drugs. They may also interfere with your ability to drive.

Other treatments

Other treatments for motion sickness include sucking ginger, although there is no convincing evidence of its effectiveness, and acupressure on the wrist by wearing a special strap (Acu Pulse Band). This is claimed to prevent nausea by applying pressure at certain acupuncture points on the wrist.

There is no convincing evidence from adequate and well controlled studies of the benefit of chlorbutol (a sedative) in relieving motion sickness. It is included in Traveltabs.

Nausea and vomiting in pregnancy

Vomiting in pregnancy is probably due to hormonal changes that occur in the early months of pregnancy. In addition, all kinds of social, emotional, physical and dietary factors may contribute to the problem. This means that a pregnant woman who is getting distressed because of vomiting needs treating as a 'whole' person: she needs understanding, advice and caring support. The last thing she needs is to be treated as if she is neurotic. Vomiting in pregnancy can be a very real and very distressing problem. It usually occurs between the 10th and 14th weeks and is worse around the 10th to 11th weeks.

Drugs that have been used to treat vomiting of pregnancy include dicyclomine (similar to hyoscine, see above) antihistamine drugs (e.g. meclozine) and phenothiazines (e.g. chlorpromazine, prochlorperazine, thiethylperazine and trifluoperazine).

Avoid drug treatment if possible

The risk of damaging an unborn baby from the use of drugs is greatest in the first 3–4 months of pregnancy, when nausea and vomiting are at their worst. It is important to remember that studies which seek to explain damage to unborn babies in terms of the drugs used in early pregnancy are very difficult to carry out and the results of such studies are even more difficult to interpret. It is therefore best *to avoid drug treatment if possible.* However, if nausea and vomiting are severe and continuous, a few days of drug treatment may occasionally be necessary in order to bring the symptoms under control. Drugs recommended for this 'emergency' purpose are promethazine (Phenergan) or thiethylperazine (Torecan).

NOTE Some women may vomit so profusely that they will require intravenous fluids and multivitamin treatment.

Vitamin B_6

Because deficiency of vitamin B_6 (pyridoxine) may occur in severe and continuous vomiting, it has been widely used to treat mild to moderate vomiting in pregnancy. Whether a deficiency of pyridoxine occurs as a result of such vomiting in pregnancy is debatable and there are no reports from adequate and well controlled studies of its benefits in preventing vomiting in pregnancy. It probably acts as a placebo but it is important to note that excessive use of high doses of vitamin B_6 may cause nerve damage.

Nausea and vomiting caused by drugs

Drugs may cause nausea and vomiting by stimulating the chemoreceptor trigger zone (e.g. morphine) or they may irritate the lining of the stomach (e.g. some anti-rheumatic drugs). Digoxin and related drugs used to treat heart failure and ipecacuanha in cough medicines probably produce both effects. Anti-cancer drugs may cause nausea and vomiting.

If a drug irritates the stomach and produces pain and indigestion it may help to take it with or after food; but if it is causing nausea and vomiting it is far better to stop the drug or to reduce the daily dosage, if possible. An alternative is to increase the time between doses and/or to use a special preparation of the drug that is made up in such a way as to reduce its potential for irritating the stomach – for example, a special coating that ensures the release of the drug further down the intestine and away from the stomach.

No drug used at present to reduce nausea and vomiting produced by another drug is entirely effective. Either they do not work very well or they produce unwanted harmful effects. Furthermore, using drugs to relieve the harmful effects of another drug is not always satisfactory because it exposes the patient to the harmful effects of yet another drug.

The groups of drugs used include:

- *Antihistamines* (see Chapter 10) – to reduce nausea and vomiting caused by morphine-related drugs
- *Domperidone* – to reduce nausea and vomiting caused by anti-cancer drugs; may also be used to treat nausea and vomiting caused by levodopa or bromocriptine in the treatment of parkinsonism
- *Metoclopramide* – to reduce nausea and vomiting caused by anti-cancer drugs.

- *Nabilone* – to reduce nausea and vomiting caused by anti-cancer drugs
- *Ondansetron* – to reduce nausea and vomiting caused by anti-cancer drugs
- *Phenothiazines* (see Chapter 41) – to reduce nausea and vomiting caused by morphine-related drugs, anti-cancer drugs.

Vomiting *after an anaesthetic* is best treated with a phenothiazine drug or with metoclopramide.

Nausea and vomiting produced by *radiation treatment* for cancer are helped by phenothiazine drugs, metoclopramide, domperidone and particularly by ondansetron.

Metoclopramide and domperidone

In addition to blocking dopamine receptors in the brain, *metoclopramide* also blocks dopamine receptors in the throat, stomach and intestine. This effect on the stomach increases its emptying and closes the inlet to the stomach from the gullet (the oesophagus). This prevents vomiting. Like other dopamine blockers (e.g. the phenothiazines), it may produce harmful effects by affecting the part of the brain responsible for posture and involuntary movement. High doses may cause abnormal movements of the muscles in the face, tongue, eyes, neck and spine, particularly in children and young adults. They may also produce parkinsonism-like effects in elderly people. Metoclopramide should not be used to relieve vomiting after surgery on the intestine because of its effects on movements of the intestine.

Domperidone, which is related to metoclopramide, does not cause the drowsiness and abnormal involuntary movements that metoclopramide and the phenothiazines cause. This is because it does not easily cross from the bloodstream into the brain.

Nabilone

A synthetic cannabis drug, nabilone is effective in relieving the nausea and vomiting produced by anti-cancer drugs. It is not known how it works.

Ondansetron (U)

Nausea and vomiting associated with disease

Nausea and vomiting produced by disorders of the stomach, gall bladder, liver and kidney failure are helped by phenothiazines or haloperidol or a related drug (see Chapter 41). However, because metoclopramide acts on the intestine it is possibly better than the phenothiazines and haloperidol at relieving nausea and vomiting due to gastro-enteritis, liver disease or gall-bladder disease.

Nausea and vomiting of migraine

In a migraine attack the emptying of the stomach is slowed down, which may cause delayed absorption of pain relievers such as paracetamol. If metoclopramide is given as soon as possible in an attack, the emptying of the stomach is increased and if a pain-relieving drug is given its absorption from the intestine into the bloodstream is speeded up.

Vertigo

The main nerve to the ear (the auditory nerve) has two components – one concerned with hearing and one concerned with balance. Any damage to the latter will produce vertigo, which is a feeling of movement of the head or of things around you. The movement may be rotatory (you feel as if the room is spinning round you) or of displacement (e.g. the floor seems to come up at an angle). Vertigo makes you feel off balance and you have to hang on to something.

In addition to some abnormality in the main nerve, vertigo may also be caused by abnormalities in certain parts of the brain or in the eyes (e.g. double vision). However, the most common cause is in the organ of balance itself – the vestibular apparatus, part of which includes the labyrinth. We may therefore refer to disorders of the organ of balance as vestibular disorders or labyrinthine disorders.

Vertigo caused by disorders of the organ of balance is referred to as peripheral vertigo in order to distinguish it from some abnormality in the brain, which is referred to as central vertigo. Peripheral vertigo may be due to some abnormality within the labyrinth – for example, Ménière's disease and benign positional vertigo. These account for about 75 per cent of all attacks of vertigo. Other cases of vertigo are due to some factor affecting the labyrinth – such as drugs, anaemia, low blood sugar, low blood pressure, virus infections or local damage caused by a middle ear disease.

Ménière's disease usually affects only one ear but can affect both. It comes on between the ages of 30 and 60. It is characterized by attacks of severe vertigo, associated with deafness and tinnitus (noises in the ear); the tinnitus in Ménière's is usually a low-pitched roaring noise. Attacks usually come in clusters and then there is a period free of attacks when balance is normal. Attacks can last for several hours and be so severe as to cause nausea and vomiting. Hearing tends to improve during periods free from attacks but over time hearing loss may get progressively worse and can become severe.

Benign positional vertigo is provoked by movements of the head. Each attack lasts for only a few seconds and there is no hearing loss. The cause may be a virus infection, injury or degeneration of the organ with age. Attacks usually stop after a few weeks or months.

Sudden vestibular failure occurs when one labyrinth stops working. There are several possible causes, which include a virus infection (e.g. shingles); there is sudden and severe vertigo, nausea and vomiting, but no hearing loss or noises in the ear (tinnitus). The vertigo persists for days or weeks and is made worse by movements of the head.

Migraine may cause episodes of vertigo similar to Ménière's disease. It is due to spasm of the arteries at the back of the neck and can be associated with dimness of vision, difficulty in talking, pins and needles in the hands and feet, and headache at the back of the head. These attacks may also occur in elderly people whose arteries are 'hardened', particularly the ones at the back of the neck which supply the back part of the brain.

Treatment of vertigo

Drugs used to treat nausea and vomiting are also used to treat vertigo. They include hyoscine, which is an anticholinergic drug, certain antihistamine drugs (e.g. cinnarizine and cyclizine) and phenothiazine drugs (e.g. chlorpromazine, prochlorperazine and thiethylperazine). Betahistine is a drug related to histamine. It is claimed that it reduces the pressure inside the organ of balance. It is used specifically to treat Ménière's disease. Other drugs include vasodilator drugs such as nicotinic acid, to improve the blood supply to the organ of balance, and diuretics, to reduce the pressure of the fluid inside the labyrinth.

There is no cure for vertigo and no drug will abort an acute attack of vertigo. During an acute attack you should keep absolutely still, and an injection or a suppository of chlorpromazine, prochlorperazine or thiethylperazine will help.

To try to reduce the number and severity of attacks of vertigo it is a matter of choosing what suits you the most. Some patients may swear by betahistine or cinnarizine, and others by prochlorperazine; it is therefore worth trying different drugs but remember that there is no cure and all the drugs do is to reduce the severity of the symptoms. This has to be balanced against the harmful effects that the drugs may produce.

Table 14.1 Drugs used to treat nausea, vomiting, motion sickness and vertigo – harmful effects and warnings*

Harmful effects

betahistine
Nausea, stomach upsets, headache, skin rash.

hyoscine
Dry mouth, drowsiness, blurred vision, constipation, difficulty in passing urine, dry skin, rapid beating of the heart, dizziness, confusion, allergic skin rashes and red eyes, impaired attention and alertness, hallucinations, agitation and disorientation (especially in children and the elderly).

antihistamines
The most common harmful effect is drowsiness. Rarely, they may cause excitement, nervousness, tremor and insomnia. They may also produce dry mouth, blurred vision, constipation and difficulty in passing urine. For other potential harmful effects see antihistamines, Chapter 10.

phenothiazines
Drowsiness, dry mouth, blocked nose, constipation, fall in blood pressure. For other potential harmful effects see Chapter 41.

metoclopramide
High doses produce abnormal movements, particularly in children and young adults. They may include spasm of the tongue, lip, face, eyelids, muscles of the arms and legs, muscles of the back and head. The majority of such reactions come on within 36 hours of starting treatment and the effects usually disappear within 24 hours of stopping the drug. Patients on prolonged treatment, particularly elderly patients, may occasionally develop parkinsonism and, rarely, a serious disorder of movement called tardive dyskinesia (see Chapter 41). It may cause enlargement of the breasts and milk to come from the breasts in both men and women because it increases the blood level of prolactin (see Chapter 60).

domperidone
Milk from the breasts and enlargement of the breasts in both men and women may occur because it increases the blood level of prolactin (see Chapter 60).

nabilone
Most common is drowsiness. Other reported harmful effects include dizziness, fall in blood pressure on standing up after lying or sitting down, rapid beating of the heart; dry mouth, vertigo, decreased appetite, cramps in the abdomen, confusion, headaches, blurred vision, depression, tremors, poor concentration and co-ordination, mood changes and hallucinations. Addiction to the drug develops with prolonged regular use.

Warnings

betahistine
Individuals with asthma or peptic ulcers should use this with caution. It should not be used by people with a phaeochromocytoma.

hyoscine
Should not be used by people with glaucoma and with caution by people who have difficulty passing urine (e.g. with an enlarged prostate gland), heart disease, narrowing of the outlet of the stomach

* For Ondansetron see Update.

Table 14.1 Drugs used to treat nausea, vomiting, motion sickness and vertigo – harmful effects and warnings (*cont.*)

(pyloric stenosis) or paralysis of the small bowel (paralytic ileus).

antihistamines
Should be used with caution by people with impaired liver function, enlarged prostate gland, glaucoma or low blood pressure. For other warnings, see antihistamines, in Chapter 10.

phenothiazines
See warnings on the use of anti-psychotic drugs in Chapter 41.

metoclopramide
Daily doses should be increased gradually and should not exceed 500 mg/kg of body weight. The dose should be reduced in anyone with impaired kidney function. Do not use for 3–4 days after surgery on the intestine. It should be used with caution in children and by young adults and elderly people.

domperidone
Should not be used to treat chronic nausea and vomiting or as a routine to treat vomiting after surgical operations. The dose should be reduced in people with impaired kidney function.

nabilone
Should not be used by people who are allergic to it or to a related drug, nor by people with severe liver disease because the drug is excreted primarily in the bile.

Risks in elderly people Hyoscine, antihistamines, phenothiazines, metoclopramide and nabilone should be used with caution by elderly people because harmful effects may be more frequent and severe. If you are 60 years of age or over, refer to Chapter 82.

Risks in pregnancy If you are pregnant or thinking of becoming pregnant, refer to Chapter 79.

Risks in breast feeding If you are breast feeding and need to take a drug to relieve nausea, vomiting, motion sickness or vertigo, refer to Chapter 80.

Risks in driving Antihistamines, phenothiazines metoclopramide and nabilone may affect your ability to drive, so do not drive until you know that it is safe to do so. The dangers are increased by alcohol, anti-anxiety drugs, sleeping drugs and anti-psychotic drugs. Hyoscine may occasionally cause confusion, in which case you should not drive. See also Chapter 88.

Risks with alcohol Antihistamines, phenothiazines, metoclopramide and nabilone may increase the effects of alcohol; therefore do not drink alcohol when taking any of these drugs.

NOTE Warnings on driving also refer to the operation of moving machinery, any hazardous occupation (e.g. working at heights), hazardous sports or flying an aircraft.

Table 14.2 Preparations used to treat nausea, vomiting, motion sickness and vertigo

Preparation	*Drug*	*Drug group*	*Dosage form*
Avomine	promethazine	Antihistamine	Tablets
Buccastem	prochlorperazine	phenothiazine	Tablets for dissolving under the tongue
Cesamet	nabilone	Cannabis-related	Capsules
chlorpromazine	chlorpromazine	Phenothiazine	Tablets, elixir
Dramamine	dimenhydrinate	Antihistamine	Tablets
Fentazin	perphenazine	Phenothiazine	Tablets, injections

Table 14.2 Preparations used to treat nausea, vomiting, motion sickness and vertigo (*cont.*)

Preparation	*Drug*	*Drug group*	*Dosage form*
Gastrese LA	metoclopramide	Antidopamine	Sustained-release tablets
Gastrobid Continus	metoclopramide	Antidopamine	Sustained-release tablets
Gastroflux	metoclopramide	Antidopamine	Tablets
Gastromax	metoclopramide	Antidopamine	Sustained-release capsules
hyoscine	hyoscine	Anticholinergic	Tablets, injection
Joy-rides	hyoscine	Anticholinergic	Tablets
Kwells	hyoscine	Anticholinergic	Tablets
Largactil	chlorpromazine	Phenothiazine	Tablets, elixir, injection
Marzine	cinnarizine	Antihistamine	Tablets
Maxolon	metoclopramide	Antidopamine	Tablets, paediatric liquid, syrup, injection
Maxolon High Dose	metoclopramide	Antidopamine	Injection
Maxolon SR	metoclopramide	Antidopamine	Sustained-release capsules
metoclopramide	metoclopramide	Antidopamine	Tablets
Metox	metoclopramide	Antidopamine	Tablets
Motilium	domperidone	Antidopamine	Tablets, suspension, suppositories
Parmid	metoclopramide	Antidopamine	Tablets, syrup
Paxadon	pyridoxine (vitamin B_6)	Vitamin	Tablets
Phenergan	promethazine	Antihistamine	Tablets, elixir, injection
Primperan	metoclopramide	Antidopamine	Tablets, syrup, injection
Scopoderm	hyoscine	Anticholinergic	Self-adhesive patch
Sea-legs	meclozine	Antihistamine	Tablets
Serc	betahistine	Histamine-related	Tablets
Stelazine	trifluoperazine	Phenothiazine	Tablets, sustained-release capsules (spansules)
Stemetil	prochlorperazine	Phenothiazine	Tablets, syrup, injection, suppositories
Stugeron	cinnarizine	Antihistamine	Tablets
Torecan	thiethylperazine	Phenothiazine	Tablets, injection, suppositories
Valoid	cyclizine	Antihistamine	Tablets, injection
Vertigon	prochlorperazine	Phenothiazine	Sustained-release capsules (spansules)

15

Indigestion and peptic ulcers

The upper and middle parts of the stomach act as a reservoir for food; the part near its outlet into the duodenum contracts and relaxes to churn and mix the food. The rate of emptying of the stomach varies with the volume of contents: the greater the volume, the faster the rate of emptying. A fatty meal delays emptying; so does an increase in stomach acidity. Some drugs increase and some decrease the rate of emptying of the stomach. Another important function of the stomach is to make digestive juice. This contains hydrochloric acid (about one and a half litres are produced every day), mucus, which protects the surface of the stomach, and an enzyme called pepsin which helps to digest protein in food.

Indigestion and dyspepsia

'Indigestion' and 'dyspepsia' are terms used to describe symptoms relating to eating. They include discomfort in the stomach, feeling full after food, belching, heartburn, nausea, loss of appetite and vomiting.

Indigestion is usually related to eating something that has upset your stomach (e.g. spicy foods), coffee, alcohol, or over-eating, smoking or anxiety. Aspirin or other anti-inflammatory drugs, corticosteroids and iron preparations may cause indigestion in some people.

Treatment of indigestion

An attack of acute indigestion usually lasts for a few days and it will help recovery if you stop smoking, stop drinking alcohol (particularly spirits) and reduce the amount of coffee and tea that you drink. Eat small regular meals and avoid food that upsets your stomach.

Antacids (see later) are effective in relieving the symptoms of indigestion; however, if the indigestion persists for more than a week or two it may be due to gastritis, acid reflux (see later) a peptic ulcer or gall bladder trouble, and you should have a medical check-up. If it is caused by the drugs you are taking, some alternative drug treatment should be considered by your doctor. *Never treat yourself for 'indigestion' for more than 2 weeks without seeking medical advice.*

Gastritis

Acute gastritis is an acute irritation and inflammation of the lining of the stomach. It is commonly caused by anti-inflammatory drugs (e.g. aspirin) and alcohol. It may produce no symptoms or it may produce nausea, pain, loss of appetite and heartburn. The treatment is to stop drinking alcohol; if it is due to the drugs you are taking, you may need to take the drug with or after food and/or reduce the dose or stop the drug.

Chronic gastritis may be caused by an auto-immune response, and may be associated with pernicious anaemia. There may be circulating antibodies to cells in the stomach lining. In some cases of chronic gastritis, bacteria have been identified (*Helicobacter pylori*), which can be confirmed by positive blood tests for antibodies against this micro-organism. Chronic gastritis may also occur in people who suffer from gastric ulcers (stomach ulcers), cancer of the stomach or in people who have had surgery on the stomach.

Chronic gastritis produces no symptoms and can be diagnosed only by X-ray (barium meal) or by examination using an instrument passed down the throat into the stomach (an endoscope). There is no specific treatment.

Peptic ulcers

The lining of the oesophagus (gullet), stomach and duodenum is covered with thick mucus which protects it from being attacked by the gastric juices. If this protective layer of mucus becomes damaged, the gastric juices may damage the underlying surface and cause an ulcer to develop. The term 'peptic ulcer' refers to ulcers in the lower end of the oesophagus (*oesophageal ulcers*), in the stomach (*gastric ulcers*) and in the duodenum (*duodenal ulcers*). Peptic ulcers occur in areas where gastric juices are present. This is why they may occur in the small intestine after surgical bypass operations of the duodenum, which allows the stomach contents to pass directly into it.

Relatively little is known about the factors that cause peptic ulcers but there is evidence that *acid* and *pepsin* in the gastric juice are principally responsible. Patients with duodenal ulcers appear to produce excessive amounts of acid and pepsin but this is not the case in patients with stomach ulcers. 'Normal' stomachs and duodenums do not develop ulcers. Therefore, the 'normal' lining must protect itself from being damaged by the acid and digested by the pepsin (an enzyme that digests protein in food). It may be something affecting this protection that predisposes certain people to develop ulcers. This protection may be related to the thick mucus that covers the surface, the ability of the lining cells of the stomach to renew themselves every few days, the nutrition of the stomach itself, its blood supply and various chemical factors. There are also other factors which may be associated with peptic ulcers such as heredity (there is often a family history), the season (there is a higher incidence in spring and autumn), drinking coffee, something in the diet, smoking, drinking alcohol, and also worry and stress (including physical stress such as burns, injury and surgery).

Peptic ulcers may cause pain, vomiting and loss of appetite. Pain from a duodenal ulcer often comes on when you are hungry and it wakes you in the night; whereas a stomach ulcer pain may come on fairly soon after food. Pain from an oesophageal ulcer may come on immediately on eating or drinking. However, pain from the various types of peptic ulcer is generally not that clear cut. Peptic ulcers may fail to cause pain or indigestion and, paradoxically, patients may develop pain and indigestion without evidence of an ulcer (non-ulcer indigestion).

Food or antacids (see later) usually relieve peptic ulcer pains. The ulcers come and go; they may be severe for a few weeks or months and then disappear for weeks, months or even years. We do not know what causes these flare-ups and quiet periods, but we do know that predisposing risk factors include smoking, over-use of coffee and alcohol, lack of vitamin C, stress, irregular rushed meals and certain drugs (e.g. aspirin and non-steroidal anti-inflammatory drugs used to treat rheumatic disorders).

Peptic ulcer is a common disease that is showing signs of decline. The extent of the disease varies according to site (e.g. stomach, duodenum), age and sex. Duodenal ulcer is four to five times more common than gastric ulcer in men, and two to three times more common in women. Duodenal ulcer has a higher incidence in men than women (2 to 1) whereas gastric ulcer has the same incidence. Duodenal ulcers usually start between the ages of 25 and 55 years, whereas stomach ulcers usually start between 40 and 70 years of age.

Warnings *Many patients with cancer of the stomach develop indigestion, and about 2–5 per cent of stomach ulcers (not duodenal ulcers) may be due to cancer. The indigestion may be associated with loss of weight, loss of appetite and blood in the motions. Although cancer of the stomach is comparatively rare when you look at the number of people who suffer from stomach ulcers, it is none the less important not to self-treat indigestion for more than a week or two without seeking medical advice. It is also important not to take treatments (see later) that are effective at relieving symptoms and healing ulcers without a thorough medical check-up, because this may delay the proper diagnosis of the underlying cause of the symptoms.*

Complications of peptic ulcers

These occur much more frequently with duodenal ulcers than gastric ulcers.

Bleeding A peptic ulcer may penetrate into a blood vessel and produce bleeding. This may result in the vomiting of blood (haematemesis) and/or blood in the motions (melaena). Aspirin and other anti-inflammatory drugs, and corticosteroids can produce acute ulcers which may bleed.

Perforation of the base of an ulcer through the wall of the stomach (or duodenum) may occur. This causes the contents of the stomach or duodenum to empty through the hole into the cavity of the abdomen (the peritoneal cavity), to produce a severe state of shock. Perforation occurs more frequently with duodenal ulcers than with stomach ulcers (gastric ulcers).

Obstruction may occur at the outlet from the stomach, due to scarring of an ulcer which narrows the outlet (stenosis). This is called pyloric stenosis.

Drugs used to treat peptic ulcers

Drugs relieve symptoms and can help to heal ulcers. No drug can cure the tendency for some people to develop peptic ulcers, but the regular use of drugs may help to prevent them in some individuals.

The main drugs used to treat peptic ulcers fall into three groups – drugs that neutralize the acid in the stomach (antacids), drugs that reduce the production of acid by the stomach cells and drugs that help to protect the stomach lining.

Drugs that neutralize the acid in the stomach – antacids

Antacids (anti-acids) have a dramatic and instant effect in relieving the pain produced by peptic ulcers and indigestion, and the pain produced by acid reflux into the oesophagus (heartburn). They neutralize the acid that is present in the stomach, and cause a reduction in its production. At high concentrations there is evidence that they also decrease the activity of pepsin. However, it is important to note that, if they only partially neutralize the acid in the stomach, they may actually cause an increase in pepsin activity. Therefore, it is important to take antacids in a high enough dose to neutralize as much of the acid as possible. In other words, if the instructions on the product say take two tablets, it could make the symptoms worse if you take only one tablet.

By neutralizing the acid in the stomach, antacids help to reduce inflammation and relieve pain. They also allow the damaged lining of the stomach to heal by preventing it from being attacked by acid and pepsin, and they therefore help ulcers to heal.

Neutralization of the acid in the stomach also causes the muscles around the junction of the oesophagus with the stomach (oesophageal sphincter) to contract. This helps to prevent reflux of the acid stomach contents up into the oesophagus. Antacids may also mop up bile acids, which are very irritant and can enter the stomach from the duodenum and wash up into the oesophagus.

The duration of action of antacids depends upon how fast the stomach empties. If the stomach is empty, an antacid will work for about half an hour; if it is taken about 1 hour after a meal it will work for up to 2 hours, and if another dose is taken after 3 hours its effects will last up to 4 hours after a meal. Some antacids increase and some decrease the muscular movements of the stomach and intestine; for example, magnesium compounds cause diarrhoea whereas aluminium compounds cause constipation.

Rebound acid production

As the effects of a dose of an antacid begin to wear off the stomach can respond by producing more acid than before. With most antacids this rebound production of acid lasts for only a short period of time but with calcium antacids it can be prolonged and intense. You will get initial relief of pain followed by an increase in the pain. They stimulate the release of gastrin, a stomach hormone that triggers the production of acid and pepsin.

Do antacids help to heal peptic ulcers?

Antacids taken in appropriate doses relieve the pain of uncomplicated peptic ulcers whether in the oesophagus, stomach or duodenum; they also relieve the symptoms of acid reflux. Whether antacids promote healing of peptic ulcers is a matter of debate. There is evidence that, if antacids are taken in sufficiently high doses at regular intervals, healing of duodenal ulcers can occur after about 4 weeks of treatment. The use of low doses at very frequent intervals (e.g. seven or eight times a day) may also have a beneficial effect on healing of duodenal ulcers. The long-term regular daily use of high doses of antacids can also prevent relapse but this is not recommended because of the risks (see later).

Antacids are not as beneficial in healing stomach ulcers as they are in healing duodenal ulcers. This may be because increased acid production is less frequent in people suffering from stomach ulcers than it is in those who suffer from duodenal ulcers. In fact, some people suffering from stomach ulcers may have normal or even low acid production. Even so, they appear to do well on a drug that reduces acid production (see later).

Antacids are effective at relieving the pain and symptoms of acid reflux (e.g. caused by a hiatus hernia) but whether they heal peptic ulcers in the oesophagus (gullet) is open to question.

Change of fashion

With the introduction of drugs that effectively block acid production (see later), antacids have gone very much out of fashion for treating peptic ulcers and chronic indigestion. They are still of course purchased in huge quantities from chemists and drug stores for the treatment of *acute indigestion* because they are very effective at relieving pain whether it is due to an ulcer or not.

Dangers of absorption of antacids into the bloodstream

The principal risk of regular daily use of antacids is the absorption of chemicals (e.g. magnesium, bismuth, aluminium) into the bloodstream, which, if they accumulate in the body over time, may be harmful. They may also cause problems in the short term; for example, the absorption of sodium may be harmful to people being treated for raised blood pressure or heart failure, in people with impaired liver or kidney function or in pregnant women. Furthermore, the absorption of very soluble antacids (e.g. sodium bicarbonate) may change the acidity of the blood.

Any antacid may cause a problem if taken regularly every day in high doses for a prolonged period of time, especially in people who are unable to excrete the absorbed chemicals effectively in their urine because they suffer from some disorder of their kidneys.

The risk from absorption of antacids into the bloodstream varies with how soluble the antacid is. *Sodium bicarbonate* reacts rapidly with the acid in the stomach to produce salt (sodium chloride), water and carbon dioxide gas. The salt is quickly absorbed, and the carbon dioxide may cause belching and distend the stomach, producing pain.

Calcium carbonate also reacts quickly with the acid in the stomach. Some of it is converted to a soluble calcium salt, which is absorbed into the blood-stream and may lead to a rise in the concentration of calcium in the blood.

If used in high doses over a prolonged period of time, the rise in blood calcium may result in the formation of kidney stones and damage to the kidneys.

When sodium bicarbonate is used along with milk and/or a calcium antacid, particularly in someone with impaired kidney function, the resulting effects are a decreased acidity of the blood (alkalosis) and a raised blood calcium level. This may produce what is called the milk–alkali syndrome – nausea, vomiting, headache, mental confusion and loss of appetite. Similar harmful effects may occur if calcium antacids are taken regularly every day over a prolonged period of time.

Aluminium hydroxide preparations vary in their solubility and their ability to neutralize acid in the stomach. If used over a prolonged period in people with impaired functioning of their kidneys, some aluminium may be absorbed and accumulate in the body, to produce toxic effects.

Magnesium hydroxide (milk of magnesia) reacts quickly with the acid in the stomach, and a small amount of the magnesium salt produced may be absorbed into the bloodstream. If used over a prolonged period of time the magnesium will accumulate in the body to produce toxic effects, particularly in people with impaired functioning of their kidneys.

Harmful effects of antacids on the stomach and intestine

Wind and distension Antacids containing sodium bicarbonate or calcium carbonate react with the acid in the stomach to produce carbon dioxide gas. This may give you wind and cause distension of the stomach and pain.

Increase in stomach acid There is a suggestion that calcium salts may actually increase the acidity of the stomach, and because of this possibility it is best not to take antacids that contain calcium salts.

Diarrhoea and constipation Antacids containing aluminium react with the acid in the stomach to produce salts that cause constipation, and antacids containing magnesium react to produce salts that cause diarrhoea. This is why antacids often contain a mixture of both aluminium and magnesium in order to balance the potential risk of diarrhoea with the potential risk of constipation.

Reduced phosphate absorption Aluminium salts decrease the absorption of phosphates into the bloodstream by binding to them in the intestine. A low blood level of phosphate may cause loss of appetite, muscle weakness and a general feeling of being unwell (malaise). It also causes release of calcium from bone, which results in increased excretion of calcium in the urine, leading to bone softening (osteoporosis). The low level of blood phosphate may also interfere with the use of vitamin D by the body, adding to the risk of bone softening.

A low blood phosphate may follow the long-term regular daily use of antacids containing aluminium salts but sometimes it may develop after only a few weeks of treatment, particularly in elderly people, in people on a low phosphate diet or in people suffering from diarrhoea. Alcoholics also appear to be at risk of developing a low blood phosphate level from taking antacids containing aluminium salts. Prolonged use of these antacids may also cause loss of calcium.

Magnesium–aluminium combinations The total neutralizing effect of magnesium–aluminium combinations is roughly equal to both the constituents added together. They have the potential for producing any of the harmful effects produced by aluminium salts and magnesium salts. They may cause accumulation of both magnesium and aluminium in the body in people suffering from kidney failure, and the aluminium may also cause a low blood phosphate level (see above). They produce less risk of diarrhoea due to the magnesium or of constipation due to aluminium, although diarrhoea still seems to occur.

Recommendations on the use of antacids

Antacids relieve the symptoms produced by peptic ulcers, indigestion not caused by an ulcer and symptoms caused by acid reflux (heartburn).

Many antacid preparations contain sodium. These should be avoided if you suffer from raised blood pressure or heart failure, impaired kidney or liver function or in pregnancy.

Sodium bicarbonate should not be used except for a very occasional single dose.

Antacids containing calcium salts should not be used.

Antacids containing aluminium salts may produce constipation, and those containing magnesium salts may produce diarrhoea; therefore, to avoid bowel trouble, it may help to use an antacid that contains both so that their effects balance each other.

Magnesium and aluminium salts are relatively insoluble in water and act for a fairly long time if they are kept in the stomach; therefore they should be taken 1–3 hours after food.

Aluminium–magnesium combinations may produce diarrhoea or constipation, but less than if each is taken separately. Avoid their long-term use because of the risk of bone softening (see earlier).

There is no convincing evidence from adequate and well controlled studies that complexes such as alexitol sodium, almasilate and hydrotalcite are any more effective than an ordinary aluminium and magnesium antacid mixture.

Antacids should only be used to treat acute symptoms of a peptic ulcer. Without medical advice, they should not be taken regularly every day in order to prevent peptic ulcers from flaring up.

A full recommended dose of an antacid should be taken 1 hour after meals and repeated in 2–3 hours (this will neutralize the acid for up to 3–4 hours). A dose should also be taken at bed-time.

Antacids should not be taken at the same time as some other drugs because the antacids may impair their absorption (see Chapter 89). Allow 2 hours between dosings.

Antacids may damage the special coating on tablets designed to resist the acid of the stomach and to release their drug in the intestine. These preparations are called enteric coated and they should be taken either 2 hours before or 2 hours after antacids.

Available antacid preparations vary enormously both in price and in their ability to neutralize the acid in the stomach and therefore to relieve symptoms.

Liquid preparations work more effectively than tablets.

Drugs that reduce the production of acid in the stomach – anticholinergic drugs

These drugs are discussed in detail in Chapter 2. One of their effects is to block those nerves in the stomach which when stimulated cause the production of gastric juices and an increase in the muscular movements of the stomach and intestine. They therefore reduce the production of acid and reduce pain caused by spasm of the muscles in the wall of the stomach.

Belladonna (from deadly nightshade) and related drugs obtained from plants have been used for years to treat peptic ulcers. They are usually mixed with antacids. Despite their popularity over the decades the gap between their ability to block acid production effectively and their harmful effects is very narrow. They easily produce blurred vision, dry mouth, constipation, difficulty in passing urine and rapid beating of the heart. These harmful effects appear with doses that produce only a mild effect in blocking acid

Table 15.1 Additives in antacid preparations

Additive	*Comments*
Sugars	Antacids containing sugars may cause tooth decay if taken regularly every day over long periods of time, particularly as they are taken between meals. They may also cause problems for diabetic patients
Dimethicone	This is a silicone used as an anti-foaming agent which lowers surface tension so that small bubbles of gas coalesce into large bubbles which help you to belch. It also helps to stop the acid contents of the stomach from frothing up into the oesophagus and causing heartburn. Activated dimethicone is a mixture of liquid dimethicone containing finely divided silicone dioxide which increases its anti-foaming properties
Oxethazaine	This is a local anaesthetic the effectiveness of which in relieving the pain of acid reflux has not been clearly demonstrated. It is included in Mucaine
Alginic acid	Alginic acid or its salts (alginates) are obtained from algae. They work as suspending or thickening agents, and, mixed with antacids, they float to the top of the stomach contents to form a raft that protects the lining. They are used to treat heartburn. NOTE Dimethicone and alginic acid produce opposite effects.
Bismuth	Bismuth salts are not effective antacids and tend to cause constipation. They may be absorbed into the bloodstream and damage the brain (see Chapter 46). They should not be used. This warning does not apply to bismuth complex (e.g. De-Nol)

Warning *Antacid preparations that contain an anticholinergic drug (e.g. belladonna, atropine, homatropine) and/or a sedative (e.g. phenobarbitone) and/or an anti-anxiety drug (e.g. chlordiazepoxide) should not be used. This is because the dose of each constituent drug cannot be changed without changing the dose of all the other drugs in the preparation.*

production. Therefore, a dose of a belladonna preparation that does not produce these harmful effects (which are not acceptable) is unlikely to have any benefit in reducing acid production.

Synthetic anticholinergic drugs (e.g. dicyclomine, poldine, propantheline) produce fewer harmful effects than anticholinergics obtained from plants, particularly on the brain. Nevertheless, at doses high enough to reduce acid production they also produce harmful effects.

Dangers of anticholinergic drugs in elderly people

The harmful effects produced by anticholinergic drugs obtained from plants (e.g. belladonna, atropine) may be particularly damaging to elderly people because they can affect the brain, producing drowsiness and confusion.

Table 15.2 Antacid preparations

Preparation	*Mineral in antacid*	*Other main active ingredients*	*Dosage form*
Actonorm	aluminium, magnesium	dimethicone	Gel
alexitol	aluminium		Tablets
Algicon	aluminium, magnesium	alginate	Tablets, suspension
almasilate	aluminium, magnesium		Suspension
Altacite Plus*	aluminium, magnesium	activated dimethicone	Tablets, suspension
Alu-Cap	aluminium (low sodium)		Capsules
Aludrox	aluminium		Gel
Aludrox Tablets	aluminium, magnesium		Tablets
Aludrox SA	aluminium, magnesium	ambutonium	Suspension
Aluhyde	aluminium, magnesium	belladonna	Tablets
aluminium hydroxide	aluminium		Tablets, mixture
aluminium hydroxide and belladonna mixture	aluminium	belladonna	Mixture
Andursil	aluminium, magnesium	activated dimethicone	Tablets, suspension
APP Consolidated	aluminium, bismuth, calcium, magnesium	homatropine, papaverine	Powder, tablets
Asilone	aluminium, magnesium	activated dimethicone	Suspension
Asilone tablets	aluminium	activated dimethicone	Tablets
Bellocarb	magnesium	belladonna	Tablets
Carbellon	magnesium	belladonna, peppermint oil charcoal (adsorbent)	Tablets
Dijex	aluminium, magnesium		Tablets, liquid
Diovol	aluminium, magnesium	dimethicone	Suspension
Gastrils	aluminium, magnesium		Pastilles

*Generic name: co-simalcite.

Table 15.2 Antacid preparations (*cont.*)

Preparation	*Mineral in antacid*	*Other main active ingredients*	*Dosage form*
Gastrocote	aluminium, magnesium, sodium	alginic acid	Tablets, suspension
Gastron	aluminium, magnesium, sodium	alginic acid	Tablets
Gaviscon	aluminium, magnesium, sodium	alginic acid	Tablets, infant powder
Gaviscon Liquid	sodium, calcium	sodium alginate	Liquid
Gelusil	aluminium, magnesium (low sodium)		Tablets
hydrotalcite	aluminium, magnesium		Suspension, tablets
Kolanticon	aluminium, magnesium	dicyclomine, activated dimethicone	Gel
Maalox	aluminium, magnesium		Tablets, suspension
Maalox Plus	aluminium, magnesium	activated dimethicone	Suspension, tablets
Maalox TC	aluminium, magnesium (low sodium)		Suspension, tablets
magaldrate	aluminium, magnesium		Suspension
magnesium carbonate	magnesium		Mixture, aromatic mixture
magnesium carbonate tablets (compound)	calcium, magnesium, sodium		Tablets
magnesium hydroxide	magnesium		Mixture
magnesium trisilicate tablets (compound)	aluminium, magnesium		Tablets
magnesium trisilicate mixture	magnesium, sodium		Mixture
magnesium trisilicate powder (compound)	magnesium, calcium		Powder
magnesium trisilicate and belladonna mixture	magnesium	belladonna	Mixture

Table 15.2 Antacid preparations (*cont.*)

Preparation	*Mineral in antacid*	*Other main active ingredients*	*Dosage form*
Malinal	aluminium, magnesium		Suspension
Mucaine	aluminium, magnesium	oxethazaine	Suspension
Mucogel	aluminium, magnesium (low sodium)		Tablets, suspension
Nulacin	magnesium	whole milk solids with dextrins and maltose	Tablets
Formula	magnesium (low sodium)		
Polycrol and Polycrol Forte	aluminium, magnesium	activated dimethicone	Tablets, gel
Pyrogastrone	aluminium, magnesium, sodium	carbenoxolone (anti-ulcer drug), alginic acid	Tablets
Pyrogastrone Liquid	sodium, aluminium, potassium	carbenoxolone (anti-ulcer drug)	Liquid
Rabro	calcium, magnesium	deglycrrhinized liquorice (anti-ulcer drug), frangula	Tablets
Roter	bismuth, magnesium, sodium	frangula	Tablets
Siloxyl	aluminium	activated dimethicone	Tablets
Siloxyl suspension	aluminium, magnesium	activated dimethicone	Suspension
Simeco	aluminium, magnesium	activated dimethicone	Tablets, suspension
sodium bicarbonate	sodium		Powder, compound tablets, paediatric mixture
Topal	aluminium, magnesium	alginic acid	Tablets
Unigest	aluminium	dimethicone	Tablets

Also, in elderly men who may suffer from an enlarged prostate gland, these drugs may so interfere with their ability to pass urine that they develop retention of urine and have to have the urine removed by catheter. In people who are prone to develop glaucoma (most of whom are elderly) these drugs may trigger an acute attack of glaucoma by producing dilatation of the pupils, which affects the drainage of fluid from the front chamber of the eye.

Because anticholinergic drugs block the nerves that normally exercise a slowing effect on the heart, they may produce rapid beating of the heart (tachycardia) which can be harmful in people who are suffering from heart disease. They also block nerves in the walls of the intestine and produce decreased muscular movements, which may cause constipation.

Although the synthetic anticholinergic drugs (e.g. dicyclomine, poldine, propantheline) are less likely to produce harmful effects on the brain, they may none the less cause constipation, difficulty in passing urine and affect the pressure of fluid in the eye (see risks of glaucoma, Chapter 35). They too should be used with utmost caution in elderly people.

Anticholinergic drugs may make acid reflux worse

Anticholinergic drugs relax the muscles at the entry of the oesophagus into the stomach (the oesophageal sphincter). This may make it easier for the acid stomach contents to wash up (reflux) into the oesophagus, which may aggravate the symptoms of reflux oesophagitis (e.g. heartburn) which occurs in disorders such as hiatus hernia.

Recommendations on the use of anticholinergic drugs

Indigestion mixtures that contain an antacid and an anticholinergic drug should not be used. The dose of one cannot be changed without changing the dose of the other, and if high doses of such a mixture are taken the dose of the anticholinergic drug may be sufficient to produce harmful effects (see earlier).

Anticholinergic drugs should not be used in people who suffer from acid reflux. Belladonna and related anticholinergics obtained from plants should not be used to treat indigestion or peptic ulcers because their potential harmful effects outweigh any possible benefit. A synthetic anticholinergic drug (e.g. poldine) may occasionally be beneficial at bed-time in order to delay emptying of the stomach during the night and to prolong the retention of an antacid in the stomach; this will give the antacid a longer time to work through the night. However, such treatment has generally been replaced by the use of an H_2 blocker at bed-time.

A selective-acting anticholinergic drug – pirenzepine (*Gastrozepin*)

The anticholinergic drugs are not selective in their actions and they produce unwanted effects on the brain, eyes, bladder, intestine, heart and many other parts of the body. Pirenzepine is an anticholinergic drug that is much more selective in reducing acid and pepsin production by the stomach. It produces fewer effects on other organs, particularly on the brain because it does not cross easily from the bloodstream into the brain. In addition to blocking acid and pepsin production, it may cause an increase in the production of bicarbonate, which is normally produced to neutralize the acid. Pirenzepine may also increase mucus production in the stomach, which in 'normal' stomachs acts as a protective coat to prevent the stomach juices from digesting its lining.

Pirenzepine is not a first drug of choice for treating peptic ulcers, although it has been shown to be as effective as the H_2 blocker cimetidine for treating stomach and duodenal ulcers; it can also be used with an H_2 blocker in patients who fail to respond to an H_2 blocker on its own.

Drugs that block the production of acid in the stomach – H_2 blockers

Histamine is one of several chemicals that are released in allergic reactions and injury. It is also involved in controlling the production of gastric juices by the stomach and it acts as a chemical messenger in the brain.

It has always been recognized that antihistamines do not block all the actions of histamine – in particular, they do not block the production of acid in the stomach. However, it was not until the 1970s that it was clearly demonstrated that there are two types of receptors to histamine in the body. Those histamine receptors that are blocked by the traditional antihistamines that relieve allergic symptoms are now labelled H_1 receptors and those that are blocked by drugs such as cimetidine and ranitidine (see later) are called H_2 receptors. The latter discovery has completely revolutionized the treatment of peptic ulcers.

H_2 blockers (H_2 receptor blockers or H_2 antagonists)

H_2 blockers (of which cimetidine was the first to be used successfully) block H_2 nerve receptors in the stomach which histamine normally stimulates in order to produce stomach juices (which includes acid). They also block the effects of the hormone gastrin, which is produced by cells in the stomach and which also stimulates the production of stomach juices. This double effect in blocking the production of stomach juices is added to by their further action in blocking the continuing effects that histamine normally has upon the production of stomach juices.

H_2 blockers stop the production of stomach juices in fasting individuals and in the night when they are asleep. They also block stomach juice production that occurs merely with the thought of food, and that produced by caffeine (e.g. in coffee and tea) and by insulin. They reduce the volume of stomach juice produced as well as its concentration of acid. The production of both pepsin and acid is therefore reduced by H_2 blockers, and it is these that are the principal factors in producing peptic ulcers.

The reduction of acid production by H_2 blockers has been shown in animals to protect them from stomach ulceration induced by stress (e.g. severe burns, head injury) and by aspirin and other anti-inflammatory drugs.

Use of H_2 blockers H_2 blockers are very effective in treating people suffering from duodenal ulcers because most of these individuals produce too much acid – not only when eating but also when fasting and in the night. By blocking acid production these drugs relieve symptoms in 1–2 weeks, and produce healing of duodenal ulcers in most patients within 4–8 weeks of regular daily treatment. They are not nearly as effective in producing healing of stomach ulcers because they may occur in the presence of normal acid production or even no acid production.

H_2 blockers are also useful for treating people suffering from acid reflux (e.g. heartburn) because they reduce the acidity of the reflux; for treating chronic indigestion without evidence of an ulcer (non-ulcer indigestion); and to prevent stomach ulcers caused by stress (e.g. which may follow severe burns or head injury) and by drugs such as aspirin and anti-rheumatic drugs. However, they do not cure the cause; they only help the ulcer to heal, and a large proportion of people develop a flare-up of their ulcer within 12 months of stopping treatment. The use of H_2 blockers in preventing relapse of peptic ulcers is discussed later.

Drugs that block the production of acid in the stomach – proton pump blockers

A complex physico-chemical process leads to the production of acid by the acid-producing cells of the stomach. This involves the exchange of nuclear particles (protons) along a chemical chain which is referred to as a proton pump. *Omeprazole* (Losec) blocks the final step of this process by blocking an enzyme. By doing this it reduces both the resting acid production (basal acid production) and the acid produced in response to food, etc. (stimulated acid production). The degree of this blockage is related to the dose used. An effective dose reduces acid production within 1 hour, and repeated in *once-daily* doses the drug reaches its maximum effect in about 4 days. Acid production returns to normal within a few days of the last dose. Omeprazole (Losec) produces more rapid and extensive healing than H_2 blockers but it is not recommended for maintenance treatment (see later).

Drugs that protect the stomach lining (cytoprotectives)

Sucralfate

Sucralfate is a complex of polyaluminium hydroxide and sulphated sucrose. It has a minimum effect in neutralizing acid in the stomach, but in the presence of acid it condenses into a sticky gel which settles on the base of peptic ulcers and protects them from acid and pepsin attack for several hours. It seems to stick more to duodenal ulcers than to stomach ulcers. It is not affected by food and antacids but protein in food sticks to it (adsorbs), to produce a further protective layer. It may also protect the stomach lining by encouraging the production of prostaglandins.

Sucralfate may cause constipation and it may interfere with the absorption of other drugs (see Chapter 89). Some aluminium is absorbed into the bloodstream, and sucralfate should be used with caution by people with kidney disease who may not be able to excrete aluminium effectively.

If given before meals, sucralfate is effective in relieving symptoms, producing healing of ulcers and preventing their recurrence. Duodenal ulcers heal better than gastric ulcers. It is considered just as good as H_2 blockers for healing peptic ulcers and for preventing relapses. However, when the drug is stopped, relapse of ulcers occurs sooner than with H_2 blockers.

Liquorice products

Liquorice wood has been included in herbal indigestion mixtures for centuries. But when, in 1948, crude powdered liquorice extracts were tried in people suffering from peptic ulcers it was found that about one in five people developed serious harmful effects, which included high blood pressure, irregular heart beat and muscle weakness. In the early 1960s, subsequent refinement produced two derivatives of liquorice which have since been used to treat peptic ulcers – these are carbenoxolone and deglycyrrhinized liquorice.

Carbenoxolone is effective in protecting the lining of the stomach and thus helping peptic ulcers to heal, but it may cause salt and water to build up in the body and a reduction in body potassium. In some people (particularly the elderly) these effects may result in weight gain and ankle swelling (due to oedema), a rise in blood pressure and heart failure.

The risks of using carbenoxolone outweigh its benefits in the elderly, in people with liver, kidney or heart disease and in people with raised blood pressure.

Deglycyrrhinized liquorice does not produce the harmful effects of carbenoxolone but it is also less effective. There are better alternatives.

Bismuth chelate

Bismuth chelate (tripotassium dicitratobismuthate, De-No, De-Noltab) is a complex bismuth compound which, in the presence of acid in the stomach, precipitates and forms a protective coating over ulcers and sticks to the base of the ulcers. It may protect the stomach lining by stimulating prostaglandin production, by blocking the effects of pepsin and by stimulating bicarbonate production to neutralize the acid. It may also kill bacteria that grow on peptic ulcers.* It is active only when the stomach contents are acid. Some bismuth is absorbed into the bloodstream and overdose in patients with impaired kidney function may cause harmful effects on the brain (encephalopathy), producing confusion, tremor and poor co-ordination of movements and also bone disorders. It blackens the motions and also makes the tongue black.

Bismuth chelate is effective in healing stomach and duodenal ulcers, and the healing is longer lasting than that produced by cimitidine. However, because of the potential dangers from the absorption of bismuth, its use should be restricted to short courses of about 1–2 months.

Prostaglandins

Misoprostol (Cytotec) is a synthetic prostaglandin that helps to protect the surface of the stomach. It stimulates production of mucus and sodium bicarbonate (the stomach's own antacid). It also reduces acid production and helps to control the flow of blood in the mucous lining of the stomach. Misoprostol helps to heal peptic ulcers. It is also used to heal and prevent ulcers caused by aspirin and non-steroidal anti-inflammatory drugs (NSAIDs). These drugs, which are used to treat rheumatoid arthritis and related disorders, block the production of prostaglandins, and their use is associated with ulceration of the stomach and intestine.

* Treatments using De-Nol and an antibiotic (e.g. metronidazole or ampicillin) are being investigated.

Table 15.3 Drugs used to heal peptic ulcers – harmful effects and warnings

bismuth chelate (De-Nol, De-Noltab)
Harmful effects include constipation, nausea and vomiting. It may cause black motions and a black tongue.

Warnings Bismuth chelate should not be used in people with severely impaired kidney function because bismuth may be absorbed into the blood and accumulate in the body, to affect the brain. Treatment

Table 15.3 Drugs used to heal peptic ulcers – harmful effects and warnings (*cont.*)

should be restricted to short courses of about 4–6 weeks.

Risks in elderly people It should be used with caution in elderly people because they may have impaired kidney function. Tests of kidney function should be carried out before treatment.

Milk should not be drunk on its own during treatment because it can stop bismuth chelate from working. Small amounts of milk in tea or coffee with meals or small amounts with cereals are permissible.

carbenoxolone (Biogastrone, Duogastrone, Pyrogastrone)
Harmful effects include the retention of sodium and water in the tissues, resulting in swelling of the tissues (e.g. ankle swelling), changes in the acidity of the blood (alkalosis), raised blood pressure and a fall in blood potassium levels.

Warnings Carbenoxolone should not be used in people with severe heart, kidney or liver failure or with a low blood potassium level. It should be used with caution in anyone in whom salt and water retention and/or a low blood potassium level could be harmful (e.g. those with heart failure, raised blood pressure, kidney disease or liver disease). Potassium supplements should be considered for those people at risk of developing a low blood potassium level. Anyone taking this treatment should be monitored regularly, including weight, blood pressure, tests of the blood chemistry particularly potassium levels and a check for fluid retention (e.g. ankle swelling). If the blood potassium falls, the drug should be stopped.

Risks in elderly people Harmful effects may be more frequent and severe; therefore it should be used with caution and in smaller doses.

cimetidine (Dyspamet, Tagamet)
Harmful effects are infrequent and usually mild. Transient diarrhoea, dizziness, skin rashes, tiredness, headache, painful joints and painful muscles may occur. Rarely, reversible mental confusion may occur, which includes agitation, depression, anxiety, hallucination and disorientation. These rare mental symptoms – which occur usually in elderly people and/or the very ill or in people with severe impaired kidney or liver function – come on within 2–3 days of starting treatment and clear up in a few days if the drug is stopped. Reversible enlargement of the breasts (gynaecomastia) may occur occasionally in both men and women after about 1 month's treatment. Very rarely, impotence has been reported when high doses are used over a prolonged period of time but not with standard dosage. Very rarely, kidney, pancreas or liver damage may occur, and damage to the bone marrow causing blood disorders. Fever and allergic reactions may, rarely, occur.

Warnings Should not use in individuals who are allergic to it. The dose should be reduced in anyone who suffers from impaired kidney or liver function. High doses by intravenous injection should not be used, particularly in people who have heart disease, because they may cause a disorder of heart rhythm.

deglycyrrhinized liquorice (Caved-S' Rabro)
Harmful effects include constipation.

Warnings It should be used with caution in people with impaired kidney function.

famotidine (Pepcid PM)
Harmful effects are infrequent and usually mild. They include headache, dizziness, constipation and diarrhoea, dry mouth, nausea and/or vomiting, skin rash, stomach discomfort and distension, loss of appetite and fatigue.

Warnings Famotidine should not be used in people who are allergic to it. In those with impaired kidney function, it should be used with caution and in smaller doses.

misoprostol (Cytotec)
Harmful effects include diarrhoea, nausea and vomiting. Reducing the dose usually

Table 15.3 Drugs used to heal peptic ulcers – harmful effects and warnings (*cont.*)

causes the symptoms to stop, and it also helps not to take another drug that may cause diarrhoea (e.g. antacids containing magnesium). It may also cause nausea, vomiting, wind, stomach cramps, indigestion and bleeding from the vagina.

Warning Misoprostol should not be used in pregnancy or in women of child-bearing age. This is because prostaglandins cause the womb to contract. It may cause vaginal bleeding or heavier periods in both pre- and post-menopausal women.

nizatidine (Axid)
Harmful effects are infrequent and usually mild. They include headache, weakness, chest pain, muscle pains, abnormal dreams, sleepiness, runny nose, sore throat, cough, itching, sweating and, rarely, may affect tests of liver function.

Warnings Nizatidine should be used with caution in people with impaired kidney or liver function.

ranitidine (Zantac)
Harmful effects are infrequent and usually mild. They include headache, dizziness, insomnia, vertigo, constipation and diarrhoea, nausea, vomiting and very rarely, mental confusion, agitation and depression – mainly in severely ill, elderly people. Liver damage, damage to the bone marrow producing blood disorders, allergic disorders (wheezing, fever and skin rashes), changes in heart rate, joint pains and breast swelling in men may occur very rarely.

Warnings Ranitidine should not be used in people who are allergic to it, and used with caution, (in smaller doses) in those with impaired kidney or liver function. It may give a false-positive test for protein in the urine.

omeprazole (Losec)
Harmful effects include nausea, headache, diarrhoea, constipation and skin rashes.

Warnings A reduced dose should be used in people with severe impairment of liver function. It should not be used during pregnancy or when breast feeding.

pirenzepine (Gastrozepin)
Harmful effects are infrequent and mild. They include dry mouth and blurred vision. There are very rare reports of its causing damage to the bone marrow, affecting white blood cell production and platelet production.

Warning Pirenzepine should not be used in people allergic to it or in individuals with an enlarged prostate gland, narrowing of the outlet from the stomach (pyloric stenosis), paralysis of the small bowel or closed-angle glaucoma. The dose should be reduced for anyone with severe impairment of kidney function.

sucralfate (Antepsin)
Harmful effects include constipation.

Warnings It should be used with caution in anyone with impaired kidney function.

Overview of the drug treatment of peptic ulcers

Treating an acute flare-up

General measures (see page 187), stopping smoking and regular antacid use should be tried first if the symptoms are mild. However, to heal peptic ulcers H_2 blockers, sucralfate and bismuth chelate are fashionable drugs at the moment.

Table 15.4 Preparations used to heal peptic ulcers

Preparation	*Main anti-ulcer drug*	*Drug group*	*Dosage form*
Antepsin	sucralfate	Protectant	Tablets, suspension
Axid	nizatidine	H_2 blocker	Capsules
Biogastrone	carbenoxolone	Protectant	Tablets
Caved-S	deglycyrrhinized liquorice	Protectant	Tablets
	bismuth subnitrate, dried aluminium hydroxide gel, magnesium carbonate, sodium bicarbonate	Antacids	
Cytotec	misoprostol	Prostaglandin	Tablets
De-Nol	bismuth chelate	Protectant	Liquid
De-Noltab	bismuth chelate	Protectant	Tablets
Duogastrone	carbenoxolone	Protectant	Capsules for duodenal release
Dyspamet	cimetidine	H_2 blocker	Chewable tablets, suspension
Gastrozepin	pirenzepine	Anticholinergic	Tablets
Losec	omeprazole	Proton pump blocker	Capsules
Pepcid PM	famotidine	H_2 blocker	Tablets
Pyrogastrone	carbenoxolone	Protectant	Tablets
	alginic acid	additive	
	aluminium hydroxide, magnesium trisilicate, sodium bicarbonate	Antacids	
Pyrogastrone Liquid	carbenoxolone	Protectant	Liquid
	aluminium hydroxide, potassium bicarbonate	Antacids	
	sodium alginate	Additive	
Rabro	deglycyrrhinized liquorice	Protectant	Tablets
	magnesium oxide, calcium carbonate	Antacid	
	frangula	Bulk-former	
Tagamet	cimetidine	H_2 blocker	Tablets, syrup, injection, intravenous infusion

Table 15.4 Preparations used to heal peptic ulcers (*cont.*)

Preparation	*Main anti-ulcer drug*	*Drug group*	*Dosage form*
Zantac	ranitidine	H_2 blocker	Tablets, dispersible tablets, injection, syrup

Of the H_2 blockers, ranitidine produces fewer harmful effects than cimetidine and there is little to choose between ranitidine, famotidine and nizatidine. Sucralfate and bismuth chelate, although just as effective as cimetidine or ranitidine, are less convenient to take.

Duodenal ulcers respond well to overnight suppression of acid production so that an H_2 blocker can be taken daily before going to bed. Duodenal ulcers should heal in 6 weeks (non-smokers) but will take longer in smokers. If treatment with H_2 blockers fails omeprazole will usually heal the ulcer in 4 weeks. Gastric ulcers need 24-hour reduction of acid and take longer to heal (8 weeks). The H_2 blocker needs to be taken in the day-time as well.

The synthetic prostaglandin misoprostol (Cytotec) is useful for treating and preventing ulcers caused by aspirin and non-steroidal anti-inflammatory drugs (see Chapter 31). (U)

Preventing recurrence

Relapses (i.e. flare-ups) of peptic ulcers appear to be more common in the first year after healing treatment than in subsequent years. Furthermore, healing treatment and maintenance preventative treatment (see below) with drugs does not appear to alter the natural history of the disease (see earlier) so that, once any treatment is stopped, you are back where you were and will go on having flare-ups and quiet periods from your ulcer independent of whatever treatment you had. One thing is clear, however: relapse is higher among smokers than non-smokers, so the first step in preventing relapses should be to stop smoking.

The really difficult questions therefore are: who should be maintained on regular daily treatment and for how long?

Maintenance treatment should be considered for anyone who has two or more flare-ups within 2 years, particularly if it results in time lost from work and/or loss of sleep. It is also indicated in people who have bled from an ulcer, and in those not fit for surgery because of their age and/or some severe heart or chest disorder.

Elderly people should also be considered for maintenance treatment because they suffer from a higher rate of complications than younger people and are more likely to develop ulcers that do not cause symptoms. They are also more likely to be taking non-steroidal anti-inflammatory drugs to treat their arthritis (see dangers, in Chapter 31)

H_2 blockers are the drugs of choice in maintenance treatment and a nightly dose reduces acid production sufficiently to prevent relapse. Any failure of treatment may mean that the individual did not take the treatment as directed or that the dose was too low to affect acid production. Smoking can cause failure, as may the regular use of aspirin and non-steroid anti-inflammatory drugs used to treat arthritis.

The duration of treatment should be for 1–2 years initially but in some people it may have to continue for many years.

Intermittent treatment

Accepting that drug treatment does not cure the cause of peptic ulcers, an alternative to regular daily long-term treatment with anti-ulcer drugs may be to use the drugs intermittently, at the earliest sign of any flare-up of the ulcer. However, continuous treatment should be considered if an individual has two or more relapses over a 2-year period. This is because recurrent flare-ups and re-treatments can result in scarring of duodenal ulcers, causing narrowing of the outlet from the stomach (pyloric stenosis).

Surgical treatment

Surgical treatment is necessary if an ulcer has perforated, bled or caused scarring and blockage to the outlet of the stomach. It is also necessary if the ulcer is due to a cancer. In other people the risks of medical treatment should be balanced against the risks of surgery but anyone with ulcers that fail to respond to medical treatment should be considered for surgery.

Reminder

Smoking both delays the healing of a peptic ulcer and increases the chance of a relapse. Should people treated for peptic ulcers agree a 'contract' – effective treatment for their ulcer provided they do not smoke?

There is no evidence that reducing stomach acid causes cancer

Food and water contain nitrates and food also contains nitrites (e.g. hot dogs and cured meats). Bacteria in the mouth and stomach can reduce nitrates to nitrites. People who produce less acid in their stomachs have an increased number of these bacteria in their stomach and, therefore, a high concentration of nitrites.

Nitrites can react with amines in food to form nitrosamines, which are capable of producing cancer. So the question is: by reducing acid in the stomach is the nitrite content of the stomach increased and does this lead to the production of potentially dangerous cancer-producing chemicals? This is an important question because it has been noted that patients who have had surgical removal of the acid producing area of their stomach have an increased level of nitrites in their stomach and an increased risk of getting cancer of the stomach.

So far there is no evidence of this risk but it is important to note that the risk applies to both medical and surgical treatment. With the increasing tendency to use acid blockers for long-term maintenance treatment this risk should be borne in mind, particularly with regard to regular daily treatment for an ulcer of the stomach which is more sensitive to such changes than other peptic ulcers.

Heartburn

The washing of stomach contents which contain acid and pepsin up into the lower end of the oesophagus (gullet) may produce inflammation of the oesophagus; this is referred to as *reflux oesophagitis*. The characteristic symptom is *heartburn* – a burning pain in the centre of the lower chest after eating a large meal, stooping or lying flat. Reflux oesophagitis is a major cause of indigestion and is linked to smoking, diet and being overweight.

The reflux of acid (acid regurgitation) from the stomach into the oesophagus is caused by a weakness in the circular muscles of the diaphragm that normally close off the top of the stomach from the oesophagus (the gastro-oesophageal sphincter) and prevent swallowed food and drink from coming back up – unless of course you vomit. This reflux of acid up into the oesophagus may be due to a *hiatus hernia*, which allows parts of the stomach to bulge upwards (herniate) into the opening (hiatus) in the diaphragm through which the oesophagus passes. However, the problem is not always a hiatus hernia and usually there is just a failure of the muscle (oesophageal sphincter) to close off completely. With this disorder, the risk of reflux of acid is obviously worse if you bend down or lie down than if you remain upright. Reflux may also occur in pregnant women, overweight patients and smokers. Drugs that relax the sphincter (see anticholinergic drugs, Chapter 2) may trigger an attack. Aspirin and non-steroidal anti-inflammatory drugs (see Chapter 31) make the condition worse.

In old people the movement of the oesophagus may be slowed down and some tablets may stick, producing irritation and even ulceration of the oesophagus; for example, aspirin and non-steroidal anti-inflammatory tablets used to treat arthritis, slow-release potassium tablets and tetracycline antibiotics. Tablets of emepronium (an anticholinergic drug used to treat incontinence) were recently taken off the market because of this problem. Elderly patients should always sit up straight or, better still, stand up when taking tablets and they should take a good drink of fluid with each tablet.

General treatment

Reflux can be reduced by sleeping propped up in bed (use three or four pillows), by avoiding too much bending down and, where appropriate, by stopping smoking, stopping alcohol and losing weight. Regular small, non-fatty meals will help and the amount of tea and coffee drunk should be regulated.

Drug treatment of heartburn

Antacids to neutralize stomach acid

Antacids are described in detail earlier in this chapter. Effective doses will neutralize the acid in the stomach and often provide instant relief from reflux symptoms.

Additives that protect the surface of the oesophagus Additives in antacid mixtures aimed at protecting the oesophagus provide additional relief. These additives include *alginic acid* or one of its salts (alginates) which are obtained from algae. They work as emulsifiers and float to the top of the gastric contents to form a 'raft' containing the antacid. This helps to protect the sensitive lining of the oesophagus from the acid in the stomach.

Another commonly used additive is the silicone *dimethicone*, which acts as an anti-foaming agent and helps to stop the acid contents of the stomach frothing up into the oesophagus. *Activated dimethicone* is a mixture of liquid dimethicone containing finely divided silicone dioxide which increases its defoaming properties. Antacid preparations containing dimethicone provide more relief from reflux symptoms than antacids alone in some people.

Alginate-containing antacids (raft-floating antacids) usually contain less antacid than ordinary antacid preparations but the raft appears to make them more effective for relieving reflux symptoms. They provide relief in some people.

Warning *A preparation containing dimethicone should never be taken with a preparation that contains alginic acid or an alginate because their actions oppose each other and the raft provided by the latter would sink.*

Antacids plus a local anaesthetic to relieve pain *Mucaine* is an antacid mixture that contains the local anaesthetic oxethazine. There is doubt about the benefits of using a local anaesthetic for this purpose but some patients experience relief from reflux symptoms.

Drugs that protect the lining of the stomach and oesophagus

Carbenoxolone added to a raft–alginate antacid (e.g. Pyrogastrone) has not been shown to be more effective than an H_2 blocker. It needs to be used with caution in older people.

Sucralfate (Antepsin) and *bismuth chelate* (De-Nol), which are effective in treating stomach and duodenal ulcers, have no special advantages when treating reflux symptoms. The synthetic prostaglandin *misoprostol* (Cytotec) may be useful.

Drugs that block acid production

H_2 blockers before meals and an alkali/alginic mixture after meals provide good relief from reflux symptoms but H_2 blockers appear to be less effective at treating peptic ulcers in the oesophagus than in the stomach or duodenum. Treatment should continue for 2 months.

If an H_2 blocker does not work, omeprazole should be tried. It may be very beneficial but it should only be taken for 2 months and then an H_2 blocker can be tried again.

Drugs that affect the gastro-oesophageal sphincter

Drugs that close the circular muscle (the gastro-oesophageal sphincter) will prevent the reflux of acid up into the oesophagus. The anti-dopamine drug *metoclopramide* is an example of these drugs, and it can work very effectively in some people.

Cisapride (Alimix, Prepulsid) is related to metoclopramide but may produce fewer harmful effects on the nervous system. It can be used with an H_2 blocker. It may cause abdominal cramps, rumbling in the stomach, diarrhoea and, rarely, headache. Convulsions have very rarely been reported. It should not be used in pregnancy or in people with bleeding from, or obstruction of, the stomach or intestine. It should be used with caution in individuals with impaired kidney or liver function and in the elderly.

Cisapride is also useful for relieving the discomfort of simple non-ulcer indigestion.

Harmful effects of metoclopramide are listed in Table 14.1. For cisapride see Update.

Warning *Anticholinergic drugs (e.g. belladonna) will have the opposite effect by relaxing the gastro-oesophageal sphincter and allowing reflux to occur more easily.*

Table 15.5 Combined drug preparations used to treat heartburn, reflux oesophagitis, hiatus hernia and indigestion due to reflux

Antacid preparations containing activated dimethicone
Actonorm (gel), Altacite Plus (tablets and suspension), Andursil (tablets and supsension), Asilone (tablets, gel and suspension), Maalox Plus (tablets and suspension), Polycrol (gel and tablets), Polycrol Forte (gel and tablets), Siloxyl (tablets and suspension) and Simeco (tablets).

Antacid preparations containing dimethicone
Diovol (suspension), Simeco (suspension) and Unigest (tablets).

Antacid preparations containing alginic acid or an alginate
Algicon (tablets and suspension), Gastrocote (tablets and liquid), Gastron (tablets), Gaviscon (tablets, liquid, infant powder) and Topal (tablets).

Other preparations
Algitec (chewable tablets and suspension) – cimetidine (an H_2 blocker) and alginic acid

Mucaine (suspension) – antacids with oxethazaine (a local anaesthetic)

Nulacin (tablets) – antacids with milk solids, dextrins and maltose

Pyrogastrone (tablets and liquid) – antacids with carbenoxolone (ulcer-healing drug) and sodium alginate

Treatment of *heartburn of pregnancy* should include general measures (see earlier) and the use of a magnesium/aluminium antacid mixed with alginic acid. Other treatments should be avoided. Very dilute hydrochloric acid may stop the reflux from the duodenum and stomach up into the oesophagus.

16

Diarrhoea

Diarrhoea is the frequent passage of liquidy motions often associated with an urgent desire to 'go' and discomfort around the anus.

Messages that make you want to open your bowels come principally from the rectum and the anus. When faeces enter the rectum from the colon they stimulate receptors in the wall of the bowel that are sensitive to being stretched. Stimulation of these receptors triggers an immediate desire to open your bowels. In addition, in the anus there are receptors that are sensitive to touch, so that when faeces make contact with the anus this also stimulates you to open your bowels. In diarrhoea the bowel content is watery, so it easily enters the rectum, triggering the stretch reflex, and makes contact with the anus, triggering the touch reflex. This double stimulation makes you want to have your bowels opened quickly and makes you keep wanting to 'go' even though you have just been!

Causes of acute diarrhoea

Diarrhoea may be due to many causes but the most common causes of acute diarrhoea in otherwise healthy people are viral, bacterial or parasitic infections, food poisoning or intolerance or allergy to certain foods. It may also be caused by some drugs (see below), following radiotherapy for cancer, and may occur in tension and anxiety.

Drug treatments may cause diarrhoea

Do not forget that many drugs may cause diarrhoea; for example, all antibiotics may produce diarrhoea, particularly the ones active against a broad spectrum of bacteria (e.g. ampicillin, cephalosporins, clindamycin, co-trimoxazole, erythromycin, lincomycin, neomycin, tetracyclines). Some antibiotics may irritate the lining of the intestine, causing diarrhoea to come on straight away. Some may knock out certain bugs in the intestine and not others; the latter multiply and spread and may trigger diarrhoea, which comes on after a few days. The diarrhoea may be so severe that it presents like colitis (inflammation of the colon), which produces severe and persistent diarrhoea. Examples of antibiotics that may produce colitis are ampicillin, cephalosporins, chloramphenicol, clindamycin, co-trimoxazole, lincomycin, metronidazole, neomycin, sulphonamides and tetracyclines.

The best treatment of diarrhoea caused by an antibiotic is to stop the antibiotic *immediately*. Colitis caused by antibiotic needs treating with an antibiotic (vancomycin) to knock out the bugs that have multiplied and spread in the colon and which produce an irritating toxin.

Warnings *Anti-diarrhoeal drugs of the morphine-type (opiates, narcotics) may prolong the diarrhoea caused by antibiotics and make it worse.*

Diarrhoea may affect the absorption of drugs from the intestine into the bloodstream. Women taking an oral contraceptive who develop diarrhoea should take additional contraceptive measures for the rest of that course.

Treatment of acute diarrhoea

Drugs used to treat diarrhoea relieve the symptoms but they do not affect the underlying disorder. It is therefore important to be aware of this fact and to make sure that any underlying cause of the diarrhoea is treated properly and that any loss of fluid and salt is corrected immediately.

Dangers from loss of water and salts

An irritated and inflamed intestine actively secretes water and salts into the motions and this loss may rapidly cause dehydration. Vomiting adds to the risk of dehydration by causing further loss of water and salts.

The priority treatment of diarrhoea (and of course diarrhoea and vomiting: gastro-enteritis) is replacement of lost water and salts. The use of a drug to stop the diarrhoea may be positively harmful unless this loss is corrected. If lost water and salts are replaced, with most commonly occurring diarrhoeas there is seldom need to take a drug anyway.

Warnings *Dehydration is dangerous and may be life threatening in babies, infants and young children, elderly people and debilitated patients.*

No anti-diarrhoeal remedy should be used to treat children under the age of 3 years; they urgently need replacement of any water and salts they may have lost.

You should seek medical advice if diarrhoea does not improve within 48 hours, if there is blood and/or pus in the motions, if you have severe abdominal pain and vomiting, if you develop a fever, if you have just returned from a foreign country, or if the diarrhoea occurs in a baby or infant, or in an elderly debilitated person.

Mild diarrhoea

Mild diarrhoea should be treated by stopping all solid foods and whole milk drinks for 12–24 hours and taking very frequent small drinks of water (or other clear fluids) in sufficient volume to balance the amount of fluids that you think you lose every time you have to go to the toilet. If you think you have lost around quarter of a litre (about half a pint) of fluid in your motions, drink a quarter litre (half pint) of water, and so on. Do not forget that for a baby's diarrhoea to produce a wet nappy he has lost a lot of fluid – this needs replacing urgently by mouth. Babies should continue to be fed as well as given rehydration fluids (see later).

Moderate diarrhoea

For moderate to severe diarrhoea, particularly if it is associated with vomiting, it is important to take in salt (sodium chloride) as well as water; and because sugar helps the absorption of salts into the bloodstream, it is very important to take a sugar/salt solution. This can be made up by adding salt and sugar to water (half a teaspoon of salt and six teaspoonfuls of sugar to a litre of water) but it is best to purchase one of the commercial preparations (see Table 16.1) because they also contain potassium and bicarbonate which may also be lost in moderate and severe diarrhoea and vomiting.

NOTE These solutions do not reduce the volume or frequency of the diarrhoea.

Severe diarrhoea

Severe diarrhoea will produce dehydration through excessive loss of fluids and people so affected will require admission to hospital in order that they may be given fluids and salts by infusion directly into a vein. This applies particularly to babies and infants, who may suddenly die if they become dehydrated. A dehydrated baby looks pale and ill, with sunken eyes, dry lips, tongue and skin, and sunken abdomen – this is an emergency!

Drugs used to relieve the symptoms of diarrhoea

Anti-diarrhoeal drugs relieve the symptom of diarrhoea – they reduce the number of times that the bowels are opened. *They have no effect on the underlying cause and may be positively harmful if they delay the giving of fluids*

Table 16.1 Electrolyte replacement preparations to treat diarrhoea

Preparation	*Salts*	*Sugars*	*Dosage form*
Dioralyte	sodium chloride, potassium chloride, sodium bicarbonate	glucose	Powder in sachets
Dioralyte Effervescent	sodium bicarbonate, potassium bicarbonate, citric acid	glucose	Effervescent tablets
Electrolade	sodium chloride potassium chloride, sodium bicarbonate, saccharin sodium	glucose	Powder in sachets
Gluco-Lyte	sodium chloride, potassium chloride, sodium bicarbonate	glucose	Powder in sachets
Rehidrat	sodium chloride, potassium chloride, sodium bicarbonate, citric acid	glucose, sucrose, laevulose	Powder in sachets

and salts– such action could prove fatal in babies and infants. Drugs used to relieve the symptom of diarrhoea work in one of two ways – on the wall of the intestine or on its contents.

Anti-diarrhoeal drugs that slow down movements of the intestine

These drugs act on nerves in the wall of the intestine, to slow down the movements that are increased in diarrhoea. There are two main groups: opiates (narcotics) and antispasmodic/anticholinergic drugs.

Warning *They should never be used until the individual is fully hydrated because they stop the movement of the intestine and may cause fluid retention in the bowel making the dehydration worse.*

Opiates

These include morphine, opium, codeine, diphenoxylate and loperamide. They reduce the movements of the intestine and tighten up the muscles of the anus. In addition, they act on the brain and help to reduce the feelings of having to 'go'. They relieve diarrhoea by reducing the propulsive movements of the intestine and therefore they reduce pain and the frequency of having to open your bowels. They slow down movement of the intestine. Except for loperamide, they all act on the brain and may cause addiction. In the doses used to treat diarrhoea they may cause drowsiness, especially in children and people with impaired liver function. They should be used with caution by elderly people because of the risk of producing a blockage of the bowels. They are useful if used occasionally to relieve symptoms in people who suffer from chronic diarrhoea.

In people whose diarrhoea is due to an infection these drugs may actually prolong the duration of the infection because they slow down the movements of the intestine. This is opposite to the body's normal response of trying to get rid of something that may be harmful. Because of this action they may also prolong an attack of diarrhoea caused by antibiotics (see earlier).

Warning *At the first sign of diarrhoea caused by an antibiotic, the drug should be stopped. Never continue with the antibiotic and take something to stop the diarrhoea.*

Anti-spasmodic/anticholinergic drugs

Anti-spasmodic drugs (see later) produce a direct relaxing effect on the muscles in the wall of the intestine. They include mebeverine and alverine, and also peppermint oil. They reduce movements of the intestine and relieve painful spasms (colic) caused by irritation of the lining of the intestine. Dicyclomine may also be used; it produces both an anticholinergic effect and a direct effect. *Anticholinergic drugs* such as atropine, mepenzolate, hyoscine and propantheline also slow down movements of the intestine and relieve spasm.

In mild diarrhoea associated with colic due to irritation of the lining of the intestine (e.g. mild dysenteries or diverticulitis), anti-spasmodics or anticholinergics may help by reducing the painful colic and reducing the number of bowel movements; but there is *no place for their routine use* to treat acute or chronic diarrhoea because in effective doses their harmful effects may easily outweigh any benefit. They should not be used to treat severe diarrhoea which may occur, for example, in ulcerative colitis (see later) or Crohn's disease (see later). They should not be used by children.

Anti-diarrhoeal drugs that alter the bowel contents

Inert powders are used to make the motions more bulky and to absorb fluids and irritant substances. These include activated charcoal, aluminium salts (e.g. kaolin), pectin (a purified carbohydrate product obtained from citrus fruits), activated attapulgite (a hydrated magnesium aluminium silicate) and calcium carbonate (chalk). They absorb fluids from the bowel contents, which makes the motions more firm and reduces the continous urge to 'go' which is caused by fluid motions.

Other drugs that increase the bulk of the motions also help to relieve mild chronic diarrhoea by absorbing water and thus making the motions firmer. They include starches and cellulose substances such as methylcellulose, ceratonia, ispaghula, sterculia and psyllium. Because they 'retain' water and increase the bulk of the motions, these drugs are also used as 'bulk laxatives' to treat constipation and in herbal slimming drugs because they cause loss of weight through loss of water (but not fat!).

Warnings *Drugs that alter the bowel contents reduce the frequency of the motions because they absorb water but they do not reduce the loss of water, salt and nutrients in the motions. This may be dangerous in infants and young children. They should not be used to treat diarrhoea in children under the age of 3 years without strict medical supervision.*

All anti-diarrhoeal drugs may produce constipation and should be taken with plenty of fluids.

Drugs used to treat infections of the intestine

Anti-bacterial drugs

It is quite unnecessary and potentially harmful to routinely use anti-bacterial drugs to treat simple acute diarrhoea not associated with chills, fever, pain and/or passing blood and/or pus in the motions. First of all, most of these attacks are self-limiting and all that is needed is to make sure that you take adequate water and salts (see above). Secondly, many are due to viral infections which do not respond to anti-bacterial drugs anyway.

People suffering from mild to moderate diarrhoea, even when due to bacterial infections (shigella and certain salmonellae), should not be treated with anti-bacterial drugs because of the risk of producing bacterial resistance to the drug. In addition, anti-bacterial drugs may alter the normal bacterial content of the intestine, which may allow fungi or other infections to take over (e.g. thrush). Also, in some bacterial infections the use of poorly absorbed anti-bacterial drugs such as neomycin, streptomycin or sulphaguanidine may actually prolong diarrhoea and the period when you can pass on the infection to another person (i.e. act as a carrier of the disease). Anti-bacterial drugs may also increase the risk of relapse and interfere with tests to determine which bacteria are causing the infection. Preparations containing clioquinol should not be used because prolonged use of high doses has been associated with nerve damage.

When to use anti-bacterial drugs

Anti-bacterial drugs should be used to treat moderately severe and severe diarrhoeas, particularly if they are associated with chills, fever, abdominal pains and blood and/or pus in the motions. However, because of over-use in the past many bacteria are resistant to available antibiotics. It is important therefore that a sample of the motions is taken so that the infecting bacteria can be cultured in the laboratory and then tested for their sensitivity to selected antibiotics. Examples of anti-bacterial drugs in fashion at the present time is given below under the treatment of travellers' diarrhoea.

Anti-protozoal drugs

The drug treatment of amoebic dysentery is discussed in Chapter 59.

Travellers' diarrhoea

It is estimated that about two out of every five people who visit a tropical climate from a temperate climate develop an attack of travellers' diarrhoea, either while they are there or upon their return home. Africa, the Middle East, Asia and Latin America are high-risk countries and so is southern Europe around the Mediterranean.

Travellers' diarrhoea may be caused by a wide range of infective organisms (viruses, bacteria, protozoa). However, in about 20–50 per cent of cases a cause cannot be established but a change in diet, temperature and excessive use of alcohol may be contributory factors.

Of the infective cases of travellers' diarrhoea that have been studied, it would appear that a species of bacteria, *Escherichia coli*, is the main culprit. These bacteria produce an instant toxin in the intestine which irritates the wall to produce diarrhoea. They are therefore referred to as enterotoxigenic bacteria.

Obviously the symptoms and severity of travellers' diarrhoea vary according to whether or not there is an infection of the intestine, and according to the type of infecting organism. Most cases involve the sudden onset of watery diarrhoea, and there may be abdominal cramps and nausea. The symptoms may last for just a day or go on for 4 or 5 days or even longer. If blood and/or pus appear in the motions this indicates that the bowel wall is not only irritated but inflamed as well and may be ulcerated.

Treatment of travellers' diarrhoea

Treatment of travellers' diarrhoea will depend upon the severity and duration of the diarrhoea, on any associated effects (e.g. blood and pus in the motions) and upon the age and general fitness of the individual – babies and infants, elderly and debilitated people are more vulnerable to the harmful effects of diarrhoea such as loss of water and salts.

Replacement of water and salts (see earlier) is essential, and increasing clear fluids (not tap water) by mouth should be beneficial if the diarrhoea is mild. However, if it is more severe, a salt/sugar solution should be taken as directed on the packet and made up using bottled water. (NOTE Always take a salt/sugar preparation with you if you are going to a hot climate.) If you do not have such a preparation, add a half teaspoon of salt and six teaspoonfuls of sugar to a litre of bottle water and drink at regular intervals in amounts according to how much fluid you think you are losing in your motions (see earlier).

Drugs to relieve the diarrhoea may be used if the diarrhoea lasts for more than a day or if it is severe, provided of course that you are taking adequate amounts of fluids. *Adsorbents* (e.g. kaolin) should not be used but an *opiate* such as codeine, diphenoxylate (in Lomotil; generic name – co-phenotrope) or loperamide (Imodium) may help. However, there are dangers associated with their use if the diarrhoea is caused by an infection (e.g. with *Shigella* or *Salmonella* bacteria). Anti-diarrhoeal drugs may prolong the infection and should not be used if there are general symptoms such as fever, chills and colicky abdominal pains.

Anti-bacterial drugs should not be used for mild attacks of travellers' diarrhoea. However, if it is moderately severe or severe – particularly if associated with abdominal cramps, blood and/or pus in the motions, fever, chills and feeling ill – it is worth trying an anti-bacterial drug such as trimethoprim (e.g. Monotrim) or ciprofloxacin (Ciproxin). It may be worth taking one of these preparations with you if you are going to a high-risk area.

Obviously it is not always wise to take anti-bacterial drugs blindly (i.e. without confirming the type and the antibiotic sensitivity of the infecting organism) but this is not always possible in certain areas of the world. However, if a microscopic examination of the motions is possible this will help considerably in deciding what is the most appropriate treatment. This examination should always be carried out *before* treatment in anyone who develops diarrhoea within a few weeks of returning home from another country.

The anti-bacterial drugs of choice for treating bacterial infections that cause diarrhoea are always changing because of the emergence of resistant strains of bacteria. At the present time, trimethoprim, ampicillin or ciprofloxacin are fashionable for treating *Shigella* infections, amoxycillin (Amoxil), or ciprofloxacin or trimethoprim for treating *Salmonella* infections and tetracyclines for treating cholera. *Campylobacter* enteritis may be treated with erythromycin or ciprofloxacin.

Preventing travellers' diarrhoea

The best treatment of travellers' diarrhoea is to prevent it. Do not forget that the infection usually spreads from someone else's faeces to your mouth through contaminated food and drink. Do not eat salads, unpeeled fruit, uncooked meats or seafoods; do not drink the tap water or use ice. Do not even clean your teeth with tap water – ALWAYS drink bottled water and use it to clean your teeth.

A daily dose of trimethoprim or doxycycline reduces the risk of developing travellers' diarrhoea but such a benefit has to be balanced against the risks of taking these anti-bacterial drugs. In general the risks will outweigh the benefits except for people who are immune deficient (e.g. AIDS) and who are visiting a high-risk area, or people who suffer from ulcerative colitis (see later). Such preventative treatment should not be taken for more than 2 weeks.

Drug treatment of chronic diarrhoeal diseases

Crohn's disease

This disease was formerly called regional enteritis or regional ileitis but the terms are too specific because the disorder can affect any part of the intestine from the mouth to the anus. In this disease, patches of inflammation develop in the lining of the intestine. The cause is unknown but it occurs more commonly between the age of 10 and 25 years in both sexes. Symptoms include loss of appetite, fever, abdominal cramps and pains after eating, nausea, vomiting and diarrhoea which may occasionally be bloody. The absorption of essential food stuffs and vitamins may be impaired (malabsorption) and the patient may lose weight. It is a chronic condition with flare-ups and quiet periods. Serious bowel and other complications may occur and people with the disease may eventually have to have surgery because they develop an obstruction, an abscess or a fistula (an unnatural communication between the bowel and some other organ, such as the bladder, or out on to the skin surface). The disease may be associated with inflammation of the eyes, skin, mouth and large joints. In children the onset may present as fever and joint pains before intestinal symptoms develop.

Treatment

There is no cure for Crohn's disease. *Food allergies* should be looked for carefully. For example, there is evidence that some people are intolerant to lactose, and the removal of lactose-rich foods from the diet will help (e.g. milk and ice cream). An increase in fibre in the diet may also help, and in others a decrease in fat intake. Special attention should always be paid to the diet, which should be nutritious and well balanced but produce minimal irritation to the inflamed bowel. Additional vitamins and minerals should also be given. In severely malnourished individuals it may be very beneficial to give total nutrition through a tube into a vein for a period of time. This helps to build the person up and also rests the bowel.

*Drug treatment**

This involves the selective use of *corticosteroids* (e.g. prednisolone) and *sulphasalazine* (Salazopyrin): for mild cases, sulphasalazine on its own and for moderate cases sulphasalazine with prednisolone; for maintenance treatment, sulphasalazine is usually used and prednisolone is added for acute flare-ups. Treatment is aimed at controlling symptoms if they are getting worse and to try to suppress acute flare-ups. It should be continued for as long as the individual shows an improvement.

NOTE Sulphasalazine is useful if the colon is involved (colitis) but is of doubtful value if the small intestine is affected.

Anti-diarrhoeal drugs such as diphenoxylate (Lomotil) or loperamide (Imodium) may be taken occasionally but they should be used with utmost caution because of the risk of producing paralysis of the small intestine and dilation of the colon (megacolon). This may be dangerous because the colon may perforate (see under 'Ulcerative colitis', below). When a large part of the small intestine is inflamed or has been removed surgically, it may help to reduce the irritant effects of the bile by taking a cholestyramine and aluminium hydroxide mixture to mop up (bind) the bile salts.

An antibiotic such as *metronidazole* (Flagyl) may help if the inflammation is severe and affecting the lower rectum and/or colon; but antibiotics should not be used with sulphasalazine

Azathioprine (Imuran), an immunosuppressive drug, may be beneficial in some individuals who are suffering from chronic active disease not responding to sulphasalazine and prednisolone. It may be used on its own or taken with prednisolone and/or sulphasalazine by mouth. It is usually used for 4–6 months.

About two in three people with the disease will improve within the first

* For Crohn's disease affecting the colon also read entry under ulcerative colitis (below)

6 months, but if treatment is continued to 12 months only about one in four will benefit.

Crohn's disease of the rectum should be treated with prednisolone suppositories or retention enemas or with sulphasalazine suppositories. *No drug prevents a flare-up of the disease during a quiet period or after surgery.*

Ulcerative colitis

This is an inflammation of the bowel which may affect just the rectum (proctitis) or part or whole of the colon (colitis). It is sometimes called proctocolitis. Unlike Crohn's disease (discussed above) the inflammation is continuous throughout the length of the affected bowel and produces loose, bloody diarrhoea containing slime (mucus) and pus. It starts most commonly between the ages of 20 and 40 years and the first attack is the worst. Subsequently the disease undergoes flare-ups and quiet periods. It is as common in men as in women. Symptoms include abdominal cramps, bloody diarrhoea, fatigue, weakness, fever, weight loss and anaemia. It may also be associated with disorders of the skin, eyes, joints, liver and blood vessels. It is not known what causes ulcerative colitis. It may be an autoimmune disease; or due to infection; or due to some food allergy. With regard to the last, there is evidence that some patients with ulcerative colitis are intolerant to lactose and the removal of lactose-rich foods (e.g. milk and ice cream) from the diet may help.

Treatment

Treatment depends upon the severity of the inflammation and the area of the bowel involved.

Diet

Special attention should always be paid to the diet, which should be nutritious and well balanced but produce minimal irritation to the bowel. Additional vitamins and minerals should also be taken. In severely malnutritioned individuals it can be very beneficial to be given total nutrition through a tube in a vein for a period of time. This helps to build up the sufferer and also rests the bowel. People with ulcerative colitis often become anaemic and will need extra iron, which may have to be given by injection because iron by mouth may upset them, particularly during an acute episode. The fibre content of the diet should be reduced in acute attacks.

Drug treatment

The main aim of drug treatment of an acute attack is to reduce the inflammation by using a *corticosteroid* (e.g. prednisolone) locally applied to the bowel in the form of suppositories or enemas and/or taken by mouth or injection. High doses are used initially for about 2 weeks and the dose is slowly tapered off. Maintenance treatment with prednisolone may be necessary in some people but there are dangers (see Chapter 62). Prednisolone by mouth is also useful for treating associated disorders of the skin, eyes, joints, liver and blood vessels.

Sulphasalazine (Salazopyrin) is also used to treat acute attacks and to prevent flare-ups. It may be taken with prednisolone. Sulphasalazine is useful for maintenance treatment to prevent flare-ups in some people but there are harmful effects to be considered (see Table 16.2).

Sulphasalazine is split in the bowel into a sulphonamide anti-bacterial drug, sulphapyridine and an anti-inflammatory aspirin-like drug, 5-aminosalicylic acid (5-ASA). Sulphapyridine is broken down in the liver before being excreted in the urine. The process of breakdown in the liver is called acetylation and some people do this quickly and some slowly. Those who do it slowly (slow acetylators) run the risk of developing toxic effects from the drug.

About one in five patients develops some harmful effects from sulphasalazine. This is due to the sulphonamide sulphapyridine, and recent research has concentrated on finding a sulphapyridine-free product because if you take 5-aminosalicylic acid (5-ASA) on its own by mouth, it does not work. This is because it is absorbed in the upper intestine, broken down and then excreted in the urine. It does not reach the colon in sufficient concentration to be effective. The following preparations are an attempt to get over this problem.

Mesalazine (Asacol, Pentasa) is an alternative to sulphasalazine for people who are allergic to sulphonamides. It consists of 5-aminosalicylic acid coated with an acrylic-based resin which releases the drug when it reaches the end of the small intestine and the beginning of the large intestine (colon).

Olsalazine (Dipentum) contains no sulphapyridine; instead, it consists of a complex of two 5-ASA molecules that remains intact until it enters the colon, where it splits to produce two separate active molecules of 5-ASA.

Other drugs that have been tried in sufferers resistant to treatment include *azathioprine* in the belief that there may be some abnormality in the body's immune system which causes it to destroy some of its own tissues (i.e. the bowel lining in this case). Azathioprine damps down the immune system.

An anti-allergy drug, *sodium cromoglycate*, has also been tried and may occasionally be helpful in some individuals whose disease is suspected of being allergic. It is given as a capsule (Nalcrom).

A *high bran fibre diet* will help people suffering from ulcerative colitis affecting the rectum (proctitis). Alternatively, a bulk-forming laxative such as methylcellulose may be used. Mild diarrhoea can be treated with codeine or loperamide but these drugs should not be used by the seriously ill nor should anti-spasmodic drugs. This is because of the risks of producing an obstruction and a ballooning of the bowel above the obstruction. This is called toxic dilation of the colon (megacolon) and it may occur in severe ulcerative colitis where there is scarring and narrowing of the colon. The use of an anti-diarrhoeal drug or an anti-spasmodic drug may aggravate this obstruction.

The drug treatment of ulcerative colitis needs careful planning in order to tailor it to the particular needs of the individual. This requires patience and time as well as a good understanding of the disease and the benefits and risks of available drug treatments. About 90 per cent of people with an acute attack should respond to drug treatment, and in about 20 per cent of these the disease will clear up for a prolonged period of time but there is always a risk that it may flare up again. Maintenance treatment with salazopyrine, mesalazine or olsalazine and/or prednisolone may have to be used in some sufferers, and of course the minimum dosage for maximum benefits should be used.

Warnings *People with chronic ulcerative colitis run a rare but higher risk than normal of developing a cancer of the colon or rectum; therefore everyone who suffers from ulcerative colitis should have an annual examination of the colon and rectum.*

Table 16.2 Drugs used to treat ulcerative colitis and Crohn's disease – harmful effects and warnings

sulphasalazine (Salazopyrin)
Harmful effects Sulphasalazine is broken down in the intestine to sulphapyridine (for harmful effects, see sulphonamides, Chapter 54) and 5-aminosalicylic acid (for harmful effects, see aspirin, Chapter 27). Individuals who break down sulphapyridine slowly are more likely to develop harmful effects. Commonly occurring harmful effects include loss of appetite, headache, nausea, vomiting, stomach upsets and raised temperature. It may, rarely, cause reduced sperm count and infertility in men (reversible), skin rashes, itching and nettle rash; and, very rarely, haemolytic anaemia (damage to red blood cells, see Chapter 47), blueness, damage to the bone marrow affecting the production of red and/or white blood cells, dermatitis, Stevens–Johnson syndrome, and other serious allergic reactions; damage to the pancreas, liver or kidneys; inflammation of the arteries, nerve damage (e.g. weakness of the arms and legs), sensitivity of the skin to sunlight, depression, insomnia, incoordination of movements, hallucinations, convulsions, damage to the hearing. Harmful effects become more common with doses above 4 g daily.

Warnings Sulphasalazine should not be used by people who are allergic to sulphasalazine or a sulphonamide drug, or to aspirin or related drugs; in anyone with

Table 16.2 Drugs used to treat ulcerative colitis and Crohn's disease – harmful effects and warnings (*cont.*)

porphyria; or in individuals with a blockage of the intestines or a blockage of the bladder. It should be used with utmost caution in people with impaired kidney or liver function, or with blood disorders; tests of liver and kidney function and blood counts should be carried out before treatment and at regular intervals during treatment. It should be used, with caution, in individuals with asthma or allergic disorders. Drink plenty of fluids each day to avoid the development of crystals in the urine. There is a risk of haemolytic anaemia in patients with glucose-6-phosphate dehydrogenase deficiency. Sulphasalazine may produce a yellow–orange coloration of the urine and skin, and it may stain contact lenses. Tests of the blood level of sulphapyridine (the sulphonamide breakdown product of sulphasalazine in the intestine) should be carried out at intervals to ensure that it does not rise unduly.

mesalazine (Asacol, Pentasa)
Harmful effects include nausea, diarrhoea, abdominal pain, headache and, occasionally, a flare-up of colitis, and very rarely kidney damage.

Warnings Mesalazine should not be used in anyone allergic to aspirin or a related drug. Use with caution in people with impaired kidney function.

olsalazine (Dipentum)
Harmful effects are infrequent and usually mild. They include diarrhoea, abdominal cramps, headache, nausea, indigestion, painful joints and skin rashes.

Warnings It should not be used in people allergic to aspirin or a related drug, or individuals with a severe impairment of kidney function.

Irritable bowel syndrome (spastic colon)

In this condition the individual complains of discomfort in the abdomen and long-standing disturbances in bowel habits – diarrhoea, constipation or a mixture of both. Diarrhoea usually occurs in the mornings and after eating. Sufferers may be tense, anxious and conscientious, and are often women aged 20–40 years. They may complain of a bloated feeling, wind, nausea, headache and tiredness and that their motions are like hard pellets or ribbons.

The greatest risk for the sufferers is to be labelled neurotic, which will be a label that may stay with them. There are probably several causes for the disease, which include food allergies, some abnormality of absorption, irritating effects of bile acids, and some disorder following a previous infection of the bowel.

Treatment

Drug treatment should be avoided if at all possible. You should try a high-fibre diet (e.g. bran) and plenty of fluids. If pain is a problem, it may be

Table 16.3 Preparations by mouth used to treat ulcerative colitis and Crohn's disease

Preparation	*Drug*	*Drug group*	*Dosage form*
Asacol †	mesalazine	Salicylate	Tablets coated with an acrylic-based resin
Azamune	azathioprine	Immunosuppressant	Tablets
Celevac	methylcellulose '450'	Bulking agent	Tablets, granules
Cellucon	methylcellulose '2500'	Bulking agent	Tablets
Deltacortril	prednisolone	Corticosteroid	Enteric-coated tablets
Dipentum	olsalazine	Salicylate	Capsules
Fybogel	ispaghula husk	Bulking agent	Sugar-free effervescent granules
Fybranta	bran	Bulking agent	Tablets
Imodium	loperamide	Opiate	Capsules, sugar-free syrup
Imuran	azathioprine	Immunosuppressant	Tablets
Isogel	ispaghula husk	Bulking agent	Granules
Metamucil	ispaghula husk	Bulking agent	Powder
Nalcrom	sodium cromoglycate	Mast cell stabilizer	Capsules
Normacol	sterculia	Bulking agent	Granules
Pentasa *	mesalazine	Salicylate	Slow-release tablets
Precortisyl	prednisolone	Corticosteroid	Tablets
Prednesol	prednisolone	Corticosteroid	Tablets
prednisolone	prednisolone	Corticosteroid	Tablets
Questran	cholestyramine	Bile acid remover	Powder
Regulan	ispaghula husk	Bulking agent	Effervescent powder, gluten-free
Salazopyrin *†	sulphasalazine	Salicylate–sulphonamide	Tablets, enteric-coated tablets, suspension, enemas
Sintisone	prednisolone	Corticosteroid	Tablets
Vi-Siblin	ispaghula husk	Bulking agent	Granules

* also an enema † also as suppositories

Table 16.4 Corticosteroid enemas

Preparation	*Drug*	*Dosage form*
Colifoam	hydrocortisone	Foam in aerosol pack
Predenema	prednisolone	Enema
Predfoam	prednisolone	Foam in aerosol
Predsol	prednisolone	Enema

worth trying a short course of an anti-spasmodic drug (see Table 16.5) such as mebeverine, alverine or a specially coated preparation of peppermint oil (e.g. Colpermin, Mintec).

Anticholinergic and anti-spasmodic drugs used to slow down movements of the stomach and intestine

Food is propelled through the stomach and intestine by rhythmic waves of muscular contractions in their walls. This is called peristalsis. Increased peristalsis in the intestine causes diarrhoea and a reduced peristalsis causes constipation. Vomiting is a reversed peristalsis of the stomach.

Muscles in the walls of the stomach and intestine are controlled by the autonomic nervous system (see Chapter 2). Stimulation of the sympathetic nerves (which use noradrenaline as a nerve messenger) causes the muscles to relax and decreases peristalsis, whereas stimulation of the parasympathetic nerves (which use acetylcholine as a nerve messenger) causes the muscles to contract and increases peristalsis.

Drugs that block acetylcholine receptors are called anticholinergic drugs. They block the effects of parasympathetic nerve stimulation and reduce peristalsis and so are used to treat diarrhoea (see earlier). Anticholinergic drugs also relieve painful spasms of muscles in the stomach and intestine (colic) and are used for this purpose. (They are also used to relieve colic in the kidneys and gall bladder, and to reduce acid production in the treatment of peptic ulcers; see Chapter 2.)

Other drugs, called anti-spasmodics, also relieve spasm of muscles in the stomach and intestine (colic) by acting directly on the muscles of the intestine and relaxing them.

Anticholinergic drugs used to relieve spasm

ambutonium bromide
atropine methonitrate
atropine sulphate
belladonna alkaloids
dicyclomine (Merbentyl)
glycopyrronium
hyoscine (Buscopan)
hyoscyamine
mepenzolate (Cantil)
pipenzolate (Piptal)
poldine (Nacton)
propantheline (Pro-Banthine)

Anti-spasmodics used to relieve spasm

alverine (Spasmonal)
mebeverine (Colofac, Colven [with ispaghula husk])
peppermint oil (Colpermin, Mintec)

Table 16.5 Preparations used to relieve painful spasm of the stomach and intestine

Preparation	*Drug*	*Drug group*	*Dosage form*
Aludrox SA	ambutonium bromide, aluminium hydroxide gel, magnesium hydroxide	Anticholinergic Antacids	Sugar-free suspension
Aluhyde	belladonna liquid extract, aluminium hydroxide, magnesium trisilicate	Anticholinergic Antacids	Tablets
aluminium hydroxide and belladonna mixture	belladonna alkaloids, aluminium hydroxide	Anticholinergic Antacid	Mixture (contains chloroform spirit)
Alvercol	alverine, sterculia	Anti-spasmodic Bulking agent	Granules
atropine sulphate	atropine sulphate	Anticholinergic	Tablets
Bellocarb	belladonna extract, magnesium carbonate, magnesium trisilicate	Anticholinergic Antacids	Tablets
Buscopan	hyoscine	Anticholinergic	Tablets, injection
Cantil	mepenzolate	Anticholinergic	Tablets, elixir
Carbellon	belladonna extract, charcoal, magnesium hydroxide, peppermint oil	Anticholinergic Adsorbent Antacid Anti-spasmodic	Tablets
Colofac	mebeverine	Anti-spasmodic	Tablets, sugar-free liquid
Colpermin	peppermint oil	Anti-spasmodic	Enteric-coated capsules
Colven	mebeverine, ispaghula husks	Anti-spasmodic Bulking agent	Effervescent granules
Eumydrin	atropine	Anticholinergic	Solution

Table 16.5 Preparations used to relieve painful spasm of the stomach and intestine (*cont.*)

Preparation	*Drug*	*Drug group*	*Dosage form*
Kolanticon	dicyclomine, aluminium hydroxide, magnesium oxide, activated dimethicone	Anticholinergic Antacids Anti-flatulent	Sugar-free gel
kolantyl	dicyclomine, aluminium hydroxide, magnesium oxide	Anticholinergic Antacids	Sugar-free gel
magnesium trisilicate and belladonna mixture	belladonna, magnesium trisilicate	Anticholinergic Antacid	Mixture
Merbentyl	dicyclomine	Anticholinergic	Tablets, syrup
Mintec	peppermint oil	Anti-spasmodic	Enteric-coated capsules
Nacton and Nacton Forte	poldine	Anticholinergic	Tablets
Piptal	pipenzolate	Anticholinergic	Tablets
Piptalin	pipenzolate activated dimethicone	Anticholinergic Deflatulent	Elixir
Pro-Banthine	propantheline	Anticholinergic	Tablets
Spasmonal	alverine	Anti-spasmodic	Capsules

17

Constipation

Constipation can mean different things to different people. Some people think they are constipated if they do not have their bowels opened every day. Other people only have their bowels opened two or three times a week and they consider this to be normal for them. In a way, being 'normal' is what you are used to and any deviation from that may be called constipation. If you are passing hard, small stools and having your bowels opened less frequently than is normal for you, you are constipated. The important thing about having your bowels opened is that it should be painless and not require too much straining and it should be satisfyingly complete.

Causes

Constipation may be a symptom of an underlying disease of the bowel or anus, of the nerves supplying the bowel (e.g. spinal cord injury), or of some other generalized disease such as an underactive thyroid gland (hypothyroidism). In these cases the treatment of the constipation is to treat the underlying disease. Constipation may also be due to general debility, lack of mobility, old age or mental deficiency. However, constipation is most often caused by a diet that does not have sufficient fibre in it and poor bowel habits (not going when you feel the urge).

Drugs may cause constipation, particularly in elderly patients. Often there is a combination of factors that come together; for example, an elderly patient with poor bowel actions on a diet low in fibre is prescribed a drug which causes constipation.

Warning *You should always seek medical advice for any change in your bowel habits that goes on for more than a week or two, particularly if there is blood in your motions.*

Drugs used to treat constipation

Drugs used to treat constipation are usually termed laxatives. Other names include cathartic, purgative, aperient and evacuant. We usually talk about a *laxative* when we wish to produce a soft, formed, easy to pass motion and a *purgative* when we wish to produce a fairly quick and fluid emptying of the bowels. However, the terms all mean the same thing and the results will depend on the type of laxative used and its dose.

There are four main groups of drugs used to treat constipation, which may be taken by mouth, and according to how they work they are referred to as stimulant laxatives, bulk-forming laxatives, osmotic laxatives and faecal softeners. Some may also be taken as suppositories or enemas.

Stimulant laxatives

These laxatives increase the movements of the large bowel by 'irritating' the lining and stimulating nerves in the bowel wall, which cause the muscles to contract. They may also increase the production of chemicals (e.g. prostaglandins) by cells in the bowel wall, which stimulates the secretion of water and salts into the bowel. How they actually produce these effects is not known but the result is that they speed up bowel movement and reduce the absorption of water and salts, which makes the motions soft and watery and also more bulky.

Harmful effects

All stimulant laxatives may cause intestinal cramps and griping pains, increased secretion of mucus and, in some people, excessive loss of water and salts (particularly potassium). Regular use may cause loss of protein and failure to absorb essential elements from food such as vitamins, which may be harmful, especially in elderly people. In addition, they may cause a weakening of the muscles of the bowel (atony of the colon) so that it does not function properly. This may actually cause constipation and the danger then is that the individual takes further doses of the stimulant laxative which only makes things worse.

Commonly used stimulant laxatives

Bisacodyl may cause intestinal cramps and, when taken by suppository, may produce soreness and irritation. To avoid irritating the lining of the stomach, bisacodyl tablets have a special protective coating (enteric coating) which does not dissolve until the tablets reach the intestine. It is structurally related to phenolphthalein (see later).

Cascara, senna and *danthron* are chemically related (they are anthraquinones). When they are taken by mouth, soluble breakdown products are absorbed from the small intestine into the bloodstream and excreted back into the bowel (colon) where they stimulate nerves in the bowel which cause the muscles to contract and speed up bowel movement. An acid breakdown product from these laxatives colours the urine red or brown according to how acid the urine is (brown if acid, red if alkaline). If taken over prolonged periods of time, they produce brown patches of pigmentation on the lining of the bowel. This is not serious and clears up in 4–12 months after the drug has been stopped. *They should not be used if you are breast feeding.* Danthron may irritate the skin in incontinent people.

It has been known for some time that *danthron* and related drugs (anthraquinones) could possibly cause cancer because they have been shown to be mutagenic (i.e. they can damage genes) and there is a relationship between this ability and the ability to produce cancer. Long-term use of high daily doses of danthron has been associated with the development of cancer in the intestines and livers of rodents. Even though there is no evidence that danthron produces cancer in humans, this once widely prescribed stimulant laxative is now reserved for treating constipation caused by morphine and related drugs used to treat pain in terminally ill patients.

A combined preparation of danthron and docusate (*co-danthrusate, Normax*) is available for this purpose. Docusate sodium is a weak laxative which softens the motions and also causes some stimulation of the bowel wall. Danthron combined with a faecal softener, poloxamer 188 is also available (co-danthramer).

Oxphyphenisatin is a stimulant laxative which should not be used regularly because it causes liver damage, producing jaundice.

Phenolphthalein is a stimulant laxative which, when taken by mouth, is absorbed from the small intestine into the bloodstream where it is taken to the liver and excreted in the bile. This means that phenolphthalein re-enters the intestine and produces a prolonged action on the intestine. After absorption into the bloodstream it is also excreted in the urine which, if alkaline, the phenolphthalein will colour red. Phenolphthalein also colours the motions red. This can be a bit alarming to the individual who may think he is passing blood in his urine and motions. Phenolphthalein may occasionally cause allergic skin rashes, protein to appear in the urine (albuminuria) and damage the red blood cells (haemoglobinaemia).

Sodium picosulphate is a powerful stimulant laxative which is used to empty the bowel before surgery or X-ray examination of the bowel.

Use of stimulant laxatives

Stimulant laxatives should be used only *occasionally* and only for a dose or two. Except in the terminally ill and/or the seriously ill, they should never be taken on a regular daily basis. They should not be used to treat children or pregnant women. They take 6–18 hours to work when taken by mouth.

Powerful stimulant laxatives should *not* be used: they include aloes, aloin, buckthorn, cassia pulp, colocynth, croton oil, euonymus, ipomoea, jalap, kaladana, podophyllum, rhubarb, tamarind and turpeth, and unstandardized preparations of cascara, frangula, rhubarb and senna.

Castor oil

Castor oil differs from other stimulant laxatives in that it is broken down in the small intestine to ricinoleic acid which causes an increase in fluid secretion from the lining of the small intestine and may possibly act as a direct irritant to the lining of the intestine. Castor oil causes the irritant contents of the intestine to move on rapidly, producing watery motions in about 3–6 hours. Because it works on the small intestine its prolonged use may result in excessive loss of nutrients, fluids and salts. It should not be used.

Bulk-forming laxatives

These are indigestible substances that increase the bulk of the contents of the bowel by absorbing water and swelling. This stimulates the bowel muscles to contract. They also encourage the growth of micro-organisms in the bowel, which increases the bulk. They are taken by mouth.

Many bulk-forming laxatives (see later) are obtained from plants (e.g. seeds, husks, and gums) and some are manufactured (e.g. methylcellulose and related compounds). Bran is a useful bulk laxative and if taken regularly every day helps to keep the bowel movements regular.

Bulk-forming laxatives are the laxatives of choice because they are not absorbed into the bloodstream and they do not interfere with the absorption of nutrients. They are slow to work and may take up to 2–3 days in some people. Indications for their use are listed in Table 17.1. The choice of bulk-forming laxatives does not really matter so long as the recommended dose is taken with a full glass of water (about 240 ml; 8 oz).

Risks of taking bulk-forming laxatives

Bulk-forming laxatives must be taken with plenty of fluids because of the risk of causing a blockage in the bowels. This is a particular danger in the elderly, in people who are debilitated from a severe illness and in people who have a disease of the bowel. Bulk laxatives may cause wind and distension of the abdomen. Some individuals may be allergic to *sterculia* and *gum preparations*, and develop a skin rash and symptoms of hayfever and asthma.

Coarse bran works better than fine bran because it retains more water, but it can interfere with the absorption of calcium, zinc and iron. *Fine bran* can be taken in cereals, bread or biscuits. Because of the risk of constipation, bran should not be used by the old elderly, the terminally ill or people with nerve disorders affecting the bowel (e.g. spinal injury). Bran should not be used by individuals with coeliac disease.

Warnings on the use of bulk laxatives

Adequate fluids must be taken each day in order to prevent obstruction to the bowel. They are not suitable for people on a restricted fluid intake and they should be used with caution by anyone taking 'water tablets' (diuretics). Bulk laxatives should not be used by individuals with weakened bowel muscles (atony) nor if there is evidence of some narrowing of the bowel. In particular, they should not be used by elderly people who have a blockage of the bowels (faecal impaction) because they will only make the blockage worse. Inhalation of the dry powder from some bulk laxatives may cause wheezing in some patients.

Osmotic laxatives (saline laxatives, health salts)

Osmotic laxatives are salts of magnesium, sodium and potassium in varying mixtures. They cause large amounts of water to be retained in the intestine instead of being absorbed. This increases the bulk of the contents and stimulates the stretch reflexes in the bowel wall. This triggers movement and the passage of a large volume of watery motions. They work in about 2 hours. Because they may produce dehydration due to excessive loss of water, they should be taken with plenty of fluids.

Osmotic laxatives should be used only occasionally as a one-off treatment for constipation.

Lactulose is a complex synthetic sugar compound made up of fructose and galactose. It is not digested in the small intestine and enters the large bowel unchanged. Here bacteria break it down into two weak acids (lactic and acetic) which draw water into the bowel by osmosis and increase the bulk of the bowel contents. The acids also encourage the growth of bacteria, which also adds to the bulk of the contents. The weak acids are absorbed in the upper colon, so the osmotic effect does not continue right through the colon. The increase in bulk of the bowel contents stimulates bowel movements. Because it makes the contents more acid it discourages the growth of those bacteria which produce ammonia and it is therefore also of use in treating people suffering from liver failure. It takes up to 48 hours to work, and may produce nausea and vomiting.

Risks of osmotic laxatives

Osmotic laxatives may produce severe loss of water and cause dehydration which may be harmful in children, in the elderly and in people who are debilitated by illness. Those that contain *magnesium* salts may be harmful because some magnesium may be absorbed into the bloodstream. In an individual with kidney disease, excretion in the urine may be defective and magnesium may accumulate in the body to produce magnesium poisoning. *Sodium* is easily absorbed into the bloodstream from those saline laxatives that contain sodium. This may be harmful to people with a raised blood pressure or heart failure and interfere with diuretic treatment aimed at reducing the body's sodium and water content. They may cause sodium and water retention in some individuals.

Faecal softeners

There are two types of softeners: *lubricants*, which cover the faeces in oil and prevent them losing water so that they remain soft and easy to pass (e.g. liquid paraffin); and *wetting agents*, which make water and solids mix more easily and make the faeces soft (e.g. docusate sodium [dioctyl sodium sulphosuccinate], poloxamers).

Liquid paraffin, if used regularly, may decrease the absorption of fat-soluble vitamins A, D, E and K from the intestine. The impaired absorption of vitamin D may decrease the absorption of calcium and phosphates and affect bone formation, and the defective absorption of vitamin K may be harmful in pregnant women. People taking anti-coagulants (anti-blood-clotting drugs) that block the production of vitamin K should not take liquid paraffin because it interferes with the absorption of vitamin K from the intestine and may therefore increase the harmful effects of these drugs.

Young or elderly and debilitated people may, rarely, inhale a few drops of liquid paraffin into their lungs when they swallow it and this may cause pneumonia (lipoid pneumonia). Small amounts may be absorbed from the intestine and may collect in lymph glands, producing swollen lymph glands in the intestinal wall, liver and spleen. It may also leak from the anus, causing irritation (pruritus ani). It should not be used in children under 3 years of age or in people with a swallowing difficulty. It should only be used occasionally.

Wetting drugs used to soften the faeces

Drugs that make water and fatty substances mix more easily (wetting agents) soften the motions and help to lubricate the lining of the bowel.

They take 24–48 hours to work. This softening allows more fluid to remain in the mixture. Examples of wetting drugs are docusate sodium and poloxamer. They are often combined with a stimulant laxative (see earlier).

Faecal softeners are of no use in treating long-standing constipation, especially in elderly or debilitated people. They may be useful for short-term treatment, for example in patients who have undergone surgical removal of haemorrhoids or other surgery around the anus.

Misuse of laxatives

Laxatives have been and still are widely misused and abused. They have become part of our folk medicine, and few adults have escaped being 'purged' in their lives, and there still is a widely held belief, particularly among elderly people, that a 'good clear out' is beneficial. This is strengthened by another belief that, to be healthy, everyone should have their bowels opened at least once every day. Of course none of this is true but around it have developed an extremely lucrative drug industry and herbal industry. Millions of pounds are made each year from people emptying their bowels and belching quite unnecessarily.

Warning *Do not use stimulant laxatives, osmotic laxatives or faecal softeners on a regular basis. The occasional use of a laxative is not harmful to health but the regular long-term use of stimulant laxatives, osmotic laxatives or faecal softeners may well be harmful. Furthermore, the regular use of these laxatives interferes with an individual's ability to have his bowels opened naturally without drugs, no matter what the manufacturers say about the 'natural' and 'gentle' effects of their laxative products!*

The laxative habit – laxative abuse

It is important for you to remember that stimulant and osmotic laxatives empty the bowel; and it is not surprising therefore that someone who has taken a stimulant or osmotic laxative every day for a week or so and then stops the laxative may go for several days without a motion. Unfortunately, this may persuade the individual that he cannot 'go' and so he takes another dose of laxative, and a vicious circle is set up leading to what is called laxative abuse.

The abuse of stimulant and osmotic laxatives is still widespread despite the fact that they cause all kinds of problems to their users – such as irritation of the lining of the bowel; excessive loss of water, nutrients and salts producing tiredness, weakness and thirst; and loss of calcium leading to bone softening.

Poor diet

We in the western world have not been helped in our bowel habits by diets that lack roughage. These diets have contributed to constipation and bowel disorders. Therefore, the sensible treatment of constipation is not to take laxatives but to make sure that your diet contains sufficient roughage e.g. insoluble fibre (cereal fibre) to prevent bowel problems developing. Insoluble fibre has two useful properties: it reaches the bowel without having been digested so that it forms roughage; and, while there, it absorbs fluid, making the motions bulky and stimulating bowel movements. However, it is not necessary to go over the top and shovel spoonfuls of bran on to everything you eat. It is the old story of moderation – eat a good sensible diet which includes adequate fruit, vegetables and cereals (e.g. wholemeal bread). This will provide adequate fibre and help to prevent constipation and bowel disease.

When to treat constipation

Table 17.1 includes a list of when and how to treat or prevent constipation. These are only *suggestions*, but remember that constipation may be very distressing in some people – such as the elderly and the seriously ill (e.g. dying from cancer) – who may have to take constipating drugs such as morphine for pain. In these individuals the use of laxatives may relieve distress. Any treatment for constipation in such people needs to be tailored to the individual's needs. This will require knowledge of available preparations and how they work.

Stopping the laxative habit

You should never take a stimulant laxative or an osmotic laxative regularly. These laxatives should be used only *occasionally* when an individual who is normally not constipated becomes constipated because of some outside factor such as going on holiday. Even then, it is better to try a bulk laxative (e.g. bran) and plenty of fluids before resorting to a stimulant or osmotic laxative.

If you are in the habit of taking a stimulant or osmotic laxative regularly, you should take steps to stop it. Try switching to a faecal softener such as docusate sodium (Dioctyl). You should stop your laxative and start with a large dose of Dioctyl; as you settle down to regular bowel movements you should gradually reduce the dose of Dioctyl over a period of several weeks and then stop it. It will help if you drink more fluids than normal each day during the first few weeks. At the same time you should make sure that your diet contains adequate fibre. If you still have a problem, it may be necessary to take a bulk laxative regularly every day (e.g. bran). If you can't take bran, try something like cellulose (methylcellulose). The latter procedure should be followed if you are in the habit of taking a faecal softener (e.g. Dioctyl) regularly every day.

NOTE You must check with your doctor whether any of the drugs you are taking may cause constipation. If they can, you should decide jointly whether you really need to be taking them, or whether you can switch to a drug or drugs that do not constipate. If either of these actions is not possible, ask your doctor to prescribe a laxative but try to avoid using a stimulant or osmotic laxatives if possible (see above).

Faecal impaction

Poor and irregular bowel movements cause incomplete emptying of the rectum, which may over time cause a mass of faeces to block the rectum – faecal impaction. It may occur in children who have defective nervous control of their rectum, in some severely mentally ill or mentally handicapped people and in the elderly, particularly if they are debilitated or confined to bed. Liquid faeces above the obstruction start to dam up and this can distend the bowel. Some of the liquid faeces may seep round the obstruction and start to leak out of the anus; this may be mistaken for diarrhoea and treated with anti-diarrhoeal drugs, which only make the condition worse. It is referred to as spurious diarrhoea. The faecal mass may also cause an ulcer at the site of the impaction.

Faecal impaction is not that uncommon in elderly people and that is why an elderly person who complains of 'leakage' should be examined most carefully by a doctor, who will need to examine the inside of the rectum by putting a finger up the anus where the mass may be felt. Sometimes the obstruction is higher up and can be felt only by pressing a hand on the abdomen.

Treatment

The treatment of faecal impaction involves the use of a suppository or an enema (see Table 17.2) and/or manual removal of the impacted mass of faeces by the patient or a doctor or nurse using gloved fingers or a special spoon.

Prevention of any future impaction is essential. Therefore, it is important to try to avoid the use of any drug that may cause constipation, and to take a bulk laxative (e.g. bran) regularly every day along with adequate fluids by mouth.

Drugs that may cause constipation

Many drugs may cause constipation and can produce particular problems in elderly people, who are prone to develop constipation anyway, and in debilitated patients. Drugs that may cause constipation include:

aluminium and calcium antacids in indigestion remedies
anticholinergic drugs
anti-parkinsonism drugs (e.g. bromocriptine)
anti-psychotic drugs
benzodiazepine anti-anxiety drugs and sleeping drugs
beta blockers may occasionally cause constipation or diarrhoea
calcium channel blockers (e.g. verapamil)
ganglion blocking drugs used to treat raised blood pressure (e.g. mecamylamine and pempidine)
iron salts
narcotic pain relievers (e.g. codeine, dextropropoxyphene, morphine, etc.)
tricyclic anti-depressant drugs
thiazide diuretics

Enemas and suppositories

Enemas

Enemas are frequently used in order to apply a laxative directly into the rectum. They include the following.

Salts (e.g. phosphates) draw water from the wall of the bowel into the contents. This increases the bulk of the motions, which stretches the bowel wall and stimulates it to empty. They are used to prepare the bowel for surgery and X-ray. They should not be used regularly because they can disturb the water and salt content of the body.

Oils (e.g. arachis oil, glycerol) lubricate hard faeces and make them easier to pass.

Softeners (e.g. docusate sodium) soften hard faeces and make them easier to pass. Docusate sodium may also have some stimulant effect.

Stimulants (e.g. bisacodyl) irritate the bowel wall and make it contract.

Soaps (e.g. soft soap enema) irritate the bowel wall and may be harmful; they should not be used.

Table 17.1 Suggestions on when to use a laxative

When to use a laxative	*Which laxative to use*
Painful and bleeding piles After surgery on the anus for piles or fissures	Try a faecal softener – e.g. docusate sodium (Dioctyl)
Bowel disorders – e.g. diverticulitis, irritable bowel syndrome, colostomy, ileostomy, ulcerative colitis	Try a higher fibre diet containing bran. If this does not work, try a bulk-forming laxative such as methylcellulose (Celevac). Must drink plenty of fluids
Pregnancy	Change to a higher fibre diet. You must drink plenty of fluids
After childbirth	Try a higher fibre diet plus plenty of fluids. A stimulant laxative – e.g. senna – may be necessary, or a softener – e.g. docusate sodium (Dioctyl)
Just after a heart attack (myocardial infarction) After an abdominal operation	Try a faecal softener – e.g. docusate sodium (Dioctyl). A stimulant laxative – e.g. senna – may be necessary or an osmotic laxative such as lactulose
Old age	Try a higher fibre diet plus plenty of fluids. Use a faecal softener – e.g. docusate sodium (Dioctyl) – or a stimulant laxative – e.g. senna (Senokot) – or try co-danthrusate (Normax). Check whether any other drugs you are taking cause constipation
Before X-ray and surgery on the bowel	A stimulant laxative is used – e.g. sodium picosulphate (Laxoberol, Picolax), bisacodyl (Dulcolax)
Occasional attacks of constipation when living habits change, such as going on holiday	Try a bulk-forming laxative – e.g. bran – every day on holiday and drink plenty of fluids, particularly if it is hot. Use a stimulant laxative only if necessary – e.g. senna (Senokot)
People debilitated by an illness (e.g. cancer) and/or receiving constipating drugs (e.g. morphine-related drugs)	Try a faecal softener – e.g. docusate sodium (Dioctyl) – or a combination of a faecal softener with a stimulant laxative – e.g. co-danthrusate (Normax) – or try a combination of lactulose (Duphalac) with a stimulant laxative – e.g. senna (Senokot)

NOTE Bulk-forming laxatives (e.g. bran) will not produce prompt emptying of the bowels; they may take a day or two to work. They are the only laxatives that may be used regularly. All other forms of laxatives should be used only for one-off treatments except in the terminally ill and in old elderly people who are immobile.

Suppositories

Suppositories offer another method of applying a laxative directly into the rectum. They may include glycerol (a lubricant laxative), bisacodyl (a stimulant laxative) or sodium acid phosphatase (an osmotic laxative).

Table 17.2 Enemas and suppositories – preparations

Preparation	*Drug*	*Drug group*
bisacodyl suppositories	bisacodyl	Stimulant laxative
Carbalax suppositories	sodium bicarbonate, sodium acid phosphate	Osmotic laxative
Dulcolax suppositories	bisacodyl	Stimulant laxative
Fletchers' Arachis Oil Retention Enema	arachis oil	Faecal softener
Fletchers' Enemette micro-enema	docusate sodium	Faecal softener
Fletchers' Phosphate Enema	sodium acid phosphate, sodium phosphate	Osmotic laxative
glycerol suppositories	glycerol, purified water	Lubricant
Micolette micro-enema	sodium lauryl sulphoacetate, sodium citrate, glycerol	Faecal softener and lubricant
Micralax micro-enema	sodium alkylsulphoacetate, sodium citrate, sorbic acid	Faecal softener, lubricant
Relaxit micro-enema	sodium citrate, sodium lauryl sulphate, sorbic acid, glycerol, sorbitol	Faecal softener, lubricant
Veripaque enema	oxyphenisatin	Stimulant laxative

Health salts

So-called health salts usually contain sodium bicarbonate (bicarbonate of soda), which gives off carbon dioxide when it mixes with the acid in the stomach; this makes you belch. They also contain magnesium and/or sodium or potassium salts which cause water to be retained in the bowel. This increases the bulk of your motions and makes you open your bowels. To put it more plainly, health salts 'give' you wind so that you can belch, and/or increase the bulk of your motions so that you have to empty your bowels. What belching and unnecessary bowel openings have to do with health is not obvious but some people seem to want to buy 'health' in a bottle – no matter whether they belch it out at one end or pass it out at the other!

Andrews Liver Salts contains citric acid, sodium bicarbonate, magnesium sulphate and 40% sugar. The preparation of Andrews for diabetics contains saccharin instead of sugar. *Eno* contains sodium carbonate and bicarbonate, citric acid and tartaric acids. *Juno Junipah Salts* contains sodium sulphate, sodium phosphate and sodium bicarbonate, saccharin and juniper oil. *Juno Junipah Tablets* contain sodium sulphate, sodium phosphate and sodium chloride, juniper oil and phenolphthalein.

Other salts that are used as laxatives include purified cream of tartar (potassium acid citrate), Epsom salts (magnesium sulphate), Milk of Magnesia (magnesium hydroxide), Rochelle salt (sodium potassium tartarate), and Glauber's salt (sodium sulphate).

Complications

Internal haemorrhoids may bleed sufficiently to cause iron deficiency anaemia due to loss of blood. They may also swell and bulge through the anus, when they are said to have prolapsed. Usually they can be pushed back in, but sometimes they become trapped and the blood inside them clots, producing thrombosed haemorrhoids.

External haemorrhoids may also thrombose and produce very painful, tender, bluish lumps in the anus. They may bleed if the thrombosed pile breaks open.

Skin tags are pieces of scar tissue covered by anal skin. They may be caused by a healed-up thrombosed external haemorrhoid or by uneven healing of the skin following injury or surgery to the haemorrhoids.

Symptoms

External haemorrhoids may itch and burn because the surface becomes irritated by moisture and faeces due to poor hygiene and, sometimes, by the applications used to treat them. Pain may occur if the overlying skin of external haemorrhoids becomes infected, inflamed or irritated. If a thrombosis develops the pain can be very severe. The overlying skin of external haemorrhoids may bleed if it is irritated and result in bright red blood on the toilet paper when the anus is wiped after defaecation.

Bleeding is usually associated with internal haemorrhoids. The blood is bright red, and may 'ooze' from the anus or occur only on defaecation when the blood covers the faeces but is not mixed with them. However, be warned – never put bleeding from the rectum down to haemorrhoids without having a careful internal examination of the rectum.

Treatment of haemorrhoids

Internal haemorrhoids that bleed and/or prolapse should be tied off at their base. After about a week the haemorrhoidal tissue sloughs off. Alternatively, the blood vessels just above the haemorrhoids can be blocked off by injecting an irritating chemical into them (sclerosing). These are not appropriate treatments for external haemorrhoids. If an *external haemorrhoid* thromboses, the clot may be removed surgically. The haemorrhoids may be removed surgically.

Local treatment

With external haemorrhoids, generally all that is needed is good local hygiene, bathing in warm water with salt added, and the avoidance of constipation by increasing the amount of fibre in the diet or by taking a bulk-forming laxative and avoiding drugs that may produce constipation.

No local application can cure piles; it can only relieve symptoms. The main group of drugs used in local applications to relieve the symptoms of haemorrhoids include the following.

Astringents dry up the surfaces – these include calamine, bismuth oxide or bismuth subgallate and zinc oxide. Hamamelis preparations (witch hazel) are often used but probably owe their effects more to the alcohol they contain than to anything else. Tannic acid is not safe because it can be absorbed into the bloodstream and damage the liver.

Lubricants make the passage of stools through the anal canal less painful – they include sodium oleate, which has detergent properties, and lauromacrogols (e.g. laureth 9). These preparations lubricate surfaces.

Protectives act as a physical barrier to protect the surface of the haemorrhoids from irritation by moisture and faecal material. These often contain soothing substances such as demulcents (e.g. glycerin) or emolients (e.g. fats and oils).

Local anaesthetics are included to relieve pain and itching. Benzocaine and lignocaine are commonly used. They are less irritant than amethocaine, cinchocaine and promoxine which may also be used in haemorrhoidal preparations. Local anaesthetic preparations should only be applied to the outside and not up into the rectum where they will have no effect but can be rapidly absorbed into the bloodstream to produce harmful effects. They may make the skin sensitive and cause irritation and should not be used regularly every day for more than 2 weeks.

Keratolytics (e.g. aluminium chlorhydroxyallantoinate) soften the skin and can get rid of debris on the surface. They should be used only on the outside skin and not inside the anus on the mucous membrane. Sulphur and resorcinol are not recommended for use in this sensitive area.

Vasoconstrictors constrict small blood vessels and are supposed to 'shrink' the haemorrhoids but there is no convincing evidence for this claim. They do, however, appear to relieve itching and swelling of the skin over the haemorrhoids. The ones most frequently used in haemorrhoidal applications include adrenaline, ephedrine or phenylephrine. If applied to the lining of the rectum (the mucous membrane), they may be absorbed into the bloodstream (see harmful effects listed in Chapter 2).

Antiseptics used in haemorrhoidal applications include hexachlorophane, chlorothymol and Peru balsam. However, since the anus and surrounding area are infected with bacteria from the bowel it is unlikely that any antiseptic will be any more effective than a good washing with soap and water. There is no evidence that the use of preparations containing an antiseptic helps to prevent infections.

Wound-healing drugs are included in some haemorrhoidal preparations despite the fact that there is no convincing evidence that they produce any beneficial effects on the 'healing' of haemorrhoids. They include live yeast cell derivatives (LYCD), also referred to as water extract of brewer's yeast, and the skin respiratory factor (SRF). There is no evidence that cod liver oil, shark liver oil or vitamins A and D have any wound-healing effects on haemorrhoids.

Counter-irritants are substances such as camphor, juniper tar and oil of turpentine which, when applied locally produce a feeling of comfort and warmth, and distract from pain coming from some deeper focus. Counter-irritants produce local inflammation and may be absorbed into the bloodstream. They are not recommended for the relief of pain from haemorrhoids.

Heparinoids are substances in local haemorrhoid applications which dissolve blood clots and reduce local swelling and inflammation. They may be of benefit in reducing the swelling of inflamed and/or irritated external haemorrhoids.

Corticosteroids relieve inflammation. They are discussed in detail in Chapter 62, and their use in skin disease is discussed in Chapter 75. They are very effective in relieving irritation. An ointment or cream containing a corticosteroid should be applied night and morning and after defaecation. They should not be used regularly every day for more than 2–3 weeks. They should not be used if thrush infection is present – this should be treated with nystatin by mouth and as a local application (see Chapter 56).

Other preparations used to treat haemorrhoids are principally herbal remedies whose effectiveness has never been proved.

How to use haemorrhoidal preparations

Haemorrhoidal preparations are intended to provide relief from itching, burning, pain, swelling, irritation and discomfort. They do not cure haemorrhoids. Vasoconstrictors and astringents reduce swelling, local anaesthetics relieve pain and corticosteroids relieve inflammation. Available preparations often contain a mixture of many drugs but it is better to use a simple one. No particular preparation can be recommended.

For maximum benefit a haemorrhoidal preparation should be used after you go to the toilet rather than before, and obviously it helps if you keep the anus clean by using moistened tissue or a cotton wool ball. Salt baths are helpful and *it is important to have regular bowel movements and not to get constipated.* A high-fibre diet helps, provided you drink plenty of fluids each day. If pain is severe a faecal softener may help.

Applications for external use should not be applied inside the anus, and they should be used sparingly.

Products for internal use that contain a vasoconstrictor should not be used if you suffer from heart disease, raised blood pressure, over-active thyroid gland or diabetes. If you have difficulty in passing urine or are taking MAOI anti-depressants (Chapter 39), you should not use an internal preparation that contains a vasoconstrictor. Pregnant women should only use internal preparations that contain a simple protective cream or ointment.

Anal fissure

An anal fissure is a tear in the surface of the anal skin caused by injury due, for example, to the passage of a large stool. The tear produces pain on defaecating and it may bleed a little. The tear (or fissure) may swell at the end and be mistaken for a haemorrhoid. Such a swelling is often referred to as 'sentinel pile' because it stands 'guard' to the tear inside the anus.

The tear is in the mid-line and can produce spasm of the anus, which produces more pain. Anal fissures usually heal spontaneously and respond to bathing, something to soften the stools (see Chapter 17) and, if necessary, a local anaesthetic ointment (Chapter 75).

Pruritus ani

Itching of the skin around the anus (pruritus ani) is a symptom, not a diagnosis. Its treatment is discussed in Chapter 75.

19

Disorders of the gall bladder

The liver secretes bile continuously and produces between 1 and 2 litres a day (see Chapter 83). Bile is a greenish-yellow fluid which enters the gall bladder via ducts from the liver. In the gall bladder it is concentrated about ten times by water and salts being absorbed into the bloodstream. The concentrated bile is released along a duct and through an opening into the duodenum. This occurs as a result of food entering the duodenum and stimulating the release of a hormone (cholecystokinin) that causes the gall bladder to contract. The opening of the gall duct into the duodenum is controlled by a circular muscle (a sphincter). This opening is in a small flask-like opening, called an ampulla; it is known as the ampulla of Vater (Vater was an anatomist who first described it).

Glyceryl trinitrate and anticholinergic drugs cause the sphincter to relax and the orifice to open up, whereas morphine and pethidine cause it to contract and the orifice to close up. Pentazocine does not close up the sphincter as much as morphine. These observations have implications for the treatment of gall bladder pain (see later).

Gall stones (cholelithiasis)

The formation of gall stones is the most common disorder that affects the gall bladder. Bile is made up of various constituents, which include bile acids and salts and bile pigments. Cholesterol is secreted into the bile by the liver and is dissolved by the bile acids. If the amount of cholesterol in the bile increases or the amount of bile acids decreases, the cholesterol clumps together in the gall bladder to form *cholesterol stones*. This type of stone accounts for about 75 per cent of all gall stones. The other 25 per cent of gall stones are principally made up of calcium salts. They are referred to as *pigment stones* because they also contain bile pigments. Inflammation and infection of the gall bladder increase the risk of developing gall stones.

Cholesterol stones are more common in women then in men, and the incidence is higher in women who have had several babies and in women who have taken an oral contraceptive pill for many years. Clearly, female sex hormones may influence their development, and possibly a diet high in cholesterol. The long-term use of the blood fat-lowering drug, clofibrate, may be associated with the production of gall stones (see Chapter 25).

Pigment stones may be black or brown. The black ones appear to be associated with advanced age and less than ideal weight, and brown ones are more common in Orientals than in Westerners. Pigment stones also occur in conditions where there is an excessive breakdown of red blood cells (see haemolytic anaemia, Chapter 47).

Symptoms

Gall stones may be present in the gall bladder for years without causing symptoms. However, they may cause recurrent colicky pain (biliary colic) in the upper abdomen and produce indigestion when the patient eats fats (fatty indigestion). They may cause an acute inflammation of the gall bladder (see later). Sometimes a gall stone may block the main duct and produce an obstruction, leading to the development of jaundice (see Chapter 83).

Treatment

Treatment for gall stones usually involves surgical removal of the gall bladder and stones. Drugs that dissolve gall stones (see below) are only of use in people with normal-functioning gall bladders who have mild symptoms and small- or medium-sized cholesterol gall stones which are not dense enough to stop X-rays passing through them (i.e. they are radiotranslucent). More dense stones (e.g. pigment stones) are unlikely to be dissolved by drugs. It takes 6–24 months to dissolve a stone and then the drug may have to be continued long term. Patients need to be on a low cholesterol diet and to attend hospital to be monitored by X-ray or ultrasound and therefore require continuous hospital supervision. After all this effort the success rate is about one in three; furthermore, gall stones recur in one in four patients within 1 year of stopping treatment.

There are two drugs used to dissolve cholesterol gall stones – chenodeoxycholic acid (Chendol, Chenofalk) and ursodeoxycholic acid (Destolit, Ursofalk). *Chenodeoxycholic acid* is a bile acid and is a normal constituent of bile. It reduces the output of cholesterol from the liver into the bile and it also increases the amount of bile acids in the bile which helps to dissolve the stones. *Ursodeoxycholic acid* produces similar effects. These drugs may have a place in the treatment of sufferers who are not fit for surgery or who refuse surgery; otherwise surgery is the best treatment.

Warning *Although these drugs reduce the amount of cholesterol entering the gall bladder they increase the amount of cholesterol in the blood.*

Another drug, *dehydrocholic acid*, may be used to improve drainage from the gall duct after surgery. It stimulates the secretion of thin watery bile.

Acute inflammation of the gall bladder (acute cholecystitis)

Acute inflammation of the gall bladder is nearly always due to obstruction to its outlet by a stone. The sufferer develops a fever with severe pain in the upper abdomen, becomes pale and restless, and vomits.

Pain is relieved by an injection of morphine and its effect on the bile duct opening into the duodenum (see earlier) is reduced by giving an atropine injection as well. Pethidine or pentazocine may be used for less severe pain. Pentazocine does not close up the gall bladder opening. In addition to pain relievers the individual will require fluids by intravenous infusion as well. Once the patient has settled down, the gall bladder should be removed surgically.

Table 19.1 Drugs used to treat gall stones – harmful effects and warnings

chenodeoxycholic acid (Chendol, Chenofalk)
Harmful effects include diarrhoea (particularly at the start of treatment and when high doses are used), itching skin, minor disorders of liver function.

Warnings Chenodeoxycholic acid should not be used if the stones are radio-opaque, if the gall bladder is not functioning, or if the individual has chronic liver disease, inflammatory disorders of the intestine or colon, or active stomach or duodenal ulcers. Avoid excessive intake of foods high in calories and cholesterol, and use a low cholesterol diet.

dehydrocholic acid
Harmful effects None reported.

Warnings Should not be used in individuals with an obstructed bile duct, chronic liver disease or acute liver disease (hepatitis) producing blockage to the flow of bile.

ursodeoxycholic acid (Destolit, Ursofalk)
Harmful effects include diarrhoea.

Warnings It should not be used if the stones are radio-opaque, if the gall bladder is not functioning, or if the individual has chronic liver disease, inflammatory disorders of the intestine or colon, or active stomach or duodenal ulcers. Avoid excessive intake of foods high in calories or cholesterol, use a low cholesterol diet.

Table 19.2 Preparations used to dissolve gall stones

Preparation	*Drug*	*Dosage form*
Chendol	chenodeoxycholic acid	Capsules, tablets
Chenofalk	chenodeoxycholic acid	Capsules
dehydrocholic acid	dehydrocholic acid	Tablets
Destolit	ursodeoxycholic acid	Tablets
Ursofalk	ursodeoxycholic acid	Capsules

20

Angina

The coronary arteries supply blood to the walls of the heart. If they are damaged because of fat deposits in the lining (see Chapter 25) or some other disorder, doctors talk about *coronary artery disease* (or coronary heart disease). This may cause a reduced blood supply to the heart on exercise, which produces pain. This is called *angina* (see below). The blood may clot over a damaged area in a coronary artery and close off the vessel. This is called a *coronary thrombosis.*

The coronary arteries are end arteries – they are rather like the branches of a tree spreading out from two main trunks, the right and left main coronary arteries. If one of the trunks gets blocked by a coronary thrombosis, a wedge-shaped area of heart wall spreading out from the site of the block suffers from a decrease in blood supply. This is called ischaemia and because it affects heart muscle (myocardium) it is referred to as *myocardial ischaemia.* If the blockage is complete, the wedge-shaped piece of heart muscle may die. This is called an infarct and because it affects heart muscle it is referred to as a *myocardial infarction.* A myocardial infarction is an acute medical emergency and is commonly referred to as an acute heart attack. A severe attack of myocardial ischaemia without producing infarction can also be an acute medical emergency and is also called an acute heart attack.

Angina

Angina (angina pectoris) is the term used to describe attacks of chest pain from the heart, of short duration and without any evidence of lasting damage to the heart muscle (i.e. ischaemia without infarction, see above). It is caused by a disorder of the coronary arteries which supply the heart. In most patients who suffer from angina the pain comes on with effort and goes off with rest. This is because on effort the heart has to pump faster and requires more oxygen than it does when at rest. If the coronary arteries are narrowed or blocked by disease they are not able to dilate in order to supply extra blood to the heart to meet its increased need for oxygen, and an imbalance develops between the oxygen the heart needs and the oxygen supplied to it. This shortage of oxygen causes chemicals to be released from the affected part of heart muscle. These produce pain from the heart – angina. As soon as the patient rests the heart has to do less work, oxygen supply meets oxygen needs and the pain goes off.

An attack of angina may occur on exercise, on exposure to the cold, during sexual intercourse, with emotion and tension, and after a heavy meal. These all put extra demand on the heart. Angina may also occur with no extra work if the coronary arteries contract and go into spasm. This reduces the oxygen supply to the heart muscle even further, to below what the resting heart requires.

Angina is a symptom and although drugs are used to reduce or prevent this unpleasant symptom they have no effect on the progression of the underlying disorder that affects the coronary arteries.

NOTE Anaemia, an over-active thyroid gland, disorders of heart rhythm and a narrowing of the aortic valve of the heart predispose to the development of angina. Amphetamines ('speed', slimming pills), adrenaline and drugs that produce adrenaline-like effects, decongestant drugs used in cough and cold remedies, thyroid drugs, ergot drugs used to treat migraine, cocaine, certain drugs that cause a fall in blood pressure (e.g. hydralazine) and several other drugs may affect the heart sufficiently to bring on an attack of angina in a susceptible person.

Types of angina

Stable angina (classic angina of effort, exertional angina) This occurs when the coronary arteries are diseased (e.g. fatty deposits in the lining of the walls: atheroma). People with this type of angina suffer an attack when the oxygen demand of the heart is increased; for example, on effort, with anxiety or emotion, after a large meal or on exposure to the cold. The attacks are predictable, last 1–3 minutes, and are usually relieved by rest and a vasodilator drug (e.g. glyceryl trinitrate).

Unstable angina People with unstable angina may suffer increasingly frequent attacks of angina with less effort, develop angina at rest and find that the pain is more difficult to relieve. It is a medical emergency and the individual should be admitted to hospital for total bed rest, investigation and treatment. It probably is due to a narrowing of a coronary artery, caused by a clot (thrombus), by platelets sticking together, or spasm.

Variant angina (Prinzmetal's angina) This is an attack of anginal pain that shows changes on electrical tracings of the heart (electrocardiograph, ECG), indicating a defective supply of blood to part of the heart. It is unpredictable and may occur at rest and often at night-time. It is due to spasm of the coronary arteries. As the spasm wears off the pain goes and the ECG reverts to 'normal'. It may be associated with weakness, sweating, shortness of breath and nausea. If the spasm is prolonged, a heart attack may develop (see later).

Acute coronary insufficiency (intermediate coronary syndrome) This causes prolonged anginal pain which is often more severe than usual.

Acute myocardial infarction This is the term used to describe irreversible damage and death to cells in a part of the heart caused by a shortage of blood (ischaemia) – see earlier.

Non-drug treatment of angina

Obviously the time to start non-drug treatment of coronary artery disease is before we get it. In other words the best treatment is prevention. This means reducing known risk factors that are associated with the development of coronary heart disease. These are discussed in Chapter 25. Very simply, we should:

- Reduce body weight to within an ideal level
- Decrease the total amount of fat in the diet whilst increasing the proportion of polyunsaturated fats
- Restrict alcohol consumption
- Stop smoking
- Reduce stress and learn to relax
- Take moderate exercise
- Be checked regularly for a raised blood pressure and be treated accordingly

This advice also applies to people who have developed coronary artery disease.

Smoking is harmful to the heart because it increases the heart rate and blood pressure. This causes the heart to work harder, increasing its oxygen need. However, smoking reduces the supply of oxygen to the heart because the carbon monoxide it contains decreases the oxygen-carrying capacity of the blood. In other words, when you smoke you reduce the supply of oxygen to the heart while increasing its oxygen needs. (Also, see Chapter 25.) *Smoking is the main avoidable risk factor in coronary heart disease.*

Exercise has not been directly related to a reduction in the number of people who develop coronary heart disease but there does appear to be an association between regular exercise and a reduced risk of developing it. However, there is no direct evidence that an increase in exercise will prevent an individual from getting a heart attack.

Drug treatment of angina

Drugs are used to treat acute attacks of angina, and to prevent attacks in the short term and in the long term. They belong to three main groups – nitrate vasodilators, beta blockers and calcium channel blockers.

Nitrate vasodilators

The drugs most commonly used are organic nitrates and nitrites and inorganic nitrates. Their basic effects are:

- To dilate small arteries (arterioles) by relaxing the muscles in their walls and therefore increasing their calibre. This reduces resistance to the flow of blood pumped out by the heart, which reduces the blood pressure. This in turn reduces the workload on the heart and, therefore, its oxygen needs.
- To dilate small veins (venules) by relaxing muscles in their walls and therefore increasing their calibre. This reduces the amount of blood returning to the right side of the heart, which reduces the volume of blood that the heart has to pump and, therefore, the workload on the heart and its oxygen needs. The reduced amount of blood entering the heart when it is at rest and filling (diastole) diminishes the resistance to the flow of blood through the coronary arteries and improves the blood supply to the heart muscle.
- To relieve any spasm of muscles in the walls of the coronary arteries which supply the heart, thereby improving the blood flow to the heart muscle and increasing the oxygen supply. This effect may help to ensure that the blood supply gets through to those parts of the heart muscle that were suffering from a poor supply of blood (ischaemia).
- Nitrate vasodilators relieve both stable and unstable angina that come on with exercise or emotion, and they relieve angina caused by spasm of a coronary artery.

Glyceryl trinitrate

This is one of the most effective drugs for producing rapid relief of angina. It is the drug of choice. To work quickly it is sucked under the tongue where it dissolves and enters the bloodstream to produce an almost immediate response. It works within 1–2 minutes and its effects last for about half an hour. This would not happen if the tablet were swallowed because after absorption from the stomach it has to pass through the liver first before getting into the general circulation. On this first pass through the liver most of it gets broken down.

Apart from relieving an attack of angina that has developed, glyceryl trinitrate is very useful for stopping an attack coming on if it is taken just before an event which normally brings on an attack – for example, going out in the cold, just before sexual intercourse, before some physical exertion. There is no limit to how many times you may take glyceryl trinitrate in any one day but if two tablets taken straight after each other do not relieve an attack of angina, you ought to check the age of the tablets (see later) and seek medical help straight away.

Preparations of glyceryl trinitrate In addition to being available in tablets to dissolve under the tongue, on the tongue or to chew, glyceryl trinitrate is also available as a mouth spray to abort an acute attack of angina.

The duration of action of glyceryl trinitrate may be increased by using it in an ointment to be rubbed into the skin. From such an application, it is slowly absorbed directly into the general circulation without first having to pass through the liver; it acts for up to 8 hours. Adhesive pads containing glyceryl trinitrate work in the same way. Slow-release preparations of glyceryl trinitrate are also available to be taken by mouth.

Harmful effects (see later) of glyceryl trinitrate include flushing, headache and a fall in blood pressure (which may produce dizziness and faintness). In general, people become tolerant to these harmful effects but it may help to spit the tablet out immediately the anginal pain has been relieved.

Tablets of glyceryl trinitrate under the tongue are still the cheapest, most effective treatment, but for those who have difficulty in dissolving these tablets a mouth spray may be more convenient to use. Slow-release preparations to be swallowed may increase the duration of action. Applications to the skin may help people who develop angina at rest or in the night.

Warning *Glyceryl trinitrate is unstable, and tablets and solutions can quickly deteriorate and rapidly lose their effectiveness. Tablets should be kept in dark glass containers with aluminium foil tops and contain no cotton wool. Unused tablets should be disposed of after 8 weeks.*

Isosorbide dinitrate and mononitrate

Isosorbide dinitrate tablets to be dissolved under the tongue and also chewable preparations are useful for relieving an acute attack of angina, particularly if attacks occur infrequently; this is because preparations of isosorbide dinitrate keep longer than tablets of glyceryl trinitrate.

Tablets of isosorbide dinitrate and isosorbide mononitrate may be taken in divided doses throughout the day to prevent attacks of angina, and special slow-release preparations to be taken by mouth can have an effect for up to

12 hours. Isosorbide mononitrate is the active breakdown product of isosorbide dinitrate produced when the drug passes through the liver, which helps to explain why it has a longer effect than glyceryl trinitrate which is broken down in the liver to inactive products.

Pentaerythritol tetranitrate

Preparations of pentaerythritol tetranitrate to be taken by mouth are used to prevent attacks of angina. They may be taken two or three times daily *in addition* to glyceryl trinitrate used when necessary to relieve an attack of angina.

Long-acting nitrates are useful if there is a risk of ischaemia without pain (silent ischaemia). Like glyceryl trinitrate, isosorbide dinitrate, isosorbide mononitrate and pentaerythritol tetranitrate may cause flushing of the face, dizziness, rapid beating of the heart and a throbbing headache.

Table 20.1 Drugs used to treat angina: nitrate vasodilator drugs – harmful effects and warnings

Harmful effects The vasodilator effects may produce flushing of the face and a throbbing headache which decreases in intensity the more frequently the drug is used. The lowering effects on the blood pressure may produce dizziness, faintness, weakness and nausea, particularly on standing up after lying down or sitting down. A rare effect of lowering the blood pressure is a reflex increase in heart rate which increases the workload of the heart and its oxygen needs. The increase in heart rate decreases the time when the heart is at rest and obtaining its own supply of blood through the coronary arteries. This may bring on an attack of angina.

Warnings Vasodilators should not be used to treat people who have just had a heart attack, who have severe anaemia or who have a raised pressure in their brain due, for example, to injury, infection, haemorrhage or a tumour. They should not be used in individuals who are allergic to nitrites or nitrates.

Risks in elderly people Harmful effects may be more frequent and severe in elderly people. They are likely to cause a marked fall in blood pressure and should be used with caution.

Risks in driving If the drug makes you feel dizzy or faint do not drive or operate moving machinery while you have these symptoms.

Risks with alcohol Alcohol may increase the risk of throbbing headaches.

General warning on use

For anyone who suffers only an occasional attack of angina, a quick-acting preparation should be used at the earliest sign of pain. A supply of glyceryl trinitrate tablets should be carried at all times and the expiry date should be carefully noted. A stinging sensation under the tongue, flushing of the face and/or headache indicate that the preparation is still active.

Keep them in the original dark glass bottle, tightly closed with no cotton wool (use aluminium foil instead). Do not transfer them to a metal or plastic container. Dispose of them after 8 weeks. A spray keeps very much longer and is useful if attacks are infrequent.

If a particular effort such as walking up stairs or sexual intercourse brings on an attack, take a dose of a quick-acting preparation a few minutes before (e.g. a glyceryl trinitrate tablet under the tongue).

Use only the smallest dose for effective relief. Regular and/or excessive use may cause the body to become tolerant to the drug's effects and this will make a standard dose less effective.

With quick-acting preparations (e.g. glyceryl trinitrate) it helps to sit down when taking the drug because this reduces the possibility of falling due to light-headedness and dizziness. If you are sensitive to these effects, spit the tablet out as soon as the anginal pain has gone.

Nitroglycerine ointment may be used at bed-time to prevent angina coming on in the night. Follow the instructions and do *not* apply it with your fingers. Do *not* rub the ointment into the skin.

Nitroglycerine patches may produce tolerance to the drug and cause it to be less effective with continuous use. Following long-term use nitrate vasodilators should be withdrawn slowly and not stopped suddenly.

Tolerance

All nitrates can induce tolerance, which may be defined as a lessened response to the effects of a drug and so a larger dose has to be given to produce a similar effect. This means that, if regular doses of a long-acting nitrate were used to prevent angina, the dose which initially produced relief may become less effective. Tolerance can occur within 24–48 hours of regular use unless a period of at least 10 hours is allowed *without* treatment. Tolerance is more likely to develop with high doses than with low doses. A period of time when there is no nitrate in the blood will help to prevent tolerance; this can be achieved at night by not taking a dose of nitrate after about 8.00 p.m. or by removing transdermal patches before bed-time. Intravenous glyceryl trinitrate should not be given continuously for more than 36 hours. People who get angina at night and need treatment at night should allow themselves a period of about 10 hours of no treatment in the daytime, and individuals who get regular attacks of angina throughout the 24 hours should take a beta blocker or a calcium channel blocker during a period of no treatment (about 10 hours) with a nitrate vasodilator.

Beta blockers used to treat angina

Beta blockers (beta adrenoreceptor blocking drugs, beta adrenoreceptor antagonists) are used in the long term prevention of angina. As stated earlier, angina occurs when the oxygen needs of the heart are greater than its oxygen supply. Whenever the heart rate increases the workload increases. Therefore in patients who have coronary artery disease, any increase in heart rate may bring on an attack of angina because the coronary arteries are not able to supply sufficient oxygen to meet increased oxygen needs. Any physical effort increases heart rate, so too do emotion (fear, panic, tension, anxiety) and drugs that produce adrenaline-like effects (see Chapter 2).

Effort and emotion activate those nerves of the sympathetic nervous system that use noradrenaline as a chemical messenger. When they are stimulated by effort or emotion, noradrenaline is released by the nerve endings on to receptors (adrenaline receptors, or adrenoreceptors) throughout the body. These receptors are of two main types – alpha and beta.

Effects produced by the stimulation of *alpha receptors* by noradrenaline include constriction of arteries (you go pale if you are scared), dilatation of the pupils, ejaculation in males, and contraction of the neck of the bladder.

Beta receptors are principally located in the heart and arteries, bronchial tubes, uterus (womb), pancreas, liver and the muscular walls of arteries that supply the muscles. Effects produced by stimulation of beta receptors include an increase in heart rate, an increase in the volume of blood pumped out by the heart, relaxation of the bronchial tubes, relaxation of the pregnant womb, dilatation of arteries that supply muscles, tremor of skeletal muscles and relaxation of the bladder.

Beta blockers protect the heart from stimulation

Drugs are available that block the effects of noradrenaline on alpha and beta receptors. The former are called alpha blockers and the latter beta blockers. Those drugs that block beta receptors (beta blockers) are used principally to treat angina, disorders of heart rhythm and raised blood pressure.

Blocking beta receptors from the effects of noradrenaline stimulation has a marked effect when the heart is being stimulated by noradrenaline during effort, excitement and anxiety and by drugs that produce adrenaline-like effects (see Chapter 2). The blocking reduces the effects of such stimulation and produces a slowing of the heart rate and a reduction in the force of contraction of the heart muscle. This reduces the workload of the heart, which reduces its oxygen needs during effort, excitement and anxiety. This helps to reduce attacks of angina. In other words, beta blockers 'protect' the heart from stimulation.

Effects of beta blockers

Beta blockers have little effect on the normal heart when the subject is at rest, but they may have a marked effect when the heart is under noradrenaline stimulation during effort, excitement or anxiety.

It is not fully understood how beta blockers work, particularly in causing a fall in blood pressure. Blood pressure is a product of the volume of blood pumped out by the heart with each beat (cardiac output) and the resistance that the flow of blood meets as it enters smaller and smaller arteries (peripheral resistance). Beta blockers increase cardiac output and reduce peripheral resistance by blocking the effects of noradrenaline stimulation. They may also have an effect on the kidneys, causing a reduction in the release of a substance (the enzyme renin) that is responsible indirectly for increasing peripheral resistance by reducing the calibre (the diameter) of arteries. Beta blockers also reduce the heart rate and slow down the conduction of impulses coming from the pacemaker of the heart. They cause retention of salt and water in the body, which may be related to changes in the blood supply to the kidneys, caused by the fall in output from the heart.

Selective and non-selective effects of beta blockers on the heart and arteries

Beta receptors are divided into two main groups – beta-1 and beta-2. Stimulation of beta-1 receptors affects principally the heart whereas stimulation of beta-2 receptors affects the bronchial tubes, uterus and blood vessels supplying the muscles of the body. Beta blocker drugs vary in the degree of blocking they produce on beta-1 and beta-2 receptors. Some are more selective for beta-1 receptors, unlike the non-selective ones which block both beta-1 and beta-2 receptors. These selective beta blockers (e.g. acebutolol, atenolol, bisopropol, metoprolol) produce most of the their effects on the heart and have a reduced effect on the bronchial tubes (see later).

Beta blockers such as propranolol which block both beta-1 and beta-2 receptors are non-selective. In addition to producing beneficial effects in people suffering from angina, they may also affect the bronchial tubes, producing wheezing (asthma). They may be harmful to individuals suffering from asthma or other wheezing disorders and should not be used by them (see later).

Beta blockers that are relatively selective in blocking beta-1 receptors are sometimes called 'cardioselective' because they produce more effects on the heart than on the bronchial tubes and therefore carry less risk of triggering asthma.

Some beta blockers partially stimulate as well as block beta receptors

Some beta blockers produce both stimulation and blocking of beta receptors.

They are said to have some intrinsic sympathomimetic activity (ISA). They are able to mimic noradrenaline. These beta blockers produce less slowing of the heart rate than the others, and they are less dangerous if the drugs are stopped suddenly. They also produce less coldness of the fingers and toes. They include acebutolol, carteolol, oxprenolol and pindolol.

Potential harmful effects of beta blockers in heart disease

The amount of exercise which a 'normal' person can do may actually be decreased by beta blockers yet increased in people with angina. This is because in someone with angina the reduction in heart rate produced by beta blockers helps the blood supply to the heart to be redistributed to areas where there is a defective supply (due to diseased coronary arteries) although over all the blood flow through the coronary arteries to the heart is decreased.

Because beta blockers slow the heart rate they may be dangerous in a person with a failing heart. They may trigger heart failure when given quickly into a vein. This is because the failing heart relies on noradrenaline stimulation to keep it beating faster in order to compensate for its poor output. Stop this stimulation with beta blockers, the heart rate slows and heart failure may be triggered. This risk is a real one because beta blockers also reduce the force of contraction of heart muscle.

Acute heart failure may occur when beta blockers are used intravenously in someone with severe heart disease; it is rare when the drugs are taken by mouth. Because beta blockers such as propranolol affect the conduction of impulses from the pacemaker of the heart, they may also be dangerous in people who have been over-dosed with digoxin and have developed a degree of blockage in the electrical pathways in the heart (heart block) (see Chapter 22).

Withdrawal symptoms

Any beta blocker that does not induce some stimulation (ISA) of the heart (see above) may produce dangerous effects if stopped suddenly after a period of treatment. This is because the heart is no longer protected against the effects of noradrenaline stimulation. Stop the beta blocker suddenly and the heart starts to beat rapidly which may trigger an attack of angina and, occasionally, a heart attack (myocardial infarction). If beta blockers are stopped suddenly in patients receiving treatment for raised blood pressure, the pressure may occasionally shoot up (rebound) to a life-threatening level. These problems may develop within hours to 1–2 days after the drug is suddenly stopped.

Effects of beta blockers on the brain

The majority of beta blockers are soluble in fat and are capable of entering the brain where they may produce harmful effects such as disturbed sleep, nightmares and mood changes. These harmful effects may be particularly disturbing in the elderly. The beta blockers atenolol, nadolol and sotalol are soluble in water and do not enter the brain easily; therefore they may produce fewer harmful effects on the brain.

Effects of beta blockers on the circulation

Beta blockers constrict small arteries and may decrease the circulation to the skin, resulting in cold hands and feet. They may produce what is termed Raynaud's phenomenon – attacks of intermittent whiteness (pallor) and blueness (cyanosis) of the hands and feet on exposure to moderate degrees of cold (see Chapter 24). Acebutolol, carteolol, oxprenolol and pindolol are less likely than the others to do this because they also partially stimulate beta receptors as well as block them (see above).

Effects of beta blockers on blood glucose levels

Propranolol and related non-selective beta blockers increase the effects of insulin in lowering the blood glucose levels by reducing those of noradrenaline which normally cause a rise in blood glucose. Therefore insulin dosage may have to be changed in diabetics. They also mask the 'adrenaline-produced' symptoms of a low blood glucose (hypoglycaemia) – for example, tremor, sweating and a rapid beating of the heart. This means that individuals may not experience some of the symptoms of hypoglycaemia, which usually act as an early warning to take some sugar. It is best for a diabetic person with angina to take selective beta blockers but they should be used with utmost caution, and not at all by anyone who has frequent attacks of hypoglycaemia.

The use of beta blockers in angina

Beta blockers protect the heart from stimulation during effort, excitement and anxiety. They relieve the symptom of angina and make life more tolerable. However, they do not alter the underlying progression of the disease.

Warnings *Treatment with beta blockers should be tapered off slowly by gradually reducing the daily dose over a period of days to weeks.*

Those beta blockers that have the ability to stimulate the heart as well as to block beta receptors (intrinsic sympathetic activity) may produce less severe withdrawal symptoms. They are sometimes referred to as cardio-protective – they protect the heart.

A serious drawback of beta blockers is that they may produce narrowing of the air passages, which may be dangerous in people with asthma or with chronic obstructive airways disease. Deaths have occurred. For this reason, their use is best avoided in such individuals unless there is no alternative, in which case a selective beta blocker should be used with utmost caution and it may be necessary to increase the dose of the bronchodilator – see discussion under 'Warnings' on the use of beta blockers.

Dangers of combined drug preparations

A new and potentially dangerous problem for asthmatic patients has developed in recent years with the introduction of combined preparations containing a diuretic drug (water tablet) and a beta blocker. These are used to treat raised blood pressure.

The danger is that the individual may not know that these preparations contain both a beta blocker *and* a diuretic, but may think of them only as blood pressure tablets. It is not surprising therefore to learn that some poor asthmatic patients are admitted to hospital every year in severe distress because they were prescribed one of these combinations for their high blood pressure.

Choice of beta blocker

There is no convincing evidence that any one of the many beta blockers available is better than all the others for treating angina. Different people react differently to any given preparation; therefore treatment should always be tailored to the individual's needs.

Beta blockers after a heart attack (myocardial infarction)

There is evidence that some beta blockers, taken daily for 2 years after a heart attack (myocardial infarction), may reduce the risk of an individual suffering another attack. Beyond 2 years it is not clear what benefit they have in preventing another heart attack. Their sudden stoppage may cause a rebound worsening of the damage to the heart muscle. There is evidence that atenolol and metoprolol, given during the acute stage, and timolol and propranolol, in the early convalescent stage, are of benefit.

Warning *Beta blockers should not be used to prevent further heart attacks in people with a low blood pressure, slow heart rate, asthma or a related wheezing disorder or heart failure that was present before the heart attack.*

Table 20.2 Drugs used to treat angina: beta blockers – harmful effects and warnings

Harmful effects of beta blockers vary between different drugs and between different individuals. They vary in frequency, severity and type. Most harmful effects produced by beta blockers are mild and are usually related to the doses used. They can easily be controlled by reducing the dose. More serious harmful effects are rare and are usually caused by high doses and/or by how a particular individual reacts. Not all of the following harmful effects have been reported with every beta blocker but they have been reported with one or more of them and should be borne in mind whenever a beta blocker is used.

Harmful effects Heart and circulation – slowing of the pulse rate, fall in blood pressure, heart failure, heart block, numbness and pins and needles in hands and feet, coldness of fingers and toes.

Brain – light-headedness, mental depression, insomnia, nightmares, drowsiness, confusion, lassitude, weakness, fatigue, visual disturbances and hallucinations. Beta blockers may also produce a reversible depression associated with disorientation in time and place, short-term memory loss, emotional ups and downs and clouded thinking.

Stomach and intestine – nausea, vomiting, stomach upsets, cramps in the abdomen, diarrhoea, constipation and very rarely thrombosis in the blood vessels supplying the intestine.

Allergy – rash, fever and sore throat, difficulty in breathing.

Chest – wheezing.

Blood – very rarely, disorders of white cell production.

Sexual function – rarely, impotence.

Miscellaneous – very rarely, loss of hair (alopecia), psoriasis-like rash of the skin, dry eyes.

Warnings Risks with asthma Non-selective beta blockers block receptors in the bronchial tubes as well as in the heart, arteries and elsewhere. Because of this action they may turn mild asthma into a serious life-threatening disorder and should not be used in anyone with asthma or obstructive airways disease. *Selective* beta blockers should not be used to treat asthma or obstructive airways disease unless it is absolutely necessary. These selective beta blockers may increase wheezing and may trigger asthma in susceptible people.

If it is absolutely necessary to use a selective beta blocker, asthmatic individuals should be advised to increase the daily doses of inhalant bronchodilator (e.g. salbutamol) or to take a slow-release theophylline drug daily by mouth. The beta blocker should be taken in divided doses throughout the day to prevent high levels in the blood.

Risks with heart failure Beta blockers should not be used in people suffering from heart failure or heart block or by anyone on the brink of developing heart failure. They slow the heart rate and depress the actions of the heart, effects that may easily tip a diseased heart into failure. The failing heart relies on some noradrenaline stimulation (see earlier), and if this is totally blocked it will go into failure.

Beta blockers that produce some noradrenaline stimulation (intrinsic sympathetic activity, ISA) of the heart may be better because they tend to cause less slowing and depression of the heart. They include acebutolol, oxprenolol and pindolol. Individuals with a history of heart failure controlled on digoxin and diuretics (see Chapter 22) may receive a beta blocker, but if heart failure persists

Table 20.2 Drugs used to treat angina: beta blockers – harmful effects and warnings (*cont.*)

or develops the beta blocker should be withdrawn. People with heart disease (e.g. valve disease) but no history of failure may be tipped into heart failure by beta blockers. At the first sign of failure they should be given digoxin and a diuretic but if the failure persists the beta blocker should be withdrawn.

Risks in diabetes Beta blockers increase the effects of insulin in lowering blood glucose and may cause a fall in blood glucose levels, resulting in hypoglycaemia (low blood glucose levels). This may be dangerous (see Chapter 65). Diabetics dependent upon insulin injections may therefore have to reduce their dose of insulin.

Beta blockers may mask some of the symptoms of a low blood glucose (hypoglycaemia) (see Chapter 65). This means that a diabetic individual may be developing hypoglycaemia without realizing it.

Beta blockers should not be used in insulin-dependent diabetic people who suffer from frequent attacks of hypoglycaemia. In other diabetics a selective beta blocker should be used (e.g. acebutolol, atenolol, betaxolol, bisoprolol, metoprolol).

Risks from stopping beta blockers suddenly in coronary heart disease Increase of angina, heart attacks and deaths have been reported when beta blockers have been stopped suddenly in people who suffer from coronary heart disease (e.g. angina). Therefore any beta blocker treatment should be reduced slowly over a week or two in such individuals.

No one taking beta blockers should stop treatment suddenly without medical advice.

Anyone taking a beta blocker should always have an extra few weeks' supply available in order to avoid the risks of sudden withdrawal.

These warnings also apply to individuals taking beta blockers for some other disorder (e.g. for raised blood pressure, migraine, thyrotoxocosis, anxiety). They should never stop the drug suddenly. The daily dose should be reduced slowly over a week or two and physical exertion should be limited during this period.

Risks with general anaesthetics and major surgery Beta blockers may increase the risk of depression of the heart in patients under a general anaesthetic. If beta blockers are continued, special caution is needed with anaesthetics that depress the heart – ether, cyclopropane and trichloroethylene. Any excessive slowing of the heart and/or fall in blood pressure should be treated with an injection of atropine.

Risks in disorders of the circulation Treatment with beta blockers reduces the volume of blood pumped out by the heart with each beat. This may aggravate the already poor supply to tissues caused by diseased arteries. Patients should be examined regularly over time to check for any deterioration.

Beta blockers may affect the healthy circulation and produce cold fingers and toes. They may even produce Raynaud's phenomenon – paleness, coldness and blueness of the fingers and toes, caused by a degree of coldness that would not affect a 'normal' person. Beta blockers that possess some ISA – for example, acebutolol, carteolol, oxprenolol and pindolol – may carry less risk of developing this disorder. If it is a problem, labetalol should be tried because, in addition to being a beta blocker, it also dilates small arteries thus increasing the blood supply to the hands and feet.

Risks of beta blockers on the brain Beta blockers may affect the brain and cause insomnia, nightmares, drowsiness, depression, disorientation and confusion. These effects may cause particular problems in the elderly. A reversible depression may develop associated with disorientation in time and place, short-term memory loss, emotional ups and downs, and clouded thinking. Elderly

Table 20.2 Drugs used to treat angina: beta blockers – harmful effects and warnings (*cont.*)

people who develop these harmful effects may be misdiagnosed as demented.

These effects on the brain may be reduced by using beta blockers that do not enter the brain so easily; for example, atenolol, nadolol and sotalol. However, because they are soluble in water they are excreted directly by the kidneys and therefore they should be given in reduced dosages in anyone suffering from impaired kidney function and to elderly people who often have some impairment of their kidney function.

Risks of allergy to beta blockers Susceptible individuals may become allergic to beta blockers and develop a skin rash, fever, sore throat and difficulty in breathing.

Risks in over-active thyroid glands Beta blockers may mask the symptoms of an over-active thyroid gland (see Chapter 63), particularly rapid beating of the heart. If the drugs are then stopped suddenly, a serious thyroid emergency may develop.

Risks in screening for glaucoma Some beta blockers are used to reduce increased pressure of fluid in the eyes (glaucoma), and there is a danger that the condition may be missed in individuals being routinely checked for glaucoma when they have a sight test. This is because a beta blocker used to treat another disorder may reduce the pressure in the eye. Always tell an optician (optometrist) what drugs you are taking.

Risks in impaired kidney function Certain diseases of the kidneys impair their function and may interfere with their ability to excrete drugs via the urine. Those drugs that are normally excreted by the kidneys may therefore increase in concentration in the bloodstream to reach toxic levels. This is always a danger in elderly people, who may have some impairment of their kidney function merely as a result of ageing, and not disease. Doses of acebutolol, atenolol, betaxolol, bisoprolol, metoprolol, nadolol, pindolol and sotalol should therefore be reduced in anyone with impaired kidney function and in the elderly.

Risks in elderly people The dose of beta blockers may have to be reduced in the elderly because harmful effects may be more frequent and severe, especially effects on the brain (see earlier). Elderly people may have impaired kidney function (see Chapter 82), so tests of kidney function should be carried out before and at regular intervals during treatment; if kidney function is impaired, the dose of the beta blocker should be reduced.

Risks with driving Because beta blockers may produce dizziness and other symptoms, do not drive or operate moving machinery until you know that it is safe to do so.

Risks with alcohol Alcohol may aggravate the effects of beta blockers in lowering blood pressure, thus producing light-headedness and dizziness. The low blood pressure may affect the heart. Be cautious about drinking alcohol if you are taking beta blockers.

Alpha/beta blockers

Labetalol (Trandate) is a non-selective beta blocker that also blocks alpha receptors. Because of its alpha effects the constriction of arteries caused by beta blocking is minimized. It reduces peripheral resistance and lowers the blood pressure, and also protects the heart from stimulation by adrenaline. It is useful for treating angina in someone who also has raised blood pressure.

Table 20.3 Alpha/beta blocker: labetalol – harmful effects and warnings

Harmful effects include transient headache, tiredness, dizziness, depressed mood, lethargy, congestion of the nose, sweating and, rarely, ankle swelling. Very rarely, there may be difficulty in passing urine, nausea and vomiting, liver damage and jaundice, muscle pains, allergic reactions (skin rashes, itching, swelling of the skin and breathlessness), blurred vision, irritation of the eyes, cramps, drug fever and lupus erythematosus.

Warnings Labetalol should not be used in patients with serious heart block, in heart conditions associated with low blood pressure or serious slowing of the heart rate. It should not be used in anyone who is allergic to it, and should be used with utmost caution in individuals with asthma or other wheezing disorders. The dose should be reduced in people with severe liver disease. Intravenous atropine should be given before a general anaesthetic. It may increase the effect of lowering blood pressure caused by the general anaesthetic halothane. Do not stop treatment suddenly. For other warnings see those for beta blockers.

Risks in elderly people Harmful effects may be more frequent and severe, so use lower doses.

Calcium channel blockers used to treat angina

Calcium is involved in the conduction of electrical impulses from the heart's pacemaker through the conduction system of the heart. It is also involved every time a heart muscle fibre contracts and relaxes. The 'electrical' activity involved every time the heart beats is therefore channelled through calcium ions. The latter mechanism is usually referred to as a 'calcium channel' and drugs that block the passage of impulses along these calcium channels are called calcium channel blockers. These drugs are therefore involved in blocking the conduction of impulses from the heart's pacemaker and blocking impulses in muscle fibres that are responsible for the contraction and relaxation of the heart with every beat. As a consequence, they improve contractility of the heart and the electrical conduction of impulses from the pacemaker through the heart is slowed down.

Calcium channel blockers also affect muscles in the walls of arteries and other tissues (e.g. the bronchial tubes and uterus), causing them to relax – this effect causes arteries to dilate and increase their calibre (*vasodilation*). This reduces the resistance to the flow of blood with the result that the blood pressure falls and the workload of the heart is reduced. Calcium channel blockers also relax the muscles in the walls of the coronary arteries, making it easier for the blood to flow through and thereby increasing the blood supply to the heart. Calcium channel blockers have little effect on muscles in veins and do not produce dilatation.

The several calcium channel blockers available differ according to the three main effects they produce – vasodilator effects, contractibility of heart muscle and reduced conduction of impulses in the heart. Their effects also vary according to how they are taken (by mouth or by injection) and by the state of the heart muscle. They all dilate the coronary arteries and increase the blood supply to the heart. They reduce the workload of the heart and lower its oxygen needs but, unlike the beta blockers, they do not greatly reduce heart rate. Calcium channel blockers are of use if attacks of angina continue to occur despite treatment with beta blockers and nitrates.

The main risks of using calcium channel blockers are related to their actions. Excessive dilatation of arteries may cause a fall in blood pressure. Rarely, the fall in blood pressure may trigger an anginal attack due to a decreased supply of blood to damaged parts of the heart muscle (myocardial ischaemia). Their effect on the strength of contraction of the heart may trigger heart failure, and their effects on the conduction of electrical impulses in the heart may affect the rate of the heart.

The calcium channel blockers at present in fashion for treating angina include amlodipine, diltiazem, nicardipine, nifedipine and verapamil.

Table 20.4 Drugs used to treat angina: calcium channel blockers – harmful effects and warnings

Harmful effects Diltiazem Infrequent and mild harmful effects include tiredness, slowness of the heart rate, a fall in blood pressure and swelling of the ankles. Very rarely, it may cause nausea, headache, dizziness, swelling of the fingers and skin rashes.

Amlodipine Infrequent and mild harmful effects include headache, flushing, dizziness and oedema (ankle swelling), nausea and fatigue.

Nicardipine Infrequent harmful effects include dizziness, headache, swelling of the ankles, flushing, palpitations, nausea, stomach upsets, drowsiness and fall in blood pressure. Rarely, it may cause allergic reactions and skin rashes, salivation and increased frequency of passing urine.

Nifedipine Infrequent harmful effects include lethargy, headache, flushing, swelling of the ankles, allergic reactions, eye pains and swollen gums; and very rarely jaundice.

Verapamil Infrequent and mild harmful effects include nausea, vomiting, constipation, flushing, fatigue and headache. Very rarely, liver damage and allergic reactions may occur. Occasionally after intravenous injection the blood pressure may fall, the heart rate slow down and, very rarely, heart block may occur and the heart may stop beating.

Warnings Amlodipine should be used with caution in individuals with impaired liver function.

Diltiazem should not be used in people suffering from severe slowness of the heart rate or heart block. It should be used with caution in individuals suffering from impaired functioning of their liver or kidneys. The dose should be reduced and tests of kidney and liver function carried out. The starting dose of diltiazem should be small and it should not be increased if the heart rate falls below 50 beats/minute. It should be used with caution in anyone with mild slowness of the pulse rate or heart block.

Nicardipine should be stopped if angina becomes worse at the start of treatment or if the dose is increased. It should be used with caution in individuals who suffer from impaired kidney or liver function.

Nifedipine should be stopped if angina occurs or becomes worse at the start of treatment. It may inhibit labour. Diabetic individuals may need to have their treatment adjusted.

Table 20.4 Drugs used to treat angina: calcium channel blockers – harmful effects and warnings (*cont.*)

Verapamil should not be used in individuals with serious heart block, slowing of the heart or heart failure. It should be used with caution in people with impaired liver or kidney function, slow heart rate, low blood pressure, mild heart block and acute phase of a heart attack. Heart failure should be controlled with digoxin or diuretics.

Risks with driving Calcium channel blockers may produce dizziness and/or other symptoms, which may affect driving ability; therefore do not drive until you know that it is safe to do so.

Guidelines on the use of drugs to treat angina

Acute recurrent attacks of stable angina

Use tablets of glyceryl trinitrate to be dissolved under the tongue when necessary. If you have difficulty with this, try a mouth spray. If attacks are not frequent, use glyceryl trinitrate mouth spray or an isosorbide preparation because they will keep longer than glyceryl trinitrate.

Preventing attacks of stable angina

It is occasionally worth trying a long-acting topical application of glyceryl trinitrate (e.g. ointment or adhesive pads) or an isosorbide preparation by mouth, but in general it is better to move on to a beta blocker.

A beta blocker by mouth should be added if attacks of angina are frequent, if many tablets of glyceryl trinitrate have to be taken, or if isosorbide by mouth is not effective. The use of a beta blocker may allow a reduction in the use of glyceryl trinitrate tablets.

A calcium channel blocker should be added if the above fails. A calcium channel blocker is an alternative if you cannot take a beta blocker because you have asthma or for some other reasons. *Verapamil* is a calcium channel blocker which affects conduction in the heart and slows the heart rate; it also causes dilatation of arteries and a fall in blood pressure. It is therefore useful for treating people who suffer from angina and raised blood pressure, so too is amlodipine.

Nifedipine and *nicardipine* are both useful for treating angina and raised blood pressure but the fall in blood pressure that they produce may cause the heart to beat fast. These two calcium channel blockers are best taken with a beta blocker that stops this reflex increase in heart rate when the blood pressure falls.

Unstable angina and variant angina

With these more serious types of angina the individual should be admitted to hospital for rest and investigations; according to the symptoms and the electrocardiograph, treatment may involve the use of a nitrate vasodilator, beta blocker and/or a calcium channel blocker by mouth or, if severe, a nitrate vasodilator (and sometimes a beta blocker) by intravenous injection. In addition, a thrombus-dissolving drug may be given (see below) and anti-thrombotic treatment with aspirin (see below).

Treatment of a heart attack

About one-half of all deaths that occur following an acute heart attack take place within about 2 hours of the first onset of symptoms. Furthermore, until the introduction of drugs that effectively dissolve a thrombus in a blocked coronary artery (see below), one-quarter of those who survived died within 4 weeks of their heart attack.

Factors that increase the risks of dying from a heart attack include delay in getting treatment, advancing age, previous damage to the heart from a myocardial infarction, evidence of heart failure and evidence of damage to the heart as indicated by a low blood pressure and pulse rate.

The main cause of sudden death is a serious disorder of heart rhythm (ventricular fibrillation, see Chapter 23). Subsequent deaths result from further damage to the heart caused by an extension of the thrombosis in the coronary arteries or a disorder of heart rhythm.

Depending upon the condition of the patient and the findings from the electrocardiograph (ECG), the immediate drug treatment may include some or all of the following.

- Oxygen by mask in order to improve the supply of oxygen to the heart and other organs
- The treatment of any disorder of heart rhythm (see Chapter 23)
- The relief of pain by giving an injection of morphine, and to prevent vomiting it may be necessary to give an injection of an anti-emetic (anti-vomiting drug) such as prochlorperazine (see Chapter 14)
- The relief of any spasm of the coronary arteries by giving a nitrate vasodilator intravenously
- The use of a thrombus-dissolving drug intravenously to dissolve the thrombus and keep the blood supply flowing (see below)
- The prevention of a recurrence of the thrombosis by starting treatment with an anti-thrombotic drug such as aspirin (see below)
- The treatment of any complications such as heart failure (see Chapter 22) or disorders of heart rhythm (see Chapter 23)

The use of thrombus-dissolving drugs (thrombolytics)

Damage to part of the heart muscle (myocardial infarction) is nearly always due to a thrombus blocking one of the coronary arteries or its branches (coronary thrombosis). Most damage occurs in the first few hours after the artery has been blocked by the thrombus.

Treatment of coronary thrombosis is therefore aimed at dissolving this blockage *as fast as possible* after it has occurred in order to keep the affected artery open and the blood supply flowing to the area of heart muscle supplied by that artery. This will limit the extent of the damage to the heart muscle, improve the function of the heart, reduce the risk of heart complications (e.g. heart failure, disorders of heart rhythm) and reduce the risk of death.

How thrombolytic drugs work

If a thrombus develops in a blood vessel, the lining of that vessel reacts by stimulating the production of an enzyme that dissolves the protein mesh (fibrin) of the thrombus. This process is called fibrinolysis (fibrin dissolving).

The active enzyme that dissolves fibrin is called plasmin. However, until it is needed (i.e. until thrombosis occurs) it is present in the blood in an inactive form as plasminogen. The latter is activated by a plasminogen activator which is present mainly in the lining surfaces of blood vessels. When thrombosis starts, it triggers the release of the activator at the site. Unfortunately the concentration of the activator in the coronary arteries is not enough to activate sufficient plasminogen to dissolve the thrombus before total blockage occurs and the heart muscle becomes damaged. It can therefore be life saving to give a drug that helps in the process of dissolving the thrombus.

The drugs used to dissolve thrombi are referred to as thrombolytics. The ones used to treat coronary thrombosis are fibrinolytics – they dissolve the fibrin that forms a thrombus. They act with plasminogen to produce an 'activator complex' that converts the inactive plasminogen into active plasmin which dissolves the fibrin in the thrombus. Their effects are short lasting and they have to be given by infusion or injection into a vein. They include the following.

Streptokinase (Kabikinase, Streptase) and *urokinase* (Ukidan) have to be given by infusion into a vein. They act generally throughout the circulation and not just specifically at the site of the coronary thrombosis – bleeding is therefore the most important harmful effect (see later).

Alteplase (Actilyse) is designed to try to prevent bleeding due to a generalized effect in the circulation. It is a bio-engineered version of the naturally occurring plasminogen activator and, unlike streptokinase and urokinase, it targets its effects directly on to plasminogen at the site of the thrombus and has a reduced effect in the general circulation, causing much less risk of bleeding. It has to be given by infusion into a vein.

Anistreplase (Eminase) is a fibrinolytic drug given by a slow intravenous injection, which is an advantage over having to give a fibrinolytic by infusion. It is a complex of streptokinase with human plasminogen (the precursor of the natural fibrinolytic enzyme, plasmin). This complex slows down the conversion of the plasminogen to plasmin in the general circulation but does not affect its binding to fibrin in the thrombus. Therefore, after intravenous injection the drug becomes bound on the thrombus *before* excess plasmin appears in the circulation. This minimizes the risk of generalized fibrinolysis and, therefore, of bleeding. Within the thrombus the complex drug is broken down, releasing plasminogen which is converted into plasmin to dissolve the thrombus.

The earlier the treatment the better

Because these drugs dissolve thrombi it is essential to give them as soon as possible after the start of symptoms (e.g. chest pain) in order to try to prevent the affected artery from being blocked completely. Treatment should be given *within 6 hours* of the first symptom but the sooner it is given the better.

Harmful effects of thrombolytic drugs

Bleeding from any site is the most serious harmful effect because the drugs dissolve thrombi anywhere in the body; for example, a wound caused by surgery or injury in the previous 10 days may start to bleed and a disorder which is prone to bleed (e.g. duodenal ulcer) may bleed. Bleeding may also occur from an injury and at the site of an injection.

Allergy is another risk with streptokinase and anistreplase because the body reacts to them as foreign proteins and produces antibodies against them. This is why repeat treatment is not recommended within a period of about 6 months. An antihistamine drug and hydrocortisone given by injection into a vein may reduce the symptoms of any allergic reaction that occurs.

Harmful effects and warnings for each individual drug are listed in Table 26.7.

The prevention of re-thrombosis

Once the effects of a thrombolytic drug have worn off there is a risk that further thrombosis will occur. This is because such treatment only dissolves the thrombus. It does not affect the underlying disease of the coronary artery that caused the blood to clot on its surface. Additional treatment is therefore necessary in order to prevent re-thrombosis: the current fashion is to give a low daily dose of aspirin by mouth, starting as soon as possible after the heart attack and continuing for many years and possibly for life.

Aspirin produces many effects on the body, and one of these is to stop platelets from clumping together at the site of damage to an artery and thus reducing the risk of thrombosis. Aspirin's effect upon a platelet is irreversible and lasts the life of that cell; therefore to prevent thrombosis, only small doses of aspirin are required and the drug need only to be taken once daily by mouth. Treatment with aspirin can be started as soon as the diagnosis of a heart attack is made. Half a tablet of aspirin (150 mg) per day is all that is needed; it can be chewed or swallowed with a glass of water. A soluble aspirin preparation is best.

Comment

The use of a thrombus-dissolving drug intravenously along with aspirin by mouth to prevent re-thrombosis has produced a dramatic improvement in the numbers of patients who survive after the first 2 hours of a heart attack. The sooner treatment is given the better, but even when delayed for several hours it can have very significant benefit.

These observations are based on patients admitted to hospital where electrocardiography and other back-up facilities are readily available. They show the importance of early diagnosis confirmed by ECG and the benefits of early treatment. They also highlight the hazards of prolonged delays which may occur before the patient is referred to hospital and the delays that may occur in an accident and emergency department once the patient has arrived at hospital. Delay in obtaining proper diagnosis and treatment is a major hazard faced by a patient who has suffered a heart attack.

Preventing another heart attack (secondary prevention)

In someone who survives a heart attack it is important to try to prevent a further attack because the risk of death will be increased according to how much the heart has been damaged. These attempts are referred to as secondary prevention.

Although there is no evidence to prove it, the following precautions may help to prevent another heart attack: reduce weight if overweight, treat raised blood pressure, reduce any increase in blood fat levels, take moderate exercise and learn to relax. *However, the single most important thing a smoker can do having survived a heart attack is to stop smoking.*

Aspirin in secondary prevention

The use of aspirin in preventing re-thrombosis following a heart attack is encouraging and a daily dose of 150 mg appears to be adequate. Treatment should be started as soon as possible after the heart attack and continued for many years and probably for life.

NOTE A standard daily dose of aspirin (300 mg) has been found beneficial in preventing a coronary thrombosis in patients who suffer from unstable angina (see earlier). This is referred to as primary prevention.

Anti-coagulant (anti-clotting) drugs in secondary prevention

These drugs are discussed in Chapter 26.

In the late fifties, patients who had a coronary thrombosis were usually put on long-term treatment with anti-coagulant drugs. But the treatment was sometimes worse than the disease in that some patients were more likely to die from the consequences of the treatment (e.g. haemorrhage) than from the damage which the thrombosis had caused to their hearts.

As usually happens in medicine the fashion then swung right the other way and for years anti-coagulant drugs were out of fashion in the treatment of a patient who had a coronary thrombosis. However, their possible benefits in preventing re-thrombosis after a heart attack is now under reconsideration both in the short term and in the long term.

Among the many complications of a myocardial infarction is the risk of damage to the lining of the heart chamber directly under the affected area. This damage can cause the development of a thrombus on the surface of the inside wall of the heart – an intramural thrombus. The risk is that a piece of the thrombus may come loose and shoot off to some other site, particularly the lungs. In such individuals the use of anti-coagulants may help to prevent complications (but see discussion on the use of heparin and aspirin in Chapter 26).

In someone who is confined to bed and who has had a coronary thrombosis there is a risk of developing a thrombus of the deep vein of the legs or pelvis, possibly resulting in pulmonary embolism. The danger is greater if the individual is elderly, overweight and/or immobile, but can be lessened by giving low doses of heparin by injection under the skin for a few days. In general, however, this risk is best avoided by getting the patient up and about as soon as possible.

Beta blockers in secondary prevention

Beta blockers appear to be beneficial in secondary prevention in some people. However, there is some controversy about who should receive beta blocker treatment, which beta blocker is the best, when they should be started and stopped, and the doses that should be used. In addition, opinion is divided as to whether they should be used more selectively. It certainly seems unnecessary to subject someone to the harmful effects of beta blockers if they had only a small heart attack and would do well without treatment.

Beta blockers should not be used in anyone with pre-existing heart failure, low blood pressure, low pulse rate, asthma or other chronic obstructive airways diseases.

Warning *Suddenly stopping a beta blocker may worsen the condition.*

Anti-arrhythmic drugs in secondary prevention

There is no convincing evidence from adequate and well controlled studies that the anti-arrhythmic drugs are of any benefit in secondary prevention.

Fish oil in secondary prevention

Fish oils reduce the blood levels of cholesterol and fats (triglycerides) and help to reduce the stickiness of platelets, thus reducing the risk of thrombosis. They comprise a suitable addition or alternative to aspirin treatment, especially in those people who cannot take aspirin because they suffer from an active peptic ulcer.

Table 20.5 Drugs used to treat myocardial infarction

Preparation	*Drug*	*Drug group*	*Dosage form*
Thrombolytic drugs			
Actilyse	alteplase	Fibrinolytic	Powder in vial
Eminase	anistreplase	Fibrinolytic	Powder in vial
Kabikinase	streptokinase	Fibrinolytic	Powder in vial
Streptase	streptokinase	Fibrinolytic	Powder in vial
Ukidan	urokinase	Fibrinolytic	Powder in vial
Anti-thrombotic drugs			
Angettes	aspirin (75 mg)	Antiplatelet	Tablets
Nu-Seals Aspirin	aspirin (300 mg)	Antiplatelet	Enteric coated tablets
Platet 300	aspirin (300 mg)	Antiplatelet	Effervescent tablets

Anti-coagulant drugs – see Chapter 26.
Intravenous nitrate vasodilators – see Table 20.1.
Beta blockers – see Table 20.2.

Table 20.6 Preparations used to treat angina

Preparation	*Drug*	*Drug group*	*Dosage form*
Adalat	nifedipine	Calcium channel blocker	Capsules
Adizem	diltiazem	Calcium channel blocker	Capsules
Adizem-SR	diltiazem	Calcium channel blocker	Substained release tablets
Angiozem	diltiazem	Calcium channel blocker	Tablets
Antipressan	atenolol	Selective beta blocker	Tablets
Apsolol	propranolol	Non-selective beta blocker	Tablets
Apsolox	oxprenolol	Non-selective beta blocker	Tablets
atenolol	atenolol	Selective beta blocker	Tablets
Bedranol SR	propranolol	Non-selective beta blocker	Sustained-release capsules
Berkatens	verapamil	Calcium channel blocker	Tablets
Berkolol	propranolol	Non-selective beta blocker	Tablets
Beta-Cardone	sotalol	Non-selective beta blocker	Tablets
Betaloc	metoprolol	Selective beta blocker	Tablets
Betaloc-SA	metoprolol	Selective beta blocker	Sustained-release tablets
Betim	timolol	Non-selective beta blocker	Tablets

Table 20.6 Preparations used to treat angina (*cont.*)

Preparation	*Drug*	*Drug group*	*Dosage form*
Blocadren	timolol	Non-selective beta blocker	Tablets
Britiazim	diltiazem	Calcium channel blocker	Tablets
Calcitat	nifedipine	Calcium channel blocker	Capsules
Cardene	nicardipine	Calcium channel blocker	Capsules
Cardiacap	pentaerythritol tetranitrate	Nitrate vasodilator	Sustained-release capsules
Cartrol	carteolol	Non-selective beta blocker	Tablets
Cedocard	isosorbide dinitrate	Nitrate vasodilator	Tablets (to dissolve under tongue or to swallow)
Cedocard-IV	isosorbide dinitrate	Nitrate vasodilator	Injection
Cedocard Retard	isosorbide dinitrate	Nitrate vasodilator	Sustained-release tablets
Coracten	nifedipine	Calcium channel blocker	Substained release capsules
Cordilox	verapamil	Calcium channel blocker	Tablets
Corgard	nadolol	Non-selective beta blocker	Tablets
Coro-Nitro	glyceryl trinitrate	Nitrate vasodilator	Aerosol
Deponit	glyceryl trinitrate	Nitrate vasodilator	Self-adhesive skin-coloured patches
Elantan	isosorbide mononitrate	Nitrate vasodilator	Tablets
Elantan LA	isosorbide mononitrate	Nitrate vasodilator	Sustained-release capsules
Emcor	bisoprolol	Selective beta blocker	Tablets
glyceryl trinitrate	glyceryl trinitrate	Nitrate vasodilator	Tablets
GTN 300	glyceryl trinitrate	Nitrate vasodilator	Tablets
Half-Inderal LA and Inderal LA	propranolol	Non-selective beta blocker	Sustained-release capsules
Imdur	isosorbide mononitrate	Nitrate vasodilator	Sustained-release tablets
Inderal	propranolol	Non-selective beta blocker	Tablets
Ismo	isosorbide mononitrate	Nitrate vasodilator	Tablets
Ismo Retard	isosorbide mononitrate	Nitrate vasodilator	Sustained-release tablets
Isoket Infusion	isosorbide dinitrate	Nitrate vasodilator	Solution for infusion
Isoket Retard	isosorbide dinitrate	Nitrate vasodilator	Sustained-release tablets
Isordil	isosorbide dinitrate	Nitrate vasodilator	Tablets

Table 20.6 Preparations used to treat angina (*cont.*)

Preparation	*Drug*	*Drug group*	*Dosage form*
Isordil Sublingual	isosorbide dinitrate	Nitrate vasodilator	Tablets to dissolve under the tongue
Isordil Tembids	isosorbide dinitrate	Nitrate vasodilator	Sustained-release capsules
Isotrate	isosorbide mononitrate	Nitrate vasodilator	Tablets
Istin	amlodipine	Calcium channel blocker	Tablets
labetalol	labetalol	Alpha/beta blocker	Tablets
Labrocol	labetalol	Alpha/beta blocker	Tablets
Lopresor	metoprolol	Selective beta blocker	Tablets
Lopresor SR	metoprolol	Selective beta blocker	Sustained-release tablets
MCR-50	isosorbide mononitrate	Nitrate vasodilator	Sustained-release capsules
metoprolol	metoprolol	Selective beta blocker	Tablets
Monit	isosorbide mononitrate	Nitrate vasodilator	Tablets
Monit LS	isosorbide mononitrate	Nitrate vasodilator	Tablets
Monit SR	isosorbide mononitrate	Nitrate vasodilator	Substained release capsules
Mono-Cedocard	isosorbide mononitrate	Nitrate vasodilator	Tablets
Monocor	bisoprolol	Selective beta blocker	Tablets
Mycardol	pentaerythritol tetranitrate	Nitrate vasodilator	Tablets
Nifedipine	nifedipine	Calcium channel blocker	Capsules
Nitrocine	glyceryl trinitrate	Nitrate vasodilator	Injection
Nitrocontin Continus	glyceryl trinitrate	Nitrate vasodilator	Sustained-release tablets
Nitrolingual	glyceryl trinitrate	Nitrate vasodilator	Aerosol spray
oxprenolol	oxprenolol	Non-selective beta blocker	Tablets
Percutol	glyceryl trinitrate	Nitrate vasodilator	Ointment
propranolol	propranolol	Non-selective beta blocker	Tablets
Sectral	acebutolol	Selective beta blocker	Capsules, tablets
Securon SR	verapamil	Calcium channel blocker	Substained release capsules
Securon	verapamil	Calcium channel blocker	Tablets
Slow-Pren	oxprenolol	Non-selective beta blocker	Sustained-release tablets
Slow-Trasicor	oxprenolol	Non-selective beta blocker	Sustained-release tablets

Table 20.6 Preparations used to treat angina (*cont.*)

Preparation	*Drug*	*Drug group*	*Dosage form*
Soni-Slo	isosorbide dinitrate	Nitrate vasodilator	Sustained-release capsules
Sorbichew	isosorbide dinitrate	Nitrate vasodilator	Chewable tablets
Sorbid SA	isosorbide dinitrate	Nitrate vasodilator	Sustained-release capsules
Sorbitrate	isosorbide dinitrate	Nitrate vasodilator	Tablets
Sotacor	sotalol	Non-selective beta blocker	Tablets
Suscard Buccal	glyceryl trinitrate	Nitrate vasodilator	Sustained-release tablets
Sustac	glyceryl trinitrate	Nitrate vasodilator	Sustained-release tablets
Tenif	atenolol	Selective beta blocker	Capsules
Tenormin	atenolol	Selective beta blocker	Tablets, sugar-free syrup
Tenormin LS	atenolol	Selective beta blocker	Tablets
Tildiem	diltiazem	Calcium channel blocker	Tablets
Trandate	labetalol	Alpha and beta blocker	Tablets
Transiderm-Nitro	glyceryl trinitrate	Nitrate vasodilator	Self-adhesive patches
Trasicor	oxprenolol	Non-selective beta blocker	Tablets
Univer	verapamil	Calcium channel blocker	Sustained-release capsules
Vascardin	isosorbide dinitrate	Nitrate vasodilator	Tablets
verapamil	verapamil	Calcium channel blocker	Tablets
Visken	pindolol	Non-selective beta blocker	Tablets

Table 20.7 Combined preparations containing a beta blocker and calcium channel blocker

Preparation	*Drug*	*Drug group*	*Dosage form*
Beta-Adalat	atenolol nifedipine	Selective beta blocker Calcium channel blocker	Capsules
Tenif	atenolol nifedipine	Selective beta blocker Calcium channel blocker	Capsules

21

Raised blood pressure (hypertension)

Blood pressure

The blood is forced around the body under pressure by the pumping action of the heart. This pressure (the blood pressure) depends principally upon the amount of blood being pumped out by the heart (the cardiac output) and the resistance it meets as it enters smaller and smaller arteries (the peripheral resistance).

The blood pressure recording consists of two readings, the upper level or *systolic pressure* and the lower or *diastolic pressure.* These are recorded in millimetres of mercury (e.g. 120/80). The diastolic blood pressure is the minimal pressure in the arteries which coincides with relaxation of the heart between each of its contractions – this period is called diastole. It is an indication of the pressure in the system and the resistance of the arterial walls. It is therefore a measure of the condition of the arteries.

The upper blood pressure reading, the systolic blood pressure, is the pressure at the point when the contraction of the heart (systole) forces a pulse wave of blood through the artery from which the pressure is being recorded (this is usually the artery at the front of the elbow).

The range of 'normal' blood pressure varies considerably between individuals, and at different times in the same individual. It is influenced by many factors; for example, age, sex, race, physical exercise, food, smoking, drugs and changes in posture. Emotion particularly may send your blood pressure up whereas sleep sends it down. Repeated blood pressure recordings when you are up and about often give lower levels over all than just a single casual recording.

Mechanisms that control the blood pressure

The blood pressure in the arteries is determined by the output from the heart (cardiac output) and the resistance to the flow of blood as it is pumped into smaller and smaller arteries; this is called the peripheral resistance. This peripheral resistance varies according to the calibre (or openness) of the arteries and the viscosity (thickness) of the blood. These are in turn controlled by the following mechanisms.

Special pressure receptors in the main arteries in the neck detect changes in blood pressure. For example, a sudden fall in blood pressure causes the pressure receptors to send messages to the blood pressure control centre in the brain which then sends messages to the heart, causing it to increase its output; the centre also sends messages to the blood vessels, causing them to constrict and reduce their calibre. The net result of this increase in output from the heart and increase in peripheral resistance is a rise in blood pressure. the reverse happens if the blood pressure rises.

In addition, the decreased blood flow to the kidneys caused by the fall in blood pressure affects the production by the kidneys of a substance called renin. This substance, which is produced in response to a fall in blood pressure, acts to produce an inactive protein (angiotensin I) which is converted in the lungs to a very powerful chemical that constricts blood vessels (angiotensin II). This chemical also causes the release of a hormone, aldosterone, from the adrenal glands which acts on the kidneys to hold back salt and water from the urine thus increasing the blood volume. The constriction of the blood vessels increases the peripheral resistance and this raises the blood pressure; the increase in volume of the blood increases the output from the heart which also helps to raise the blood pressure.

Renin release is activated by a reduced blood supply to the kidneys which, apart from a fall in blood pressure, can be caused by narrowing of arteries supplying the kidneys. This narrowing of the arteries can occur in people with high blood pressure and so in these individuals there is a vicious circle of events that raises the blood pressure even further – narrowing of the arteries causes release of renin by the kidneys which causes a further increase in the blood pressure. This damages the arteries even further, causing them to become more narrowed, which in turn causes more release of renin and so on!

Heart muscle and muscles in blood vessels can also exert their own control over the blood pressure; for example, an increase in the volume of blood in the heart increases the force of contraction of heart muscle, which sends up the pressure. Similarly, a rise in blood volume in arteries causes their muscle walls to contract and increase the pressure inside them. Both these mechanisms can affect the blood pressure.

Raised blood pressure (hypertension)

As stated earlier, the diastolic blood pressure (the lower reading) is a measure of the condition of the arteries. This is important to understand because it is damage to the arteries caused by a raised blood pressure that gives rise to complications (see later). An individual should be considered to have a raised blood pressure (hypertension: raised tension) only if the diastolic pressure is consistently raised above accepted 'normal' levels for his or her age in the absence of any factors that may cause a temporary increase during the recording. It is the *sustained* level of the blood pressure that is important. This means that no decision should be based on a casual reading but *only* as the result of several readings (at least three) taken on separate days.

There are two types of hypertension. One is very common and accounts for about 95 per cent of all cases of hypertension, and because we do not know what causes it we call it *essential*, or *idiopathic, hypertension*. The other type is *secondary hypertension* and accounts for about 5 per cent of cases. It is called secondary hypertension because it develops secondarily to a known disorder such as kidney disease, toxaemia of pregnancy, narrowing of the main artery from the heart or of an artery supplying a kidney or to a tumour (phaeochromocytoma) of the sympathetic nervous system found most often in the adrenal glands.

Some drugs may cause hypertension

Certain drugs may cause a significant rise in blood pressure. They include amphetamines; adrenaline and related drugs such as those used as decongestants to treat coughs and colds; ergot preparations used to treat migraine; tricyclic anti-depressant used with adrenaline-related drugs; carbenoxolone used to treat peptic ulcers; and oral contraceptives. Note the dangers of MAOI anti-depressants when taken with certain other drugs and foods (see page 595).

Grading hypertension

There is a wide variation in blood pressure levels among people diagnosed as having hypertension, and the present medical fashion is to allocate them roughly into three main groups – mild, moderate and severe hypertension. However, this grading should apply only to patients under the age of 70 years because above that age there are additional factors to consider (see Chapter 82).

With regard to grading, there is controversy over what level of hypertension should be regarded as mild, moderate or severe. The following ranges appear to be acceptable.

- *Mild hypertension:* a sustained diastolic blood pressure of 90–109, without evidence of complications (see later)
- *Moderate hypertension:* a sustained diastolic blood pressure of 110–129

- *Severe hypertension:* a sustained diastolic blood pressure of 130 or above

NOTE Although these gradings may help in studies of the incidence and management of hypertension, they do not help in the actual treatment. Each person should always be treated individually according to their particular needs and response to treatment.

Developing hypertension

The blood pressure taken in the arms of young adults in the sitting or lying position at rest is about 120/80 (millimetres of mercury). Since the blood pressure is determined by the volume of blood pumped out by the heart with each stroke (cardiac output) and the resistance to the flow of that blood in the arteries as they get progressively smaller (the peripheral resistance), obviously the blood pressure is affected by any condition that influences either or both of these. Emotion, for example, increases the heart rate and output from the heart and hence the blood pressure. It may therefore be difficult to record a 'true' level in someone who is nervous and tense. In general, an increase in output from the heart (cardiac output) increases the systolic pressure, whereas an increase in peripheral resistance increases the diastolic pressure. Both the systolic and diastolic pressures rise with age, but the systolic pressure increase is greater than the diastolic. An important cause of the rise in systolic blood pressure with age is the decrease in the 'give' of the arteries because their walls become rigid with advancing age. This means that, at the same level of output from the heart, the systolic blood pressure is higher in the elderly than in younger people. In other words, the arteries cannot accommodate the same volume of blood because they are narrow and cannot dilate.

Early in the course of hypertension, rises in blood pressure are intermittent and are exaggerated in response to emotion or cold. This suggests that the muscles controlling the calibre of arteries are overactive, producing spasm of the artery walls resulting in narrowing and an increase in resistance to the flow of blood so that more pressure is required to pump the blood round. Later on, the rises in blood pressure become maintained as the body's control mechanism becomes adjusted (or re-set) to a higher level. Eventually the repeated or continuous spasm of the muscles in the arteries causes their walls to thicken. This produces further narrowing of the arteries. At this stage even a normal response to exercise, exertion or cold produces a rise in blood pressure.

During the early years of hypertension the individual usually experiences no symptoms, although sudden increases may cause a throbbing headache and/or dizziness. After being untreated for years the raised blood pressure may then start to affect certain organs, to produce complications and symptoms associated with these complications (see below).

Risks from hypertension

We are interested in hypertension because there is an increased risk of heart attacks and strokes in people with a blood pressure raised above 'normal'. Sustained high blood pressure is also associated with kidney damage, which in turn causes an increase in blood pressure because damaged kidneys may produce a chemical that raises the blood pressure (see later). High blood pressure may also damage the blood vessels in the eye.

An idea of the damage that high blood pressure can produce in arteries is seen when the backs of the eyes (the retinae) are examined with a light (ophthalmoscope). According to how high the blood pressure is, the small arteries in the retinae show progressive changes from looking normal and healthy to looking narrow and hardened, and eventually to being so damaged that they leak blood and fluid into the retina.

Risk factors

Blood pressure increases with age; in early life the pressure is higher in men than in women but from middle age (around about 45 years) the pressure becomes higher in women than in men. However, men are much more likely than women to develop complications from a raised blood pressure, and the higher the pressure the greater is the risk of premature death.

Hereditary factors and age predispose an individual to develop hypertension; and enviromental factors make a contribution – alcohol, smoking, being overweight, lack of exercise, anxiety, tension and a diet with high salt (particularly a high sodium to potassium ratio), low calcium and high fat have all been linked with hypertension. These are often referred to as high risk factors. (See discussion of risk factors in atherosclerosis, Chapter 25.)

Treating hypertension

As stated earlier, the blood pressure is affected by many factors and in any given group of people some will have low blood pressures, the majority will be in the middle and some will have high blood pressures.

If those people with high levels are part of a natural distribution, why bother to treat them? The reason why doctors treat these individuals is because of the known complications that a raised blood pressure can produce (see above). Complications caused by hypertension account for many deaths, particularly in men.

The trouble with having hypertension is that there is no cure; we can only control it. The blood pressure can be kept down to reasonable levels using drugs on a regular daily basis. There is no doubt that in people with severe hypertension, regular daily drug treatment reduces the risks of heart failure, kidney failure and strokes. It may also reduce the risks of getting a heart attack. The same also applies to the treatment of moderate hypertension. So there does appear to be a relationship between the level of the blood pressure and the damage it produces, and the reduction of this damage by the selective use of drugs.

Who should be treated?

Evidence collected over the years on the life expectancy of people with severe hypertension indicates that it is serious and life threatening unless the individual is immediately put on drug treatment to bring the pressure down and to maintain it at a reasonable level of safety (i.e. around 90). Of those people with moderate hypertension, evidence suggests that they are at risk unless they get effective drug treatment. Of those people with mild hypertension (95–109), evidence is not at all clear (see later).

People who definitely need drug treatment

Anyone with a raised blood pressure (whether mild, moderate or severe) definitely needs treatment if he/she has:

- Signs that the heart is under strain
- A history of angina which indicates that the coronary artery circulation is damaged
- Signs that the blood supply to the brain is defective (cerebral ischaemia)
- Evidence of high blood fat levels (hyperlipidaemia) which is associated with premature death from coronary artery disease
- Evidence of kidney damage which will make the blood pressure worse
- Evidence from X-rays and ECG of enlargement of the heart
- Evidence that the blood pressure has damaged the small blood vessels in the back of the eyes (hypertensive retinopathy)

Individuals with any of these problems appear to benefit if their blood pressure is reduced and maintained at around about a diastolic of 90.

Even where there are no signs of complications, evidence of the benefits of effective drug treatment for moderate or severe hypertension is still convincing, whereas there are some difficulties in drawing a conclusion on the overall benefits of the drug treatment of mild hypertension (at levels below 100). What makes it difficult is a lack of scientifically valid studies that have attempted to compare the outcome over time for a treated group and a non-treated group. Without evidence from such trials it really is not possible to state that all patients with mild hypertension should be treated with drugs (but see later, page 297).

Any drug used to treat hypertension may produce harmful effects as well as benefits. Once people start treatment for mild hypertension they may go from feeling well and having no symptoms to developing unpleasant symptoms such as nausea and lassitude from a beta blocker or loss of libido from a diuretic. Because these two groups of drugs are the ones most commonly used to treat mild and moderate hypertension such individuals must really wonder about the price they are paying to prevent some future event which may never happen. It is not surprising that many people do not take their drugs as directed. Because of forgetfulness or for many other reasons at least one in three patients (and probably many more) do not take drug treatments as directed. They miss out doses or even a whole day's treatment. Collections of unused drugs from patients' homes confirm this and show that there is much waste of prescribed drugs. This failure of people to take drugs as directed adds to the difficulties in interpreting findings from studies of the drug treatment of hypertension.

Failure to take a drug according to instructions is called 'non-compliance' and it is often an indication of poor communication between the doctor and the patient and/or between the pharmacist and the patient. The doctor or pharmacist may fail to take time to explain to the patient the benefits and risks of treatment and the risks of no treatment. Yet if you are put on a drug which presumably must be taken for the rest of your life, you need to be as informed as possible about the benefits and risks of no treatment, about non-drug treatments and about the benefits and risks of available drug treatments. You should be able to contribute to the decision on whether to treat or not and which drug to take.

How good are doctors at treating hypertension?

Knowing the risks of untreated hypertension, how effective are doctors at identifying people with hypertension (i.e. a diastolic above 90 in middle age) and how effectively do they use drug treatments? The answers are depressing and are expressed in what doctors themselves call 'the rule of halves'. This expresses the under-diagnosis, under-treatment and poor control of raised blood pressure in the population. They accept that half the people with hypertension are not identified; of the ones that are picked up, only about half get treatment; and of those that do, only about a half get effective treatment. In other words, doctors claim that only about one-eighth of all people with hypertension get proper treatment. If this is the case and if drug treatment of moderate and severe hypertension is so effective in preventing complications and increasing life expectancy, something should be done about it. For a start there should be routine screening of everyone over the age of 40 years. Those individuals identified as suffering from moderate or severe hypertension should be treated, and those with mild hypertension should be given useful advice on non-drug treatments and their progress carefully monitored. Where relevant, all patients should be advised to stop smoking, lose weight and reduce alcohol intake.

Non-drug treatments of hypertension

Lose weight For someone who is overweight and has mild hypertension it is important to lose weight before starting on any form of drug treatment. The blood pressure can fall significantly for every 6 kg in weight lost up to a loss of about 18 kg. This loss, which should be gradual over several weeks, could easily be sufficient to take the individual out of the danger levels.

Restrict salt There is much controversy about the relationship between the amount of salt in the diet and hypertension. There are experts who argue in favour of reducing the daily amount we take in and those who argue that it would make no difference. There is no doubt that people in the West take in far more salt than they need but we have no evidence that reducing salt intake helps to prevent hypertension in those individuals who are prone to develop it. Moreover, there is no convincing evidence that salt restriction is helpful and leads to a reduction in dosage of drugs in people being treated for hypertension, although it may possibly be beneficial in those with severe hypertension who are elderly and/or black.

It may help if *excessive* salt intake is reduced. This may be achieved by not adding salt to food while cooking or at the table and keeping an eye on processed foods high in salt. We need much more research on the significance of the sodium to potassium ratio in the diet and on the role of calcium.

Reduce alcohol intake There is a definite association between the amount of alcohol taken in each day and the level of the blood pressure. Therefore it may help to significantly reduce the daily intake of alcohol before anyone suffering from mild to moderate hypertension and who is a moderate or heavy drinker goes on to drug treatment.

Change diet There is an association between hypertension, fatty damage to the arteries and premature death from a heart attack or stroke. A high level of animal fats in the diet has been identified as an important risk factor associated with these causes of death; therefore it makes sense to reduce the overall amount of fat in the diet and to increase the proportion of vegetable fats (polyunsaturates) over animal fats. Vegetarians have a lower blood pressure than non-vegetarians, but note that a diet low in dairy produce may reduce the calcium intake and this has been associated with a rise in blood pressure.

Stop smoking Because of the association between tobacco smoking and premature death from coronary heart disease, it is important to stop smoking. Smoking may also be associated with fatty damage to arteries.

Other general measures such as taking more exercise and learning to relax may help some people but in general there is no convincing evidence of their benefits.

This is fairly tough advice, but if it were taken there could well be a reduction in the number of people with mild hypertension who require drug treatment.

NOTE The risk factors just discussed are *not* the causes of hypertension; they are what are called associated factors.

Start non-drug treatment when your blood pressure is normal

The best time to take this advice on non-drug treatment is when you are told that your blood pressure is normal.

Drugs used to treat raised blood pressure (hypertension)

There are five main groups of drugs used to treat hypertension:

1. Diuretics (water tablets)
2. Drugs that act on the nerves that control blood pressure
3. Drugs that dilate blood vessels (vasodilators)
4. Angiotensin-converting enzyme inhibitors
5. Calcium channel blockers

Diuretics (water tablets) used to treat raised blood pressure

How do they work?

Diuretics (water tablets, see Chapter 22) act upon the urine excretory system of the kidneys to produce an increased output of sodium salt in the urine. The amount of salt in the urine determines the amount of water in the urine; if the salt level is high, larger amounts of water pass from the blood into the urine, and vice versa. These drugs therefore make the body lose salt and water. This increases the volume of the urine (diuresis) and reduces the volume of blood that the heart has to pump round the body (cardiac output). It therefore reduces the blood pressure. However, with the regular daily use of diuretics the dose needed to keep the blood pressure reduced is less than the daily dose normally used to increase the volume of the urine and reduce the volume of the blood, and they have other actions.

Following regular daily treatment with diuretics over 2–3 weeks, the blood volume returns nearly to what it was before treatment was started, while the blood pressure remains reduced and the resistance to the flow of blood through the small arteries (peripheral resistance) falls. The effects of diuretics in producing this fall in blood pressure are not fully understood. They may produce a reduction in the salt content of the walls of the smaller blood vessels, making them easier to dilate. In other words, they relax the walls of the arteries – they are vaso-relaxant. This will increase the calibre of the arteries, reduce the resistance to the flow of blood and therefore reduce the blood pressure. This effect on peripheral resistance may well be a secondary effect of their diuretic effect, which causes a change in the salt (sodium) balance in the body, which affects the walls of the blood vessels.

Choice of diuretic

The best diuretics to reduce the blood pressure are the thiazide diuretics. There is no point in using the stronger diuretics such as frusemide because in the long-term treatment of blood pressure we want not a more powerful diuretic effect (loss of water and salt from the body) but rather a steady blood pressure lowering effect. This is why the dose of a diuretic used to treat hypertension is less than the dose used to treat the fluid retention that occurs, for example, in heart failure.

Potassium-sparing diuretics (e.g. amiloride, triamterene) may be used to treat people with hypertension who have a low blood potassium for some other reason or in whom a low blood potassium could be harmful.

Risks of using thiazide diuretics

Harmful effects of thiazide diuretics are listed in Table 22.9. The principal risks from using them to treat hypertension are: loss of potassium; excessive loss of water and salts; an increase in uric acid levels in the blood, which may trigger an attack of gout in a susceptible person; a rise in the blood suger level and sugar in the urine in diabetics and in anyone prone to develop diabetes; and effects on sexual function, which include loss of libido and failure to attain or maintain an erection.

The thiazide diuretics may cause an increase in blood fat levels (plasma lipids); because the latter may be associated with coronary artery disease we need to know much more about the long-term risks of using these drugs to treat hypertension. Certainly, it is a warning to use as small an effective daily dosage as possible.

Warning *Individuals given a diuretic drug for the treatment of hypertension should have their blood chemistry tested after 3–4 weeks of treatment in order to check whether the blood potassium level is normal. If it is low, the dose of diuretics should be reduced. In people in whom a low blood potassium could cause problems (see below) these tests should also be carried out* ***before*** *treatment is started and at regular intervals during treatment (every 6 months).*

When to use potassium supplements

Because thiazide diuretics cause a loss of potassium in the urine, it may be necessary to give potassium supplements to some individuals (for a discussion of the use of potassium salts in people taking diuretic drugs, see Chapter 22). Potassium loss is clearly an important factor to consider when diuretics are used to treat excessive fluid in the tissues, as occurs, for example, in heart failure. However, the doses of diuretics used to treat hypertension should be much less than those used to treat fluid retention and therefore there is seldom any need to give potassium supplements in otherwise healthy people except to advise them on their diet. Potassium supplements should only be given to people being treated for raised blood pressure with diuretics if a low blood potassium could cause problems – patients with coronary artery disease, disorders of heart rhythm, severe liver disease, disorders of the intestine producing excessive fluid loss (e.g. colitis) and diabetes.

Drugs that act on the nerves that control blood pressure

Before reading this section you are advised to read Chapter 2.

The nerves supplying the heart and blood vessels are not under voluntary control; they are under the control of a self-governing system called the autonomic nervous system. This system is in two parts, the sympathetic nervous system and the parasympathetic nervous system. These two systems oppose each other but a very careful balance between them is maintained by centres in the brain. The sympathetic nervous system is an important regulator of the heart and circulation, especially in response to physical or emotional stress. The end result of stimulating the sympathetic nervous system is the release of noradrenaline from nerve endings which stimulate the adrenaline receptors in the heart, blood vessels and elsewhere. Also, in response to stress, the adrenal medulla releases adrenaline, which is transported through the bloodstream and stimulates adrenaline receptors. You therefore have adrenaline and noradrenaline acting on the heart and arteries, causing an increase in heart rate, increased output of blood from the heart and an increase in blood pressure.

One aspect of the drug treatment of hypertension is therefore aimed at blocking these adrenaline-like effects on the heart and blood vessels. There are four groups of drugs that are capable of doing this. They act on the blood pressure control centre in the brain and/or on the nerves supplying the heart and blood vessels.

1. Drugs that act on the blood pressure control centre in the brain – central alpha stimulants.
2. *Drugs that block receptors in the heart and arteries from being stimulated by noradrenaline. These include: (a) beta receptor blockers (beta blockers); (b) alpha receptor blockers (alpha blockers); and (c) alpha and beta receptor blockers (alpha/beta blockers).
3. *Drugs that block adrenergic nerve endings which supply the heart and blood vessels – adrenergic neurone blockers.
4. *Drugs that block the main nerve junctions (ganglia) of the autonomic nervous system – ganglion blockers.

*NOTE These effects are not just selective on the heart and arteries but affect many other organs and tissues in the body.

Drugs that act on the blood pressure control centre in the brain (central alpha stimulants)

Methyldopa It is not too clear how this drug works but the current idea is that it affects the blood pressure control centre in the brain. Once it has entered the bloodstream it is taken to the liver and converted into an adrenaline-like chemical called methylnoradrenaline which then acts as a false nerve messenger. It stimulates alpha receptors in the control centre which then reacts as if there were a lot of noradrenaline being released throughout the body. The centre attempts to correct this by reducing the release of noradrenaline from the nerves supplying the heart and arteries (and of course other tissues and organs in the body). This causes the arteries to dilate, which reduces the resistance to the flow of blood (peripheral resistance) and the output from the heart to decrease. These effects cause a fall in the blood pressure. The advantage of methyldopa is that it reduces the blood pressure equally whether the patient is standing, sitting, lying down or exercising; this is not the case with some of the other drugs. It has the advantage of being safe to use in people with asthma or heart failure and in pregnant women.

Clonidine Like methyldopa, this drug also directly stimulates alpha receptors in the control centre of the brain which are responsible for reducing the release of noradrenaline by the nerves supplying the heart and blood vessels and other tissues and organs in the body. It also reduces the output of noradrenaline from the endings of these nerves.

Drugs that block receptors in the heart and arteries from being stimulated by adrenaline

Beta blockers block the effects of adrenaline and noradrenaline on beta receptors in the heart, arteries and elsewhere. These drugs (e.g. propranolol) are discussed in detail in Chapter 20. All of the beta blockers are equally effective in lowering raised blood pressure if given in appropriate dosages. Their effects in reducing blood pressure are complex: they block beta receptors and lower blood pressure by reducing the output from the heart (cardiac output), reducing renin production by the kidneys, and by altering the sensitivity of blood pressure monitoring nerves. They also have an effect on the blood pressure control centre in the brain and they block adrenaline receptors in the arteries. They produce a fall in blood pressure when taken regularly every day. Differences in effects between the various beta blockers have not been shown to be of any particular advantage when treating people for raised blood pressure.

Alpha blockers These drugs block the effect of adrenaline and noradrenaline on alpha receptors in arteries. This blocking produces dilatation of the arteries, which increases their calibre. This reduces the resistance to the flow of blood and produces a fall in blood pressure. However, because they do not block beta receptors, noradrenaline can still work on noradrenaline receptors in the heart and cause a rapid heart rate which is unaffected by non-selective alpha blockers (e.g. phenoxybenzamine). The alpha blockers that selectively block alpha-1 receptors and not alpha-2 receptors produce little or no reflex increase in heart rate. They also produce some beneficial effects on blood fat levels. Selective alpha-1 blockers include doxazosin, indoramin, prazosin and terazosin.

Alpha/beta blockers Labetalol is a selective alpha and non-selective beta blocker. It therefore combines the effects of beta blocking with alpha blocking. It reduces blood pressure by producing dilatation of arteries, which increases their calibre and reduces the peripheral resistance. Heart rate and output are a little affected. Labetalol may produce a fall in blood pressure on standing up from sitting or lying down (postural hypotension).

Drugs that block adrenergic nerve endings which supply the heart and blood vessels – adrenergic neurone blockers

This group of drugs (bethanidine, debrisoquine, guanethidine) prevents the release of the chemical messenger, noradrenaline, from the nerves that supply blood vessels. This causes the blood vessels to dilate and their calibre to increase. The resistance to the flow of blood through arteries is decreased, which produces a fall in blood pressure and a reduction in output from the heart. The volume of blood in veins is increased because they dilate and this causes a reduction in the volume of blood returned to the heart. These drugs may cause a marked fall in blood pressure on standing up after lying or sitting. They do not lower the blood pressure when the individual is lying down.

Reserpine and related drugs (rauwolfia alkaloids) Reserpine is an alkaloid from rauwolfia plants. About 50 other rauwolfia alkaloids are known. Reserpine has been widely used as a sedative to treat mental illness in the past but it may produce severe depression. It has also been widely used to treat people suffering from hypertension over the past 30 years. It depletes the storage of noradrenaline in the brain, in the adrenal glands and at nerve endings, which means that less noradrenaline is available to act as a chemical messenger when the nerves are stimulated. This produces dilatation of the arteries, a decrease in resistance to the flow of blood and a fall in blood pressure. A fall in blood pressure on standing up after lying or sitting down is a problem because the drug blocks the normal reflex control.

The worst harmful effects of reserpine are on the brain, producing drowsiness, nightmares and depression, and its use to treat raised blood pressure is no longer fashionable in Britain.

Drugs that block the main nerve junctions (ganglia) of the autonomic nervous system – ganglion blockers

These drugs include hexamethonium, mecamylamine, pemipidine, pentolinium and trimetaphan. They block the chemical messenger (acetylecholine) in the main switchboxes (ganglia) of the sympathetic nervous system (see Chapter 2). They therefore produce many unwanted effects on both the sympathetic and the parasympathetic systems. These effects include blurred vision, dry mouth, constipation, difficulty in passing urine, impotence and failure to ejaculate. A serious harmful effect is a severe fall in blood pressure on standing up from lying or sitting (postural hypotension). They are no longer used, except for trimetaphan which is used to produce a low blood pressure during certain surgical procedures.

Drugs that dilate arteries (vasodilators)

These drugs (diazoxide, hydralazine, minoxidil, sodium nitroprusside) act directly on the muscles in arteries, producing dilatation leading to a drop in resistance to the flow of blood and a fall in blood pressure. We do not know how they work. The body's control centres try to compensate for the fall in blood pressure by increasing the output from the heart, increasing the rate of the heart (tachycardia), and by retaining water and salt in the body. These effects almost counteract the blood pressure lowering effects of these drugs; therefore they have to be given with other drugs, such as a beta blocker to reduce the heart rate and output of the heart and a diuretic drug to reduce the water and salt retention.

Dangers of hydralazine

Some people break down hydralazine more slowly than others who receive the same dose. Those who break down hydralazine slowly run the risk of getting high toxic levels of the drug in the blood. This characteristic is inherited, About one in ten individuals may develop a severe reaction to hydralazine. This is like the disorder lupus erythematosus, which is characterized by painful muscles, painful joints and fever. More rarely, skin rashes, swollen glands, chest pain, weakness and enlargement of the spleen and liver may occur. This syndrome occurs after about 2 months of treatment in those people who break down the drug slowly, particularly during the summer season and when the dose is 200 mg daily or more. The syndrome usually disappears within 6 months of stopping the drug but the rheumatoid arthritis-like symptoms may persist for years.

Angiotensin-converting enzyme inhibitors (ACE inhibitors)

The renin–angiotensin system has been described earlier. ACE inhibitors block the enzyme that converts angiotensin I to angiotensin II. This causes dilatation of arteries, a decrease in the resistance to the flow of blood and a fall in blood pressure. The actions of these drugs also result in a reduced production of the hormone aldosterone by the adrenal medulla. This reduces the salt-retaining effects of this hormone on the kidneys and causes an increased loss of salt and water in the urine, which reduces the blood volume, the output from the heart falls and contributes to a fall in blood pressure. The reflexes for controlling the blood pressure on changing posture are retained, so a fall in blood pressure on standing up after lying or sitting is rare.

Calcium channel blockers (calcium antagonists)

These drugs are discussed in detail in Chapter 20. They relax the muscles in arteries, causing them to dilate. This reduces peripheral resistance and causes a fall in blood pressure. Nicardipine and nifedipine affect the heart less than verapamil and may be used along with beta blockers to treat hypertension.

Recommended drug treatments for hypertension

The goal of drug treatment is to try to keep the diastolic blood pressure at about 90 or below, and certainly below 100, without dropping it so far that it is going to cause symptoms or is going to adversely affect the blood supply to the kidneys, brain and heart.

Hypertension is usually a life-long disease that causes few symptoms until it is well advanced. To try to keep the blood pressure down to what is regarded as an acceptable level involves the use of expensive, and potentially harmful, drugs on a regular daily basis for life. The important decision is therefore whether or not to treat with drugs. This decision will be influenced by many factors; for example, the level of the blood pressure and the age and sex of the individual, the presence or absence of any complications caused by the blood pressure, and the presence of other diseases (e.g. coronary artery disease).

Mild hypertension

The benefits of treating the lower levels of mild hypertension with drugs appear to be small; perhaps a stroke may be prevented in a few men and women if they take their treatment regularly over a 20-year period.

A major cause of premature death among men is a heart attack caused by coronary artery disease. The drug treatment of mild hypertension may reduce the rate of heart attack in non-smokers but not in smokers. Therefore, it would surely be cheaper and more effective if people with mild hypertension who smoke were to stop smoking. This would significantly reduce their risks of heart attack.

Which patients with mild hypertension would benefit from treatment?

Anyone diagnosed as having mild hypertension (90–109) should be advised to follow the guidelines on non-drug treatment listed earlier for at least 6 months and should have their blood pressure checked every month. If the blood pressure remains at 100 or above, drug treatment should be started. In those in whom it remains *below 100* but at 95 or above, they should be seen every 3–6 months and their blood pressure checked, and every year they should have a complete medical to check for early signs of complications from their raised blood pressure. If complications appear, they should be treated with drugs to lower blood pressure. When their blood pressure remains below 95, no drug treatment should be given but their blood pressure should be checked every 6–12 months.

Mild to moderate hypertension

For a consistent diastolic of *100 or over*, a beta blocker appears to be of value in people who do not have asthma and who are under 50 years of age, white and have a rapid resting pulse rate without evidence of arterial disease. Beta blockers are also useful in individuals with gout (see 'Risks of using thiazide diuretics', earlier) and if there is evidence that coronary artery disease is affecting the oxygen supply to the heart muscle (myocardial ischaemia) producing angina. Beta blockers should not be given to anyone with heart failure, asthma or other wheezing disorders, or heart block.

No one beta blocker has been shown to be better than all the others, so the choice is not critical. Labetalol is useful if the individual also suffers from angina.

Thiazide diuretics are equally effective for treating people with an average diastolic or 100 or over, and are appropriate for the elderly, blacks and anyone suffering from congestive heart failure, kidney failure or who cannot take a beta blocker. They should not be used in people with diabetes or gout. It is important to use the minimum effective dose and to check the blood chemistry (particularly potassium) before treatment, after 4 weeks of treatment and at regular intervals in anyone in whom a low potassium may cause problems. No one thiazide has been shown to be better than the others at lowering blood pressure; therefore the choice is not critical.

Moderate to severe hypertension

With sustained blood pressure of *110 and above*, a single drug (e.g. a thiazide diuretic or a beta blocker) does not usually work. The next step is to try two drugs (e.g. a diuretic plus a beta blocker) and if this fails to add in a third drug, such as a selective alpha blocker (e.g. prazosin: Hypovase) or a vasodilator (e.g. hydralazine: Apresoline), to the treatment. Alternatively, methyldopa (e.g. Aldomet) may be added. This method of treatment is usually referred to as a 'step-wise' approach – treatment goes up in steps.

The use of a beta blocker and a vasodilator together often causes fluid retention and loss of effectiveness. Therefore the addition of a diuretic is sensible. Vasodilator drugs that affect the arteries in preference to the veins may cause rapid beating of the heart and affect the kidneys; these effects can be reduced by the addition of a beta blocker. Therefore drug treatment with a beta blocker, a diuretic and a vasodilator together is often necessary to control moderate to severe hypertension. In severe hypertension, the addition of minoxidil (Loniten) may sometimes be necessary.

Calcium channel blockers (e.g. nifedipine) are as effective as thiazide diuretics or beta blockers, and are becoming increasingly popular even though their long-term safety has not been established. It is now fashionable to use them when an individual cannot take a beta blocker and/or a diuretic or when combined beta blocker and diuretic treatment has failed to control blood pressure. Nifedipine and nicardipine may be combined with a beta blocker but verapamil should *never* be combined with a beta blocker.

Similarly, ACE inhibitors (e.g. captopril, enalapril) are becoming popular and may be combined with a thiazide diuretic in someone who cannot take a beta blocker, or used as an additional step in the treatment of severe hypertension, but the dose of any diuretic should be reduced before starting an ACE inhibitor.

Comment Beta blockers and diuretics are the drugs of first choice for treating uncomplicated hypertension. They have been studied over many years, whereas we lack evidence of the long-term benefits of ACE inhibitors, calcium channel-blockers and alpha blockers. These should remain as second choice drugs until there is sufficient evidence of their long-term benefits over beta blockers and/or diuretics.

Diazoxide (Eudemine) is given by injection in a crisis – when the blood pressure goes really high and must be treated quickly.

Failure to respond to treatment

Failure to take drugs to lower high blood pressure as directed (see above) is a main reason for lack of response to treatment. High salt intake may be another reason for lack of response, so too may be a raised blood pressure secondary to some other disease (see earlier).

To help us to 'comply' with treatment it is important that treatment regimens be as simple as possible – for example, once or twice a day; but this should not necessarily be an excuse to prescribe combined preparations containing more than one drug.

Unfortunately when some people are prescribed drugs to lower their high blood pressure, they may be left on the same drug or drugs in the same daily dosage year in and year out; yet it would be beneficial if, after being well controlled for 6 months or more, attempts were made to slowly reduce the daily dosage or the number of drugs in order to achieve the important long-term goal – maximum benefits for minimum dosage and risks.

Warnings *A risk with the step-wise approach to treatment is that patients may be given more and more drugs, without the doctor really knowing whether the failure of the blood pressure to fall is or is not due to failure of the patient to take the drugs as directed.*

It is important to understand the benefits and risks of drugs used to lower blood pressure, both separately and together, and to recognize the necessity to reduce the blood pressure slowly over several weeks.

Take your own blood pressure and take care of yourself

If you are taking drug treatment for hypertension it will help if you buy an electronic blood pressure machine and keep records of your blood pressure. Readings taken at home are often more representative than a reading carried out by a doctor during a busy surgery.

Stop smoking if you smoke, reduce alcohol intake if you drink moderately or to excess, keep weight at ideal level, watch the fat in your diet, do not add salt when cooking or at the table, take regular exercise and learn to relax. *Avoid isometric exercises* (body building, weight lifting, push-ups) because these can send your blood pressure up. Do *isotonic exercises* – walking, bicycling, swimming.

After 6 months of treatment you should (in consultation with your doctor) attempt to reduce the amount of drug treatment that you are taking, slowly over several weeks. If your blood pressure remains reduced then stay on the reduced treatment for another year and repeat the exercise the next year. It is surprising how many patients can actually stop treatment after several months of reduced treatment.

Treatment of a raised systolic blood pressure

As stated earlier, the decision to treat someone with a raised blood pressure is principally based upon the level of the diastolic blood pressure. This is because it is more directly related to the state of the arteries than is the systolic blood pressure. The systolic blood pressure is usually not considered to be raised until it is over 160 while the diastolic is 95 or below. This isolated rise in the systolic blood pressure occurs in about one in four people aged over 70 years. Any attempt to treat it may result in more harm than good in some people, particularly in old elderly people whose systolic blood pressure easily goes high in response to effort or emotion and falls on standing up after sitting or lying down (see below).

It is a different story in someone being treated for hypertension (a raised diastolic pressure), because a rise in systolic blood pressure is a bad sign that indicates damage to the arteries caused by the hypertension. It may be a predictor of a stroke or heart attack. In such people, attempts should be made to control the systolic pressure as well as the diastolic blood pressure.

Treatment of raised blood pressure in the elderly

Elderly people (i.e. those aged 65 years or over) may develop either a high systolic blood pressure or a high diastolic blood pressure, or both. There are no accurate figures on the extent and levels of raised blood in the elderly population.

Elderly people may also develop a fall in systolic blood pressure on standing up after sitting or lying down. This fall may be sufficient to make them dizzy, faint or light-headed; therefore it is very imporant that elderly people have their blood pressure taken when they are *standing up*, and it is this level that should determine whether drug treatment is given or not. If drugs are given to treat a high blood pressure recorded with an elderly person sitting down, that individual may develop a serious fall in blood pressure on standing up and, apart from suffering faint feelings and light-headedness, may actually fall to the ground and sustain an injury.

There is much controversy over what constitutes a raised blood pressure that requires drug treatment in elderly people. At the present time, elderly people under 80 years of age with a systolic pressure of 160 or above and a diastolic of 90 or above should be considered for drug treatment provided these are *sustained* levels (i.e. the results of several recordings) and provided they are taken with the patient *standing*.

There is further controversy about which drugs should be taken by the elderly, if treatment is indicated. Because elderly people with a raised diastolic blood pressure also tend to have a raised systolic, it is fashionable to use diuretics which brings down both systolic and diastolic blood pressure. It is also fashionable to use a beta blocker and follow a step-wise approach. However, it is important that the elderly person as a whole is treated; not just the high blood pressure. Not treating a high systolic level and dropping the diastolic level too low may increase the risk of a stroke in an elderly person.

NOTE A fall in blood pressure on standing up after sitting or lying down (postural hypotension) may be made worse by hot weather, alcohol, by some drugs used to treat raised blood pressure, by water tablets (diuretics) used to treat heart failure, and by a low level of salt in the body. When getting out of bed, elderly people should sit up and then count to ten before they stand up. If they stand up and feel dizzy and weak, they should sit or lie down immediately in order to avoid fainting, and try again once the symptoms have worn off.

Raised blood pressure in pregnancy

Raised blood pressure in pregnancy may be due to already existing hypertension or to a specific type of hypertension that occurs in pregnancy and is associated with fluid retention (oedema), causing swollen ankles and hands and protein in the urine. This group of symptoms is called toxaemia of pregnancy. We do not know what causes it. Toxaemia develops in the last 3 months of pregnancy and it can affect the growth of the baby and increase the risk of a stillbirth. In the mother it can cause fits, kidney and heart failure and a stroke. The best drug to use in treating toxaemia of pregnancy is methyldopa. The beta blocker atenolol and the alpha and beta blocker labetalol are also safe to use in pregnancy. Hydralazine may be used in emergencies. Diuretics should not be used because they may reduce the blood supply to the baby through the placenta.

Table 21.1 Preparations used to treat raised blood pressure (U)

Preparation	*Drug*	*Drug group*	*Dosage form*
Accupro	quinapril	ACE inhibitor	Tablets
Acepril	captopril	ACE inhibitor	Tablets
Adalat Retard	nifedipine	Calcium channel blocker	Sustained-release tablets
Aldomet	methyldopa	Central alpha stimulant	Tablets, suspension, injection
Antipressan	atenolol	Selective beta blocker	Tablets
Apresoline	hydralazine	Vasodilator	Tablets, injection
Aprinox	bendrofluazide	Thiazide diuretic	Tablets
Apsolol	propranolol	Non-selective beta blocker	Tablets
Apsolox	oxprenolol	Non-selective beta blocker	Tablets
Arelix	piretanide	Loop diuretic	Sustained-release capsules
Arfonad	trimetaphan	Ganglion blocker	Injection
atenolol	atenolol	Selective beta blocker	Tablets
Baratol	indoramin	Selective alpha-1 blocker	Tablets
Baycaron	mefruside	Thiazide-like diuretic	Tablets
Bedranol SR	propranolol	Non-selective beta blocker	Sustained-release capsules
Bendogen	bethanidine	Adrenergic neurone blocker	Tablets
bendrofluazide	bendrofluazide	Thiazide diuretic	Tablets
Berkolol	propranolol	Non-selective beta blocker	Tablets
Berkozide	bendrofluazide	Thiazide diuretic	Tablets
Beta-Cardone	sotalol	Non-selective beta blocker	Tablets
Betaloc	metoprolol	Selective beta blocker	Tablets
Betaloc-SA	metoprolol	Selective beta blocker	Sustained-release tablets
bethanidine	bethanidine	Adrenergic neurone blocker	Tablets
Betim	timolol	Non-selective beta blocker	Tablets
Blocadren	timolol	Non-selective beta blocker	Tablets
Calcitrat	nifedipine	Calcium channel blocker	Capsules
Capoten	captopril	ACE inhibitor	Tablets

Table 21.1 Preparations used to treat raised blood pressure (*cont.*)

Preparation	*Drug*	*Drug group*	*Dosage form*
Carace	lisinopril	ACE inhibitor	Tablets
Cardene	nicardipine	Calcium channel blocker	Capsules
Cardura	doxazosin	Selective alpha blocker	Tablets
Catapres	clonidine	Central alpha blocker	Tablets, perlongets (sustained-release capsules), injection
Centyl	bendrofluazide	Thiazide diuretic	Tablets
Cordilox 160	verapamil	Calcium channel blocker	Tablets
Corgard	nadolol	Non-selective beta blocker	Tablets
Coversyl	perindopril	ACE inhibitor	Tablets
Decaserpyl	methoserpidine	Rauwolfia alkaloid	Tablets
Declinax	debrisoquine	Adrenergic neurone blocker	Tablets
Dibenyline	phenoxybenzamine	Non-selective alpha blocker	Capsules
Diurexan	xipamide	Thiazide-like diuretic	Tablets
Dopamet	methyldopa	Central alpha blocker	Tablets
Dryptal	frusemide	Loop diuretic	Tablets
Emcor	bisoprolol	Selective beta blocker	Tablets
Enduron	methyclothiazide	Thiazide diuretic	Tablets
Esbatal	bethanidine	Adrenergic neurone blocker	Tablets
Esidrex	hydrochlorothiazide	Thiazide diuretic	Tablets
Eudemine	diazoxide	Vasodilator	Tablets, injection
frusemide	frusemide	Loop diurectic	Tablets
hydralazine	hydralazine	Vasodilator	Tablets
Hydrenox	hydroflumethiazide	Thiazide diuretic	Tablets
HydroSaluric	hydrochlorothiazide	Thiazide diuretic	Tablets
Hygroton	chlorthalidone	Thiazide-like diuretic	Tablets
Hypovase	prazosin	Selective alpha-1 blocker	Tablets
Hytrin	terazosin	Selective alpha-1 blocker	Tablets
Inderal	propranolol	Non-selective beta blocker	Tablets
Inderal LA and Half-Inderal LA	propranolol	Non-selective beta blocker	Sustained-release capsules

Table 21.1 Preparations used to treat raised blood pressure (*cont.*)

Preparation	*Drug*	*Drug group*	*Dosage form*
Innovace	enalapril	ACE inhibitor	Tablets
Ismelin	guanethidine	Adrenergic neurone blocker	Tablets, injection
Istin	amlodipine	Calcium channel blocker	Tablets
Kerlone	betaxolol	Selective beta blocker	Tablets
labetalol	labetalol	Alpha/beta blocker	Tablets
Labrocol	labetalol	Alpha/beta blocker	Tablets
Lasix	frusemide	Loop diuretic	Tablets
Loniten	minoxidil	Vasodilator	Tablets
Lopresor	metoprolol	Selective beta blocker	Tablets
Lopresor SR	metoprolol	Selective beta blocker	Sustained-release tablets
Medomet	methyldopa	Central alpha stimulant	Capsules, tablets
Metenix	metolazone	Thiazide-like diuretic	Tablets
methyldopa	methyldopa	Central alpha blocker	Tablets
Monocor	bisoprolol	Selective beta blocker	Tablets
Natrilix	indapamide	Thiazide-like drug (vasorelaxant)	Tablets
Navidrex	cyclopenthiazide	Thiazide diuretic	Tablets
Neo-NaClex	bendrofluazide	Thiazide diuretic	Tablets
Nephril	polythiazide	Thiazide diuretic	Tablets
Nipride	sodium nitroprusside	Vasodilator	Powder for injection
oxprenolol	oxprenolol	Non-selective beta blocker	Tablets
Prescal	isradipine	Calcium channel blocker	Tablets
propranolol	propranolol	Non-selective beta blocker	Tablets
reserpine	reserpine	Rauwolfia alkaloid	Tablets
Rogitine	phentolamine	Non-selective alpha blocker	Injection
Saluric	chlorothiazide	Thiazide diuretic	Tablets
Sectral	acebutolol	Selective beta blocker	Capsules, tablets
Securon	verapamil	Calcium channel blocker	Tablets
Securon SR	verapamil	Calcium channel blocker	Sustained-release tablets
Serpasil	reserpine	Rauwolfia alkaloid	Tablets

Table 21.1 Preparations used to treat raised blood pressure (*cont.*)

Preparation	*Drug*	*Drug group*	*Dosage form*
Slow-Pren	oxprenolol	Non-selective beta blocker	Sustained-release tablets
Slow-Trasicor	oxprenolol	Non-selective beta blocker	Sustained-release tablets
sodium nitroprusside	sodium nitroprusside	Vasodilator	Solution for intravenous injection
Sotacor	sotalol	Non-selective beta blocker	Tablets
Tenormin	atenolol	Selective beta blocker	Tablets, sugar-free syrup
Tenormin LS	atenolol	Selective beta blocker	Tablets
Trandate	labetalol	Alpha/beta blocker	Tablets
Trasicor	oxprenolol	Non-selective beta blocker	Tablets
Tritace	ramipril	ACE inhibitor	Capsules
Univer	verapamil	Calcium channel blocker	Sustained-release capsules
verapamil	verapamil	Calcium channel blocker	Tablets
Visken	pindolol	Non-selective beta blocker	Tablets
Zestril	lisinopril	ACE inhibitor	Tablets

Blood pressure emergencies

In some cases of rapidly advancing hypertension (accelerated or malignant hypertension), a high diastolic pressure above 140 in severe toxaemia of pregnancy and in people who develop heart failure (left ventricular failure) there may be a risk to life and it may be necessary to drop the blood pressure fairly quickly but bearing in mind that a sudden fall in blood pressure (particularly below 90) may cause a stroke, impairment of kidney function or impairment of blood supply to the heart (myocardial ischaemia).

Drugs used for this purpose include atenolol (a beta blocker), labetalol (an alpha/beta blocker), nifedipine (a calcium channel blocker) and hydralazine (a vasodilator). Drugs used intravenously include sodium nitroprusside or labetalol by infusion and diazoxide or hydralazine by slow injection. Sodium nitroprusside is the first drug of choice; it is usually given by mouth and rarely by intravenous injection. The blood pressure should be dropped to 120 in the first 24 hours and then more gradually after that. Intravenous drugs should be used only in serious cases.

Table 21.2 Combined preparations used to treat raised blood pressure

Preparation	*Drug*	*Drug group*	*Dosage form*
Acezide	captopril hydrochlorothiazide	ACE inhibitor Thiazide diuretic	Tablets
Beta-Adalat	atenolol nifedipine	Selective beta blocker Calcium channel blocker	Capsules
Capozide	captopril hydrochlorothiazide	ACE inhibitor Thiazide diuretic	Tablets
Centyl-K	bendrofluazide potassium	Thiazide diuretic Potassium supplement	Sustained-release tablets
Co-Betaloc	metoprolol hydrochlorothiazide	Selective beta blocker Thiazide diuretic	Tablets
Co-Betaloc SA	metoprolol hydrochlorothiazide	Selective beta blocker Thiazide diuretic	Sustained-release tablets
Corgaretic 40 and 80	nadolol benzthiazide	Non-selective beta blocker Thiazide diuretic	Tablets
Dyazide	hydrochlorothiazide triamterene	Thiazide diuretic Potassium-sparing diuretic	Tablets
Hydromet	methyldopa hydrochlorothiazide	Central alpha blocker Thiazide diuretic	Tablets
Hygroton K	chlorothalidone potassium	Thiazide-like diuretic Potassium supplement	Sustained-release tablets
Hypertane	hydrochlorothiazide amiloride	Thiazide diuretic Potassium-sparing diuretic	Tablets
Inderetic	propranolol bendrofluazide	Non-selective beta blocker Thiazide diuretic	Capsules
Inderex	propranolol bendrofluazide	Non-selective beta blocker Thiazide diuretic	Sustained-release capsules
Kalspare	chlorthalidone triamterene	Thiazide-like diuretic Potassium-sparing diuretic	Tablets

Table 21.2 Combined preparations used to treat raised blood pressure (*cont.*)

Preparation	*Drug*	*Drug group*	*Dosage form*
Kalten	atenolol	Selective beta blocker	Capsules
	amiloride	Potassium-sparing diuretic	
	hydrochlorothiazide	Thiazide diuretic	
Lasipressin	penbutolol	Non-selective beta blocker	Tablets
	frusemide	Loop diuretic	
Lasilactone	frusemide	Loop diuretic	Capsules
	spironolactone	Potassium-sparing diuretic	
Lopresoretic	metoprolol	Selective beta blocker	Tablets
	chlorthalidone	Thiazide diuretic	
Moducren	timolol	Non-selective beta blocker	Tablets
	amiloride	Potassium-sparing diuretic	
	hydrochlorothiazide	Thiazide diuretic	
Moduret 25	hydrochlorothiazide	Thiazide diuretic	Tablets
	amiloride	Potassium-sparing diuretic	
Moduretic	hydrochlorothiazide	Thiazide diuretic	Tablets, solution
	amiloride	Potassium-sparing diuretic	
Navidrex-K	cyclopenthiazide	Thiazide diuretic	Sustained-release tablets
	potassium	Potassium supplement	
Navispare	cyclopenthiazide	Thiazide diuretic	Tablets
	amiloride	Potassium-sparing diuretic	
Neo-NaClex-K	bendrofluazide	Thiazide diuretic	Sustained-release tablets
	potassium	Potassium supplement	
Normetic	hydrochlorothiazide	Thiazide diuretic	Tablets
	amiloride	Potassium-sparing diuretic	
Prestim	timolol	Non-selective beta blocker	Tablets
	bendrofluazide	Thiazide diuretic	
Prestim Forte	timolol	Non-selective beta blocker	Tablets
	bendrofluazide	Thiazide diuretic	

Table 21.2 Combined preparations used to treat raised blood pressure (*cont.*)

Preparation	*Drug*	*Drug group*	*Dosage form*
Secadrex	acebutolol	Selective beta blocker	Tablets
	hydrochlorothiazide	Thiazide diuretic	
Serpasil Esidrex	reserpine	Rauwolfia alkaloid	Tablets
	hydrochlorothiazide	Thiazide diuretic	
Sotazide	sotalol	Non-selective beta blocker	Tablets
	hydrochlorothiazide	Thiazide diuretic	
Tenif	atenolol	Selective beta blocker	Capsules
	nifedipine	Calcium-channel blocker	
Tenoret 50	atenolol	Selective beta blocker	Tablets
	chlorthalidone	Thiazide diuretic	
Tenoretic	atenolol	Selective beta blocker	Tablets
	chlorthalidone	Thiazide diuretic	
Tolerzide	sotalol	Non-selective beta blocker	Tablets
	hydrochlorothiazide	Thiazide diuretic	
Trasidrex*	oxprenolol	Non-selective beta blocker	Sustained-release tablets
Triamco	hydrochlorothiazide	Thiazide diuretic	Tablets
	triamterene	Potassium-sparing diuretic	
Vasetic	hydrochlorothiazide	Thiazide diuretic	Tablets
	amilonide	Potassium-sparing diuretic	
Viskaldix	pindolol	Non-selective beta blocker	Tablets
	clopamide	Thiazide diuretic	

* Co-prenozide is the generic name for Trasidrex.

Table 21.3 Drugs used to treat raised blood pressure: adrenergic neurone blockers – harmful effects and warnings

bethanidine (Bendogen, Esbatal)
Harmful effects include a fall in blood pressure on standing up after sitting or lying (may produce light-headedness and faintness), failure to ejaculate, fluid retention (e.g. ankle swelling), blocked nose, muscle weakness.

Warnings Should not be used in anyone

Table 21.3 Drugs used to treat raised blood pressure: adrenergic neurone blockers – harmful effects and warnings (*cont.*)

who suffers from kidney failure, and with caution in people who suffer from peptic ulcer.

Risk in elderly people Harmful effects may be more frequent and severe; a drop in blood pressure on standing after sitting or lying may cause elderly people to fall.

debrisoquine (Declinax)
Harmful effects include a fall in blood pressure on standing up and after sitting or lying down (may produce light-headedness and faintness), failure to ejaculate, fluid retention (e.g. ankle swelling), blocked nose, muscle weakness, malaise, nausea, headache, sweating, frequency of passing urine, rarely diarrhoea.

Warnings It should not be used in individuals who have had a recent heart attack or stroke, or who are allergic to it. It should be used with caution in anyone with impaired kidney function.

Risks in elderly people Harmful effects may be more frequent and severe; a drop in blood pressure on standing after sitting or lying may cause an elderly person to fall.

guanethidine (Ismelin)
Harmful effects include fall in blood pressure on standing up after sitting or lying (may produce light-headedness and faintness), dizziness, weakness, lassitude, failure to ejaculate, fluid retention (e.g. ankle swelling), blocked nose, diarrhoea.

Warnings It should not be used in individuals who suffer from kidney failure. It should be used with caution in people who suffer from peptic ulcers.

Risks in elderly people Harmful effects may be more frequent and severe; a drop in blood pressure on standing after sitting or lying may cause an elderly person to fall.

Table 21.4 Drugs used to treat raised blood pressure: ACE inhibitors – harmful effects and warnings

captopril (Acepril, in Acezide, Capoten, in Capozide)
Harmful effects include persistent dry cough, loss of taste, soreness and ulcers of the mouth, loss of weight, stomach upsets, skin rashes, itching, flushing, allergic reactions, sensitivity of the skin to sunlight, fall in blood pressure on standing up after sitting or lying (may produce light-headedness and faintness), rapid beating of the heart, pins and needles in the hands, serum sickness, wheezing, swollen glands, blood disorders, protein in the urine and increase of waste products in the blood (e.g. urea), increased potassium levels in the blood (therefore do not use a salt substitute that contains potassium). Liver damage may occur very rarely. Harmful effects are more frequent and severe in patients with impaired kidney function.

Warnings Captopril should not be used in anyone with aortic stenosis or who is allergic to it, it should not be used in severe heart failure; use with caution in individuals with impaired kidney function. A white blood cell count should be carried out if an individual develops an infection, sore throat and/or fever. Urine tests for protein should be carried out at regular intervals during treatment. The first and second dose may cause a marked fall in blood pressure within 3 hours in anyone who is also taking a diuretic drug, who is on a low sodium diet or who is having kidney dialysis.

Risks in elderly people Harmful effects may be more frequent and severe; therefore, use with caution.

enalapril (Innovace)
Harmful effects include persistent dry cough, dizziness, headache, fatigue, weakness, low blood pressure on standing up after sitting or lying, alteration of taste, nausea, diarrhoea, muscle cramps, skin

Table 21.4 Drugs used to treat raised blood pressure: ACE inhibitors – harmful effects and warnings (*cont.*)

rash, angiodema, increase in waste products in the blood (e.g. urea) – more common in people with kidney impairment. Allergic reactions may occur and occasionally be serious.

Warnings Enalapril should not be used in people allergic to the drug. The dose of any diuretic being taken should be reduced, if possible. The first dose may cause a marked fall in blood pressure, especially in anyone taking a diuretic, on a low sodium diet, on kidney dialysis, or who is dehydrated. The dose should be reduced in anyone who has impaired kidney function. It should be used with caution with general anaesthetics in patients undergoing major surgery. Black patients may show a reduced response.

Risks in elderly people Harmful effects may be more frequent and severe; therefore it must be used with caution.

lisinopril (Carace, Zestril)
Harmful effects include a fall in blood pressure, allergic skin rash and angioedema, dizziness, headache, nausea, diarrhoea, cough, fatigue, chest pain, weakness, palpitations. It may cause kidney failure in people suffering from severe congestive heart failure or kidney disease.

Warnings Lisinopril should not be used in anyone with aortic stenosis or chronic chest disease associated with heart failure (*cor pulmonale*). It should be used with caution in individuals with impaired kidney function; tests of kidney function should be carried out before and at regular intervals during treatment.

perindopril (Conversyl)
Harmful effects include nausea, abdominal pain, fatigue, weakness, malaise, headache, cough, itching, flushing, skin rashes and, rarely, blood disorders and impairment of kidney function.

Warnings Perindopril should be used with caution in individuals with impaired kidney function, a low blood pressure that is producing symptoms or a raised blood pressure due to kidney disease. Potassium-sparing diuretics and potassium supplements should be used with caution.

Risks in elderly people Harmful effects may be more frequent and severe; therefore it must be used with caution and tests of kidney function should be carried out before and at regular intervals during treatment.

quinapril (Accupro)
Harmful effects include headache, nausea, indigestion, dizziness, running nose, cough, fatigue, painful muscles, pain in the chest and stomach, and a fall in blood pressure. Rarely, it may cause an allergic reaction producing patchy swellings of the skin (angioedema). If this happens the drug should be stopped immediately.

Warnings Quinapril should be used with caution in individuals with severe heart failure or impaired kidney function; tests of kidney function should be carried out before treatment and at regular intervals during treatment.

Risks in elderly people Harmful effects may be more frequent and severe; tests of kidney function must be carried out as above.

Table 21.5 Drugs used to treat raised blood pressure: alpha blockers – harmful effects and warnings

Selective alpha blockers

doxazosin (Cardura)
Harmful effects include headache, dizziness, fatigue, weakness, a fall in blood pressure on standing up after lying or sitting down (postural hypotension) and, occasionally, swelling of the ankles.

Table 21.5 Drugs used to treat raised blood pressure: alpha blockers – harmful effects and warnings (*cont.*)

indoramin (Baratol)
Harmful effects Sedation may occur in some people and is related to dose. Less commonly, dizziness, depression, failure to ejaculate, dry mouth, blocked nose, increase in weight and parkinsonism-like effects may occur.

Warnings Indoramin should not be used in individuals suffering from heart failure until it is controlled with digoxin and diuretics. It should be used with caution, in people suffering from depression, impaired kidney or liver function, epilepsy or parkinsonism.

Risks in elderly people Harmful effects may be more frequent and severe; use smaller doses or less frequent doses.

Risks when driving It may affect your ability to drive; therefore do not drive until you know that it is safe to do so.

Risks with alcohol It may increase the effects of alcohol; therefore do not drink alcohol if you are taking this drug.

prazosin (Hypovase)
Harmful effects Most commonly occurring harmful effects are mild and transient. They include dizziness, headaches, drowsiness, lack of energy, weakness, nausaa, vomiting, diarrhoea, constipation and palpitations. Low blood pressure on standing up after sitting or lying (may cause light-headedness, dizziness and faintness) and increased heart rate may occur. Rarely, the following harmful effects have been reported: transient loss of consciousness, fluid retention (swelling of ankles) and aggravation of angina (therefore use with a diuretic and a beta blocker), breathlessness, nervousness, vertigo, hallucinations, depression, numbness and pins and needles in the arms and legs, skin rashes, itching, loss of hair, increased frequency of passing urine, impotence, incontinence of urine, dry mouth, red eyes, stuffy nose, ringing in the ears, sweating, blurred vision.

Warnings The first dose may occasionally cause collapse due to the sudden fall in blood pressure; therefore, lie down after the first dose or take it at bedtime. People who suffer from impaired kidney function should be given a reduced initial dosage.

Risks in elderly people Harmful effects, particularly a fall in blood pressure, may be more frequent and severe; therefore use with caution. Use smaller doses and start with smallest effective dose.

Risks with driving Your ability to drive may be affected; therefore do not drive until you know that it is safe to do so.

terazosin (Hytrin)
Harmful effects include dizziness, lack of energy, ankle swelling, fall in blood pressure on standing up after sitting or lying (which may produce dizziness, light-headedness and fainting), rapid beating of the heart and palpitations.

Warnings If fainting feelings occur, you should lie flat. This effect occurs at the start of treatment and small starting doses should always be used. Terazosin should not be used in people who suffer from fainting, blackouts, stroke, myocardial infarction, angina, peptic ulcers, alcoholism or liver disease.

Risks in elderly people Harmful effects of alpha blockers may be more frequent and severe in elderly people; therefore use with caution.

Risks with driving Your ability to drive may be affected; therefore do not drive until you know that it is safe to do so.

Non-selective alpha blockers

phenoxybenzamine (Dibenyline)
Harmful effects include a fall in blood pressure on standing up after sitting or lying (may produce light-headedness and faintness), increase in heart rate, stuffy nose, failure to ejaculate, lassitude, stomach upsets, constriction of the pupils.

Warnings Phenoxybenzamine should not be used in individuals who have had a stroke or within 3–4 weeks of a heart

Table 21.5 Drugs used to treat raised blood pressure: alpha blockers – harmful effects and warnings (*cont.*)

attack; and used with caution in people who suffer from heart disease or disorders of their circulation, angina or impaired kidney function.

Risks in elderly people Harmful effects may be more frequent and severe; therefore use with caution.

phentolamine (Rogitine)
Harmful effects include a fall in blood pressure on standing up after sitting or lying (may produce light-headedness, dizziness and faintness), rapid beating of the heart, nausea, vomiting, diarrhoea, stuffy nose, weakness, flushing, disorders of heart rhythm.

Warnings Phentolamine should not be used in anyone suffering from severe raised blood pressure. The fall in blood pressure may trigger angina, or a heart attack in patients with coronary artery disease or a stroke in patients with disease of the arteries supplying the brain. Heart rate and blood pressure should be carefully monitored.

Risks in elderly people Harmful effects may be frequent and severe; therefore use with caution.

Table 21.6 Drugs used to treat raised blood pressure (hypertension): central alpha stimulants (clonidine and methyldopa) – harmful effects and warnings

clonidine (Catapres)
Harmful effects Mild, transient harmful effects include drowsiness lethargy and dry mouth. Infrequent harmful effects include mental depression, fluid retention (e.g. ankle swelling), slow heart rate, coldness of the fingers and toes, headache, difficulty with sleeping, nausea, a feeling of extreme well-being (euphoria), skin rashes, constipation, impotence (rarely), and agitation on stopping long-term treatment.

Warnings Clonidine should be used with caution in people suffering from mental depression or who have disorders of the circulation. Sudden withdrawal may produce a severe rise in blood pressure, therefore the daily dosage should be reduced slowly over several days to weeks.

Risks with driving It may cause drowsiness, so do not drive until you know that it is safe to do so.

methyldopa (Aldomet, Dopamet, in Hydromet)
Harmful effects Mild, transient harmful effects related to dose include drowsiness, headache and weakness. Other harmful effects are infrequent; they include dry mouth, depression, nightmares, weakness, diarrhoea, fluid retention (e.g. ankle swelling), failure to ejaculate, breast enlargement and milk production, liver damage, haemolytic anaemia, systemic lupus erythematosus, slow heart rate, aggravation of angina, fall in blood pressure on standing up after sitting or lying, increase in weight, nausea, vomiting, abdominal distension, constipation, flatulence, colitis, blood disorders, skin rashes, fever, stuffy nose, rise in waste products in the blood (e.g. urea), pain in muscles and joints.

Warnings Methyldopa should not be used in people who suffer from active liver disease, or in anyone with a history of mental depression. People who suffer from impaired kidney function should be started on lower doses. About 20 per cent of individuals taking methyldopa develop a positive laboratory test for haemolytic anaemia (Coombe's test). Regular tests of liver function and blood counts should be carried out during treatment. Suddenly stopping methyldopa may cause agitation, insomnia, rapid heart rate and aggravate angina.

Risks in elderly people Harmful effects may be more frequent and severe; therefore Methyldopa should be used with caution – there is the risk of increased dizziness,

Table 21.6 Drugs used to treat raised blood pressure (hypertension): central alpha stimulants (clonidine and methyldopa) – harmful effects and warnings (*cont.*)

unsteadiness, fainting and falling.

Risks with driving It may cause drowsiness; therefore do not drive until you know that it is safe to do so.

Table 21.7 Drugs used to treat raised blood pressure: ganglion blockers – harmful effects and warnings

trimetaphan (Arfonad)
Harmful effects include rapid beating of the heart, depression of breathing, constipation, difficulty passing urine, dilatation of the pupils, dry mouth and nose and, rarely, low blood sugar and low blood potassium.

Warnings Trimetaphan should not be used in people suffering from severe heart disease, arteriosclerosis or narrowing of the outlet from the stomach (pyloric stenosis). It must be used with caution in individuals who suffer from disease of the blood vessels supplying the brain (cerebral artery disease) or heart (coronary artery disease), diabetes, impaired kidney or liver function or impaired adrenal function (e.g. Addison's disease), degenerative brain disease, enlarged prostate gland, glaucoma or in anyone who suffers from allergies.

Risks in elderly people Harmful effects may be more frequent and severe; therefore use with caution.

Table 21.8 Drugs used to treat raised blood pressure (hypertension): reserpine and related drugs (rauwolfia alkaloids) – harmful effects and warnings

Not all of the following harmful effects have been reported with every rauwolfia alkaloid but they have been reported with one or more of them and should be borne in mind whenever one of them is used.

Harmful effects include vomiting, diarrhoea, nausea, loss of appetite, dryness of the mouth, disorders of heart rhythm, fainting, slowing of the heart rate, chest pain (like angina), swelling of the ankles, breathlessness, blocked nose, nose bleeds, disorders of movement like parkinsonism, dizziness, headache, depression and sometimes a paradoxical anxiety, nervousness, nightmares, drowsiness, muscle pains, milk from the breasts and enlargement of the breasts, impotence, difficulty passing urine, decreased libido, weight gain, blurred vision, difficulty with hearing, red eyes and allergic reactions (skin rash, itching).

Warnings Rauwolfia alkaloids should not be used in people who are allergic to these drugs, or who have mental depression, active peptic ulcers or ulcerative colitis or Parkinson's disease. Stop immediately if there are any signs of depression developing (e.g. depressed mood, early morning wakening, impotence, self-deprecation). Depression may be severe, even to the point of suicide and it may persist for months after the drugs are stopped.

Risks in elderly people Harmful effects may be more frequent and severe; therefore use with utmost caution.

Risks with driving They affect ability to drive; therefore drive only when you know that it is safe to do so.

Risks with alcohol They may increase the effects of alcohol; therefore do not drink alcohol if you are taking one of these drugs.

Table 21.9 Drugs used to treat raised blood pressure: vasodilators – harmful effects and warnings

diazoxide (Eudemine)
Harmful effects include rapid beating of the heart, increase in blood sugar levels which may seriously aggravate diabetes, and fluid retention (e.g. ankle swelling) which may cause heart failure in someone prone to develop heart failure. Rarely, there may be growth of hair on forehead, back and limbs, loss of appetite, nausea, vomiting, diarrhoea, transient loss of taste, headache, weakness, anxiety and dizziness; very rarely there may be blood disorders, skin rashes, blurred vision and cataracts (which clear up when the drug is stopped).

Warnings Diazoxide should not be used in people who are allergic to it. It should be used with utmost caution in individuals with coronary artery disease, women in labour, or in anyone with impaired kidney function. Blood counts (white blood cells and platelets) should be carried out at regular intervals during treatment. Regular tests of blood glucose level and tests of urine for glucose should be carried out during treatment. Thiazide diuretics will help to reduce the fluid retention but rises in blood glucose level and uric acid level may be made worse.

Risks in elderly people Harmful effects may be more frequent and severe in elderly people; therefore use with caution.

hydralazine (Apresoline)
Harmful effects include headache, loss of appetite, nausea, vomiting, diarrhoea, palpitations, rapid beating of the heart, flushing, runny eyes, blocked nose, allergic reactions, breathlessness and fluid retention (ankle swelling). Very rarely, nerve damage (e.g. numbness and pins and needles in the arms and legs) may occur which is reversed by taking vitamin B_6 (pyrridoxine) or by stopping the drug. Rarely, after prolonged treatment lupus erythematosus may occur. Other rare harmful effects include fever, skin rash, liver damage, kidney damage, anxiety, depression and blood disorders.

Warnings Hydralazine should not be used in people who are allergic to it. It should be used with utmost caution in anyone suspected of having coronary artery disease – it may trigger angina or a heart attack – and used with caution in those with disordered circulation to the brain, who are prone to develop a stroke. Reduced dosage should be used in individuals with impaired kidney or liver function and in anyone who develops depression, disorientation, anxiety or difficulty in passing urine. Systemic lupus erythematosus may develop in patients on long-term treatment with a dose of 100 mg or more daily (less in women).

minoxidil (Loniten)
Use diuretics and a salt-restricted diet in all patients on treatment with this drug.

Harmful effects include stomach upsets, increase in weight, fluid retention (e.g. ankle swelling) which may aggravate heart failure, rapid beating of the heart, excess growth of hair, tenderness of the breasts, stomach upsets and, rarely, skin rashes.

Warnings Minoxidil should not be used in people who have fluid retention (oedema). It may aggravate heart failure and angina, and may trigger angina in someone with coronary artery disease. Patients on kidney dialysis should have a lower dose.

Risks in elderly people Harmful effects may be more frequent and severe; therefore use with caution.

sodium nitroprusside (Nipride)
See Table 22.9.

22

Heart failure

In the failing heart the volume of blood in the heart chambers increases when it is relaxed. This causes the heart muscles to stretch, which weakens the pumping action of the heart. More blood accumulates in the heart, which causes a back-pressure to build up in the blood vessels returning blood to the heart. On the left side of the heart this back-pressure causes congestion in the lungs, producing breathlessness. This is called left-sided heart failure. On the right side of the heart (where blood from all over the body except the lungs is returned) the back-pressure builds up right back into the tissues of the body. This produces an increase of fluid in the tissues called oedema (dropsy). This is called congestive heart failure. A person with congestive heart failure will have swollen ankles because the excess fluid in the tissues gravitates downwards; when confined to bed such people will develop swelling at the bottom of their backs (sacral oedema).

Heart failure may be produced by any disorder that affects the heart muscle; for example, a poor blood supply due to disease of the coronary arteries which supply the heart. Also, any disorder that puts an extra workload on the heart may produce heart failure. Such disorders include raised blood pressure (the commonest cause), disease of the heart valves, disorders of heart rhythm, severe anaemia (because of the reduced number of red blood cells to carry oxygen, the heart has to work harder in order to maintain a supply of oxygen to the tissues) and an over-active thyroid gland (which causes the body to burn up energy faster than normal and therefore the heart has to pump faster to keep energy supplies going). Chronic diseases of the lungs may also produce heart failure by causing a back-pressure in the blood vessels coming from the heart.

In someone prone to develop heart failure it may be triggered by a failure to take treatment as directed, a failure of the doctor to give adequate treatment, disorders of heart rhythm, severe infections (particularly a chest infection), anaemia, over-active thyroid gland, obesity and pregnancy.

Certain drugs may trigger heart failure in a susceptible person. These include beta blockers, corticosteroids and non-steroidal anti-inflammatory drugs.

Drug treatment of heart failure

In addition to treating the underlying causes of the heart failure where possible (e.g. anaemia, raised blood pressure, valvular diseases and overactive thyroid gland), the signs (e.g. ankle swelling) and symptoms (e.g. breathlessness) of heart failure can be relieved by drugs.

There are five main groups of drugs used to treat heart failure.

1. Drugs used to remove salt and water from the body in order to reduce the excess fluid in the tissues (oedema) and to decrease the volume of blood that the heart has to pump round the body and therefore reduce the workload on the heart. These drugs are known as *diuretics* (water tablets)
2. Drugs used to improve the heart's pumping action; these drugs work directly on the heart muscle. They belong to a group of drugs known as *cardiac glycosides* (e.g. digoxin)
3. Drugs used to dilate the blood vessels in order to reduce the resistance to the flow of blood and therefore reduce the pressure required to pump the blood round the body. This reduces the workload on the heart. These drugs are know as *vasodilators*
4. Drugs that improve the heart's pumping action and also dilate blood vessels. These reduce both the pre-load and the after-load on the heart
5. Drugs that stimulate the heart

Diuretics (water tablets)

The kidneys exercise a most delicate and complex control over the amount of salts (mainly potassium and sodium) and water in the body. As urine is produced by the kidneys, salts first enter the urine but are subsequently reabsorbed back into the bloodstream according to the body's needs. The amount of salts in the urine governs the amount of water present. If the concentration of salts is high, a large amount of water will pass out into the urine; if it is low, a reduced amount of water passes into the urine. These mechanisms are used in order to keep the body's salts and water balance at an optimal level. This balance can be disturbed in patients with heart failure, liver failure or kidney failure. In these conditions salts, and therefore water, are retained in the body. The water level in the body increases, producing swelling of the tissues (oedema); this usually shows up as a swelling of the ankles.

The urine-producing system in the kidneys is called a nephron and each kidney has about 1.5 million nephrons. Each nephron starts with a filter (glomerulus) where blood coming to the kidney is filtered. Then comes a long stem (tubule) from which most of the fluid and salts that have gone through the filter are reabsorbed back into the bloodstream. The part that stays in the tubule is the urine. Cells in the lining of the tubule can also secrete substances (solvents) directly into the urine. The beginning (or proximal) part of the tubule is all twisted and curled (convoluted), the middle part forms a big loop (the loop of Henle) and the end bit is called the distal tubule, which is also convoluted. Several distal tubules connect to collecting ducts which all join up to drain into the beginning of the ureter which is the tube that connects the kidney to the bladder.

Drugs that work upon the kidneys to increase the output of sodium salt and water in the urine are called diuretics (water tablets), and the increase in the volume of urine is called diuresis.

The main use of diuretics is in the treatment of oedema (fluid retention) caused by heart, kidney or liver failure. They are also used to treat raised blood pressure. There are several groups of diuretic drugs that work at different sites in the nephron.

Types of diuretics

Osmotic diuretics

These diuretics work by osmosis – they prevent water leaving the urine and going back into the blood. *Mannitol* and *urea* are examples of osmotic diuretics. These are rarely used except in people who have taken an overdose of certain drugs. They are then given to increase the volume of the urine in order to wash the drug from the body. They are also used to reduce swelling of the brain which may occur after a head injury.

Carbonic anhydrase inhibitors

At the beginning of the nephron (proximal tubule) an enzyme – carbonic anhydrase – is responsible for exchanging hydrogen ions for sodium ions in the urine. There is a group of drugs that block the action of carbonic anhydrase so that the sodium concentration in the urine increases and this takes water with it. These are called carbonic anhydrase inhibitors and include *acetazolamide* and *dichlorphenamide*. They are only weak diuretics and are no longer used to treat fluid retention (oedema). However, they are used to treat glaucoma, which is caused by a build up of fluids in the front chambers of the eyes. These drugs reduce the formation of this fluid.

Reports of the value of these drugs to relieve the symptoms of mountain sickness (altitude sickness) are not convincing. The best treatment for mountain sickness is to get down the mountain!

Loop diuretics (or 'high ceiling' diuretics)

Bumetanide, ethacrynic acid, frusemide and *piretanide* cause salt to concentrate in the urine, which takes large volumes of water with it. Their site of action is on the loop in the nephron, so they are known as *loop diuretics*. They are powerful diuretics and have a rapid onset of action which quickly reaches a high peak of effectiveness (this is why they are also referred to as 'high-ceiling' diuretics). By mouth they are effective within 1 hour and their effects have worn off in about 6 hours, so they can be given twice daily without interfering with sleep. By injection into a vein they work within half an hour.

Their effect is directly related to the dose given. They are used to treat fluid retention (oedema) due to kidney, heart or liver disease. They are also used to treat fluid on the lungs (pulmonary oedema) due to heart failure.

The *main harmful effects* of loop diuretics include a fall in the level of potassium in the body, a fall in the level of sodium, dehydration (loss of water), a fall in the level of magnesium and calcium, and a rise in the level of uric acid which may trigger an acute attack of gout in a susceptible person. They also cause a rise in the blood glucose level, which may trigger diabetes in a susceptible person, and cause problems for individuals on anti-diabetic drug treatment. If taken in large doses by people with impaired kidney function, frusemide may cause deafness and bumetanide may cause deafness and muscle pains.

Thiazide diuretics and related drugs

Thiazide diuretics and related drugs act on the distal part of tubules to prevent the re-absorption of salt. This increases the amount of salt in the urine which carries large volumes of water with it. They are moderately strong, are active when given by mouth and are very useful for long-term treatments. When given by mouth they work within about 1–2 hours and their effects last about 12–24 hours. They are used to treat oedema (fluid retention), and in low doses they are used to treat people suffering from raised blood pressure.

Harmful effects of thiazide diuretics include loss of potassium, sodium and water in the urine, producing low blood levels of potassium and sodium, and loss of water from the body (dehydration). They also produce a fall in the concentration of magnesium in the blood. They cause the blood sugar to increase, which may trigger diabetes in a susceptible person or cause problems in people taking anti-diabetic drugs. They also cause an increase of uric acid in the blood (hyperuricaemia), which may trigger an acute attack of gout in a susceptible individual. The excretion of calcium may, very rarely, be reduced by the prolonged use of thiazide diuretics, leading to a raised blood level of calcium (hypercalcaemia). They may also cause a rise in blood fat levels (e.g. cholesterol).

Potassium-sparing diuretics

Spironolactone and potassium canrenoate Further down the distal convoluted tubules, sodium is actively reabsorbed back into the bloodstream in exchange for potassium and hydrogen ions. These effects are under the control of the hormone aldosterone, produced by the adrenal glands. Drugs that block the effect of aldosterone are called aldosterone antagonists. They cause sodium (and therefore water) to stay in the urine, and potassium to pass back into the blood. They include spironolactone and potassium canrenoate (which is a breakdown product of spironolactone in the body). They are given by mouth to treat fluid retention (oedema) caused by liver disease (e.g. cirrhosis of the liver), kidney disease and heart failure. They are also used to treat Conn's syndrome, a disease of the adrenal glands that causes over-production of aldosterone. They may be used as additional treatment in people taking a thiazide or loop diuretic, in an attempt to reduce the loss of potassium that occurs with these drugs.

A serious risk with these drugs is a raised blood potassium, which causes abnormalities in the electrical activity of the heart. These show up on electrical tracings of the heart (ECG). They may produce swelling of the breasts (gynaecomastia), impotence and menstrual disturbances.

Amiloride and triamterene These two drugs work at the same site as aldosterone antagonists, and produce similar effects although they do not block aldosterone. They are used as moderately effective diuretics. They cause retention of potassium and are useful alternatives to having to give additional potassium to people taking thiazide or loop diuretics (see later).

Misuse of diuretic drugs in elderly people

Most harmful effects produced by diuretic drugs occur in elderly people, who may be kept on daily treatment with a diuretic drug for years on end without tests of their blood chemistry and full medical check-ups. Harmful effects of a low concentration of sodium in the body include weakness, giddiness and confusion. A fall in blood pressure on standing up after sitting or lying down may occur and cause faintness, dizziness and the risk of falling. Transient weakness of an arm or leg may occur (like a stroke) and a low potassium may trigger kidney failure in an elderly person with impaired kidney function, and also increase the risk of disorders of heart rhythm, especially with digoxin (see later). They may also trigger incontinence of urine.

Main risks of diuretics

Potassium loss

Potassium loss may cause serious dangers to individuals on diuretic treatment if large and frequent doses of diuretics are taken; if the diet is low in potassium (a particular hazard in elderly people); or if a person is taking other drugs that may produce a low potassium concentration in the blood (e.g. corticosteroids or carbenoxolone). Potassium loss produces muscle weakness, constipation, loss of appetite and changes in the electrical activity of the heart producing disorders of heart rhythm.

Severe effects of low potassium produced by diuretics may occur in people who are already losing potassium because of some longstanding disorder of the bowel (e.g. chronic diarrhoea). Acute vomiting and diarrhoea or taking laxatives every day may also produce potassium loss.

Warnings *Stimulant or osmotic laxatives cause loss of water and salts in the motions; therefore they should not be used regularly, particularly by anyone who is taking diuretic drugs.*

Potassium loss may be particularly harmful to people who are taking digoxin or a related drug for heart failure or a disorder of heart rhythm. The low potassium in the blood increases the toxic effects of digoxin and related drugs on the heart, producing dangerous disorders of heart rhythm.

Potassium excess

To reduce potassium loss, it is common practice to give a potassium salt along with a diuretic or to use a potassium-sparing diuretic. These practices are not without their danger. In people with impaired kidney function, the excretion of potassium may be poor and there is a risk of producing high blood levels of potassium if a potassium supplement or a potassium-sparing diuretic is also given. Equally, kidney function in elderly people may be impaired and therefore potassium supplements and potassium-sparing diuretics should be used with similar caution. This warning also applies to salt substitiutes that contain potassium.

High blood potassium may cause pins and needles in the hands and feet, listlessness, mental confusion, weakness and a fall in blood pressure and disorders of heart rhythm and rate. These harmful effects may be hazardous to elderly people because they may be put down to 'old age' and the treatment continued.

Dehydration

High doses of diuretics may cause a large amount of salt and water to be lost from the body, producing dehydration. The individual becomes lethargic and sleepy, and the blood pressure falls. The kidneys fail to work properly and the concentration of waste products increases in the blood (e.g. the blood urea increases), producing further problems.

Long-term salt loss

The long-term use of diuretics may lead to a fall in body salt (sodium chloride), producing lethargy, weakness, slowing down, loss of appetite and nausea. In the elderly it is therefore important to check the blood levels of sodium and potassium at regular intervals (every 3–6 months) and to decide whether the individual really needs to take a diuretic or not.

Is there a need to take extra potassium when diuretics are used to treat fluid retention (oedema)?

In patients being treated with diuretic drugs for fluid retention (oedema) due to liver, kidney or heart disease, the regular daily dosage of diuretic is often sufficiently high to cause a daily loss of potassium in the urine. This usually exceeds the amount of potassium that is in the diet and these people, particularly the elderly, may develop a deficiency of potassium. This loss of potassium may produce serious risks in the elderly, and in people taking digoxin or related drugs (see later). In these people it is important that they take additional potassium in an adequate dose (divided throughout the day) and to make sure that they have regular blood tests (every 3 months) to measure the blood sodium and potassium levels. An alternative is to use a potassium-sparing diuretic instead of one that causes potassium loss (see earlier).

Is there a need to take extra potassium when diuretics are used to treat raised blood pressure?

When diuretic drugs are used to treat raised blood pressure the daily dose should not be high enough to produce potassium loss. Therefore, otherwise healthy people on long-term treatment with a diuretic for blood pressure do not need additional potassium. They need sensible advice on potassium-rich foods. However, certain individuals may need to take potassium supplements (see earlier).

Combined preparations of a diuretic plus a potassium salt

From the preceding brief discussion of when to give potassium supplements, it is evident that they are not necessary in otherwise healthy people being treated over the long term with a thiazide diuretic in the doses necessary to treat a raised blood pressure, nor are they necessary in anyone on maintenance treatment with a thiazide diuretic following an attack of mild heart failure. Despite this advice, thousands of combined preparations containing a thiazide diuretic and a potassium salt (see later) are prescribed every day at a significant cost to the health service.

Combined preparations of a diuretic drug plus a potassium salt do not supply enough potassium for anyone who needs additional potassium and they are not necessary in those people who do not.

In those individuals who need additional potassium these combinations are too inflexible and do not give the opportunity to vary the dose of potassium without also varying the dose of the diuretics. In people who need extra potassium it is better to give the diuretic and the potassium separately. Of course this may cause problems for some because they have to remember to take two lots of tablets at different times of the day.

In people being treated for fluid retention and who are taking doses of a diuretic over a long period of time, potassium loss may be minimized by maintaining a good intake of potassium in the diet and by the intermittent use of the diuretics – for example, every other day or three times a week. If potassium supplements are required, they are best given separately in a liquid preparation as chloride salt (as chloride is lost in the urine along with potassium).

Harmful effects of potassium supplements

When taken by mouth some potassium salts (e.g. potassium chloride) may produce nausea, vomiting, diarrhoea and stomach cramps. They may also cause ulceration of the intestine, particularly those tablets with a special coating (enteric coated) that are designed to resist the acid in the stomach and dissolve only when they get through to the small intestine. There are numerous reports of intestinal ulceration, sometimes with bleeding and perforation caused by enteric-coated potassium chloride tablets. In some individuals the late formation of a scar has caused narrowing of the intestine (a stricture), leading to an obstruction. Ulceration of the stomach may occur and ulceration of the intestine has also followed the use of sustained-release (i.e. slow-release) preparations. Slow-release potassium tablets may 'stick' in the throat and cause ulceration of the gullet (oesophagus).

Combining diuretics

The need for potassium supplements may be avoided by the use of a potassium-sparing diuretic given along with a thiazide diuretic – for example, a thiazide plus spironolactone, amiloride or triamterene; or frusemide, bumetanide or ethacrynic acid plus spironolactone. But these combinations require special knowledge and understanding because such products may increase the blood potassium level, which may be as harmful if not more harmful than a low blood potassium level.

Drugs that improve the pumping action of the heart

Digoxin and related drugs (cardiac glycosides)

These drugs belong to a group that have been used for centuries to treat 'dropsy'. They are called *cardiac glycosides*, and are found in a number of plants (e.g. digoxin is obtained from the leaves of white foxglove). They are sometimes referred to as *digitalis* drugs. These drugs produce similar actions and effects on the body but differ in the rate at which they start to act and in the duration of their effects. They act mainly on the muscle of the heart.

Digoxin is the most commonly used cardiac glycoside and therefore in this chapter I will refer only to digoxin although the comments are equally applicable to the others.

The effects produced by digoxin

In heart failure, digoxin causes the heart muscle to work more efficiently; this improves the pumping action of the heart and increases output. This reduces the back-pressure and decreases the size of the heart. A secondary effect is to reduce the volume of the blood by improving the circulation to the kidneys, causing an increased output of urine.

Digoxin reduces the rapid beating of the heart which occurs in heart failure in an attempt to keep up the output of the heart. It does this by reducing the effects of adrenaline stimulation and by making the heart more sensitive to the stimulation of the vagus nerve which normally opposes the action of adrenaline. It also slows down the rate of transmission of electrical impulses from the heart's pacemaker to the rest of the heart muscle.

Digoxin is effective in relieving fluid retention (e.g. ankle swelling), breathing difficulties and fatigue associated with heart failure. It increases the individual's capacity to do exercise and initially increases the output of urine. It is also used to treat atrial fibrillation, a disorder of heart rhythm (see Chapter 23).

Harmful effects of digoxin

Digoxin is a very effective drug if used sensibly; however, it accumulates in the body and may produce dangerous and sometimes fatal harmful effects. These are particularly likely to occur if the daily dosage of digoxin is too high and/or if the individual's kidneys are not working efficiently. Therefore measurements of kidney function should be carried out routinely. The results should be used as a guide to treatment, and if there is any evidence of impaired kidney function the daily dosage of digoxin should be reduced. This applies especially to elderly people whose kidneys may not be working efficiently. This is why the dose of digoxin for an elderly person should always be the smallest effective dose possible, because any interference with the excretion of digoxin in the urine will easily lead to toxic levels of the drug in the body.

Too large a dose of digoxin produces loss of appetite, nausea, vomiting, diarrhoea, headache and fatigue. It may make elderly people confused.

A particular danger of digoxin is its effect on the heart rate. Too big a daily dose for too long a time may produce serious effects which are made worse if the individual is also taking diuretic drugs (water tablets). These may cause a fall in the blood potassium level, which makes the heart more sensitive to the toxic effects of digoxin (see Table 22.7).

Warnings *Digoxin is excreted by the kidneys; if their function is impaired, the drug may accumulate in the blood and produce harmful effects. Digitoxin, which is broken down in the liver, is an alternative in such cases.*

The risks of using diuretics with digoxin are increased in the elderly; therefore elderly people should not be kept on regular daily treatment with a diuretic drug and digoxin for long periods of time without regular medical check-ups of their progress.

Treatment should be individualized

Using standard doses of digoxin may cause problems because different patients may react differently to digoxin and therefore the 'right' dose must be established for each individual patient. People taking digoxin should be regularly checked for signs and symptoms of toxicity (physical examination plus electrocardiograph of the heart) until their condition is stable and the most appropriate daily dose worked out. Periodic tests of the blood level of the drug should be carried out, particularly in anyone with impaired kidney function. The blood sample should be taken not less then 6 hours after the last dose.

Long-term use of digoxin

Until fairly recently, if you were put on digoxin you were on it for life. It is now time, though, that we questioned the need to continue digoxin treatment in people who have got over an attack of heart failure, because it may be stopped in some individuals without any untoward effect, particularly in the elderly.

Regular daily treatment with digoxin should be stopped if the person is well and the heart failure was due to some treatable disorder (e.g. severe anaemia). It may also be stopped if the individual is well, having no symptoms, and if the level of digoxin in the blood is lower than the recommended effective level. The latter usually shows that he or she did not need to be kept on the drug anyway.

Vasodilator drugs that reduce the workload of the heart

As the amount of blood pumped out by the failing heart falls, the small arteries around the body begin to constrict in order to maintain the blood pressure; but as the failure of the heart increases it finds it more and more difficult to pump out blood against this increased resistance. In addition, the back-pressure in the veins returning blood to the heart builds up and this adds to the failure. In order to reduce the workload on the heart, drugs are used that dilate the blood vessels. These are called vasodilators; by increasing the calibre of the blood vessels they reduce the amount of work that the heart has to do (see below).

Vasodilators used to treat heart failure include the following.

1. Nitrate vasodilators that principally dilate veins

These dilate small veins and allow the blood to pool in the veins of the body. This causes a reduction in the amount of blood returning to the heart and therefore reduces the work that it has to do. This is called reducing the 'pre-load' on the heart. However, nitrate vasodilators also dilate arteries which helps to reduce the 'after-load' on the heart (see below).

2. ACE inhibitors and hydralazine

These drugs principally dilate the arteries, increasing their calibre and reducing the resisitance to the flow of blood from the heart. This reduces the work of the heart because it has to pump against less resistance. This is called reducing the 'after-load' on the heart. ACE inhibitors also reduce excess body fluids by improving the loss of sodium and water in the urine.

3. Nitroprusside and prazosin (an alpha blocker)

These drugs produce *both* effects listed above, dilating both veins and arteries about equally, and help to reduce 'pre-load' and 'after-load' on the heart.

Drugs that stimulate the heart

Enoximone (Perfan) and *milrinone* (Primacor). They block an enzyme in the heart muscle (phosphodiesterase) to produce stimulation. They are of use in the short-term treatment of severe congestive heart failure. *Dopexamine* (Dopacord) is used to treat heart failure associated with heart surgery. It stimulates beta receptors in the heart and improves blood flow through the kidneys. *Dobutamine* (Dobutrex) and *dopamine* (Intropin) act on beta receptors in heart muscle; they improve contraction of the heart but have little effect upon its rate. They are used to stimulate the heart to beat when it fails suddenly.

Isoprenaline increases both the heart rate and the contraction of the heart and may be used to stimulate the heart in heart block.

Xamoterol (Corwin) is a partial stimulant of beta receptors which should be used *only* to treat chronic mild heart failure in patients who are not breathless at rest and only get breathless on exertion. It should be used only in hospital under strict medical supervision.

Recommendations on the drug treatment of heart failure

The specific drug treatment of heart failure involves the use of a diuretic, a vasodilator and digoxin singly or together in various combinations.

Diuretics are usually the first line of treatment: a thiazide diuretic by mouth for mild to moderate heart failure, and a loop diuretic such as frusemide for moderate to severe heart failure by injection in the acute stage and then later by mouth. Long-term maintenance treatment should be with a thiazide diuretic by mouth or, if there is no improvement, with a loop diuretic such as frusemide.

Because people on long-term treatment with thiazide or loop diuretics run the risk of losing potassium in their urine, chemical tests of the blood should be carried out at regular intervals (every 3 months). If the blood potassium is low, indicating a loss of potassium, it will be necessary to add a potassium supplement to the treatment or to add a potassium-sparing diuretic.

The next step in treatment is to add a vasodilator if the individual fails to respond to diuretics. Sometimes a vasodilator is used to start treatment. One that principally dilates veins (e.g. a nitrate vasodilator) will be helpful to someone whose main symptoms are due to congestion, particularly of the lungs, producing breathlessness, whereas one that principally dilates arteries (e.g. an ACE inhibitor) will help those patients whose symptoms are due to poor output from the heart (e.g. fatigue). People with chronic heart failure who have had a poor response to other treatments will often benefit from a vasodilator that dilates both veins and arteries (e.g. sodium nitroprusside).

The ACE inhibitors are particularly useful for this purpose. They stop the production of angiotensin II in the body which causes marked constriction of arteries. This causes the small arteries (arterioles) to dilate and the resistance to the flow of blood to be reduced, which reduces the workload of the heart (the after-load). They also improve the blood supply to the kidneys, which causes a reduced production of the chemical and an increased production of urine, resulting in a fall in the volume of the blood which also reduces the workload of the heart.

Combined treatment with a diuretic and an ACE inhibitor will help to reduce breathlessness, reduce fluid retention, reduce fatigue and improve ability to exercise. Diuretics do not improve the output from the heart and this may trigger the angiotensin reflex. This is stopped by adding an ACE inhibitor.

Digoxin is best used to treat individuals with heart failure who have a disorder of heart rhythm called atrial fibrillation (see Chapter 23). Only about half of the patients with a normal heart rhythm will benefit from the use of digoxin.

Harmful effects from digoxin occur in about 1 in 5 people, particularly the elderly. They are usually produced by too large a daily dosage of digoxin given for too long a period of time without measuring the level of the drug in the blood to see whether it has reached toxic levels. When heart failure symptoms are mild, it is far better to start off with a small daily dose of digoxin and slowly increase the dose upwards rather than the old practice of giving a high starting dose and then slowly reducing it. This latter method is all right for moderate or severe heart failure provided the individual is examined carefully before each dose and particular attention is paid to the rate and rhythm of the heart. If there is any doubt, an electrical tracing of the heart (ECG) should be carried out before the next dose is given and a sample of blood sent off to the laboratory to test whether the concentration of digoxin in the blood is at a toxic level.

Enoximone (Perfan) and milrinone (Primacor) offer an additional choice in patients with severe congestive heart failure.

Non-drug treatment of heart failure

In addition to drug treatments, people with chronic heart failure should limit their amount of activity, reduce their weight if they are overweight, stop smoking if they smoke and reduce their daily salt intake by using no added salt in cooking or at the table.

Table 22.1 Preparations used to treat heart failure: diuretics

Preparation	*Drug*	*Drug group*	*Dosage form*
Aldactone	spironolactone	Potassium sparing	Tablets
Aluzine	frusemide	Loop	Tablets
Aprinox	bendrofluazide	Thiazide	Tablets
Baycaron	mefruside	Thiazide-like	Tablets
bendrofluazide	bendrofluazide	Thiazide	Tablets
Berkamil	amiloride	Potassium sparing	Tablets
Berkozide	bendrofluazide	Thiazide	Tablets
Burinex	bumetanide	Loop	Tablets, sugar-free liquid, injection
Centyl	bendrofluazide	Thiazide	Tablets
Diatensec	spironolactone	Potassium sparing	Tablets
Diurexan	xipamide	Thiazide-like	Tablets
Dryptal	frusemide	Loop	Tablets
Dytac	triamterene	Potassium sparing	Capsules
Edecrin	ethacrynic acid	Loop	Tablets, injection
Enduron	methyclothiazide	Thiazide	Tablets
Esidrex	hydrochlorothiazide	Thiazide	Tablets
frusemide	frusemide	Loop	Tablets
Frusid	frusemide	Loop	Tablets
Hydrenox	hydroflumethiazide	Thiazide	Tablets
HydroSaluric	hydrochlorothiazide	Thiazide	Tablets
Hygroton	chlorthalidone	Thiazide-like	Tablets
Laractone	spironolactone	Potassium sparing	Tablets
Lasix	frusemide	Loop	Tablets, injection, paediatric liquid

Table 22.1 Preparations used to treat heart failure: diuretics (*cont.*)

Preparation	*Drug*	*Drug group*	*Dosage form*
Metenix	metolazone	Thiazide-like	Tablets
Midamor	amiloride	Potassium sparing	Tablets
Navidrex	cyclopenthiazide	Thiazide	Tablets
Neo-NaClex	bendrofluazide	Thiazide	Tablets
Nephril	polythiazide	Thiazide	Tablets
Saluric	chlorothiazide	Thiazide	Tablets
Spiretic	spironolactone	Potassium sparing	Tablets
Spiroctan	spironolactone	Potassium sparing	Tablets, capsules
Spiroctan-M	potassium canrenoate	Potassium sparing	Injection
Spirolone	spironolactone	Potassium sparing	Tablets
spironolactone	spironolactone	Potassium sparing	Tablets

Table 22.2 Combined diuretic preparations used to treat heart failure

Preparation	*Drug*	*Drug group*	*Dosage form*
Aldactide 25 and 50	spironolactone hydroflumethiazide	Potassium sparing Thiazide	Tablets
Amilco	amiloride hydrochlorothiazide	Potassium sparing Thiazide	Tablets
Burinex A	bumetanide amiloride	Loop Potassium sparing	Tablets
Dyazide*	triamterene hydrochlorothiazide	Potassium sparing Thiaizide	Tablets
Dytide*	triamterene benzthiazide	Potassium sparing Thiazide	Capsules
Frumil	amiloride frusemide	Potassium sparing Loop	Tablets
Frusene*	triamterene frusemide	Potassium sparing Loop	Tablets
Hypertane	amiloride hydrochlorothiazide	Potassium sparing Thiazide	Tablets
Kalspare*	triamterene chlorthalidone	Potassium sparing Thiazide	Tablets
Lasilactone	spironolactone frusemide	Potassium sparing Loop	Capsules
Lasoride	frusemide amiloride	Loop Potassium sparing	Tablets
Moduret 25	hydrochlorothiazide amiloride	Thiazide Potassium sparing	Tablets

Table 22.2 Combined diuretic preparations used to treat heart failure (*cont.*)

Preparation	*Drug*	*Drug group*	*Dosage form*
Moduretic	amiloride hydrochlorothiazide	Potassium sparing Thiazide	Tablets, solution
Normetic	amiloride hydrochlorothiazide	Potassium sparing Thiazide	Tablets
Triamco*	triamterene hydrochlorothiazide	Potassium sparing Thiazide	Tablets
Vasetic	hydrochlorothiazide amiloride	Thiazide Potassium sparing	Tablets

*May cause urine to look blue in some lights.

Table 22.3 Combined diuretic and potassium preparations used to treat heart failure

Preparation	*Drug*	*Drug group*	*Dosage form*
Burinex K	bumetanide potassium chloride	Loop Potassium supplement	Sustained-release tablets
Centyl-K	bendrofluazide potassium chloride	Thiazide Potassium supplement	Sustained-release tablets
Diumide-K Continus	frusemide potassium chloride	Loop Potassium supplement	Tablets
Hygroton K	chlorthalidone potassium chloride	Thiazide-like Potassium supplement	Sustained-release tablets
Lasikal	frusemide potassium chloride	Loop Potassium supplement	Sustained-release tablets
Lasix K	frusemide potassium chloride	Loop diuretic Potassium supplement	Tablets Sustained-release tablets
Navidrex-K	cyclopenthiazide potassium chloride	Thiazide Potassium supplement	Slow-release tablets
Neo-NaClex-K	bendrofluazide potassium chloride	Thiazide Potassium supplement	Sustained-release tablets

Table 22.4 Potassium supplement preparations

Preparation	*Dosage form*
Kay-Cee-L	Sugar-free syrup
Kloref	Effervescent tablets
Leo K	Sustained-release tablets
Nu-K	Sustained-release capsules
potassium chloride tablets, effervescent	Effervescent tablets
Sando-K	Effervescent tablets
Slow-K	Sustained-release tablets

Table 22.5 Preparations used to treat heart failure: digoxin and related drugs (cardiac glycosides)

Preparation	*Drug*	*Dosage form*
Cedilanid	lanatoside C	Tablets
digitoxin	digitoxin	Tablets
digoxin	digoxin	Tablets, paediatric injection
Lanoxin	digoxin	Tablets, injection
Lanoxin-PG	digoxin	Tablets, elixir

Table 22.6 Preparations used to treat heart failure: vasodilators

Preparation	*Drug*	*Drug group*	*Dosage form*
Accupro	quinapril	ACE inhibitor	Tablets
Acepril	captopril	ACE inhibitor	Tablets
Apresoline	hydralazine	Vasodilator	Tablets, injection
Capoten	captopril	ACE inhibitor	Tablets
Carace	lisinopril	ACE inhibitor	Tablets
Cedocard	isosorbide dinitrate	Nitrate	Tablets
Elantan	isosorbide mononitrate	Nitrate	Tablets
Hypovase	prazosin	Selective alpha blocker	Tablets
Innovace	enalapril	ACE inhibitor	Tablets
Ismo	isosorbide mononitrate	Nitrate	Tablets
Isoket Infusion	isosorbide dinitrate	Nitrate	Ampoules for intravenous infusion
Isordil	isosorbide dinitrate	Nitrate	Tablets; and Isordil Sublingual (tablets to dissolve under the tongue)

Table 22.6 Preparations used to treat heart failure; vasodilators (*cont.*)

Preparation	*Drug*	*Drug group*	*Dosage form*
Isotrate	isosorbide mononitrate	Nitrate	Tablets
Nipride	sodium nitroprusside	Vasodilator	Powder ampoules for intravenous infusion
Nitrocine	glyceryl trinitrate	Nitrate	Injection
Nitronal	glyceryl trinitrate	Nitrate	Injection
Suscard Buccal	glyceryl trinitrate	Nitrate	Sustained-release tablets
Tridil	glyceryl trinitrate	Nitrate	Injection
Vascardin	isosorbide dinitrate	Nitrate	Tablets
Zestril	lisinopril	ACE inhibitor	Tablets

Table 22.7 Digoxin and related drugs – harmful effects and warnings

Harmful effects include nausea, vomiting and loss of appetite. These are the most common harmful effects and the earliest signs of overdosage. In addition, diarrhoea, stomach pains, salivation and sweating may occur. Rarely, some patients may develop symptoms caused by toxic effects on the brain; these include headache, drowsiness, depression, disorientation, mental confusion, delirium and hallucinations. Pain in the face, malaise, fatigue and visual disturbances may occur. Colour vision may be affected with everything appearing yellow or green or, less frequently, red, brown, blue or white. Allergic skin rashes, blood disorders and enlargement of the breasts may occur very rarely. The most serious dose-related harmful effects are on the heart, producing disorders of rhythm and rate.

Warnings Digoxin and related drugs should not be used in individuals who have a disorder of the heart rate called Wolff–Parkinson–White syndrome (see Chapter 23) because of the harmful effects on the conduction of electrical impulses in the heart. They should be used with caution in anyone with impaired kidney function, low blood potassium level, raised blood calcium, low blood magnesium, thyroid disorder (over- or under-active), or who has suffered from a recent heart attack (myocardial infarction). Premature infants and newborn babies are particularly sensitive to digoxin and related drugs.

Risks in elderly people Harmful effects of digoxin and related drugs may be more frequent and severe in the elderly, particularly if they have an impairment of kidney function. Smaller doses should always be used in elderly people and tests of their kidney function should be carried out.

Table 22.8 Diuretics – harmful effects and warnings

Thiazide diuretics

Harmful effects of thiazide diuretics vary between different drugs and between different individuals. They vary in frequency, severity and type. Most harmful effects produced by thiazide diuretics are mild and are usually related to the doses used. They can easily be controlled by reducing the dose. More serious harmful effects are rare and are usually caused by high doses and/or by how a particular individual reacts. Not all of the following

Table 22.8 Diuretics – harmful effects and warnings (*cont.*)

harmful effects have been reported with every thiazide diuretic but they have been reported with one or more of them and should be borne in mind whenever a thiazide diuretic is used.

Harmful effects include loss of appetite, stomach upsets, nausea, vomiting, diarrhoea, a fall in blood sodium, potassium and magnesium, dehydration, changes in the acidity of the blood, raised blood uric acid levels, raised blood sugar, and an increase in blood cholesterol levels. They may, rarely, cause a rise in blood calcium levels. Occasionally, thiazide diuretics may cause skin rashes, impotence, liver damage with jaundice, sensitivity of the skin to sunlight, muscle spasm, weakness, restlessness, blurred vision, allergic reactions (particularly in people who are prone to allergy or who suffer from asthma) and blood disorders.

Warnings Thiazide diuretics should not be used in people who suffer from kidney failure or from high blood calcium levels. They may cause a low blood potassium level and, because of their effects on increasing the blood sugar level, they may trigger diabetes in a susceptible person and they may cause problems in the treatment of diabetes. Because of their effects on increasing blood uric acid levels, they may trigger an acute attack of gout in a susceptible individual. They may worsen any impairment of kidney or liver function and trigger liver coma in someone suffering from advanced cirrhosis of the liver. Potassium supplements should be given to anyone who is taking high and regular doses of thiazides and/or when the diet is low in potassium.

Risks in elderly people Harmful effects of thiazide diuretics may be more frequent and severe in elderly people, especially if used in high doses and/or regularly every day for prolonged periods of time. Elderly people are particularly sensitive to changes in the body's water and salts; therefore regular tests of the chemistry of their blood should be carried out with particular emphasis on blood sodium and potassium levels. These tests of blood chemistry should be carried out before treatment starts, after 1 month of treatment and then preferably every 3–6 months during treatment.

Loop diuretics

Harmful effects include a fall in blood sodium, potassium, magnesium and calcium; dehydration, increase in blood sugar and uric acid; loss of appetite, nausea, vomiting, stomach upsets, diarrhoea, constipation, malaise; very rarely, skin rashes, jaundice due to liver damage, and damage to the bone marrow producing blood disorders. Frusemide and bumetanide may damage the ears, producing noises in the ears (tinnitus) and deafness when given to people with impaired kidney function or when given with aminoglycoside antibiotics, which may also damage hearing. Bumetanide may also cause painful muscles (myalgia). Ethacrynic acid injections are painful. Piretanide rarely causes nausea, vomiting, diarrhoea or rashes, but in high doses it may cause painful muscles (myalgia).

Warnings Loop diuretics should not be used in individuals who are low in body salts (e.g. sodium and potassium) or who have cirrhosis of the liver, nor in anyone showing signs of overdosing with digoxin or related drugs.

Because they may cause an increase in blood sugar they may trigger an attack of diabetes in susceptible individuals, and may cause problems in diabetics receiving anti-diabetic drugs. Moreover, because they may cause an increase in blood uric acid they may trigger an attack of gout in a susceptible person. They may lower the blood calcium level and, rarely, trigger tetany. They may cause a rise in nitrogen waste products in the blood (e.g. urea).

Loop diuretics should be used with great caution in people with severe kidney failure. They may increase the risk of retention of urine in anyone who suffers from an enlarged prostate gland or other difficulty in passing urine.

Table 22.8 Diuretics – harmful effects and warnings (*cont.*)

Tests of blood chemistry should be carried out before treatment starts and at regular intervals during treatment. People on long-term treatment should have tests of their blood chemistry every 3–6 months. High doses should not be used in anyone suffering from kidney failure caused by drugs or in people with kidney failure and severe liver failure. Individuals who are allergic to sulphonamide drugs may be allergic to frusemide.

Risks in elderly people Harmful effects may be more frequent and severe in the elderly, particularly disturbances of the chemistry of the blood (e.g. sodium and potassium). Loop diuretics may also cause problems with passing urine.

Potassium-sparing diuretics

Harmful effects Amiloride may, rarely, cause headache, weakness, fatigue, confusion, nausea, loss of appetite, vomiting, diarrhoea, abdominal pain, constipation, dizziness, cough and breathlessness, and impotence. Very rarely, it may cause pain in the heart and chest, jaundice, skin rashes, itching, loss of hair, joint pains, tremor, pins and needles, nervousness, decreased libido, visual disturbances, nasal congestion and difficulty with passing urine.

Potassium canrenoate may cause nausea, vomiting and confusion when given in high doses. It may produce pain and irritation at the site of the injection. Other possible harmful effects are listed under spironolactone (below) but because potassium canrenoate is given only by injection in acute cases, and not for long-term regular daily use, no such harmful effects have been reported.

Spironolactone may cause enlargement of the breasts, stomach upsets, stomach cramps, diarrhoea, drowsiness, lethargy, headache, skin rashes, mental confusion, fever, incoordination of voluntary movements, inability to attain or maintain an erection, irregular periods or loss of periods, bleeding from the vagina after the menopause, hairiness and deep voice, and blood disorders.

Triamterine may cause stomach upsets, diarrhoea, nausea and vomiting, weakness, headache, dry mouth, allergic reactions and sensitivity of the skin to sunlight.

Warnings Potassium-sparing diuretics should not be used in anyone whose kidney function is severly impaired, nor in individuals known to be allergic to the particular drug or who have a raised blood potassium level. More than one of these drugs should never be taken together because such a combination may cause a dangerous rise in blood potassium levels. They cause an increase in blood potassium, so do not take potassium supplements or a high potassium diet or use salt substitutes that contain potassium. If the blood potassium goes above normal levels the drugs should be stopped. These diuretics may cause a low blood sodium, producing a dry mouth, lethargy and drowsiness, and they may cause a rise in nitrogen waste products in the blood (e.g. urea). Every 3–6 months patients should have a check on the chemistry of their blood, particularly sodium, potassium and nitrogen waste products (e.g. urea). Regular checks of kidney and liver function should also be carried out.

Amiloride and triamterine should be used with caution in people suffering from diabetes or cirrhosis of the liver. Spironolactone and potassium canrenoate cause cancer in rats, and therefore they should be used with caution over the long term, particularly in young people. They should be used with caution in anyone with mild or moderate kidney failure or with liver failure.

Risks in elderly people Harmful effects may be more frequent and severe in the elderly; therefore potassium-sparing diuretics should be used with caution. Elderly patients should have regular checks of the chemistry of their blood and tests of their liver and kidney function.

Table 22.9 Drugs used to treat heart failure: vasodilators – harmful effects and warnings

ACE inhibitors
See Table 21.4

nitrate vasodilators
See Table 20.1

prazosin
See alpha blockers, Table 21.5

hydralazine
See vasodilators, Table 21.9

Sodium nitroprusside (Nipride)
Harmful effects include headache, dizziness, nausea, retching, stomach pains, sweating, palpitations, apprehension and restlessness.

Warnings Sodium nitroprusside should be used with caution in those individuals with under-active thyroid gland or who have impaired blood circulation to the brain; the level of cyanide in the blood should be measured at regular intervals. It should not be used in people who suffer from severe liver or kidney disease or vitamin B_{12} deficiency.

Risks in elderly people Harmful effects may be more frequent and severe in the elderly; therefore use caution.

Table 22.10 Other drugs used to treat heart failure – harmful effects and warnings

dobutamine (Dobutrex)*
Harmful effects The most common harmful effect is rapid beating of the heart. Overdose will cause a marked rise in systolic blood pressure.

Warnings Dobutamine should be used with caution if there is a severe drop in blood pressure.

dopamine (dopamine hydrochloride, dopamine hydrochloride in dextrose solution, Intropin)*
Harmful effects include nausea, vomiting, rapid beating of the heart, fall or rise in blood pressure, constriction of arteries producing a cold, pale skin.

Warnings Dopamine should not be used in people with rapid heart rate or phaeochromocytoma. Low doses produce dilatation of arteries and increase the blood flow through the kidneys, but high doses cause constriction of arteries and can trigger heart failure in someone who has had a heart attack.

enoximone (Perfan)
Harmful effects include drop in blood pressure, headache, insomnia, and stomach and bowel upsets. It may, rarely, cause chills, fever, reduced production of urine, pains in the arms and legs, and inability to pass urine. Very rarely, it may cause a drop in blood platelets, changes in the chemistry of the blood, and impaired liver and kidney function.

Warnings Enoximone should be used with caution in patients with impaired kidney or liver function; blood counts, tests of liver and kidney function, and tests of the chemistry of the blood should be carried out before and at regular intervals during treatment.

isoprenaline (Saventrine)*
Harmful effects include rapid beating of the heart, sweating, tremor, palpitations, headache, disorders of heart rhythm.

Warnings Isoprenaline should be used with caution in patients with coronary heart disease, diabetes or over-active thyroid.

metaraminol (Aramine)*
Harmful effects include rapid beating of the heart, disorders of heart rhythm and

Table 22.10 Other drugs used to treat heart failure – harmful effects and warnings (*cont.*)

reduced flow of blood to the kidneys.

Warnings Metaraminol should not be used in an individual who has had a heart attack (myocardial infarction) or in pregnancy. Leakage from the site of injection may damage surrounding tissues.

methoxamine (Vasoxine)*

Harmful effects include slowing of the heart rate, headache and rise in blood pressure.

Warnings Methoxamine must not be used in someone who has had a severe coronary thrombosis. It should be used with caution in people with over-active thyroid and in pregnant women.

noradrenaline (Levophed)*

Harmful effects include slowing of heart rate, palpitations and headache.

Warnings Noradrenaline should not be used in someone who has had a heart attack (myocardial infarction) or in pregnancy. Leakage from the site of the injection may damage surrounding tissues.

phenylephrine

Harmful effects include headache, a rise in blood pressure, palpitations, rapid beating of the heart, coldness and tingling of the skin and headache. Occasionally, the heart rate may slow down.

Warnings Phenylephrine should not be used in someone who has had a heart attack (myocardial infarction) or in pregnancy. Do not use in people with over-active thyroid or severe raised blood pressure.

xamoterol (Corwin)

Harmful effects include stomach and bowel upsets, dizziness, headache and, occasionally, palpitations, chest pains, muscle cramps and skin rashes.

Warnings Xamoterol should not be used in severe heart failure or in breast-feeding mothers. It should be used with caution in patients with disorders of heart rhythm, obstructive airways disease or in pregnant women. The dose should be reduced if kidney function is impaired. In low concentrations it stimulates beta$_1$ receptors but in high concentrations it blocks beta$_1$ and beta$_2$ receptors and can be dangerous (see earlier).

* For use in sudden acute heart failure see Table 2.6, page 25

For dopexamine and milrinone, see Update.

23

Disorders of heart rhythm and rate

The heart contains two upper chambers (the atria) and two lower chambers (the ventricles). The pumping action of the upper and lower chambers are co-ordinated by electrical impulses from the pacemaker (the sinoatrial node or SA node) of the heart, which is located in the right atrium. The frequency of impulses coming from the pacemaker determines the heart rate.

Electrical impulses spread out from the pacemaker of the heart through all the muscle cells of the upper chambers (the atria) and then come together to be conducted by a special conduction centre (the atrio-ventricular node or AV node) down special pathways (the bundle of His) to the lower chambers of the heart (the ventricles). This means that contraction of the upper chambers of the heart is followed by contraction of the lower chambers in a regular manner. The rhythm of the normal heart is therefore regular and determined by the pacemaker. However, the activity of the heart is also dependent upon the nerves from the autonomic nervous system. Stimulation of parasympathetic nerves (the vagus nerve) releases acetylcholine which slows down the heart rate, and stimulation of the sympathetic nerves releases noradrenaline which makes the heart beat faster.

The electrocardiograph (ECG) is a surface recording of the electrical impulses as they pass through the heart. The ECG measures the rate, rhythm and form of the electrical impulses (the waves) and is used to diagnose damage or disease of the heart.

Abnormal rates and rhythms

If the co-ordination of electrical impulses spreading from the upper to the lower chambers breaks down, the heart may beat abnormally – which may be irregular or faster or slower than usual. The heart's rhythm can be affected by any disorder that affects its control mechanisms (see below). In addition, certain disorders (e.g. over-active thyroid gland, anxiety states) and drugs (e.g. drugs that produce an adrenaline-like action) may affect the heart rate (see later).

In certain disorders of the heart, other 'areas' in the heart may compete with the pacemaker and set off their own beats. These are usually referred to as ectopic beats, and they set in motion what are called ectopic rhythms –

rhythms not coming from the pacemaker but arising elsewhere in the heart. They may be regular or irregular, and are classified according to their site of origin in the heart. For example, ectopic beats coming from the upper chambers (the atria) are called atrial ectopic beats and those coming from the lower chambers (the ventricles) are called ventricular ectopic beats.

Changes in heart rate may come from the upper or lower chambers. Slow beating of the heart is called bradycardia and fast beating of the heart is called tachycardia. Fast beating of the heart coming from the upper chambers (the atria) is called atrial tachycardia and fast beating coming from the lower chambers is called ventricular tachycardia.

Disorders affecting the upper chambers (the atria)

Extra beats

Ectopic beats are common and usually do not imply any underlying heart disease. The individual may not notice anything or may feel pauses in the regular beating of the heart (missed beats) or extra bumps of the heart (e.g. extra beats, or extra-systoles). No specific treatment is usually needed. They are often associated with a high caffeine intake due to drinking too much tea and/or coffee. They are also associated with drinking alcohol, smoking tobacco, emotional stress, fatigue and anxiety.

Heart drugs may actually cause ectopic beats – for example, digoxin and diuretic drugs (water tablets) used to treat heart failure.

Rapid beats

Rapid beating of the heart when an individual is resting may be due to heart failure, over-active thyroid gland or fever. It comes from the pacemaker (the sinoatrial node) and is therefore called sinus tachycardia.

Drugs that produce adrenaline-like effects in the body (sympathomimetic drugs) and are used as slimming drugs, in cold and cough remedies or to treat asthma may cause rapid beating of the heart.

Some attacks of rapid beating of the heart may come on suddenly and stop suddenly. This is called paroxysmal tachycardia. It is usually not related to heart disease and is brought on by drinking too much caffeine in tea, coffee or colas, by alcohol and tobacco, by an over-active thyroid gland or by the over-use of thyroid drugs. Anxiety and stress may also cause paroxysmal tachycardia. Usually no specific treatment is needed except for pressing on one of the main arteries in the neck (the carotid arteries);

or some other which manoeuvre will slow the heart rate down and abort the attack. If, however, it persists, there are several drugs available to bring the rate under control.

Irregular beats

Sometimes an ectopic rhythm may bypass the pacemaker and make the heart beat very fast and sometimes irregularly. An example of this is the Wolff–Parkinson–White syndrome in which an abnormal short conducting pathway opens up between the upper and lower chambers of the heart. It has to be treated by giving drugs that reduce the rate of conduction of electrical impulses in the bypass and also prolong the period of time when the heart muscle cells cannot discharge (the refractory period). These drugs include amiodarone, disopyramide and quinidine.

Rapid beating of the heart may occur in patients in whom the rate of conduction of impulses from the upper to the lower chambers is slowed down or blocked (atrio-ventricular, or AV, block) by drugs. It is called paroxysmal tachycardia with heart block. This is usually caused by using digoxin with diuretic drugs to treat people suffering from heart failure. The diuretics cause a fall in blood potassium, which increases the toxic effects of digoxin on the heart. The treatment consists of stopping the digoxin and giving potassium salts.

Chaotic rhythms

In certain diseases of the heart – for example, rheumatic heart disease (especially mitral valve disease), coronary artery disease and over-active thyroid gland – the upper chambers of the heart (the atria) may race away on their own while the lower chambers (the ventricles) pick up beats at irregular intervals. This produces a chaotic heart rhythm which is not one bit regular. In fact, it is often described as being irregularly irregular. This condition is called atrial fibrillation. Treatment involves treating the underlying disorder. In mitral valve disease, digoxin is used to slow down the conduction of impulses from the rapidly beating upper chambers down into the lower chambers. In the absence of such an obvious cause, amiodarone, disopyramide and quinidine may help to control the abnormal rhythm.

Dangerous rhythms

What is called atrial flutter may occur with heart disease (coronary artery disease, raised blood pressure, mitral valve disease). The upper chambers (atria) beat so fast that the conducting pathways to the lower chambers cannot cope and only about one in two or one in four impulses gets through. It is a very unstable rhythm and digoxin is the drug of choice for treatment. Alternatives are quinidine or disopyramide.

Disorders affecting the lower chambers (the ventricles)

Extra beats

Ectopic beats coming from the lower chambers of the heart (ventricular ectopic beats) arise from an irritable focus in one of the ventricles. They are often seen in healthy people and they occur more frequently with advancing age. They may also occur in coronary artery disease and other heart diseases. In otherwise healthy people they may be triggered by fatigue, anxiety, tension, alcohol, smoking, and caffeine in tea, coffee or colas. Tricyclic anti-depressant drugs and a low blood potassium level caused by diuretic drugs may cause ectopic beats.

Any underlying cause of extra beats should be treated. The use of lignocaine to treat ventricular ectopic beats in people who have had a heart attack (myocardial infarction) has not been shown to improve survival.

In people with 'normal' hearts the best treatment is preventive before resorting to such drugs as quinidine, beta blockers, disopyramide or mexiletine. But of course some people may find it easier to take a drug than to take advice – particularly if it means stopping alcohol, stopping smoking, stopping caffeine drinks (tea, coffee and colas), learning to relax, taking more exercise and losing weight! There is little doubt which would be more beneficial.

Rapid beats

Rapid beating of the heart (tachycardia) originating in the ventricles rather than coming from the pacemaker is a very serious disorder. This *ventricular tachycardia* may be a complication of a heart attack (myocardial infarction) or some other serious disorder of the heart. It may also be produced by digoxin, tricyclic anti-depressants, drugs that produce adrenaline-like effects on the body and quinidine.

Emergencies

Ventricular tachycardia requires emergency treatment: intravenous lignocaine is the drug of choice accompanied by measures to treat any low blood potassium and magnesium levels and to reduce the acidity of the blood by giving intravenous sodium bicarbonate. Other drugs may be used (e.g. mexiletine or disopyramide). However, instead of trying this drug and that drug, it may be better to apply an electric shock to the heart, bearing in mind of course that if the ventricular tachycardia is due to digoxin toxicity, it will do no good at all. Following this emergency treatment, the patient should be given disopyramide, mexiletine or quinidine by mouth.

Ventricular fibrillation is another disorder of rhythm arising from the ventricles. It may be life threatening. In ventricular fibrillation there is a loss of organized electrical activity of the heart muscle. Each muscle fibre does its own thing, resulting in an inability of the ventricles to pump blood around the body. It is the commonest immediate cause of death in patients who have had a heart attack (myocardial infarction). The application of a direct electric shock to the heart using a defibrillator can be life saving. Everything must be done to maintain the circulation, and in addition the increased acidity of the blood should be treated with intravenous sodium bicarbonate.

If the ventricles of the heart stop beating (ventricular asystole), sudden death will occur unless the ventricles are stimulated to start beating again by cardiac massage or by a sudden blow to the chest. It may be due to a local fault in the conduction of impulses through the ventricles and a sudden blow on the chest may just correct this. However, it may be due to extensive damage to the ventricles caused by a coronary thrombosis, in which case very little can be done.

Cardiac arrest

Cardiac arrest is the sudden and complete loss of function of the heart. It is a much over-used term and these days you are often not allowed to die in hospital without being diagnosed as having a 'cardiac arrest' and being subjected to all manner of heroic and useless interventions. In one sense, everybody who dies has a cardiac arrest – in other words the heart stops beating. The label 'cardiac arrest' should be reserved for special situations where immediate resuscitation could save a person's life (e.g. following drowning, electrocution or some other accident) or following a sudden heart attack (e.g. coronary thrombosis). Such resuscitation must be carried out immediately because the brain will undergo irreversible damage if it is without oxygen for more than 2–3 minutes. However, an inevitable consequence of this advice is that many patients who do not require cardiac massage and mouth-to-mouth breathing (or mechanical respiration using a ventilating machine) will receive it, and some patients who have undergone irreversible brain damage will survive because of the resuscitation.

Diagnosing disorders of heart rhythm and rate

The onset of a disordered rhythm (arrhythmia) may be without any symptoms and can be diagnosed only by an electrocardiograph (ECG) tracing. On the other hand, some people may complain of palpitations and they may feel dizzy, faint and develop a pain in their chest with breathlessness. It is obvious therefore that the only way to diagnose a disorder of rhythm is by an ECG. This is why patients in coronary care units have the electrical activity of their hearts monitored continuously – so that an early diagnosis can be made and appropriate treatment given. In patients up and about and who have intermittent symptoms it may be necessary to use a mobile monitoring device that is strapped on for 24 hours and transfers the electric impulses onto a tape. The messages on the tape are then transcribed into an ECG back at the hospital.

A specialized technique involves inserting electrodes up the veins in the arms or legs, into the heart. These monitor the electrical activity of the heart and apply an electric stimulus when necessary. However, this system may actually cause ventricular fibrillation in some patients.

From this brief overview of the types of disordered heart rhythms and rates it is possible to identify some major causes.

- A defective supply of blood to the heart (ischaemic heart disease), caused by disease of the coronary arteries
- Congenital abnormalities of the heart's conducting pathways
- Acquired abnormalities of the heart – e.g. mitral valve disease caused by rheumatic fever
- Over-use of diuretic drugs (water tablets), causing a fall in the blood potassium levels
- Disturbance in the chemistry of the blood – e.g. increased acidity, low oxygen

Treatment of disorders of heart rhythm

In people who develop a disordered rhythm of their heart (cardiac arrhythmia) the decision to treat, the urgency of such treatment and the type of treatment given will depend upon the type of dysrhythmia and the general condition of the individual.

Non-drug treatments

These include the following:

Direct current electrical shock to the heart (direct current cardioversion) using what is called a defibrillator or DC shock. This is effective in about nine out of ten patients. The electric current stops the heart for a second or two, and when it starts to beat again the rhythm reverts to normal in most cases. For arrhythmias that are not urgent the patient is given an anaesthetic and the shock is timed to be synchronous with the appropriate point on the electrocardiogram.

Digoxin increases the risk of other arrhythmias after shock treatment; therefore it should preferably be stopped 36 hours before the shock is due. Procainamide may be tried immediately before the shock and lignocaine and phenytoin should be available in case an ectopic rhythm starts in the ventricles.

In people who have had atrial fibrillation and flutter for a long time, the conversion to a normal rhythm by shock treatment may loosen a clot from the inside of the upper heart chambers which may then shoot off and wedge somewhere, producing serious problems (e.g. in the lungs). These individuals should be given anti-blood-clotting drugs (anti-coagulants) for 3 weeks before the shock.

Artificial pacemakers are available which can control the upper chambers (the atria), the lower chambers (the ventricles) or both. They can be used to control slow and fast heart rates. Implantable automatic defibrillators have shown some success in people prone to develop severe attacks of ventricular fibrillation or tachycardia.

Drug treatment

The use of drugs to treat disorders of rhythm requires knowledge of the individual and the type of arrhythmia from which that person is suffering. It is important that the whole patient is treated and not just the electric tracing of the heart (ECG). Any underlying disorder should be treated: for example, a low blood potassium level or over-active thyroid gland. Depending on the disorder of heart rhythm, all that may be needed is sound advice on stopping smoking and reducing the amount of alcohol, tea and coffee that is drunk each day. Alternatively, in serious cases, non-drug treatments such as DC shock (DC cardioversion) or a pacemaker may be necessary.

There are several groups of drugs available to treat arrhythmias and attempts have been made to classify them according to their main actions and effects on the heart. However, in practice, doctors tend to use them according to their own experience and observations (i.e. empirically). Nevertheless, the increasing number of drugs available to treat arrhythmias means that there should be some sort of classification in the hope of providing guidelines on their use.

Most anti-arrhythmic drugs depress the function of the heart and must be used with caution in anyone with heart failure or conduction defects. Such drugs may increase the disordered rhythm and they may produce harmful effects on other organs and tissues.

Balancing the benefits and risks

In addition to knowledge of the individual and the disorder, it is important that the doctor has knowledge of the actions and effects of anti-arrhythmic drugs, knowledge of how to achieve adequate concentrations of the drug at the target site (the heart) and knowledge of their harmful effects. With this knowledge the doctor should be able to balance the benefits to risks of a particular drug treatment in a particular patient. This is important because most of the currently available anti-arrhythmic drugs may actually predispose patients to the risks of a disordered rhythm if used inappropriately.

Treatment should be tailored to the individual's needs

To be effective at the target site (the heart) these drugs have to reach a certain level of concentration in the blood, and there is often a narrow margin between the blood concentration required to correct the arrhythmia and the concentration that will produce harmful effects. Guidelines are available and the monitoring of blood levels of these drugs should be carried out on patients receiving treatment. Nevertheless, it is important to remember that different people react differently to any given drug or doses of a drug. By this I mean that all treatments should be tailored to the individual's needs – they should be individualized and not standardized.

To use blood level monitoring measures effectively it is important to know how the drugs are absorbed from the intestine, distributed around the body, broken down in the liver and excreted by the kidneys. For example any impairment of liver function may affect the breakdown of drugs, and any impairment of kidney function may affect the excretion of a drug. These impairments may cause the concentration of the drug in the blood to rise to toxic levels unless a reduced dose is given. This applies particularly to elderly people, in whom liver and/or kidney function may be decreased. In addition, the elderly develop more disorders of the heart and circulation than do younger people, which may affect the distribution of the drug around the body and also alter the sensitivity of the heart to drugs. A low blood potassium puts patients at particular risk.

Because different people react differently to drugs it is sometimes necessary to 'test' the effects of a drug by monitoring the electrical activities of the heart (e.g. ECG). This is called 'directed' treatment and may be useful in someone with recurrent attacks of ventricular disorders of rhythm. This seems a very sensible approach, rather than waiting to treat the next attack which may cause death.

Dangers when given with other drugs

With drugs used to treat disorders of rhythm (arrhythmias) there is usually a narrow margin between the dose required to produce beneficial effects and the dose that will produce harmful effects. There is also a risk that one drug can react harmfully with another (drug interactions), and a large number of such interactions have been reported. Any interaction that results in an increase in the blood level of an anti-arrhythmic drug will increase its toxic effects, and any interaction that reduces its blood level will decrease its effectiveness. The risks of such interactions are real ones because people who develop an arrhythmia often require treatment for some other disorder, such as diabetes, raised blood pressure or disorders of the heart and circulation.

Many drug interactions offer no real danger, but some do and it is important to be aware of these because there is a tendency to use more than one anti-arrhythmia drug at a time (see Chapter 89).

Classification

Drugs used to treat disorders of heart rhythm show a wide variation in their chemical structures, their sites of actions in the body and their uses. In addition, some drugs have more than one action. They are often grouped into four classes, but on the whole this does not help all that much.

Class I contains those drugs that possess local anaesthetic properties and which affect the surfaces of the cells (membrane-stabilizing properties) in the conducting system, causing a reduction in the excitability of the heart muscle and the 'triggering' of spontaneous beats. Drugs in this group include disopyramide, flecainide, lignocaine, mexiletine, phenytoin, procainamide, propafenone, quinidine and tocainide.

Class II drugs reduce the potential for disordered rhythm which occurs in response to stimulation of the heart by adrenaline-like chemicals. These include the beta blockers, which block the effect of these chemicals, and bretylium, which blocks the release of adrenaline-like substances.

Class III drugs prolong the resting phase of the heart. These include amiodarone and disopyramide.

Class IV drugs are calcium channel blockers. They depress the passage of impulses through the conducting system of the heart, particularly the atrio-ventricular (AV) node which transfers impulses from the upper chambers to lower chambers (see earlier).

Digoxin does not come in any of the above groups but it is the drug of choice for treating attacks of atrial fibrillation and atrial flutter. However, in the long-term treatment of atrial fibrillation it is now being replaced by such drugs as verapamil or disopyramide.

Atropine may be used to treat slow heart rate (bradycardia) after a heart attack or when caused by beta blockers.

Table 23.1 Drugs used to treat disorders of heart rhythm and rate: anti-arrhythmics – harmful effects and warnings

amiodarone (Cordarone X)
Used to treat Wolff–Parkinson–White syndrome and as a second choice drug when other drugs cannot be used.

Harmful effects The following harmful effects are rare but should be borne in mind when used for prolonged treatment with high doses (the level of the drug in the blood should be carefully monitored): deposits in the cornea of the eyes and nerve damage producing numbness and pins and needles in the hands and feet, sensitivity of the skin to sunlight, a slate-grey discoloration of the skin, disorders of thyroid function, inflammation of the lungs, liver damage, nausea, vomiting, metallic taste in the mouth, tremor, nightmares, dizziness, headaches, sleeplessness and inflammation of part of the testicles with high doses (epididymitis).

Warnings Amiodarone should not be used in anyone with a slow pulse rate or certain types of heart block, or in individuals who are allergic to iodine or who have thyroid disorders. It interferes with tests of thyroid function. Tests of liver function and thyroid function should be carried out before and at regular intervals during treatment.

Risks in elderly people Harmful effects may be more frequent and severe; therefore use with caution.

bretylium (Bretylate)
Used as a second choice to treat disorders of ventricular rhythm.

Harmful effects include nausea, vomiting and low blood pressure, particularly on standing up after sitting or lying; this may cause dizziness, light-headedness, vertigo and faintness.

Warnings Anyone taking bretylium should not be given noradrenaline or other sympathomimetic drugs nor digoxin or a related drug. Patients should be kept lying down until they become tolerant to the blood pressure lowering effects; this may take several days.

Risks in elderly people Harmful effects may be more frequent and severe; therefore use with caution.

disopyramide (Dirythmin SA, Rythmodan, Rythmodan Retard)
Used to treat disorders of rhythm affecting the ventricles, especially after a heart attack (myocardial infarction) and to treat disorders of rhythm and rate coming from above the ventricles.

Harmful effects include dry mouth, blurred vision, difficulty with passing urine, low pulse rate, low blood pressure and, rarely, heart block.

Warnings Disopyramide should be used with caution in individuals with glaucoma, heart failure, enlarged prostate

Table 23.1 Drugs used to treat disorders of heart rhythm and rate: anti-arrhythmics – harmful effects and warnings (*cont.*)

gland, myasthenia gravis or digoxin intoxication. It may be ineffective if the blood potassium is very low. Anyone with impaired kidney function should be given a reduced dose.

Risks in elderly people Harmful effects may be more frequent and severe in the elderly; therefore kidney function should be checked, and the dosage reduced if necessary. Elderly people may develop difficulty passing water and opening their bowels.

flecainide (Tambocor)
Used to treat disorders of rhythm affecting the ventricles and the heart above the ventricles.

Harmful effects include dizziness and light-headedness; occasionally there are visual disturbances (e.g. double vision, blurred vision), nausea and vomiting and, very rarely, jaundice.

Warnings Flecainide should not be used in people with heart failure, chronic coronary heart disease or heart block, and used with caution in anyone with pacemakers. Individuals with impaired kidney function should be given reduced doses. Any disturbance of chemicals (electrolytes) in the blood should be corrected before treatment.

Risks in elderly people Harmful effects may be more frequent and severe; therefore use with caution.

lignocaine (Xylocard)
Used to treat disorders of rhythm affecting the ventricles, especially after a heart attack (myocardial infarction).

Harmful effects Transient dizziness, pins and needles in the hands and feet, and drowsiness may occur when injections are given too rapidly. Other occasional harmful effects include confusion, convulsions, noises in the ears (tinnitus), disorientation, blurred vision, tremor, depressed breathing, low blood pressure and slow heart rate (may rarely cause the heart to stop).

Warnings Lignocaine should not be used in people who are allergic to it or who have heart block or heart failure not due to a disorder of rhythm. The dose should be reduced in heart failure, in liver failure and following heart surgery.

Risks in elderly people Harmful effects may be more frequent and severe in the elderly, particularly if they have heart failure which may reduce the excretion of the drug from the kidneys. The dose should be reduced.

mexiletine (Mexitil, Mexitil Perlongets)
Used to treat disorders of rhythm affecting the ventricles, especially after a heart attack (myocardial infarction).

Harmful effects are mainly related to the concentration in the blood and may be reduced by reducing the speed of injection or by delaying the next dose by mouth and by reducing the dose. These dose-related harmful effects include nausea, vomiting, indigestion, unpleasant taste, hiccoughs, light-headedness and drowsiness, and, rarely, confusion, dizziness, blurred vision, double vision, flickering of the eyes (nystagmus), difficulty with speech, incoordination of movements, tremor, numbness and pins and needles in the arms and legs, convulsions, mental symptoms, low blood pressure, slow pulse rate and palpitations. Very rarely, skin rashes, jaundice and blood disorders may occur.

Warnings Mexiletine should not be used in anyone with a slow heart rate or heart block. Very careful monitoring is needed in anyone who suffers from conduction defects of the heart, mild to moderate slowing of the heart rate, or kidney or liver failure. It may increase the tremor of parkinsonism. Checks of kidney and liver function should be carried out at regular intervals during treatment.

Risks in elderly people There are no specific reports on harmful effects in elderly people; nevertheless, use with caution.

Table 23.1 Drugs used to treat disorders of heart rhythm and rate: anti-arrhythmics – harmful effects and warnings (*cont.*)

phenytoin sodium (Epanutin Parenteral)
Used to treat disorders of rhythm affecting the ventricles or above the ventricles, especially those caused by over-dosage with digoxin and related drugs.

Harmful effects include slow heart rate, low blood pressure, confusion. It may stop the heart beating (asystole).

Warnings Phenytoin sodium should not be used in anyone suffering from heart block. It must not be given with lignocaine, nor to treat rapid heart beat caused by digoxin overdose.

procainamide (Procainamide Durules, Pronestyl)
Used to treat disorders of rhythm affecting the ventricles, especially after a heart attack (myocardial infarction), and to treat disorders of rhythm from above the ventricles.

Harmful effects The following harmful effects are rare but should be borne in mind particularly in relation to people on prolonged treatment with high doses (the level of the drug in the blood should be carefully monitored): loss of appetite, nausea, vomiting, diarrhoea, flushing, allergic reactions, skin rashes, itching, depression, vertigo, serious mental symptoms with hallucinations, shivering, fever, joint pains, muscle pains, bitter taste in the mouth, muscle weakness, a lupus erythematosus-like syndrome and blood disorders.

Warnings Procainamide should not be used in people who are allergic to it or in anyone suffering from heart block, heart failure or low blood pressure. It should be used with utmost caution in individuals with asthma, myasthenia gravis or kidney failure. Accumulation of the drug in the body causes liver and kidney damage.

Risks in elderly people Harmful effects may be more frequent; therefore use with caution.

propafenone (Arythmol)
Used to treat disorders of rhythm affecting the ventricles.

Harmful effects include dizziness, headache, fatigue, nausea, vomiting, bitter taste in the mouth, constipation and diarrhoea; occasionally it may cause allergic skin rashes, slowness of heart rate and heart block.

Warnings Propafenone should not be used in anyone with uncontrolled congestive heart failure, severe slowing of the heart rate, certain types of heart block, severe chronic obstructive disease of the bronchi or disturbed blood sodium and potassium levels. It should be used with caution in people with impaired kidney or liver function or heart failure.

Risks in elderly people Use with caution in elderly people with a pacemaker.

quinidine (Kiditard, Kinidin Durules)
Used to prevent disorders of rhythm affecting the ventricles and rapid heart beat coming from above the ventricles (supraventricular tachycardia).

Harmful effects Common harmful effects which are dose-related include nausea, vomiting and diarrhoea. Allergic reactions to quinidine may occasionally occur; they include nettle rash, purpura, asthma, reduced platelet count and haemolytic anaemia. It may cause disorders of heart rhythm and, very rarely, liver damage. Overdosing may cause cinchonism – blurred vision, dizziness, flushing, fever, confusion, vertigo, abdominal pain, headache, ringing and buzzing in the ears (tinnitus).

Warnings Quinidine should not be used in anyone with heart block or who has an acute infection. People who are allergic to it should not take quinidine (they can be tested for allergy using a 200 mg dose by mouth). It should be used with caution in people with partial heart block, heart failure, digoxin overdose, heart wall damage, myasthenia gravis or impaired kidney function.

Risks in elderly people Harmful effects may be more frequent and severe; therefore use with caution.

Table 23.1 Drugs used to treat disorders of heart rhythm and rate: anti-arrhythmics – harmful effects and warnings (*cont.*)

tocainide (Tonocard)
Used to treat disorders of rhythm affecting the ventricles.

Harmful effects are usually mild and transient; they include tremor, dizziness, light-headedness, numbness and pins and needles in the arms and legs, visual hallucinations, mental disorders, convulsions, nausa, vomiting, skin rashes and fever. Intravenous injection may cause slow heart rate, low blood pressure, and very rarely, blood disorders, scarring of the lungs and a lupus erythematosus-like syndrome, have been reported.

Warnings It should not be used in anyone who suffers from heart block, or who is allergic to procainamide or related amide drugs. It should be used with caution in people with severe liver or kidney impairment, or heart failure. Weekly blood counts should be carried out for the first 12 weeks and then every month. Tests of liver and kidney function should be carried out before treatment starts and the dose adjusted accordingly.

Risks in elderly people Harmful effects may be more frequent and severe; therefore use with caution.

Table 23.2 Preparations used to treat disorders of heart rhythm and rate

Preparation	*Drug*	*Drug group*	*Dosage form*
Angilol	propranolol	Non-selective beta blocker	Tablets
Apsolol	propranolol	Non-selective beta blocker	Tablets
Apsolox	oxprenolol	Non-selective beta blocker	Tablets
Arythmol	propafenone	Class I anti-arrhythmic	Tablets
atropine	atropine	Anticholinergic	Injection
Berkatens	verapamil	Calcium channel blocker	Tablets
Berkolol	propranolol	Non-selective beta blocker	Tablets
Beta-Cardone	sotalol	Non-selective beta blocker	Tablets
Betaloc	metoprolol	Selective beta blocker	Tablets, injection
Bretylate	bretylium	Class II anti-arrhythmic	Injection
Cordarone X	amiodarone	Class III anti-arrhythmic	Tablets
Cordilox	verapamil	Calcium channel blocker	Tablets; injection (Cordilox IV)
Corgard	nadolol	Non-selective beta blocker	Tablets
digitoxin	digitoxin	Cardiac glycoside	Tablets
digoxin	digoxin	Cardiac glycoside	Tablets, paediatric injection

Table 23.2 Preparations used to treat disorders of heart rhythm and rate (*cont.*)

Preparation	*Drug*	*Drug group*	*Dosage form*
Dirythmin SA	disopyramide	Class I anti-arrhythmic	Sustained-release tablets
disopyramide	disopyramide	Class I anti-arrhythmic	Capsules
Epanutin Parenteral	phenytoin sodium	Class I anti-arrhythmic	Injection
Inderal	propranolol	Non-selective beta blocker	Tablets, injection
Kiditard	quinidine	Class I anti-arrhythmic	Sustained-release capsules
Kinidin Durules	quinidine	Class I anti-arrhythmic	Sustained-release tablets
Lanoxin	digoxin	Cardiac glycoside	Tablets, injection
Lanoxin-PG	digoxin	Cardiac glycoside	Tablets, elixir
lignocaine	lignocaine	Class I anti-arrhythmic	Injection
Lopresor	metoprolol	Selective beta blocker	Tablets
Mexitil	mexiletine	Class I anti-arrhythmic	Capsules, injection
Mexitil Perlongets	mexiletine	Class I anti-arrhythmic	Sustained-release capsules
oxprenolol	oxprenolol	Non-selective beta blocker	Tablets
Procainamide Durules	procainamide	Class I anti-arrhythmic	Sustained-release tablets
Pronestyl	procainamide	Class I anti-arrhythmic	Tablets, injection
propranolol	propranolol	Non-selective beta blocker	Tablets
quinidine sulphate	quinidine	Class I anti-arrhythmic	Tablets
Rythmodan	disopyramide	Class I anti-arrhythmic	Capsules, injection
Rythmodan Retard	disopyramide	Class I anti-arrhythmic	Sustained-release tablets
Sectral	acebutolol	Selective beta blocker	Capsules
Securon	verapamil	Calcium channel blocker	Tablets; injection (Securon IV)
Sotacor	sotalol	Non-selective beta blocker	Tablets, injection
Tambocor	flecainide	Class I anti-arrhythmic	Tablets, injection

Table 23.2 Preparations used to treat disorders of heart rhythm and rate (*cont.*)

Preparation	*Drug*	*Drug group*	*Dosage form*
Tenormin	atenolol	Selective beta blocker	Tablets, sugar-free syrup, injection
Tonocard	tocainide	Class I anti-arrhythmic	Tablets, injection
Trasicor	oxprenolol	Non-selective beta blocker	Tablets
verapamil	verapamil	Calcium channel blocker	Tablets
Xylocard	lignocaine	Class I anti-arrhythmic	Injection, intravenous infusion

24

Disorders of the circulation

Regulation of the circulation

Regulation of the circulatory system ensures that the entire body is provided with enough blood not only when you are resting but also when you are exercising. This requires at all times a minimum supply of blood to all organs and tissues, and on exercise a redistribution of the blood to active organs (e.g. the muscles) at the expense of other organs that are resting (e.g. the intestine). This redistribution of blood on exercise is essential because the heart could not cope with having to supply a maximum amount of blood to all organs and tissues at all times.

Regulation of the blood flow to the various organs and tissues in the body is achieved principally by alterations in the diameter (calibre) of the blood vessels. At rest, the muscles in the walls of arteries are in a state of tension: they are partially contracted, causing some reduction in the diameter of the blood vessel. If the nerves to these muscles are cut the arteries partially dilate and their diameter increases. This local control (or auto-regulation) helps to keep the blood flow to the organ constant in the face of changes in blood pressure. It also helps to control the blood flow in response to local chemical changes, which are also independent of the blood presure. This local control or autoregulation responds, for example, to changes in oxygen supply, carbon dioxide levels in the blood and to chemicals released locally in response to injury or allergy. Arteries supplying the heart (coronary arteries) and the brain (cerebral arteries) are almost totally under the control of local changes in oxygen supply, carbon dioxide levels and changes in acidity of the blood.

Nervous control of arteries, principally the smaller arteries (arterioles), is by the sympathetic nervous system which uses noradrenaline as a chemical messenger. There are two main groups of receptors in the body which are stimulated by noradrenaline; they are called *alpha receptors* and *beta receptors* because their locations are different and because their stimulation produces different effects. Noradrenaline stimulation of alpha receptors in arteries produces constriction (reduction in diameter) and stimulation of beta receptors produces dilatation (an increase in diameter).

Alpha receptors are predominant in arteries in the kidneys and skin, so noradrenaline stimulation will produce constriction of the arteries in these organs (you go pale when you are scared). In the arteries in muscles (the skeletal or voluntary muscles) there are more beta receptors than alpha receptors. Noradrenaline stimulation of beta receptors in muscles causes the arteries to dilate so that the blood supply is increased (this gets your muscles ready for what is called 'fight or flight'). In this state of readiness for 'fight or flight' the adrenal glands also pump out adrenaline into the bloodstream and the receptors in the arteries in muscles respond more to this circulating adrenaline than to the direct nervous stimulation from noradrenaline.

There are about equal numbers of alpha and beta receptors in the blood vessels of the stomach and intestine and in the coronary arteries supplying the heart.

Centres in the brain co-ordinate responses both locally and generally so that, for example, if a group of muscles is activated (e.g. you start to run) the centres in the brain will activate the sympathetic nervous system and stimulate the heart to beat faster and dilate the arteries in the muscles, etc. However, local needs (e.g. oxygen deficiency) will produce 'instant' dilatation of arteries because such a deficiency will always take priority over noradrenaline stimulation via the sympathetic nerves.

Because the skin is concerned with maintaining the body temperature, the blood supply to the skin is largely under the control of centres in the brain. Nevertheless the blood supply to the skin is sensitive to adrenaline stimulation; 'lie detectors' rely on changes in blood flow and skin temperature in the fingers.

Drugs used to treat disorders of the circulation

Drugs that improve the circulation act by blocking the stimulation of alpha receptors, by stimulating beta receptors and/or by acting directly on the muscle walls of arteries. The net result is that they increase the diameter of the arteries (vasodilatation) and therefore increase their calibre.

Drugs used to improve the blood supply principally to the arms and legs

Alpha blockers

Alpha blockers (e.g. prazosin, thymoxamine) block the noradrenaline receptors in those arteries that constrict in response to noradrenaline stimulation. They therefore dilate. However, this interferes with the normal regulation of the circulation and may cause a fall in blood pressure on standing up from sitting or lying down (postural hypotension) and reflex rapid beating of the heart.

Nicotinic acid and derivatives

Nicotinic acid (a member of the B group of vitamins) and its derivatives produce vasodilatation by a direct action on the arteries. They cause a marked flushing in the blush areas (face and neck) but their vasodilator effect is less in the arms and legs. Nicotinic acid derivatives such as nicofuranose, inositol nicotinate and nicotinyl alcohol produce fewer harmful effects than nicotinic acid.

Calcium channel blockers

The calcium channel blockers nifedipine and nimodipine reduce contraction of the muscular walls of arteries by blocking the calcium channels. This causes the muscles to relax and the vessels to dilate. Nifedipine produces beneficial effects on the circulation to the arms and legs and it is used to treat Raynaud's phenomenon (see later). Nimodipine produces its main effects on the circulation to the brain and it is used to relieve the spasm of arteries supplying the brain, which may occur reflexly following a haemorrhage into the lining of the brain (subarachnoid haemorrhage).

Cinnarizine

This antihistamine drug also produces some calcium channel blocking effect, causing dilatation of the arteries. It may be beneficial in some patients suffering from disorders of the circulation to the arms and legs.

Other drugs

The following drugs may improve the circulation to the arms and legs and the brain in some people.

Naftidrofuryl improves the use of oxygen and glucose by cells and reduces the production of harmful chemicals (e.g. lactic acid) which may be produced by cells when their blood supply is reduced (ischaemia). It also dilates arteries. It is referred to as a *cell activator*.

Cyclandelate maintains the pliability of the walls of red blood cells and stops platelets sticking together; these effects may help to maintain the flow of blood in narrowed arteries. It also has a direct effect on reducing spasm of small arteries. It is called a *calcium overload regulator* because of its effect on the use of calcium by cells.

Oxpentifylline produces dilatation of arteries, probably by a direct action on the muscles of the arteries.

The benefits of using drugs to treat circulatory disorders of the arms and legs

Most serious disorders of the circulation affecting the arms and legs are due to a blockage or spasm of the arteries that supply the arms and legs. Drugs that dilate arteries may improve the blood supply at rest, but there is no evidence from adequate and well controlled studies of their benefits on exercise (e.g. when walking). Furthermore, they are rarely of benefit in relieving pains that come on at rest.

The use of *alpha blockers* (e.g. prazosin and thymoxamine) to treat circulatory disorders to the skin and muscles is disappointing except in disorders that are reversible and are caused by spasm of arteries (see Raynaud's disease, later). Exercise is the best treatment for improving the circulation to muscles.

Alpha blockers should not be used in serious arterial disease of the arms and legs because these drugs may have more effect in dilating less affected arteries than severely affected ones and therefore they may 'steal' blood away from the worse affected sites to less affected sites.

Nicotinic acid and its derivatives produce more dilatation of the arteries in the face and neck (blush area) than in the arms and legs. They have not been shown to produce a consistent increase in blood flow to the skin and muscles of the arms and legs. They may affect the blood clotting system, reduce the stickiness of blood and affect blood fat levels.

The *calcium channel blocker* nifedipine is a useful drug for treating arterial spasm in Raynaud's disease (see later).

With *other drugs* used to treat disorders of the circulation (see earlier) there is some controversy about whether they produce much benefit over and above that provided by the body's own circulatory regulation system.

NOTE The best treatment for people who smoke is to stop smoking.

Atherosclerosis

Atherosclerosis is a degenerative disorder of arteries which involves patchy deposits of fat in the walls of large and medium-sized arteries. Most commonly affected are the main artery from the heart (the aorta), the main arteries that supply the legs and the arteries that supply the heart (coronary arteries) and the brain (cerebral arteries).

These fatty deposits develop over decades, probably from childhood. Eventually they scar and ulcerate. This may cause a clot (thrombus) to develop at the site. The clot obstructs the flow of blood in the artery, which causes a defective blood supply to the limb (ischaemia). This causes the area affected (e.g. the foot) to go cold, blue and swollen. Atherosclerosis and its treatment are discussed in detail in Chapter 25.

Atherosclerosis obliterans

A severe form of atherosclerosis – atherosclerosis obliterans – may affect the main blood vessels that supply the limbs, usually the legs. It affects males more than females and usually occurs after the age of 50 years and is more common in diabetic patients and smokers. It produces coldness of the feet and legs, and pains in the legs on exercise (intermittent claudication). The blood supply to the feet becomes severely limited, and ulceration and gangrene (death of the tissues) may develop.

Drugs that improve the circulation should not be used to treat people suffering from atherosclerosis obliterans because they may divert blood away from the affected site and make it worse. The long-term use of anti-coagulant drugs is of very questionable value, and drugs that dissolve clots (thrombi) (see Chapter 26) appear to help only a few people in whom the disease is of recent onset. Surgery to remove a block in an artery may be necessary. Cutting the nerves supplying the blood vessels may be considered in cases with severe complications; this will remove the natural tendency of the blood vessels to constrict and cause them to dilate.

Smokers should stop smoking, the overweight should lose weight and diabetes, if present, should be treated. Cold should be avoided, the skin should be protected against injury and any skin infection should be treated immediately. Regular exercise should be encouraged.

Buerger's disease (thromboangiitis obliterans)

This is a disease that causes obstruction to the flow of blood in arteries and veins. It is caused by inflammation of the walls of medium- and small-sized arteries and veins in the legs and arms. The cause is unknown but there is a very strong association with tobacco smoking, particular of cigarettes. It mainly affects young males between the ages of 20 and 40 years, and there is a high incidence of the disorder in Israel, the Orient and the Indies compared with the USA and western Europe.

The lining of the arteries and veins is damaged by inflammation, and clots (thrombi) develop at the sites of damage. The vessels of the legs are most commonly affected, and the reduced blood supply leads to pain, coldness, ulceration and gangrene of the toes. A high proportion of sufferers have to undergo amputation of their toes or feet.

Treatment

Treatment involves stopping smoking and general protective care of the legs and feet. If some of the arteries are in spasm, cutting the sympathetic nerves to the affected leg may cause the affected arteries to dilate and this may help. Drugs are of little use except to relieve any transient spasm in some of the arteries.

Raynaud's disease

Raynaud's disease is an intermittent paleness and blueness of the fingers and toes brought on by a degree of coldness that would not affect a normal person. It is caused by spasm of the arteries supplying the fingers and toes, and is also brought on by emotion. It occurs nine times more commonly in women than in men and affects the fingers more commonly than the toes. On exposure to cold the fingers may go cold, pale and blue, feel numb, tingle and burn. There may be pain as well as numbness and not every change occurs each time. On re-warming, the fingers go very red. These reactions are referred to as *Raynaud's phenomenon* (see later).

The cause of Raynaud's disease is not known. The coldness and paleness are due to the small arteries closing off (vasoconstriction), the blueness is due to lack of oxygen in the blood because of the poor circulation, and the redness on warming up is due to dilatation of the arteries. Severe Raynaud's disease may result in damage to the skin of the fingers, and ulcerations.

Raynaud's syndrome

The symptoms and signs of Raynaud's disease may also develop secondarily to some other disorder, and are usually then referred to as Raynaud's syndrome or as secondary Raynaud's disease. It may occur in arterial diseases of the limbs, in diseases such as rheumatoid arthritis and scleroderma, due to repetitive damage to the hands (e.g. in pneumatic drill operators) and in disorders of the nerves supplying the arms and hands. It may occur in certain blood clotting disorders, and may be caused by overuse of ergot drugs taken to treat migraine (ergotamine and methysergide) and by exposure to chemicals such as polyvinyl chloride. Beta blocker drugs (particularly propranolol) may produce cold fingers and toes, and, in some people, may occasionally give rise to the syndrome.

Raynaud's phenomenon

The symptoms and signs described under Raynaud's disease and which also occur in secondary Raynaud's disease (or Raynaud's syndrome) are referred to as Raynaud's phenomenon.

Non-drug treatment of Raynaud's phenomenon

Protective measures, such as warm clothing to all the body as well as to the hands and feet, are most important. This is necessary because exposure to cold on other parts of the body (e.g. the face) can produce a reflex narrowing of the arteries supplying the hands and feet.

Sufferers should wear thermal underwear, fur-lined boots and hats, and use electrically heated gloves and socks. Smokers should stop smoking because smoking causes constriction of the arteries to the skin. Biofeedback techniques may help some people to increase the blood supply to the fingers and toes, and whirling the arms round and round at about 80 circles per minute for 10 minutes may help to abort an attack. Some individuals find that certain foods may bring on an attack (e.g. dairy produce), so it makes sense to keep a careful note of your diet and its relationship to attacks.

NOTE Although cold weather is the main trigger factor, an attack can come on with any sudden change in temperature, even in summer! The treatment of Raynaud's syndrome is to treat or prevent the underlying disorder and to treat the phenomenon as necessary (see below).

Drug treatment

People with mild to moderate Raynaud's disease whose skin is not damaged should not be treated with drugs to improve the circulation. They should take protective measures, as described above.

In severe cases of Raynaud's disease, drug treatment may be necessary, in addition to protective measures, particularly in those individuals who have developed damage to the skin of their fingers or toes. The aim of drug treatment is to dilate the arteries and to increase the resting blood supply to the fingers and toes so that there is less reduction of the blood supply on exposure to the cold – this may reduce the severity and duration of an attack.

Drugs that dilate arteries

No drug works specifically on the arteries in the hands or feet – they affect all arteries throughout the body and may affect the heart rate and blood pressure. Therefore any treatment is always a balance between local benefits to the hands and feet and risks to the heart and circulation in general.

Nitrate vasodilators

Glyceryl trinitrate ointment applied locally dilates the arteries but its effects are so short-lived that it is of little benefit.

Calcium channel blockers

The calcium channel blocker nifedipine is fashionable at the moment. It appears to reduce the frequency and severity of attacks in some people.

ACE inhibitors

The ACE inhibitor captopril is under investigation and appears to reduce the frequency and severity of attacks in some people.

Other drugs aimed at improving the circulation have been tried but without much success. They include the drugs discussed earlier under disorders of the circulation to the limbs. There is no convincing evidence from adequate and well controlled studies that high doses of various vitamins, fish oils or evening primrose oil are beneficial.

Prostaglandins

Prostaglandins produce four effects that may be beneficial to patients suffering from Raynaud's disease – they dilate arteries; stop platelets clumping together; affect the surface of red blood cells, making them more flexible so that they can pass through narrowed vessels; and make the blood less viscous (sticky). Unfortunately, at present they have to be given by intravenous injection and they may produce severe dilatation of arteries, causing flushing, a drop in blood pressure and faintness.

Drugs that affect the stickiness of the blood

Stanozolol is an anabolic steroid that breaks down thrombi and may help in severe cases of Raynaud's disease, where thrombi have developed in small blood vessels because of the poor circulation. It may help to improve circulation and heal ulcers in some men and post-menopausal women with normal liver function. It should not be used by women of child-bearing age.

Drugs that stop platelets clumping together are also under investigation; they include dazoxiben, which blocks an enzyme that makes platelets sticky. The drug ketanserin blocks the constriction of arteries produced by the neuro-transmitter 5-hydroxytryptamine (serotonin) and is also under investigation.

Thyroid drugs

A thyroid drug, tri-iodothyronine has been used to increase the body's burning up of energy. The 'heat' of the body is increased, which causes the arteries in the skin to dilate in order to regulate the temperature. This helps to improve the blood supply to the hands and feet, but it is like taking a sledge-hammer to crack a nut.

Local applications

Apart from the transient effect produced by glyceryl trinitrate there is no local application that is of benefit.

Drugs of choice

Nifedipine is the first drug of choice at the present time. However, drugs do not cure the disorder and their benefits must always be balanced against their risks. There is no doubt that preventive measures (as discussed earlier) should be the priority.

Acrocyanosis

This is a rare disorder which produces a persistent blueness and coldness of the hands and, less often, the feet. Its cause is unknown, and it is more common in men than in women. It usually starts in young adulthood or early middle age. No drug treatment is necessary. Protection from the cold is the best treatment.

Livedo reticularis

This is a lacy blue discoloration of the skin, of unknown cause, that occurs in young adults. Apart from stopping smoking (which constricts blood vessels in the skin) and ensuring protection from the cold, no treatment is necessary.

Erythromelalgia

This is a disorder of the circulation which produces episodes of painful hot redness of the skin of the feet and, less often, the hands. The disease may occur at any age. Treatment involves the avoidance of heat. In an attack the feet should be raised and cooled. Aspirin by mouth may relieve an attack. Drugs that constrict arteries have been tried (e.g. propranolol) but are usually not necessary.

Chilblains (pernio)

This is an inflammatory condition of the toes and fingers, induced by cold. Redness, itching and ulceration may occur. They usually occur before the age of 20 years, and women are more affected than men. Warm surroundings such as central heating have dramatically reduced the incidence of chilblains. Sensible warm clothing, stopping smoking (because smoking constricts the arteries that supply the skin), and exercise are usually all that is needed. Attempting to improve the circulation by taking vasodilator drugs by mouth is not recommended nor is the application of creams and ointments aimed at improving the circulation. Simple protective ointments (e.g. Vaseline petroleum jelly) are best but the important thing is to avoid getting chilblains by keeping the feet and hands warm and protected from the cold. It is important to keep the whole of the body warm because coldness in for example the face can cause a reflex constriction of arteries in the hands and toes, making them go cold.

Sudden blocking of an artery

An artery may be blocked suddenly by a thrombus (a clot) or an embolus (a piece of a thrombus from another site). Treatment is by surgical removal and/or anti-clotting drugs according to the size and position of the artery that is blocked off.

Thrombophlebitis

Thrombophlebitis or phlebitis are terms used to describe thrombosis in a vein, which may or may not be accompanied by inflammation of the adjoining walls of the vein.

A thrombosis in a vein is caused by a slowing down in the flow of blood (e.g. when a person is immobile for a prolonged period of time), when the lining surface of the vein is damaged, and/or when there is some change in the clotting mechanisms. Pregnancy and the use of oral contraceptive drugs affect both the flow of blood and the clotting mechanisms, and predispose to the development of thrombosis. Other disorders that predispose to thrombosis include heart disease, immobilization in bed (e.g. due to paralysis or after major surgery), varicose veins and immobility (e.g. during a long car or aeroplane trip). Inflammation of the walls of veins may be caused by certain drugs (e.g. anti-cancer drugs given into a vein), infections and certain types of cancer.

Treatment of superficial thrombophlebitis

Thrombophlebitis affecting superficial veins may be helped by giving an anti-inflammatory drug such as indomethacin. Otherwise there is no specific drug treatment.

Treatment of thrombophlebitis of deep veins

This is a serious condition because of the risk of a piece of the thrombus coming loose and travelling to the lungs where it may block a main artery in the lungs – a pulmonary embolism. The treatment is with anti-clotting drugs (see Chapter 26).

Drugs used to improve the blood supply to the brain

Mental function may be affected when the blood supply to the brain is inadequate. This may occur if the arteries that supply the brain are narrowed by disease. The two commonly occurring diseases of these arteries are arteriosclerosis (hardening of the arteries with advancing age) and atherosclerosis (patchy deposits of fat in the arteries).

Muscles in the walls of the arteries that supply the brain are very sensitive to local chemical changes in the brain – particularly a fall in oxygen supply, a rise in carbon dioxide and a rise in acidity. Any of these changes will trigger an immediate response in the walls of the arteries, causing the muscles to relax and dilate the arteries in order to increase their diameter and increase the amount of blood flowing through them to the brain. This response takes precedence over any stimulation of the arteries by the nervous system, which means that local mechanisms are continuously in control of maximizing the blood supply to the brain if it is diminished as a result of damage to the arteries by disease.

It is against this background that the use of drugs to improve the circulation to the brain should be judged. Their use may dilate healthy arteries and increase the blood supply to parts of the brain that are *not* suffering from a defective blood supply, but they may have little effect on diseased arteries which are already stretched to their maximum as a result of local control mechanisms. The overall result could be that blood is 'stolen' from those parts of the brain that have a deficient blood supply and diverted to parts of the brain that have a healthy blood supply, and this could be harmful.

The use of drugs to improve the circulation of blood to the brain in order to improve mental and other brain functions in elderly people is subject to much research. Obviously it is very difficult to assess mental function in the elderly, comparing the results of drug treatment with no treatment, particularly in the long term. Therefore claims for any benefits from drug treatment need to be carefully assessed.

Claims for the benefits of drug treatment in people suffering from senile dementia (dementia that may develop in old age) also need careful assessment, as do claims for the benefit of drug treatment in anyone suffering from pre-senile dementia (dementia that comes on between the ages of 30 and 60 years). The latter group includes people who develop Alzheimer's disease.

Drugs marketed to improve mental function in elderly people include:

- *co-dergocrine* (Hydergine tablets), which is related to ergot and is claimed to improve the use of oxygen and glucose by the cells in the brain
- *cyclandelate* (Cyclobral capsules, Cyclospasmol tablets, capsules and powder for suspension), see page 354
- *naftidrofuryl* (Praxilene capsules, Praxilene Forte injections), see page 354

Table 24.1 Drugs used to improve the circulation – harmful effects and warnings

cinnarizine (Stugeron Forte)
Harmful effects It may cause drowsiness and, rarely, dry mouth and blurred vision. For other potential harmful effects of antihistamine, see Table 10.2.

Warnings See antihistamines, Table 10.2. Cinnarizine should be used with caution in people with low blood pressure.

Risks in elderly people Harmful effects may be more frequent and severe; therefore use with caution.

Risks in driving It may impair your ability to drive, particularly if taken with alcohol.

Risks with alcohol It increases the effects of alcohol; do not drink alcohol when you are taking this drug.

co-dergocrine (Hydergine)
Harmful effects are infrequent and usually mild. They include stomach and bowel upsets, flushing, skin rashes, stuffiness of the nose, abdominal cramps, headache, drop in blood pressure on standing up after sitting or lying (may produce light-headedness, dizziness and faintness), allergic reactions.

Warnings Co-dergocrine should not be used in anyone allergic to the drug, and used with caution in people with a slow heart rate.

Risks in elderly people Harmful effects may be more frequent and severe; therefore use with caution.

cyclandelate (Cyclobral, Cyclospasmol)
Harmful effects Very high doses may cause nausea, flushing, weakness, stomach and bowel upsets and dizziness.

Warnings Cyclandelate should not be used in anyone suffering from the early stages of a stroke.

Risks in elderly people Harmful effects may be more frequent and severe; therefore use with caution.

naftidrofuryl (Praxilene)
Harmful effects May occasionally cause nausea and stomach pains.

Warning Naftidrofuryl should not be given by injection to people with heart block; nor given to anyone who is allergic to it.

nicotinic acid derivatives: nicofuranose (Bradilan); inositol nicotinate (Hexopal); nicotinyl alcohol (Ronicol)
Harmful effects The most commonly occurring harmful effects include flushing, dizziness and nausea. Nicotinic acid may cause both a rise in blood glucose, and aggravate diabetes, and a rise in blood uric acid level, and aggravate gout.

Warnings The dose should be tailored to individual response. Do not take before going to bed or going in a hot room because flushing may be excessive. Do not take within 24 hours of a surgical operation.

Risks in elderly people Harmful effects may be more frequent and severe; therefore use with caution.

Risks with alcohol The harmful effects (flushing, etc.) may be made worse by alcohol.

nifedipine (Adalat)
See Table 20.4

oxpentifylline (Trental)
Harmful effects include nausea, malaise, stomach upsets, dizziness, flushing and allergic reactions.

Warnings Oxpentifylline should not be used in people who are allergic to it. It should be used with caution in anyone who suffers from low blood pressure or severe coronary artery disease or severe kidney disease.

Risks in elderly people Harmful effects may be more frequent and severe; therefore use with caution.

prazosin (Hypovase)
See Table 21.5

thymoxamine (Opilon)
Harmful effects include nausea, diarrhoea, headache, dizziness and flushing of the face.

Warnings Thymoxamine should be used with caution in anyone who suffers from diabetes or from coronary artery disease (e.g. angina).

Table 24.2 Preparations used to treat disorders of the circulation

Preparation	*Drug*	*Drug group*	*Dosage form*
Adalat	nifedipine	Calcium channel blocker	Liquid in capsules
Bradilan	nicofuranose	Nicotinic acid derivative	Enteric-coated tablets
Cyclobral	cyclandelate	Calcium overload regulator	Capsules
Cyclospasmol	cyclandelate	Calcium overload regulator	Capsules, tablets, suspension
Hexopal	inositol nicotinate	Nicotinic acid derivative	Tablets, suspension; also Hexopal Forte tablets
Hydergine	co-dergocrine	Ergot alkaloid cell activator	Tablets
Hypovase	prazosin	Selective alpha blocker	Tablets
Nimotop	nimodipine	Calcium channel blocker	Tablets, infusion
Opilon	thymoxamine	Selective alpha blocker	Tablets
Praxilene	naftidrofuryl	Cell activator	Capsules
Praxilene Forte	naftidrofuryl	Cell activator	Injection
Ronicol	nicotinyl alcohol	Nicotinic acid derivative	Tablets
Ronicol Timespan	nicotinyl alcohol	Nicotinic acid derivative	Sustained-release tablets
Stugeron Forte	cinnarizine	Antihistamine	Capsules
Trental	oxpentifylline	Xanthine	Sustained-release tablets

25

Deposits of cholesterol and fats in arteries (atherosclerosis)

Control of blood fats (lipids)

The daily intake of animal and vegetable fats varies considerably between individuals. The major portion (90 per cent) consists of what chemists call triglycerides, a combination of glycerol with three different fatty acids. The rest consist of cholesterol and other fatty substances. NOTE Fats that occur in living tissues are usually referred to as lipids.

Cholesterol is a waxy substance that is present in all animal cells and is involved with their functioning. It is used in the production of steroid hormones and is present in high concentrations in the adrenal glands. The level of cholesterol in the blood is fairly constant for each individual but shows a variation between individuals (see later).

Triglycerides in food are broken down to smaller particles before absorption by an enzyme in the intestine (called lipase) and by bile salts. Those fat particles that are relatively soluble in water then enter the bloodstream and are taken directly to the liver. The larger insoluble particles come together again in the wall of the intestine and are picked up by transporter proteins. These minute globules of fat and protein are called chylomicrons (see later) and they are responsible for making the blood serum look 'milky' for up to half an hour after a meal.

Cholesterol in food is absorbed from the intestine and is taken to the liver where it may be excreted in the bile, converted into bile salts or incorporated into lipoproteins and transported to the tissues. In addition to dealing with triglycerides and cholesterol from food, the liver also manufactures new triglycerides and cholesterol.

Triglycerides and cholesterol (lipids) do not circulate free in the blood but are bound to transporter proteins as complexes known as *lipoproteins*. The major groups of lipoproteins include the following:

- *Chylomicrons* – These are the largest lipoproteins and carry lipids *from the intestine* to be deposited in fat cells (adipose tissue) or to be broken down to fatty acids and burned as energy in muscle cells. The remnants of chylomicrons and unused fatty acids in the blood are removed by the liver and used in many chemical processes.

- *Very low density lipoproteins (VLDL)* transport cholesterol and triglycerides *made in the liver* to the tissues. Some of the lipids are removed for storage or to be used as energy, leaving lipoprotein complexes intermediate (IDL) and then of low density (*low density lipoproteins, LDL*). These LDLs circulate in the blood and are mostly removed by receptors in the liver and other tissues.
- *High density lipoproteins (HDL)* – These act as the main transporters of cholesterol back from the tissues to the liver.

About 25 per cent of cholesterol is transported as HDL and 75 per cent as LDL. A raised level of cholesterol in the blood can result from an increased conversion of VLDL to LDL or a defective clearance of LDL from the blood. Increased release of VLDL by the liver may occur in obesity, in diabetes or from a genetic disorder. This results in an increased level of LDL and cholesterol in the blood and an increase in triglycerides. Failure to get rid of LDL from the blood may be due to some malfunction of LDL receptors in the liver and tissues.

Cholesterol from food goes straight to the liver and causes an increased concentration in the cells of the liver. This suppresses the function of LDL receptors, resulting in an increased release of LDL and cholesterol into the bloodstream. *Saturated fats (e.g. animal fats)* from food have a similar effect and cause an increase of cholesterol and LDL in the blood.

The concentration of LDL in the blood is directly related to the development of fatty deposits in arteries (atheromatous plaques, see below). This risk is increased if the levels of VLDL, total cholesterol and total triglycerides are also high. A raised HDL level may be an indication of reduced risk.

Lipoproteins act as reservoirs from which triglycerides and cholesterol can be drawn at any time. Triglyceride breakdown products (free fatty acids) act as a very high energy source for the body; this breakdown is controlled by an enzyme (lipase) that is present in the lining of the blood vessels in many organs and tissues. It splits fatty acids from triglycerides. The free fatty acids that are produced are transported in the bloodstream on albumin proteins and taken to muscles and other cells where they are burned for energy. They are also taken to fat depots and converted back into triglycerides (fats) and stored in fat cells for future use.

Fatty deposits in arteries (atherosclerosis)

Atherosclerosis is a patchy thickening of the walls of arteries, caused by deposits of cholesterol along with some fats – atheromatous plaques. Over time the lining of the artery that covers the deposits may become scarred and break down, producing ulcers on the surface. The blood then starts to stick to the ulcer to form a clot (or thrombus), which increases in size and eventually closes off the affected artery – partially or completely. Atheromatous plaques are often widespread throughout the body. They particularly affect large and medium-sized arteries, especially the main artery from the heart (the aorta), the main arteries that supply the legs and the arteries that supply the heart (coronary arteries) and the brain (cerebral arteries). Thrombosis is discussed in Chapter 26.

We are not at all certain how or why atheromatous plaques develop in arteries but we do know from post-mortem findings that they are associated with the formation of thrombi (clots in blood vessels) which are a major cause of premature death (i.e. death before 65 years of age). We also know from post-mortem findings that deposits of fats in arteries can be present from a very early age in otherwise healthy people.

These deposits (atheromatous plaques) in arteries lead to narrowing and to thrombosis and are a major cause of heart attacks due to thrombosis affecting a coronary artery (coronary thrombosis) and of strokes due to thrombosis affecting an artery supplying the brain (cerebral thrombosis). Deposits may also cause blockages in the arteries of the limbs, particularly of the legs.

The formation of a deposit (atheromatous plaque) is due to some imbalance between the laying down and the removal of cholesterol and fats, and this imbalance is related to the ratios of lipoproteins in the blood. These ratios can therefore be used as indicators of risk (see earlier).

Many factors come together to cause the patchy laying down of deposits of fats in arteries and we are able to recognize some of them which we call risk factors.

Factors associated with an increased risk of developing atherosclerosis (risk factors)

There are several risk factors associated with the development of atherosclerosis. They include the following.

Age

The risk of developing atherosclerosis and death from heart attacks or strokes increases with age. This is not directly related to ageing but the older you get the more exposed you are to factors that may produce these deposits in the arteries. Nevertheless, atherosclerosis is a major cause of premature death (death before the age of 65 years).

Sex

The risks are higher in men than in women, and higher in women after menopause than before it.

Blood pressure

There is an important association between raised blood pressure, atherosclerosis and premature death from heart attack and stroke (see Chapter 21).

Cigarette smoking

There is a direct relationship between the number of cigarettes smoked and atherosclerosis, leading to heart attacks, strokes and disorders of circulation in the legs. Cigarette smoking lowers HDL and increases the risk of thrombosis. Passive smokers inhale sidestream smoke from burning cigarettes and run a similar risk.

Glucose

Inability of the body to handle carbohydrates effectively (e.g. in diabetes), causing a raised level of glucose in the blood and/or in the urine, is a risk factor in the development of atherosclerosis.

Obesity

Being 20 per cent or more overweight carries a significantly increased risk of developing atherosclerosis. Associated with being overweight are the additional risk factors of raised blood pressure and diabetes. In men under 50 years of age, a 20 per cent increase in weight is regarded as a significant risk on its own.

A high level of cholesterol and/or triglycerides in the blood

It is well recognized that there are many factors which may contribute to the formation of atheromatous plaques in arteries; however, the levels of cholesterol and/or triglycerides in the blood are an important indicator of risk.

A high cholesterol level is said to be present when it is above an arbitrary normal limit of 6.5 mmol/litre, and a high triglyceride level when it is above 5.6 mmol/litre. Evidence from research suggests that if raised cholesterol and/or triglyceride levels are reduced to 'normal', the risk of developing atherosclerosis is also reduced, thus lowering the risk of heart attacks, strokes and disorders of the circulation.

Diseases that cause high cholesterol and/or triglyceride levels

Diseases that cause high levels of cholesterol and/or triglycerides in the blood may be either primary or secondary to some other disease such as diabetes, under-active thyroid gland, kidney disease, obstruction to the bile system or inflammation of the pancreas. Primary causes of raised cholesterol and triglycerides in the blood may be divided into two major groups: those that are clearly inherited and are due to a specific genetic defect (see below); and those that appear to be a consequence of weakly inherited genetic abnormalities combined with environmental factors such as a diet high in animal fats, smoking and heavy drinking in a susceptible person.

Risk groups

People with a specific inherited defect in how their bodies handle cholesterol and/or triglycerides account for only about 5 per cent of all cases of raised blood cholesterol/triglyceride levels (*hyperlipidaemia*). These individuals suffer from familial hyperlipidaemia (raised levels that runs in families). Some of these people suffer from hypercholesterolaemia (raised cholesterol). They have raised levels of low density lipoproteins (LDLs) due to a deficiency of LDL receptors in the body. Others suffer from raised lipoprotein levels due to a combination of factors.

Half of these individuals will develop coronary heart disease by the time they are 50 years old. When such a person is diagnosed as suffering from a raised blood cholesterol/triglycerides level, each member of the family should also be investigated.

People with weakly inherited genetic abnormalities have a predisposition to develop raised levels of cholesterol and/or triglycerides in the blood and atherosclerosis when exposed to the various risk factors discussed earlier. This disorder is relatively common.

Another group of people who may develop raised levels of cholesterol and/or triglycerides and who develop atherosclerosis are those who are overweight and/or who easily develop a raised level of glucose in the blood and urine in response to sugar intake. The latter is referred to as carbohydrate intolerance. Another group at risk are those who have a raised blood uric acid level.

NOTE All known risk factors taken together account for only about one-half of all cases of atherosclerosis and subsequent death from heart attacks or strokes, so there is much we do not understand at present about the factors that cause this disease.

Preventing atherosclerosis

Three important steps in preventing atherosclerosis and therefore in preventing premature deaths from heart attacks and strokes are:

- Identify and treat raised blood pressure (see Chapter 21)
- Stop smoking
- Reduce blood cholesterol/triglyceride levels if they are raised

Reducing levels of cholesterol and triglycerides in blood

Reduce weight

If your blood cholesterol and/or triglyceride are raised, the first step is to *reduce weight* if you are overweight.

Reduce the amount and change the types of fats in the diet

A major factor in food that affects the levels of cholesterol and triglycerides in the blood is the amount and type of fat in the diet. A diet high in fat pushes up the blood cholesterol and fat levels, particularly if it contains foods high in *saturated fatty acids* – for example, dairy produce (milk, cream, butter) and fatty red meats. On the other hand, *polyunsaturated fats* tend to lower LDLs and total cholesterol. Foods high in these polyunsaturated fats include fish oils, margarine (soft polyunsaturated), corn oil, soya bean oil and sunflower seed oil. Fish oils are particularly beneficial; not only do they lower cholesterol and triglycerides but they also reduce the stickiness of platelets – lowering the risk of thrombosis – and dilate small arteries.

Sensible advice is therefore to *reduce the overall amount of fats that you eat and to eat foods that contain proportionally more polyunsaturates than saturates.* Use margarine instead of butter. Reduce the amount of cream and ice cream that you eat; drink skimmed or semi-skimmed milk. Eat less fatty red meat and replace some of it with chicken, and eat oily fish (e.g. mackerel, herring) twice a week. Cut the fat off red meat. Grill instead of fry. Reduce the overall amount of cheese that you eat and proportionally increase the amount of cottage cheese over hard cheese. Reduce your fat intake by eating fewer chocolates, cakes, biscuits, pastries and puddings. Use unsaturated oils (e.g. corn oil, sunflower oil, olive oil) for cooking. Eat proportionally more vegetables, fruit, cereals, and wholemeal bread, rice and pasta.

Fibre intake

A diet high in *soluble fibres*, e.g. vegetables, fruit, pulses, oats, may help to reduce blood cholesterol levels, but note that a diet high in *bran fibre* will not have this effect.

Drug treatment of raised blood cholesterol and triglyceride levels

Drugs to lower high levels of cholesterol and triglyceride in the blood should not be used routinely. Diet treatment should always be tried first and, in addition, smokers should stop smoking, a raised blood pressure should be treated, the overweight should lose weight down to normally accepted levels, and heavy alcohol drinkers should bring their drinking down to minimal levels. Regular exercise may also help and any contributory disease should be treated specifically; for example, diabetes or underworking of the thyroid gland. Drugs should be considered as a last resort if all these efforts fail, and even then they must only be used along with a strict diet, weight control, control of blood pressure and no smoking. It is a nonsense to take drugs to lower blood cholesterol and triglyceride levels if you are overweight and continue to drink heavily and to smoke.

Drugs that lower blood cholesterol and/or triglyceride levels

Harmful effects and warnings on the use of drugs used to lower blood cholesterol and triglyceride levels are listed in Table 25.1.

About one in four adults has a raised level of cholesterol and/or triglyceride but only a small proportion of these require treatment with drugs. Evidence of raised levels should be confirmed by a blood test after a 14-hour fast. This should be repeated two or three times before finally deciding whether an individual actually has a raised blood cholesterol/triglyceride level sufficient to warrant treatment with drugs. Drugs that lower LDL and raise HDL may reduce the progression of atherosclerosis and may cause atheromatous plaques to shrink. However, they do not correct the underlying disorder that leads to these deposits and therefore they usually have to be taken indefinitely. If they are stopped, the blood cholesterol and trigylercides almost always return to their previous high level.

Nicotinic acid group of drugs

Nicotinic acid reduces both cholesterol and triglyceride levels by principally blocking their manufacture in the liver. It also increases HDL. It produces intense flushing of the skin with itching, particularly of the face and upper part of the body. These reactions slowly wear off over several weeks and may be helped by taking one aspirin tablet half an hour before taking a nicotinic acid tablet. It also helps to start with a small dose and slowly increase it. *Nicofuranose* produces similar effects but causes less flushing than nicotinic acid. These drugs may increase the levels of glucose and uric acid in the blood, effects that clear up when the drugs are stopped.

Clofibrate group of drugs

Bezafibrate, clofibrate and *fenofibrate* lower triglyceride and VLDL and LDL levels by affecting their production in the liver and their breakdown in the tissues. They also raise HDL level.

Gemfibrozil is chemically related to clofibrate and produces similar effects.

Drugs that bind bile acids in the intestine

Cholestyramine and *colestipol* are resins that are not absorbed into the bloodstream when they are taken by mouth. In the intestine they bind to bile acids (which are formed from cholesterol in the liver) and increase their excretion in the motions. The re-cycling of bile acids back to the liver is reduced and the liver responds by increasing the conversion of cholesterol into bile acids, which causes the blood level of cholesterol to fall. However, they may cause an increase in triglycerides, VLDL and IDL. The long-term effects of these drugs is to reduce the total body content of cholesterol.

These resins often produce stomach upsets and constipation which may be troublesome. They also interfere with the absorption of fats and, in particular, may affect the absorption of fat-soluble vitamins A, D, E and K. Therefore bran (to help the constipation) and vitamin supplements are recommended in anyone taking regular high daily doses of these drugs. The resins also bind to other drugs and prevent their absorption (see Chapter 89), so any other drug should be taken at least 1 hour before or 4 hours after taking one of these resins that lower cholesterol.

Probucol is unrelated to the above drugs. It increases the excretion of bile acids in the motions, impairs the absorption of fats from the intestine, and increases the conversion of cholesterol to bile acids in the liver although probucol is not an ion exchange resin. In the body it attaches itself to fat and can stay in the body for months after the individual has stopped taking it. It decreases cholesterol and may have a beneficial effect on atheromatous plaques despite the fact that it lowers HDL and does not lower triglycerides.

Fish oils

Fish oils (marine triglycerides) reduce blood levels of cholesterol and triglycerides, probably by blocking the production of VLDL in the liver. They may also increase the activity of lipase, which breaks fats down to fatty acids. An element of fish oil may also help to reduce the stickiness of platelets, which may reduce the risk of thrombosis.

Simvastatin

Simvastatin reduces the synthesis of cholesterol in the liver by blocking an enzyme (reductase) responsible for the final stage of a twenty-five step process in its production. However, the enzyme is not totally blocked and so does not interfere with the manufacture of steroids from cholesterol and the use of cholesterol in maintaining the walls of cells. In addition, simvastatin increases the breakdown of cholesterol in the tissues by altering receptors that pick up low density lipoproteins (LDLs) which are high in cholesterol. It is a 'prodrug' which is inactive until it enters the liver, where it is converted into its active form.

Pravastatin

Pravastatin has similar effects but is more selective on liver cells. (U)

The screening of blood cholesterol and triglycerides

A single test result that shows your cholesterol and triglycerides levels to be within a normal range may be of some significance but an isolated result that shows them to be raised is of little value. If they are raised, it is important to have at least three further estimates taken on different days and preferably after 12–14 hours of fasting. This will give a more constant indication of whether your blood cholesterol and blood fats are raised.

Guidelines on levels and treatment

	Desirable	*Borderline*	*High*	*Very high*
Total cholesterol (in mmol/litre)	<5.2	5.2–6.5	6.5–7.8	>7.8
Total fats (triglycerides) (in mmol/litre)	<2.3	2.3–5.6	5.6–10.0	>10.0

NOTE A low LDL and a high HDL are regarded as beneficial and these should also be considered.

If your cholesterol is at a desirable level, now is the time to start preventative non-drug treatment: stop smoking if you smoke, reduce alcohol intake if high, lose weight if overweight, take an adequate amount of physical exercise, reduce the amount of saturated fats in your diet and proportionally increase the amount of polyunsaturated fats, and eat oily fish twice a week.

If your cholesterol is borderline, be even more rigid about the above advice and even more strict about your diet.

If your cholesterol is high or very high, in addition to the above you should be referred to a special blood fat clinic (lipid clinic) and be given appropriate drug treatment as well.

NOTE If you suffer from coronary artery disease (e.g. angina) then you should be even more conscientious about your non-drug treatments.

If your blood triglycerides are raised, you should follow the advice given above for non-drug treatment of high blood cholesterol as well as having treatment for any disorder that may cause a rise in your blood triglyceride levels (e.g. diabetes).

NOTE High alcohol intake and certain drugs may increase your blood fat levels. The drugs include oestrogens (e.g. in the pill), thiazide diuretics (water tablets) used to treat raised blood pressure and heart failure, and beta blockers used to treat angina and raised blood pressure. You should reduce alcohol intake and, where appropriate, take advice on alternative drug treatment for your disorder.

If your triglycerides are high or very high, you should be referred to a lipid clinic where you may be given drugs in addition to rigid non-drug treatment.

Table 25.1 Drugs used to lower blood fat levels – harmful effects and warnings

bezafibrate (Bezalip, Bezalip-Mono)
Harmful effects are infrequent; they include nausea, fullness in the stomach and, rarely, itching, impotence, allergic reactions (e.g. nettle rash) and painful muscles.

Warnings Blood fat levels should be measured before and at regular intervals during treatment. Bezafibrate should not be used in anyone who is allergic to it or who has severe kidney or liver impairment, low blood protein levels or gall bladder disease. The dose should be reduced in individuals with moderately impaired kidney function.

Risks in elderly people Harmful effects may be more frequent and severe; therefore the dosage should be reduced.

cholestyramine (Questran)
Harmful effects include constipation, flatulence, heartburn, nausea, diarrhoea (with large doses), stomach upsets, skin rashes and, rarely, fat in the faeces (steatorrhoea) with high doses.

Warnings Blood fat levels should be measured before and at regular intervals during treatment. Cholestyramine should not be used in anyone with a blocked bile duct. With prolonged use of high doses, supplements of fat-soluble vitamins A, D, E and K and folic acid should be given, particularly in children.

Risks in elderly people Harmful effects may be more frequent and severe; therefore use with caution.

clofibrate (Atromid-S)
Harmful effects are infrequent and usually mild and transient; they include nausea, vomiting, loose stools, indigestion, wind and distension of the abdomen, headache, dizziness, fatigue, impotence. Rarely, there may be: allergic reactions (e.g. skin rash, nettle rash), itching; muscle aches and pains and weakness, dry brittle hair and loss of hair (alopecia); gall stones; and occasional changes in liver function tests.

Warnings Clofibrate should not be used in people with severe liver, kidney or gall bladder disease or who are allergic to it. There is an increased risk of developing gall stones and complications from gall stones. Individuals with mild or moderate impairment of kidney function should be given reduced doses.

Risks in elderly people Harmful effects may be more frequent and severe; therefore reduce the dosage.

colestipol (Colestid)
Harmful effects are usually mild and transient; they include nausea, constipation, heartburn, flatulence, nausea and vomiting. Very rarely, there may be allergic reactions (nettle rash, dermatitis), muscle and joint pains, headache, dizziness, anxiety, vertigo, drowsiness, loss of appetite, fatigue and diarrhoea.

Warnings Colestipol should not be used in people who are allergic to it or who have a blocked bile duct. It may make pre-existing constipation worse causing a blockage (faecal impaction). Blood fat levels should be measured before and at regular intervals during treatment. With high doses, supplements of fat-soluble vitamins A, D, E and K and folic acid should be given, particularly to children.

Risks in elderly people Treatment should be tailored to the individual's needs and response; therefore use with caution.

fish oils (marine triglycerides, Maxepa)
Harmful effects include nausea and belching.

Warnings Fish oils should be used with caution in anyone with bleeding disorders.

gemfibrizol (Lopid)
Harmful effects include diarrhoea, nausea, vomiting, wind and stomach pains. Very rarely, there have been reports of dry mouth, loss of appetite, constipation, itching, allergic reactions, nettle rash,

Table 25.1 Drugs used to lower blood fat levels – harmful effects and warnings (*cont.*)

dermatitis, headache, dizziness, blurred vision, impotence, swollen joints, muscle pains, back pains, gall stones, blood disorders, fatigue and malaise.

Warnings Gemfibrizol should not be used in individuals who suffer from alcoholism, impaired liver function, gall stones, severe impairment of kidney function or in anyone who is allergic to it. A full blood count, liver function tests and measurement of blood fat levels should be carried out before treatment and at regular intervals during treatment. People on long-term treatment should also have an eye examination every year and tests of their kidney functions.

fenofibrate (Lipantil)
Harmful effects include stomach upsets, headache, fatigue, dizziness and, rarely, muscle cramps and impotence.

Warnings It should not be used by anyone with severe impairment of kidney or liver function or gall bladder disease. It should be used with caution by individuals with mild or moderate impairment of kidney function – the dose should be reduced.

Risks in elderly people Harmful effects may be more frequent and severe; therefore use with caution. Kidney function should be checked and, if impaired, the dose reduced.

Risks in pregnancy Do not use in pregnancy.

Risks in breast feeding Do not use in breast-feeding mothers.

nicotinic acid and nicofuranose (Bradilan)
See Table 24.1

probucol (Lurselle)
Harmful effects are usually mild to moderate and transient; they include nausea, vomiting, flatulence, diarrhoea and stomach pains. Very rarely, there may be allergic reactions, headache, dizziness, blood disorders, skin rashes, itching, impotence, blurred vision and changes on electrical tracings of the heart (ECG).

Warnings

Risks in elderly people Harmful effects may be more frequent and severe; therefore use with caution.

simvastatin (Zocor)
Harmful effects are infrequent and usually mild. They include nausea, indigestion, wind, constipation, stomach cramps and pains, diarrhoea, fatigue and, rarely, skin rash. Rarely, muscle damage producing muscle weakness may occur and treatment should be stopped if the blood level of a muscle enzyme is raised (creatinine phosphokinase).

Warnings Simvastatin should not be used in anyone with active liver disease. Tests of liver function should be carried out before treatment starts and at 4- to 6-week intervals during treatment. A check on the eyes should be carried out every 12 months.

Comment

Most findings on treatment aimed at lowering blood cholesterol and triglycerides are based on the drug treatment of men at high risk. We need to know much more about the effects of diet alone and diet plus not smoking, and also about the risks and benefits in women.

Table 25.2 Preparations used to lower blood cholesterol and fat levels

Preparation	*Drug*	*Dosage form*
Atromid-S	clofibrate	Capsules
Bezalip	bezafibrate	Tablets
Bezalip-Mono	bezafibrate	Tablets
Bradilan	nicofuranose	Enteric-coated tablets
Colestid	colestipol	Granules
Lipantil	fenofibrate	Capsules
Lipostat	pravastatin	Tablets (U)
Lopid	gemfibrozil	Capsules
Lurselle	probucol	Tablets
Maxepa	fish oils	Capsules, liquid
nicotinic acid	nicotinic acid	Tablets
Olbetam	acipimox	Capsules
Questran	cholestyramine	Powder
Questran A		Powder (low sugar)
Zocor	simvastatin	Tablets

26

Bleeding disorders and thrombosis

A *blood clot* is a semi-solid mass produced by coagulation of blood. It consists of a mesh of fibrin in which are trapped red and white blood cells and platelets.

Fibrin is an insoluble protein formed from a soluble protein (fibrinogen) in the plasma. An enzyme, thrombin, in the blood converts fibrinogen to fibrin. This formation of fibrin is an essential process in blood clotting.

Platelets are very small blood cells that produce chemicals which make them stick to each other and to the walls of blood vessels. They also produce other chemicals that are involved in clotting. Platelets therefore have an important function in blood clotting and also form an important part of blood clots, particularly in arteries (see later).

Blood clotting or *coagulation* is the process of clotting or coagulation of whole blood. It comprises a series of very complex reactions.

Arrest of bleeding

Three mechanisms help to stop bleeding: the injured blood vessels close up (go into spasm) to try to stop further bleeding; platelets in the blood clump together and to the walls of the damaged blood vessels to try to stem the flow of blood; the blood itself clots.

The blood vessels

The shutting down of the blood vessels is temporary but it is an important first and immediate step to stop bleeding. It provides time for the other steps to take place. If these do not develop properly, bleeding will recur (called secondary bleeding) when the blood vessels open up again.

The platelets

When blood vessels are injured, they release a chemical that causes platelets to stick to the injured wall. This stimulates the platelets to release further chemicals that cause them to stick to each other and to the wall of the injured vessel. They also release factors which, together with vitamin K, act on a substance called fibrinogen in the blood to convert it to an insoluble protein called fibrin.

Clotting factors

The end point of a very complex chemical process is the formation of a fibrin mesh around the platelets, which forms a blood clot and blocks off the injured vessels.

There are 13 major factors in the blood involved in producing fibrin and the formation of a blood clot. The one we know the most about these days is factor VIII because it is used to treat haemophilia.

Factor VIII is collected from pooled blood obtained from hundreds of donors. If one or more of these donors were infected with hepatitis virus or the AIDS virus at the time they gave blood, the infections might be transmitted to haemophiliac patients who receive treatment with the infected factor VIII blood product. Most virus-infected factor VIII blood products have come from the USA. As a consequence of this contamination, several hundred haemophiliac patients have been infected with hepatitis and/or AIDS. This risk has now been greatly reduced because all blood products are sterilized before use.

Mechanisms that counter blood clotting

In addition to the above mechanisms that cause clotting there are counter-mechanisms in the blood that ensure that clotting goes on only where it is needed and does not continue unnecessarily. These include the *fibrinolytic system*, which is responsible for converting an inert substance (plasminogen) in the blood into an active substance (plasmin) that digests fibrin and other factors and dissolves clots. Also in the blood circulation there are *clotting inhibitors*, which neutralize clotting factors in the blood in vessels away from the site of injury; they stop blood from clotting in normal uninjured blood vessels.

Bleeding disorders

Disorders of bleeding may occur for the following reasons.

Defects in blood vessels These include a group of disorders known as *purpuras*, which show themselves as minute bleedings and bruising in the skin and lining of the mouth due to damage to small blood vessels. This damage may be caused by diseases (e.g. typhoid, measles, meningitis); by drugs (e.g. aspirin, ergot, frusemide, indomethacin, phenobarbitone, phenylbutazone, phenytoin, quinine); by severe allergic reactions; in some liver and kidney diseases; by a hereditary disease; and by vitamin C deficiency (scurvy).

Damage to the bone marrow, resulting in reduced platelet production may cause purpura. It is characterized by a low platelet count (thrombocytopenia), purpura (minute bleedings and bruisings in the skin and mouth), a prolonged bleeding time, abnormal clot formation and, sometimes, an enlarged spleen. This thrombocytopenic purpura may be caused by several disorders and also by drugs such as chlordiazepoxide, chlorothiazide, frusemide, indomethacin, phenylbutazone, sulphonamides and tolbutamide. Excessive exposure to X-rays and radioactive substances may also damage platelet production.

Disorders of the clotting mechanisms There are several disorders that affect clotting but the most commonly known is *haemophilia*, which is caused by a deficiency of blood clotting factor VIII (the anti-haemophilia factor). Haemophilia is hereditary and produces a life-long tendency to excessive bleeding and a very prolonged time before the blood clots. The daughters of haemophiliacs may carry the trait and there is a 50 per cent chance that their sons will have haemophilia and that 50 per cent of their daughters will carry the trait. Treatment is based on adequate replacement of factor VIII. Unfortunately, it has a short life in the body and has to be given frequently until a bleeding episode stops (e.g. the removal of a tooth).

The factor VIII preparation must be of the right blood group for the patient and should be negative for hepatitis and AIDS. Unfortunately, many patients have developed hepatitis and/or AIDS from contaminated blood (see earlier). In addition, the frequent giving of factor VIII preparations to haemophiliacs appears to weaken the immune system against infections.

Thrombosis

Thrombosis refers to the clotting of blood inside a blood vessel or the heart. A thrombus is a blood clot which is formed and remains in a blood vessel or the heart.

Factors that predispose to thrombosis

In health, the blood is kept fluid by various complex mechanisms. However, the blood can clot and form a thrombus inside a blood vessel or the heart under certain circumstances. These include abnormalities that affect the lining of blood vessels (e.g. fat deposits in the lining – atherosclerosis) and any injury or damage to the lining caused, for example, by an injection into a vein. Similarly, damage to the lining of the heart may predispose to thrombosis in the heart; for example, damage to the lining caused by death of an area of heart muscle as a result of a coronary thrombosis.

Abnormalities that affect blood flow may also cause thrombosis. For example, immobility and lack of muscular exercise can cause thrombosis in a vein, which is why people who are confined to bed are more likely to develop thrombosis than someone who is up and about. Pressure on a vein may also cause thrombosis; for example, sitting in one position on a long journey may cause thrombosis in a leg vein that is being squeezed. Thrombosis may also occur if the blood is thickened by any disease that causes an excess number of blood cells (e.g. leukaemia). And finally any disorder that affects the many factors that cause blood clotting may cause thrombosis.

Thrombosis may produce two types of thrombi: white and red. A *white thrombus* occurs in arteries where the blood is fast flowing. It is composed principally of platelets stuck together and to the wall of the vessel and held together by layers of fibrin. It can build up and totally block an artery (e.g. coronary thrombosis). A *red thrombus* consists of a lot of fibrin and blood cells but relatively few platelets. It is formed mainly in veins where the blood flow is relatively slow. A red thrombus may also form behind a white thrombus in an artery where the blood flow starts to slow down due to the blockage. Red thrombi are fragile and pieces can easily break off and travel in the bloodstream to block a blood vessel elsewhere. The piece of the thrombus that comes loose is called an embolus and the process is called embolism. If the embolus sticks in a blood vessel in the brain, it is called a cerebral embolus; if it sticks in a blood vessel in the lungs, it is called a pulmonary embolus, and so on.

Thrombosis in the arteries that supply the heart (coronary thrombosis) or the brain (cerebral thrombosis) is a major cause of death and disability. thrombosis is usually due to disease of the arteries. Thrombosis in veins is usually less serious but thrombi in the deep veins of the legs or pelvis may be fatal if a piece of a thrombus comes loose and lodges in a blood vessel in the lungs (pulmonary embolism).

Drugs that stop blood from clotting

Drugs that stop the blood from clotting may be divided into two groups: those that act directly by interfering with the process of blood clotting and have to be given by injection (heparin and ancrod), and those that act indirectly and may be given by mouth. The former can stop blood clotting outside of the body (e.g. in a test tube) whereas the latter only work in the body by interfering with the production in the liver of factors involved in blood clotting. The drugs that act directly are rapidly effective whereas those that act indirectly take several days to produce their maximum effects.

Anti-blood-clotting drugs (anti-coagulants) that act directly and are given by injection

Heparin

Heparin is made up of large molecules that cannot be absorbed from the stomach and intestine, so it has to be given by injection (see later). Injections into muscles should be avoided because of the risk of bleeding into the muscle. Heparin acts directly on the blood by preventing the formation of thrombin, a protein involved in the formation of a blood clot. It also blocks the involvement of thrombin in forming a blood clot and reduces the stickiness of platelets which are also involved. It works almost immediately but its effects quickly wear off and it has to be given at regular intervals or continuously. Heparin is broken down in the liver and excreted in the urine; therefore its effects will last longer in patients who suffer from severe liver or kidney disease.

Because heparin is broken down rapidly in the body it has to be given by continuous infusion into a vein or injected at regular intervals which must not exceed 6 hours. Full doses by infusion into a vein are given to prevent thrombosis in patients having heart surgery on kidney dialysis. Low doses are injected under the skin to prevent thrombosis after surgery in patients at risk; for example, those who are elderly, are overweight or have a previous history of thrombosis.

Clotting time (coagulation time) The normal time taken for blood to clot on glass (the clotting time) is about 5–7 minutes. If heparin is to be effective in stopping clotting in blood vessels the dose has to be adjusted to keep the clotting time outside of the body above 15 minutes. Both heparin and anti-coagulant (anti-blood-clotting) drugs by mouth are started at the same time. After about 3 days, when the latter drugs will be producing their maximal effect (see later), the heparin is stopped. If heparin has to be continued because the patient cannot, for example, take anti-coagulants by mouth, tests are carried out to measure the clotting of the blood.

Allergy to heparin Heparin is obtained from the lungs of oxen and the intestines of oxen, pigs and sheep; some people may be allergic to certain animal proteins and develop allergic reactions such as chills, fever and nettle rash (urticaria). Allergic reactions to the preservatives used in heparin preparations may also occur in some individuals, producing both an allergic reaction at the site of injection and a generalized allergic reaction.

The risk of bleeding Bleeding is the most common harmful effect produced by heparin. Lack of careful selection of individuals for treatment, failure to control the dosage effectively and failure to monitor blood clotting times may lead to unnecessary bleeding. Before being given heparin, patients should be examined carefully for any signs of a bleeding disorder or any disorder that might bleed (e.g. duodenal ulcer, stomach ulcer). Aspirin increases the effects of heparin, so anyone being given heparin should avoid all medicines containing aspirin.

White clot syndrome Rarely, patients may develop new thrombus formation associated with a fall in blood platelets. This results in the formation of white clots which can block off various blood vessels, resulting in death of patches of skin, gangrene of the toes and/or fingers, heart attack, stroke or an embolism in the lungs. The drug must be stopped immediately if an individual develops new thrombosis associated with a fall in blood platelets. This syndrome is more likely to occur with heparin from ox lungs than with that from pigs' intestines. *It is important to check the blood platelet level regularly in people on long-term heparin treatment.*

Stopping bleeding Bleeding caused by heparin can be controlled by stopping the drug and, if severe, by giving a specific antidote – protamine sulphate. This is a protein from the sperm of certain salmon fish and it forms a complex with heparin, making it inactive.

Ancrod

Ancrod is an enzyme prepared from the venom of the Malayan pit viper. It acts directly upon fibrinogen and interferes with the proper formation of fibrin – the protein mesh that holds a clot together. It may cause large amounts of unstable fibrin to develop in the bloodstream and therefore infusion into a vein should be slow. Its effects are monitored by observing the size of blood clot after a sample of blood has been allowed to stand for about 2 hours. The aim is to predict a dose that produces a blood clot of 2–3 mm in size. An alternative is to measure the concentration of fibrinogen in the blood. As with heparin the main harmful effect of ancrod is bleeding, and it may take up to 24 hours after stopping ancrod for fibrinogen to return to normal function. Therefore, if bleeding is severe, the patient has to be given ancrod anti-venom as a specific antidote. Some individuals may develop an acute allergic reaction to the anti-venom and full resuscitative equipment and treatment should be available when the drug is given. An alternative antidote is to give freeze-dried fibrinogen or fresh-frozen plasma. The only common use of ancrod has been in the treatment and prevention of deep vein thrombosis but it offers no advantage over heparin.

Anti-coagulant drugs that are taken by mouth (oral anti-coagulants)

Anti-coagulant drugs which can be taken by mouth (oral anti-coagulants) act in the liver by blocking the formation of anti-clotting factors from vitamin K. They are therefore also known as vitamin K antagonists. There is a time lag of about 36–48 hours between taking them and the appearance of their effects. This varies between the different products. For immediate anti-clotting treatment, people are started off on heparin by injection at the same time as starting an anti-coagulant by mouth.

Two groups of drugs are available: coumarins (e.g. nicoumalone and warfarin) and indanediones (e.g. phenindione).

The main uses of oral anti-coagulants are: to treat thrombosis in a deep vein; in people with an uncontrolled disorder of heart rhythm (atrial fibrillation) in whom there is a risk of a thrombus forming in the heart and pieces shooting off (embolism); and in people with artificial heart valves where there is a similar risk.

Factors that may increase the effects of oral anti-coagulants

The effect of oral anti-coagulant drugs is increased by a deficiency of vitamin K. This may occur because of a poor diet, disease of the small bowel from which vitamin K is normally absorbed, and any disorder of the bile system which delivers bile to the intestine. This is because bile salts help to digest fats and vitamin K is soluble in fats. If absorption of fats is defective, less vitamin K is absorbed.

Liver disease may increase the effect of oral anti-coagulants because it may impair the production of blood clotting factors. The effect of these anti-coagulant drugs is also increased in people suffering from fever and overactive thyroid gland (hyperthyroidism). In these conditions the body's use of energy is increased, and this may increase the breakdown of clotting factors – including those dependent upon vitamin K for their production; such individuals will require a reduced dose of anti-coagulant drug. Their effects may also be increased by heart failure and by diarrhoea (which may affect the absorption of vitamin K).

Factors that may decrease the effects of oral anti-coagulants

The response to oral anti-coagulants may be decreased in pregnancy because there is an increase in activity of other blood clotting factors. However, this only occurs in the mother and not in the baby, so the baby may be very sensitive to the dose of oral anti-coagulants given to the mother. This is because the drugs pass into the baby and its liver has only a limited ability to produce clotting factors (see 'Risks in pregnancy', later). Some individuals inherit an increased use of vitamin K and a resistance to anti-coagulant drugs.

The risk of bleeding

Bleeding is the main problem caused by the use of oral anti-coagulants. It may occur when these drugs are used to treat people who should not be given them; for example, people who suffer from a duodenal ulcer or stomach ulcer, or from kidney or liver disease. Too large a starting dose often produces unnecessary bleeding, as may failure to adjust the dose according to laboratory reports.

With long-term use, bleeding is rare provided that careful control is kept on the dosage and that other drugs that may cause trouble are avoided. The risk of bleeding is associated with the length of time that treatment is continued and also the extent of anti-clotting effects that are produced.

Controlling the dose of oral anti-coagulants

Treatment with oral anti-coagulants by mouth is monitored by the *prothrombin time.* Prothrombin (factor II) is one of the factors involved in blood clotting. Its production is reduced by oral anti-coagulants. The prothrombin time test gives an indication of this reduction by comparing clotting of 'normal' blood with that of the patient's blood. The difference is reported using an international normalized ratio (INR) to compare these differences. The treatment range for this ratio is 2–2.5 but may be as high as 3–4.5 according to the seriousness of the disorder being treated. The INR should be measured on the second or third day of treatment and then every other day until it is stable and then at less frequent intervals.

Prothrombin tests should be carried out at regular intervals because numerous factors, alone or in combination, can affect response – travel, change of diet, physical state, other diseases (e.g. liver disease) and other drugs. If bleeding occurs and the INR rises the next dose of drug should be stopped and the INR measured. Treatment will then depend on the following guidelines:

No bleeding; INR 4.5–7	Stop drug for 1 or more days according to INR
No bleeding; INR greater than 7	Stop drug and probably give antidote (vitamin K_1) 5–10 mg by mouth
Bleeding; INR less than 4.5	Give fresh-frozen plasma and check the cause
Severe bleeding; INR greater than 2	Give intravenous vitamin K_1 slowly plus factors II, IX and X (or fresh-frozen plasma); check the cause

NOTE Vitamin K_1 (phytomenadione) will take up to 12 hours to work and will stop oral anti-coagulants from working for several days to weeks.

Risks of anti-coagulant drugs in the elderly

The risks of harmful effects from anti-coagulants are increased in elderly people, who are more sensitive to the drugs than are younger adults. The elderly are more likely to be suffering from other diseases and be receiving other drug treatments that may interfere with their response.

Risks from heparin can be reduced by giving it by continuous intravenous infusion rather than by repeated intravenous injections, by careful monitoring of clotting time, by getting the individual up and about as soon as possible, and by stopping it as soon as possible.

The risks from anti-coagulant drugs by mouth can be reduced by using smaller doses and by monitoring their effects on the blood at regular intervals.

Risks in pregnancy

Oral anti-coagulants may damage the unborn baby, so they should not be used in the first 3 months of pregnancy. Nor should they be used in the last 4 weeks of pregnancy because they may cause bleeding in the baby (see earlier). Women of child-bearing age on long-term treatment should be aware of the risks of taking oral anti-coagulants if they get pregnant. If pregnancy occurs, oral anti-coagulants should be stopped immediately and heparin injections under the skin given instead. This method of treatment should be used until the end of the 16th week of pregnancy. The woman may then resume taking oral anti-coagulants until the 36th week and then go back on to heparin until after delivery of the baby. After delivery she can revert to oral anti-coagulants by mouth.

Risks in breast feeding

There is a risk that phenindione may cause bleeding in the baby, and it should not be used. Nicoumalone and warfarin appear to be safer but the baby should be give vitamin K_1. Heparin is safe because it is not excreted in breast milk.

Interaction with other drugs

Many drugs interact with oral anti-coagulants, and either increase or decrease their effects (see Chapter 89). You should always check to see whether any drug you are prescribed or about to purchase interferes with the action of the oral anti-coagulant you are taking.

A need for better education

The long-term use of oral anti-coagulants requires specialist supervision, the availability of hospital laboratory facilities and good education of both people taking the drugs and their nearest carer.

Always carry a treatment card with you

If you are taking an oral anti-coagulant drug you should carry a drug treatment card around with you at all times. This should include details of your drug treatment, laboratory test results, details of potential harmful effects, and detailed warnings and precautions on the use of the drug and on any other drugs that you may take.

Unfortunately, patients themselves are often the cause of failure of treatment or for problems with treatment. This is because they may fail to stick to the recommended doses and warnings. However, this may be the result of poor communication and education by the doctor and/or pharmacist and the lack of appropriate oral and written instructions about the treatment.

If you are taking oral anti-coagulants you should try to keep details each day of the doses you have taken, preferably by keeping a diary or a treatment calendar.

The use of anti-coagulants

To prevent thrombosis in veins

The main use of anti-coagulants is to prevent thrombosis from occurring in veins. They are also used to prevent the extension of a thrombus that has already developed.

There is an increased risk of people developing thrombi in the deep veins of the legs and pelvis if they are in bed, immobile and elderly, particularly if they are undergoing surgery, especially on hip joints, the womb or the prostate gland. Medical conditions such as severe heart failure, coronary thrombosis, cancer and being overweight also predispose to the risk of thrombosis. Individuals who have previously had a thrombus are at greater risk.

In order to prevent deep vein thrombosis and to prevent the risk of pulmonary embolism, injections of low doses of heparin under the skin are used as long as the patient is immobile. Dextran is an alternative to heparin in patients undergoing bone and joint surgery but in hip surgery it may be necessary to use anti-clotting drugs by mouth as well (e.g. warfarin).

There are additional non-drug treatments to prevent thrombosis; e.g. the use of inflatable 'stockings' which can be used to produce intermittent pulses of pressure on the muscles in the legs in order to keep the blood in the veins moving.

For patients undergoing heart surgery or kidney dialysis, heparin is used in full dosage during the procedures.

Treatment of thrombosis in veins

Thrombosis in a deep vein of the legs or pelvis is dangerous because of the risk of pulmonary embolism (see earlier). The aim of treatment is to prevent an extension of the thrombus, to prevent the thrombus spreading and closing off other veins, and to prevent pulmonary embolism. Treatment usually starts with heparin by continuous infusion into a vein, and an anti-coagulant drug (e.g. warfarin) is added by mouth on the same day or the next day. Heparin should be continued until laboratory tests show that an appropriate dose of the oral anti-coagulant has been reached. The oral anti-coagulant is then continued for 2–3 months before it is stopped.

Warning *The use of anti-coagulant drugs in someone who has developed a thrombus does not necessarily prevent a pulmonary embolism. They do not dissolve the thrombus, they only prevent it from extending and they prevent thrombosis in some other blood vessel. The body's own mechanisms will slowly dissolve the thrombus.*

Treatment of pulmonary embolism

Pulmonary embolism occurs when a piece of thrombus from a vein or the heart comes loose and travels in the bloodstream to lodge in one of the arteries of the lungs. It may block a main artery and produce sudden death or it may block a smaller artery and cause death of the lung tissue supplied by that blocked artery (pulmonary infarction). The individual develops severe pain in the chest, coughs up blood and becomes breathless. Treatment involves the use of intravenous heparin initially and then anti-coagulant drugs by mouth (e.g. warfarin). Treatment should continue for 6 weeks to 6 months, according to circumstances. An alternative treatment is to use drugs that dissolve the embolus (e.g. streptokinase or urokinase). This treatment certainly dissolves the embolus but we need more evidence that it actually increases the chances of survival.

Treatment of stroke

A stroke may occur if the blood supply to part of the brain is cut off due to a thrombus in one of its arteries. It may also occur if the blood vessel bursts and there is a haemorrhage into the brain tissue.

Thrombosis in an artery supplying the brain is usually associated with disease of the arteries in which fat deposits are laid down in the lining (atherosclerosis). The fatty deposits scar, ulcerate and narrow the arteries; this may lead to the development of a thrombus, resulting in a blockage of an artery and death of the brain tissue supplied by that artery (cerebral infarction).

There is an association between disease of the arteries supplying the brain and those supplying the heart (coronary arteries).

Little can be done to reverse the effects of a thrombus although, rarely, it may be removed surgically. Medical treatment is aimed at minimizing the extent of brain death. The use of drugs that improve the circulation (vasodilators) may do more harm than good because they may cause blood to be 'stolen' from the damaged part of the brain and diverted to the healthy parts.

Dextran solution in glucose into a vein every 12 hours for 3 days may help to reduce early death but it has no lasting benefit. It reduces the stickiness of the platelets.

Anti-coagulants have no place in the treatment of a stroke due to thrombosis, and thrombus-dissolving drugs have not been shown to be of benefit.

Treatment of coronary thrombosis (heart attack)

The treatment of coronary thrombosis is discussed in Chapter 20.

Preventing strokes

In patients who show signs that a stroke is actually developing, anti-coagulant drugs may stop the progression but treatment has to be long term and there is always a risk of producing a haemorrhage into the brain. Dextran is an example of a drug that may help to prevent a stroke developing but we need more evidence about its long-term effects.

Some people with disease of the arteries may experience transient attacks of reduced blood supply to parts of their brain, causing multiple infarcts that result in minor strokes. These individuals can be helped by taking one aspirin tablet daily. The aspirin helps to prevent thrombosis and will thus reduce the risk of further strokes.

Long-term use of anti-coagulants

Deep vein thrombosis

Treatment for deep vein thrombosis should be continued for at least 6 months whether the individual had a pulmonary embolism or not.

People who keep getting a deep vein thrombosis may need life-long treatment.

Atrial fibrillation

Individuals with atrial fibrillation due to narrowing of the mitral valve (mitral stenosis) are at risk of developing thrombosis in the left atrium of the heart; small pieces of the thrombus (emboli) may come loose and travel in the bloodstream to wedge in a small artery – causing, for example, a stroke. To prevent this thrombo-embolism they should be kept on an anti-coagulant for life. Anyone with atrial fibrillation due to other causes (e.g. over-active thyroid gland) should also be kept on long-term anti-coagulant treatment.

Artificial heart valves

People with artificial heart valves are usually kept on treatment because there is a risk of thrombosis and embolism. Tissue heart valves are less likely to cause trouble.

Table 26.1 Anti-coagulants – harmful effects and warnings

Injections

ancrod (Arvin)
Harmful effects include bleeding, allergic skin rash (nettle rash); some individuals who suffer from migraine may develop a headache after an injection; when given by catheter into a vein it may cause local swelling and redness at the injection site. A second or subsequent course of treatment may not work as well as the first in some people.

Warnings Ancrod should not be used in anyone with severe infections, coronary thrombosis, a low platelet count or a diffuse clotting in the blood. It should not be used in anyone with a bleeding disorder or who is being given dextrans to expand the blood volume. The first intravenous injection should not be given in less than 4 hours in order to avoid thickening the blood due to the accumulation of fibrin breakdown products. Its effect on breaking up fibrin may result in complications in people with damage to the blood vessels at the back of the eye caused by disorders such as a raised blood pressure or diabetes. Ancrod may cause bleeding, kidney pain and kidney stones in anyone with impaired kidney function. It may also cause problems in those who have had a stroke due to a brain haemorrhage or who have had an operation on their brain.

Anti-venom The antidote to ancrod may cause serious allergic reactions; therefore a test dose should be given. Full resuscitative treatment must be immediately to hand. Alternatives to anti-venom are fibrinogen or fresh-frozen plasma.

heparin
(For preparations, see Table 26.2)

Harmful effects include bleeding from various sites. Early signs of overdose include nose bleeds, red blood cells in the urine and bruising. Any underlying diseased organ (e.g. a stomach ulcer) may bleed and, rarely, local bleeding may cause serious problems; for example, bleeding into the adrenal glands may cause signs of acute adrenal failure. Injections may cause irritation at the site of injection with redness, pain, bruising and occasional ulceration. Allergic reactions may be generalized and include chills, fever, nettle rash and sometimes wheezing, runny nose, runny eyes, nausea and vomiting. Rarely, anaphylactic shock may occur. Itching and burning of the skin, especially on the soles of the feet, may also occur. A fall in blood platelets may occur which, very rarely, may result in the development of thromboses in blood vessels – producing death of patches of skin (necrosis), gangrene of the toes and fingers, heart attack or stroke. Long-term use of high doses of heparin may cause softening of bone (osteoporosis), loss of hair (alopecia), chronic erection of the penis (priapism), rebound rise in blood fat levels when the drug is stopped and, rarely, changes in liver function tests.

Warnings Heparin should not be used in anyone with a severe reduction in blood platelets or who is allergic to it (unless the condition is life threatening). It may be used only with extreme caution where there is a risk of bleeding and/or where bleeding could be a serious complication. It should also be used with extreme caution in patients with severe blood pressure or infection of the lining of the heart (endocarditis); during or just after surgery on the brain, spinal cord, eyes, major surgery, during spinal anaesthesia; in patients with bleeding disorders (e.g. haemophilia), stomach ulcers, duodenal ulcers, ulcerative colitis, severe liver disease affecting blood clotting, or during menstruation. Resistance to heparin may develop during a fever, following a heart attack (myocardial infarction), with certain cancers and following surgery. Blood platelets should be monitored at regular intervals.

heparin antidote Protamine sulphate injection may cause flushing, a fall in blood pressure and a slow heart rate. An overdose may interfere with blood clotting.

Table 26.1 Anti-coagulants – harmful effects and warnings (*cont.*)

By mouth (oral anti-coagulants)

nicoumalone (Sinthrome)
Harmful effects Rarely, it may cause nausea, loss of appetite, headache and giddiness. Like other anti-coagulants, it may, very rarely, cause patches of damage to the skin (necrosis), particularly after childbirth or the menopause.

Warnings Nicoumalone should not be used in people who suffer from haemophilia or any other disorder of bleeding, peptic ulcers, severe raised blood pressure, severe infection of the heart valves or severe liver failure. It should not be used during surgery (especially on the brain).

Risks in elderly people Harmful effects may be more frequent and severe; therefore use lower doses.

phenindione (Dindevan)
Harmful effects include skin rashes, patches of damage to the skin (necrosis) particularly after childbirth or the menopause, fever, reduction in the number of white blood cells in the blood, diarrhoea and, rarely, liver damage and kidney damage. The urine may be coloured pink or orange.

Warnings Phenindione should not be used in anyone suffering from kidney or liver damage, any disorder of bleeding or severe high blood pressure; nor should it be used within 24 hours of surgery or childbirth. The dose must be reduced if weight loss occurs, in acute illnesses, if kidney function is impaired, if intake of vitamin K in the diet is not adequate, or if the diet is low in fats and oils. Increased dose may be necessary if there is a gain in weight, stomach upsets (vomiting and/or diarrhoea), or increased vitamin K or fats and oils in the diet.

Risks in elderly people Harmful effects may be more frequent and severe; therefore use lower doses.

warfarin (Marevan, Warfarin WBP)
Harmful effects The main harmful effect is bleeding. Other harmful effects are uncommon but include skin rashes, loss of hair, and diarrhoea. Patches of damage to the skin (necrosis) may occur a few days after starting the treatment, particularly in overweight elderly women. Rarely, purple toes have been reported.

Warnings Warfarin must not be used in anyone with disorders of bleeding, peptic ulcers, severe high blood pressure, bacterial infection of the heart valves, severe kidney or liver disease, or within 24 hours of surgery or childbirth. The dose should be reduced if weight loss occurs, in acute illness, impaired kidney function, or if there is reduced intake of vitamin K or fats and oils in the diet. Increased dosage may be necessary if there is a gain in weight, stomach upsets (vomiting and/or diarrhoea), or increased intake of vitamin K, or fats and oils in the diet.

Risks in elderly people Harmful effects may be more frequent and severe; therefore use with caution.

Anti-platelet drugs

Platelets are small cells that circulate in the blood and contribute to the formation of a thrombus inside a blood vessel. They stick to each other and to the walls of the blood vessel and they also produce important substances that are involved in clotting. They are more involved in the formation of thrombi in arteries than in veins.

Table 26.2 Heparin injections: preparations

Preparation	*Drug*	*Preparation*	*Drug*
Calciparine	heparin calcium	Monoparin Calcium	heparin calcium
heparin injection	heparin sodium *or* heparin calcium	Multiparin	heparin sodium
		Pump-Hep	heparin sodium
Minihep	heparin sodium	Unihep	heparin sodium
Minihep Calcium	heparin calcium	Uniparin	heparin sodium
Monoparin	heparin sodium	Uniparin Calcium	heparin calcium

Table 26.3 Heparin flushes used to keep catheters and cannulae open

Preparation	*Drug*	*Dosage form*
Heparinised Saline	heparin sodium	Solution
Hep-Flush	heparin sodium	Solution
Hepsal	heparin sodium	Solution

Table 26.4 Heparin antidote

Preparation	*Drug*	*Dosage form*
protamine sulphate injection	protamine sulphate	Injection

Table 26.5 Anti-coagulant preparations

Preparation	*Drug*	*Dosage form*
Dindevan	phenindione	Tablets
Marevan	warfarin sodium	Tablets
Sinthrome	nicoumalone	Tablets
Warfarin WBP	warfarin sodium	Tablets

Drugs that prevent platelets from sticking together and from sticking to the walls of the blood vessels are referred to as anti-platelet drugs or anti-thrombotic drugs; they are used principally to prevent thrombi occurring in arteries and in the heart. This is because thrombi that develop in fast-flowing blood in arteries consist mainly of platelets enmeshed in layers of fibrin. Because a thrombus in a vein consists more of fibrin than of platelets, anti-platelet drugs have little effect and are not used to prevent thrombi in veins.

There are several anti-platelet drugs being used and/or tested at the present time; examples include aspirin, dipyridamole and epoprostenol.

Aspirin

Even though aspirin is excreted from the body within a few hours, a single dose can reduce the stickiness and clumping together of platelets, for the life of those platelets. This helps to prevent thrombosis occurring in blood vessels.

The use of aspirin following a heart attack is discussed in Chapter 20, and in preventing strokes in Chapter 26. Aspirin is also used to prevent thrombosis in people with artificial heart valves and in patients undergoing hip surgery.

Dipyridamole (Persantin)

Dipyridamole interferes with the stickiness of platelets. It is used with warfarin to prevent thrombosis in patients undergoing heart valve replacement; it is being tested in diabetic patients who have developed eye complications due to micro-thrombi in the small arteries of the eyes.

epoprostenol (prostacyclin, Flolan)

A naturally occurring prostaglandin produced by the lining of blood vessels. It is used to prevent clotting in heart–lung bypass surgery, kidney dialysis and liver dialysis. It is given alone or with heparin. It works for only a few minutes and has to be given by continuous infusion into a vein.

Table 26.6 Anti-platelet drugs – harmful effects and warnings

aspirin
See Chapter 27

epoprostenol
Harmful effects include flushing of the face, headache, nausea, vomiting, abdominal colic, jaw pain, dry mouth, lassitude, reddening over the site of infusion, chest pain and tightness in the chest, and a fall in blood pressure following intravenous injection.

Warnings Epoprostenol dilates arteries and causes flushing and a fall in blood pressure; these effects disappear within about half an hour of stopping the drug. Infusion may cause a rise in blood sugar.

dipyridamole (Persantin)
Harmful effects include dizziness, faintness, indigestion and diarrhoea. It produces dilatation of blood vessels and may cause a throbbing headache.

Warnings Dipyridamole should be used with caution in anyone with angina, or who has suffered a recent heart attack, or in people with blood-clotting defects. It may increase the effects of oral anti-coagulants. Antacids (in indigestion mixtures) may reduce its absorption from the intestine and reduce its effectiveness.

Drugs that dissolve thrombi

Drugs that dissolve thrombi are known as thrombolytic drugs. Those used most commonly dissolve fibrin in a thrombus and are referred to as fibrinolytics. They are discussed under the treatment of heart attack (Chapter 20).

The anabolic steriod, stanozolol, may have some effect in dissolving fibrin, and has been used to treat Raynaud's disease (see Chapter 24) complicated by scarring and narrowing of small arteries in which thrombosis may occur.

Anti-fibrinolytic drugs

An increase in the production of fibrin-dissolving substances (e.g. plasmin) may occur in the body in response to exercise, stress and drugs that produce adrenaline-like effects, but this is of no significance. However, the condition may be inherited and be associated with bleeding complications in childbirth. It may also occur and cause problems in certain cancers and in severe shock from bleeding.

Bleeding due to a localized dissolving of fibrin in thrombi may occur in surgery on the prostate gland or bladder, due to the presence of the fibrinolytic urokinase in the urine. Localized dissolving of a thrombus may also occur after a sub-arachnoid brain haemorrhage and should be considered as a possible cause of re-bleeding.

Tranexamic acid (Cyklokapron) acts as an antidote for an overdose of a thrombus-dissolving drug (fibrinolytic drug). It blocks the activation of plasminogen and blocks the action of plasmin which prevents the premature dissolving of a thrombus and helps to stop bleeding. It is also used in people who produce too much thrombus-dissolving chemicals themselves and run the risk of bleeding spontaneously. Tranexamic acid is useful for stopping bleeding after tooth extraction in a haemophiliac patient, to treat heavy menstrual periods, and to treat bleeding after surgical removal of the prostate gland and surgery on the bladder (see above). It may also be used to reduce bleeding caused by an intra-uterine contraceptive device which triggers bleeding due to fibrinolysis in some women.

Other drugs used to prevent bleeding

Aprotinin (Trasylol) inactivates plasmin and is used to prevent severe bleeding due to a rise in the blood level of plasmin in certain leukaemias and thrombolytic treatments.

Ethamsylate (Dicynene) is used to stop bleeding from very small blood vessels (capillaries). It blocks prostaglandins, improves the stickiness of platelets and affects the walls of capillaries. It may be used to treat heavy menstrual periods and bleeding caused by intra-uterine contraceptive devices. It is also used to prevent bleeding in low birth weight infants.

Vitamin K is necessary for the formation of blood-clotting factors (II and VII, IX and X). Its deficiency may occur in certain disorders of the intestine that interfere with the absorption of vitamin K, which is soluble in fat. Deficiency may also occur in liver disease and diseases of the gall bladder. These disorders are treated with a vitamin K preparation that dissolves in water and does not rely on fat for its absorption; menadiol sodium phosphate (Synkavit) is used for this purpose.

Newborn babies may develop a deficiency of vitamin K because their intestines lack the bacteria that normally manufacture vitamin K in the intestine. This deficiency is treated with phytomenadione (vitamin K_1, Konakion) by intramuscular injection.

Overdose of oral anti-coagulants that block the use of vitamin K in the production of blood-clotting factors in the liver is treated with vitamin K.

Table 26.7 Fibrinolytic drugs – harmful effects and warnings

alteplase (Actilyse)
Used to dissolve the thrombus in someone who has had a coronary thrombosis (see Chapter 20). An initial dose is given by intravenous injection over 1–2 minutes followed by a slow infusion over 3 hours.

Harmful effects include nausea, vomiting and bleeding (may be localized or, rarely, into the brain) and, rarely, disorders of heart rhythm during infusion.

Warnings Alteplase should not be used in anyone suffering from diseases of the arteries that supply the brain (e.g. stroke), uncontrolled hypertension, bleeding disorders, an active peptic ulcer, acute pancreatitis or severe liver disease, within 10 days of bleeding from whatever cause, or within 10 days of surgery or injury. It must be used with caution in people with diabetes or severe impairment of kidney function.

anistreplase (Eminase)
Used to dissolve the thrombus in someone who has had a coronary thrombosis (see Chapter 20). It is given by a single slow intravenous injection over 4–5 minutes.

Harmful effects include bleeding, flushing, slowness of the heart rate, fall in blood pressure, nausea, vomiting, fever and allergic reactions.

Warnings Anistreplase should not be used within 10 days of surgery or injury, nor in anyone with active peptic ulcers, stroke, severe hypertension or a brain tumour. It must be used with caution in people with embolic disorders or disorders of heart rhythm. Do not repeat the treatment within 6 months.

streptokinase (Kabikinase, Streptase)
Used to dissolve the thrombus in someone who has had a coronary thrombosis (see Chapter 20). It is given by a single intravenous infusion over 3 hours. It is also used to treat deep vein thrombosis, pulmonary embolism, thrombo-embolism and thrombosis in arteries in the arms or legs or the eyes.

Harmful effects include a rise in temperature; allergic reactions may occur and be mild (e.g. nettle rash) or, very rarely, they may be severe (e.g. anaphylaxis). These reactions can be

Table 26.7 Fibrinolytic drugs – harmful effects and warnings (*cont.*)

controlled by prior treatment with a corticosteroid (e.g. prednisolone by mouth). Oozing of blood may occur at the site of injection; rarely, bleeding may occur.

Warnings Streptokinase should not be used in anyone who has had an allergic reaction to streptokinase on recent treatment (more than 5 days and less than 3 months), nor in people who have had surgery or severe injury in the past 10 days, a recent streptococcal sore throat, bleeding from the stomach or intestines in the past 6 months, disorders of blood clotting, liver or kidney disease, arteriosclerosis, a stroke due to a brain haemorrhage, severe raised blood pressure, ulcerative colitis, severe bronchitis, diabetes, recent abortion or childbirth, cancer of an internal organ, or during a heavy menstrual period. It should be used with caution in someone with auricular fibrillation or mitral valve disease.

Risks in elderly people The risk of a stroke from a brain haemorrhage is increased in elderly people; therefore use with caution.

urokinase (Ukidan)
Used to treat thrombosis in the blood vessels of the eyes and to remove clots from dialysis machines and blood shunts.

Harmful effects include bleeding and fever.

Warnings Urokinase should not be used if there has been recent bleeding or surgery or needle biopsy in the previous 72 hours.

Table 26.8 Anti-fibrinolytic preparations

Preparation	*Drug*	*Dosage form*
Cyklokapron	tranexamic acid	Tablets, syrup, injection
Dicynene	ethamsylate	Tablets, injection
Trasylol	aprotinin	Injection

Table 26.9 Anti-fibrinolytic drugs – harmful effects and warnings

aprotinin (Trasylol)
Harmful effects include allergic reactions.

tranexamic acid (Cyklokapron)
Harmful effects include nausea, vomiting, diarrhoea and giddiness after too rapid an injection into a vein.

Warnings Tranexamic acid should be used with caution: in anyone with impaired kidney function – reduced doses should be given according to the results of kidney function tests; in someone bleeding from the kidneys (e.g. in haemophilia) because obstruction to the ureters may occur; in individuals who have recently had a thrombosis.

Other drugs used to stop bleeding
ethamyslate (Dicynene)

Harmful effects include nausea, headache, skin rash, transient fall in blood pressure following intravenous injection.

Table 26.10 Vitamin K preparations – harmful effects and warnings

menadiol (Synkavit)	phytomenadione (vitamin K_1, Konakion)
Harmful effects include damage to the red blood cells (haemolytic anaemia) which may cause excessive bile pigment in the blood, which may in turn damage the brain in newborn babies. This damage to red blood cells (haemolysis) may occur if there is a deficiency of glucose-6-phosphate dehydrogenase in the red blood cells or low levels of alpha-tocopherol in the blood. *Warnings* Menadiol must not be used in newborn babies, especially if premature, nor just before, during or after childbirth. Use vitamin K_1 (Konakion) instead. *Risks in pregnancy* Use with caution in first 6 months. If used at the end of pregnancy, there is a risk of haemolysis and jaundice in the newborn baby (kernicterus).	*Harmful effects* include flushing of the face, sweating, allergic reactions, tightness in the chest and blue coloration of the skin and lining of the mouth. Collapse of the circulation may occur if given too quickly in too large a dose into a vein. Damage to the skin and tissues at the site of intravenous injections may occur with regular use in people with impaired liver function. Some individuals may be severely allergic to a castor oil derivative in the preparation. *Warnings* Phytomenadione should not be used in people who are allergic to it. Intravenous injections should be given slowly. *Risks in elderly people* Harmful effects may be more frequent and severe; therefore use lower doses.

27

Pain

We all experience pain at some time or another, and each of us varies in the amount of pain we can tolerate. Severe, continuous or unusual pain needs explaining and relief. If we have sprained an ankle, we can understand the cause of the pain and it is reasonable to take a pain reliever. But all too often we take pain relievers for pain, particularly headaches, without attempting to identify the cause. Pain is only a symptom, and therefore you should always try to determine the cause. If you have toothache, do not just take pain relievers – go to your dentist. If you get recurrent headaches try to think what brings them on – noise, smoking, worry, something in the diet, and so on. Very often pain produces fear and anxiety – somebody with chest pain may worry that he has a bad heart and somebody with headache may worry about a brain tumour. If you have a pain that is continuous or unusual for you or if you find yourself becoming anxious or worrying about a pain, these are sufficient reasons to consult your doctor.

We have much to learn about the relationships between the mind and the body when it comes to understanding pain. The feeling of pain is not just the pain itself, we actually 'suffer' from pain, and how much we suffer depends on many factors – particularly our mood (whether we are anxious or depressed), our fears (e.g. fear about what is causing the pain, fear of losing our job, fear of death), and our beliefs (e.g. in the treatment, in the future and our religious belief).

The mechanisms of pain

Nerve endings, highly sensitive to pain, are widely distributed throughout various tissues of the body. These respond to pressure or stretching that produces the sensation of pain. They are also very sensitive to chemicals released in response to injury and inflammation.

The area of pain can usually be identified. For example, *superficial pain* is felt in or just beneath the skin or on the surface of the mouth or the gullet (oesophagus). *Intermediate pain* is felt in muscles, ligaments, bones or joints, and *deep pain* is felt in an internal organ, such as the stomach or bowels.

The relief of these various types of pain need not necessarily rely on pain-relieving drugs – cold water applied to a skin burn may relieve the pain, heat or massage may relieve muscle pain, and an alkali mixture may relieve the pain of a duodenal ulcer. It must be obvious, therefore, that the best way to treat pain is to attempt to relieve the underlying cause.

Acute pain means that tissue damage has occurred. It has a protective function – it warns you that something is wrong. It is therefore most unwise to take something to relieve the pain and then to put that injured tissue back under stress. For example, it may be harmful for an injured footballer to receive a pain-relieving injection for acute pain due to an injury caused on the field. This will mask the pain and could easily allow further injury to occur without the footballer knowing until later, when the effect of the pain injection has worn off.

Warning *Permanent, long-term injury may be caused to muscles, ligaments and joints by relieving the pain at the time of first or subsequent injury and then proceeding to put that injured tissue under further stress.*

Chronic pain is quite a different matter and may be associated with continuing damage to the affected tissue; for example, joint damage in arthritis, or pain from a tumour that continues to grow and put pressure on surrounding tissues. Also, chronic pain is often associated with anxiety or depression and disturbance of sleep. Treatment of chronic pain is not therefore just a matter of giving a pain reliever. The whole person needs treating in terms of his or her physical, emotional, social and spiritual needs. In addition to the use of pain relievers, complementary treatments for pain relief should be considered: for example, surgery, radiotherapy and/or anti-cancer drugs for pain from cancer; the relief of underlying inflammation with corticosteroid drugs or anti-inflammatory drugs; blocking with a local anaesthetic or cutting the nerves that supply an affected painful area; or applying electrical nerve stimulation through the skin (transcutaneous electrical nerve stimulation, TENS) which may break the passage of pain impulses up the spinal cord to the brain where they are 'felt'. Acupuncture may work in a similar way and also stimulate release of the body's own pain relievers (e.g. endorphins). Other possibilities include hypnosis, behaviour therapy and psychiatric treatment.

Pain-relieving drugs

Drugs that depress the functions of the brain to produce stupor and sleep are called narcotics. The term covers general anaesthetics, sleeping drugs and morphine-related drugs, but is usually used to describe morphine-related drugs. *Narcotic pain relievers* refer to morphine-related drugs. Aspirin, paracetamol, anti-inflammatory drugs used to relieve pain (e.g. ibuprofen), benorylate and nefopam are *non-narcotic pain relievers*. These terms serve no real purpose except to highlight the important difference between the two groups in that morphine-related pain relievers produce addiction whereas aspirin, paracetamol etc. do not.

Morphine and several related pain relievers are obtained from opium and they used to be called opiates. However, an increasing number of morphine-like pain-relieving drugs have been synthesized in recent years and therefore the term 'opioid' has been introduced to refer to all drugs with morphine-like actions whether derived from opium or not. The term 'opioid' is also used to describe drugs that oppose the actions of morphine-like drugs in the body, some of which also relieve pain (see later). The terms 'narcotic pain relievers' and 'opioid pain relievers' refer to the same group of drugs.

Non-narcotic pain relievers

Anti-inflammatory drugs (see Chapter 30) relieve the pain of inflammation. They act locally to block the production of chemicals such as prostaglandins that cause inflammation. There are many anti-inflammatory pain relievers on the market and they are frequently used to relieve pain and inflammation affecting muscles, ligaments, bones and joints.

Aspirin is used to relieve mild pain (e.g. headache). It is also an effective anti-inflammatory drug (Chapter 30) that is used extensively to treat rheumatic disorders.

Paracetamol is a mild pain reliever that has no anti-inflammatory properties and does not appear to act locally at the site of injury or inflammation. It is thought to act on the brain and nervous system by blocking prostaglandin production.

Nefopam is a mild to moderate pain reliever that is related to morphine and produces no anti-inflammatory effects.

Narcotic pain relievers

In response to pain, the body produces substances called opiopeptins (e.g. endorphins and enkephalins), which lessen the perception of pain by acting on special receptors (opioid receptors) in the brain, spinal cord, gut and elsewhere. Narcotic pain relievers act on these receptors.

Narcotic pain relievers vary widely in their potency. Codeine and dextropropoxyphene are mild pain relievers, and are discussed in the section or mild pain relievers. Morphine, methadone and other narcotics are much stronger and are used to treat severe pain, and are discussed under the section 'Narcotic pain relievers used to treat moderate to severe pain'.

Testing the effectiveness of pain relievers

Numerous factors make us feel pain more at one time than at another. We feel pain much more if we are tense, anxious, worried or depressed, and of course the reverse applies too. For these reasons, the testing of pain relievers in animals and on volunteer 'patients' under laboratory conditions often gives no real indication of the pain-relieving potential of a drug on 'real' patients in pain.

We all vary in our response to pain-relieving drugs, and about two in five of us will get relief of pain from placebo (dummy) tablets or injections. This is an interesting phenomenon but the placebo effect soon wears off with repeated doses of dummy drugs. A pain-relieving drug must therefore be tested on people suffering from pain. Narcotic pain relievers are usually tested on post-operative pain after abdominal surgery, and anti-inflammatory drugs are tested on rheumatic or arthritic pain.

Drugs used to relieve mild to moderate pain

Mild to moderate pains include simple headache, toothache, muscle pains, joint pains and painful menstrual periods. The drugs used to treat mild to moderate pain include aspirin and other anti-inflammatory drugs (e.g. ibuprofen), paracetamol, benorylate and nefopam and the narcotic pain relievers codeine and dextropropoxyphene.

Non-narcotic pain relievers

Aspirin

Aspirin is acetylsalicylic acid and belongs to a group of drugs known as the salicylates. It relieves mild to moderate pain, brings down a raised temperature (anti-pyretic effect) and relieves inflammation. In addition, it has many other complex effects on the body. It reduces the stickiness of platelets and in high doses it can interfere with blood clotting. Aspirin can affect the excretion of uric acid by the kidneys, increase the blood sugar, stimulate breathing, increase the burning up of oxygen by cells in the body, and make the blood acidic.

Its anti-infammatory and anti-pyretic effects are due to its ability to block the production of certain chemicals (e.g. prostaglandins) that are responsible, among many other actions, for producing inflammation when a tissue is injured. The blocking effect of aspirin on inflammation-producing chemicals may also contribute to its pain-relieving properties because it may make nerve endings less sensitive to these chemicals. It may also have some effects in the brain and reduce the perception of pain.

Aspirin relieves mild to moderate pain, and because of its anti-inflammatory actions it is particularly effective against pain associated with inflammation (e.g. muscle and joint pain). Aspirin is effective against toothache and headache but not against internal pain (e.g. bowel pain). Aspirin is also effective for relieving pain in other conditions thought to be associated with the release of prostaglandins; for example migraine and vascular headaches and painful menstrual periods. Taken regularly every day, aspirin can also relieve the pain and inflammation of rheumatoid arthritis (see Chapter 30).

NOTE Aspirin relieves the symptoms of inflammation but it does *not* cure the underlying cause.

Aspirin causes bleeding from the stomach The most common harmful effects produced by aspirin are nausea and indigestion. It may also cause vomiting. Damage to the lining of the stomach, producing ulceration and bleeding, is common. Very slight blood loss occurs in many people who take aspirin. It is worse with high regular doses. There may be no warning of the bleeding because the individual may not experience any symptoms. Taking alcohol along with aspirin may increase the risk of bleeding, and a significant proportion of people admitted as emergencies to hospital suffering from vomiting blood have taken alcohol and aspirin together.

Regular daily use of aspirin over several weeks or months may cause a sufficient loss of blood from the damaged lining of the stomach to produce a deficiency of iron, leading to anaemia. This can be particularly harmful in elderly people who may not be on a nutritious diet containing sufficient iron for their normal needs, in women who have heavy periods, and in debilitated patients who may already be anaemic.

Aspirin erodes the lining of the stomach, leading to bleeding because it directly damages the normally protective surface. This damage allows the acid in the stomach to attack the cells underneath the surface. This damage is probably due to aspirin's ability to block the production of chemicals (e.g. prostaglandins) that normally stimulate the production of mucus in the stomach. This mucus provides a natural protective coating to the surface of the stomach, and if its production is blocked the surface of the stomach will not be as well protected against acid attack.

Aspirin may also cause existing ulcers to bleed, so it should be avoided by anyone who has an active peptic ulcer of the oesophagus, stomach or duodenum. Aspirin and non-steroidal anti-inflammatory drugs are an important cause of bleeding ulcers in the elderly, and for this reason they should be used with utmost caution in people over 65 years of age.

Aspirin and the nervous system In high doses, aspirin may produce noises in the ears (tinnitus), dizziness, deafness, sweating, nausea, vomiting, headache and mental confusion. This is referred to as 'salicylism' and clears up if the dose of aspirin is reduced or stopped. Very high doses may affect the breathing centre in the brain, producing rapid breathing which may alter the acidity of the blood.

Allergy to aspirin Some people are allergic to aspirin, particularly if they suffer from asthma or drug allergies. It may cause wheezing, angioedema and urticaria (nettle rash). Rarely, an acute allergy to aspirin may produce a rapid fall in blood pressure and collapse. Some individuals may develop a reaction to aspirin over time, and develop a blocked and running nose (see page 68).

Warnings *Deaths from aspirin and related drugs have, albeit very rarely, occurred due to severe attacks of wheezing and breathlessness, particularly in people who already suffered from asthma.*

Anyone allergic to aspirin may also be cross-allergic to tartrazine (an orange dye used to colour medicines, foods and drinks) and to other non-steroidal anti-inflammatory drugs (NSAIDs) used to treat rheumatoid arthritis and related disorders (see Table 30.1).

Aspirin and bleeding Aspirin affects several of the processes involved in blood clotting and may produce bleeding. It should not be used by anyone who suffers from haemophilia or who is taking anti-blood-clotting drugs.

Avoid using aspirin in children Aspirin should not be given to children under the age of 12 years who are suffering from an acute viral infection (e.g. influenza, chickenpox). This is because there is a rare risk of producing brain and liver damage, resulting in severe vomiting, impaired consciousness, delirium and coma (Reye's syndrome). This is a severe complication: 50 per cent of those affected die and some survivors have brain damage. Reye's syndrome may also occur in teenagers treated with aspirin for acute viral infections.

Other harmful effects of aspirin Aspirin in a daily dose of 2 g or less usually decreases the excretion of uric acid in the urine and increases the blood uric acid level, whereas with doses greater than 4 g daily it increases the excretion of uric acid in the urine and decreases the blood uric acid level. (See Chapter 32 for a discussion on the treatment of gout.)

Aspirin may, very rarely, cause liver damage, especially in people with rheumatoid arthritis.

Aspirin may reduce the output of urine from the kidneys in people with kidney disease. Very rarely, this may occur in someone with normal functioning kidneys.

Aspirin is not a harmless homely remedy Aspirin is an effective drug for relieving mild to moderate pain, particularly if it is due to inflammation. But it is not a harmless homely remedy and it should be used like any other effective drug – sensibly and with caution. It should be kept out of reach of children, preferably in a child-proof container. Hundreds of people (particularly children) are accidentally or intentionally overdosed every year and some of them die.

Preventing damage to the stomach It may help to prevent aspirin from damaging the lining of the stomach if it is not taken on an empty stomach. Take it after food, with a large drink of fluid other than alcohol. If aspirin has to be taken regularly every day, special aspirin preparations aimed at reducing damage to the stomach are available (see Chapter 30).

Other non-steroidal anti-inflammatory drugs (NSAIDS)

Other anti-inflammatory drugs used to relieve mild to moderate pain are discussed in Chapter 30.

Warning *Any benefit obtained from the use of non-steroidal anti-inflammatory drugs to relieve mild to moderate pain must be balanced against the risk of damaging the lining of the stomach, producing ulceration and bleeding, and against the risk of allergy, particularly in patients who are allergic to aspirin and/or who suffer from asthma.*

Table 27.1 Aspirin – harmful effects and warnings

Harmful effects include stomach upsets, nausea, indigestion, vomiting, irritation of the lining of the stomach producing ulcers and bleeding, iron deficiency anaemia due to chronic loss of blood, allergic reactions (nettle rash, skin rashes, wheezing, angioedema, runny nose and, occasionally, death from a severe attack of wheezing and breathlessness) and interference with blood clotting mechanisms. Repeated, large doses of aspirin produce salicylism – dizziness, noises in the ears, deafness, sweating, nausea, vomiting, headache and mental confusion. Symptoms from higher doses include over-breathing, fever and

Table 27.1 Aspirin – harmful effects and warnings (*cont.*)

restlessness. Aspirin may, rarely, damage the liver and cause Reye's syndrome (see earlier).

Warnings Do not use aspirin if you suffer from peptic ulcers (e.g. stomach or duodenal ulcers) or chronic indigestion, haemophilia or other bleeding disorder, if you are allergic and/or develop asthma to aspirin or some other non-steroidal anti-inflammatory drug, or if you are taking anti-coagulant drugs. Do not give aspirin to children under the age of 12 years.

Use with caution if you have impaired kidney or liver function – take a smaller dose – or if you suffer from asthma or other wheezing disorder, nasal polyps, vasomotor rhinitis or gout. Buffered aspirin and effervescent preparations are high in sodium; do not take any of these if you are being treated for heart disease or raised blood pressure and/or if you are on a salt-restricted diet.

Risks in elderly people Harmful effects may be more frequent and severe; therefore use with caution. Aspirin in the elderly is likely to cause hidden bleeding in the stomach; therefore watch for blood in the stools, which produces a colour like tar.

Risks with alcohol There is an increased risk of damage to the stomach lining, producing ulceration and bleeding.

Paracetamol

Paracetamol is thought to work principally by reducing prostaglandin production in the brain. It is an effective mild to moderate pain reliever; it also brings down a raised temperature.

As a pain reliever, paracetamol is a suitable alternative to aspirin. However, it is not effective in reducing the symptoms of inflammation, so is of less value in those conditions where the pain is caused by inflammation (e.g. muscle and joint pains) and other conditions, such as painful menstrual periods, where pain is thought to be due to the release of inflammatory chemicals (e.g. prostaglandins).

Dangers of overdose with paracetamol Acute overdose of paracetamol is dangerous because the individual may appear to be improving for 2–3 days and then goes into liver failure and dies. Acute kidney damage may occasionally occur following overdose.

Paracetamol is not a harmless homely remedy Paracetamol is useful for relieving mild to moderate pain. It is widely used as a homely remedy but, like any other drug, it should be used with respect. It should be kept out of reach of children, preferably in child-proof containers. There are now more overdose problems from paracetamol in children than from aspirin.

Table 27.2 Examples of non-steroidal anti-inflammatory drugs (NSAIDs) used to relieve mild to moderate pain

Preparation	*Drug*	*Dosage form*
Apsifen	ibuprofen	Tablets
Brufen	ibuprofen	Tablets, syrup
Dolobid	diflunisal	Tablets
Ebufac	ibuprofen	Tablets
Femafen	ibuprofen	Sustained-release capsules
Fenbid	ibuprofen	Sustained-release capsules
Fenopron	fenoprofen	Tablets
Ibular	ibuprofen	Tablets
Ibumetin	ibuprofen	Tablets
ibuprofen	ibuprofen	Tablets
Inabrin	ibuprofen	Tablets
Laraflex	naproxen	Tablets
Librofem	ibuprofen	Tablets
Lidifen	ibuprofen	Tablets
Maxagesic	ibuprofen	Tablets
mefenamic acid	mefenamic acid	Capsules
Migrafen	ibuprofen	Tablets
Motrin	ibuprofen	Tablets
Naprosyn	naproxen	Tablets, suspension, granules, suppositories
naproxen	naproxen	Tablets
Novaprin	ibuprofen	Tablets
Nurofen	ibuprofen	Tablets
Pacifene	ibuprofen	Tablets
Paxofen	ibuprofen	Tablets
Ponstan	mefenamic acid	Tablets, dispersible tablets, capsules, paediatric suspension
Proflex	ibuprofen	Sustained-release capsules
Progesic	fenoprofen	Tablets
Relcofen	ibuprofen	Tablets
Seclodin	ibuprofen	Capsules
Suspren	ibuprofen	Sustained-release capsules
Synflex	naproxen	Tablets

Table 27.3 Paracetamol – harmful effects and warnings

Harmful effects are very rare; they include skin rashes and other allergic reactions, and blood disorders.

Warnings Paracetamol should not be taken by anyone who is allergic to it. It should be used with caution in people who have chronic malnutrition, impaired kidney function or whose liver function is impaired particularly by alcohol or drugs (e.g. barbiturates).

Benorylate – an aspirin–paracetamol compound

Benorylate is a compound of aspirin and paracetamol which, once it is absorbed into the bloodstream, is taken to the liver where it is split into aspirin and paracetamol. It thus acts as a mild to moderate pain reliever. Because it contains aspirin, it also relieves inflammation and may be used to treat rheumatic disorders and painful menstrual periods.

Because it contains aspirin it should not be given to children under 12 years of age and the dose should be reduced in elderly people. *Harmful effects and warnings* listed under aspirin and paracetamol apply to benorylate. If you are taking benorylate, do not take any other pain reliever that contains aspirin or paracetamol.

Nefopam

Nefopam (Acupan) is an effective mild to moderate pain reliever. It is not a morphine-related drug nor is it an anti-inflammatory drug like aspirin.

Harmful effects include nausea, vomiting, blurred vision, drowsiness, sweating, insomnia, headache and rapid beating of the heart. It may, very rarely, cause confusion and hallucinations.

Warnings Nefopam should not be used in anyone with a history of convulsions nor as a pain reliever by someone who has had a heart attack. It should be used with caution in people with impaired kidney or liver function. Harmful effects may be more frequent and severe in the elderly, so it should be used with caution. Information on its safety in children is not available, so do not use it in children under 12 years of age. Some individuals may experience difficulty in passing urine.

Narcotic pain relievers used to relieve mild to moderate pain

There is a gap between such drugs as aspirin, ibuprofen and paracetamol that are effective in relieving mild to moderate pain and those narcotic pain relievers that are effective against moderate to severe pain. This gap is inadequately filled by a group of narcotic pain relievers that are less powerful than morphine. Two drugs from this group are frequently used to relieve mild to moderate pain. They are *codeine* and *dextropropoxyphene*. Each is used more often in combination with aspirin or paracetamol than on its own (see Tables 27.5–27.6). They act on specific receptors in the brain and nervous system, which are part of the body's own pain control system (see earlier).

The *addition of aspirin* to preparations containing codeine or dextropropoxyphene increases the risks of taking such a preparation regularly every day because the aspirin may produce damage to the stomach lining and cause bleeding (see earlier).

The *addition of paracetamol* to preparations containing codeine or dextropropoxyphene may cause problems if one of these combined preparations is taken in overdose.

Risk of addiction to codeine and dextropropoxyphene

Codeine and dextropropoxyphene are morphine-related drugs and preparations containing them should not be treated as simple homely remedies. They should not be taken regularly every day for more than 2 weeks without strict medical supervision. They may give you a lift in mood (euphoria), and because of this effect you may begin to rely on them to 'get you through' the day. If you continue taking them regularly every day you may become dependent on them. This means that you will find yourself in a position of having to go on taking the drugs every day because of the 'let down' feelings you get if you try to stop taking them. It is possible to become physically dependent on these drugs, such that you will develop unpleasant withdrawal symptoms if you stop them suddenly. These are similar to the symptoms produced by the withdrawal of morphine (see later).

Dihydrocodeine relieves moderate to severe pains; it is discussed later.

Pentazocine (*Fortral*) is also discussed later. It is a narcotic pain reliever that relieves moderate pain when taken by mouth and severe pain when given by injection. It acts like morphine and yet can block the action of morphine. When taken by mouth it is absorbed into the bloodstream and taken straight to the liver, where much of it is broken down. This is why it is only effective against moderate pain when taken by mouth. When given by injection it avoids this first pass through the liver and is as effective as morphine.

Table 27.4 Codeine and dextropropoxyphene – harmful effects and warnings

Harmful effects
Codeine may cause constipation, nausea, vomiting, dizziness, drowsiness, difficulty in passing urine, flushed face and tiredness. Very rarely, it may produce a skin rash in people allergic to codeine and sometimes sensitivity of the skin to sunlight.

Dextropropoxyphene may cause dizziness, drowsiness, nausea, vomiting, constipation, abdominal pain, tiredness, headache, a feeling of extreme well-being (euphoria), insomnia, visual disturbances and skin rashes. High daily doses (above 720 mg) may produce delusions, hallucinations, confusion and convulsions. It may, rarely, cause liver damage.

Warnings Codeine and dextropropoxyphene are related to morphine and are potential drugs of addiction (see earlier). Anyone allergic to these drugs should not take any preparation that contains them. They should be used with caution in people with impaired kidney function.

Risks in elderly people Harmful effects such as constipation, drowsiness and dizziness may be more of a problem in elderly

Table 27.4 Codeine and dextropropoxyphene – harmful effects and warnings (*cont.*)

people; therefore their regular daily use should be avoided.

Risks in driving Because codeine and dextropropoxyphene may produce dizziness and drowsiness, you should not drive until you know that it is safe to do so. See additional dangers when taken with alcohol and other drugs below.

Risks with alcohol Codeine and dextropropoxyphene increase the effects of alcohol. You should not drink alcohol while taking any preparation that contains codeine or dextropropoxyphene.

Combined preparations of non-narcotic and narcotic drugs used to treat mild to moderate pain

Pain-relieving preparations that contain a narcotic pain reliever (e.g. codeine, dextropropoxyphene) combined with a drug such as paracetamol or aspirin are very popular, although there is little convincing evidence from adequate and well controlled studies that they are more effective than an appropriate dose of one of the drugs on its own.

Their popularity may be due to the users' reliance on a daily dose of codeine or dextropropoxyphene which gives them a 'lift'. This may possibly explain why they are considered by some individuals to be more effective at relieving mild to moderate pain than aspirin or paracetamol used separately.

Dihydrocodeine (DF 118, DHC Continus) relieves moderate to severe pain. It is included in a small dose combined with paracetamol in Co-dydramol (Paramol).

Pentazocine (Fortral) when taken by mouth relieves moderate pain, and is combined with paracetamol in Fortagesic.

Risks of long-term use of combined pain relievers

The daily use of combined pain relievers over several years has been associated with addiction (see above) and with kidney damage. The mechanisms by which these preparations cause kidney damage (analgesic nephropathy) is not understood. It has been associated with the use of phenacetin in these mixtures. Phenacetin was included in combined pain relievers up to the late sixties, when it was considered to be the cause of kidney damage and taken off the market in many countries. However, the position is still unclear and the best advice is not to take any combined pain reliever regularly every day for more than a week or two without medical advice.

Both dihydrocodeine and pentazocine are more powerful pain relievers than codeine and dextropropoxyphene, and the warnings on potential harmful effects and the risks of addiction with long-term use apply equally to combined preparations that contain either one of these drugs.

The possible problems of adding caffeine to pain relievers

Several combined pain relievers have caffeine added. This may cause an additional problem because caffeine lifts mood and some individuals may feel a need to take them regularly every day. What is more, when they stop they may get a caffeine-withdrawal headache, which convinces them that they really need the pain reliever. There is no convincing evidence that including caffeine in pain-relieving preparations increases their ability to relieve pain. It may, however, increase the damaging effects of aspirin on the lining of the stomach.

Table 27.5 Combined aspirin preparations

Preparation	*Drug*	*Dosage form*
Actron	aspirin, paracetamol, caffeine, citric acid, sodium bicarbonate	Effervescent tablets
Alka-Seltzer	aspirin, citric acid, sodium bicarbonate	Effervescent tablets
Anadin Maximum Strength Capsules	aspirin, caffeine	Capsules
Anadin Soluble Tablets	aspirin, caffeine	Effervescent tablets
Anadin Tablets	aspirin, caffeine, quinine sulphate	Tablets
Antoin	aspirin, codeine, caffeine	Dispersible tablets
Askit	aspirin, caffeine, aloxiprin, aluminium glycinate	Tablets, powders
Aspav	aspirin, papaveretum	Dispersible tablets
aspirin, paracetamol and codeine tablets	aspirin, paracetamol, codeine	Tablets
Beecham's Powders	aspirin, caffeine	Powders
Beecham's Powders Tablets	aspirin, caffeine	Tablets
Co-codaprin	aspirin, codeine	Tablets
Co-codaprin Dispersible	aspirin, codeine	Soluble tablets
Codis	aspirin, codeine	Soluble tablets
Cojene	aspirin, codeine, caffeine	Tablets
Doloxene Co	aspirin, caffeine, dextropropoxyphene	Capsules

Table 27.5 Combined aspirin preparations (*cont.*)

Preparation	*Drug*	*Dosage form*
Equagesic	aspirin, meprobamate, ethoheptazine	Three-layer tablets
Fynnon Calcium Aspirin	aspirin, calcium carbonate	Tablets
Hypon	aspirin, caffeine, codeine	Tablets
Migravess and Migravess Forte	aspirin, metoclopramide	Effervescent tablets
Mrs Cullen's Powders	aspirin, caffeine calcium phosphate, saccharin, sodium lauryl sulphate	Powders
Nurse Sykes Powders	aspirin, paracetamol, caffeine, light kaolin	Powders
Phensic	aspirin, caffeine	Tablets
Powerin	aspirin, paracetamol, caffeine	Tablets
Robaxisal Forte	aspirin, methocarbamol	Tablets
Veganin	aspirin, paracetamol, codeine	Tablets

Table 27.6 Drugs used to treat mild to moderate pain: combined paracetamol preparations

Preparation	*Drug*	*Dosage form*
Cafadol	paracetamol, caffeine	Tablets
Co-codamol	paracetamol, codeine	Tablets, dispersible tablets
Codanin	paracetamol, codeine	Tablets
Co-dydramol	paracetamol, dihydrocodeine	Tablets
Co-proxamol	paracetamol, dextropropoxyphene	Tablets
Cosalgesic	paracetamol, dextropropoxyphene (co-proxamol)	Tablets
DeWitt's Analgesic Pills	paracetamol, caffeine	Tablets
Distalgesic	paracetamol, dextropropoxyphene (co-proxamol)	Tablets

Table 27.6 Drugs used to treat mild to moderate pain: combined paracetamol preparations (*cont.*)

Preparation	*Drug*	*Dosage form*
Doan's Backache Pills (Extra Strength)	paracetamol, sodium salicylate	Tablets
Femerital	paracetamol, ambucetamide	Tablets
Fenning's Adult Cooling Powders	paracetamol, caffeine	Powders
Lobak	paracetamol, chlormezanone	Tablets
Medised	paracetamol, promethazine	Tablets, suspension
Migraleve	paracetamol, codeine, buclizine	Tablets
Panadeine	paracetamol, codeine	Tablets
Paracodol	paracetamol, codeine	Effervescent tablets, capsules
Paradeine	paracetamol, codeine, phenolphthalein	Tablets
Parahypon	paracetamol, codeine, caffeine	Tablets
Parake	paracetamol, codeine	Tablets
Paralgin	paracetamol, caffeine, codeine	Tablets
Paramol	paracetamol, dihydrocodeine (co-dydramol)	Tablets
Pardale	paracetamol, codeine, caffeine	Tablets
Paxalgesic	paracetamol, dextropropoxyphene (co-proxamol)	Tablets
Persomnia	paracetamol, codeine	Tablets
Propain	paracetamol, codeine, diphenhydramine, caffeine	Tablets
Solpadeine	paracetamol, codeine, caffeine	Effervescent tablets
Solpadol	paracetamol, codeine	Effervescent tablets
Syndol	paracetamol, codeine, caffeine, doxylamine	Tablets
Tramil	paracetamol, caffeine	Capsules
Tylex	paracetamol, codeine	Capsules

Table 27.6 Drugs used to treat mild to moderate pain: combined paracetamol preparations (*cont.*)

Preparation	*Drug*	*Dosage form*
Unigesic	paracetamol, caffeine	Capsules
Zefringe Sachets	paracetamol, caffeine	Sachets of effervescent granules

Narcotic pain relievers used to treat moderate to severe pain

The narcotic pain relievers that relieve moderate to severe pain and severe pain (see Tables 27.7–27.9) are more likely to produce addiction than the less potent ones such as codeine that are used to relieve mild to moderate pain. They are therefore subjected to legal controls, with regard to their storage, prescribing, dispensing and administration.

Because of this risk of addiction, much work has gone into trying to develop drugs that would relieve severe pain but would not produce addiction. This exercise has centred around drugs that are known to block *some* of the actions of morphine. It was hoped that such drugs would compete with morphine-related drugs on opioid receptors and reverse some of their effects not involved in relieving pain.

Several drugs are now available that block the effects of morphine on opioid receptors to varying degrees. Naloxone blocks all the actions of morphine and is therefore used to treat patients suffering from overdose of morphine or some other opioid. It is referred to as a pure *opioid antagonist*. Other drugs are available that block some of the actions of morphine but not the relief of pain. They act partially like morphine and are referred to as *partial antagonists*. They include pentazocine and buprenorphine.

Unfortunately, initial hopes that partially acting opioids would not be addictive have not been fulfilled, and there are reports of individuals being addicted to them.

Effects of narcotic pain relievers on the body

All narcotic pain relievers produce actions and effects similar to those produced by morphine. They produce their major effects on the brain and the intestine, and include not only pain relief but also drowsiness, mood changes, depression of breathing, suppression of cough, tolerance, addiction, nausea, vomiting and a slowing down of movements of the intestine producing constipation. They may also cause retention of urine, and injections may cause pain and damage to the tissues at the site of injection. The different narcotic pain relievers produce these effects to a lesser or greater degree and individuals vary in how they respond to them. Different people may experience different harmful effects, and someone who is up and about may develop more harmful effects than another person who is confined to bed. The effectiveness of narcotic pain relievers varies according to whether they are taken by mouth or by injection. Effectiveness also varies according to their speed of onset and duration of action.

It is important to note that an individual may develop increased sensitivity to pain after the effect of a narcotic pain reliever (opioid) has worn off, and that the duration but not the degree of pain relief produced increases progressively with age. Harmful effects of narcotic pain relievers are listed later.

Tolerance and addiction

All narcotic pain relievers can produce tolerance, which may be defined as a lessened response to the effects of a drug so that an ever-larger dose has to be taken to produce similar effects. They can also produce addiction – some rarely (e.g. codeine), and some frequently (e.g. heroin). This is discussed later.

The use of narcotic pain relievers

Strong narcotic pain relievers are used to relieve internal pain (e.g. pain from an acute heart attack), post-operative pain, pain following severe injury and the pain of certain cancers.

They may not be the most effective drugs for treating severe pain from bones or joints. These pains may respond better to anti-inflammatory drugs (see earlier). Some doctors talk about opioid-sensitive pain and opioid non-sensitive pain; this can be a useful distinction because there is no point in filling a patient with morphine if it is not going to achieve pain relief.

Morphine is the narcotic pain reliever of choice for relieving severe pain that is opioid sensitive. The availability of other narcotic pain relievers for moderate to severe and severe pain offers an opportunity for change according to the patient's needs. The real problem is not a lack of effective pain relievers but the fact that they may not be used effectively.

Ineffective use of narcotic pain relievers

Narcotic pain relievers are all effective if used properly and according to the patient's needs. However, in relieving severe pain none of them is superior to the original one – morphine. It still remains the standard against which new pain relievers are measured. Unfortunately, it may sometimes not be used effectively. Patients who are dying and in severe pain may be given too small a dose too infrequently and so they may be left to suffer. Pain relief in children may also be inadequate. Instead of being given doses of morphine at short fixed intervals of time, some patients are left to 'demand' the next dose, having unnecessarily experienced – and then dreaded – the return of pain.

The relief of severe and continuous pain

Because of some rather inadequate animal studies on morphine addiction in the past rather than from observations in human patients suffering from severe and continuous pain, some doctors in the past were hesitant to use morphine in sufficiently high and/or regular dosage because of fear of producing addiction. This was an exaggerated fear because less drug is needed to prevent a recurrence of pain than to relieve it once it has been allowed to return. Each person should be treated individually and the dose of narcotic pain reliever varied according to that person's needs and response. Furthermore, treatment should be tailored to changing needs of the individual. This means that the drug, dose, time between doses and route of administration (by mouth, rectum, injection, intravenous infusion etc.) should be varied in order to provide maximum benefits at all times for the patient being treated. The effective relief of pain requires time, patience, knowledge and compassion. The expanding hospice care services for dying patients is, in part, a recognition that such care is not always adequately provided.

No patient should be denied round-the-clock relief from pain, and preparations of morphine and related pain relievers now make this possible. Of particular value to someone in severe, continuous pain is a device that allows a constant infusion of morphine under the skin using a battery-operated syringe driver which the patient can control according to his needs.

Another problem with the use of narcotic pain relievers is that unpleasant harmful effects may also need relieving. For example, in patients who are in severe and continuous pain and who need morphine, nausea may be treated with an anti-nausea/vomiting drug (e.g. cyclizine, chlorpromazine); however, it is safer to use the anti-nauseant drug separately than in a combined preparation with morphine because you cannot increase the dose of morphine without overdosing with the anti-nauseant. Constipation may be treated by giving a laxative. Additional treatments such as a nerve block or selective radiotherapy should be used where appropriate. No patient should want to die because of pain.

Pain after surgical operations

Pain after a surgical operation may be worse than it should be in some patients because fixed doses of pain relievers are used 'as needed' instead of the dose and frequency of dosage being adjusted to the needs of the particular patient. In the end it is always a balance of benefits to risks in each individual. To improve the benefits and reduce the risks requires knowledge both of the patient and his disorder and of the drugs that are available.

The routine use of narcotic pain relievers before a surgical operation in pain-free patients is difficult to justify and an anti-anxiety drug such as diazepam (Valium) would be better for reducing apprehension.

Narcotic pain relievers

Morphine is the first drug of choice. It may be given by mouth, injection or suppository. It frequently causes nausea and vomiting, euphoria and a detached mental state.

Buprenorphine partially antagonizes the effects of narcotic pain relievers such as morphine, and has a longer duration of action than morphine. It can be given by mouth, under the tongue or by injection. Because it partially blocks some of the effects of narcotic pain relievers such as morphine, it may trigger pain and withdrawal effects if given to someone who has become dependent on one of these drugs.

Because buprenorphine blocks some of the effects of narcotic pain relievers such as morphine, the antagonist naloxone (see earlier) will not work so well if buprenorphine is taken in overdose. Doxapram (Dopram), a respiratory stimulant, has to be used to relieve the depression of rate and depth of breathing that may result from such an overdose.

Codeine is used to relieve mild to moderate pain (see earlier). It causes too much constipation to be of any value in long-term treatment of pain. It may be given by mouth or injection.

Dextromoramide produces less drowsiness than morphine but is shorter acting. It may be given by mouth, injection or as a suppository.

Dextropropoxyphene is used to treat mild to moderate pain (see earlier). It is given by mouth.

Diamorphine (heroin) is an effective pain reliever but is more likely to produce euphoria and addiction than is morphine. However, it causes less nausea, constipation or fall in blood pressure. It is more soluble than morphine and can be injected in smaller volumes, which is important in very thin patients. It may be used by injection in patients dying from cancer who are in severe pain but cannot tolerate morphine.

Dihydrocodeine is used to treat moderate to severe pain. It may cause dizziness as well as constipation. It may be given by mouth or by injection.

Dipipanone produces less drowsiness than morphine but is shorter acting. Diconal is the only preparation available that contains dipipanone; it also contains the anti-nauseant drug cyclizine.

Fentanyl (Sublimaze, Thalamonol) and *alfentanil* (Rapifen) are short-acting narcotic pain relievers used with general anaesthetics such as thiopentone in order to provide relief from pain during surgery and to add to the effects of the anaesthetic. They are given by intravenous injections.

Levorphanol produces less drowsiness than morphine and lasts longer; because of this it should not be given more than twice daily, otherwise it may accumulate in the body to produce harmful effects. It may be given by mouth or injection.

Meptazinol has less effect than morphine in depressing the rate and depth of breathing but it may produce nausea and vomiting. It is sometimes used to relieve pain during and after surgery. It may be given by mouth or injection.

Methadone produces less drowsiness than morphine and lasts longer; because of this it should not be given more than twice daily, otherwise it may accumulate in the body to produce harmful effects. It may be given by mouth or injection.

Nalbuphine may produce less nausea and vomiting than morphine. It may be given by injection.

Papaveretum (mixed opium alkaloids) has no advantage over morphine. It is sometimes used to relieve pain before (pre-medication), during and after surgery. It is given by injection.

Pentazocine has some blocking effects on narcotic pain relievers (it is a partial antagonist, see earlier) and should not be used in anyone who has become dependent on narcotic pain relievers such as morphine because it will trigger pain and withdrawal symptoms. By mouth, it relieves moderate pain but much of it is broken down as it passes through the liver; it is therefore more effective by injection. It should *not* be used to relieve the pain of an acute heart attack (myocardial infarction) because it may increase the work of the heart. It may be given by mouth, injection or suppository.

Pethidine is less effective and shorter acting than morphine and is used to relieve pain in childbirth because it affects the newborn baby's breathing less than morphine: this is probably because it is less effective than morphine! It is also used to treat pain from gall bladder disease because it has less effect than morphine on the muscular opening of the bile duct into the duodenum. It is also used to relieve pain caused by kidney stones. It may be given by mouth or injection.

Phenazocine is less effective than morphine but is used to treat gall bladder pain because it has less effect than morphine on the muscular opening of the bile duct into the duodenum. It may be taken by mouth – swallowed or dissolved under the tongue (if nausea and vomiting are problems).

Phenoperidine is short acting, and is used to relieve pain during surgery and to add to the effects of an anaesthetic. It is given by injection.

Table 27.7 Narcotic pain relievers – harmful effects and warnings

Harmful effects
Harmful effects include light-headedness, drowsiness, dizziness, nausea, vomiting, flushing and sweating. These are more common in people who are up and about and not experiencing severe pain; in such cases lower doses should be used and if necessary the individual should lie down. Other harmful effects include clouding of the mind, weakness, headache, insomnia, disorientation, visual disturbances, agitation, a feeling of extreme well-being (euphoria) or a feeling of being unwell and restless (dysphoria); slowness of the pulse, palpitations, faintness; constipation, loss of appetite and dry mouth; and difficulty in passing urine, or inability to pass urine (urinary retention) and reduced libido. Allergic reactions include itching, skin rashes, itching nose and swelling of the skin (oedema). They make the pupils go small and cause stiffness of the muscles in the back.

Tolerance All narcotic pain relievers can produce tolerance, which may be defined as a lessened response to the effects of a drug so that ever-larger doses have to be taken to produce effects similar to those produced at the start of treatment.

Addiction Addiction to a narcotic pain reliever (e.g. heroin) causes an overwhelming desire to continue taking the drug, a tendency to increase the dose in order to obtain the same or greater effects, and a total preoccupation with obtaining a supply of the drug. Physical dependence develops, and stopping the drug suddenly may produce withdrawal symptoms which include yawning, runny eyes, runny nose, sneezing, small pupils, shivering, headache, weakness, sweating, anxiety, irritability, difficulty with sleeping, orgasm, loss of appetite, nausea, vomiting, loss of weight, dehydration, loss of body fluids leading to dehydration, pain in bones, abdominal cramps, muscle cramps, rise in temperature, goose pimples (cold turkey), increase in heart rate, increased rate of breathing and a rise in blood pressure.

The severity of the withdrawal symptoms will depend upon the degree of physical dependence that has developed. The speed of onset, the intensity and the duration of withdrawal symptoms depend upon which narcotic pain-relieving drug is used and how long it stays in the body. With morphine and heroin, withdrawal symptoms usually start within about 6–10 hours after the last dose. The effects peak in about 36–48 hours and by the fifth day most symptoms have cleared up, but some may last for months. With pethidine, many of the withdrawal symptoms clear up in about 24 hours whereas with methadone they may last up to 2 weeks. This slowness in producing withdrawal effects is the reason why methadone is given as a substitute for heroin – it produces less immediate and less intense withdrawal symptoms.

Warnings
Head injury Narcotic pain-relieving drugs should be used with caution in someone who has suffered a head injury. This is because they may adversely affect breathing and raise the pressure of the fluid inside the brain. They may also mask important signs of head injury such as the reaction of the pupils to light.

Asthma and bronchitis Narcotic pain-

Table 27.7 Narcotic pain relievers – harmful effects and warnings (*cont.*)

relieving drugs should be used with caution in people who suffer from asthma, chronic bronchitis and other chronic chest complaints. This is because they make the breathing centre less responsive to the level of carbon dioxide in the blood. They also suppress cough.

Low blood pressure Narcotic pain-relieving drugs may cause a fall in blood pressure, which may be harmful to an individual whose blood pressure is already low because of loss of blood through a haemorrhage or to someone who is given certain anaesthetics that lower blood pressure.

Acute abdominal pains If a narcotic pain-relieving drug is given to relieve acute abdominal pain before a diagnosis is made, it may mask a serious underlying problem – for example, a perforated bowel.

Special risk groups Narcotic pain-relieving drugs should be used with caution and in reduced dosages in the elderly (see later), in debilitated patients, and in anyone with impaired liver or kidney function, Addison's disease, under-active thyroid gland, difficulty in passing urine (e.g. due to an enlarged prostate gland), low blood pressure, or a history of drug abuse. People with acute liver disease should not be given narcotic pain relievers.

Patients who are up and about Patients who are up and about may experience more harmful effects than if they are confined to bed (see earlier). One problem is that narcotic pain-relieving drugs may cause a fall in blood pressure on standing up after lying or sitting down, which can produce light-headedness, dizziness, nausea and faintness. In addition, the drugs may impair the physical and mental activities needed to drive or to operate moving machinery.

Risks in elderly people Harmful effects from narcotic pain-relieving drugs may be more frequent and severe in the elderly, particularly drowsiness, dizziness, unsteadiness and constipation. They should therefore be used with caution and in reduced doses.

Risks in pregnancy At the end of pregnancy and during labour the stronger narcotics may depress the baby's breathing. Also in labour, they may cause the mother to vomit and slow down movements in her stomach. An added risk is that she may inhale vomit into the lungs which could produce pneumonia. Babies born to narcotic-addicted mothers will also suffer from addiction at birth.

Risks in breast feeding Regular daily use of high doses of a narcotic pain-relieving drug may produce addiction in the baby.

Risks in driving Narcotic pain-relieving drugs may produce drowsiness and affect your ability to drive; therefore do not drive until the effects have worn off. The dangers are increased by alcohol and certain other drugs (see Chapter 89).

Risks with alcohol Narcotic pain-relieving drugs increase the effects of alcohol; therefore do not drink if you are taking one of these drugs.

Warning *Combined preparations of a narcotic pain-relieving drug and an anti-vomiting drug are not suitable for regular daily use because, if the daily dose is increased in order to improve pain relief, there is a risk of overdosing with the anti-vomiting drug. An example of such a combination is Diconal (dipipanone and cyclizine).*

Table 27.8 Narcotic pain relievers used to treat moderate to severe pain

Preparation	*Drug*	*Dosage form*
Diconal	dipipanone, cyclizine (anti-nauseant)	Tablets
dihydrocodeine	dihydrocodeine	Tablets, elixir, injection
DF 118	dihydrocodeine	Tablets, elixir, injection
Fortral	pentazocine	Capsules, tablets, injection, suppositories
Meptid	meptazinol	Tablets, injection
Narphen	phenazocine	Tablets
Nubain	nalbuphine	Injection
Pamergan P100	pethidine, promethazine (anti-nauseant)	Injection
pethidine	pethidine	Tablets, injection
pentazocine	pentazocine	Capsules, tablets, injection, suppositories
Temgesic	buprenorphine	Tablets for dissolving under the tongue, injection

Table 27.9 Narcotic pain relievers used to treat severe pain

Preparation	*Drug*	*Dosage form*
Cyclimorph	morphine, cyclizine (anti-nauseant)	Injection
diamorphine (heroin)	diamorphine	Injection
morphine	morphine salts	Injection, suppositories, elixir
MST Continus	morphine	Sustained-release tablets
Nepenthe	morphine	Oral solution, injection
Omnopon	papaveretum	Injection
Oramorph	morphine	Oral solution, concentrated sugar-free oral solution
Oxycodone		Suppositories
Palfium	dextromoramide	Tablets, injection, suppositories
Physeptone	methadone	Tablets, injection

28

Local anaesthetics

Local anaesthetics are drugs that block the transmission of impulses in nerve tissues when applied locally in appropriate concentrations. Their effects are reversible and they are used to produce loss of pain in a part of the body without loss of consciousness – they could be called local pain relievers. They act on any part of the brain and nervous system and on every type of nerve fibre; they can block pain sensation but they can also cause paralysis. Small nerve fibres are more susceptible to the actions of local anaesthetics than are large nerve fibres. Pain is the first sensation to disappear, followed by cold, warmth and then deep pressure. The local anaesthetics in common use have been selected because they do not irritate the tissues to which they are applied and cause no permanent nerve damage. They are soluble in water and the solutions can be sterilized. Their choice depends upon the speed with which they work, their duration of action and their potential harmful effects when absorbed into the bloodstream.

Use of local anaesthetics

Local anaesthetics may be administered in several different ways according to the drug being used.

Surface or topical anaesthesia (as a solution, jelly or lozenges) blocks pain in nerve endings in the skin or mucous membranes, and to do this the local anaesthetic must have good powers of penetration.

Local or infiltration anaesthesia is produced by injection directly into an area. To be effective the drug must not be absorbed too quickly into the bloodstream, otherwise its effects wear off. Injections of local anaesthetics are also used to cut off pain sensation in an area (e.g. a nerve block as used by dentists); this is called a regional nerve block.

Epidural anaesthesia is a nerve block produced by injecting the anaesthetic into the space between the lining membranes (the dura) of the spinal cord; it is commonly used in childbirth.

Caudal anaesthesia is an injection into the space between the membranes at the lower end of the spinal cord where the main nerves from the spinal cord run together before leaving the spine to supply the pelvis and legs (caudal means 'like a tail').

Spinal anaesthesia is produced by injecting the local anaesthetic inside the covering membrane of the spinal cord, causing temporary paralysis of the nerves with which it comes into contact. The area affected is determined by the specific gravity of the drug (i.e. the rate at which it drops down the fluid inside the spinal cord) and by tipping the patient up or down according to the area which is to be anaesthetized. It may be used in people who are not suitable for a general anaesthetic.

Choice of local anaesthetic

The choice of local anaesthetic depends upon many factors but in particular upon the risk of absorption into the bloodstream and the production of dangerous harmful effects.

Injectable local anaesthetics in common use include *bupivacaine, lignocaine* and *prilocaine. Procaine* is seldom used. *Amethocaine* is used principally as a surface anaesthetic in solution (e.g. eye drops) and in lozenges for the throat. *Benzocaine* is used in lozenges for sore throats and in ointments used to treat haemorrhoids. *Cinchocaine* is also used as a surface anaesthetic. *Cocaine* solutions are used for application to the nose, throat, eyes and larynx before surgery on these areas. Other local anaesthetics included in eye drops are *lignocaine, oxybuprocaine* and *proxymetacaine.*

Benefits and risks of using local anaesthetics

Harmful effects and warnings on the use of local anaesthetics appear in Table 28.1.

The benefits and risks of using local anaesthetics are determined by the preparation that is used, its concentration and the duration of its use. The techniques involved in delivering it as accurately as possible to its target site will also influence the balance of benefits and risks.

Local anaesthetics applied to surfaces, particularly the lining of the nose, mouth or throat, can be rapidly absorbed into the bloodstream to produce general harmful effects. Patients should therefore spit out any excess solution in order to prevent absorption.

The danger of infiltrating a local anaesthetic by injection into a site is that large doses have to be used and so in major surgery the risks of producing harmful effects outweigh the benefits.

The balance between the amount of local anaesthetic given and the risks from absorption into the bloodstream applies also to nerve blocks. Increasing the concentration of the drug will increase the risks, particularly in areas with a good blood supply. The safe and effective use of nerve blocks requires an understanding of the local anaesthetics that are available and how the body deals with them, and the type of nerve to be blocked. The amount and concentration of a local anaesthetic used should depend upon which nerves are to be blocked, the type of nerves, the required duration of action, the size of area to be anaesthetized and the rate of blood flow to the site. The age, weight and general physical condition of the patient are also important.

Risks when mixed with adrenaline

The effects of local anaesthetics quickly wear off when the drug is removed from its site of action, and for this reason it is common practice to mix a local anaesthetic with a drug that constricts arteries (vasoconstrictor drug), thus delaying the 'washing away' of the local anaesthetic into the bloodstream. The principal drug used for this purpose is adrenaline. The use of these mixtures is not without danger; for example, if such a mixture is used to block pain in a finger, the constriction of the arteries may so reduce the circulation to the finger end as to cause the tissues to die (gangrene). Therefore, they should not be used near terminal arteries, as in the fingers, toes, ears, nose and penis. Some of the adrenaline may enter the bloodstream and cause both an increase in heart rate and chest pain which may be harmful to someone with raised blood pressure or angina. It may be necessary to block these effects with a beta blocker. Cocaine constricts arteries and therefore helps to maintain its concentration locally.

Warnings *Maximum concentration of a local anaesthetic in the blood occurs about 10–30 minutes* ***after*** *injection, so patients should always be kept under observation for the first half an hour after an injection.*

Spinal anaesthesia *may produce alarming harmful effects because the local anaesthetic may affect the sympathetic nerves, producing dilatation of arteries and veins – resulting in a fall in blood pressure and a decreased output of blood from the heart.*

In ***epidural anaesthesia*** *(used in childbirth) the local anaesthetic enters the mother's bloodstream and may cross into the baby's circulation. The baby is not able to break down the drug effectively and may suffer from the effects of the local anaesthetic for up to 48 hours after birth.*

When ***applied to the eye***, *the protective blink reflex is lost and particles blown into the eye may damage the 'window of the eyes' (the cornea); therefore a protective cover should always be worn for half a day over an eye that has had anaesthetic drops applied.*

Table 28.1 Local anaesthetic injections – harmful effects and warnings

Harmful effects are rare and are usually due to excessively high levels of local anaesthetic in the blood, which may occur if too big a dose is used and/or if there is rapid absorption into the bloodstream from the site of injection. Occasionally an individual may be allergic or idiosyncratically sensitive to a local anaesthetic.

Harmful effects on the brain and nerves include anxiety, restlessness, excitement and nervousness, dizziness, blurred vision, tremors, yawning and twitching; these may lead on to drowsiness, fits, unconsciousness and arrest of breathing. Initial excitement may be transient or absent and the first sign may be drowsiness going straight into unconsciousness and arrest of breathing.

Harmful effects on the heart and circulation include a fall in blood pressure, pallor, sweating, slowing of the heart rate, irregular heart beats and, rarely, arrest of the heart. There may be wheezing or vomiting due to the harmful effects on the sympathetic nerves that supply the muscles in the bronchial tubes and intestine, respectively.

People allergic to a local anaesthetic may develop skin rashes, asthma and, very rarely, a severe allergic reaction (anaphylactic reaction) which may be fatal. Allergy occurs most commonly with the local anaesthetics amethocaine, benzocaine, cocaine, oxybuprocaine, procaine and proxymetacaine. These are chemically related and are referred to as ester-type local anaesthetics. Allergy occurs less often with bupivacaine, cinchocaine, lignocaine, mepivacaine and prilocaine, which are amide-type local anaesthetics. The preservative in local anaesthetic solutions may also produce allergic reactions in some people.

The *safety* of local anaesthetics depends upon the balance between the rate at which they enter the bloodstream and the rate at which they are destroyed. The former can be reduced by including a vasoconstrictor in the solution (see earlier).

Prilocaine and other ester-type local anaesthetics used in spinal anaesthesia are destroyed by an enzyme (cholinesterase) in the blood and the liver (see Chapter 2). The enzyme is not present in spinal cord fluid. If one of these drugs is injected into the spinal cord fluid its effects last until it has been cleared from the spinal cord into the bloodstream.

Lignocaine and other amide-type local anaesthetics are broken down in the liver and so they should be used with caution in anyone with liver disease. These local anaesthetics are transported around the blood attached to proteins. The concentration of these proteins in the blood may be decreased by oral contraceptive drugs and increased by smoking and injury – factors that may influence the harmful effects of these local anaesthetics. The lungs also take up these drugs and affect their activity.

Warnings Resuscitative equipment and anti-allergic drugs (see Chapter 10) should be immediately available whenever a local anaesthetic injection is used. The smallest volume needed to produce anaesthesia of the area should be used. Overdose should be avoided. They must not be used in people who are allergic or sensitive to local anaesthetics. They should be used with caution in anyone who suffers from allergies (e.g. asthma, eczema, hayfever), or from epilepsy, heart block, slow heart rate, severe chest disorders, impaired liver function, myasthenia gravis, or if the dose or site of injection may result in high levels of the drug in the blood. People with a low plasma cholinesterase or who are taking an anticholinesterase drug should not be given an ester-type local anaesthetic (see Chapter 2). The risks of harmful effects from local anaesthetics may be reduced by including adrenaline in the preparation (see earlier). Prilocaine or mepivacaine solutions do not require the addition of adrenaline, and may be used where adrenaline should not be employed – for example, to anesthetize a finger (see earlier for harmful effects).

Risks in elderly people Harmful effects may be more frequent and severe in elderly people; therefore use reduced doses.

Table 28.2 Local anaesthetic preparations

Drug	*Preparation*
amethocaine	amethocaine eye drops, Minims amethocaine eye drops, in Eludril Spray, in Noxyflex powder for solution
benzocaine	benzocaine lozenges, in compound benzocaine lozenges, in AAA Mouth and Throat Spray, Intralgin, Medilave Gel, Merocaine, Transvasin and Tyrozets
bupivacaine	in Marcain preparations
cinchocaine	Nupercainal, in Proctosedyl, Scheriproct, Ultraproct, Uniroid
cocaine	cocaine eye drops, cocaine and homatropine eye drops
lignocaine	in Betnovate Rectal Ointment, Bradosol Plus, in Calgel, Depo-Medrone with Lidocaine, EMLA, Instillagel, Minims lignocaine and fluorescein, Xylocaine, Xyloproct (Xylocard is used to treat disorders of heart rhythm)
mepivacaine	in Estradurin
oxybuprocaine	Minims Benoxinate eye drops, Opulets Benoxinate eye drops
prilocaine	Citanest injection, in EMLA cream
procaine	procaine injection
proxymetacaine	Ophthaine eye drops

29

Migraine

The term 'vascular headache' is applied to a headache associated with a group of symptoms that appear to be due to changes in the calibre of blood vessels supplying the head and brain. Most vascular headaches occur only on one side of the head, and usually (but not always) they are throbbing in character. They may recur over months or years.

The causes of vascular headaches are not fully understood. For example, in migraine (see later) several complex chemical changes affecting the blood vessels are thought to occur in response to certain chemicals in food or drink or to some other trigger factor (e.g. anxiety, physical exercise). The chemicals produced by the body in response to these factors include adrenaline, serotonin and histamine. These are released into the bloodstream and affect the blood vessels supplying the head and brain, producing constriction initially and then dilatation of arteries. These changes are associated with headaches and other symptoms.

Why the body reacts to trigger factors in this way and why the arteries that supply the head and brain react in this way are not known. It is obviously associated with our genetic make-up and emotions; but vascular headaches must be triggered by *something* – they just cannot come on their own. Therefore it is very important to seek trigger factors, and to try to avoid them if possible and take positive steps to reduce them (e.g. learn relaxation if you are tense).

Factors that may bring on an attack of migraine

- Psychological – e.g. anxiety, tension, worry, emotion, depression, shock, excitement
- Physical – e.g. over-exertion, lifting, straining, bending, heading a football
- External factors – e.g. sunlight, weather, travelling, change of routine, staying in bed, watching television, noise, smells, smoking, drugs
- Dietary – e.g. irregular meals, fasting, certain foods such as cheese, onion, cucumber, bananas, chocolate, fried foods, pastry, cured meats that contain sodium nitrates and nitrites (e.g. hot dogs, ham, bacon), alcohol

Classic migraine

Classic migraine comes on in four stages. The *first stage* is the warning stage (prodromal stage) when you may feel a change in mood, hunger, thirst or drowsiness. This is followed by the *second stage* when the arteries supplying the brain and scalp constrict and affect the blood supply to certain parts of the brain, producing, for example, partial loss of vision, flashing lights and black spots in front of the eyes, weakness and/or pins and needles in a hand or foot or down one half of the body, or difficulty with speech. These nerve symptoms may not be followed by a headache in elderly people, in which case they are thought to be equivalent to migraine and are therefore called migraine equivalent. They may easily be mistaken for the early signs of a stroke.

The *third stage* of migraine comes on when the arteries dilate. The nerve symptoms start to disappear, a one-sided throbbing headache develops on the side opposite to the side affected by the nerve symptoms. The headache is frequently accompanied by nausea, vomiting, diarrhoea, sensitivity to light, sensitivity to noise and generally not feeling well. The headache may last for a few hours or for the whole day and it often goes off by vomiting or going to sleep. The *fourth stage* is when the headache has gone off and the individual feels worn out and the scalp may feel tender to touch on the side where the headache was. Any sudden movement of the head can bring the headache back.

Common migraine (migrainous headache)

Common migraine is similar to classic migraine except that the nerve symptoms are absent. It is usually a recurrent, throbbing, one-sided headache associated with nausea and/or vomiting and sensitivity to light. It often begins in childhood, affects women more than men and runs in families. Attacks can be caused by oral contraceptive drugs and vasodilator drugs (e.g. glyceryl trinitrate).

Cluster headaches

Cluster headaches are brief attacks of severe, acute one-sided headaches that occur in bouts for a few weeks, disappearing for months or years on end. They affect men more than women, and mostly occur in middle age. Clusters usually come on in spring and autumn and last for 3–8 weeks. They can occur several times during the day and particularly at night. They last for 30 minutes to 2 hours, and start with a cutting pain in the nose and behind one eye and then spread to involve the forehead. During an attack, the affected side of the nose may run and get blocked, and the affected eye may water. During the time when the headaches are occurring, alcohol will bring on an attack but not between clusters. We do not know what causes them and treatment is unsatisfactory. (U).

Other vascular headaches

In some people a brief throbbing headache on both sides of the head may occur during orgasm. Physical exertion may bring on a vascular headache in some people, so too can a hangover. Nitrates (e.g. in hot dogs) can trigger a throbbing one-sided headache in some individuals, and monosodium glutamate (e.g. in soy sauce) can cause the 'Chinese restaurant syndrome' – headache, tightness in the face and head, giddiness and diarrhoea. Do not forget that monosodium glutamate is a flavour enhancer present in many convenience foods.

Treatment of migraine

The most important treatment is *prevention*. This means attempting to identify the factors that bring on an attack and avoiding them in the future. Go through a list of possible trigger factors (see above) and cross off the ones you cannot directly relate to your attacks. Then systematically go through the other trigger factors until you have identified one or more that bring on your attacks and then avoid them. It may be something simple such as having to avoid certain cheeses and nuts, or something more difficult such as learning how to relax. Whatever it is, prevention is better than waiting until an attack comes on and then taking drugs.

Drugs used to treat acute attacks of migraine

The important point about using drugs to treat an acute attack of migraine is to anticipate an attack – at the earliest possible sign that you are going to develop an attack you should take whichever drug suits you the best.

Drugs available to treat an acute attack include the following.

Mild pain relievers

The choice of mild pain reliever is usually between *aspirin* or *paracetamol*. The addition of *codeine* may help (see combined pain relievers, Chapter 27).

Aspirin and other anti-inflammatory drugs (e.g. *ibuprofen*) are very useful because they block the production of chemicals (e.g. prostaglandins) which are thought to contribute to the pain and symptoms of migraine. Paracetamol may also block the production of prostaglandins in the brain and nervous system; a herbal remedy, the plant feverfew (*Chrysanthemum parthenium*), is thought to work in a similar way. Codeine blocks opioid receptors and reduces the perception of pain by the brain. There is no convincing evidence from adequate and well controlled studies that adding caffeine to combined mild pain relievers helps to improve their effectiveness.

Helping pain relievers to work and relieving vomiting

One problem in an acute attack of migraine is that the movements of the stomach are reduced, producing a delay in the emptying of the stomach contents into the intestine. This interferes with the absorption of any drug that is absorbed into the bloodstream from the small intestine (e.g. mild pain relievers), so they do not work as quickly or as effectively as when the stomach is functioning normally. One solution to this is to take soluble preparations of aspirin or paracetomol dissolved in a glass of water; this will help their absorption. An alternative is to take a pain reliever in the form of a suppository.

If *nausea and/or vomiting* is a problem another solution is to take a drug such as metoclopramide which not only relieves nausea and vomiting but also increases the movements of the stomach and speeds up the emptying of its contents into the small intestine. This will improve the absorption into the bloodstream of pain-relieving drugs taken by mouth. It is therefore helpful to take metoclopramide by mouth (tablets or syrup) at the earliest sign of an impending migraine attack, followed in about 10 minutes by a pain reliever by mouth such as soluble paracetamol or soluble aspirin. If the vomiting is severe you may vomit the tablets up, so it will help if you have an injection of metoclopramide into a muscle about quarter of an hour before you take the pain reliever by mouth.

An alternative treatment for the nausea and vomiting is to use one of the anti-vomiting drugs listed in Table 14.2; for example, prochlorperazine, which may be given by injection into a muscle or via the rectum as a suppository.

Combined anti-vomiting/mild pain-relieving preparations

Preparations are available that contain the anti-vomiting drug metoclopramide with soluble aspirin in an effervescent preparation (e.g. Migravess) or with soluble paracetamol in an effervescent preparation (e.g. Paramax). Some people find these preparations helpful, but if you are vomiting a lot it may be necessary to give the metoclopramide by injection into a muscle first, followed by a dose of aspirin or paracetomol by mouth some 10–15 minutes later because combined preparation by mouth may be vomited straight back.

Warning *If metoclopramide is given by injection, you could overdose with it if you then take a combined preparation by mouth. Another problem with such combined preparations is that you cannot vary the dose of one drug without varying the other, and there are added risks from both drugs if you take more than the recommended dose of the combined preparation.*

Ergotamine and related drugs

Ergotamine

Ergotamine and related drugs are obtained from ergot, which is a fungus that affects grasses, especially rye. Ergotamine is an extract from ergot. It causes the walls of arteries to constrict (vasoconstriction) but how it works in relieving migraine is not known. It could act in several ways, including blocking the chemicals that are released in the body during a migraine attack. This would help to reduce the dilatation of the arteries that occurs in migraine.

The use of ergotamine Ergotamine is available in sugar-coated tablets, suppositories, an aerosol inhalation and tablets for sucking under the tongue. In repeated doses it may cause nausea, vomiting, muscle cramps and abdominal pains. Regular users can come to rely on it and may over-use it. It may produce ergot poisoning (see later), and deaths have been reported from its use. Overdose with ergotamine may actually produce headaches, and so may rapid withdrawal of the drug. You should take no more than 6–8 mg of ergotamine during any one attack and no more than 10–12 mg of ergotamine in any one week. You should not repeat treatment with ergotamine within 4 days of the last course of treatment.

Ergotamine should never be taken regularly every day in order to prevent an attack of migraine coming on because it causes constriction of the arteries and may cause gangrene in the fingers or toes. It should be used only by people whose migraine attacks do not respond to pain relievers; but it must be remembered that ergotamine may make nausea and vomiting worse and that it does not relieve the warning (prodromal) symptoms (e.g. flashing lights, pins and needles).

The benefits of ergotamine should be balanced against the risks (Table 29.1) in an individual. Ergotamine must be given as early as possible, and with an anti-vomiting drug if it produces nausea and vomiting. Opinion is divided as to the most effective method of taking ergotamine, and different people may prefer different methods – it is really what the individual prefers. The addition of caffeine may improve the absorption of ergotamine from the intestine.

Dihydroergotamine produces less nausea and vomiting than ergotamine but is less effective.

Other drugs

Isometheptene is a sympathomimetic drug (see Chapter 2) that constricts arteries and may reduce the dilatation that occurs in migraine. It is available combined with paracetamol in Midrid. There are risks in using combinations of drugs because the dose of one of the drugs cannot be varied according to the individual's needs. Also such combinations can cause serious problems if an overdose is taken.

A *benzodiazepine* (see Chapter 40) such as diazepam, if given as a one-off dose, may help to relieve muscle spasm in the head and neck, and also anxiety and tension.

Drugs used to prevent attacks of migraine

It is far safer to search for trigger factors (see earlier) than to use any drug. Do not forget that oral contraceptives may trigger attacks of migraine or make them worse. If migraine attacks increase in frequency or severity or become localized in any part of the head, oral contraceptives should be stopped immediately and alternative methods of preventing conception should be used.

If someone develops more than one severe attack of migraine per month and all other methods of prevention have failed, one of the following treatments may be tried – bearing in mind that they do not cure anything, they merely relieve the symptoms.

Pizotifen

Pizotifen blocks the production of chemicals (e.g. serotonin and histamine) that are released in the body in response to some migraine trigger factors and which cause constriction of the arteries supplying the brain. Pizotifen blocks their action and helps to prevent the constriction. It is referred to as a serotonin blocker (or 5 HT blocker) but it also produces some sedative, anti-depressant and antihistamine effects.

Harmful effects include dry mouth, blurred vision, constipation, difficulty in passing urine, drowsiness, weight gain, nausea, dizziness and muscle pain.

Warnings *Pizotifen must not be used in anyone with closed-angle glaucoma, or with enlarged prostate gland or obstruction to the flow of urine – may cause inability to pass urine, leading to retention. Harmful effects may be more frequent and severe in the elderly, so it should be used with caution. It may interfere with your ability to drive, so do not drive until you know that it is safe to do so. The effects of alcohol are increased, so do not drink alcohol while taking pizotifen.*

Beta blockers

(See Chapter 20). The beneficial effects of propranolol (a beta blocker) were noted incidentally in patients being treated for angina. In people suffering from classic or common migraine beta blockers are effective in reducing the number of attacks and/or reducing the intensity of attacks. They may change the balance between the constriction and dilatation of arteries in the brain which cause the symptoms of migraine. Beta blockers used to prevent migraine include atenolol, metoprolol, nadolol, propranolol and timolol. They are equally effective.

NOTE the dangers of beta blockers, which cause coldness of the hands and feet, interacting with ergotamine or methysergide, which may also cause a serious reduction in the blood supply to the hands and feet.

Amitriptyline

Amitriptyline is a tricyclic anti-depressant drug (see Chapter 39) that may be effective in preventing attacks of migraine in some people. This effect appears to be independent of its anti-depressant effects but it is not understood how it works.

Calcium channel blockers

Nifedipine and verapamil are examples of calcium channel blockers (see Chapter 39) that may be effective in preventing attacks of migraine in some people. These effects may be directly related to their dilating actions on the arteries supplying the brain.

Cyproheptadine

Cyproheptadine is an antihistamine (see Chapter 10) that produces some calcium channel blocking effects (see Chapter 39). It may dilate the arteries in the brain and be helpful to some people.

Clonidine

Clonidine is a centrally acting alpha stimulant that dilates arteries. It has been used to treat raised blood pressure (Chapter 21). It is of doubtful value in migraine.

Methysergide

Methysergide is a drug obtained from ergot, a fungus that grows on grasses, particularly rye. It is chemically related to LSD. How it works in migraine is not understood but its effects may be related to its ability to block certain chemicals (e.g. serotonin) produced in the body in response to factors known to trigger migraine. (These chemicals act on the arteries supplying the brain, and methysergide may block their actions.) It has been found useful in preventing attacks of migraine and other vascular headaches, but is of no value once an acute attack of migraine has begun. It takes about 2 days to take effect, and its effects last for about 2 days after the drug has been stopped.

A most serious harmful effect produced by methysergide is an inflammatory scarring (fibrosis) affecting the coverings of various organs. For example, it may produce severe scarring of tissues at the back of the abdomen (retro-peritoneal fibrosis), of the covering of the lungs (pleura) and the lung tissues (pleuro-pulmonary fibrosis), of the coronary arteries and of the lining of the heart (endocardial fibrosis). This scarring usually disappears after the drug is stopped but in some people it does not. Persistent scarring of the inside of the heart and of the heart valves has been reported.

Because of the serious harmful effects that methysergide may produce, it should be used only under strict hospital supervision. Treatment should be interrupted for at least 1 month or more every 6 months. Treatment should be gradually reduced over a period of 2–3 weeks.

Comments on the use of drugs to prevent migraine

It is better to prevent attacks of migraine than to treat them after they have developed, and it is clearly better not to take drugs if possible. An important part of prevention is to try to identify trigger factors and avoid them (see earlier).

When it comes to the use of drugs to prevent migraine, a major problem in assessing effectiveness of drugs is that reports of successful drug treatments often do not make it clear whether the drugs were used to treat classic migraine or common migraine, which is important because the former is usually more difficult to relieve than the latter.

No one drug used by doctors to prevent migraine helps all sufferers, so it is often a matter of trying different drugs and working out the benefits and risks of treatment for a particular individual. Of the drugs available to prevent migraine, a beta blocker such as propranolol is the best and should be tried first. If it does not work, pizotifen or amitriptyline may be tried. Nifedipine should be tried if these fail. Methysergide should rarely be used and then only in special migraine clinics in hospitals and provided the patient fully understands the very serious risks involved in using this drug.

Table 29.1 Ergot-related drugs – harmful effects and warnings

ergotamine
Harmful effects include nausea, vomiting, headache, abdominal pain, weakness in the legs and muscle pains. Regular daily use of high doses, particularly in anyone with impaired kidney or liver function may cause chronic ergotism – chronic ergot poisoning. This consists of coldness of the hands and feet, coldness of the skin, muscle pains, angina, changes in heart rate and blood pressure, and gangrene of the fingers and toes. Other symptoms include headache, nausea, vomiting, diarrhoea, dizziness, weakness of the legs, constriction of the pupils (affecting vision), confusion, drowsiness, strokes and convulsions. Sudden withdrawal may produce headaches.

Dihydroergotamine injections may cause nausea, chest pain, coldness and pins and needles in the hands and feet.

Warnings Ergotamine or dihydroergotamine must not be used in anyone with coronary heart disease, raised blood pressure, disorders of the circulation, sepsis, overactive thyroid, or impaired kidney or liver function. If numbness or pins and needles develop in the hands and/or feet the drug should be stopped immediately.

methysergide
Harmful effects include nausea, drowsiness, dizziness, mood changes, fluid retention (e.g. ankle swelling), tremor, fall in blood pressure on standing up after sitting or lying down (may produce light-headedness and faintness), rapid beating of the heart, and cold hands and feet. Scarring (fibrosis) of internal tissues may occur with prolonged use (see earlier).

Warnings Methysergide must not be used in anyone who suffers from kidney, liver, heart or lung disease or 'rheumatic' diseases. It should be used with caution in people with peptic ulcers; avoid stopping the drug suddenly. Use for only 6 months at a time (see earlier), and only

Table 29.1 Ergot-related drugs – harmful effects and warnings

under hospital supervision.
Risks in elderly people Harmful effects may be more frequent and severe; therefore use with caution.

Table 29.2 Preparations used to treat acute migraine

Preparation	*Drug*	*Drug group*	*Dosage form*
Cafergot	ergotamine caffeine	Ergot-related drug Xanthine	Tablets, suppositories
Dihydergot	dihydroergotamine	Ergot-related drug	Injection
Lingraine	ergotamine	Ergot-related drug	Tablets
Medihaler Ergotamine	ergotamine	Ergot-related drug	Aerosol
Midrid	isometheptene paracetamol	Adrenaline-like drug Mild pain reliever	Capsules
Migraleve	buclizine paracetamol codeine	Antihistamine Mild pain reliever Narcotic pain reliever	Tablets
Migravess and Migravess Forte	metoclopramide aspirin	Antidopamine (anti-vomiting) Mild pain reliever	Effervescent tablets
Migril	ergotamine cyclizine caffeine	Ergot-related drug Antihistamine Xanthine	Tablets
Paramax	paracetamol metoclopramide	Mild pain reliever Antidopamine (anti-vomiting)	Tablets, effervescent sugar-free powder in sachets
Propain	codeine diphenhydramine paracetamol caffeine	Narcotic pain reliever Antihistamine Mild pain reliever Xanthine	Tablets

Table 29.3 Preparations used to prevent migraine

Preparation	*Drug*	*Drug group*	*Dosage form*
Angilol	propranolol	Non-selective beta blocker	Tablets
Apsolol	propranolol	Non-selective beta blocker	Tablets
Berkolol	propranolol	Non-selective beta blocker	Tablets
Betaloc	metoprolol	Selective beta blocker	Tablets
Betaloc SA	metoprolol	Selective beta blocker	Sustained-release tablets
Betim	timolol	Non-selective beta blocker	Tablets
Blocadren	timolol	Non-selective beta blocker	Tablets
Corgard	nadolol	Non-selective beta blocker	Tablets
Deseril	methysergide	Serotonin-blocker	Tablets
Dihydergot	dihydroergotamine	Ergot-related drug	Injection
Dixarit	clonidine	Centrally acting alpha blocker	Tablets
Half-Inderal LA	propranolol	Non-selective beta blocker	Sustained-release capsules
Inderal	propranolol	Non-selective beta blocker	Tablets, injection
Inderal-LA	propranolol	Non-selective beta blocker	Sustained-release capsules
Lingraine	ergotamine	Ergot-related drug	Tablets
Lopresor	metoprolol	Selective beta blocker	Tablets
Medihaler Ergotamine	ergotamine	Ergot-related drug	Aerosol
propranolol	propranolol	Non-selective beta blocker	Tablets
Sanomigran	pizotifen	Serotonin blocker	Tablets, sugar-free elixir
verapamil	verapamil	Calcium channel blocker	Tablets

30

Rheumatoid arthritis

Arthritis means inflammation of a joint, and this can be due to many causes from an injury to an infection. When the arthritis is due to wear and tear we call it *osteoarthritis* or osteoarthrosis, and of course this is more common the older we get. It commonly affects joints of the spine, of the fingers and particularly weight-bearing joints such as the knees and hip joints. Osteoarthritis is discussed in Chapter 31.

Rheumatoid arthritis may affect one joint or many joints, particularly those in the fingers, wrists, elbows, shoulders, ankles and knees. It is an inflammation of joints, possibly caused by the body reacting against something in its own tissues (auto-immunity, see Chapter 9). It may last for a few days or for many years, sometimes for life, with periodic flare-ups and quiet periods. It may also be associated with generalized effects such as weakness, fatigue, poor appetite and fever; and inflammation of other tissues; for example, in the blood vessels, heart, skin, lungs, spleen, nerves and eyes. Rheumatoid arthritis may be mild, moderate or severe. It causes painful swellings of joints, with stiffness – which may lead to wasting of the muscles around the joint, resulting in instability of the affected joint and deformity. About one in ten patients undergoes a spontaneous recovery within 6 months to 2 years of the onset of rheumatoid arthritis.

Rheumatoid arthritis starts with a severe inflammation of the lining covering the inner surfaces of the affected joint (the synovial membrane). The lining swells, inflammatory fluids fill the joint space and the joint becomes red, swollen and painful. The lining then becomes scarred and the scar tissue spreads over and under the shiny cartilage that protects the ends of the bones. Eventually, the space within the joint becomes filled with scar tissue, underlying bony surfaces become damaged and deformed, and the muscles around the joint become inflamed and wasted.

Drug treatment of rheumatoid arthritis

The aim of drug treatment in rheumatoid arthritis is to relieve pain and stiffness, to maintain mobility of the affected joints and, hopefully, to prevent deformity. There are two main approaches to drug treatment:

- To relieve symptoms
- To attempt to modify, reduce or stop the progressive destruction of joints

Relief of symptoms in rheumatoid arthritis

The two main groups of drugs used to relieve the symptoms of rheumatoid arthritis are non-steroidal anti-inflammatory drugs (NSAIDs) and steroidal anti-inflammatory drugs.

Non-steroidal anti-inflammatory drugs (NSAIDs)

Inflammation involves pain, swelling (because fluid leaves the blood vessels to enter the tissues), and redness and heat due to an increase in blood supply. It is caused by the release of chemicals from the tissues in response to injury or infection. There are many chemicals involved but the group that have been studied the most are known as prostaglandins, and it is now well documented that, if you can block the production of prostaglandins, inflammation and pain can be reduced.

We do not understand how anti-inflammatory drugs work but we do know that aspirin and other anti-inflammatory pain relievers (see later) have the ability to block the release of prostaglandins by injured tissues and reduce inflammation. But note that they only relieve the symptoms of inflammation; they do nothing to slow down, stop or prevent the underlying injury to the tissues which causes that inflammation. In fact, some doctors argue that, by relieving the symptoms of inflammation, the joints are used more than they should be and this may contribute in part to the progressive damage that occurs to joints in rheumatoid arthritis.

Aspirin and related drugs and other anti-inflammatory drugs are known as non-steroidal anti-inflammatory drugs (NSAIDs) to distinguish them from steroidal drugs (corticosteroids) that are also used to reduce inflammation.

NSAIDs in treating rheumatoid arthritis

Apart from their effects in relieving inflammation there is nothing specific about the actions of NSAIDs in the treatment of rheumatoid arthritis. In fact, in recent years we have often allowed ourselves to be misled about the importance of blocking prostaglandin production and its relevance to the treatment of rheumatoid arthritis. A drug's ability to block prostaglandins in the laboratory is not necessarily related directly to the drug's effectiveness in people suffering from rheumatoid arthritis. It is more than evident from research findings that complex processes are involved in producing the inflammation of rheumatoid arthritis. This may in part explain why different people react differently to any one anti-inflammatory drugs. This observation highlights the difficulties in evaluating the effectiveness of these drugs and the need to treat the usually exaggerated claims for a new NSAID with great caution. Furthermore, reports from trials of these NSAIDs are often conflicting because of different methods used to compare the effectiveness of one drug against another. Dosages used may be different, methods of assessment may be different and the numbers of patients used may be too small to draw any significant conclusion.

Regard claims for wonder drugs with caution

Headlines in the news media about a new 'wonder drug' to treat rheumatoid arthritis should always be regarded with caution: it is usually only a matter of months before it is realized that the so-called wonder drug is either no more effective or is actually more harmful than the drugs already in common use.

As yet there is no wonder drug and there is no cure for rheumatoid arthritis. Available NSAIDs can relieve symptoms of pain and swelling and reduce suffering but they should be only part of a comprehensive treatment programme which should include physiotherapy, splinting where appropriate, and special fittings in the home to make life easier. Also, more attention should be paid to the diet of patients suffering from rheumatoid arthritis. This should be well balanced and nutritious and include supplementary vitamins and minerals; and it should be carefully examined in order to identify the presence or absence of elements that may affect the arthritis for better or worse.

NSAIDs relieve both pain and inflammation. If taken when necessary, they relieve mild to moderate pain; for example headache, period pains, soft tissue pain (e.g. sprains and strains), backache and pain following surgery. However, if an NSAID is taken in recommended doses *regularly* every day it will also reduce the swelling, redness and heat produced by inflammation. NSAIDs are therefore of particular value in treating disorders such as rheumatoid arthritis which is characterized by continuous pain and inflammation of joints. They are also of value in treating other muscle and joint disorders that are associated with inflammation (e.g. acute gout).

Different patients respond differently

Different patients react differently to NSAIDs and it is important for you to remember that these drugs only relieve symptoms, they do not cure the disease or prevent its getting worse. Any one of these preparations is worth trying but, if it does not relieve pain within about 1 week and reduce swelling of joints within about 3 weeks, it is not going to work. Simple points, such as can it be taken just twice a day instead of three times a day or can it be taken by rectum as a suppository at night, are important in selecting one of these drugs.

There are so many NSAIDs on the market that it makes selection difficult. They are usually more like each other than different, in so far as if they produce similar beneficial effects, they usually produce similar harmful effects. So there really is nothing to choose between them except for an individual's preference.

Aspirin and related drugs in treating rheumatoid arthritis

Aspirin is discussed in detail in Chapter 27. Although some medical experts talk about aspirin being the first drug of choice to treat rheumatoid arthritis, many doctors do not agree. This is because relieving the pain and swelling of rheumatoid arthritis requires regular daily use of high doses of aspirin, which may cause unacceptable harmful effects. A particularly dangerous problem with aspirin is that it may cause ulcerations of the stomach and duodenum, with bleeding, which may occur with any dose or preparation of aspirin. These are especially dangerous in elderly people.

Special aspirin preparations Preparations of aspirin for *regular daily use* are available which are manufactured with the specific aim of trying to reduce damage to the stomach lining by delaying the release of aspirin until the product has passed out of the stomach and into the intestine. Techniques include putting the aspirin inside lots of small capsules (micro-encapsulation), which protect the aspirin as it passes through the stomach and then allow the slow release of the aspirin in the intestine. Another method is to cover tablets of aspirin with a special coat that resists the acid of the stomach; this is called enteric coating (e.g. Nu-Seals). An alternative is to mix the aspirin with a base resistant to the acid of the stomach (e.g. Caprin) or the aspirin can be mixed with a base to neuturalize (or buffer) the acid (e.g. aloxiprin, Palaprin Forte).

Salsalate (Disalcid) is an aspirin-related drug preparation that is insoluble in stomach juice and therefore produces less risk of damage to the stomach; it is slower acting but lasts longer than aspirin.

Choline magnesium trisalicylate (Trisilate) is another aspirin-related drug preparation, which is claimed to produce less risk of bleeding. It only needs to be taken twice daily.

Diflunisal (Dolobid) is also related to aspirin and need only to be taken twice daily. It produces fewer harmful effects than aspirin but is also less effective.

NOTE Unfortunately the above preparations do not appear to be safer nor are suppositories any safer.

Benorylate (Benoral) is an aspirin/paracetamol compound. It produces less irritation of the stomach because it is absorbed unchanged into the bloodstream where it is taken directly to the liver and broken down into aspirin and paracetamol. It has a longer duration of action than aspirin or paracetamol given separately.

Steroidal anti-inflammatory drugs (corticosteroids)

Corticosteroids relieve the symptoms of inflammation, and the benefits and risks of using them are discussed in detail in Chapter 62. In rheumatoid arthritis they relieve symptoms; they do not cure. They do not alter the progressive destruction of the joints which occurs in the disease. If used in high doses (more than 10 mg of prednisolone or equivalent daily) over a prolonged period of time (3 months or more), the risks of use may easily outweigh any benefit.

Enthusiasm in the past for corticosteroids by mouth or injection to treat rheumatoid arthritis has now given way to the acceptance that there is only a limited place for their use. This should be restricted to individuals in whom all other treatment has failed and in whom the disease is still progressive and crippling. In these people, corticosteroids by mouth or injection will relieve symptoms and make life more bearable, but any such benefit needs carefully balancing with the risks (see Chapter 62).

The maximum daily dose by mouth of a corticosteroid should not exceed 7.5 mg of prednisolone or its equivalent in order to prevent the adrenal glands from being 'knocked out'. It should preferably be taken in the mornings or, where possible, in a higher dose on alternate days in order to have a minimal effect on the glands. Intermittent courses of treatment should always be used when possible. This means using corticosteroids for acute flare-ups and reducing or stopping them slowly during quiet phases. However, the use of high doses by intravenous infusion once a month in severe acute cases needs critical assessment before it can be recommended.

Do not stop corticosteroids suddenly

When long-term use of corticosteroid by mouth is to be stopped, the daily dose of the drug should be reduced gradually over a period of weeks to months depending upon the previous daily dose and duration of the treatment. This is to prevent withdrawal symptoms by giving the pituitary and adrenal glands time to return to normal function. It will also prevent a sudden flare-up of the disease, which may occur if any anti-inflammatory treatment is stopped suddenly.

Corticosteroids injected into joints

Injections of a corticosteroid directly into an affected joint may help to relieve the heat, pain and swelling of inflammation in the joint, increase mobility and help to reduce deformity. However, repeated injections into the same joint may result in a painless destruction of the joint and local wasting of muscles. Local injections of corticosteroids should be given only occasionally, and sterile techniques should be used in order to avoid introducing an infection into the joint. For these injections it is customary to use an almost insoluble and long-acting preparation of a corticosteroid (see Table 30.2).

Drugs that may modify, reduce or stop the destruction of joints (anti-rheumatic drugs)

Sulphasalazine

Sulphasalazine (Salazopyrin) is used to treat ulcerative colitis and Crohn's disease. It is also of benefit in some individuals suffering from rheumatoid arthritis because of its anti-inflammatory effects. When taken by mouth it is hardly absorbed, and when it reaches the large bowel, bacteria break it down into a sulphonamide drug – sulphapyridine – and an anti-inflammatory drug – 5-aminosalicylic acid which is related to aspirin. Only about a quarter of this aspirin-like drug is absorbed into the bloodstream whereas sulphapyridine is well absorbed and probably accounts for the harmful effects which sulphasalazine produces (see Chapter 16).

Gold

Gold (e.g. Myocrisin) has been in and out of fashion for the past fifty years. It is now back in fashion because it is accepted that NSAIDs produce no effect on the progressive destruction of the joints that occurs in rheumatoid arthritis. As stated earlier, they only relieve symptoms; they do not cure or slow down the process.

When to use gold

Gold can be very toxic if used inappropriately; therefore it is very important to try to minimize the risks of producing harmful effects by careful selection of patients for treatment and by strict supervision of its use. This has not always happened in the past and often it has been given too late in the disease to be of any real value. You cannot heal the destruction of joints once it has occurred. Therefore, some experts now consider that gold should be given earlier in the disease, in the hope of slowing down and temporarily stopping the progress of the disease in some individuals. This is the present day approach to the use of gold but it must be noted that any improvement is only temporary and this must be balanced against the risks of gold treatment.

Harmful effects on the use of gold

Harmful effects and warnings on the use of gold are listed in Table 30.4. Gold is particularly damaging to the skin and to the lining of the mouth and intestine.

The serious harmful effects produced by gold are not common and may often be avoided if the drug is stopped at the earliest possible sign of damage. This means that patients taking gold need very careful monitoring. They must have a complete physical examination, including blood and urine tests, at regular intervals. It also helps if gold is started in small doses at first and then the dose gradually increased over a period of weeks.

Gold is also available in a preparation that can be given by mouth: *auranofin* (Ridaura). It is marginally less effective than injections but, except for diarrhoea, harmful effects are fewer. Blood and urine tests should be carried out monthly.

Penicillamine

Penicillamine (Distamine, Pendramine) is a drug used to treat patients suffering from copper, mercury or lead poisoning because it chemically bonds with the metal to form an inactive compound (i.e. it is a chelating agent). Discovery of its benefits in the treatment of rheumatoid arthritis was purely by chance and we do not know how it works. It is probably as effective as gold. People taking penicillamine should have regular complete physical examinations, including blood and urine tests. Particular attention should be paid to looking for evidence of liver damage, fever and allergic reactions – see harmful effects and warnings in Table 30.4.

Chloroquine and hydroxychloroquine

Chloroquine (Nivaquine) and hydroxychloroquine (Plaquenil) are two anti-malarial drugs that, like penicillamine, were found by chance to have anti-inflammatory effects in rheumatoid arthritis. Like gold and penicillamine, there is some evidence that they may slow down or stop the progress of the disease in some individuals. However, their use is limited because of the harmful effects they may produce – particularly eye damage (see below). They are slow to work and take up to 4 weeks to produce any beneficial effect. Only about half of those people treated show any signs of improvement.

A serious harmful effect produced by these drugs are deposits of pigment in the cornea of the eyes, producing misty vision and haloes around bright lights. This occurs at high doses and may develop after only 4 weeks of treatment. They disappear within 3 months if the drug is stopped. Damage to the back of the eyes (the retina) may also occur but is rare unless high doses are used for over a year. This damage may be irreversible.

Levamisole

This drug is used to treat worm infections but it also stimulates the body's resistance to infection (immune responses). It appears to stimulate a depressed response but stimulation above normal does not occur. In rheumatoid arthritis it is an alternative to gold and penicillamine but it may produce serious harmful effects. It is not used in the UK.

Immunosuppressant drugs

There is some evidence that the selective use of drugs that block the body's immune response may help some individuals suffering from severe and disabling rheumatoid arthritis in whom other treatments have failed to produce any improvement. Four drugs are used – *azathioprine* (Azamune, Berkaprine, Immunoprin, Imuran), *chlorambucil* (Leukeran), *cyclophosphamide* (Endoxana) and *methotrexate* (Emtexate, Maxtrex). However, the benefits of using them to treat rheumatoid arthritis may easily be outweighed by the risks (see Chapter 9).

NOTE Azathioprine (Azamune, Berkaprine, Immunoprin, Imuran) and methotrexate (Maxtrex) may provide some relief in people who develop severe arthritis as a complication of psoriasis (see Chapter 75).

Overview of the drug treatment of rheumatoid arthritis

Drugs that relieve symptoms

Non-steroidal anti-inflammatory drugs (NSAIDs) all produce similar beneficial effects but also produce similar harmful effects. No one drug is better than all the others and the one chosen is a matter of personal preference. This is because different people may react differently to the same NSAID. If an NSAID does not relieve pain within about 1 week or reduce swelling of joints within about 3 weeks, it is not going to work and another drug should be tried.

It is important to remember that anti-inflammatory drugs relieve symptoms; they do not cure or affect the progress of the disease. In some individuals they may aggravate the damage to the joints by making the joints more mobile. Therefore what short-term benefits they produce need to be carefully balanced against the short-, medium- and long-term risks of their use.

Some specialists may start off treatment with aspirin or a related drug, often using a preparation specially designed for absorption in the small intestine rather than in the stomach (see earlier); others may start off treatment with ibuprofen or a related drug. The latter group of drugs are not superior to aspirin in relieving inflammation but they are generally better tolerated. More powerful NSAIDs such as indomethacin offer a useful additional choice. However, no one drug can be recommended over all the others, and treatment should always be tailored to an individual's needs and response to treatment.

The main risks of using NSAIDs

Irritation of the stomach and/or intestine, producing ulceration, perforation and bleeding is a problem with all NSAIDs, particularly in the elderly.

Allergic reactions may occasionally occur, and may, very rarely, produce severe wheezing and death. These allergic reactions are more likely to occur in someone who suffers from asthma and/or is allergic to aspirin. There is cross-allergy between these drugs, and someone allergic to aspirin may be allergic to other NSAIDs. Also, people allergic to tartrazine, an orange dye in foods and drinks (e.g. orange squash) may be cross-allergic to aspirin and also to other NSAIDs.

Blurred and/or diminished vision and changes in colour vision may, rarely, occur. If someone develops eye symptoms while taking an NSAID, the drug should be stopped and the individual should be examined by an eye specialist.

Fluid retention resulting in weight gain and ankle swelling may occur occasionally; therefore NSAIDs should be used with caution in anyone suffering from heart failure or raised blood pressure.

NSAIDs may, rarely, interfere with the ability of blood platelets to stick together to prevent bleeding. As a consequence they may *prolong the bleeding time* and should be used with caution in individuals suffering from disorders of blood clotting or anyone taking anti-blood-clotting drugs.

NSAIDs *reduce fever and inflammation* and may therefore mask an underlying painful condition.

NSAIDs may occasionally produce *abnormal liver function tests*; therefore individuals with evidence of impaired liver function should have tests of their liver function carried out before and at regular intervals during treatment. Very rarely, NSAIDs may cause liver damage with jaundice, and deaths have occurred; therefore at the earliest signs of liver damage (see Chapter 78) an NSAID should be stopped.

Very rarely, NSAIDs may *damage the kidneys*, producing blood and protein in the urine and, occasionally, nephrotic syndrome (see Chapter 33). Another form of kidney damage may also occur very rarely, due to the blocking of prostaglandins in the kidneys. This may cause a reduced blood supply in the kidney tissues and trigger kidney failure in people who already have impaired kidney or liver function, who are suffering from heart failure, who are taking diuretic drugs or who are elderly. The problem clears up if the NSAID is stopped. Individuals with evidence of impaired kidney function should have tests of their kidney function before and at regular intervals during treatment.

The risks from NSAIDs appear to be related to the dose and the duration of use, and they can be particularly dangerous in elderly people, in whom any harmful effect may be much more serious. However, the numbers of reported harmful effects from NSAIDs are very small compared with the millions of prescriptions issued every year. Nevertheless, they do suggest a need for caution. They should not be used by people with an active peptic ulcer (e.g. stomach, duodenal or oesophageal ulcer) or a history of a peptic ulcer or with ulcerative bowel disease (e.g. ulcerative colitis), nor by anyone allergic to aspirin or to one of the other NSAIDs, particularly if they suffer from asthma. In the elderly, NSAIDs should be used *only when absolutely necessary* and they should be used in the smallest effective dose for the shortest possible duration of time. They should also be used with utmost caution in anyone with impaired liver, kidney or heart function; NSAIDs are more dangerous in these conditions.

Reducing the risk of NSAIDs

To reduce the risks of NSAID treatment, everyone with impaired kidney, liver or heart function and all elderly people should have tests of their kidney and liver function, blood counts and tests of their blood chemistry carried out *before* treatment *and* at regular intervals during treatment. Any evidence of impairment from these tests is an indication for using a smaller dose or for not using an NSAID. Furthermore, people who suffer from these disorders and particularly the elderly are often taking other drugs (e.g. diuretics); therefore they should be aware of any dangers of the drugs interacting with each other (see Chapter 89).

To prevent harmful effects that NSAIDs may have in blocking prostaglandin production in various organs (e.g. the stomach, producing ulceration and bleeding) it is probably safer to use short-acting preparations when possible in order to allow some recovery between doses. Short-acting ones include ibuprofen, diclofenac, ketoprofen, and flurbiprofen; medium-acting ones include diflunisal, naproxen, fenbufen and sulindac; and long-acting ones include azapropazone and piroxicam.

To protect the lining of the stomach from damage by NSAIDs it helps if they are taken with a non-alcoholic drink (e.g. milk) during or just after a meal. Attempts to reduce the risk of damage by using specially coated preparations designed to release the active drug further down the intestine (e.g. enteric-coated preparations) do not appear to have succeeded. Similarly, the use of suppositories or pro-drugs (preparations in which the active drug is released when it reaches the liver) may still produce harmful effects in the stomach and intestine. This is probably due to the fact that NSAIDs produce general prostaglandin-blocking effects throughout the body, including the stomach and intestine, rather than producing a local effect by direct contact.

In those people in whom there is a risk of damage to the stomach and intestine but for whom there is no alternative to the use of an NSAID, it may be appropriate to take an additional drug each day in the hope of reducing the damage. For example, a prostaglandin drug such as misoprostol (Cytotec) may help to prevent ulcers, and so may drugs that reduce acid production in the stomach – for example, an H_2 blocker such as ranitidine (Zantac). A proton pump blocker such as omeprazole (Losec) is useful for treating ulcers caused by NSAIDs. These drugs are used to treat peptic ulcers, and are discussed in Chapter 15. The value of honey for this purpose needs further investigation.

The use of steroidal anti-inflammatory drugs

Corticosteroid drugs (e.g. prednisolone) by mouth produce a dramatic relief of symptoms but they do not cure or alter the progress of the disease. They should be used very selectively for treating those patients in whom all other treatments have failed and in whom the disease is still acute, progressive and crippling. They should be added to treatment and used in the smallest effective dose for the shortest time possible in order to control acute flare-ups of inflammation that may further limit mobility in an already damaged joint.

Corticosteroid injections into joints should be used with caution.

Drugs that may modify, reduce or stop the destruction of joints (anti-rheumatic drugs)

Drugs most commonly used for this purpose include gold, chloroquine, and hydroxychloroquine and penicillamine. They may take several months (over a year in some people) to produce any beneficial effect. It is difficult to determine in advance which patients will benefit most from which drug, and no drug appears to be of much long-term benefit.

Anti-rheumatic drugs should be considered if an individual's symptoms are not relieved by adequate doses of an NSAID and/or if there is evidence from medical examination, blood tests and X-ray examinations that the disease is getting worse and causing a lot of damage to joints and/or if the patient has developed other complications from the disease (e.g. damage to arteries or the lungs).

Gold by deep intramuscular injection is often the first drug of choice to add to NSAID treatment. After a test dose, an injection is given weekly until there is improvement. It is then given monthly for up to 5 years. If relapse occurs, the frequency should be revised to once weekly and then gradually reduced back to once monthly. A complete relapse should be avoided because once a course of gold has been stopped, a second course is usually of little benefit. Gold by mouth should be given daily, starting with a small daily dose and then slowly increasing the dose to the maximum recommended by the manufacturer. If there is no response after 9 months, the drug should be stopped. Gold treatment should be stopped if blood disorders develop or signs of kidney damage (e.g. protein in the urine) occur.

Penicillamine is an effective alternative to gold and needs a trial period of 6–12 months. *Chloroquine* and *hydroxychloroquine* are also alternatives. A trial period of about 6 months is necessary. After 12 months of treatment with chloroquine or hydroxychloroquine there is a rare risk of eye damage.

Immunosuppressive drugs should be used only when NSAID treatment combined with an anti-rheumatic drug has failed to provide relief. They are used in an attempt to prevent further destruction of joints, deformity and immobility. There is no convincing evidence that any one immunosuppressive drug works better than the others. The choice of drug is not critical; rather it is the decision to use such a drug that is critical and they should be used only in specialized units that have full back-up laboratory facilities to check for bone marrow damage and other harmful effects (see Chapter 9).

NOTE Drug treatment of rheumatoid arthritis should only be a part of its treatment and not *the* treatment. All patients should be given the opportunity to experience the benefits of physical and other treatments (e.g. physiotherapy, hydrotherapy) and particular attention should always be paid to good nutrition and the use of vitamin and mineral supplements as well as exploring the diet for possible factors that may make the condition worse. The role of fish liver oils or ginger needs further research before they can be recommended, as does the role of oil of evening primrose.

Table 30.1 Non-steroid anti-inflammatory drugs (NSAIDs) used to treat rheumatoid arthritis

Preparation	*Drug*	*Dosage form*
Alrheumat	ketoprofen	Capsules
Apsifen	ibuprofen	Tablets
Artracin	indomethacin	Capsules
aspirin	aspirin	Tablets, soluble tablets
Brufen	ibuprofen	Tablets, syrup
Caprin	aspirin	Enteric-coated tablets
Clinoril	sulindac	Tablets
Disalcid	salsalate	Capsules
Dolobid	diflunisal	Tablets
Ebufac	ibuprofen	Tablets
Feldene	piroxicam	Capsules, suppositories, dispersible tablets
Fenbid	ibuprofen	Sustained-release capsules (spansules)
Fenopron	fenoprofen	Tablets
Flexin Continus	indomethacin	Sustained-release tablets
Froben	flurbiprofen	Tablets, suppositories; sustained-release capsules (Froben SR)
ibuprofen	ibuprofen	Tablets
Imbrilon	indomethacin	Capsules, suppositories
Indocid	indomethacin	Capsules, sugar-free suspension, suppositories
Indocid-R	indomethacin	Sustained-release capsules
Indolar SR	indomethacin	Sustained-release capsules
indomethacin	indomethacin	Capsules, suppositories
Indomod	indomethacin	Sustained-release capsules
Laraflex	naproxen	Tablets
Lederfen	fenbufen	Tablets, capsules
Lederfen F	fenbufen	Effervescent tablets
Lidifen	ibuprofen	Tablets
Lodine	etodolac	Capsules, tablets
Mobiflex	tenoxicam	Tablets
Motrin	ibuprofen	Tablets
Naprosyn	naproxen	Tablets, suspension, granules, suppositories
Nu-Seals	aspirin	Enteric-coated tablets
Orudis	ketoprofen	Capsules, suppositories
Oruvail	ketoprofen	Sustained-release capsules, injection
Palaprin Forte	aloxiprin	Tablets
Paxofen	ibuprofen	Tablets

Table 30.1 Non-steroid anti-inflammatory drugs (NSAIDs) used to treat rheumatoid arthritis (*cont.*)

Preparation	*Drug*	*Dosage form*
Ponstan	mefenamic acid	Capsules, dispersible tablets, paediatric suspension; tablets (Ponstan Forte)
Progesic	fenoprofen	Tablets
Relifex	nabumetone	Tablets, suspension
Rheumox	azapropazone	Capsules, tablets
Rhumalgan	diclofenac	Enteric-coated tablets
sodium salicylate	sodium salicylate	Mixture
Solprin	aspirin	Soluble tablets
Surgam	tiaprofenic acid	Tablets, granules in sachets; sustained-release capsules (Surgam SA)
Synflex	naproxen	Tablets
Tolectin	tolmetin	Capsules
Trilisate	choline magnesium trisilicate	Tablets
Volraman	diclofenac	Enteric-coated tablets
Voltarol	diclofenac	Enteric-coated tablets, injection, suppositories, paediatric suppositories, dispersible tablets; sustained-release tablets (Voltarol Retard)

Table 30.2 Corticosteroid preparations for injecting into joints

Preparation	*Drug*	*Preparation*	*Drug*
Adcortyl	triamcinolone acetonide	hydrocortisone acetate	hydrocortisone acetate
Decadron	dexamethasone sodium phosphate	Hydrocortistab	hydrocortisone acetate
Deltastab	prednisolone acetate	Kenalog	triamcinolone acetonide
Depo-Medrone with Lidocaine	methylprednis-olone acetate, lignocaine hydrochloride	Lederspan	triamcinolone hexacetonide

Table 30.3 Non-steroidal anti-inflammatory drugs (NSAIDs) – harmful effects and warnings*

aspirin
Harmful effects include stomach upsets and irritation of the stomach and intestine, with ulceration and bleeding. Regular use of high doses may produce hearing disturbances and noises in the ears (rarely, leading to deafness), dizziness and confusion. Rarely, allergic skin reactions and wheezing may occur and, very occasionally, blood disorders. For other potential harmful effects see Chapter 27.

Warnings Aspirin must not be used in people with peptic ulcers, haemophilia or who are taking anti-coagulant drugs, nor in children under the age of 12 years. It should be used with caution in anyone who suffers from allergies, asthma, severe impairment of kidney function or dehydration. For other warnings, see Chapter 27.

azapropazone
Harmful effects Like all NSAIDs, it may cause stomach upsets and ulceration and bleeding from the stomach as well as allergic reactions. Occasionally, it may cause fluid retention (e.g. ankle swelling) and sensitivity of the skin to sunlight, and, very rarely, scarring of the lungs and a positive test for haemolytic anaemia (Coombe's test, see Chapter 26).

Warnings Azapropazone must not be used in people allergic to phenylbutazone or oxyphenbutazone. It should be used with caution in anyone with impaired kidney or liver function, stomach ulcers, blood disorders, allergies, asthma or allergy to aspirin or other NSAIDs.

benorylate
Harmful effects Benorylate is broken down to aspirin and paracetamol (see Chapter 27).

choline salicylate
See aspirin (Chapter 27).

diclofenac sodium
Harmful effects Like all NSAIDs, it may cause stomach upsets, ulceration and bleeding from the stomach and intestine, and allergic reactions. Mild, transient effects include belching, stomach pains, nausea, diarrhoea, headache and dizziness. Occasionally, tiredness, insomnia irritability and fluid retention (ankle swelling) may occur and, very rarely, liver damage, kidney damage and blood disorders. Local injections may cause pain, hardness and abscesses at sites of injections. Suppositories may produce itching, burning and frequency of bowel movements.

Warnings Diclofenac must not be used in people with peptic ulcers or bleeding from the stomach or intestine, in anyone allergic to diclofenac or in asthmatics allergic to aspirin or other NSAIDs. Suppositories must not be used in individuals with inflamed and/or ulcerative disorders of the anus, rectum or colon. It should be used with caution in anyone with a history of bleeding from the stomach or intestine, ulcerative colitis, Crohn's disease, or disorders of bleeding. People with severe liver, heart or kidney failure should be monitored carefully, and anyone on long-term treatment should have regular tests of their kidney and liver function, and blood counts.

diflunisal
Harmful effects Like all NSAIDs it may cause stomach upsets, ulceration and bleeding from the stomach and intestine, and allergic reactions. Mild effects include indigestion, diarrhoea, nausea, skin rashes and headache. Occasionally, there may be sleepiness, vomiting, constipation, wind, loss of appetite, insomnia, dizziness, noises in the ears (tinnitus), fatigue and tiredness, and, very rarely, jaundice, itching, skin rashes, sensitivity of the skin to sunlight, inflammation of the mouth, Stevens–Johnson syndrome, nervousness, depression and vertigo. Allergic reactions may be serious, with wheezing and fever. Blood disorders and damage to the kidneys

* See also the main risks of using NSAIDs, page 447.

Table 30.3 Non-steroidal anti-inflammatory drugs (NSAIDs) – harmful effects and warnings (*cont.*)

or liver may occur very rarely.

Warnings Diflunisal must not be used in individuals with severe kidney disease, or who are allergic to the drug or who have had acute asthma due to aspirin or an NSAID, nor in anyone with active bleeding from the stomach or intestine or peptic ulcers, or who is taking anti-coagulant drugs. The dose should be reduced in patients with impaired kidney function. Anyone on long-term treatment should have regular tests of liver and kidney function, blood counts and eye examinations.

etodolac
Harmful effects Like all NSAIDs, it may cause stomach upsets, ulceration and bleeding from the stomach and intestine, and allergic reactions. Mild effects include nausea, stomach pains, diarrhoea, indigestion, heartburn, wind, constipation, headache, dizziness, drowsiness, noises in the ears (tinnitus) and fatigue.

Warnings It must not be used in people who are allergic to it, or who develop asthma and other allergic symptoms to aspirin or other NSAIDs, nor in anyone with active peptic ulcers or bleeding from the stomach or intestine or with a history of peptic ulcers or bleeding.

fenbufen
Harmful effects Like all NSAIDs, it may cause stomach upsets, ulceration and bleeding from the stomach and intestine, and allergic reactions. Skin rashes are the most common and may occasionally be serious. Rarely, allergic lung damage and blood disorders may occur.

Warnings It must not be used in people who are allergic to it or to aspirin or other NSAIDs, nor in anyone with active peptic ulcers or bleeding from the stomach or intestine. Fenbufen should be used with caution in anyone with a history of peptic ulcers or chronic inflamed intestinal disorders.

fenoprofen
Harmful effects Like all NSAIDs it may cause stomach upsets, ulceration and bleeding from the stomach and intestine, and allergic reactions. Occasionally, it may cause indigestion, constipation, diarrhoea, ulcers in the mouth, nausea, vomiting and loss of appetite and, very rarely, kidney damage, liver damage with jaundice, blood disorders, allergic rections (itching, skin rashes, nettle rash, Stevens–Johnson syndrome), headache, sleepiness, dizziness, tremor, confusion, insomnia, noises in the ears (tinnitus), reduced hearing, blurred vision, palpitations, sweating, nervousness and fluid retention (e.g. ankle swelling).

Warnings Fenoprofen must not be used in people who are allergic to it or to aspirin or other NSAIDs; it may trigger an asthma attack in someone with a history of asthma or allergic disorders. It should not be used in anyone with active peptic ulcers or bleeding from the stomach or intestine, and with caution in someone with a history of peptic ulcers or chronic inflamed intestinal disorders. Because of the risk of fluid retention, it should be used with caution in people with heart failure or raised blood pressure. Tests of liver and kidney function should be carried out at regular intervals in patients on long-term treatment. Regular blood counts (including haemoglobin) should be carried out.

flurbiprofen
Harmful effects Like all NSAIDs it may cause stomach upsets, ulceration and bleeding from the stomach and intestine, and allergic reactions. Diarrhoea, ulcers of the mouth, nettle rash and skin rashes may occur, and, very rarely, liver damage, blood disorders and nerve damage. Suppositories may cause local itching and diarrhoea.

Warnings Flurbiprofen must not be used in people who are allergic to it or to aspirin or other NSAIDs; it may trigger an asthma attack in someone with a history of asthma or allergic disorders. It should not be used at all in patients with active

Table 30.3 Non-steroidal anti-inflammatory drugs (NSAIDs) – harmful effects and warnings (*cont.*)

peptic ulcers or bleeding from the stomach or intestine, and with caution in anyone with a history of peptic ulcers or chronic inflamed intestinal disorders, or who has impaired kidney function. Tests of liver and kidney function should be carried out at regular intervals in patients on long-term treatment. Regular blood counts (including haemoglobin) should be carried out.

ibuprofen
Harmful effects Like all NSAIDs it may cause stomach upsets, ulceration and bleeding from the stomach and intestine, and allergic reactions. Occasionally, skin rashes may occur and rarely blood disorders (thrombocytopenia).

Warnings Ibuprofen must not be used in people who are allergic to it or to aspirin or other NSAIDs; it may trigger an asthma attack in someone with a history of asthma or allergic disorders. It should not be used at all in patients with active peptic ulcers or bleeding from the stomach or intestine, and with caution in patients with a history of peptic ulcers or chronic inflamed intestinal disorders. Because of the risks of fluid retention, it should be used with caution in anyone with heart failure or raised blood pressure. In patients on long-term treatment, regular blood counts (including haemoglobin) should be carried out.

indomethacin
Harmful effects The most common harmful effects include diarrhoea, abdominal pains, constipation, loss of appetite, wind and bloating. Ulceration of the oesophagus, stomach, duodenum or intestine may occur, sometimes with bleeding. Very rarely, there may be liver damage with jaundice, headache, dizziness, vertigo, sleepiness, depression, fatigue, anxiety, muscle weakness, insomnia, muzziness in the head, mental symptoms, confusion, drowsiness, light-headedness, fainting, numbness, and pins and needles in the hands and feet. They are usually transient and clear up if the dose is reduced. Aggravation of epilepsy and parkinsonism, coma, convulsions, and noises in the ears (tinnitus) may occur very rarely, as may deposits in the cornea of the eyes, disturbances of the retina of the eyes, blurred vision and hearing disturbances, raised blood pressure, chest pain, rapid beating of the heart, heart failure, palpitations, fluid retention (e.g. ankle swelling), flushing and sweating, rise in blood sugar levels, itching, skin rashes, loss of hair, Stevens–Johnson syndrome, blood disorders, allergic reactions, and enlargement and tenderness of the breasts. Suppositories may cause irritation, pain on emptying the bowels and irritation of the rectum with itching and bleeding.

Warnings Indomethacin must not be used in people who are allergic to it or to aspirin or other NSAID, or who have active peptic ulcers or disorders of the intestine. It should be used with caution in anyone with disorders of bleeding, impaired kidney or liver function, asthma or a history of allergies, parkinsonism or psychotic illness. If blurred vision develops, the drug should be stopped and a complete specialist eye examination carried out. Regular eye tests and tests of liver and kidney function and blood counts should be carried out during prolonged treatment. The dose should be reduced or stopped if headaches develop.

Risks in driving It may cause drowsiness and impair driving ability; therefore drive only when you know that it is safe to do so.

ketoprofen
Harmful effects Like all NSAIDs, it may cause stomach upsets, ulceration and bleeding from the stomach and intestine, and allergic reactions. Mild and usually transient harmful effects include indigestion, constipation, diarrhoea, nausea and heartburn. Occasionally, it may cause headache, dizziness, confusion, vertigo, drowsiness, ankle swelling, mood changes and insomnia. Very rarely, it may

Table 30.3 Non-steroidal anti-inflammatory drugs (NSAIDs) – harmful effects and warnings (*cont.*)

cause blood disorders, kidney or liver damage and skin rashes.

Warnings Ketoprofen must not be used in people who are allergic to it or to aspirin or other NSAIDs; it may trigger an asthma attack in someone with a history of asthma or allergic disorders. It should not be used at all in patients with active peptic ulcers or bleeding from the stomach or intestine, and used with caution in patients with a history of peptic ulcers or chronic inflamed intestinal disorders. Because of the risks of fluid retention, it should be used with caution in anyone with heart failure or raised blood pressure. In patients on long-term treatment, regular blood counts (including haemoglobin) should be carried out.

mefenamic acid
Harmful effects it may, occasionally, cause diarrhoea, skin rashes, allergic wheezing and, rarely, liver damage, blood disorders, kidney damage, drowsiness and dizziness.

Warnings Mefenamic acid must not be used in anyone in whom it has previously caused diarrhoea, skin rashes or wheezing, or in individuals with active peptic ulcers and bleeding from the stomach or intestine. It should be used with caution in patients with a history of peptic ulcers or chronic inflamed intestinal disorders or with impaired kidney or liver function. Patients should have a blood count before and at regular intervals during treatment.

nabumetone
Harmful effects include diarrhoea, indigestion, nausea, constipation, abdominal pain, wind, headache, dizziness, skin rashes and drowsiness.

Warnings Nabumetone must not be used in people who are allergic to aspirin or other NSAIDs or who have active peptic ulcers, inflamed intestinal disorders or severe liver disorders. It should be used with caution in anyone with impaired kidney function or a history of peptic ulcers. Individuals with impaired kidney function should have reduced doses and tests of their kidney function carried out at regular intervals during treatment.

Risks with driving It may interfere with your ability to drive; therefore drive only when you know it is safe to do so.

naproxen
Harmful effects Like all NSAIDs, it may cause stomach upsets, ulceration and bleeding from the stomach and intestine, and allergic reactions. It may cause constipation, heartburn, abdominal pain, nausea, indigestion, diarrhoea, and, occasionally, sore mouth and gums, headache, dizziness, drowsiness, light-headedness, vertigo, itching, skin rashes, sweating, noises in the ears (tinnitus), hearing disturbances, visual disturbances, fluid retention (e.g. ankle swelling), breathlessness, palpitations and thirst. Very rarely, it may cause liver damage with jaundice, kidney damage, blood disorders, depression, inability to concentrate, insomnia, malaise, painful and weak muscles, loss of hair and allergic reactions.

Warnings Naproxen must not be used in individuals who are allergic to it or to aspirin or other NSAIDs nor in anyone with active peptic ulcers or bleeding from the stomach or intestine. It should be used with caution in people with a history of peptic ulcers or chronic inflamed intestinal disorders. Because of the risk of fluid retention, it should be used with caution in anyone with heart failure or raised blood pressure. The drug is excreted by the kidneys; therefore tests of kidney function should be carried out at regular intervals in patients on long-term treatment and a reduced dose should be used in patients with any impairment of kidney function. Naproxen may prolong bleeding; therefore it should be used with caution in people with disorders of bleeding or who are taking anti-coagulant drugs.

salsalate
Harmful effects include stomach upsets and

Table 30.3 Non-steroidal anti-inflammatory drugs (NSAIDs) – harmful effects and warnings (*cont.*)

ulceration of the stomach with bleeding. High doses may cause hearing disturbances and noises in the ears (rarely, leading to deafness), dizziness and confusion. It may, rarely, cause allergic skin rashes, allergic wheezing and swelling of the throat, and blood disorders. For other harmful effects, see aspirin (Chapter 27).

Warnings Salsalate must not be used in people with peptic ulcers, with haemophilia or who are taking anti-coagulant drugs, nor in children under the age of 12 years. It must not be used in someone who is allergic to aspirin. It should be used with caution in people who suffer from allergies, asthma, severe impairment of kidney function or dehydration.

sodium salicylate
Harmful effects include stomach upsets and irritation of the stomach and intestine with ulceration and bleeding. Regular use of high doses may cause hearing disturbances and noises in the ears (rarely, leading to deafness), dizziness and confusion. It may, rarely, cause allergic skin rashes and allergic wheezing, angioedema and blood disorders. For other harmful effects, see aspirin (Chapter 27).

Warnings Sodium salicylate should not be used in people with acute kidney failure, with peptic ulcers, with haemophilia or who are taking anti-coagulant drugs, nor in children under the age of 12 years or anyone who is allergic to aspirin. It should be used with caution in people who suffer from allergies, asthma, severe impairment of kidney function or dehydration, or who are on a low sodium diet and/or who have heart failure. Do not use in acute kidney function.

sulindac
Harmful effects are usually mild and often respond to a reduction in dosage. The most frequently occurring harmful effects include stomach and bowel upsets. Very rarely, it may cause peptic ulcers with bleeding; liver damage with jaundice; skin rashes, blood disorders, kidney stones and kidney damage; vertigo, sleepiness, insomnia, weakness, depression; blurred vision, metallic or bitter taste or loss of taste, sore tongue, raised blood potassium and allergic reactions which may be very serious and be associated with wheezing, fever, skin rashes, blood disorders, damage to the liver and other organs, and painful joints.

Warnings Sulindac must not be used in people who are allergic to it or to aspirin or other NSAIDs, nor in individuals with active peptic ulcers or bleeding from the stomach or intestine. It should be used with caution in anyone with a history of kidney stones or peptic ulcers or chronic inflamed intestine disorders, or because fluid retention may occur in anyone with heart failure or raised blood pressure. Tests of liver function should be carried out at regular intervals in patients with impaired liver function. The drug is excreted by the kidneys; therefore tests of kidney function should be carried out at regular intervals in patients on long-term treatment and a reduced dose should be used in anyone with any impairment of kidney function. Sulindac may prolong bleeding; therefore it must be used with caution in patients with disorders of bleeding or in anyone taking anti-coagulant drugs. You should drink plenty of fluids while on this treatment.

tenoxicam
Harmful effects Like all NSAIDs it may cause stomach upsets, ulceration and bleeding from the stomach and intestine and allergic reactions. Other harmful effects include constipation, diarrhoea, fluid retention, headaches, dizziness; rarely there may be blood disorders, changes in tests of liver function and visual disturbances.

Warnings Tenoxicam must not be used in people with active peptic ulcers,

Table 30.3 Non-steroidal anti-inflammatory drugs (NSAIDs) – harmful effects and warnings (*cont.*)

bleeding from the stomach or intestine, severe gastritis, allergy to aspirin or NSAIDs. It should be used with caution in the elderly and in anyone with impaired kidney or liver function.

tiaprofenic acid
Harmful effects Like all NSAIDs it may cause stomach upsets, ulceration and bleeding from the stomach and intestine, and allergic reactions. Harmful effects include indigestion, nausea, abdominal pain, vomiting, loss of appetite, heartburn, sore mouth, constipation, diarrhoea, wind; rarely, there may be headache, drowsiness, skin rash, sensitivity of the skin to sunlight, itching, allergic reactions and loss of hair.

Warnings Tiaprofenic acid must not be used in individuals who are allergic to the drug or with active peptic ulcers or inflammation of the intestine. It should be used with caution in anyone with a history of peptic ulcers, severe impairment of liver or kidney function, asthma or allergy to aspirin or other NSAIDs.

tolmetin
Harmful effects Like all NSAIDs it may cause stomach upsets, ulceration and bleeding from the stomach and allergic reactions. It may, rarely, cause headache, fluid retention (e.g. ankle swelling), skin rashes and blood disorders.

Warnings Tolmetin must not be used in people who are allergic to it or to aspirin or other NSAIDs, nor in individuals with active peptic ulcers or ulceration of the intestine. It should be used with caution in anyone with a history of peptic ulcers or chronic inflammatory intestinal disorders. It may prolong the bleeding time; therefore it should be used with caution in people with disorders of bleeding or who are taking anti-coagulant drugs. The drug is excreted by the kidneys; therefore tests of kidney function should be carried out at regular intervals in anyone on long-term treatment and a reduced dose should be used for individuals with any impairment of kidney function.

Table 30.4 Anti-rheumatic drugs – harmful effects and warnings

chloroquine and hydroxychloroquine
Harmful effects include nausea, vomiting and headache. *Doses used to treat malaria are usually well tolerated, but the* high doses *used to treat rheumatoid arthritis may cause harmful effects, some of which are occasionally serious.* They include itching, skin rashes, severe mental symptoms, convulsions, fall in blood pressure, changes in electrical tracings of the heart (ECG), double vision and difficulty in focusing. Prolonged use of high doses may cause deposits in the cornea of the eyes and damage to the retina. These changes may occur long after the individual has stopped taking the drug. Pigmented deposits and opacities in the cornea are often reversible if the drug is stopped at the earliest possible sign of any eye trouble. However, damage to the retina at the back of the eye, which causes defective vision, loss of colour vision and blind spots, is often not reversible after the drug has been stopped. This damage to the retina appears to be due to the overall dose taken in a course of

Table 30.4 Anti-rheumatic drugs – harmful effects and warnings (*cont.*)

treatment. Rare harmful effects include loss of hair, sensitivity of the skin to sunlight, skin rashes, noises in the ears (tinnitus), reduced hearing due to damage to the nerve supply to the ears, muscle weakness, bleaching of the hair, bluish-black pigmentation of the skin and lining of the mouth, and blood disorders.

Warnings An eye examination should be carried out before treatment and at regular intervals (3–6 months) during treatment. Chloroquine or hydroxychloroquine must not be used in anyone with eye disease or any visual defect or who is allergic to this group of drugs. They must be used with caution in people with impaired kidney or liver function. Harmful effects are more likely to occur in alcoholics therefore use with caution. Everyone on prolonged treatment should have regular complete medical examinations and regular blood counts should be carried out. If it is used to treat a patient who is also suffering from psoriasis, the drug may cause a severe flare-up of the psoriasis. It may also cause a flare-up of symptoms in patients suffering from porphyria.

Risks in elderly people Harmful effects may be more frequent and severe; therefore use with caution.

Risks with driving Damage caused to the eyes may make you unfit to drive.

gold (sodium aurothiomalate) by injection (Myocrisin)

Harmful effects may be largely prevented by carefully adjusting the dose and monitoring for harmful effects. They include mouth ulcers, skin rashes (dermatitis), fluid retention, protein in the urine and kidney damage, blood disorders (which may be sudden and fatal), scarring of the lungs, colitis and damage to nerves (producing numbness and pins and needles).

Warnings Gold must not be used in anyone with severe impaired function of the kidneys or liver, a history of blood disorders, severe dermatitis or active colitis. It should be used with utmost caution in individuals with a history of nettle rash, eczema or colitis. Urine should be tested for protein before each injection, the skin should be examined carefully and a full blood count including a platelet count should be carried out and the results made available before each injection. Blood disorders are more likely to occur when a dose of 400 mg to 1 gram has been given or between the 10th and 20th weeks of treatment but they may also occur with as little as 40 mg in total or after only 2–4 weeks of treatment.

Risks in elderly people Harmful effects may be more frequent and severe; therefore use with caution.

gold (auranofin) by mouth (Ridaura)

A gold salt that can be taken by mouth.

Harmful effects include sore mouth, diarrhoea, abdominal pain, nausea, ulceration of the intestine, itching, rashes, loss of hair, conjunctivitis and disturbances of taste. Very rarely, it may cause blood disorders, kidney damage and lung damage.

Warnings Auranofin should not be used in individuals with severe ulceration of the intestine, scarring of the lungs (fibrosis), severe dermatitis (exfoliative dermatitis), damage to the bone marrow producing serious blood disorders, serious kidney or liver disease, or systemic lupus erythematosus. It should be used with caution in people with impaired kidney or liver function, inflammatory disorders of the intestine or a history of bone marrow damage. Blood counts and urine tests for protein should be carried out before treatment and at monthly intervals whilst on treatment.

penicillamine

Harmful effects Vary in incidence and severity according to the dose that is used and the disorder being treated. Reported harmful effects include allergic reactions,

Table 30.4 Anti-rheumatic drugs – harmful effects and warnings (*cont.*)

nettle rash, redness of the skin if the temperature goes above 41°C, nausea, vomiting, loss of appetite, loss of taste (for about 6 weeks), mouth ulcers, bleeding into the skin, protein in the urine, kidney damage, blood disorders which may be serious, muscle weakness, fever and systemic lupus erythematosus.

Warnings Penicillamine must not be used in anyone who is allergic to penicillamine or who suffers from impaired kidney function, depressed bone marrow function or lupus erythematosus, nor in individuals receiving gold treatment, chloroquine, hydroxychloroquine or immunosuppressive drugs. It should be used with caution in people with impaired kidney function. Regular tests of kidney function, urine tests and blood counts should be carried out in individuals on long-term treatment. In rheumatoid arthritis no improvement will occur for 6–12 weeks. If improvement occurs after this period treatment should continue for six months and then be slowly reduced a little every 12 weeks. Nausea may be prevented by taking the drug with food or on going to bed, and if starting doses are small and then gradually increased. Rashes are common. Those that occur in the first few months usually clear up if the drug is stopped and then started at a lower dose and increased gradually. Rashes developing late in treatment are more difficult to clear up and usually require the drug to be stopped.

Risks in elderly people Do not use.

Rheumatic rubs

Rheumatic rubs contain chemicals that are referred to as counter-irritants – they *counter* pain in an underlying tissue by *irritating* sensory nerve endings in the area of skin supplied by nerves that link up in the spinal cord with nerves that supply the underlying tissue or organ. Their ability to counter pain may be due to nervous stimuli from the skin blocking painful stimuli from the underlying tissue as they enter the spinal cord. In other words, they 'crowd out' the painful stimuli. Massage and warmth probably produce a similar blocking effect by the sensations that they produce in the overlying skin and tissues.

Counter-irritants may also cause a reflex stimulation of the nerves that supply the muscular walls of small arteries in the underlying tissues. This stimulation may cause the muscles in the artery walls to relax, producing dilatation and an increase in blood supply to the affected tissue. This may wash away inflammatory chemicals that have been released in response to injury or disease.

Counter-irritants stimulate the nerve endings in the skin by producing local inflammation (heat and redness). Drugs that produce these effects on the skin are often referred to as rubefacients. The intensity of the inflammation will depend upon the chemical used, how irritant it is, its concentration, the solvent that it is dissolved in and the period of contact that it has with skin.

Many preparations contain more than one counter-irritant, which may add to their effectiveness but may also increase their harmful effects.

NOTE It is irrational to combine a counter-irritant with a local anaesthetic or anti-itching drug. This is because the latter drugs depress pain and other receptors in the skin, and these actions would oppose the stimulation of nerve receptors produced by the counter-irritants.

Preparations

The type of vehicle used to prepare a rheumatic rub is important because you want the preparation to stay on the surface of the skin but not to penetrate the skin. Preparations include liniments, gels, lotions and ointments.

Liniments are solutions or mixtures of various substances in oil, alcoholic solutions of soap or emulsions. They are rubbed into the skin. Oily preparations are useful when massage is desired.

Gels are semi-solid jelly preparations which spread easily but may also penetrate the skin more easily and should not be used in excess.

Lotions may be water or alcoholic suspensions. They spread easily on the surface, dry off and leave a coating of counter-irritant on the surface of the skin.

Ointments are semi-solid preparations which are useful if massage is desired.

Harmful effects and warnings on the use of rheumatic rubs

Some rheumatic rubs may be very dangerous if swallowed accidently (e.g. methyl salicylate, camphor). Preparations should therefore be labelled for *External use only* and kept well out of reach of children. Contact with the eyes should be avoided and they should not be applied to large areas of skin nor to wounds or damaged skin. They should not be applied inside the mouth or nose, and should not be used in children under the age of 2 years because they can absorb them into the bloodstream more easily than adults. Rheumatic rubs should be used only for the *temporary* relief of minor aches and pains in muscles and joints, and not regularly every day. The principal harmful effects produced by rheumatic rubs include rashes, blisters and allergic reactions.

Refrigerants

A number of compressed and liquefied gases are used as refrigerants. Many of them previously contained fluorocarbons but, because of their hazardous effects on the atmosphere, their use is now restricted. They cool the skin and numb the ends of pain-sensitive nerves, and constrict the blood vessels in the skin. They provide a very brief relief of local pain and should be used only to reduce a sudden and transient pain caused by a kick or a minor muscle sprain or strain – provided the overlying skin is intact.

Warning *Pain is a useful warning sign of injury, and the over-enthusiastic use of these preparations in sporting injuries may do more harm than good. By allowing a transient relief of pain they may allow an individual to carry on, thus running the risk of making the injury worse.*

The use of applications containing an NSAID

Topical preparations containing a non-steroidal anti-inflammatory drug (NSAID) may be useful for relieving local pain and swelling in an inflamed or injured joint, muscle or tendon. The NSAID penetrates the local tissues in a concentration sufficient to relieve local pain and inflammation but only a small amount is absorbed into the bloodstream and so the risk of harmful effects elsewhere in the body is significantly reduced. Nonetheless, they can still cause allergy, asthma and stomach upsets.

These preparations should not be applied on broken skin, on the lips or eyes, or on sites of infection. They should not be used in people known to be allergic to aspirin or other NSAIDs. They should not be used in children, in pregnancy and in breast-feeding mothers. They may irritate the skin and produce redness, itching and a rash. They may also discolour the skin. Rheumatic rubs containing an NSAID include Diflam cream (benzydamine) Feldene gel and Sports gel (piroxicam), Proflex cream (ibuprofen), Traxam gel (felbinac) and Voltarol Emulgel (diclofenac).

The use of rheumatic rubs

Conditions for which rheumatic rubs are often used include:

- *Rheumatism* – a general term used to describe any painful condition of muscles, joints or bones
- *Fibrositis* – a general term used to describe any painful condition affecting the fibrous tissues in the skin, muscles, tendons and structures around joints; it is a form of rheumatism that does not affect joints

- *Lumbago* – a general term for pain affecting the joints and muscles of the lower part of the back; many cases are due to damage of a lumbar disc in the spine
- *A sprain* – caused by a stretching or twisting injury to the muscles, ligaments or tissues around joints, which is not sufficient to actually rupture the structures but which can produce a tear causing pain, bruising and swelling
- *A strain* – caused by over-stretching a muscle, ligament or tissues around a joint; it produces pain on movement.

31

Osteoarthritis, chronic back pain and Paget's disease

Osteoarthritis

The term 'osteoarthritis' (or osteoarthrosis) refers to a chronic arthritis of joints usually associated with degeneration of the joints and advancing age. It is not, like rheumatoid arthritis, accompanied by some general debility. It may affect any joint, particularly weight-bearing joints such as the spine, hips and knees. It may also follow injury to a joint or a condition such as rheumatoid arthritis, or it may be due to failure of a joint to develop properly. There are many disorders that may result in osteoarthritis.

Osteoarthritis is the most common disease of joints and a major cause of disability among elderly people.

Whatever the cause of osteoarthritis the net result is that the shiny, smooth cartilage of the affected joint gets worn away, exposing the underlying bone which becomes hardened (eburnated) and nobbly. There is pain and stiffness in the affected joint (due to muscle spasm), and, as the disease progresses, movement becomes limited because the capsule of the joint becomes scarred (fibrosed) and the surface of the bones within the joint becomes uneven due to new bone developing in some parts and not in others. Minor twists or injuries may cause fluid to collect in the joint and the muscles around the joint start to waste, resulting in the joint becoming very unstable. In this state it can easily 'give way' and is more prone to injury from just a simple accident. Pain in an osteoarthritic joint can be very severe because of minor fractures of the bone surfaces inside the joint, damage to the capsule of the joint and/or damage to the ligaments and tissues surrounding the joint.

In some middle-aged women, osteoarthritis may affect the end joints of the fingers, resulting in the formation of cysts and bony outgrowths (Heberden's nodes) – it is called nodal osteoarthritis. In some of these women similar bony nodules (nodes) may affect the base of the thumb, the spine, hips and knees.

Treatment of osteoarthritis

Drug treatment

There is no drug that will stop, reverse or prevent the progressive destruction of a joint affected by osteoarthritis. Drugs may, however, be used to relieve symptoms such as pain, stiffness and painful muscle spasms.

Osteoarthritis is a chronic disorder which may slowly get worse and which may be subjected to flare-ups of pain and stiffness followed by long episodes of only mild discomfort. It is therefore important to try to avoid regular long-term treatment with drugs, and to use them only during a flare-up of symptoms.

Non-steroidal anti-inflammatory drugs (NSAIDs) are the first drugs of choice for treating acute flare-ups, and a *mild pain reliever* (e.g. paracetamol) may be added to the treatment if necessary. However, NSAIDs should be used with utmost caution in the elderly, who are the principal sufferers from oesteoarthritis. *Narcotic pain relievers* (e.g. codeine) should also be used with caution because of the risk of constipation and addiction.

Corticosteroids by mouth should not be used to treat osteoarthritis, and local injections of a corticosteroid into an affected joint should be used with utmost caution. *Muscle relaxants* occasionally help to prevent muscle spasm and may be used in conjunction with physiotherapy (see discussion later on the use of muscle relaxants in treating chronic back pain).

There is no convincing evidence of the benefits of special diets or fish oils.

Non-drug treatment is important

The important part of treatment of osteoarthritis is to achieve a balance between resting and exercising the affected joint. Loss of weight in someone who is overweight is essential. Any injury or undue stress to the joint should be avoided – which may mean using a walking stick, wearing a support or a built-up shoe or whatever and, if appropriate or possible, changing to a less physical occupation. Non-weight-bearing exercises such as swimming or hydrotherapy may be helpful. In some severe cases hip or knee replacement may be necessary.

Chronic back pain

There are several groups of drugs used to treat chronic backache but in general they are of limited use.

Drugs that relieve mild to moderate pain

This group of drugs is discussed in detail in Chapter 27.

Paracetamol is effective in relieving mild pain but of limited use in treating chronic back pain.

Codeine, dihydrocodeine and dextropropoxyphene are of limited use on their own in relieving bone and joint pains. They all produce nausea, sedation, dizziness and constipation, and are potentially addictive.

Pentazocine relieves moderate pain when taken by mouth, and severe pain when given by injection.

Codeine, dihydrocodeine, dextropropoxyphene and pentazocine are related to morphine and may produce drowsiness and affect the ability to drive a motor vehicle or operate moving machinery. They all increase the effects of alcohol.

The regular daily use of these drugs to relieve backache is not recommended nor is the use of compound pain-relieving preparations containing aspirin or paracetamol combined with codeine, dihydrocodeine or dextropropoxyphene (see Tables 27.5 and 27.6). Their long-term use may cause addiction. They are useful if taken for a few days at a time for acute episodes of pain, when they may be given along with an anti-inflammatory drug (see below) but constipation may be a problem, particularly in the elderly.

Non-steroidal anti-inflammatory drugs (NSAIDs)

NSAIDs are discussed in detail in Chapter 30. They are usually more like each other than different in that if they are similarly effective in relieving the symptoms of inflammation they usually produce similar harmful effects – which include ulceration and bleeding of the stomach and intestine. They also produce allergic reactions, particularly in people who are sensitive to aspirin or who suffer from asthma. NSAIDs are of use in treating acute episodes of pain. If taken at night they may help to reduce pain and stiffness in the morning; suppository preparations are useful for this purpose. These drugs should be used intermittently to treat acute episodes of pain, and for no more than a few weeks at a time.

Aspirin (see pages 403 and 442) is a very effective anti-inflammatory drug but its regular daily use produces problems, especially ulceration and bleeding of the stomach and duodenum. Some people may be allergic to aspirin and cross-allergic to other anti-inflammatory drugs and to tartrazine (an orange dye used in foods, drinks and medicines). Preparations include various types of slow-release and buffered formulations. *Benorylate* (an aspirin/paracetamol compound) is worth considering for the treatment of acute episodes of back pain, but see page 442.

Indomethacin is a potent anti-inflammatory drug that may be very effective in relieving back pain. However, it is harmful to the stomach and intestine, causing ulceration and bleeding. It may produce headache, dizziness, drowsiness and mental confusion, particularly in elderly people. It should only be used for the treatment of an acute episode of back pain.

Phenylbutazone has been taken off the market because of the harmful effects but it is an effective drug for relieving back pain. It is reserved for treating patients who suffer from ankylosing spondylitis but may be used only under the supervision of a hospital specialist.

Skeletal muscle relaxants

Painful spasms in skeletal muscles and stiffness caused by back trouble may be relieved by *diazepam* (e.g. Valium) or a related benzodiazepine if given in anti-anxiety doses. Because of the potential harmful effects of these drugs they should be given in the smallest possible dose for the shortest duration of time (read Chapter 40, on anti-anxiety drugs).

Baclofen (Lioresal) produces similar effects to diazepam. It depresses the transmission of painful stimuli up the spinal cord and their perception by the brain. High doses will produce drowsiness and floppy muscles. Its harmful effects are listed in Table 31.1.

Dantrolene (Dantrium) acts more directly on the muscles and produces fewer effects on the brain. Its harmful effects are listed in Table 31.1.

Other skeletal muscle relaxants include *carisprodol* (Carisoma), *chlormezanone* (in Lobak) and *methocarbamol* (Robaxin, in Robaxisal Forte). These act mostly within the spinal cord. *Orphenadrine* (Norflex) is an anticholinergic drug that produces some muscle relaxation.

The combination of a muscle relaxant with a mild to moderate pain reliever in one preparation is not recommended because the dose of one drug cannot be varied according to the individual's needs without altering the dose of the other drug.

Mood-altering drugs

Backache may affect mood, and mood may affect backache. *Diazepam* (Valium) relaxes muscles and also relieves the symptoms of anxiety, so it may occasionally be of use in some individuals in the smallest possible dose for as short a time as possible. Anti-depressant drugs may help some people but it is not appropriate to use these drugs to treat backache alone, unless the individual is depressed.

Rheumatic rubs

These are discussed in Chapter 30.

Coolant sprays

These have no place in the treatment of chronic back pain.

Table 31.1 Skeletal muscle relaxants – harmful effects and warnings

baclofen
Harmful effects include nausea, vomiting, drowsiness, dizziness, weakness, fatigue, fall in blood pressure, floppy muscles and confusion. These are related to dose and may be reduced by lowering the dose. Occasionally, baclofen may cause headache, insomnia, constipation or diarrhoea, frequency of passing urine, impotence, sweating, mood changes, hallucinations, tremors, visual disturbances, allergies, skin rashes, itching, impaired liver function. It may worsen serious mental illness and epilepsy.

Warnings Baclofen must not be used in people with active peptic ulcers, or who are allergic to it.

Abrupt withdrawal of baclofen may cause visual hallucinations, convulsions and heart complications; to prevent these complications the drug must be withdrawn gradually, reducing the daily dose slowly over several days to weeks. It must be used with caution and in reduced doses in anyone with impaired kidney function or with epilepsy, or in whom muscle spasticity helps to maintain posture. Patients with strokes do not benefit from the drug.

Risks in elderly people Harmful effects may be more frequent and severe in elderly people, particularly during the early stages of treatment.

Risks with driving It may affect your ability to drive; therefore do not drive until you know that it is safe to do so.

Risks with alcohol It may increase the effects of alcohol; do not drink while taking this drug.

carisoprodol
Harmful effects include drowsiness, dizziness, nausea, light-headedness, headaches, lethargy, dryness of mouth, jaundice, skin rashes and allergic reactions.

Warnings Carisoprodol must not be used in anyone who is allergic to it. It must be used with caution in people with impaired kidney or liver function.

Risks in elderly people Harmful effects may be more frequent and severe; therefore use with caution.

Risks with driving May interfere with ability to drive; therefore do not drive while on treatment.

Risks with alcohol Do not drink alcohol while taking this drug.

dantrolene
Harmful effects include drowsiness, dizziness, weakness, general malaise, fatigue and diarrhoea. Rarely, it may cause rashes and jaundice.

Warnings Dantrolene must not be used in anyone in whom muscle spasm helps to maintain posture or who has impaired liver function. Liver function tests should be carried out before and at 6 weeks after start of treatment and then at regular intervals. Dantrolene must be used with caution in people with chronic chest disorders or heart disease.

Risks in elderly people Harmful effects may be more frequent and severe; therefore use with caution.

Table 31.1 Skeletal muscle relaxants – harmful effects and warnings (*cont.*)

Risks with driving It may interfere with your ability to drive; therefore do not drive until you know how the drug affects you.

diazepam
See benzodiazepines (Chapter 40).

ketazolam
See benzodiazepines (Chapter 40).

methocarbamol
Harmful effects include drowsiness and, rarely, restlessness, anxiety, vertigo, tremor, confusion, convulsions, light-headedness, dizziness, nausea and vomiting. Rarely, there may be allergic reactions, which include nettle rash, skin rashes and swellings of the skin (angioedema).

Warnings Methocarbamol must not be used in individuals who are allergic to it, or in anyone with epilepsy, brain damage, myasthenia gravis, coma or pre-coma.

Risks in elderly people Harmful effects may be more frequent and severe; therefore use with caution and in reduced dosage.

Risks with driving It may affect your ability to drive; therefore do not drive until you know how the drug is affecting you.

Risks with alcohol It may increase the effects of alcohol, so do not drink alcohol while on treatment with this drug.

orphenadrine
Harmful effects include dry mouth, blurred vision, dizziness and restlessness. High doses may cause palpitations, rapid beating of the heart, difficulty passing urine, weakness, nausea, headache, constipation, drowsiness, confusion, hallucinations, agitation, tremor and irritation of the stomach. Rarely, skin rashes and allergic reactions may occur.

Warnings Orphenadrine must not be used in people who are allergic to it or who have glaucoma, retention of urine due to enlarged prostate gland or some other mechanical cause, narrowing of the outlet of the stomach or myasthenia gravis. It should be used with caution in anyone with a rapid heart beat, heart disease or impaired kidney or liver function.

Risks in elderly people Harmful effects may be more frequent, particularly confusion; therefore use with caution and reduce the dose.

Paget's disease of bone (osteitis deformans)

This disease causes softening, enlargement and deformity of bones. We do not know what causes it. It is rare before the age of 40 years but becomes more common with advancing age. Men are most commonly affected and it may 'run' in families.

In Paget's disease, bone is laid down and dissolved rapidly, and there is increased flow of blood to the bones so that they feel warm to touch. The rapid turnover of bone produces deformity, with enlargement of the bones in some parts and erosion in others. The sufferer may have aching pains or no symptoms at all. The deformity (e.g. bowing of the legs) can result in arthritis in the joints. It may affect the pelvis, leg bones, lumbar spine and/or skull. If Paget's disease affects the skull it may produce enlargement of the skull and deafness because the enlarged bones may press on the nerves to the ears. Involvement of the spine may press on nerves to the legs producing weakness or paralysis. If it affects the arms or legs, there is a risk of fractures.

Table 31.2 Drugs used to relax spasm of skeletal muscles

Preparation	*Drug*	*Dosage form*
Alupram	diazepam	Tablets
Atensine	diazepam	Tablets
Carisoma	carisoprodol	Tablets
Dantrium	dantrolene	Capsules
Diazemuls	diazepam	Injection
diazepam	diazepam	Capsules, tablets, elixir
Lioresal	baclofen	Tablets, sugar-free liquid
Lobak	chlormezanone paracetamol	Tablets
Norflex	orphenadrine	Injection
Robaxin	methocarbamol	Tablets, injection
Robaxisal Forte	methocarbamol aspirin	Tablets
Solis	diazepam	Capsules
Stesolid	diazepam	Injection, rectal solution
Tensium	diazepam	Tablets
Valium	diazepam	Tablets, sugar-free syrup, suppositories, injection

Treatment

Calcitonin obtained from the thyroid glands of pigs (pork calcitonin: Calcitare) or from salmon (salcatonin: Calsynar, Miacaleic) is used by injection to relieve the bone pains of Paget's disease. It regulates the laying down and dissolving of bone (bone turnover), and may help to reduce nerve damage caused by the pressure from enlarged bones.

Disodium etidronate (Didronel tablets) is also used to relieve pain in the treatment of Paget's disease. It is a diphosphonate that prevents the resorption (dissolving) of bone.

Table 31.3 Drugs used to treat Paget's disease – harmful effects and warnings

calcitonin (calitare, Miacaleic) and salcatonin (Calsynar)
Harmful effects include nausea, vomiting, flushing of the face, tingling of the hands, unpleasant taste in the mouth and inflammation of the site of injection.

Warnings In patients with a history of allergies (e.g. hayfever, eczema, asthma) a test dose of pork calcitonin should be given by using a scratch of the skin or an injection into the skin. A similar test should be carried out to test for allergy to gelatin in the preparation. Some people may develop antibodies to pork calcitonin but these do not appear to cause problems. Following injections of pork calcitonin the blood calcium level may

Table 31.3 Drugs used to treat Paget's disease – harmful effects and warnings (*cont.*)

initially fall; this may cause problems in people taking digoxin or related drugs.

disodium etidronate (Didronel)
Harmful effects include nausea, diarrhoea, metallic taste and transient loss of taste. High doses may actually cause an increase in bone pain and an increased risk of fracture.

Warnings Do not use in people with severe impairment of kidney function. Dose should be reduced in mild and moderate impairment, and tests of kidney function should be carried out at regular intervals. Use with caution in individuals with inflammatory intestinal disorders. Intake of calcium and vitamins should be adequate. Stop if fractures occur.

Risks in elderly people Harmful effects may be more frequent and severe; therefore use with utmost caution.

32

Gout

The term 'gout' is used to describe a mixed group of diseases in which crystals of uric acid salts are deposited in or near joints and cause recurrent attacks of acute inflammation of the joints and the surrounding tissues. In some people these crystals form white clumps (tophi) in and around the joints and cause destruction of the joints, with severe deformity. This particularly affects the hands and feet. Also, in patients with gout, crystals deposited in the kidneys may cause damage to the kidney tissues and be deposited in the urine leading to the development of kidney stones (uric acid stones). Individuals who suffer from gout may develop all or some of these complications in varying degrees of severity.

Gout principally affects males after the age of puberty and is rare in females (certainly before the menopause). Its incidence in males increases with advancing age.

Uric acid levels

Deposits of uric acid salts in the tissues are a consequence of excessive amounts of uric acid in the blood (hyperuricaemia). These excessive amounts appear to be determined by the age, sex and body weight of the individual and also by some inherited predisposition (i.e. a genetic factor). In a susceptible person, a high level of uric acid in the blood appears to be associated with a diet high in certain proteins (see later) and with being overweight.

A raised blood uric acid is arbitrarily defined as a level above 0.42 millimoles per litre (mmol/l) in adult males and 0.36 mmol/l in adult females. Not everybody who has a raised blood uric acid develops gout – a raised blood uric acid level without symptoms is ten times more common than gout, which occurs in about 6 out of every 1,000 people.

Uric acid production in the body

In the body, proteins are broken down in the liver to nitrogen-containing substances and excreted by the kidneys as urea, ammonium salts, uric acid and other substances. Uric acid comes particularly from the breakdown of purines, and normally its daily excretion is very small. Purines are breakdown products of proteins from animal cells, both from inside the body and from food.

In humans, the end product of purine breakdown is uric acid which forms insoluble salts, whereas in animals the end product is a soluble chemical called allantoin which is excreted in the urine. This is why most animals do not get gout. It is the insoluble salts of uric acid (urates) in humans that cause problems in those people who produce too much uric acid and/or do not excrete it effectively in the urine.

The concentration of uric acid (as urates) in the blood is a balance between the absorption of purines from foodstuffs and the breakdown of cells in the body on the one hand and the breakdown of purines by the liver and excretion of uric acid (as urates) in the urine on the other.

Primary gout refers to gout caused by the body's over-production of uric acid, or its decreased excretion by the kidney, or by both mechanisms. *Secondary gout* refers to an over-production of uric acid and/or a decreased excretion by the kidneys as a consequence of some other disorder or drug treatment.

Excessive production of uric acid

Primary causes of excessive production of uric acid

In a minority of individuals who suffer from gout the raised blood uric acid level is caused by excessive production of uric acid. A rare hereditary type of gout is a consequence of a specific enzyme defect resulting in an increased level of uric acid in the blood. Such a rare defect should be considered if gout develops at an unusually early age, if there is a family history of gout developing at an early age, and/or if uric acid kidney stones are the first sign that an individual has gout.

Secondary causes of excessive production of uric acid

Secondary causes of over-production of uric acid include an excessive turnover of purines in the body which may occur when the body is producing and breaking down cells to excess – for example, in disorders of the blood or blood-forming tissues in the bone marrow (e.g. leukaemia) or the use of some anti-cancer drugs which destroy cells (see below).

Excretion of uric acid

In normal subjects, about one-third of the uric acid produced in the body is excreted through the bile into the intestine and also directly from cells in the wall of the intestine; about two-thirds is excreted by kidneys.

Primary causes of decreased excretion of uric acid

Impaired excretion of uric acid by the kidneys is the problem in the majority of people who suffer from gout. In most of these individuals there appears to be some genetic abnormality that affects the functioning of the kidneys.

Secondary causes of decreased excretion of uric acid

Uric acid excretion may be impaired in kidney failure, by drugs affecting the kidney (see below), by chemicals (e.g. lead), by disorders that may affect the kidneys (e.g. raised blood pressure), or by a disturbance in the chemistry of the blood, called lactic acidosis, which may occur in starvation, with excessive vomiting or on exercise.

Certain drugs may cause gout

Gout may develop in people who are taking drugs that increase the production of uric acid. For example, anti-cancer drugs used to treat leukaemia kill off cells at a rapid rate and the breakdown of these cells in the body causes an increase in purines and therefore an increase in the uric acid level in the blood. This may cause gout in predisposed individuals. Drugs may also increase the blood uric acid level by decreasing its excretion by the kidneys. This may be due to direct damage to the kidneys or by their actions in blocking the secretion of uric acid (as urates) into the urine. This latter effect is produced by diuretic drugs such as thiazide diuretics and loop diuretics. Aspirin in low doses may reduce uric acid secretion into the urine, and aspirin, phenylbutazone and probenecid may interfere with the transport of uric acid by proteins in the blood, causing more free uric acid to be present in the blood.

Acute attacks of gout

In an acute attack of gout the affected joint becomes hot, red and swollen, the overlying skin becomes hot and shiny and the pain may be excruciating.

Acute attacks may be associated with fever and sometimes are preceded by loss of appetite and nausea. Sometimes an acute attack may affect the tissues surrounding the joint rather than the joint itself.

If untreated, an acute attack may last days or weeks but eventually subsides. As the joint recovers there may be itching and scaliness of the overlying skin.

Some sufferers may have only an isolated attack of acute gout whereas others may get recurrent acute attacks over months or years. Occasionally, the attacks may be so frequent that they merge into one another and the individual suffers a prolonged attack of what is called sub-acute gout – i.e. neither acute nor chronic but in between.

Chronic gout

Recurrent attacks of acute gout result in progressive destruction of the affected joint, causing impaired function and deformity of the joint. Tophi (see above) are frequently found in tendon sheaths, around joints and in the cartilage of the ear lobes. Other complications of chronic gout include the development of uric acid (urate) kidney stones and damage to the kidney tissue.

Gout is often associated with other disorders; for example, obesity, raised blood fat levels, diabetes, hypertension and coronary heart disease.

Treatment of gout

Drugs are used to relieve the pain and inflammation of an acute attack of gout and to prevent attacks of gout. Drug treatment is also aimed at preventing or reversing complications that may result from deposits of uric acid salts in the joints and kidneys and also at preventing the formation of kidney stones.

In addition to drug treatment, weight reduction, diet and reduced alcohol intake may help.

Weight reduction is important in an individual who is overweight. However, fasting should be avoided because it may raise the blood uric acid level. Loss of weight should therefore be gradual.

Diet may be important because purines present in food make a significant contribution to the production of uric acid in the body. A purine-restricted diet may cause a fall in blood uric acid level in normal people and in those individuals who cannot excrete uric acid efficiently in the urine. However, drug treatment is so effective that a strict diet is not necessary. Foods rich in purines include liver, kidneys, sweatbread, sardines, anchovies, fish and yeast extract.

Fluid intake People with gout should drink at least 3 litres of fluid every day.

Excessive alcohol consumption should be avoided in anyone with gout. Alcoholic drinks contain purines.

Drugs used to treat acute attacks of gout

Non-steroidal anti-inflammatory drugs (NSAIDs)

Non-steroidal anti-inflammatory drugs (NSAIDs) relieve the pain, redness and swelling; when given promptly during an acute attack of gout, they provide relief within about 6–12 hours and complete recovery within 3 days. They are considered to be the first drugs of choice by many medical authorities. NSAIDs relieve pain and inflammation but they do not affect the blood level of uric acid.

The NSAIDs now in fashion for treating acute attacks of gout include azapropazone, diclofenac, indomethacin, naproxen, piroxicam and sulindac (see Table 32.1).

Although *aspirin* is a very effective anti-inflammatory drug it is best not to use it to treat acute attacks of gout. This is because in doses that relieve mild pain (1–2 g daily) aspirin may reduce the excretion of uric acid by the kidneys. In high doses (over 5 g per day) aspirin may increase the excretion of uric acid while relieving pain and inflammation but often at the price of unacceptable harmful effects.

Colchicine

Colchicine relieves inflammation in gout. It may be used to relieve acute symptoms and also to prevent attacks. It is obtained from the autumn crocus and has been used to treat gout for over 200 years. It does not affect the level of uric acid in the blood.

When taken by mouth it is absorbed into the bloodstream, taken to the liver and partly broken down. The drug and its breakdown products are then excreted back into the intestine through the bile and through secretion from glands in the lining of the intestine. In this way about 80 per cent of a dose of colchicine is excreted in the faeces; the rest is excreted in the urine.

Use of colchicine

The main harmful effects produced by colchicine are nausea, vomiting and diarrhoea, which develop within a few hours of taking a dose. They are not related directly to the dose used or to how it is taken, but seem to be related to variations in response between individuals. Different people react differently and therefore it requires patience to work out the right dose that will relieve an individual's symptoms and not produce nausea, vomiting and diarrhoea. If these harmful effects occur, the drug must be stopped immediately. Colchicine stays a long time in the body and repeated doses may produce serious harmful effects (see later).

Colchicine should be started as soon as possible in an acute attack (within the first 12 hours), when it will provide rapid relief in about 90 per cent of sufferers.

Some doctors prescribe colchicine in small doses every hour until the pain and swelling in the inflamed joints are relieved or until nausea, vomiting and diarrhoea develop. Others give it every 2–3 hours. No more than 10 mg in total should be given in any one course, and a course of treatment should never be repeated within less than 3 days. An injection of colchicine into a vein may produce immediate beneficial effects but the drug is very irritating to the tissues if it leaks from the site of injection.

An interesting point about colchicine is that its use is *specific* to gout and an individual's response to colchicine is diagnostic. If a patient's painful and swollen joints improve dramatically with colchicine, he or she is definitely suffering from gout.

Colchicine is more popular in the USA than in the UK for treating acute attacks of gout, and its long-term use in low doses is also popular in the USA for preventing recurrent acute attacks of gouty arthritis.

Steroidal anti-inflammatory drugs

Very occasionally an acute attack of gout may not respond to treatment with an NSAID (e.g. indomethacin or naproxen) or to colchicine. In these cases it may occasionally be necessary to use a steroidal anti-inflammatory drug (e.g. an intramuscular injection of corticotrophin). This may produce a dramatic improvement. However, after this improvement, an acute attack of gout may come back (this is called a rebound attack). It is wise to try to prevent this rebound attack by taking an NSAID or colchicine (in low dose) daily for 1 week after the injection. Corticotrophin should be used only occasionally and never for long-term use.

Aborting an acute attack of gout

An NSAID (e.g. indomethacin, naproxen) or colchicine may be used to abort an attack of gout if the recommended daily dose is taken at the very first sign of an impending attack. People with long-standing gout should always have a supply of one of these drugs to hand for such purposes.

Drugs used to prevent attacks of gout

The prolonged use of drugs that lower the levels of uric acid in the blood and tissues should always be considered once an individual has recovered from an acute attack of gout, especially in someone who suffers from associated kidney disease, recurrent acute attacks of gouty arthritis, tophi and/or evidence of chronic gouty arthritis or who suffers from gout and has a very high level of uric acid in the blood.

Two groups of drugs are used for this purpose: those that increase the excretion of uric acid in the urine (e.g. probenecid, sulphinpyrazone or azapropazone); and those that block its formation (e.g. allopurinol).

Drugs used to increase the excretion of uric acid in the urine

Drugs that increase the excretion of uric acid in the urine are referred to as uricosuric drugs. They act directly on the kidneys to block the reabsorption or uric acid from the urine and, therefore, to increase its rate of excretion. When the rate of excretion of uric acid in the urine is greater than the rate at which uric acid is formed, its level in the blood falls. Continuous daily use of these drugs not only prevents new deposits of uric acid salts in tissues but also causes old deposits to shrink.

Probenecid and *sulphinpyrazone* promote the excretion of uric acid (urates) in the urine by reducing its reabsorption from the urine back into the bloodstream. They are of no use in treating an acute attack of gout and may actually trigger an acute attack in the first few weeks of treatment as the uric acid salt deposits in joints are broken down and uric acid re-enters the bloodstream. Therefore, treatment with these drugs should not be started during an acute attack of gout, but they may be continued if they had already been started before the attack began. Probenecid or sulphinpyrazone are best suited to sufferers who are under 60 years of age and who have good kidney function and no kidney stones. They should be started in small doses divided throughout the day in order not to trigger an acute attack.

People taking a uricosuric drug should drink plenty of fluids and take sodium bicarbonate or potassium citrate to lower the acidity of the urine in order to reduce the risk of developing kidney stones or other kidney problems caused by deposits of uric acid salts in the kidneys.

NOTE Aspirin blocks the actions of these drugs and should *not* be used.

Regular daily doses of an anti-inflammatory drug (see above) or colchicine (in low dosage) should be taken for the first few months of treatment to prevent further acute attacks of gout and until the blood uric acid level is down to normal.

Azapropazone is an NSAID that is useful for treating an acute attack of gout. It is also useful for preventing attacks because, like probenecid and sulphinpyrazone, it increases the excretion of uric acid by the kidneys.

Drugs that block the formation of uric acid

Allopurinol is an effective drug for treating high blood levels of uric acid whether due to a defect in protein breakdown (primary gout), secondary to other disorders, or as a result of other drug treatments (e.g. thiazide diuretics, anti-cancer drugs). It blocks the production of uric acid by blocking the enzyme (xanthine oxidase) responsible for the formation of uric acid, which is the end breakdown product of purines. The chemicals that go to form uric acid are much more soluble than uric acid and are easily excreted in the urine. Allopurinol causes the blood level of uric acid to fall and the collections of uric acid salts in joints and skin to dissolve. This prevents both the development and the progression of gouty arthritis. Also, uric acid stones in the kidneys do not develop and the risk of kidney damage is reduced. During the first few weeks or months of treatment, acute attacks of gout may increase but later they are reduced and generally prevented.

Allupurinol is of no benefit in treating acute attacks of gout and it should not be started until all symptoms of acute arthritis have subsided. It is particularly useful in gouty patients who suffer from impaired kidney function and/or kidney stones, who cannot take drugs that increase the excretion of uric acid (see above).

Allergy to allopurinol is a rare harmful effect; some individuals may become allergic to it after months or even years of regular daily treatment. Allergy may cause skin rashes with fever, malaise and aching muscles. These attacks are more frequent in people with kidney disease.

Kidney stones

The risks of developing uric acid kidney stones is reduced by allopurinol treatment but it is also wise to drink plenty of fluids as well. Treatment should be started with a low daily dose and increased slowly over several weeks in order to avoid triggering an acute attack of gout. Allopurinol should be taken once a day to start with but if the dose goes above 300 mg daily, this should be divided and given twice daily (morning and night).

Warnings *It is very important to understand that the drugs used to treat acute attacks of gout act quite differently from those that are used to prevent attacks. Except for azapropazone, drugs used to prevent gout will worsen and prolong an acute attack of gout.*

NOTE A raised level of uric acid in the blood without symptoms of gout is not usually treated unless there is a family history of gout and/or if the level is high, in which case allopurinol is the drug of choice.

Table 32.1 Drugs used to treat acute attacks of gout – harmful effects and warnings

Anti-inflammatory drugs
Harmful effects Anti-inflammatory drugs are used in high doses for only a few days to treat an acute attack of gout. The most commonly used include azapropazone, diclofenac, indomethacin, naproxen, piroxicam and sulindac. Because these drugs are used for only a few days at a time, harmful effects are few; nevertheless they can be serious and include nausea, vomiting, diarrhoea, ulceration of the stomach with bleeding, allergic reactions and fluid retention. For other potential harmful effects see Chapter 30.

Warnings These drugs should not be used to treat acute attacks of gout in people with active peptic ulcers, and should be used with utmost caution in individuals who are allergic to aspirin or one of the other anti-inflammatory drugs, and/or who suffer from asthma. For other warnings on their use see Chapter 30.

colchicine
Harmful effects include nausea, vomiting and abdominal pain, which may occur whether the drug is given by mouth or by injection. Large doses may, rarely, cause severe diarrhoea, bleeding from the intestine and, very rarely, muscle weakness, skin rashes, kidney and liver damage, dehydration, loss of hair and nerve damage. Damage to the bone marrow, knocking out red and/or white cell production, may rarely occur with prolonged treatment. Thrombophlebitis may develop at the site of injection.

Warnings Colchicine must be used with caution in people with impaired kidney, liver or heart function, peptic ulcers, ulcerative colitis or other disorders of the stomach or intestine.

Risks in elderly people Harmful effects may be more frequent and severe; therefore use with caution.

corticotrophin
This is given in a dose of 80 units by intramuscular injection, repeated in 2 days if necessary. In these one-off doses harmful effects are unlikely.

General principles on the drug treatment of gout

There is no place for 'standard' treatment regimens in someone who suffers from gout. Each person needs treatment tailored to his or her particular needs and response. This may often be a matter of trial and error until a suitable treatment schedule is worked out.

An *acute attack* of gout will usually respond to an NSAID or to colchicine but, rarely, it may be necessary to use a steroidal anti-inflammatory drug (e.g. corticotrophin). After an acute attack of gout has settled down, minor symptoms may continue for a few months and therefore, in addition to using a drug that reduces the level of uric acid in the blood and tissues, it may be necessary to continue with regular daily doses of an NSAID or low doses of colchicine for a few months to prevent any flare-up. In the USA a common practice is to use low doses of colchicine daily until the blood uric acid level is below an agreed level and until that patient has not had an acute attack for 6–12 months.

There is controversy about when to treat a patient who has a raised blood uric acid level. Some experts point out that many first attacks of gout are not followed by recurrent attacks of acute gout. They suggest long-term treatment to lower blood uric levels only when a patient has had two or more attacks of acute gouty arthritis, has evidence of tophi or chronic gouty arthritis, of kidney disease or of gout with a markedly raised blood uric acid level. Other experts suggest a more aggressive approach with long-term treatment starting after the first attack of gouty arthritis or kidney stones in order to reduce the risk of kidney damage and to prevent the formation of tophi in joints or elsewhere. In making a decision whether or not to take preventative treatment it is important to note that a raised blood uric acid level is often present for 10–20 years before an acute attack of gout develops, even though joint and kidney damage may already have occurred.

NOTE Measurements of the amount of urates in a 24-hour collection of urine may help to identify those individuals who are over-producing uric acid and excreting it at a high level in the urine. These people are best treated with allopurinol. Anyone with high blood uric acid level who shows an under-excretion of urates in the 24-hour collection of urine is best treated with a uricosuric drug (e.g. probenecid, sulphinpyrazone).

Table 32.2 Drugs used to prevent gout – harmful effects and warnings

allopurinol
Harmful effects are rare and usually mild. Their frequency and severity are increased in patients with impaired kidney and/or liver function. The harmful effects include nausea, vomiting, skin rashes, drowsiness, headache, vertigo, malaise, disturbance of taste, raised blood pressure and, occasionally, loss of hair. Skin rashes are the most common harmful effect; they

Table 32.2 Drugs used to prevent gout – harmful effects and warnings (*cont.*)

may be mild or severe and occur at any time during treatment. Serious skin rashes may occur with a generalized allergic reaction involving fever and swollen glands, and can be associated with inflammation of the liver and, rarely, the kidneys.

Warnings Allopurinol should not be used in individuals who are allergic to it nor to treat an acute attack of gout. An NSAID or colchicine should be used in the first few months of treatment to prevent an acute attack. Plenty of fluids should be drunk (3 litres per day). It must be used with caution in people with liver disease, and in reduced dosage for anyone with impaired kidney function.

Risks in elderly people Harmful effects may be more frequent and severe; therefore use with caution.

azapropazone
Harmful effects Occasionally there may be skin rashes, sensitivity of the skin to sunlight producing an allergic skin rash (photo-allergy) and fluid retention (e.g. ankle swelling). The fluid retention may trigger heart failure in a susceptible person. Stomach upsets, nausea and bleeding from the stomach may occur occasionally, and, very rarely, scarring of the lungs and positive tests for haemolytic anaemia.

Warnings Azapropazone should not be used in anyone with severe impairment of kidney function or who is allergic to phenylbutazone and related drugs. It should be used with caution in people with mild to moderate impairment of kidney function, peptic ulcers, allergic disorders, asthma or blood disorders, or who are allergic to aspirin and other anti-inflammatory drugs.

Risks in elderly people Harmful effects may be more frequent and severe; therefore use with caution.

probenecid
Harmful effects are infrequent and include headache, loss of appetite, nausea, vomiting and frequency of passing urine. Very rarely, there may be allergic reactions, including anaphylaxis, dermatitis, itching, fever, sore gums, flushing, dizziness, blood disorders, kidney damage and liver damage. A flare-up of gout may occur and, rarely, kidney stones with or without blood in the urine and pain in the kidneys.

Warnings Probenecid should not be used in people who are allergic to it, or who have a history of blood disorders, kidney stones, or during an acute attack of gout. It should be used with caution in anyone with peptic ulcers or kidney or liver disorders. Sufferers should drink plenty of fluids to reduce the acidity of the urine. Any flare-up of the gout should be treated with an NSAID or colchicine.

Risks in elderly people Harmful effects may be more frequent and severe; therefore use with caution. Kidney function should be checked before treatment and at regular intervals during treatment.

sulphinpyrazone
Harmful effects are usually mild and transient. They include nausea, vomiting, diarrhoea and stomach pains. Occasionally, there may be skin rash, flare-up of peptic ulcers and allergic reactions, and, very rarely, blood disorders, bleeding from the stomach and impaired kidney function. An acute attack of gout may be triggered.

Warnings Sulphinpyrazone should not be used in individuals who are allergic to phenylbutazone, azapropazone or related drugs or who have severe liver disease or peptic ulcers. It should be used with caution in people with impaired kidney function, a history of peptic ulcers or allergy to aspirin and other anti-inflammatory drugs. A gradually increasing daily dose should be used in anyone with a raised blood uric acid level, a history of kidney stones or kidney colic, and if the treatment has been stopped and then re-started. Tests of kidney function and blood counts should be carried out before and at regular intervals during

Table 32.2 Drugs used to prevent gout – harmful effects and warnings (*cont.*)

treatment. Because it causes salt and water retention in the body, it must be used with caution in someone prone to develop heart failure. To prevent kidney problems, drink plenty of fluids to reduce the acidity of the urine.

Risks in elderly people Harmful effects may be more frequent and severe; therefore use with caution. It is important to check kidney function before and at regular intervals during treatment; smaller doses must be used if there is evidence of kidney impairment.

Table 32.3 Preparations used to prevent gout

Preparation	*Drug*	*Drug group*	*Dosage form*
allopurinol	allopurinol	Xanthine oxidase inhibitor	Tablets
Aluline	allopurinol	Xanthine oxidase inhibitor	Tablets
Anturan	sulphinpyrazone	Uricosuric	Tablets
Benemid	probenecid	Uricosuric	Tablets
Caplenal	allopurinol	Xanthine oxidase inhibitor	Tablets
Cosuric	allopurinol	Xanthine oxidase inhibitor	Tablets
Hamarin	allopurinol	Xanthine oxidase inhibitor	Tablets
Rheumox	azapropazone	Uricosuric and NSAID	Capsules
Zyloric	allopurinol	Xanthine oxidase inhibitor	Tablets

33

Disorders of the urinary tract

Urine is produced by the kidneys, passes down the ureters and is stored in the bladder. As the volume of urine in the bladder increases, the bladder wall stretches and stimulates nerve endings that are sensitive to the stretching. It also puts pressure on pressure-sensitive nerves near the outlet from the bladder. Stimulation of these nerves produces the desire to pass urine. However, the ring of muscle around the bladder neck normally keeps the bladder outlet closed until it is consciously relaxed when you go to pass urine.

The term 'urinary tract' refers to the whole system – kidneys, ureters, bladder and urethra. In males it also includes the prostate and seminal vesicles. A number of disorders can affect the urinary tract and the most common include infections of the urinary tract; urgency and frequency of passing urine; incontinence of urine and bed wetting; and retention of urine.

Infections of the urinary tract

'Urinary tract infection' is a term used to describe an infection in the urine and/or in the tissues of any of the structures in the urinary tract – kidneys, ureters, bladder, prostate and urethra. Bacteria are the most common infecting micro-organisms. Rarely, a urinary tract infection may be caused by yeasts, fungi or viruses. The term covers a wide range of symptoms and describes conditions from inflammation of the bladder (cystitis) to a severe infection of the kidneys (acute pyelonephritis). The infection may be located to a particular site; for example, the urethra (urethritis), bladder (cystitis), kidney (acute or chronic pyelonephritis) or prostate (prostatitis). On the other hand, the urine may be infected with bacteria without any symptoms (asymptomatic bacteruria).

A major problem with infections of the urinary tract is that sufferers may get recurrent infections which can eventually damage the kidneys.

The normal urinary tract is free from bacteria except for some organisms near the outlet (the urethra) which contaminate it. Infection of the urinary tract usually comes from outside and spreads upwards through the urethra into the bladder. It is most frequently caused by bacteria that are normally present in the large bowel and spread into the urethra from faeces which contaminate the skin around the anus and genitals. This spread of infection from the anus into the urethra and then upwards into the bladder is more common in women because their urethras are short.

Sometimes urinary tract infections may be triggered by a blockage in the urinary tract, caused, for example, by a kidney stone or an enlarged prostate gland, by the presence of a catheter, by nerve damage to the bladder so that it does not empty properly, or by disease of the kidneys due to some other disorder (e.g. diabetes). Very rarely, bacteria from the bowel may spread via the bloodstream to infect the urinary tract but only if the kidneys are damaged by disease.

Urinary catheters

A catheter to draw off urine from the bladder is a major source of infection of the urinary tract, particularly a catheter that is left in place (indwelling catheter).

The insertion of a catheter into the bladder is a common cause of urinary infection; when this is done in hospital, there is a risk of infection from hospital bacteria which are often resistant to the commonly used antibiotics.

Honeymoon cystitis

The so-called 'honeymoon cystitis' in women is associated with sexual activity in previously non-sexually active women. Repeated thrusting of the penis into the vagina may irritate the back wall of the bladder and subsequently make it difficult to pass urine after intercourse. During intercourse, bacteria from the anus may spread up into the vagina and into the urethra and they may enter the bladder. Passing urine straight after intercourse helps to get rid of these bacteria. In women who find it difficult to pass urine straight after intercourse the bacteria may multiply to cause an infection of the urethra and/or bladder.

Contraceptive diaphragms (caps) may cause irritation and interfere with the ability to pass urine straight after intercourse and so increase the risk of infection. Spermicides may also cause irritation.

Post-menopausal women who do not produce sufficient secretions from their vagina to provide lubrication during sexual intercourse, may also be susceptible to urinary infections.

Risks of urinary tract infections in pregnancy

Pregnant women may develop a urinary tract infection early in pregnancy, which may develop into a serious kidney infection later in pregnancy. This kidney infection may be associated with anaemia, premature birth and still-birth. Therefore early diagnosis and proper treatment of urinary infections in pregnant women is essential even though they may have no symptoms.

Risks of urinary tract infections in elderly people

Some elderly women are prone to get urinary infections because they may have lax vaginal muscles, which causes the outlet from the bladder to sag. Elderly men who have enlarged prostate glands are also prone to urinary infection. It may be triggered by a doctor inserting an instrument to examine the inside of the bladder.

Symptoms of urinary tract infections

Symptoms of a urinary tract infection include passing urine frequently; burning, stinging and pain when the urine is passed; and pain or discomfort in the bladder. A fever may be present and blood may appear in the urine – which may be cloudy.

Diagnosis of a urinary tract infection is made from laboratory tests of the urine; X-rays may be necessary to look for an abnormality in the urinary tract.

Warning *Any urinary tract infection in a child should be fully investigated and treated by a specialist, in order to prevent kidney complications when the child grows up.*

Anti-bacterial drug treatment of urinary tract infections

The aim of drug treatment is to clear the urine of bacteria in order to relieve symptoms and to prevent kidney damage.

Infections of the urinary tract without symptoms

In pregnant women Any bacterial infection of the urine without symptoms (asymptomatic bacteruria) in early pregnancy should be treated as a matter of urgency in order to prevent the development of a kidney infection (pyelonephritis) and other problems later in the pregnancy (see earlier). Penicillins, cephalosporins or nitrofurantoin are safe to use in pregnancy.

Warning *Co-trimoxazole, sulphonamides, nalidixic acid and tetracyclines should* **not** *be used to treat urinary tract infections in pregnancy.*

In non-pregnant women In non-pregnant women, opinion is divided about the value of anti-bacterial drug treatment of asymptomatic urinary infection. This is because of the high level of re-infections that occur. It should be treated if there is evidence of some abnormality in the urinary tract affecting the urethra, bladder, ureters or kidneys.

In elderly people Elderly people run a risk of repeated infections of the urine without symptoms. In these individuals, the harmful effects of available drugs may be far worse than the risks from the infection. However, if they are incontinent, if they have to keep passing urine or if they are confined to bed, they should be given a course of anti-bacterial drugs (see Table 33.2).

Infections of the urinary tract that produce symptoms

Infections of the urethra (urethritis) and bladder (cystitis) that produce symptoms should be treated adequately with an appropriate anti-bacterial drug by mouth (e.g. ampicillin or amoxycillin, co-trimoxazole, trimethoprim, nitrofurantoin or nalidixic acid). Because many of these anti-bacterial drugs are used to treat other infections and because most bacteria that cause urinary tract infections are from the bowel, there is a risk that the infecting bacteria may become resistant to one or more of these drugs. Therefore it is important that the doctor sends off a sample of urine to the laboratory to be cultured for bacteria and that the sensitivity of these bacteria is tested against recommended anti-bacterial drugs.

Because of the problem of bacterial resistance, a sample of urine should be sent to the laboratory *before* treatment starts with any of these drugs. When the laboratory report is back, the drug may be continued if tests have shown that the bacteria are sensitive to it. If they are not, treatment should be changed to one of the other anti-bacterial drugs that have been shown to be effective. Treatment should be continued for 2 weeks.

In uncomplicated infections of the urinary tract, anti-bacterial drugs in common use include carfecillin, cinoxacin, ciprofloxacin, co-trimoxazole, nalidixic acid, nitrofurantoin and trimethoprim. Other antibiotics that may be used according to antibiotic sensitivity tests of identified bacteria in the urine include ampicillin, cephalosporins and tetracyclines.

Bacterial resistance to certain drugs has occurred because of the widespread use of anti-bacterial drugs to treat urinary tract infections without knowledge of the type of bacterial infection and the anti-bacterial drug to which it is most sensitive. Individuals may also encourage bacterial resistance and the recurrence of urinary tract infections by not taking antibacterial drugs *as directed*, particularly by failing to *complete* a full course of treatment. For a further discussion of bacterial resistance to anti-bacterial drugs, see Chapter 48.

When anti-bacterial drug treatment is effective, bacteria should disappear from the urine within 24 hours. It is important therefore to send off a repeat urine test after about 3 days. If the urine is still infected, a check should be made as to whether the patient is taking the drug as directed. If he/she is, the drug should be changed. A final laboratory test on the urine should be carried out after about 1 week. If this procedure were followed, much of the suffering caused by urinary tract infections might well be reduced dramatically.

Recurrent urinary infections

Recurrence of a urinary tract infection after a few weeks usually means that the focus of infection has not been cleared up effectively. Later recurrent attacks are usually due to re-infection. This problem occurs particularly in women. If recurrent infections are frequent, regular daily doses of an anti-bacterial drug should be given in order to prevent further attacks. A single dose of erythromycin, doxycycline, co-trimoxazole or some other anti-bacterial drug should be given daily at bed-time for 3–6 months; this is usually effective. If, however, infection again recurs, there is probably some abnormality in the urinary tract, or the bacteria have become resistant to the drug, or the patient has forgotten to take the drug as directed and/or the patient is re-infecting him/herself with faecal material from around the anus.

Improving the effectiveness of anti-bacterial drug treatment

Making the urine more acid (acidifying the urine) helps the following anti-bacterial drugs to work more effectively – tetracyclines, nitrofurantoin and cloxacillin. Ascorbic acid (vitamin C) and ammonium chloride may be used for this purpose.

Making the urine less acid (making it alkaline) helps the following anti-bacterial drugs to work more effectively – streptomycin, gentamicin, clindamycin, lincomycin and cephalosporins. Potassium citrate, sodium bicarbonate and sodium citrate may be used for this purpose.

Catheter infections

The use of anti-bacterial drugs to prevent urinary tract infections in patients with catheters in their bladders will only encourage the development of resistant bacteria. Therefore anti-bacterial drugs should be used only to treat infections that have developed.

Bladder wash-outs may be of benefit in preventing infections. The simplest and safest is sterile salt solution but an antiseptic solution such as chlorhexidine may also be of value. Any wash-out, particularly those containing an anti-bacterial drug, should be used with utmost caution because of the danger of the drug being absorbed into the bloodstream and producing harmful effects.

Patients with damaged heart valves always run a serious risk if any infection gets into their bloodstream. This is because the infection can easily settle on the damaged heart valves. These individuals should always be given anti-bacterial drugs to cover the period when they are undergoing a procedure that may introduce bacteria into the blood – for example, inserting an instrument into the bladder. In such circumstances it is advisable to give a cephalosporin or gentamicin by mouth or by injection.

Preventing recurrence of urinary tract infections

After an acute episode of a urinary tract infection has been treated with full course of an anti-bacterial drug and the urine shown to be clear, treatment should then be continued on a low daily dose for 3 months. People who suffer from recurrent infections should have this treatment continued for 6 months, with their urine being tested every 2–3 months. With long-term treatment the dose of the drug should be taken at night after passing urine so that it can concentrate in the urine overnight and work more effectively.

Anyone taking anti-bacterial drugs for a urinary tract infection should drink plenty of fluids and pass urine frequently. Women who suffer from recurrent urinary tract infections should pass urine and wash their genitals and anus just before and just after sexual intercourse and also use a lubricant jelly to avoid injury. They should always wipe their vagina *separately* from their anus (or from front to back), and during sexual activity attempts should be made to avoid the spread of bacteria from the anus to the vagina. It is also important to avoid the use of vaginal deodorants, bubble baths and gels because they may irritate the urethra. They should not use contraceptive diaphragms (caps), or spermicides. Tight tights should not be worn and the genitals and anus should be washed night and morning.

Risks in patients with kidney failure

In people with kidney failure due to some kidney disease, the excretion of certain anti-bacterial drugs in the urine may be impaired. The concentration of these drugs in the blood increases, which increases the risk of harmful effects. Because of this risk, tetracyclines, hexamine and nitrofurantoin should be avoided in these patients, and other anti-bacterial drugs should be used with utmost caution by monitoring their levels in the blood.

Anti-bacterial drugs used specifically to treat urinary infections

Anti-bacterial drugs used to treat urinary tract infections are taken by mouth and are absorbed into the bloodstream, taken to the kidneys and concentrated in the urine where they act on bacteria by preventing their growth.

Hexamine (methenamine) was used for years to treat uncomplicated urinary tract infections but it has now gone out of fashion because it only stops bacteria from multiplying and does not kill them. It requires the urine to be made acid and it produces harmful effects on the skin, stomach and bladder. In acid urine, hexamine is broken down into formaldehyde, which is an effective antiseptic. The urine needs to be acid and therefore hexamine is usually given in a form that produces both an acid and formaldehyde – hexamine hippurate produces formaldehyde and hippuric acid, and hexamine mandelate produces formaldehyde and mandelic acid in the urine. Hexamine has been used to suppress urinary infections in people who suffer from recurrent attacks.

Nalidixic acid is a 4-quinolone anti-bacterial drug. Along with its active breakdown product, hydroxynalidixic acid, it is concentrated in the urine to produce useful anti-bacterial effects. Nalidixic acid may cause some serious harmful effects (see Table 33.1). It should be used with caution and only against bacteria that have been shown to be sensitive to it. Bacteria become rapidly resistant to nalidixic acid. Therefore if an individual does not improve or if laboratory tests show that the infection still persists, an alternative drug should be used. For example, *cinoxacin* and *ciprofloxacin* are 4-quinolone anti-bacterial drugs that are effective against a wide range of bacteria (see pages 759, 761).

Nitrofurantoin has anti-bacterial effects against some of the bacteria that cause urinary tract infections. Rapid excretion of nitrofurantoin by the kidneys prevents toxic levels developing in the blood. It works more effectively in acid urine and, its breakdown products may colour the urine brown. It is concentrated in the urine but in anyone whose kidneys are not working effectively because of disease, the clearance of nitrofurantoin from the blood into the urine is defective and the concentration of the drug in the blood may increase to toxic levels, which produces harmful effects. These harmful effects may be serious and are likely to occur in people who have been on treatment for a long time, particularly if they are elderly. The most serious harmful effects are damage to the blood, liver, lungs and nervous system.

Table 33.1 Anti-bacterial drugs used to treat urinary tract infections – harmful effects and warnings

carfecillin (Uticillin)
Harmful effects are similar to those of the penicillins (Chapter 49); it may also occasionally cause nausea, diarrhoea and skin rash.

Warnings see penicillin (Chapter 49). Carfecillin must not be used in anyone who is allergic to penicillin, nor in individuals with severe impairment of kidney function because the level of carfecillin in the urine may not reach an effective concentration.

cinoxacin (Cinobac)
Harmful effects include loss of appetite, nausea, vomiting, stomach cramps and diarrhoea. Rarely, allergic reactions which include skin rashes, itching and swelling of the hands, feet and mouth may occur. Occasionally, it may cause dizziness, headache, discomfort on looking into the light, noises in the ears, burning feeling in the anal–genital area (the perineum) and changes in liver function tests.

Warnings Cinoxacin must not be used in people who are allergic to it, or whose kidney function is severely impaired. It should be used with caution in anyone with mild or moderate impairment of kidney function.

Risks in elderly people Harmful effects may be more frequent and severe; therefore use with caution.

hexamine (Hiprex)
Harmful effects include skin rashes, irritation of the stomach, irritation of the bladder and blood and/or protein in the urine.

Warnings Hexamine must not be used in people who are dehydrated, who have acidity of the blood or who have impaired liver or kidney function. Urine must be kept acid.

Risks in elderly people Harmful effects may be more frequent and severe in the elderly; therefore use with caution.

nalidixic acid (in Mictral)
Harmful effects include nausea, vomiting and diarrhoea. Rarely, it may damage red blood cells (haemolytic anaemia) in someone with glucose-6-phosphate dehydrogenase deficiency and, very rarely, it may cause allergic reactions including skin rashes, nettle rash, itching, fever, joint pains with stiffness and swelling, muscle pains and weakness, sensitivity of skin to sunlight (redness and blisters), jaundice and visual disturbances. Very rarely, high doses may cause convulsions and severe mental symptoms (toxic psychosis).

Warnings Nalidixic acid must not be used in people who are allergic to it or who have a history of convulsions or brain disorders. It should be used with caution in anyone with impaired kidney or liver function, or disorders of the arteries supplying the brain; they should avoid strong sunlight. If painful joints develop the drug should be stopped immediately. It must be used with caution in children who have not reached puberty because of theoretical risks of damage to joints of weight-bearing bones.

Risks in elderly people Harmful effects may be more frequent and severe; therefore use with caution. Tests of kidney and liver function and blood counts should be carried out at regular intervals if the drug is taken for more than 2 weeks.

nitrofurantoin (Furadantin, Macrodantin)
Harmful effects Nausea and vomiting may occur and are related to the dose. Long-term treatment (6 months or more) may, rarely, cause damage to nerves (producing numbness and pins and needles in arms

Table 33.1 Anti-bacterial drugs used to treat urinary tract infections – harmful effects and warnings (*cont.*)

and legs), rashes, fever, liver damage and destruction of red blood cells (haemolytic anaemia), in people who suffer from glucose-6-phosphate dehydrogenase deficiency. Very rarely, acute allergic reactions may occur and affect the lungs, producing fever, chills, cough, chest pain, breathlessness and damage to the lung tissue. This is related to the duration of treatment (6 months or more) and may start with feeling unwell, cough and breathlessness on exertion.

Warnings Nitrofurantoin should not be given to individuals who are allergic to it or who have glucose-6-phosphate dehydrogenase deficiency or impaired kidney function. It is ineffective in alkaline urine. Treatment should be stopped immediately if numbness or pins and needles develop in any part of the body. Factors that predispose to nerve damage include impaired kidney function, anaemia, diabetes, disturbed chemistry of the blood, vitamin B deficiency and debilitating illness.

Risks in elderly people Harmful effects may be more frequent and severe; therefore use with caution.

Table 33.2 Anti-bacterial drugs used to treat urinary tract infections

Preparation	*Drug*	*Dosage form*
Cinobac	cinoxacin	Capsules
Furadantin	nitrofurantoin	Tablets, suspension
Hiprex	hexamine	Tablets
Macrodantin	nitrofurantoin	Capsules
Mictral	nalidixic acid, anhydrous citric acid, sodium citrate, sodium bicarbonate	Effervescent granules in sachets
Negram	nalidixic acid	Tablets, suspension
nitrofurantoin	nitrofurantoin	Tablets
Uriben	nalidixic acid	Suspension
Uticillin	carfecillin	Tablets

Table 33.3 Anti-bacterial solutions for instillation into the bladder

Preparation	*Drug*	*Dosage form*
Noxyflex (anti-bacterial/ anti-fungal)	noxythiolin and amethocaine (local anaesthetic)	Solution – powder for reconstitution
Noxyflex S (anti-bacterial/ anti-fungal)	noxythiolin	Solution – powder for reconstitution

Drugs used to relieve pain in urinary tract infections

Potassium citrate has been used for decades to relieve the discomfort of inflammation of the bladder (cystitis) and of the urethra (urethritis). It reduces the acidity of the urine (i.e. makes it alkaline), which makes it less stinging. Other drugs used to make the urine less acid include sodium bicarbonate, sodium citrate and potassium citrate. A commonly used preparation in the past included a mixture of potassium citrate and hyoscyamus (an anticholinergic drug).

Warning *There is a serious risk in using preparations to make the urine less acid: they only relieve the stinging, they cure nothing and the real danger is that an underlying infection of the urinary tract may go untreated or not be treated adequately. Note that potassium salts may be dangerous in people whose kidney function is impaired.* ***Do not self-treat urinary tract infections.***

Table 33.4 Drugs used to change the acidity of the urine – harmful effects and warnings

ammonium chloride mixture
Makes the urine *acid*.

Harmful effects Large doses may cause nausea, vomiting, thirst, headache, overbreathing, drowsiness and acidity of the blood. Acidification of the urine soon wears off.

Warnings It must not be used in patients with impaired kidney or liver function.

ascorbic acid (vitamin C)
Makes the urine *acid*. For harmful effects and warnings, see Chapter 45.

potassium citrate
Makes the urine *alkaline*.

Harmful effects include irritation of the stomach, increased volume of urine and a rise in blood potassium levels.

Warnings Blood potassium levels must be monitored, particularly in people with impaired kidney function.

sodium bicarbonate
Makes the urine *alkaline*.

Harmful effects include belching due to release of carbon dioxide in the stomach; prolonged use may reduce the acidity of the blood.

Warnings It should be used with caution in patients with impaired kidney function or who are on a low sodium diet, and in pregnant women.

sodium citrate
Makes the urine *alkaline*.

Harmful effects include mild increase in volume of urine produced.

Warnings It should be used with caution in pregnancy.

Table 33.5 Drugs used to change the acidity of the urine

Preparation	*Drug*	*Drug Group*	*Dosage form*
ammonium chloride mixture	ammonium chloride	Acidifying drug	Solution
ascorbic acid	ascorbic acid	Acidifying drug	Tablets
Effercitrate	potassium citrate	Alkalizing drug	Effervescent tablets
potassium citrate	potassium citrate	Alkalizing drug	Solution
Redoxon	ascorbic acid	Acidifying drug	Tablets, effervescent
sodium bicarbonate	sodium bicarbonate	Alkalizing drug	Powder
Urisal	sodium citrate	Alkalizing drug	Granules

Pain relievers

Phenazopyridine is used to relieve the pain of the urinary tract infection. It may colour the urine red, and in people with impaired kidney function it may reach toxic levels in the blood and damage the red blood cells. It relieves symptoms, it does not cure. The danger is that any underlying infection may go untreated or not be treated adequately. It is combined with a sulphonamide drug, sulphacarbamide, in Uromide.

Local anaesthetic preparations

The applications of a local anaesthetic gel (e.g. lignocaine gel) around the entrance of the urethra may help to relieve urethral pain but the trouble is that local anaesthetics may themselves produce irritation. Proprietary preparations include Instillagel, Xylocaine gel and Xylocaine Antiseptic gel (lignocaine with chlorhexidine).

Urgency and frequency of passing urine

Having to pass urine urgently (*urgency*) and having to pass it frequently (*frequency*) can be a serious problem in some people, particularly the elderly. It may be due to many causes – increased fluid intake (e.g. in diabetes, alcoholism), inflammation of the bladder and/or its outlet (the urethra), partial obstruction to the outlet of the bladder caused by an enlarged prostate gland in men, weakness of the outlet from the bladder caused by vaginal prolapse, or damage to the nerves supplying the bladder. It may also be due to psychological problems: some people who are nervous or tense have to pass urine frequently, and of course it can be a habit.

The desire to empty the bladder is caused by the increasing volume of urine stretching the bladder wall and stimulating stretch-sensitive nerves and by the pressure of urine on pressure-sensitive nerves near the outlet from the bladder. *Anticholinergic drugs* block this stimulation so that the bladder can hold more urine – it can be stretched more and can resist more pressure before it contracts. The most commonly used anticholinergic drug for this purpose is propantheline (Pro-Banthine). However, in effective doses, anticholinergic drugs may produce unacceptable harmful effects which include dry mouth, blurred vision and constipation, and they may trigger glaucoma in a susceptible individual.

Terodiline (Micturin) is a drug that produces anticholinergic effects and also some calcium channel-blocking effects, and may be beneficial in some people.

Flavoxate (Urispas) is an anti-spasmodic that relaxes the muscles of the bladder and may also be of benefit to some people.

Anti-depressant drugs (amitriptyline, imipramine and nortriptyline) have also been used to treat urgency and frequency probably because they also produce some anticholinergic effects.

Incontinence of urine

Incontinence of urine refers to lack of control over emptying the bladder. Incontinence of small or large volumes of urine may occur in people who are confused (e.g. in senile dementia). Other causes of incontinence of urine include damage to nervous tissues in the brain, spinal cord or the nerves supplying the bladder, weakness at the outlet of the bladder (see 'Stress incontinence' below) or as a result of retention of urine which causes an overflow of urine with dribbling (retention overflow). Severe inflammation of the bladder (cystitis) may sometimes cause incontinence.

Stress incontinence

Stress incontinence is when your urine 'leaks' for example, if you laugh, sneeze or cough. It occurs more often in women and may be 'normal' in young women and girls when they are laughing. In older women it is often the consequence of childbirth having caused some damage to the walls of the vagina. In later life this causes the outlet from the bladder to sag, which may cause a lack of control over the outflow of urine. The incidence of stress incontinence in both men and women increases with advancing age as the muscles around the outlet from the bladder get weaker. In stress incontinence only small volumes of urine escape but there is a feeling of urgency and of 'bursting to go'.

Drugs may cause incontinence

Water tablets (diuretics) are prescribed frequently to elderly people to treat their heart failure and/or blood pressure. This makes the kidney pass out large volumes of urine, which may easily trigger incontinence in a susceptible person. These drugs are usually taken in the morning in order to avoid problems in the night, but some elderly people get so worried that they stop drinking from lunch-time onwards because they are scared of wetting the bed. This may aggravate the harmful effects of these drugs on the body's water and salts.

Incontinence of urine is distressing

Urinary incontinence in elderly people is often mismanaged; yet it is very embarrassing for them to keep wetting themselves. They do not like to mention it, not even to the doctor. They stop going out and mixing socially, and quite often become isolated in their homes because of the problem.

Incontinence of urine in women may affect their sex lives. It may put them off sex and it may cause them to wet themselves during intercourse and/or during orgasm.

Incontinence of urine is not a symptom that should be just ignored. People with incontinence should be referred to a special incontinence clinic for a complete check-up. Quite often there is much that can be done to help. For example, exercises to strengthen the muscles in the floor of the pelvis may help to reduce stress incontinence, and so may surgery to tighten up any stretched ligament. It is also useful to know that regular emptying of the bladder may help to reduce urgency.

Drug treatment of incontinence

Drugs may relieve the 'symptom' of incontinence, they do nothing to help the underlying disorder. It is clearly better, therefore, to treat, if possible, the cause of the incontinence rather than resort to drugs, which in many cases are useless.

NOTE Drug treatment is unlikely to benefit individuals who have incontinence due to loss of nerve control of the bladder.

Drugs that may be of use in some individuals with incontinence include anticholinergics, some anti-depressants, sympathomimetics and anti-spasmodics.

Anticholinergic drugs

Anticholinergics block parasympathetic nerves that supply the bladder. These nerves stimulate the muscles of the bladder to contract in response to stretching and pressure on the wall of the bladder as the volume of urine inside it increases. By blocking this stimulation – particularly the pressure responses coming from a very sensitive area just near the neck of the bladder – they may help to reduce the leakage of urine.

Anticholinergic drugs used to treat incontinence (e.g. propantheline) may produce harmful effects, which include dry mouth, blurred vision, constipation and rapid beating of the heart. Terodiline (Micturin) produces anticholinergic effects and also some calcium channel-blocking effects, and may be beneficial in some individuals suffering from incontinence.

Certain *anti-depressant* drugs may also be tried (e.g. amitriptyline, imipramine or nortriptyline). They may work because they produce some anticholinergic effects on the bladder.

Sympathomimetic drugs

Sympathomimetic drugs (see Chapter 2), e.g. ephedrine, phenylpropanolamine, pseudoephedrine, also make the bladder less sensitive to stretching and pressure, so more urine can be retained in the bladder without the leakage and urgency that occur in incontinence. They do not block the nerves that cause the bladder to contract but they counteract the effects of these nerves.

Anti-spasmodic drugs

Flavoxate (Urispas) is an anti-spasmodic drug that relaxes the muscle of the bladder. It may be of benefit in some people suffering from incontinence.

Table 33.6 Drugs used to treat incontinence of urine and urinary frequency – harmful effects and warnings

flavoxate (Urispas)
Harmful effects include headache, nausea, fatigue, blurred vision, dry mouth and diarrhoea.

Warnings must not be used in people with disease of the oesophagus, or with poor emptying of their stomach or with obstructive disease of the bowel or urinary tract. It must be used with caution in individuals with glaucoma.

propantheline (Pro-Banthine)
Harmful effects include dry mouth, blurred vision, dry skin (risk of heat stroke), increased heart rate, difficulty in passing urine and constipation. For other harmful effects produced by anticholinergic drugs, see Chapter 2.

Warnings Propantheline must not be used to treat individuals who are allergic to any anticholinergic drug or who have obstructive disease of the stomach or intestine, narrowing of the outlet of the stomach (pyloric stenosis), paralysis of the small intestine, ulcerative colitis, hiatus hernia with acid reflux, glaucoma or myasthenia gravis. It must be used with caution in people with impaired kidney or liver function, over-active thyroid gland, heart disease, enlarged prostate gland or high blood pressure.

Risks in elderly people Harmful effects may be more frequent and severe; therefore use with caution.

Risks in driving It may produce drowsiness and blurred vision and therefore affect your ability to drive. Do not drive until you know that it is safe to do so.

Table 33.6 Drugs used to treat incontinence of urine and urinary frequency – harmful effects and warnings (*cont.*)

terodiline (Micturin)
Harmful effects include dry mouth, blurred vision, dry skin (risk of heat stroke), increased heart rate, difficulty in passing urine and constipation. For other harmful effects produced by anticholinergic drugs, see Chapter 2.

Warnings Terodiline must not be used in individuals who are allergic to any anticholinergic drug or who have obstructive disease of the stomach or intestine, narrowing of the outlet of the stomach (pyloric stenosis), paralysis of the small intestine, ulcerative colitis, hiatus hernia with acid reflux, glaucoma or myasthenia gravis. It must be used with caution in people with impaired liver or kidney function, over-active thyroid gland, heart disease, enlarged prostate gland or high blood pressure.

Risks in elderly people Harmful effects may be more frequent and severe; therefore use with caution.

Anti-depressant drugs

For the harmful effects and warnings on the use of anti-depressant drugs amitriptyline, imipramine and nortriptyline, see Chapter 39.

Bedwetting in children

Bedwetting is obviously quite normal in babies and infants but becomes a problem when it persists or comes on again in older children. About 5 per cent of 10-year-olds still wet the bed, and in some children a severe emotional upset may cause a recurrence.

The best treatment is reassurance, support and counselling along with bladder training. Any form of punishment or criticism will only make the child worse. The use of an alarm system which sets a bell ringing the second a drop of urine is passed on to a pad placed beneath the bottom may be helpful. The bell wakes the child and he or she can then go and pass urine in the toilet. A reward system may also help: for example, a star chart whereby the child gets a star for every dry night and a present when there are a certain number of stars on the chart; however, whatever method is used, the child must not be made to feel a failure.

Drug treatment should have little if any place in treating bedwetting

Drug treatment should never be used in children under 7 years of age, and it is doubtful if it should ever be used in children over 7 years, except when visiting a friend or going on holiday or to prove that they can actually go all night without wetting the bed.

Anti-depressant drugs used to treat bedwetting

Anti-depressants used to treat bedwetting (nocturnal enuresis) include amitriptyline (Tryptizol), imipramine (Tofranil) and nortriptyline (Allegron). They produce anticholinergic effects, which are normally regarded as harmful effects when the drugs are used to treat depression. These effects block the nerves that produce contraction of the bladder in response to stretching and pressure on its walls due to the volume of urine in the bladder. Beyond this we do not know how anti-depressant drugs work in preventing bedwetting. Nor do we know whether bedwetting is associated with those changes in mood which doctors would label depression.

Anti-depressant drugs may produce serious harmful effects in children. They do not cure the problem, and bedwetting can recur when they are stopped. These doubtful benefits have therefore to be balanced against the harmful effects of using them, particularly the dangers of producing changes in behaviour and effects on the heart to which children are especially vulnerable. Because of these harmful effects on the heart, treatment should not be continued for more than 3 months without carrying out an electric tracing of the heart (ECG). These drugs may, very rarely, trigger fits in children.

Anti-depressants are very dangerous in overdose in children and should be kept well out of their reach.

Stimulant drugs used to treat bedwetting

Stimulant drugs used to treat bedwetting (e.g. ephedrine) are *sympathomimetic drugs* i.e. they produce adrenaline-like effects on the body (see Chapter 2). They counteract the nerves that make the bladder contract, so more urine can be retained in the bladder before having to empty it. They also stimulate the brain and lessen the depth of sleep, so the child responds to the urge to empty his or her bladder more easily. Any possible benefit from the treatment should be carefully balanced against the risk of harmful effects (see later).

In the doses used to treat bedwetting they may cause dry mouth, drowsiness, sweating and itching. For other harmful effects and warnings, see Chapter 2.

Desmopressin In some individuals who regularly wet the bed there may possibly be a deficiency of vasopressin, the hormone that stops urine production. It is produced by the pituitary gland and acts as an anti-urine-producing (anti-diuretic) hormone. Desmopressin is related to vasopressin and produces the same effects. It may be taken by nasal spray. A single dose stops urine production for about 10–12 hours, sufficient to allow a dry night. It should not be used in children aged 5 years or under. It should be used for no more than 3 months and then there should be a break of at least 1 week to check if the child is all right without treatment. For harmful effects and warnings, see Chapter 60.

Retention of urine

Inability to pass urine causes retention of urine in the bladder. This may occur because of an obstruction to the outflow of the urine from the bladder (e.g. an enlarged prostate gland in an elderly man). It may also be the result of damage to the nerves supplying the bladder (e.g. spinal injury).

Retention of urine may actually cause incontinence because the bladder fills up and then starts to overflow. This causes the patient to dribble all the time. It is called retention with overflow and is easily diagnosed as retention because the bladder is full and often tender. Anticholinergic drugs and sympathomimetic drugs will make the retention of urine worse.

Drugs may cause inability to pass urine

Certain drugs may cause retention of urine in people who already have some partial obstruction (e.g. elderly men with enlarged prostate glands) for example, any drug with anticholinergic effects and morphine-related drugs. Patients who are recovering from surgery may develop retention of urine due to prolonged effects of the anaesthetic.

Treatment of retention of urine

Acute retention of urine is painful, and initial treatment is to draw off the urine by inserting a catheter into the bladder but there is always a risk of causing an infection.

Carbachol by mouth or *bethanechol* (Myotonine) by mouth or injection may relieve retention by stimulating the bladder muscles to contract. They act like acetylcholine, the parasympathetic nerve messenger (see Chapter 2), and may be used to stimulate emptying of the bladder after a surgical operation when a general anaesthetic has been given.

Distigmine (Ubretid) may help individuals who have retention of urine because of nerve damage. It prolongs the action of the nerve messenger acetylcholine (see Chapter 2) that stimulates the nerves supplying the muscles of the bladder, causing them to contract. It is used to treat retention of urine following a surgical operation and also to help the bladder contract in people who have lost nervous control of the bladder (e.g. following a spinal injury).

Neostigmine (Prostigmin) prolongs the actions of the nerve messenger acetylcholine that stimulates the nerve supplying the muscles of the bladder, causing them to contract. It is used to treat retention of urine following a surgical operation when a general anaesthetic has been given.

Benign prostatic hypertrophy

Benign prostatic hypertrophy is an enlargement of the prostate gland. It affects about 50 per cent of men between the ages of 50 and 60, and about 90 per cent of men aged 80 years or over. The enlargement interferes with the flow of urine, resulting in difficulty in getting started (hesitancy), a poor stream due to reduced pressure, dribbling when finished and retention of urine in the bladder. These symptoms occur because of the blockage to the flow of urine caused by the enlarged prostate gland. However, they may also occur due to spasm of muscles in and around the prostate gland. Drugs that block nerves supplying these muscles cause them to relax and therefore have less obstructive effect on the flow of urine. Drugs used for this purpose are called alpha blockers because they block alpha receptors (see discussion of their use under vasodilators used to treat raised blood pressure, Chapter 21). They reduce the degree of obstruction and help to increase the volume of urine passed. They also reduce the need to pass urine in the night. The ones in fashion include prazosin (Hypovase) and indoramin (Doralese). Their harmful effects and warnings on their use are listed in Table 21.5.

Table 33.7 Drugs used to treat retention of urine – harmful effects and warnings

bethanecol (Myotonine)
Harmful effects include nausea, vomiting, blurred vision, abdominal cramps, sweating, decreased heart rate, wheezing, fainting, diarrhoea and salivation.

Warnings Bethanecol must not be used in people with acute iritis, obstruction of the stomach or intestine, obstruction to the flow of urine (e.g. enlarged prostate gland), recent heart attack or recent intestinal surgery, asthma, severe slow pulse rate, low blood pressure, epilepsy or parkinsonism. It must be used with caution in individuals with over-active thyroid gland or active peptic ulcers.

carbachol
Harmful effects which are more frequent than with bethanecol, include nausea, vomiting, blurred vision, abdominal cramps, decreased heart rate, wheezing, fainting, diarrhoea and excessive salivation.

Warnings See under bethanecol.

distigmine (Ubretid)
Harmful effects include nausea, vomiting,

Table 33.7 Drugs used to treat retention of urine – harmful effects and warnings (*cont.*)

blurred vision, abdominal cramps, decreased heart rate, wheezing, fainting, diarrhoea and excessive salivation. The harmful effects are mild but are more prolonged than with bethanecol.

Warnings Distigmine must not be used in severe shock following surgery, collapse of the blood circulation or in people with intestinal or urinary obstruction and used with caution in people with asthma, heart disease, peptic ulcers, epilepsy or parkinsonism. In myasthenia gravis it may be necessary to reduce the dose of their treatment.

neostigmine (Prostigmin)
Harmful effects include nausea, vomiting, increased salivation, diarrhoea and stomach cramps.

Warnings Because of the risk of an acute allergic reaction, atropine and drugs for treating an acute allergic reaction along with facilities for resuscitation should be immediately available. Neostigmine must not be used in people with an obstruction of their intestine or bladder (e.g. enlarged prostate), nor during anaesthesia with cyclopropane or halothane. It should be used with caution in individuals with asthma, slow pulse rate, recent heart attack, epilepsy, low blood pressure, peptic ulcer, parkinsonism and over-active thyroid gland.

prazosin (Hypovase)
See Table 21.5.

indoramin (Doralese)
Harmful effects and warnings are similar to those for prazosin – see Table 21.5.

34

Sexually transmitted diseases

Sexually transmitted diseases are a diverse group of infections caused by various micro-organisms that are transmitted by sexual contact. In this context I use the term 'sexual' to cover the full range of heterosexual and homosexual behaviour including genital, genital–anal, oral–genital and oral–anal contact.

Sexually transmitted diseases are associated with promiscuity because it is the number of different sexual partners an individual has that increases his/her risk of getting such an infection. Furthermore, a high proportion of infected individuals suffer from more than one sexually transmitted disease, which also gives an indication of contact with a number of different sexual partners. Oral–anal or oral–penile–anal contact produces an additional risk of transmitting other diseases such as bowel infections and hepatitis.

The commonest sexually transmitted diseases are non-gonococcal (or non-specific) urethritis, gonorrhoea and herpes. The spread of hepatitis by sexual contact is on the increase and so is AIDS. Syphilis is now comparatively rare. There are many other sexually transmitted diseases but they are beyond the scope of this book.

Sexually transmitted diseases may cause infection of any part of the urinary and genital tract: for example, of the urethra (urethritis), of the vagina (vaginitis), of the cervix (cervicitis), of the fallopian tubes (salpingitis), of the testes (epididymitis) and of the penis. In addition, they may cause infection of the anus, rectum and throat and affect other organs such as the liver (hepatitis) and the joints (arthritis). Late complications (apart from those produced by AIDS) occur mainly in women. These may produce infertility or ectopic pregnancies due to damage to the fallopian tubes. These late complications may occur many years after the infection was contracted and the women may not even have had any symptoms.

An important part of treatment of sexually transmitted diseases is to try to reduce the spread of infection by tracing and treating contacts of infected persons. Prevention is also important in terms of reduced sexual activity outside of a stable relationship and the wearing of a protective condom during sexual intercourse. Early drug treatment is very effective in certain sexually transmitted diseases and is important in preventing early and late complications.

Non-gonococcal urethritis (non-specific urethritis, NSU)

Non-gonococcal urethritis is the commonest sexually transmitted disease. In men it presents like gonorrhoea, with a discharge from the penis and pain on passing urine; laboratory tests fail to identify gonorrhoea micro-organisms and most infections are found to be due to infection with *Chlamydia trachomatis* or *Ureaplasma urealyticum*. In about one in five individuals no infectious micro-organism is detected.

In women the infection may produce no symptoms but it can infect the cervix, so it is important that women partners of infected men are examined carefully and treated. The infection may spread upwards into the womb and fallopian tubes and therefore it is essential that women are treated early and effectively. A women with an infection of the neck of her womb (cervix) can infect her baby at birth, causing the baby to develop an eye infection or a throat or lung infection.

Treatment

A course of tetracycline antibiotics for 10–21 days is the first line of treatment (e.g. oxytetracycline). Cure rates of NSU are lower than those of gonorrhoea. An alternative treatment is erythromycin. For harmful effects of tetracyclines see Chapter 51, and for erythromycin see Chapter 53.

Warning *Note that, unlike gonorrhoea, non-gonococcal urethritis does not respond to a single dose of antibiotic. The antibiotic* ***must*** *be taken as directed and the full course of treatment* ***must*** *be completed.*

Sexual partners should be treated if they are infected. Treatment fails in about one in five due to a flare-up of the infection; to failure to take the treatment as directed; or from re-infection by an infected sexual partner.

One important difficulty with non-gonococcal urethritis is that the acute symptoms resolve on their own in some patients, which may make it difficult to assess the effects of treatment.

Reiter's disease

Reiter's disease is a non-gonococcal urethritis associated with conjunctivitis and arthritis. It occurs very much more frequently in men than in women and is the commonest form of inflammatory arthritis in young men. About 1–2 per cent of patients with non-gonococcal urethritis develop Reiter's disease.

The onset of the disease may be acute, starting 2–3 weeks after sexual exposure to an infected partner. The infected patient develops urethritis, arthritis of a main weight-bearing joint (e.g. knee) and conjunctivitis (in about 5 per cent). In addition there may be fever, weight loss and coldness of the feet.

Sometimes the onset may be slow and present only as an inflamed joint or tendon which may be associated with inflammation of the tip of penis (balanitis). Occasionally the infection may affect the inside of the eyes as well as causing conjunctivitis. The arthritis may clear up in 2–3 months but may recur, and chronic low back pain and stiffness may develop.

The treatment of Reiter's disease will vary according to stage and with the severity of the disease. The urethritis is treated with tetracycline antibiotics, the arthritis may be treated with anti-inflammatory pain relievers (NSAIDs) and the conjunctivitis may require corticosteroid eye drops. There is no cure, and treatment only relieves symptoms. The disease fades away in the majority of patients but in a few (one in ten) it may last for years, particularly the arthritis and the eye disorders.

Gonorrhoea

The micro-organisms that cause gonorrhoea can infect the penis or vagina by genital contact, the rectum by anal–penile contact, the throat by oral–genital contact and the eyes of newborn babies (ophthalmia neonatorum) from contact with their mother's genital tract during childbirth. A gonorrhoeal infection of the rectum resulting from penile–anal sex often causes no symptoms.

In men the genital infection causes an inflammation of the urethra, producing a discharge and pain on passing urine. In females, infection of the urethra and neck of the womb (cervix) may cause a vaginal discharge and pain on passing urine but about half of infected women have no symptoms.

In males, gonorrhoeal infections may spread upwards from the urethra to the testicles, and in women it may spread upwards to produce inflammation of the fallopian tubes (salpingitis) and other organs. These are serious complications because they may lead to late complications such as sterility and ectopic pregnancies. Rarely, gonorrhoea may cause fever and arthritis when the bacteria enters the bloodstream.

Treatment

Treatment of gonorrhoea consists of a single dose of one of the following mixtures: a single injection into a muscle of procaine penicillin plus probenecid by mouth; or ampicillin and probenecid by mouth. The probenecid reduces the excretion of the antibiotic in the urine and the amount in the blood increases.

Patients who are allergic to penicillin may be given co-trimoxazole by mouth in a single dose. Alternative antibiotics include spectinomycin or cefuroxime.

Herpes simplex infection

This condition is due to the herpes simplex virus type 2 (see discussion under anti-viral drugs, Chapter 57). The infection is spread by sexual contact and produces sores on the genitals and anus. It resembles cold sores on the lips, which are also caused by a herpes simplex virus.

The infection produces tiny blisters and ulcers (sores) on the genitals and there may be an associated fever and swollen glands in the groin. In homosexual men the anus may be affected and this may occur rarely in heterosexual females who have had penile–anal sex with an infected partner.

The initial illness lasts for 2–4 weeks and in about half of infected individuals the attacks of blisters and ulcers keep recurring. Each attack lasts for 2–4 days. A herpes infection of the vagina in a pregnant women may infect her baby during childbirth, producing an infection of the baby's eyes.

NOTE There is a possible link between sexually transmitted genital herpes and subsequent development of cancer of the cervix in later life.

Treatment

The use of anti-viral drugs to treat herpes is discussed in Chapter 57. Bathing the affected area with salt solution will help, and any secondary bacterial infection of the herpes sores should respond to co-trimoxazole by mouth.

Hepatitis

Hepatitis is discussed in Chapter 83. It can be sexually transmitted.

AIDS

AIDS stands for acquired immune deficiency syndrome. 'Immune deficiency' implies a weakness in the body's defence system against infection, and the term 'syndrome' means a distinct group of symptoms and signs. A symptom is something that you feel, like a pain or itching, and a sign is something that you can see or touch, like a skin rash or a swollen gland. The disease is acquired and not inherited, although a baby can be born with AIDS by acquiring it from its mother during pregnancy.

AIDS is caused by a virus known as the human immuno-deficiency virus, or HIV for short. The virus has been found in blood, in semen, in the vagina from secretions produced by the cervix (the neck of the womb), and in tears, saliva, urine, breast milk and in the fluid in the brain and spinal cord (cerebro-spinal fluid). However, except for blood, semen and possibly secretions from the cervix, the concentration of the virus in other body fluids is probably too small for the infection to spread from one person to another.

The spread of HIV

The commonest way of acquiring HIV is through anal intercourse with an infected person. Other important ways of catching the infection is by vaginal intercourse and by receiving HIV-infected blood through a blood transfusion or by receiving an HIV-infected blood product (e.g. factor VIII to treat haemophilia). HIV can also spread among drug addicts who share needles, syringes and other equipment contaminated with HIV-infected blood. Babies may become infected from their HIV-infected mothers during pregnancy and possibly during their birth. The virus may possibly spread via infected semen donated for use in artificial insemination, and via infected organs donated for transplanting (e.g. cornea, skin, bone marrow, kidneys, heart valves).

AIDS cannot spread from person to person by ordinary everyday contact nor can it spread by sharing cups or glasses, from toilet seats, from cooking utensils or from swimming pools. Nor is there any evidence that it can spread from person to person by mosquito bites, lice or bed bugs.

The AIDS epidemic in the West has occurred mostly among homosexual men and drug addicts, and has spread into the heterosexual population principally via infected bisexual men and drug addicts.

The virus can spread by sexual intercourse from men to men, from men to women, and from women to men but, so far, in the West, only a very small proportion of women are infected and most of them are drug addicts who have been infected by HIV-contaminated blood on shared needles and syringes. However, the picture is different in Africa where, among those who are infected with HIV, nearly as many women as men are infected and there is a high level of HIV infection among male and female prostitutes. There is also a risk of HIV being transmitted via contaminated blood transfusions and contaminated needles and syringes used for medical purposes.

Increased risk of infection

People with HIV are most infective at the early stages of the disease before they have produced antibodies, that is *before* they know from blood tests whether they have been infected (i.e. they are antibody-positive, see later). They are also more infective around the time when they develop the AIDS disease (see later).

Any tears, cuts, abrasions, sores, ulcers, infection or other injury or damage to the surface of the penis, lips, mouth, throat, skin, anus, vagina or neck of the womb increase the risk of catching HIV from direct contact with contaminated blood, semen or other body fluids from an HIV-infected person. Without injury or damage the surface of some tissues may be more resistant to the virus than others – for example, the lining of the vagina appears to be more protective against HIV infection than is the lining of the anus. Also, the lining of the anus may be torn more easily during penile–anal sex than is the vagina during penile–vaginal sex, thus increasing the risk of transmission of the virus from infected semen or blood.

Tests for HIV infection

Tests for HIV infection depend upon testing the blood for antibodies against the virus. Infected individuals produce these HIV antibodies some 3 weeks to 3 months after first contracting the infection. The conversion from a negative blood test (or serum test) for antibodies to a positive test is often referred to as *sero-conversion*, after which such people may be referred to as being HIV-positive. This means that they have contracted the HIV infection and produced antibodies. They are infectious and can transmit the disease but they do not have AIDS.

Tests for HIV antibodies are carried out against proteins obtained from a sample of purified HIV virus. The tests may be against the 'whole' virus or against individual proteins obtained from the surface of the HIV virus (the virus envelope). When the blood of newly infected individuals is tested at intervals it is found that their antibody level rises, as does the range of antibodies produced to the various proteins on the surface of the HIV.

In addition to blood (see above), other body fluids (e.g. semen) may also be used to test for antibodies; the use of saliva to test for HIV antibodies is under investigation.

Direct tests for HIV or proteins on the wall of the virus are available. They may be of use in double-checking the diagnosis in newborn babies in whom antibody production may not be fully developed. Positive tests for HIV (rather than antibodies) in patients with advanced AIDS may indicate that their immune-deficiency is interfering with their production of antibodies against the virus. Tests for HIV may possibly be useful for monitoring the response to anti-viral drug treatment – if the drug is working there should be a reduction in the numbers of the virus and an increase in the number of immune cells (T lymphocytes).

The HIV attacks cells involved in the body's defence against infection

HIV enters the host's blood concealed in white blood cells (T lymphocytes) passed into them from HIV-infected blood, semen, etc. (see earlier) of an infected person. Once inside the host's bloodstream the viruses burst out of their cells and enter the host's blood and immediately start targeting themselves onto the host's T lymphocytes. These T lymphocytes carry a special protein on their surfaces that HIV can recognize and use as receptors. When contact is made, a protein on the surface of the virus locks onto the special protein (CD4) on the T lymphocyte and the virus is then able to get inside the T lymphocyte. CD4 is also present on the surface of some other white blood cells (e.g. monocytes and macrophages) involved in fighting infections. These cells are also entered by the virus.

HIV contains a special enzyme (reverse transcriptase) which enables the viruses to make replicas of themselves (replication) by integrating their own genetic material into the genetic material of the host T lymphocyte. They are then able to use the lymphocyte as a virus factory. The lymphocytes die prematurely and the new viruses are released into the bloodstream to attack other T lymphocytes. They may also pass directly from one T lymphocyte to another and thus avoid detection by the body's immune system, which produces antibodies against the viruses but cannot detect them when they are inside the host cells.

The lymphocytes attacked by HIV are special T lymphocytes ('helper' or 'inducer' T lymphocytes), which play a central role in the immune response. They are sometimes referred to as 'leaders of the immunological orchestra' because they set in motion many activities that ultimately result in the development of killer cells, antibodies and large white cells (macrophages) which are activated to move in and destroy those invading micro-organisms that have triggered the immune response (see Chapter 9). Destruction of helper/inducer T lymphocytes by HIV leaves the individual with a seriously reduced resistance to infection from bacteria, viruses, fungi and protozoa. Their destruction also interferes with the body's control over the growth of any abnormal cells (e.g. cancer cells), which makes an HIV-infected person susceptible to the development of certain types of cancer (see later).

Acute stage of HIV infection

During the first few weeks after contracting an HIV infection there may be no symptoms or the individual may develop vague symptoms like those seen in glandular fever. These symptoms may occur around the time that the individual starts producing antibodies to the virus (see earlier) and include sore throat, malaise, mild fever, swollen glands, and aching muscles and joints. Also about the time when antibody tests become positive, an individual may, rarely, develop symptoms and signs of an acute brain infection (encephalitis) which include fever, fatigue, changes in mood, disorientation, personality changes, loss of memory and fits. The individual usually recovers after about a week. Other transient disorders which may, occasionally, occur at this time include acute meningitis producing headaches, nausea, vomiting and discomfort on looking in the light; acute inflammation of the spinal cord (myelopathy) producing weakness, numbness and pins and needles of the legs; and inflammation of nerves (neuropathy) producing pain and weakness in the arms and legs and various other parts of the body.

Chronic stage of HIV infection

Following the stage when antibodies are produced, the disease may enter either a latent stage without any symptoms or a chronic stage during which several disease entities may occur. These include: persistent generalized adenopathy, AIDS-related complex and opportunistic infections.

Persistent generalized lymphadenopathy (PGL)

Lymphadenopathy means a disease of the lymph glands (nodes) which causes them to be enlarged. To be diagnosed as suffering from PGL the individual must have enlarged glands of more than 1 cm in diameter affecting two or more sites (e.g. armpits, neck) other than the groin for at least 3 months in the absence of any other illness or drug treatment known to produce enlarged glands. Long-term follow-up to date indicates that 10–30 per cent of patients with PGL go on to develop AIDS.

AIDS-related complex (ARC)

Months or years after being infected with HIV, some people will develop what is referred to as AIDS-related complex or ARC. The symptoms and signs of ARC include PGL (see above), fatigue, reduced ability to do physical exercise, an intermittent or continuous fever, night sweats, weight loss and intermittent or continuous diarrhoea. ARC may be diagnosed if the individual has two or more of these problems which have lasted for 3 months or more along with two or more abnormal blood tests such as anaemia, reduced white blood count, raised gammaglobulins, and signs of damage to cells involved in the immune system. Of those individuals who develop ARC some may and some may not go on to develop fully blown AIDS (see later).

Opportunistic infections

Opportunistic infections may occur in chronic HIV infection because the individual's resistance to infection is weakened. These infections are usually more severe in AIDS; they include bacterial, viral, fungal and protozoal infections (see later).

AIDS disease

We do not really know how many people infected with HIV go on to develop AIDS. However, it appears that the longer HIV-positive individuals are followed-up the higher is the overall proportion who develop AIDS. Nevertheless, not everyone who is HIV positive will develop AIDS.

So far, with our limited knowledge of the natural progression of the disease, it appears that the period of time from first becoming infected with HIV to the development of AIDS (the incubation period) is 2–5 years. However, it still remains difficult to identify those HIV-positive individuals who will go on to develop AIDS and those who will not. Warning signs include persistent fever, malaise, diarrhoea, weight loss, shingles, thrush of the mouth, anaemia and positive blood tests that indicate damage to cells involved in the immune system. Hairy leucoplakia is an additional warning sign; it consists of white warty lumps on the side of the tongue and inside of cheeks. The main manifestations of AIDS are infections and cancers.

Infections in AIDS

As people's HIV infection progresses over the years, their resistance to infection may become reduced and they become highly vulnerable to all kinds of infections in addition to the HIV infection from which they are suffering. We refer to these infections as opportunistic because they take the opportunity to attack an individual whose resistance is low. They include bacteria, viruses, fungi and protozoa. People with AIDS may develop several different infections at the same time and about half of them develop pneumonia. Their intestines and brains are commonly infected and their skin, kidneys and liver may also become infected by various micro-organisms.

Common general symptoms produced by the disease and by the opportunistic infections include fever, diarrhoea, weight loss, swollen glands, wasting, cough and breathlessness. Infections of the skin include fungal infections (e.g. ringworm, thrush) and impetigo, cold sores, shingles and dermatitis.

Dental decay and abscesses may occur and the gums may ulcerate. Thrush of the mouth or oesophagus (gullet) may cause discomfort in the mouth and difficulty in swallowing. Herpes infections may cause ulceration of the mouth, oesophagus, stomach and duodenum; infections of the intestines may cause intermittent or continuous diarrhoea, leading to malabsorption of nutrients, wasting and weight loss. Ulcers and bleeding from the intestines may occur. Inflammation of the liver (hepatitis) may cause fever and a painful enlarged liver.

Serious infections of the lungs frequently occur in people suffering from AIDS, causing breathlessness, cough and fever.* The infections may be bacterial (including tuberculosis), viral and/or fungal.

About one-third of AIDS patients suffer from encephalitis (infection of the brain). It may develop gradually and cause forgetfulness, inability to concentrate and to think quickly, loss of balance, weakness of the legs, loss of libido, deterioration in hand-writing and incoordination of movement. The illness may progress to dementia over weeks or months and the patient may become incontinent and bed-ridden. Rarely, encephalitis may develop suddenly and cause fever, confusion and convulsions. Encephalitis may be caused directly by the HIV infection or by invading viruses such as shingles.

Meningitis may also occur in AIDS, causing headaches, nausea, vomiting and discomfort on looking into the light. It is preceded by fever, fatigue and loss of weight. It is most often caused by a fungus infection.

Spread of infections to the brain, producing abscesses, may cause signs and symptoms similar to those of a brain tumour, such as headache, confusion, lethargy and weakness, and paralysis of arms and legs according to which site of the brain is affected. Thrush, tuberculosis and toxoplasmosis are the commonest cause of brain abscesses in AIDS.

A rare virus infection (papovavirus) may cause nerve damage affecting

* Often due to pneumonia caused by *Pneumocystis carnii* (PCP).

speech, walking and movements. Other virus infections may damage nerves and muscles; toxoplasmosis may damage the retina of the eye, affecting vision.

From this brief description it is evident that brain and nerve damage may occur at different times. The damage may vary in intensity and affect a few or many sites in the brain, spinal cord and nerves. The extent of brain or nerve damage may therefore vary from just a headache to blindness, deafness, paralysis, incontinence and severe dementia.

Cancers in AIDS

The immune system of the body is always on the look-out for cancer cells and it produces killer cells that identify and destroy them. This ability to watch out for and kill cancer cells is impaired in AIDS so that, in addition to opportunistic infections, the second major problem in AIDS is the development of cancers.

The two most common types of cancer in AIDS are Kaposi's sarcoma and malignant lymphoma. Other cancers may possibly be associated with AIDS; for example, cancer of the lining of the mouth and cancer of the lining of the rectum.

Kaposi's sarcoma is the most common cancer in AIDS. It consists of malignant tumours (swellings) developing from cells that form the lining of blood vessels and the lining of lymph vessels. The latter form a network that drains fluids from tissues and organs back into the bloodstream.

The tumours spread rapidly and may affect any part of the skin as well as internal organs. They start as tiny, flat, dusky red patches which grow into small nodules. They may occur on the face, arms, legs and trunk, and may also grow on the roof of the mouth.

Internal organs commonly affected by Kaposi's sarcoma include the lungs, stomach and intestine. Wherever the tumours block blood vessels or lymph vessels they may cause fluids to enter the surrounding tissues, producing local swellings; for example, tumours on the face may cause swelling around the eyes.

Most AIDS patients do not die from Kaposi's sarcoma – they die as a consequence of their immune deficiency. Very rarely, a Kaposi's sarcoma of the lung or intestine may ulcerate and bleed.

Malignant lymphomas 'Lymphoma' is a general term used to describe new growths arising from various tissues and cells in the immune system. They are usually divided into two main groups – Hodgkin's lymphoma and non-Hodgkin's lymphoma. The former is a malignant growth of the lymph glands (lymph nodes) whereas the latter is a malignant growth of lymphoid cells (usually B but occasionally T cells). The condition may be widespread and affect lymph nodes, bone marrow, spleen and other organs such as the stomach, rectum and thyroid gland. The classification is difficult because lymphomas merge with cancers of white blood cells (e.g. lympathic leukaemia affecting lymphocytes).

In AIDS there is an increased incidence of B cell lymphomas, which are very malignant and occur mainly in homosexual men. The lymphomas in AIDS affect lymphoid tissue in the bone marrow, brain and nervous system, stomach and intestine (including rectum) and tissues in the mouth. They may, rarely, affect lymph nodes. The disease causes fever and loss of weight, and the outcome of treatment of AIDS patients suffering from malignant lymphomas is very poor.

Non-Hodgkin's lymphoma may also occur in patients who suffer from PGL (see earlier).

Treatment

People who are HIV positive need expert help, counselling and advice, as do their family and friends. They need to be assured of strict confidentiality and they should have a comprehensive medical examination every 3 months to check for any signs or symptoms that indicate an opportunistic infection or the development of Kaposi's sarcoma or malignant lymphomas. Regular blood tests should be carried out to spot any early signs of immune deficiency, underlying infection or anaemia. They will need advice on diet, exercise, dental care and skin care and advice on how to reduce the risks of transmitting the virus to other people. They may also need advice on insurance and work.

Individuals who develop acute illnesses at the start of the disease will, in addition, require good nursing care where appropriate, drug treatment to relieve any symptoms and reassurance that they will recover quickly and are at no greater risk from developing AIDS than if they had not developed any symptoms. Where appropriate, patients who develop a chronic stage of the disease (see earlier) will require drug treatment along the lines discussed below.

Drug treatment of AIDS

The mainstays of treatment are social support, good nursing care, drug treatment of any symptoms, drug treatment of any opportunistic infections, specific drug treatment for the HIV infection and radiation and/or drug treatment for any cancers.

Drug treatment of opportunistic infections Because patients suffering from

AIDS have little defence against infections, they are very vulnerable and are likely to develop serious and debilitating illnesses from infections caused by bacteria, viruses, fungi and/or protozoa. They are also unable to respond to anti-infective drug treatments as effectively as if their immune systems were not deficient. Even with the selection of the most appropriate anti-infective drug or drugs, it is often possible only to suppress an infection rather than eradicate it. This means that an infection may easily flare up again once treatment has stopped, and to try to prevent flare ups it is often necessary to give long-term treatment. However, some of the drugs used to treat acute flare ups are not suitable for long-term preventative treatment because of the risk of harmful effects. This produces obvious difficulties in the treatment of people with immune deficiency. The treatment of each AIDS patient must therefore be tailored to the individual's particular needs and response. The expected benefits and risks from anti-infective drug treatment must be carefully assessed in each individual in order to provide maximum relief of pain and suffering.

The drug treatment of opportunistic infections involves the selection and effective use of the most appropriate anti-bacterial, anti-viral, anti-fungal and/or anti-protozoal drug and the careful monitoring of the patient for any improvement or deterioration in his or her condition, and the early recognition of any serious harmful effects from the drugs being used.

Specific drug treatment of the HIV infection

Several approaches to the drug treatment of HIV infections are in progress in various research centres around the world. These include:

- Attempts to prevent the HIV virus from making replicas of itself by blocking certain enzymes or regulator genes involved in this process
- Attempts to block virus receptors on lymphocytes and other cells by attaching antibodies to them
- Attempts to stop replication by using interferons
- Attempts to neutralize HIV by injecting a soluble preparation of CD4 protein or to destroy them by injecting CD4 protein attached to an antibody

To stop HIV from replicating *Zidovudine* (Retrovir) formerly called azidothymidine or AZT is now the most commonly used anti-viral drug. It stops the viruses replicating and gives the immune system an opportunity to recover. It reduces the risk of death and severe illness in some people suffering from AIDS or from ARC. It reduces the incidence and severity of opportunistic infections and improves well-being by reducing some of the signs and symptoms of the disease, and causes an improvement in the immune system.

The most serious harmful effect that zidovudine may produce is damage to the bone marrow, knocking out red blood cell production, causing anaemia, and knocking out white blood cell production, causing a greater reduction in the resistance to infection. People with the severest forms of AIDS are at the greatest risk from these harmful effects and yet they are the ones who may benefit from treatment. It is a matter of balancing benefits against risks.

The damage to the bone marrow usually comes on slowly and can be picked up from regular blood tests. The anaemia may develop as early as 2–4 weeks after the start of treatment and the reduced white cell count after 4–8 weeks. Reduction in dose or temporarily stopping the drug and blood transfusions for the anaemia may be required. Recovery of bone marrow function occurs quickly (within 2 weeks) and the drug can be re-started at a lower dose. Only a few patients have had to stop the drug altogether.

Harmful effects and warnings on the use of zidovudine are listed in Table 57.1.

Zidovudine may prevent AIDS dementia complex by blocking viral replication in the brain. Its use in HIV-positive individuals without symptoms is under investigation.

To neutralize HIV by injecting CD4 protein CD4 is the special protein on the surface of T lymphocytes and certain other white blood cells (e.g. macrophages) on which HIV lock themselves before entering into the cells to replicate. By bio-engineering it is now possible to manufacture a soluble preparation of the protein CD4 which can be given by injection into the bloodstream. Once it is in the blood the HIVs start attaching themselves to the CD4 proteins and it therefore offers an opportunity to mop up the viruses in the blood and prevent them from attacking T lymphocytes, etc. Unfortunately, the body quickly gets rid of the CD4 protein and so it has to be given twice daily in order to maintain an effective concentration in the blood.

A possible risk of using CD4 is that the body may produce antibodies against it and these CD4-specific antibodies could then start to destroy T lymphocytes and other cells that have a CD4 protein on their surfaces.

To neutralize HIV by injecting CD4 protein attached to an antibody In an attempt to prolong the effects of CD4 protein and to prevent it from being destroyed by specific antibodies produced by the immune system, tests are being carried out using a method of 'tagging' the CD4 to an antibody (a gammaglobulin protein). This prolongs the life of the CD4 protein because antibodies last longer in the body. It looks as if two injections a week should keep the CD4 at an effective level. This *hybrid antibody* may also possibly stimulate the immune system to produce cells to attack HIV. It would have to be given twice weekly for life but, so far, harmful effects do not appear serious.

To destroy HIV by injecting CD4 antibody A problem with HIV infections is that more T lymphocytes die than appear to be infected with HIV. A possible explanation is that proteins on the surface of HIV may break off and lock on to CD4 proteins on T lymphocytes – these tagged T lymphocytes are then 'seen' as foreign and are destroyed by the body's immune system. A further problem with HIV is that the arrangement of proteins on the surface of the viruses undergo changes, which may explain why the body's own antibodies fail to eliminate the virus.

The next step in treatment could therefore be to 'design' a CD4 antibody in such a way that one end (the CD4 protein) locks on to the virus and the other end (the antibody) links up with certain immune factors to kill the virus.

Drug treatment of cancers

Treatment of Kaposi's sarcoma varies according to the extent, size and location of tumours and whether they ulcerate or bleed. It usually involves the use of irradiation locally to tumours in order to shrink them. Rapidly spreading Kaposi's sarcoma is treated with anti-cancer drugs or interferons. The treatment of lymphoma is by anti-cancer drugs, which may produce a beneficial response while the drugs are taken but the disease soon recurs after treatment is stopped.

Because irradiation and anti-cancer drugs may knock out cells involved in the body's immune system, the expected benefits and risks must be carefully balanced in people who are already suffering from an immune deficiency because of their disease. An indication of the degree of their immune deficiency is the severity and extent of any opportunistic infection from which they are suffering.

Preventing AIDS

Homosexual and bisexual men, drug addicts who share needles and syringes, and individuals who have had sexual contacts in parts of Africa are at the greatest risk of being infected with HIV; so too are haemophiliacs who have received HIV-contaminated blood products in the past. The sexual partners of these individuals are also at risk. In addition, anyone who has casual sex is at risk, particularly if they have multiple partners.

Prevention of AIDS involves the use of safer sexual practices, using a condom for penetrative sex and reducing the number of sexual partners.

Except for HIV-negative individuals who have a stable relationship and do not have sex outside of that relationship, everyone who engages in sexual activities needs to practise safer sex. Males should always wear a condom for penetrative sex whether anal or vaginal, and sexual partners should avoid any sexual activity that tears or damages tissues and draws blood and they should avoid sharing sex toys.

Wet kissing, licking the anus (cunnilinction) and urinating over each other (water sports) may carry a risk, so may sucking the penis (felatio), particularly if the seminal fluid is ejaculated (comes) into the mouth. Masturbating each other, dry kissing and body rubbing appear to be low risk; however, to repeat the warning, *any activity that tears or damages tissues and draws blood should be avoided.*

Risk of spreading HIV infection is increased if any infected blood, semen, vaginal secretion or other body fluid (e.g. urine) comes directly into contact with any tears, cuts, abrasions, sores, ulcers, infection (e.g. other sexually transmitted diseases, see earlier) or other injury or damage to the surface of the penis, lips, mouth, throat, skin, anus or vagina.

Drug addicts should not share needles and syringes and other paraphernalia that may become contaminated with HIV-infected blood. They should practise safer sex (see above) and be aware of the dangers of male and female prostitution, which some addicts may resort to for the money to keep their drug habits going.

Prevention of the spread of AIDS via blood and donor organs

All blood donors should be screened for HIV antibodies and any HIV-positive blood discarded. For extra safety, all blood products (e.g. factor VIII for haemophiliacs) should be heat treated to destroy viruses.

To prevent transmission of HIV infection via blood and blood products the following people should not give blood:

- Men who have had sex with another man at any time since 1977
- Drug abusers (male or female) who have injected drugs at any time since 1977
- Haemophiliacs who have received untreated blood products at any time since 1977
- People who have lived in or visited Africa south of the Sahara at any time since 1977 and have had sex with men and/or women living there
- Sexual partners of people in the above groups. This includes single contacts as well as regular relationships

All donors for transplant should be screened for HIV infection before their semen or organs are used.

Pregnancy and breast feeding

It is estimated that up to 50 per cent of HIV-positive pregnant women will infect their unborn babies. HIV-infected mothers can also pass the virus to their baby through breast feeding and so they should bottle feed.

Travellers

In many parts of the world HIV screening of blood donors is not carried out and blood for transfusion may be HIV-contaminated, as may be needles and syringes used for medical purposes. If you are travelling to one of these countries it is advisable to take a sterile pack of needles and so on for use in an emergency.* If a blood transfusion is needed, your embassy may be able to advise whether HIV-screened blood for transfusion is available.

Immunization against AIDS

Vaccination and immunization are discussed in Chapter 11.

The difficulty in immunizing against AIDS is that HIV damages the immune system, yet it is this system that has to be stimulated by any vaccine in order to produce antibodies to provide protection against that infection. A further problem with HIV is that different strains keep emerging and vaccines can only be prepared against specific strains that have been identified. To get round this problem, research is endeavouring to prepare a vaccine made from certain proteins contained on the surface of the virus (the virus envelope), the ones that lock on to the CD4 protein on T lymphocytes. An alternative is to try a CD4 antibody.

Although the body produces antibodies to HIV (see 'Tests for HIV infection', earlier) the disease still progresses despite the presence of antibodies from as early as 3–12 weeks after first being infected. The antibodies we test for obviously do not stop the progression of the disease in most HIV-infected individuals, so the fundamental question is: why should immunization be beneficial if it too relies on the body producing antibodies against HIV? No one knows the answer to this, nor is it known what effects antibody production would have in *preventing* someone from getting the disease. In other words, will pre-existing immunity brought about by immunization (as measured by the level of HIV antibodies) protect against HIV infection?

* Contact the Medical Advisory Service for Travellers Abroad (MASTA), London School of Hygiene and Tropical Medicine, Keppel Street, London WC1E 7HT.

An added complication is the association between HIV infection and AIDS – vaccination may protect against HIV infection but will it protect against AIDS? This association cannot be tested in animals because HIV has not been shown to cause AIDS in animals. Some monkeys and apes may be transiently infected with HIV but no case of AIDS has been reported.

35

Eye diseases

Anti-bacterial drugs applied to the eyes

Anti-bacterial drugs are discussed in detail in Chapter 48. Only anti-bacterial drugs (antibiotics) that are never, or seldom, taken internally should be applied topically to the eyes. This is to reduce the risk of the person becoming allergic to an antibiotic and then subsequently running the risk of a serious allergic reaction if that drug is then taken by mouth or injection at some future date. Antibiotics with a wide spectrum of activity against bacteria are used locally. They include chloramphenicol, framycetin, gentamicin and neomycin. Gentamicin and tobramycin are effective against a particularly nasty infection caused by *Pseudomonas*, and fusidic acid is useful against bacteria that also cause boils (*Staphylococcus*).

Anti-bacterial drugs may enter the bloodstream

Some of the anti-bacterial drug in eye applications may be absorbed directly from the eyes into the bloodstream. In addition, eye drops may run down into the nose and mouth and be absorbed, and young children may touch their eyes and lick any ointment off their fingers.

The old-fashioned *mercuric oxide eye ointment* (Golden eye ointment) should not be used because mercury may be absorbed into the bloodstream.

Brolene (propamidine) can be bought from pharmacists and is suitable for treating minor infections of the eyelids (blepharitis) and inflammation of the conjunctivae (conjunctivitis).

Anti-viral drugs applied to the eyes

The herpes simplex virus that produces cold sores can also infect the eyes, producing ulcers of the cornea; so too can the herpes zoster virus that causes shingles. Three anti-viral drugs are available for treating herpes infections of the eyes: *acyclovir*, *idoxuridine* and *vidarabine* (see Chapter 57).

Anti-fungal drugs applied to the eyes

Anti-fungal drugs are discussed in Chapter 56. Fungal infections of the eyes are rare but they can occur in patients who are taking drugs used to suppress the immune system. Anti-fungal drugs are usually taken by mouth but special preparations to apply to the eyes may be obtained on request from special centres.

Corticosteroid drugs applied to the eyes

The most effective anti-inflammatory drugs used to treat inflammatory conditions of the eyes are the corticosteroids (see Chapter 62). They may be used as local applications, local injections under the conjunctivae or by mouth.

Unfortunately, corticosteroid eye applications are sometimes used to treat minor disorders of the eyes and also in ignorance to treat potentially serious disorders such as virus infections (e.g. herpes). The application of a corticosteroid to a virus infection of the eye may have serious consequences for the patient. This is because the corticosteroid suppresses the inflammation but has no effect on the virus infection, which may spread painlessly into the eye and result in scarring and perforation of the cornea. This warning on treating a virus infection of the eye applies to corticosteroids used alone or in combination with an anti-bacterial drug. Another important risk in using corticosteroid applications is that they can increase the pressure inside the eyes and may trigger an attack of glaucoma in a susceptible person (see later). This 'steroid glaucoma' may come on several weeks after treatment was started.

If corticosteroids are taken by mouth in high dosage (e.g. more than 15 mg of prednisolone daily or the equivalent dosage of one of the other corticosteroids) over a prolonged period of time (several years), they may produce cataracts. See discussion on recommended daily dosages of corticosteroids in patients on long-term treatment (Chapter 62).

Warnings *Different strengths, different solubilities (soluble in fat or water), and different formulations of corticosteroids (eye drops as solutions or suspensions, or as ointments) will pass through the cornea (the window of the eye) to different extents, and the extent of this penetration will be determined by the degree of damage or inflammation on the surface of the eye. It is therefore difficult to make standard comparisons of the effectiveness of the various preparations that are available but it makes sense to use a low-potency corticosteroid such as fluorometholone or clobetasone (see Chapter 62) for the shortest duration of time possible, particularly in those patients with glaucoma or who run a risk of developing it (see later).*

It is very important to restrict the use of corticosteroid eye preparations and not use them to treat acute red eye (e.g. allergic or viral conjunctivitis) or inflammation of the eyelids. A corticosteroid should be used ***only*** *after a full eye examination has been carried out (including sight test) and fluorescein eye drops have been inserted in the eye to check for any ulcers or scarring of the cornea. If these are present the individual should be referred to an eye specialist. The patient should also see an eye specialist if there is no improvement after 1–2 weeks of treatment.*

Anti-inflammatory drugs applied to the eyes

Oxyphenbutazone (Tanderil) eye ointment is a non-steroidal anti-inflammatory drug (see Chapter 30) occasionally used to reduce inflammation in the surface of the outer coat of the eye (the sclera – the white part).

Antihistamine drugs applied to the eyes

Eye drops containing an antihistamine may help to relieve the redness and itching of allergic conjunctivitis but they should be used only for a few days at a time; for example, antazoline combined with a decongestant xylometazoline (Otrivine-Antistin). Opticrom eye drops, which contain sodium cromoglycate (see Chapter 10) may be useful for preventing allergic eye disorders.

Local anaesthetics applied to the eyes

Amethocaine, cocaine, oxybuprocaine and proxymetacaine are used as local anaesthetics on the eyes. They may be applied as drops or by injection. They may produce stinging of the eye; oxybuprocaine may be better for children because it produces less stinging when applied.

Other drugs applied to the eyes

Anti-itching preparations

These should not be used. They may contain aspirin-related drugs, camphor or menthol, and, because they relieve pain, they may mask the fact that some dust has entered the eye. Delay in recognizing this may lead to damage of the cornea and the formation of ulcers.

Other anti-infective preparations

Silver protein products should not be used. They may stain the conjunctivae black. Mercurial compounds should not be used because mercury can be absorbed. Also, the effectiveness of these preparations has never been demonstrated. Sulphacetamide (10%) is not very effective and may cause allergic reactions and the development of resistant strains of bacteria.

Astringent preparations

Astringents dry up the surfaces and relieve swelling and inflammation. They are used to relieve *minor irritation* of the eyes. In high doses they are irritating.

Zinc sulphate (0.25%) eye drop solution is the only astringent that should be used on the eyes, but note that it does not relieve congestion.

Lubricant eye applications (tear substitutes)

Lubricant preparations are included in eye drops if tear production is defective. They include hypromellose, polyvinyl alcohol, polyethylene glycol and acetylcysteine. They are often referred to as artificial tears.

Decongestant eye applications

Sympathomimetic drugs such as ephedrine, naphazoline or phenylephrine constrict blood vessels (see Chapter 2) and will help to relieve the irritation, redness, swelling and watering of the eyes that occur with hayfever. They should be used only for short courses of treatment and *not* regularly every day for more than 10 days at a time. They can be absorbed into the bloodstream from the eye and also run down into the nose and mouth, from which they are absorbed. They may produce a rise in blood pressure, a rapid pulse and nervousness, and may be harmful to children, patients with angina, raised blood pressure or over-active thyroid gland. Regular long-term use of decongestant eye drops may cause rebound congestion of the eyes, which may be worse than before treatment was started (see problems with rebound nasal congestion after using nasal decongestants, in Chapter 7).

Eye washes

Eye washes should contain *no* active ingredient and they should be used *only* for bathing and flushing the eyes if they have been exposed to some toxic substance. They should contain only a preservative such as benzalkonium, a buffer to make the eye wash the same acidity as tears, and a chemical that ensures that the salt content is the same as tears. The inclusion of any other ingredient is unnecessary and potentially harmful.

Combined eye preparations containing a corticosteroid and anti-bacterial drug

There are several eye preparations available that contain an anti-bacterial drug and a corticosteroid in the same preparation (see Table 35.5). Although convenient for the patient and very effective if used sensibly, these preparations may, none the less, cause serious problems if used inappropriately (see above). Because of the damage produced by their widespread use in the past it is now recommended that they be used only under the supervision of an eye specialist.

Anti-infective drugs by mouth

In severe infections of the eyes, anti-infective drugs are given by mouth or by injection in addition to applications to the eyes. This is to ensure that a sufficient concentration of drug gets into the affected eyes. The drugs used will depend upon the type and severity of the infection. An anti-infective drug may be injected directly under the conjunctiva in order to achieve a high enough dose of the drug in the eye.

Drugs that dilate the pupils

Drugs that dilate the pupils are called mydriatics. They cause the pupil to dilate by paralysing the circular muscle of the iris or by stimulating it to contract, or by a mixture of both actions. Those that paralyse the circular muscle may be referred to as cycloplegics and they may produce prolonged effects.

Anticholinergic drugs (see Chapter 2) are used in eye drops to dilate the pupils. Short-acting anticholinergic drugs such as tropicamide are used by eye specialists to dilate the pupils so that they can examine the inside of the eyes more easily. Longer acting anticholinergic drugs are used to rest the pupil in patients who have an infection of the pupil. The effects of tropicamide last about 3 hours; lachesine about 4–6 hours; cyclopentolate, hyoscine and homatropine last for about 24 hours, and the effects of atropine may last for over a week.

Phenylephrine is a sympathomimetic drug (see Chapter 2) which may be used in eye drops along with an anticholinergic drug to dilate the pupils.

Thymoxamine (Minims Thymoxamine Hydrochloride) may be used to reverse the dilatation of the pupil caused by sympathomimetic drugs (e.g. adrenaline, phenylephrine).

Table 35.1 Anti-bacterial eye preparations

Preparation	*Drug*	*Dosage form*
Achromycin	tetracycline	Oil suspension drops
Albucid	sulphacetamide	Drops, ointment in a greasy basis, ointment in a water-miscible basis
Aureomycin	chlortetracycline	Ointment
Brolene drops	propamidine	Drops
Brolene ointment	dibromopropamidine	Ointment
chloramphenicol	chloramphenicol	Drops
Chloromycetin	chloramphenicol	Ointment, drops (Chloromycetin Redidrops)
Cidomycin	gentamicin	Drops, ointment
framycetin	framycetin	Drops, ointment
Framygen	framycetin	Drops, ointment
Fucithalmic	fusidic acid	Drops (slow release)
Garamycin	gentamicin	Drops
gentamicin	gentamicin	Drops
Genticin	gentamicin	Drops, ointment
Graneodin	neomycin, gramicidin	Ointment
Isopto Cetamide	sulphacetamide, hypromellose (lubricant)	Drops
Minims Chloramphenicol	chloramphenicol	Drops
Minims Gentamicin	gentamicin	Drops
Minims Neomycin	neomycin sulphate	Drops
Minims Sulphacetamide	sulphacetamide sodium	Drops
neomycin	neomycin	Drops
Neosporin	neomycin, gramicidin, polymyxin B	Drops
Opulets Chloramphenicol	chloramphenicol	Drops
Polyfax	polymyxin B, bacitracin	Ointment
Polytrim	polymyxin B, trimethoprim	Drops
Sno Phenicol	chloramphenicol	Drops
Soframycin	framycetin	Drops, ointment
sulphacetamide	sulphacetamide	Drops
Tobralex	tobramycin	Drops

Table 35.2 Corticosteroid anti-inflammatory eye preparations

Preparation	*Drug*	*Dosage form*
Betnesol	betamethasone	Drops, ointment
Eumovate	clobetasone	Drops
FML	fluorometholone	Drops
hydrocortisone	hydrocortisone	Drops
Maxidex	dexamethasone with hypromellose (lubricant)	Drops
Minims Prednisolone	prednisolone	Drops
Pred Forte	prednisolone	Drops (long-acting)
Predsol	prednisolone	Drops
Vista-Methasone	betamethasone	Drops

Table 35.3 Non-steroidal anti-inflammatory eye preparation

Preparation	*Drug*	*Dosage form*
Tanderil	oxyphenbutazone	Ointment

Table 35.4 Anti-viral eye preparations

Preparation	*Drug*	*Dosage form*
Idoxene	idoxuridine	Ointment
idoxuridine	idoxuridine	Drops, ointment
Kerecid	idoxuridine	Drops
Zovirax	acyclovir	Ointment

Table 35.5 Combined corticosteroid/anti-bacterial eye preparations

Preparation	*Drug*	*Drug group*	*Dosage form*
Betnesol-N	betamethasone neomycin	Corticosteroid Anti-bacterial	Drops, ointment
Chloromycetin Hydrocortisone	hydrocortisone chloramphenicol	Corticosteroid Anti-bacterial	Ointment
Eumovate-N	clobetasone neomycin	Corticosteroid Anti-bacterial	Drops
FML-Neo	fluorometholone neomycin	Corticosteroid Anti-bacterial	Drops
Framycort	hydrocortisone framycetin	Corticosteroid Anti-bacterial	Drops, ointment

Table 35.5 Combined corticosteroid/anti-bacterial eye preparations (*cont*)

Preparation	*Drug*	*Drug group*	*Dosage form*
Maxitrol	dexamethasone neomycin polymyxin B	Corticosteroid Anti-bacterial Anti-bacterial	Drops, ointment (drops also contain hypromellose, a lubricant)
Neo-Cortef	hydrocortisone neomycin	Corticosteroid Anti-bacterial	Drops, ointment
Predsol-N	prednisolone neomycin	Corticosteroid Anti-bacterial	Drops
Sofradex	dexamethasone framycetin gramicidin	Corticosteroid Anti-bacterial Anti-bacterial	Drops, ointment
Vista-Methasone-N	betamethasone neomycin	Corticosteroid Anti-bacterial	Drops

Table 35.6 Anti-allergic eye preparations

Preparation	*Drug*	*Drug group*	*Dosage form*
Opticrom	sodium cromoglycate	Mast cell stabilizer	Drops, ointment
Otrivine-Antistin	antazoline xylometazoline	Antihistamine Sympathomimetic decongestant	Drops
Vasocon-A	antazoline naphazoline	Antihistamine Sympathomimetic decongestant	Drops

Table 35.7 Local anaesthetic eye drops

Preparation	*Drug*	*Preparation*	*Drug*
amethocaine	amethocaine	Minims Benoxinate	oxybuprocaine
cocaine	cocaine	Minims Lignocaine and Fluorescein	lignocaine, fluorescein
Cocaine and Homatropine Eye-drops	cocaine, homatropine	Ophthaine	proxymetacaine
Minims Amethocaine	amethocaine	Opulets Benoxinate	oxybuprocaine

Table 35.8 Lubricant eye drops – artificial tears

Preparation	*Drug*	*Preparation*	*Drug*
Hypotears	polyethylene glycol polyvinyl alcohol	Isopto Plain	hypromellose
		Lacri-Lube*	liquid paraffin
hypromellose	hypromellose	Liquifilm Tears	polyvinyl alcohol
Ilube	acetylcysteine, hypromellose	Minims Artificial Tears	hydroxyethylcellulose sodium chloride
Isopto Alkaline	hypromellose	Minims Castor Oil	castor oil
Isopto Frin	phenylephrine hypromellose	Sno Tears	polyvinyl alcohol
		Tears Naturale	dextran 70 hypromellose

* Eye ointment

Table 35.9 Eye drops that dilate the pupils – harmful effects and warning

Harmful effects Eye drops that contain an anticholinergic drug (see Chapter 2) may produce a contact dermatitis of the eyelids and surrounding skin, and they may be absorbed into the bloodstream to produce harmful effects such as dry mouth, constipation, rapid beating of the heart and difficulty in passing urine. These harmful effects may occur particularly in very young children and elderly people. Not only may the drugs be absorbed directly into the bloodstream from the eyes but the eye drops may also run into the nose and down the cheeks into the mouth to be absorbed. Young children may lick their cheeks or get the eye drops on their fingers and then suck them.

Warnings *Risks in elderly people* Eye drops that contain an anticholinergic drug may trigger an acute attack of glaucoma in a susceptible elderly person. (See also risks by mouth, later.) Eye drops that contain a sympathomimetic drug (e.g. phenylephrine) should not be used in people with narrow-angle glaucoma, raised blood pressure, coronary artery disease or over-active thyroid.

Risks in driving Dilated pupils may affect your vision, so you should not drive until these effects have worn off.

Table 35.10 Drugs used to dilate the pupils

Preparation	*Drug*	*Dosage form*
atropine	atropine	Drops, ointment
homatropine	homatropine	Drops
hyoscine	hyoscine	Drops
Isopto Atropine	atropine, hypromellose (lubricant)	Drops
lachesine	lachesine	Drops
Minims Atropine	atropine	Drops
Minims Cyclopentolate	cyclopentolate	Drops
Minims Homatropine	homatropine	Drops

Table 35.10 Drugs used to dilate the pupils (*cont.*)

Preparation	*Drug*	*Dosage form*
Minims Phenylephrine	phenylephrine	Drops
Minims Tropicamide	tropicamide	Drops
Mydriacyl	tropicamide	Drops
Mydrilate	cyclopentolate	Drops
Opulets Atropine	atropine	Drops
Opulets Cyclopentolate	cyclopentolate	Drops
phenylephrine	phenylephrine	Drops

Drugs that constrict the pupils

Drugs that cause the pupils to constrict (go small) are called *miotics*. They are cholinergic drugs that produce an effect opposite to that of anticholinergic drugs. They constrict the muscle that works the iris, which makes the pupil go small and opens up the drainage canal in the front chamber of the eye. Miotics are used to constrict the pupil after someone has had a mydriatic applied to dilate the pupil for an eye examination, particularly in anyone over the age of 40 years in order to avoid the risk of triggering an attack of glaucoma. They are also used to treat open-angle glaucoma in order to reduce the pressure in the front of the eye (see later under 'Glaucoma').

Cholinergic drugs (see Chapter 2) that are used to constrict the pupils include drugs that act like acetylcholine (e.g. carbachol and pilocarpine) and drugs that delay the breakdown of acetylcholine (e.g. physostigmine and ecothiopate).

Miotics applied to the eyes may be absorbed directly into the blood-stream. Also, when applied as eye drops, they may run down the nose and down the cheek into the mouth and be absorbed into the bloodstream. They may therefore produce generalized harmful effects, which include increased salivation, loss of appetite, nausea, vomiting, stomach pains and diarrhoea. Local effects of miotics include difficulty with focusing and allergic reactions.

Table 35.11 Drugs used to constrict the pupils

Preparation	*Drug*	*Dosage form*
Isopto Carbachol	carbachol, hypromellose (lubricant)	Eye drops
Isopto Carpine	pilocarpine, hypromellose (lubricant)	Eye drops
Minims Pilocarpine	pilocarpine	Eye drops

Table 35.11 Drugs used to constrict the pupils (*cont.*)

Preparation	*Drug*	*Dosage form*
Ocusert Pilo	pilocarpine	Ocular inserts: sustained release
Opulets Pilocarpine	pilocarpine	Eye drops
physostigmine	physostigmine	Eye drops
physostigmine and pilocarpine	physostigmine pilocarpine	Eye drops
pilocarpine	pilocarpine	Eye drops
Sno Pilo	pilocarpine	Eye drops

Glaucoma

'Glaucoma' is a term used to describe an increase in pressure inside the eye and the damage that it produces. About 1 person in 100 over 40 years of age develops glaucoma and about 5 in 100 of those over 65 years.

In glaucoma the pressure of the fluid in the front chamber of the eyes (between the lens and the cornea) is raised due to a defective draining away of the fluid while the inflow remains steady. The increase in pressure affects the transparency of the cornea (the window of the eye) and compresses the blood vessels that supply the main optic nerve that links the eye to the brain. The latter may produce irreversible damage to the optic nerve, resulting in a permanent loss of vision. This loss of vision may come on suddenly over a few days or may develop slowly over years. There are two principal types of glaucoma – open-angle and closed-angle glaucoma.

Open-angle glaucoma (chronic simple glaucoma)

This is the most common type of glaucoma. It comes on slowly and is commonest in elderly people. The increase in pressure is caused by a decreased outflow from the front chamber of the eye, which probably results from a degeneration of the outlet mechanisms. It causes no early symptoms but may lead to a slow and progressive reduction in the outer fields of vision (the peripheral vision) and eventually to blindness. Both eyes are usually involved, although one eye may be affected more severely than the other and the loss of vision may not be noticed for months or years. There is no pain with open-angle glaucoma and no sudden onset of symptoms. It accounts for about 1 in 10 of all new entries in the blind register. Relatives are at greater risk, so are diabetic and short-sighted people.

Closed-angle glaucoma (narrow-angle glaucoma, acute glaucoma, congestive glaucoma)

Closed-angle glaucoma develops when the drainage of fluid from the front chamber of the eye is blocked *suddenly*. This may occur when the pupil dilates because the circular muscles of the iris become more bulky and may block the narrow angle between the iris and the lens, and interfere with the drainage of fluid. A large number of drugs (see Chapter 2) may close this angle by causing dilatation of the pupil and may trigger an acute attack of glaucoma in a susceptible person (e.g. someone with a small eyeball).

When the angle is blocked the pressure in the front chamber of the eye builds up rapidly and the individual complains of a sudden onset of blurred vision, perhaps preceded by seeing halos around objects, severe pain in the affected eye and usually some headache, nausea and vomiting. There is a loss of vision, the eye is red and the pupil looks cloudy. It may be very serious and requires *immediate treatment* from an eye specialist.

Warning *Elderly, long-sighted people are at particular risk of developing closed-angle glaucoma.*

Drugs that may trigger an attack of closed-angle glaucoma in susceptible people

anticholinergic drugs (e.g. atropine and hyoscine)
antihistamines
chlorpropamide used to treat diabetes
corticosteroids
cough and cold remedies containing anticholinergic drugs and/or antihistamines
fenfluramine used as a slimming drug
ganglion blocking drugs used to treat raised blood pressure (e.g. hexamethonium)
indomethacin used to treat rheumatoid arthritis
monoamine oxidase anti-depressants
oral contraceptives
tricyclic and cyclic anti-depressants

Warnings *Because glaucoma may produce blindness, early diagnosis and treatment are essential. It is therefore important to remember that some elderly people, instead of developing the fully blown symptoms of closed-angle glaucoma,* *may just develop headache, nausea and vomiting and one eye may be that bit redder than the other. These individuals should be referred to an eye specialist.*

Drugs used to treat glaucoma and how they work

Miotic eye drops (e.g. carbachol, pilocarpine) constrict the pupil and open up the drainage area; this decreases the pressure in the front chamber of the eye by improving the drainage of the fluid. They may produce blurring of vision in young people and an aching in the brow.

Adrenaline eye drops help to improve the drainage of fluid in the front chamber of the eye and may decrease its rate of production. The net result is a reduction in the pressure in the eye. Adrenaline may produce severe smarting and redness of the eye, and it should not be used in closed-angle glaucoma (see earlier) because adrenaline dilates the pupil and this may interfere with drainage.

Dipivefrin (Propine) eye drops are formulated to pass quickly through the cornea and enter the fluid in the front chamber of the eye where the dipivefrine is converted into adrenaline.

Guanethidine is used to treat raised blood pressure. It is applied to the eye as drops to treat glaucoma because it helps to reduce the pressure inside the eye by reducing the rate of production of the fluid in the front chamber of the eye and increasing its drainage. It has a slow constricting effect on the pupil although at first it may cause the pupil to dilate. It increases and prolongs the effects of adrenaline.

Beta blockers are discussed in detail in Chapter 20. Several are now in fashion as eye drops for treating glaucoma. They are thought to reduce the pressure inside the eye by reducing the rate of production of the fluid in the front chamber of the eye.

Like any drug applied to the eyes, beta blockers may be absorbed directly into the bloodstream and also from the nose and mouth if the drops run into them. This absorption may produce harmful effects particularly in people who suffer from asthma; in individuals with a slow heart rate because these drugs slow down the heart rate; and in patients with heart failure because they may make the condition worse. Sufficient amounts of drug may also be absorbed to interact with other drugs; for example, with the drug verapamil used to treat angina and disorders of heart rhythm. The absorbed beta blocker may interact with the verapamil to cause a fall in blood pressure, heart failure and may, very rarely, stop the heart from beating. Beta blocker eye drops may produce dry eyes, conjunctivitis and allergic inflammation of the eyelids.

NOTE The general effects of eye drops may be reduced by closing the eyes for several minutes after applying the drops. This stops the drops running down the tear passages into the nose.

Diuretics (water tablets)

Diuretics are discussed in detail in Chapter 22. One of these drugs, *acetazolamide*, is used to reduce the pressure in the eye. It reduces the secretion of fluid in the front chamber of the eye. *Dichlorphenamide* produces similar effects but is longer lasting than acetazolamide.

Harmful effects of acetazolamide and dichlorphenamide include headaches, drowsiness, dizziness, depression, fatigue, numbness and pins and needles in the hands and feet, and loss of appetite. They may cause a fall in levels of potassium in the blood.

Drug treatment of open-angle (chronic simple) glaucoma

In this condition drugs are used to reduce the pressure inside the eye and to maintain this pressure at a normal level, usually for the rest of the individual's life. Effective drug treatment (if taken as directed) prevents further deterioration in vision, but of course it cannot restore any damage that has already occurred and this is why early diagnosis is important.

Treatment usually starts with *beta blocker* eye drops to reduce the rate of production of fluid in the eye; then a drug that constricts the pupil and improves drainage of fluid from the eye may be added. *Pilocarpine* is one of the most commonly used drugs for this purpose and it is often preferred in older patients. However, younger people and short-sighted people may find that the constriction of the pupil produced by pilocarpine affects their vision, whilst other people may find that the drops actually help them to focus. Over time it may be necessary to add *adrenaline* to the beta blocker and pilocarpine.

Because pilocarpine constricts the pupils, individuals with a disorder of the lens (e.g. early cataract) may find that their vision is further impaired. In these people it is best to try a beta blocker first and then add in adrenaline eye drops if necessary.

If these treatments are not beneficial, the addition of *acetazolamide* by mouth may add to the effects produced by the eye drops; it is also useful until laser treatment or surgery can be undertaken to improve drainage of fluid from the eye.

NOTE Ophthalmic opticians (optometrists) carry out routine measurements of the pressure in the eyes by using an instrument that blows air on the cornea; this is one reason why it is important to consult an ophthalmic optician at regular intervals (every 1 or 2 years) if you are over the age of 40 years

Drug treatment of acute (closed-angle) glaucoma

A person who has developed acute glaucoma needs urgent medical treatment in order to prevent loss of vision. Drugs are used to bring down the pressure in the eyes and then laser treatment or surgery may be carried out to provide drainage of the fluid and to prevent a recurrence of the problem. It is not common for drug treatment to be continued for any length of time.

Acetazolamide is usually the first drug to be given, at first by injection and then by mouth. Eye drops to constrict the pupil are then applied at frequent intervals, and occasionally a thiazide diuretic is given by mouth to draw fluid out of the tissues by osmosis (see thiazide diuretics, in Chapter 22).

Warning *Glaucoma causes blindness, yet despite this risk one of the main hazards of drug treatment is the failure of some patients to use eye drops as directed.*

Inflammation of the eyelids (blepharitis)

Blepharitis causes the eyelids to be itchy, red and scaly. It is usually due to an infection spreading from the roots of the eyelashes. The treatment is to apply one of the ointments listed in Table 35.1 to the eyelids.

Inflammation of the conjunctivae (conjunctivitis)

Conjunctivitis is an inflammation of the clear covering of the eye – the conjunctiva. The eyes become red and may feel sore and gritty, and there may be a discharge that causes the eyelids to stick together overnight. It is commonly caused by a viral or a bacterial infection. *Chloramphenicol* eye drops in the day-time and ointment at night will usually clear up a bacterial infection in 2–3 days. If it does not then the infection is probably due to a virus and there is no specific treatment. For allergic conjunctivitis see page 107. Corticosteroid eye drops must not be used without an antibiotic. For herpes infections see page 789.

Inflammation of the pupil (iridocyclitis)

In iridocyclitis the sufferer complains of a sore red eye with loss of vision and the pupil is irregular, small and sticky. Treatment is urgent and should include dilating the pupil with atropine or cyclopentolate and giving a corticosteroid by mouth or locally into the affected eye. Anyone with this condition should be referred immediately to a specialist eye clinic.

Table 35.12 Drugs used to treat glaucoma – harmful effects and warnings

acetazolamide (Diamox)
Harmful effects are usually transient and related to the dose. They include transient short-sightedness, flushing, thirst, headache, drowsiness, dizziness, fatigue, irritability, excitement, thirst and passing large volumes of urine, numbness and tingling in the arms, legs and face, incoordination of movements, loss of hearing, over-breathing and stomach upsets (loss of appetite, vomiting). Acetazolamide is a sulphonamide derivative and it may, rarely, produce sulphonamide-type harmful effects (see Chapter 54). They include fever, blood disorders, skin rashes, kidney stones and colic.

Warnings Acetazolamide must not be used in people who are allergic to sulphonamides, nor in people suffering from impaired kidney function, Addison's disease or in individuals who are losing sodium and potassium in their urine. It should be used with caution in people with impaired liver function, or who have difficulty in passing urine due to some obstruction (e.g. enlarged prostate gland). Avoid long-term use in patients with chronic closed-angle glaucoma. In patients on long-term treatment, blood counts should be carried out at regular intervals.

Risks in elderly people Harmful effects may be more frequent and severe; therefore use with caution.

adrenaline (Epifrin, Eppy, Isopto Epinal, Simplene)
Harmful effects include stinging and redness of the eyes, pigmentation of the eyes, headache and irritation of the skin. Rarely, there may be rapid beating of the heart, pallor, palpitations, trembling, sweating and raised blood pressure.

Warnings It must not be used in individuals with narrow-angle glaucoma. It should be used with caution in anyone suffering from heart disease, over-active thyroid gland, rapid heart rate or raised blood pressure.

betaxolol (Betoptic)
Harmful effects include discomfort, watering of the eye and, rarely, redness, itching and discomfort on looking in the light. Rarely, corneal damage may occur. For general harmful effects of beta blockers, see Chapter 20.

Warnings It must be used with caution in people with asthma or other wheezing disorders, slow heart rate or heart failure.

carbachol (Isopto Carbachol)
Harmful effects include redness of the eye, headache, decrease in vision, salivation, fainting, irregular heart beat, stomach cramps, vomiting, diarrhoea and wheezing. It may, rarely, cause detachment of the retina in susceptible people.

Warnings Carbachol must not be used in people who are allergic to the drug, or who have had a recent heart attack or recent surgery on the intestine, or who have a bowel obstruction or difficulty in passing urine due to some obstruction. It should be used with caution in individuals who have some injury to the cornea, acute heart failure, bronchial asthma, active peptic ulcer, over-active thyroid gland, epilepsy or parkinsonism. Do not use when wearing soft contact lenses. Avoid overdose. It may cause difficulty with seeing in the dark; therefore avoid any hazardous occupation in poor light.

Risks in elderly people Harmful effects may be more frequent and severe; therefore use with caution.

Risks in driving Affects vision in the dark therefore avoid night-time driving.

carteolol (Teoptic)
Harmful effects include dry eye, allergic reactions to the eye, irritation and redness, burning pain and blurred vision. Rarely, corneal damage may occur. For general harmful effects of beta blockers, see Chapter 20.

Warnings Carteolol must not be used in people with severe heart failure, asthma or other wheezing disorders. Do not use when wearing soft or gas-permeable contact lenses.

Table 35.12 Drugs used to treat glaucoma – harmful effects and warnings (*cont.*)

dichlorphenamide (Daranide)
Harmful effects include stomach upsets (loss of appetite, nausea, vomiting), loss of weight, constipation, frequency of passing urine, kidney stones and colic, skin rashes, itching, blood disorders, headache, weakness, nervousness, feeling of suffocation (as if there is a ball in the throat), sedation, lassitude, confusion, disorientation, dizziness, incoordination of movements, tremor, noises in the ears, numbness and pins and needles in the hands, feet and tongue.

Warnings Dichlorphenamide must not be used in people who suffer from liver failure, kidney failure, adrenal failure, low blood sodium or potassium levels, chronic closed-angle glaucoma, chronic lung disease or who are allergic to the drug; it may cause a fall in blood potassium levels, decreased kidney function and changes in the acidity of the blood.

Risks in elderly people Harmful effects may be more frequent and severe; therefore use with caution.

Risks in driving Harmful effects may affect your ability to drive. Do not drive until you know how the drug affects you.

dipivefrin (Propine)
Harmful effects include stinging, allergic reactions and rebound redness of the eyes when the drug is stopped.

Warnings Dipivefrine must not be used in anyone with closed-angle glaucoma.

ecothiopate
Harmful effects include aching brow, stinging and redness of the eyes and blurring of vision at start of treatment; they usually clear up after 5–10 days. Very rarely, opacities in the lens may develop in adults; paradoxical increase in pressure in the eye, cysts on the iris, conjunctivitis, blockage of tear ducts and detachment of the retina have been reported.

Warnings Ecothiopate must not be used in people who are allergic to it, have inflammation of the eye or have closed-angle glaucoma (most cases). Pilocarpine eye drops are used for 2 months before high strength ecothiopate is given in adults. Stop the drug temporarily if persistent diarrhoea, incontinence of urine, profuse sweating, muscle weakness or irregularities of the heart rate occur. Ecothiopate should be used with caution in anyone with peptic ulcer, slow heart rate, low blood pressure, recent heart attack, epilepsy, parkinsonism, eye infections or in anyone with a history of detached retina. If used just before eye surgery, it may increase the risk of bleeding into the eye chamber. Harmful effects may be increased by exposure to certain insecticides and pesticides (carbamate or organophosphate types) due to absorption through the skin; wear a mask and change clothes frequently if you work with these products.

gaunethidine (Ganda [with adrenaline], Ismelin)
Harmful effects include redness of the eyes, drooping eyelid, slight constriction of the pupil on prolonged high dose, and irritation.

Warnings Guanethidine must not be used in anyone with closed-angle glaucoma or who is allergic to the drug. Do not wear soft contact lenses during treatment.

levobunolol (Betagan)
Harmful effects include irritation of the eyes, headache and dizziness. For general harmful effects of beta blockers, see Chapter 20.

Warnings Levobunolol should not be used in anyone with severe heart failure, asthma or other wheezing disorders.

metipranolol (Glauline, Minims Metipranolol)
Harmful effects include discomfort, watering, itching and redness of the eyes.

Table 35.12 Drugs used to treat glaucoma – harmful effects and warnings (*cont.*)

For general harmful effects of beta blockers, see Chapter 20.

Warnings Metipranolol must not be used in anyone who suffers from asthma or related wheezing disorders or heart block. It should be used with caution in people with slow heart rate or heart failure.

physostigmine
Harmful effects include salivation, loss of appetite, nausea, vomiting, stomach cramps, diarrhoea, fast heart rate and rise in blood pressure.

Warnings Physostigmine must not be used in individuals with an obstruction of the intestine or obstruction to the flow of urine (e.g. enlarged prostate). It should be used with caution in anyone with a slow heart rate, asthma, heart disease, epilepsy, low blood pressure or parkinsonism.

pilocarpine (Isopto Carpine, Minims Pilocarcipine, Ocusert Pilo, Opulets Pilocarpine, Sno-Pilo)
Harmful effects include redness of the eyes, short-sightedness and headache over the brow or sides of the head (particularly in younger people at the start of treatment), reduced vision in poor light (particularly in older people with cataracts); very rarely, detached retina and lens opacities may develop with prolonged use.

Warnings Pilocarpine must not be used in people who are allergic to it, or who have acute iritis. Avoid hazardous work in poor light.

Risks with driving It interferes with vision in the dark; therefore do not drive at night.

timolol (Timoptol)
Harmful effects include irritation, conjunctivitis, sore eyelids (blepharitis), visual disturbance, double vision, drooping eyelids and, rarely, damage to the cornea. It may increase the pressure in the eye. For general harmful effects of beta blockers, see Chapter 20.

Warnings Timolol must not be used in people who suffer from asthma or a related wheezing disorder, slow pulse rate, heart block, heart failure, or who are allergic to the drug. It should be used with caution in anyone with severe heart disease.

Ulcers on the eye

Ulcers on the cornea of the eye produce a painful red eye. They are frequently caused by a virus infection that causes 'cold sores' (herpes simplex) or shingles (herpes zoster). Anti-viral drugs used to treat these disorders is discussed in Chapter 57.

Allergic reactions in the eyes

To drugs

People may become allergic to drugs or to other constituents in eye preparations applied to the eyes and they develop red eyes and a rash on the eyelids. The preparation must be stopped and corticosteroid drops applied, but this decision must be left to an eye specialist because the

Table 35.13 Drugs used to treat glaucoma

Preparation	*Drug*	*Drug group*	*Dosage form*
Betagan	levobunolol	Beta blocker	Eye drops
Betoptic	betaxolol	Beta blocker	Eye drops
Daranide	dichlorphenamide	Carbonic anhydrase inhibitor	Tablets
Diamox	acetazolamide	Carbonic anhydrase inhibitor	Sustained-release capsules (Diamox Sustets), tablets, powder (for oral use), powder for injection
Epifrin	adrenaline	Sympathomimetic	Eye drops
Eppy	adrenaline	Sympathomimetic	Eye drops
Ganda	guanethidine adrenaline	Adrenergic neurone blocker Sympathomimetic	Eye drops
Glauline	metipranolol	Beta blocker	Eye drops
Ismelin	guanethidine	Adrenergic neurone blocker	Eye drops
Isopto Carbachol	carbachol hypromellose	Cholinergic Lubricant	Eye drops
Isopto Carpine	pilocarpine hypromellose	Cholinergic Lubricant	Eye drops
Isopto Epinal	adrenaline hypromellose	Sympathomimetic Lubricant	Eye drops
Minims Metipranolol	metipranolol	Beta blocker	Eye drops
Minims Pilocarpine	pilocarpine	Cholinergic	Eye drops
Ocusert Pilo	pilocarpine	Cholinergic	Ocular insert, sustained release
Opulets Pilocarpine	pilocarpine	Cholinergic	Eye drops
physostigmine	physostigmine	Cholinergic	Eye drops
physostigmine and pilocarpine eye drops	physostigmine pilocarpine	Cholinergic Cholinergic	Eye drops
pilocarpine	pilocarpine	Cholinergic	Eye drops
Propine	dipivefrine	Sympathomimetic	Eye drops
Simplene	adrenaline	Sympathomimetic	Eye drops
Sno-Pilo	pilocarpine	Cholinergic	Eye drops
Teoptic	carteolol	Beta blocker	Eye drops
Timoptol	timolol	Beta blocker	Eye drops in Ocumeter metered dose

regular use of most drops are for the treatment of a serious condition such as glaucoma.

To eye make-up

Some individuals may develop an allergic conjunctivitis and/or an allergic rash on their eyelids due to contact with eye make-up. They should stop using that make-up, and antihistamine eye drops may help; for example antazoline plus xylometazoline (Otrivine-Antihistin) used two or three times daily – but only for a few days.

In hayfever

People who suffer from allergy to pollens, house mites and other particles may develop conjunctivitis which may be very troublesome. Simple eye drops (e.g. zinc sulphate) or eye drops containing an antihistamine (see later) may help. It may be worth trying special eye drops (e.g. sodium cromoglycate; Opticrom) to prevent an allergic reaction, but it must be remembered that this drug only *prevents* allergic reactions, it does not relieve an attack once it has started. For the treatment of hayfever, see Chapter 10.

Dry eyes

Dry eyes may be due to defective production of tears. This may, rarely, occur in rheumatoid arthritis and with chronic inflammation of the conjunctivae. Dry eyes produce soreness and irritation, which may be helped by applying artificial tears – these consist of hypromellose, liquid paraffin, acetylcysteine (a drug that dissolves mucus) or polyvinyl alcohol (see Table 35.8).

Drugs that cause dry eyes

The first beta blocker on the market (practolol) caused serious dry eye problems, leading to damage to the conjunctivae and the cornea (the window of the eye). It was withdrawn from general use because it also produced other serious problems. *Propranolol* may occasionally cause dry eyes in some people because it produces a narrowing of the opening in the eyelids where tears are secreted. The anti-viral drug *idoxuridine*, used to treat herpes of the eyes, may cause similar troubles, as may *anticholinergic drugs* (e.g. atropine) and *ganglion blocking drugs* used to treat blood pressure (e.g. hexamethonium). Reduced tear production has also been noted with *chlorpromazine* and related anti-psychotic drugs used to treat schizophrenia and other serious mental disorders.

Cataracts

The lens is a transparent structure without blood vessels. If it is damaged through injury, radiation or ageing it becomes opaque and interferes with vision.

A cataract is an opacity of the lens of an eye, which causes a gradual loss of vision. If the outer parts of a cataract are clear, it is called 'immature' and if it is completely opaque is called 'mature'. An 'over-mature' (hypermature) cataract causes the pupil to look white.

German measles affecting the mother during pregnancy may cause cataracts in the newborn (congenital cataracts). Acquired cataracts may be due to injury, radiation or some metabolic disorder (e.g. a low blood calcium). Diabetes appears to accelerate the development of cataracts in susceptible individuals.

Some drugs may cause cataracts

The following are examples of drugs that may occasionally cause cataracts – usually following their prolonged use in high doses.

busulphan and related anti-cancer drugs
chlorambucil, an anti-cancer drug
chlorpromazine, thioridazine and trifluoperazine and other anti-psychotic drugs
corticosteroids
corticotrophin (ACTH)

Trachoma

Trachoma is an infectious disease of the eyes, affecting the conjunctivae and cornea, which eventually produces scarring and blindness. It is prevalent in Africa and Asia, and is responsible for millions of people being blind.

Trachoma is caused by a micro-organism (*Chlamydia*) that is more like a bacterium than a virus but, like viruses, *Chlamydia* 'live' inside cells.

Tetracycline or chlortetracycline eye ointment applied twice a day for 5 days every 6 months may help to reduce the progression of the disease. For specific treatment of an individual, two approaches are recommended – a sulphonamide (e.g. sulphadimethoxine) or erythromycin by mouth plus tetracycline eye ointment. The latter is usually recommended for children.

36

Parkinson's disease and parkinsonism

Parkinsonism is a disorder of the nervous system in which voluntary movements are slow and shaky and it is difficult for the individual to control and start movements, there are uncontrollable movements of the head and limbs, the muscles are stiff and rigid, the face is expressionless and the person stoops and walks with a shuffle. This group of signs and symptoms is termed 'Parkinson's syndrome' or 'parkinsonism' because they resemble those seen in Parkinson's disease which was first described by Parkinson in 1887 as paralysis agitans or the shaking palsy. There are several causes of parkinsonism and the severity of the disorders varies between patients.

Parkinson's disease (paralysis agitans) is due to degeneration of parts of the brain responsible for the co-ordination of movements. The cause of this disease is unknown and therefore it is sometimes referred to as idiopathic parkinsonism.

Parkinsonism may also occur secondary to some other disorder which 'damages' the parts of the brain responsible for co-ordinating movements. One cause of secondary parkinsonism is the long-term after effects of a severe widespread epidemic (pandemic) of inflammation of the brain (encephalitis lethargica) which occurred in the early 1920s. This type of parkinsonism is referred to as post-encephalitic parkinsonism. Parkinsonism may also be produced by the harmful effects of anti-psychotic drugs used to treat schizophrenia and other severe mental illnesses. When caused by these drugs it is often referred to as drug-induced parkinsonism or pseudo-parkinsonism. Parkinsonism may develop after carbon monoxide poisoning or manganese poisoning. It may occur in association with some serious nervous diseases (e.g. Altzheimer's disease) and it may also be caused when there is a poor blood supply to the brain due to narrowing and hardening of the arteries in old age (arteriosclerosis).

Parkinsonism has also developed in people who have taken 'designer drugs' due to a chemical called MPTP which may contaminate illegally manufactured drugs related to the narcotic pethidine. Post-mortem examinations in these individuals have shown damage to the parts of the brain that are affected in Parkinson's disease and with a similar degeneration of certain cells.

Damage to the brain's co-ordinating centre for movement causes the signs and symptoms of parkinsonism

Our ability to control and co-ordinate movements of our limbs and other parts of our body is under the control of two systems in the brain which balance each other. These systems are located in part of the brain called the basal ganglia. One system is dominant and uses the chemical *acetylcholine* to transmit messages. The other system provides a balance and uses the chemical *dopamine* to transmit messages. To put it simply, we talk about the 'acetylcholine system' being dominant and the 'dopamine system' opposing it in order to create a balanced effect.

In Parkinson's disease there is damage to nerve tracks in the basal ganglia, causing a defective production of dopamine. This results in an under-functioning of those parts of the brain that rely on dopamine and allows those parts that rely on acetylcholine to become more dominant. This imbalance reduces the ability of the patient to control and co-ordinate movements in the arms, legs, facial muscles, muscles responsible for posture and other muscles in the body.

Carbon monoxide, MPTP and manganese also damage these tracks. Anti-psychotic drugs used to treat severe mental illness block the action of dopamine and have the same effects by reducing the control that the dopamine system has over the acetylcholine system.

Drug treatment of parkinsonism

Any weakening of the dopamine system allows the acetylcholine system to dominate, and this is what produces the symptoms of parkinsonism. The drug treatment of parkinsonism therefore relies on drugs which either 'improve' the dopamine system or reduce the effects of the acetylcholine system.

NOTE Remember that people who suffer from parkinsonism are not intellectually impaired – there is no need to raise your voice and boss them around. They understand everything and are probably more intelligent than you are but they are trapped in a 'chemical prison' and so they cannot give the appropriate expression on their face or speak or act as quickly as you.

Drugs that improve the dopamine system (dopaminergic drugs)

Dopamine levels in the brain cannot be boosted by giving dopamine by mouth because it is poorly absorbed from the intestine and it cannot enter the brain from the bloodstream. Other methods of boosting dopamine in the brain have therefore to be used:

- To give *levodopa*, the chemical from which dopamine is naturally produced by nerve cells and which is well absorbed into the bloodstream when taken by mouth. Levodopa increases the amount of dopamine available in the brain and restores the balance with acetylcholine. Levodopa is referred to as a *dopamine* precursor.
- To give *amantadine* which stimulates the production and release of dopamine from stores in the brain and also blocks the removal of dopamine from its sites of action. Amantadine is referred to as a *dopaminergic drug*.
- To give *bromocriptine* or *lysuride*, which stimulate dopamine receptors. These drugs are referred to as *dopaminergic receptor agonists* or stimulants.
- To give *selegiline*, which selectively blocks the B iso-enzyme of monoamine oxidase, to stop the breakdown of dopamine, ensuring that it has a longer time to work. Selegiline is referred to as *selective MAO blocker*.

Levodopa

The discovery that dopamine was a nerve messenger (neurotransmitter) and that there was a deficiency of dopamine in the brain of individuals suffering from parkinsonism led to the testing of levodopa in the early 1960s. The body makes dopamine from levodopa (a precursor of dopamine) and its use presented doctors with an exciting opportunity to improve the dopamine system instead of just trying to damp down the acetylcholine system.

Unfortunately, there is a major problem: when levodopa is given by mouth it is absorbed into the bloodstream and carried round the body where it is rapidly converted into dopamine, and only a small amount of levodopa enters the brain to be converted into dopamine in the brain. The dopamine formed in the body from levodopa may cause nausea and vomiting and a fall in blood pressure, and it cannot cross from the bloodstream into the brain to produce its beneficial effects. To get sufficient levodopa to enter the brain before it is converted into dopamine in the body and wasted, it is necessary to give very high doses – which may cause many harmful effects.

A solution to this problem is to give levodopa along with a drug that blocks its conversion to dopamine in the body. This allows the concentration of levodopa in the blood to rise to a level at which it is capable of passing from the blood into the brain where it is converted into dopamine.

Benserazide and carbidopa are drugs that block the effects of an enzyme called dopa-decarboxylase, which is responsible for the manufacture of dopamine from levodopa. They block the enzyme dopa-decarboxylase in the body but they do not affect the manufacture of dopamine from levodopa in the brain. When either of these drugs is given along with levodopa, it is not converted to dopamine in the body, the blood concentration of levodopa increases and it enters the brain to be converted into dopamine by nerve cells in the brain.

An effective use of these drugs is to give a dose of levodopa along with a dose of benserazide or carbidopa. This means that a lower dose of levodopa can be given to produce the same desired effects. If given separately, there is always a risk that too high a dose of levodopa is given; therefore fixed-dose combined preparations are used – for example, benserazide and levodopa (co-beneldopa, Madopar) or carbidopa and levodopa (co-careldopa Sinemet).

These combinations allow the effective dose of levodopa to be reduced by about 75 per cent, thus reducing harmful effects *outside* of the brain (e.g. nausea, vomiting, fall in blood pressure). The benefits take effect quicker than if levodopa is given alone, and the response to treatment is more steady rather than being up and down. However, harmful effects on the brain are *not* reduced and abnormal involuntary movements and mental disorders tend to occur earlier in treatment with these combinations than with levodopa alone.

Levodopa preparations (Madopar and Sinemet) produce an improvement in about three out of four patients. Slowness of movement and muscle rigidity improve more quickly than the shaking but if treatment is kept going for several months this may also improve. These effects help to improve general mobility and ability to do things and mood may also improve. Treatment should always be started with small doses and the daily dose slowly increased every 2–3 days just so long as the beneficial effects outweigh any harmful effects.

Harmful effects of levodopa

Most patients experience some harmful effects from levodopa, which are usually directly related to the dose and clear up if the drug is stopped or the dose reduced. However, different patients react differently. Elderly people in particular are easily upset by high doses of levodopa.

Early harmful effects of levodopa preparations occur mainly in the body (away from the brain) and include nausea, vomiting, fall in blood pressure and disorders of heart rhythm.

Long-term harmful effects of levodopa preparations principally affect the brain. Occasionally, these may be very disturbing and include abnormal uncontrollable movements of the tongue, lips, face and limbs and severe mental disturbances.

Interactions of levodopa with other drugs

Pyridoxine (vitamin B_6) increases the activity of the enzyme dopa-decarboxylase, so more levodopa is converted to dopamine outside of the brain. Therefore, if pyridoxine (which is present in many multivitamin preparations) is given to a patient who is taking levodopa, the beneficial effects of levodopa are reduced. Obviously, this does not occur when the levodopa is given along with carbidopa in Sinemet or with benserazide in Madopar.

Anti-psychotic drugs (e.g. chlorpromazine) block the action of dopamine on dopamine receptors and so reduce the beneficial effects of levodopa. They should *not* be used to treat mental illness in people who are taking a levodopa preparation, nor should they be used to treat the nausea and vomiting produced by levodopa. In anyone who develops parkinsonism it is important to consider whether the patient has been taking anti-psychotic drugs because these may cause parkinsonism. If the patient has been taking them for a short period of time, the symptoms should improve if the drugs are stopped. However, if the anti-psychotic drugs have to be continued, anticholinergic drugs should be used to treat the parkinsonism because they act on the acetylcholine system and not on the dopamine system.

Monoamine oxidase inhibitors (MAOIs) used to treat depression interfere with the inactivation of dopamine, so levodopa should not be given until at least 2 weeks after the patient has stopped taking the MAOI drug. The combination may produce a dangerous rise in blood pressure.

Anticholinergic drugs used to treat parkinsonism (see later) improve treatment with levodopa. They are particularly helpful in reducing shaking. However, large doses of an anticholinergic drug slow down the movements of the stomach and intestine. This may delay levodopa leaving the stomach and entering the small intestine where it is absorbed into the bloodstream, with a result that not enough is absorbed to produce a beneficial effect.

Amantadine

Amantadine was introduced as an anti-viral drug for the prevention of influenza, and by chance it was found to improve symptoms in some people suffering from parkinsonism. It produces some improvement in shaking, rigidity and slowness of movement (bradikinesia) in a small proportion of people. Its benefits last only a short period of time.

Harmful effects produced by amantadine are usually mild and short lasting. They clear up completely if the drug is stopped. However, if the dose goes above 200 mg daily, harmful effects increase and become severe. When amantadine is given with an anticholinergic drug, harmful effects such as hallucinations, confusion and nightmares increase. These may also increase in people who also suffer from some underlying mental illness.

Bromocriptine and lysuride

Bromocriptine is a derivative of ergot. It stimulates dopamine receptors throughout the body, producing effects on the brain, the heart and circulation, the pituitary gland and the stomach and intestine. In Parkinson's disease and parkinsonism it stimulates surviving dopamine receptors in the co-ordinating centre in the brain, and by this action it helps to reduce rigidity and slowness of movements and improves gait.

The harmful effects produced by bromocriptine may be separated into two groups – those that occur when treatment is first started and those that develop when treatment has been continued for months to years. Like levodopa, *initial harmful effects* are in the body and outside of the brain; they include nausea, vomiting and a fall in blood pressure when standing up after being seated or lying down (postural hypotension). Rarely, a patient may collapse with the very first dose of bromocriptine, due to a sudden drop in blood pressure.

The *long-term harmful effects* of bromocriptine include mental symptoms (confusion, hallucinations), involuntary movements, a blue mottling of the skin (livedo reticularis), dry mouth, leg cramps, fluid retention (e.g. ankle swelling) and fluid on the lungs (pleural effusion). It also stops the production of the milk-producing hormone, prolactin, and is used to stop milk production after childbirth. It is also used to treat infertility.

Lysuride produces effects similar to those of bromocriptine.

Selegiline

Nerve messengers (neurotransmitters) that work on the brain and nervous system are broken down and got rid of at a rate that balances their production. Obviously this has to happen or else the body would fill up with nerve messengers. Protein substances called enzymes catalyse these breakdowns. Adrenaline-like chemicals and dopamine are broken down by an enzyme called monoamine oxidase. Type A of this enzyme (or iso-enzyme) is responsible for the breakdown of adrenaline-like chemicals and type B iso-enzyme is responsible for the breakdown of dopamine.

For many years monoamine oxidase inhibitor drugs (MAOIs) have been used to treat depression. They block type A monoamine oxidase iso-enzyme from breaking down adrenaline-related chemicals. Selegiline blocks type B monoamine oxidase iso-enzyme and *reduces* the breakdown of dopamine. It is referred to as a monoamine oxidase B inhibitor. It may also have a blocking effect on dopamine receptors.

Selegiline is selective in blocking the breakdown of dopamine, particularly in the brain where there is a preponderance of type B monoamine oxidase iso-enzyme compared with the rest of the body. Because selegiline blocks the breakdown of dopamine in the brain, it adds to the effects of levodopa – which means that the dose of levodopa can be reduced and the risk of harmful effects is reduced. A list of *harmful effects* produced by selegiline appears in Table 36.1. Unlike monoamine oxidase A inhibitors, it does not affect the breakdown of adrenaline-like chemicals and therefore it does not produce a dangerous rise in blood pressure when taken with certain drugs or foods (see MAOIs, Chapter 39).

Table 36.1 Drugs that improve the dopamine system – harmful effects and warnings

amantadine (Symmetrel)
Harmful effects The drug is well tolerated but harmful effects may occur in some people. They include agitation, restlessness, depression, nervousness, inability to concentrate, insomnia, confusion, hallucinations, feelings of detachment, dizziness, loss of appetite, nausea, constipation, blue mottling of the skin (livedo reticularis), dry mouth and swelling of the ankles. Rarely, skin rashes and a reduced white blood count may occur.

Warnings Amantadine must not be used in patients who suffer from epilepsy or peptic ulcers or severe impairment of kidney function. It should be used with caution in people with heart, liver or kidney disease, raised blood pressure, recurrent eczema or serious mental illness (psychosis). Avoid stopping the drug suddenly; reduce the daily dose slowly.

Risks in elderly people Harmful effects may be more frequent and severe; therefore use with caution.

bromocriptine (Parlodel)
Harmful effects Nausea is the most common harmful effect; occasionally, there may be vomiting, constipation, headache, dizziness, fall in blood pressure on standing after sitting or lying down (this may produce dizziness, light-headedness and faintness). Rarely, the drug may cause drowsiness, confusion,

Table 36.1 Drugs that improve the dopamine system – harmful effects and warnings (*cont.*)

hallucinations, disorders of movement, dry mouth, leg cramps, fluid in the lungs (pleural effusion), cold fingers and toes in cold weather, red painful swollen feet and blue mottling of the skin (livedo reticularis).

Warnings Fall in blood pressure may be a problem in the first few days of treatment, producing light-headedness, dizziness and fainting. Bromocriptine should be used with caution in individuals suffering from mental illness, heart or circulatory disease. Women receiving it over a long period of time should have a cervical smear and examination of the womb every 2 years. Anyone on long-term treatment should have regular check-ups including blood pressure, electrical tracing of the heart (ECG), blood counts and tests of liver and kidney function.

Risks in elderly people Harmful effects may be more frequent and severe; therefore use with caution.

Risks with driving It may produce drowsiness and dizziness; therefore do not drive until you know that it is safe to do so.

Risks with alcohol It may increase effects of alcohol; therefore do not drink when taking bromocriptine.

levodopa (Brocadopa, Larodopa, Madopar [with benserazide], Sinemet [with carbidopa])

Harmful effects The most common harmful effects are related to the dose; they include involuntary movements, spasm of the eyelids and muscle twitching. Other harmful effects that may occur rarely include mental symptoms (hallucinations, insomnia, nightmares, delusions, anxiety, confusion, paranoia, depression, suicidal tendencies, dementia), palpitations, fall in blood pressure on standing after sitting or lying down (may produce dizziness, light-headedness and faintness), loss of appetite, nausea, vomiting, bleeding from the stomach, high blood pressure, blood disorders, lethargy, sedation, fatigue, malaise, stomach and bowel upsets, excessive salivation, bitter taste, dry mouth, sweating, ankle swelling, loss of hair, skin rashes, unpleasant body odour, leg cramps, problems with breathing, retention of urine, incontinence, dark urine, persistent erections (priapism), double and/or blurred vision, hot flushes, changes in the size of the pupils, weight gain or loss and flushing.

Warnings Levodopa must not be used in patients who are allergic to levodopa or who have closed-angle glaucoma, nor in anyone with a melanoma because it may activate a malignant melanoma (cancer of the pigment cells in the skin). It should be used with caution in patients with open-angle glaucoma, chest disease, peptic ulcers, heart disease, diabetes or mental illness. During prolonged treatment, patients should have regular tests of liver and kidney function, blood counts, electrical tracings of the heart (ECG) and a full medical and psychiatric check-up. The drug should be stopped 8 hours before a surgical operation because of the risk of producing irregular heart rates. Individuals should be advised to resume 'normal' activities gradually.

Risks in elderly people Harmful effects may be more frequent and severe; therefore use with caution.

lysuride (Revanil)

Harmful effects include nausea, vomiting, dizziness, headache, lethargy, drowsiness, constipation, skin rashes, fall in blood pressure and pains in the abdomen. Occasionally it may cause mental symptoms and, rarely, Raynaud's syndrome.

Warnings Lysuride should not be used in people with disorders of the circulation or coronary artery disease. It should be used with caution in individuals with a pituitary tumour.

Table 36.1 Drugs that improve the dopamine system – harmful effects and warnings (*cont.*)

selegiline (Eldepryl) *Harmful effects* include a fall in blood pressure on standing up after lying or sitting (may produce dizziness and light-headedness), nausea, vomiting, confusion, agitation and, rarely, serious mental symptoms. Involuntary movements may occur (the dose of levodopa preparation should be reduced if this occurs). *Warnings* Selegiline may increase the harmful effects of levodopa; therefore the dose of a levodopa preparation should be reduced by 20–50 per cent. *Risks in elderly people* Harmful effects may be more frequent and severe.	

Drugs that reduce the effects of the acetylcholine system (anticholinergic drugs)

Anticholinergic drugs block the action of acetylcholine in the brain and at nerve endings in the parasympathetic nervous system. They block acetylcholine receptors and make acetylcholine ineffective. In people suffering from parkinsonism this action has a moderate effect in reducing shaking and stiffness, and it also reduces dribbling (sialorrhoea) by drying up the secretions of the salivary glands. Anticholinergic drugs do not improve the slowness of movement which occurs in parkinsonism (see later).

People with mild early symptoms often improve on anticholinergic drugs before they need to take a levodopa preparation. Patients with post-encephalitic parkinsonism appear to respond better to anticholinergic drugs than do patients with idiopathic Parkinson's disease. These drugs also reduce the signs and symptoms of drug-induced parkinsonism (see later), and an anticholinergic may be given intravenously when there is a severe flare-up of symptoms triggered by an infection (e.g. influenza) or when severe parkinsonism is produced by anti-psychotic drugs.

When an anticholinergic drug is given with levodopa, the two drugs act together on the acetylcholine system and the dopamine system respectively to produce a greater response than each drug given alone – an action that is termed synergism.

The harmful effects produced by anticholinergic drugs are listed later.

The anticholinergic drugs selected to treat parkinsonism work principally on the brain but they may still produce effects on the body such as dry mouth, blurred vision, constipation and difficulty in passing urine. These harmful effects may produce problems for the elderly; in particular, their effects on the brain may produce confusion, sleepiness, delirium and hallucinations. The drugs used most commonly are benzhexol, benztropine, biperiden, methixene, orphenadrine and procyclidine.

Table 36.2 Anticholinergic drugs used to treat parkinsonism – harmful effects and warnings

Harmful effects Common harmful effects include blurred vision, nausea, vomiting, constipation, dryness of the mouth and dizziness. Infrequent harmful effects include rapid heart rate, palpitations, allergic reactions, drowsiness, mental slowness, restlessness, excitement, confusion, delusions, hallucinations, weakness, and mood changes. These harmful effects are more likely to occur when high doses are used in people who are sensitive to anticholinergic drugs.

Warnings Anticholinergic drugs should not be used in patients who have developed tardive dyskinesia due to the use of anti-psychotic drugs. They should be used with caution in people who suffer from glaucoma, heart disease, impaired kidney or liver function, difficulty in passing urine (e.g. elderly men with enlarged prostate glands) or peptic ulcers (e.g. stomach or duodenal ulcers). Patients should be started off on a low daily dosage and the doses gradually increased over a period of several days.

Risks in elderly people Harmful effects may be more frequent and severe; therefore smaller doses should be used. There is a risk of producing confusion.

Risks in driving These drugs may produce drowsiness and other effects on the brain; therefore do not drive until you know that it is safe to do so.

Risks in alcohol Alcohol produces increased drowsiness; therefore, you should not drink alcohol when you are taking anticholinergic drugs.

Table 36.3 Drugs used to treat parkinsonism

Preparation	*Drug*	*Drug group*	*Dosage form*
Akineton	biperiden	Anticholinergic	Tablets
Arpicolin	procyclidine	Anticholinergic	Syrup
Artane	benzhexol	Anticholinergic	Tablets
Bentex	benzhexol	Anticholinergic	Tablets
benzhexol	benzhexol	Anticholinergic	Tablets
Biorphen	orphenadrine	Anticholinergic	Oral solution
Brocadopa	levodopa	Dopamine precursor	Capsules
Broflex	benzhexol	Anticholinergic	Syrup
Cogentin	benztropine	Anticholinergic	Tablets, injection
Disipal	orphenadrine	Anticholinergic	Tablets
Eldepryl	selegiline	Monoamine oxidase B inhibitor	Tablets
Kemadrin	procyclidine	Anticholinergic	Tablets, injection
Larodopa	levodopa	Dopamine precursor	Tablets
levodopa	levodopa	Dopamine precursor	Capsules, tablets
Madopar	levodopa benserazide	Dopamine precursor Dopa decarboxylase inhibitor	Capsules, dispersible tablets; Madopar CR (sustained-release capsules)
Mantadine	amantadine	Dopaminergic	Capsules
Parlodel	bromocriptine	Dopamine stimulant	Capsules, tablets
Revanil	lysuride	Dopamine stimulant	Tablets

Table 36.3 Drugs used to treat parkinsonism (*cont.*)

Preparation	*Drug*	*Drug group*	*Dosage form*
Sinemet	levodopa	Dopamine precursor	Tablets
	carbidopa	Dopa decarboxylase inhibitor	
Symmetrel	amantadine	Dopaminergic	Capsules, syrup
Tremonil	methixene	Anticholinergic	Tablets

Overview of the drug treatment of parkinsonism

Levodopa preparations

As stated earlier, levodopa relieves many of the symptoms of parkinsonism, particularly rigidity and slowness of movement. It may also reduce shaking, difficulty in swallowing, dribbling from the mouth and difficulties with maintaining posture. Treatment greatly helps some patients with Parkinson's disease. Their facial expression, walking, writing, speaking, breathing and swallowing all improve. In addition, their mood improves, their energy returns and they become more alert. Unfortunately, in some patients, particularly the elderly, the treatment may occasionally cause unpleasant harmful effects which include insomnia, anxiety, depression, nightmares, confusion and serious mental symptoms such as hallucinations, paranoia and mania.

Combining levodopa with benserazide (Madopar) or carbidopa (Sinemet) reduces the speed of breakdown of levodopa in the body. This enables more levodopa to get into the brain to be converted to dopamine and produce its beneficial effects. It also allows a smaller dose of levodopa to be used, which reduces the risks of harmful effects. These benefits have to be balanced against the risks of using levodopa because it does not stop the progression of the disease, it only relieves symptoms.

Levodopa treatment should be stopped for 12 hours before changing the drug from levodopa to Madopar or Sinemet.

Unfortunately, the majority of people with Parkinson's disease who take levodopa develop some harmful effects from the drug. The intensity and type of harmful effect varies from person to person and at different stages in the disease. These are generally directly related to dose and may be reduced or stopped if the dose of the drug is reduced or the drug is stopped. This is why treatment with levodopa should start with low doses and gradually increase by small amounts every 2 or 3 days. The final dose will represent a balance between benefits and harmful effects.

Nausea and vomiting produced by levodopa preparations may be controlled by starting with small daily doses and then increasing the daily dose slowly over several weeks (see earlier). It may also help to reduce nausea and vomiting if levodopa preparations are taken *after* meals. Domperidone, an anti-nausea and anti-vomiting drug, may help if the nausea and vomiting are severe.

Response to levodopa preparations

A combined preparation of levodopa with benserazide (Madopar) or with carbidopa (Sinemet) is a first treatment of choice for individuals disabled by idiopathic Parkinson's disease. The elderly and people who have had the disease for many years may not tolerate high doses of levodopa to relieve their disability. Levodopa preparations are less effective in treating patients suffering from post-encephalitic parkinsonism and they should not be used to treat anyone suffering from parkinsonism caused by treatment with anti-psychotic drugs.

One-third of patients treated with levodopa do very well and about one-third do less well. The remainder seem not to be able to tolerate the harmful effects and they fail to respond. In those patients who do respond, there should be a slow improvement over the first 16–18 months which may be maintained for up to 2 years. After this period, patients may start to get worse and fail to respond to levodopa. They may also develop 'on–off' effects and 'wearing-off' effects.

'On-off' effects

A difficult problem with levodopa treatment is the on–off phenomenon where, for no reason, the drug suddenly loses its effectiveness and symptoms such as weakness and freezing of movements may develop. These attacks come without warning and may last for 2–4 hours. They may occur frequently throughout the day and cause real problems for the individual.

'Wear-off' effects (end-of-dose effects)

The trouble with levodopa is that after several months or years its effects wear off and serious symptoms begin to return, particularly slowness of movements. Wearing-off effects come particularly towards the end of each inter-dose period (i.e. just before the next dose is due).

End-of-dose deterioration and on–off effects may be helped by reducing fluctuations and peaks in the concentration of the drug in the blood. This may be achieved by giving small doses at more frequent intervals throughout the day, or by using sustained-release preparations. Unfortunately, any increase in daily dose will increase the risk of developing abnormal movements, so the harmful effects of treatment may soon outweigh any beneficial effects.

Treatment with levodopa preparations should not be stopped quickly – the daily dose should be reduced slowly over several weeks in order to prevent a sudden flare-up of the disability. Also, as a patient gets older the daily maintenance dose may need to be reduced gradually.

Because the appearance of unpleasant harmful effects such as movement disorders and variations in response (on–off effects) are related to the duration of treatment, there is some disagreement among specialists as to when levodopa preparations should be started. Some point out that harmful effects are related more to the progression of the disease than to the duration of the treatment, and recommend that treatment with levodopa preparations should start early in the disease. Others argue that it is better to use levodopa preparations later in the disease when a lot of disability has developed. Either way, whenever levodopa preparations are used, they make life for many patients much more tolerable for several years.

The value of the idea that stopping all drugs (a drug 'holiday') will help to make the sites of action of dopamine more sensitive or improve the benefits from a course of treatment has not been clearly demonstrated.

Bromocriptine and lysuride

Bromocriptine and lysuride have no advantages over levodopa. They may help to reduce rigidity and slowness of movement but their use is limited because of their harmful effects.

Bromocriptine or lysuride are of value in those patients who cannot tolerate levodopa or in whom the effects of levodopa are wearing off. In these individuals partial replacement of levodopa with bromocriptine or lysuride may be helpful but their use is often limited when given with levodopa because of serious harmful effects such as hallucinations, involuntary movements and confusion. It may be worth trying bromocriptine or lysuride in the earlier stages of the disease in untreated patients before treatment with levodopa is considered or in those individuals who cannot tolerate the harmful effects of levodopa. They have a long duration of action and may be useful at bed-time as a single dose in those people whose symptoms are worse in the early morning. It may also help to add bromocriptine or lysuride to levodopa treatment if the patient develops 'on–off' attacks as the disease progresses.

Amantadine

Amantadine (Symmetril) produces fewer harmful effects than bromocriptine or levodopa but it is also less effective. It reduces mild rigidity, shaking and slowness of movement. Only a small proportion of patients benefit from amantadine, and in those individuals its beneficial effects may wear off over just a few weeks to months.

Amantadine offers an alternative treatment in the less disabled patient before it is decided to give levodopa or in those in whom the beneficial effects of levodopa are wearing off and/or the harmful effects are not being tolerated.

Selegiline

Selegiline increases and prolongs the effects of levodopa in the treatment of parkinsonism. It helps to relieve the fluctuations in response to levodopa and reduces the 'wear-off' effects and the 'on–off' effects. It allows the dose of levodopa to be reduced by nearly one-third; it has a long duration of action and needs to be taken only once daily. Selegiline should be added to levodopa treatment when patients are experiencing wearing off or on–off effects with levodopa. It may be used alone in early untreated patients when it may delay the onset of disability and the need for levodopa. It may improve symptoms, and exert a protective effect against external toxins. It should be started in low doses at the earliest sign of parkinsonism.

Anticholinergic drugs

Anticholinergic drugs improve shaking and rigidity but have little effect on slowness of movement. They dry up the mouth and help to reduce dribbling, and may add to the beneficial effects of levodopa preparations. They also reduce symptoms of parkinsonism caused by anti-psychotic drugs. Patients with mild early symptoms often improve on these drugs *before* they need to take levodopa. Patients with post-encephalitic parkinsonism appear to respond better to anticholinergic drugs than patients with idiopathic Parkinson's disease.

Different people may respond differently to any one of the anticholinergic drugs; therefore if one drug does not work, it is worth trying another.

The need for individualized treatment

The drug treatment of parkinsonism relieves symptoms, it does not alter the underlying progression of the disease. Because of this and because patients vary in how they will respond, it is essential that treatment is always tailored to an individual patient's needs and is in the hands of someone who really understands the disease and how available drugs work. This is particularly so if several drugs are used together. For example, it is very important that doctors should individualize initial and maintenance treatment with levodopa. At the start of treatment with levodopa the daily dose should be increased very slowly (every 2–3 days) in order to keep harmful effects to a minimum. The same applies to maintenance treatment in which the benefits and risks should be carefully balanced and treatment tailored to the individual's response. With careful control, improvement may last for 2 years or more.

Stopping treatment should also be carried out with great care, and the daily dose of the drugs should be reduced slowly at regular intervals (every 2–3 days) over a period of weeks. In elderly patients, the daily dose may need to be kept low in order to lessen the risk of harmful effects.

37

Epilepsy

'Epilepsy' is a general term for a group of disorders of the brain which produce sudden and transitory attacks or seizures that may affect various parts of the brain. The attacks are caused by an excessive or disordered 'electrical' discharge from nerve cells in the affected part of the brain. Electrical tracings of the brain (EEGs) show that epileptic attacks are due to electrical discharges spreading outwards from a focus. If such a focus affects the part of the brain that controls movements, it produces a convulsion; if it affects the part that controls behaviour, it produces abnormal behaviour; and if it affects a sensory area then it may produce increased sensations (e.g. an abnormal sense of smell).

In most cases of epilepsy the cause is unknown and they are referred to as primary or idiopathic epilepsies. Where there is a cause such as a tumour, infection or injury they are called secondary or symptomatic epilepsies.

Definitions

When discussing epilepsy the term *seizure* (or *fit*) refers to an 'episode' or an 'attack' of epilepsy caused by an excessive amount of electrical activity in parts of the brain. Such an episode may or may not produce a convulsion.

A *convulsion* is a violent involuntary contraction of the muscles, which may be prolonged or occur in spasms. Depending upon the type of seizure, it may affect a few muscles (e.g. just in the thumb) or many muscles (e.g. the whole body).

Clonus (a *clonic* state) refers to repetitive contractions of a muscle or muscles, producing jerking movements.

Tonus (a *tonic* state) refers to a state of partial or continuous contraction of muscles, producing rigidity.

Tonic/clonic refers to a state of tonic rigidity of muscles followed by clonic jerking of the muscles.

Myoclonus (myoclonic contraction) is a sudden shock-like contraction of a muscle or muscles.

Opisthotonos is a spasm (tonus) of the back muscles, causing the back to arch backwards.

Classification of seizures

The classification of seizures keeps changing; the following is an example of one in fashion at present.

Partial seizures (local or focal seizures)

Most partial seizures cause a sudden disturbance of the senses or muscle spasms without loss of consciousness.

Simple partial seizures are seizures occurring without loss of consciousness. They may present as a local convulsion affecting, for example, a single limb (Jacksonian epilepsy). They may affect sensation producing, for example, pins and needles in one area of the body; the autonomic nervous system producing, for example, nausea, vomiting and abdominal pain (abdominal epilepsy seen in childhood); or they may produce psychic symptoms such as fear or rage.

Complex partial seizures Partial seizures are called complex when they are associated with some loss of consciousness, confused behaviour and a wide range of other effects.

Both simple and complex partial seizures can evolve into a major convulsion (secondary tonic/clonic convulsions).

Generalized seizures (convulsive or non-convulsive)

Convulsive seizures

Clonic seizures produce loss of consciousness with rhythmic jerking of muscles which may be localized (Jacksonian epilepsy).

Tonic seizures cause arching of the back (opisthotonos) with loss of consciousness and some autonomic nervous system effects (e.g. emptying the bladder).

Tonic/clonic seizures (grand mal epilepsy) cause major convulsions with loss of consciousness. There is usually a warning sensation such as flashing lights or a noise followed by a sudden loss of consciousness during which convulsions occur and individuals may wet themselves and foam at the mouth. These seizures usually last for a few minutes but they may last for over an hour. A prolonged attack, which may last up to 1 hour, is usually referred to as *status epilepticus*

Non-convulsive seizures

Absence seizures (petit mal epilepsy) most commonly affect children. There are no convulsions, but there is a brief, abrupt loss of consciousness producing a blank stare with some jerking of the eyelids and other muscles in the body.

Atypical absence seizures are like absence seizures but they come on more slowly and last longer, and they may be associated with confusion.

Myoclonic seizures cause isolated twitching of muscles in the face, arms, legs or trunk.

Atonic seizures are 'drop' attacks due to loss of tone of muscles. Just the head may drop forward or the individual may drop to the floor due to a sudden loss of muscle control.

Drug treatment of epilepsies

Normally there is a relatively low level of electrical activity in the brain but in a seizure there is a build-up of excessive electrical activity starting in one place (or focus) and spreading outwards, causing uncontrolled stimulation of other parts of the brain; for example, stimulation of brain cells that bring about movement will cause increased activity of those muscles under the nervous control of those brain cells – this will cause the muscles to twitch and go rigid (a convulsion). Most anti-epileptic drugs (or anti-convulsant drugs) damp down the electrical activity of brain cells and prevent excessive build-up of electrical activity which could result in a seizure.

An epileptic attack may be stopped by any drug that depresses the brain function (e.g. a sleeping drug or an anaesthetic). Drugs selected to treat epilepsies should block the electrical discharges but produce as little depression of the brain as possible – you don't want a drug that controls seizures but sends you to sleep or changes your behaviour. Epileptics must have their seizures controlled and yet be able to go to work or school as normal. This is a particularly important point because the first aim of treatment is to prevent attacks.

Benefits of drug treatment

Effective treatment of the epilepsies requires knowledge of the benefits and risks of available anti-epileptic drugs, knowledge of the different types of seizure that may affect an individual, and detailed knowledge of the person to be treated and the type of seizure or seizures from which he or she is suffering. It also requires the availability of up-to-date methods of diagnosis and monitoring. In other words, someone suffering from epilepsy should have access to specialist services.

When treatments with anti-epileptic drugs are tailored to the particular needs and responses of each individual, about four out of five of those suffering from generalized seizures and about half of those suffering from partial seizures will remain completely free from such attacks while on the drug treatments. Other people will be significantly helped.

Starting drug treatment

Initial treatment of most epilepsies should be with a single drug used properly. Some people suffer from more than one type of seizure, in which case more than one drug may be required to control their seizures; occasionally, some patients may require more than one drug to control their single type of seizure.

It is important that patients are started off on a *single* drug, starting with a *low* daily dosage and building up the daily dosage until the desired effect is achieved. This is because some harmful effects are directly related to daily dosage and it is necessary to get the dose as right as possible for the individual in order to achieve the correct balance between the desired effects and the risk of producing harmful effects. When starting treatment, high doses should be used only if the risks of the seizures are greater than the risks produced by high doses.

Getting the daily dose right

The daily dosage of the selected drug should be slowly increased every few weeks until adequate control of seizures is achieved or until the harmful effects of the drug limit any further increase or may actually warrant a reduction of dosage. Where possible, measurement of the concentration of the drug in the blood should help to get this balance right. It will also give an indication as to whether the patient is taking the drug as directed.

The frequency of dosage throughout the day depends on how long the drug remains at an effective concentration in the blood. Most anti-epileptic drugs need to be taken at least twice daily in order to keep the concentration in the blood topped up. Some are long acting (e.g. phenytoin and phenobarbitone) and may be given once a day (e.g. at bed-time); others may produce dangerously high levels if given in high dosage, and so they need to be given in smaller doses more often (e.g. three times daily). Young children break down and get rid of anti-epileptic drugs faster than adults; therefore they need more frequent dosages throughout the day and a higher dose for their weight than adults.

Do not stop drugs suddenly

If a single drug does not control seizures, it should be replaced with another one. However, no drug should be stopped suddenly because this can trigger a severe attack of epilepsy (status epilepticus, see 'Epileptic emergencies' later). Therefore, the daily dosage of any drug should be reduced slowly over a period of weeks while an alternative drug is started at low daily dosages and then slowly increased.

When it is decided to stop anti-epileptic drug treatment the daily dose of the drug should be reduced slowly over a matter of months. This warning applies particularly to barbiturates.

Using more than one drug

Using a combination of anti-epileptic drugs may increase the harmful effect of treatment without reducing seizures. It may also subject the individual to the risks of one drug interacting with another. This is because several of the available anti-epileptic drugs work against each other (drug–drug interactions, see Chapter 89). For example, phenytoin may reduce the concentration of carbamazepine in the blood, and phenobarbitone, phenytoin, primidone and carbamazepine may increase each other's rate of breakdown, resulting in a reduction in their concentration in the blood and, therefore, in their effectiveness. There is no point in combining some drugs – for example, primidone with phenobarbitone. This is because primidone is broken down in the liver to phenobarbitone, which acts as the anti-epileptic drug – you might as well just give phenobarbitone on its own!

Nevertheless, the current fashion for trying to use just one drug should not override the patient's needs. Every treatment should be tailored to the individual and occasionally a patient may well require the use of more than one drug, particularly if the seizures continue despite evidence from blood tests that the first drug is at an appropriate concentration in the blood or has reached a toxic concentration.

A partnership between doctor and patient

To achieve control of seizures requires patience, care and knowledge by doctors. It also requires full co-operation from patients and/or their carers. It helps if patients keep a diary of attacks (a seizure chart) and they must be conscientious about their treatment and make frequent visits to an epilepsy clinic in the first few months of treatment. Equally, long-term regular daily treatment requires patients to be absolutely conscientious about taking their anti-epileptic drugs as directed. It also requires that doctors maintain their interest in their patients and arrange full medical examinations and investigations (including EEG) at regular intervals in order to monitor the progress of the disease, to assess the effectiveness of treatment and to watch out for harmful effects from the drugs.

The drug treatment of epilepsy should be a partnership between patients (or their carers) and their doctors. Patients and/or their carers should be as informed as possible about epilepsy and its treatment. They should also be well informed about the benefits of diet and the avoidance of alcohol.

Where appropriate, doctors should periodically carry out blood tests to check the concentration of the drug(s) in the blood. This may give a warning about the risks of the treatment and it will also help to check whether patients are actually taking the drug(s) as directed. Blood tests are particularly important in people taking more than one drug who develop harmful symptoms. A blood test that measures the concentration of each drug in the blood will identify the drug responsible for the harmful effects.

Failure of treatment

Patients with epilepsy usually benefit greatly from drug treatment but they may also suffer unnecessarily from bad drug treatment. Common causes of failure of treatment are the wrong diagnosis of the type of seizure, wrong choice of drug, stopping drugs too quickly, chopping and changing drugs, giving the wrong combination of drugs, failing to examine the patient regularly, failing to carry out special tests such as an EEG and failing, where appropriate, to carry out estimations of the concentration of the drug(s) in the blood.

Patients themselves are often responsible for making sure that treatment is not effective. They forget or purposely do not bother to stick closely to the instructions for taking their drugs. They may miss clinic appointments and fail to report any new symptoms, which may be due to the harmful effects of the drugs they are taking.

Stopping drug treatment

It is very important for people who suffer from epilepsy to know whether they must take anti-epileptic drugs every day for the rest of their life. Unfortunately, medical opinion is divided. Some doctors suggest that if the patient has not had a seizure for 2 years or more, the daily dose should be very slowly reduced (every 1–2 weeks) over a period of months and if a seizure does not occur during that time then the drug can be stopped. Others suggest that in about three out of ten patients the seizures return, and point to the problems such patients may then have with regard to their jobs and their licence to drive motor vehicles. The latter is an important point because anyone who has had a seizure while awake will not be allowed to drive for a further 2 years. If a decision is taken to slowly reduce and stop treatment, the patient should not drive during that period and for 6–12 months after stopping the anti-epileptic drugs.

Risks of drug treatment

Several different drugs are used to treat different types of seizure, and their harmful effects and warnings on their use are listed in Table 37.1. The risks of harmful effects are increased by using too high dosages too frequently, by using two or more drugs together and by lack of adequate monitoring of the patient's response.

Risks in elderly people

Harmful effects of anti-epileptic drugs are more frequent and severe in elderly people; therefore the drugs should be used with caution, starting with smaller doses than normal and slowly increasing the daily dosage over a period of several weeks.

Risks in pregnancy

There is a risk of damage to the baby if anti-epileptic drugs are taken during pregnancy (see Chapter 79), but this risk must be balanced against those to the baby of inadequately controlled seizures in the mother. The risk is greater with generalized seizures than partial ones, and with status epilepticus.

Requirements for anti-convulsant drugs during pregnancy may change because blood levels may fall and cause an increase in frequency of seizure. It is important, therefore, to have regular estimations of the blood levels of the drug during pregnancy and to have the dose adjusted accordingly, in order to keep it within effective and safe limits.

Risks in breast feeding

Anti-epileptic drugs should be used with caution in breast-feeding mothers (see Chapter 80), particularly barbiturates (e.g. phenobarbitone, methyl-phenobarbitone) and primidone (which is converted to phenobarbitone in the body).

Risks in driving

Do not drive or operate machinery if the drug makes you drowsy or until you know that it is safe to do so. People who suffer from epilepsy may hold an ordinary driver's licence but they are not allowed to drive a heavy goods vehicle or public service vehicle. An ordinary driving licence is issued provided that they have not had a fit for 2 years or more. If they suffer from fits only when they are asleep, they must state this and also that they have never had an attack when awake over the previous 3 years.

Risks with alcohol

Alcohol may decrease the effects of some anti-epileptic drugs and increase the drowsiness produced by others (see Chapter 87).

Interaction of anti-epileptic drugs with other drugs

For a discussion of drug interactions, see Chapter 89.

NOTE that the measurement of the levels of an anti-epileptic drug in the blood is a useful indication of whether other drugs are interacting with it and producing an increase or decrease in its concentration in the blood.

Recommendations

Different types of seizures are caused by different mechanisms and therefore different drugs are effective in relieving them. Anti-epileptic drug treatment should be tailored to the individual's needs and based upon the findings from a detailed medical examination and investigations.

It is better to use only one drug and use it effectively than to use several drugs ineffectively in the same individual. Nevertheless, some people will only benefit from the use of more than one drug.

Where possible the dose and frequency of taking a drug should be worked out from measures of the concentration of the drug in the blood.

The failure of patients to take anti-epileptic drugs as directed is a major cause of failure to control seizures. The ability of a patient to stick to a prescribed treatment schedule (compliance) may be helped if the schedule is as simple as possible – for example, twice a day is better than three times a day, and some of the long-acting drugs (e.g. phenobarbitone) need only be taken once daily on going to bed.

If large doses of a drug have to be taken, it is best to divide them into three dosages each day to prevent high and potentially toxic levels in the blood.

Anti-epileptic drugs should not be withdrawn suddenly; the daily dosage should be reduced slowly, step by step over weeks to months. There is the risk of rebound seizures if an anti-epileptic drug is stopped suddenly.

If you are taking anti-epileptic drugs, you should stick to the prescribed dosage schedule and inform your doctor if you are not able to take the drug because of vomiting or surgery or for some other reason.

You should always check whether any other drug or alcohol interacts with the drug or drugs you are taking, and discuss this problem with your doctor.

If you develop a skin rash you should consult your doctor immediately.

Good dental hygiene is important, particularly if you are taking phenytoin or one of the other anti-epileptic drugs that may cause an overgrowth of the gums.

Epileptic emergencies

Repeated and prolonged epileptic seizures without recovery of consciousness between attacks are called status epilepticus. It is an emergency because, if it is not treated, the patient may die. The immediate treatment is to give a dose of diazepam or clonazepam directly into a vein (intravenous). If it is not possible to get a needle into a vein, diazepam may be given as a solution into the rectum. Diazepam or clonazepam should work effectively in about nine out of ten patients. If they do not work, chlormethiazole should be injected into a vein or phenytoin sodium given by slow intravenous injection (with ECG monitoring). Paraldehyde by injection into a muscle or by rectum was popular in the past and is still used occasionally; so too is phenobarbitone sodium, but it is slow to act.

Diazepam, clonazepam and chlormethiazole may depress breathing. Facilities for keeping the airways open and for mechanical respiration should be available to the doctor giving treatment. Diazepam and clonazepam may cause thrombophlebitis at the site of injection into a vein.

Convulsions in feverish children (febrile convulsions)

A very small proportion of children (2–3 per cent) may develop a convulsion when they have a fever. If it is brief (lasts only for a minute or two), they need sponging all over with tepid water and a dose of paracetamol to bring the temperature down; and if they are feverish in future, they should be sponged down and given a dose of paracetamol at the start of the fever in order to be on the safe side.

If the convulsion lasts for 10–15 minutes, or if there is a history of convulsions, diazepam should be given by slow injection into a vein or into the rectum as a matter of urgency because there is a risk of brain damage from a convulsion that lasts 15 minutes or more.

Opinion is divided as to whether children who have had a severe convulsion due to fever (febrile convulsion) should be kept on long-term regular daily treatment with an anti-epileptic drug. It is generally considered necessary for children under the age of about 14 months and/or if they have other signs of damage to the brain and nervous system, or if the convulsion lasted for 15 minutes or more and was complex in nature. These factors increase the risk of children subsequently developing epilepsy, but there is no evidence that daily treatment with anti-epileptic drugs actually reduces this risk. Nevertheless, some suggest that such children should be given an anti-epileptic drug (e.g. phenobarbitone or sodium valproate) daily as a preventive over a period of 2 years.

Table 37.1 Drugs used to treat epilepsy – harmful effects and warnings

acetazolamide (Diamox)
Harmful effects are usually transient and related to the dose. They include transient short-sightedness, flushing, headache, drowsiness, dizziness, fatigue, irritability, excitement, thirst and passing large volumes of urine, numbness and tingling in the arms, legs and face, incoordination of movements, loss of hearing, over-breathing and stomach upsets (loss of appetite, vomiting). Acetazolamide is a sulphonamide derivative and it may, rarely, produce sulphonamide-type harmful effects. They include fever, blood disorders, skin rashes, kidney stones and colic.

Warnings Acetazolamide must not be used in anyone who is allergic to sulphonamides, nor in people suffering from impaired kidney function, Addison's disease or who are losing sodium and potassium in their urine. It should be used with caution in individuals with impaired liver function, or who have difficulty in passing urine due to some obstruction (e.g. enlarged prostate gland). Long-term use should be avoided in people with chronic (closed-angle) glaucoma. If anyone is on long-term treatment, blood counts should be carried out at regular intervals.

Risks in elderly people Harmful effects may be more frequent and severe; therefore use with caution.

carbamazepine (Tegretol)
Harmful effects The most commonly occurring harmful effects include dizziness and double vision; these are related to the dose and can be avoided if the daily dose of the drug is increased gradually. Less frequent harmful effects include drowsiness, visual disturbances, stomach and intestinal upsets (often associated with peak blood levels), a generalized red rash, serious blood disorders, low blood sodium and fluid retention (e.g. ankle swelling) with high doses and, rarely, jaundice and kidney damage.

Warnings Carbamazepine must not be used in anyone who is allergic to it, nor in people with conduction defects of the heart or porphyria. It should be used with caution in people with impaired liver function. Regular blood counts should be carried out in the first few months of treatment. It may reduce the effectiveness of oral contraceptives.

Risks in elderly people Harmful effects may be more frequent and severe; therefore use with caution.

chlormethiazole (Heminevrin)
See Chapter 38.

Table 37.1 Drugs used to treat epilepsy – harmful effects and warnings (*cont.*)

clobazam (Frisium)
See benzodiazepines (Chapter 40).

clonazepam (Rivotril)
See benzodiazepines (Chapter 40).

diazepam (Diazemuls, Stesolid, Valium)
See benzodiazepines (Chapter 40)

ethosuximide (Emeside, Zarontin)
Harmful effects are usually mild and transient, and occur at the start of treatment. They include nausea, vomiting, loss of appetite, abdominal pains, apathy, drowsiness, headache, dizziness, incoordination of movements and mood changes. Rarely, it may cause liver damage, skin rashes, systemic lupus erythematosus, redness of the skin and blood disorders. Serious mental illness may be made worse; disturbed sleep, night terrors, aggressiveness and inability to concentrate may, rarely, occur.

Warnings Ethosuximide must not be used in anyone who is allergic to it or similar chemicals or who suffers from porphyria. It should be used with caution in people who suffer from liver or kidney disease. Regular tests of kidney and liver function and blood counts should be carried out during treatment.

Risks in driving It may affect your ability to drive, so do not drive until you know that it is safe to do so.

lorazepam (Ativan)
See benzodiazepines (Chapter 40).

methylphenobarbitone (Prominal)
See barbiturates (Chapter 38).

paraldehyde
Harmful effects Paraldehyde is now used only in emergencies. It decomposes on storage, and corrosive poisoning, causing death, may (rarely) occur following the use of such preparations. It has an unpleasant taste and makes the breath smell. By mouth it may irritate the stomach and by suppository it may irritate the rectum. Intramuscular injections are painful and may cause nerve damage and sterile abscesses. Intravenous use may cause thrombophlebitis and may damage the heart and cause fluid and bleeding into the lungs. It may cause skin rashes.

Warnings Paraldehyde should not be used in anyone with a chronic chest disorder, and used with caution in people with impaired liver function or stomach disorders (e.g. stomach ulcers). It must not be given rectally to individuals with colitis. It must be well diluted before use by mouth or rectum. Do not use old preparations.

Risks in elderly people Harmful effects may be more frequent and severe; therefore use with caution.

Risks in pregnancy Use only in an emergency, with caution.

Risks in breast feeding Use only in an emergency, with caution.

Risks with driving It may affect your ability to drive, so do not drive until the effects of the drug have worn off.

Risks with alcohol It increases the effect of alcohol, so do not drink alcohol on the same day that you receive this drug.

phenytoin (Epanutin)
Harmful effects Mild harmful effects at the start of treatment include nausea, vomiting, mental confusion, dizziness, headache, tremor, insomnia, nervousness, loss of weight and unsteadiness. Sleepiness, slurred speech and blurred vision may occur with high doses. Coarse expressions of the face, acne and excessive growth of the gums may occasionally occur in young people. Allergic reactions, fever, skin rashes, joint pains, liver damage, blood disorders (including megaloblastic anaemia) and lupus erythematosus may, rarely, occur.

Warnings Phenytoin must not be used in anyone who is allergic to the drug or related drugs or who is suffering from porphyria. A reduced dose should be used in people with impaired kidney function. The drug should

Table 37.1 Drugs used to treat epilepsy – harmful effects and warnings (*cont.*)

be stopped gradually. It may cause a fall in blood calcium levels, which may cause bone softening (oesteomalacia) in adults and rickets in children.

Risks in elderly people Harmful effects may be more frequent and severe; therefore use with caution.

primidone (Mysoline)
Harmful effects Drowsiness and listlessness are common at the start of treatment. Other transient harmful effects include incoordination of movements, nausea, headache, vomiting and visual disturbances. These harmful effects may be severe in people who are sensitive to the drug and so the drug has to be stopped. Rarely, allergic skin rashes, severe mental symptoms, swelling of the legs, thirst, increased output of urine, impotence, megaloblastic anaemia and other blood disorders may occur.

Warnings Primidone must not be used in anyone suffering from acute intermittent porphyria. Smaller doses are required for children, elderly debilitated patients or those with impaired functioning of their kidneys, liver or lungs. Long-term treatment may produce addiction.

Risks in elderly people Harmful effects may be more frequent and severe; therefore use with caution and in reduced dose.

Risks in driving It interferes with your ability to drive, therefore, drive only when you know that it is safe to do so.

Risks with alcohol It increases the effects of alcohol, so do not drink alcohol when you are taking this drug.

sodium valproate (Epilim)
Harmful effects Liver damage, sometimes causing death, may rarely occur; those at greatest risk are children under the age of 3 years, and those with brain damage, seizures and mental retardation, and certain metabolic disorders. The risk of liver damage occurs mainly in the first 6 months of treatment (maximum period of risk 2–12 weeks) and usually involves the use of more than one anti-epileptic drug. Laboratory tests are not very useful for predicting which individuals will be at risk nor are they very useful for spotting the early signs of trouble. It is best to rely on early signs and symptoms of liver damage. Routine tests of liver function should be taken before and at regular intervals during the first 6 months of treatment; if there is any suggestion of impaired liver function, the patient should be kept under very close observation by the doctor. The drug should be stopped immediately upon the onset of an acute illness, especially within the first 6 months; indications for stopping include vomiting, lethargy, weakness, drowsiness, loss of appetite or jaundice or loss of seizure control. A transient rise in blood ammonia without liver damage may occur, causing vomiting, incoordination of movement and clouding of the consciousness; the drug should be stopped *immediately*. Rarely, damage to the pancreas (pancreatitis) may occur in the first 6 months of treatment, which may produce severe stomach pains. Very rarely, there may be damage to the bone marrow, affecting red cell and white cell production and the stickiness of platelets, which will cause the bleeding time to be prolonged and result in easy bruising and bleeding. It may cause an increase in appetite and weight, and some patients may develop stomach upsets at the start of treatment. Transient loss of hair may occur, which does not appear to be related to the dose; regrowth of hair starts about 6 months later, and the hair may be more curly than previously. Occasionally, it may cause skin rashes, incoordination of movements, tremor, lethargy, confusion, stupor and hallucinations, aggression, increased alertness, hyperactivity, disorders of behaviour and absence of menstrual period.

Warnings Sodium valproate must not be used in patients with active liver disease. It should be used with utmost caution in children and adults with a history of liver disease. Tests of liver function should be

Table 37.1 Drugs used to treat epilepsy – harmful effects and warnings (*cont.*)

carried out before treatment and at regular intervals (every 2 weeks) during the first 6 months of treatment, particularly in individuals with a history of liver disease or in children with severe epilepsy associated with brain damage. The drug may cause a false positive urine test for diabetes. A blood count and platelet count should be carried out at regular intervals, particularly before any surgical or dental procedures.

Risks in elderly people Blood levels of the drug should be interpreted with caution.

Table 37.2 Drugs used to treat epilepsies

Type of epilepsy	*Drugs used*
Generalized tonic/clonic seizures (grand mal)	carbamazepine (Tegretol) phenytoin (Epanutin) sodium valproate (Epilim) phenobarbitone primidone (Mysoline) clonazepam (Rivotril)
Partial seizures (focal, local seizures)	carbamazepine (Tegretol) phenytoin (Epanutin) phenobarbitone primidone (Mysoline) sodium valproate (Epilim) clonazepam (Rivotril) clobazam (Frisium) acetazolamide (Diamox)
Absent seizures (petit mal)	ethosuximide (Emeside, Zarontin) sodium valproate (Epilim)
Myoclonic seizures (myoclonic jerks)	sodium valproate (Epilim) clonazepam (Rivotril) ethosuximide (Emeside, Zarontin)
Atypical absence, atonic and clonic seizures	phenytoin (Epanutin) sodium valproate (Epilim) clonazepam (Rivotril) ethosuximide (Emeside, Zarontin) phenobarbitone

NOTE Estimations of the concentration of an anti-epileptic drug in the blood enables the dose to be adjusted in order to achieve maximum benefits from the smallest dose and ensure that the risk of harmful effects are kept to a minimum. These estimates are useful with drugs such as ethosuximide, phenytoin and carbamazepine but are of less value with barbiturates (phenobarbitone, and drugs that are converted into phenobarbitone in the body – e.g. methylphenobarbitone and primidone) because the body develops a tolerance to these drugs so that, over time, a higher dose is needed to produce the same effects as the initial dose. Blood level estimates are not useful with sodium valproate because they are not a good indicator of effectiveness.

Table 37.3 Preparations used to treat epilepsy (U)

Preparation	*Drug*	*Dosage form*
Ativan	lorazepam	Injection
carbamazepine	carbamazepine	Tablets
clobazam	clobazam	Capsules
Diamox	acetazolamide	Tablets
Diamox Parenteral	acetazolamide	Powder in vial for reconstitution
Diazemuls	diazepam	Emulsion injection
Emeside	ethosuximide	Capsules, syrup
Epanutin	phenytoin sodium	Capsules, suspension
Epanutin Infatabs	phenytoin sodium	Chewable tablets
Epanutin Parenteral	phenytoin sodium	Injection
Epilim	sodium valproate	Crushable tablets, sugar-free liquid, syrup, enteric-coated tablets
Epilim Intravenous	sodium valproate	Powder in vial
ethosuximide	ethosuximide	Capsules, elixir
Frisium	clobazam	Capsules
Heminevrin IV Infusion	chlormethiazole	Intravenous infusion
Mysoline	primidone	Tablets, suspension
paraldehyde	paraldehyde	Injection, enema
phenobarbitone	phenobarbitone	Tablets, elixir
phenobarbitone sodium	phenobarbitone sodium	Tablets, injection
phenytoin sodium	phenytoin sodium	Tablets
Prominal	methylphenobarbitone	Tablets
Rivotril	clonazepam	Tablets, injection
Stesolid	diazepam	Rectal solution, injection
Tegretol	carbamazepine	Tablets, sugar-free liquid, chewable tablets
Tegretol Retard	carbamazepine	Sustained-release tablets
Valium	diazepam	Injection
Zarontin	ethosuximide	Capsules, syrup

38

Sleep disorders

The functions of sleep

We really know very little about sleep and its function. It may be related to various anatomical structures in the brain and to certain chemical changes. It produces electrical changes in the brain, eyes and muscles. These can be measured by electrical tracings of muscles (electromyograph, EMG), eye movements (electro-oculograph, EOG) and brain waves (electro-encephalograph, EEG). From these tests two main kinds of 'normal sleep' activity have been defined: a stage of non-rapid eye movements (NREM) sleep) which is followed by a stage of rapid eye movements (REM sleep). NREM sleep is called orthodox sleep and is the stage when we 'think'; REM sleep is called paradoxical sleep and is the stage when we 'dream'. It seems that both stages of sleep are essential for health.

Sleep requirements

Sleep requirements vary from person to person and so 'normal' sleep is what suits you under ordinary everyday circumstances. The amount of sleep you need is as much a part of you as your appetite or your conscience. If your sleep is disturbed for only a night or two, this is usually of no consequence; but if the disturbance persists for two or more weeks then you have a sleep problem and need to take action.

Insomnia really means sleeplessness but nowadays it is used to describe most sleeping difficulties. These include difficulty in getting off to sleep, inability to stay asleep, frequent wakenings, restless sleep – often with nightmares, early morning wakening and sleep which is not refreshing (you wake up and feel as exhausted as you did when you went to bed).

Causes of poor sleep

There are many causes of sleep disturbance – these may be social, physical or mental. Among social causes are changes in your environment such as a strange bed or bedroom, changes in temperature, noise, motion and changes of routine like going on night work. Pain from any cause, irritation of the skin, discomfort from indigestion and muscle cramps are some of the physical causes of disturbed sleep. Cat-napping in the day is often a cause of insomnia in elderly people. Emotional disorders (e.g. anxiety, tension, depression) are a common cause of persistent insomnia. However, remember that social, physical and mental factors are all interrelated. Problems at work may produce anxiety which may produce insomnia. Persistent noise at night may interfere with sleep which may cause you to worry about lack of sleep, which may then produce tension and irritability resulting in further difficulty in sleeping. The death of a close friend or relative, the loss of a job, failure at work or in a examination may trigger psychological symptoms, a prominent one of which may be disturbed sleep.

Insomnia must always be regarded as a symptom of some underlying disorder. This is of particular importance in psychological disorders, especially in people who feel anxious, tense and/or miserable. In such individuals insomnia will be just one of a group of mental or physical symptoms that they may experience.

Many drugs can cause insomnia

Drug misuse is a common cause of insomnia. For example, caffeine in tea, coffee, cocoa and colas may keep you awake, particularly as you get older. Regular alcohol drinkers may find themselves waking early and people who take heroin or morphine may find their sleep impaired. Amphetamines, most slimming drugs and some anti-depressant drugs may keep you awake. So may some drugs used in decongestant cough and cold remedies.

Prescribing of sleeping drugs

The widespread use of sleeping drugs over the past 50 years has caused many problems. The situation may now be improving but, even so, millions of tablets and capsules of sleeping drugs are still prescribed every year, with little control over their use by some people, many of whom are able to pick up repeat prescriptions without ever seeing a doctor for months on end.

Up to the early seventies most prescribed sleeping drugs were barbiturates, whose harmful effects were well documented and the dangers of addiction and overdosage well recognized; yet their 'generous' prescribing by doctors ensured that thousands upon thousands of people were addicted to them and/or suffered from incapacitating changes in mood. In addition, they were frequently taken – accidentally or intentionally – in overdose and were responsible for many deaths, particularly when taken with alcohol.

Not only were sleeping drugs widely used in the community, they were also used extensively in hospitals. Some people actually started their addiction to sleeping drugs while in hospital because up to the mid-seventies many patients were routinely given a nightly dose of a sleeping drug during their stay. It became a standard joke – 'wake up, Mr Smith, and take your sleeping pill'. Do not forget that the thalidomide tragedy occurred because pregnant women were prescribed it to relieve minor sleep disturbances, whether they were in hospital or at home.

In the early to middle seventies the barbiturates were progressively replaced by the benzodiazepines (e.g. Mogadon) because they are safer than the baribiturates and other sleeping drugs when taken in overdose. Unfortunately, they were prescribed extensively and were easily available on repeat prescriptions to thousands of patients for years on end, many of whom became addicted to them (see later).

Doctors are one of the biggest causes of insomnia

As stated earlier, insomnia is a symptom that should not be treated in isolation. Yet one of the biggest causes of 'insomnia' in the population is doctors. By keeping patients on sleeping drugs for months and years on end, they guarantee that these people will not be able to sleep if they stop taking sleeping drugs.

After nightly use of a sleeping drug for a few weeks it may take 6–12 weeks without drugs before you can sleep 'normally' again without drugs. During this period you will suffer withdrawal effects (see later) and your sleep may be disturbed, you may have nightmares and you may feel anxious in the day-time. It is not surprising that you think you must go on taking the drugs because you think you are suffering from insomnia.

The sad thing about the use of sleeping drugs is that some doctors have turned a particularly vulnerable group of people into 'psychological addicts'. About three-quarters of all sleeping drugs are prescribed to elderly people, who may have been prescribed sleeping drugs at the time of their spouse's death without counselling and support and then kept on sleeping drugs for years on end. For people living alone it must be very difficult to face the prospect of about 6–12 weeks of disturbed sleep in a lonely house if they try to come off sleeping drugs. It is not surprising that some elderly patients are loath to stop them.

Sleep produced by drugs may be comforting in the first few days of bereavement but not if they have to be continued for weeks on end. What is more, after a few months of nightly use of sleeping drugs, sleep may become disturbed again. So any beneficial effects wear off but the 'need' to go on taking sleeping drugs remains strong.

Warnings on the use of sleeping drugs in elderly people

All sleeping drugs depress brain function and can produce intoxication, tolerance and addiction. They can cause hangover and affect mood. They may be particularly harmful in elderly people, who are sensitive to their depressing effects on the brain and they may easily become confused. If old elderly people (i.e. over 75 years of age) are prescribed too high a dose, they may wet the bed and suffer hangover effects for most of the next day. These hangover effects occur more frequently with long-acting sleeping drugs than with short-acting ones and high doses will produce more hangover effects than small doses. Furthermore, long-acting drugs may stay in the body for days on end so that each dose helps to build up the amount that is already in the body, which explains why old elderly people may easily become intoxicated because their liver and kidneys cannot get rid of the drugs as fast as a young fit person.

When to take sleeping drugs

Very occasionally it may be appropriate to take sleeping drugs for a night or two during severe periods of stress (e.g. after a bereavement) or after prolonged periods of intense work when you just cannot relax, or intermittently through long periods of stress or when travelling overnight or working shifts. In such circumstances they should be taken for only a few nights in a row, because the sleeping drug habit is a real risk after a few weeks of drug-induced sleep.

Have you an emotional problem?

Do not forget that emotional problems are a common cause of sleep disturbance and these may produce many symptoms in addition to insomnia; for example, frequent headaches, feeling anxious or tense, sad, depressed or tearful, backaches, pains in the chest, indigestion, dizziness, no energy, feeling fed up, feeling irritable, fears about your health or about going out by yourself, loss of appetite, loss of interest in sex, loss of weight, palpitations, feelings of guilt, feeling not wanted or feeling that other people are talking about you. These are only some of the group of symptoms that would suggest that you are suffering from a psychological disorder and need appropriate treatment. Remember also that tension may produce anxiety in the day-time and insomnia at night.

Are you depressed?

If you have a change in mood, the use of sleeping drugs or sedatives may aggravate your condition – especially if you are feeling sad or miserable. It is important to recognize what are labelled 'depressive symptoms'. These include characteristic sleep disturbances such as difficulty in getting to sleep, restless sleep and early morning wakening. Fatigue is a particularly important symptom if you are depressed, and no matter how long you stay in bed you still feel exhausted. Sleeping drugs will not help; in fact they can make you feel worse if you are depressed. However, anti-depressant drugs may be very effective in relieving these symptoms. This again highlights the importance of not just treating insomnia on its own. You need to consider as many factors as possible for the cause of your insomnia. After all, the symptoms are telling you that there is something wrong in your life, and advice and counselling may be more effective than sleeping drugs which solve nothing – they only temporarily relieve the symptom of insomnia.

Use non-drug treatments for insomnia

There are safer alternatives to sleeping drugs, such as a hot bath before retiring, reading a book, taking a walk, not having too large an evening meal, cutting out coffee, tea or cocoa in the evening, reducing smoking, reducing alcohol intake, trying to get some regular exercise and fresh air during the day and – probably most important of all – being taught how to relax. The ritual just before going to bed may condition you to go to sleep – undressing, washing, etc. A milk–cereal drink may help you sleep more peacefully.

Breaking the sleeping drug habit

Tests have shown that all sleeping drugs disrupt normal sleeping patterns although you may feel that you sleep well. They suppress what is called paradoxical sleep (i.e. the period of sleep when you dream a lot). This means that when you stop your sleeping drugs you will find it difficult to sleep, and when you do manage to sleep you will dream a lot and your sleep will be restless and you may have nightmares. This is why you may easily become convinced that you can't sleep without taking a sleeping drug; but the very fact that you have disturbed sleep if you stop them is why you should stop them. It shows that the drugs are affecting your normal brain function. In addition to experiencing difficulties with sleep, you may also experience other withdrawal symptoms if you try to suddenly stop taking sleeping drugs.

Most sleeping drugs these days are benzodiazepines and the effects of sudden withdrawal and methods of withdrawal are discussed in detail in Chapter 40. But whatever the sleeping drug, the same advice applies.

Gradually reduce the dose of your sleeping drug

If you have been taking a sleeping drug every night for several weeks or more and try to stop it suddenly, you may get disturbed sleep, dreams and nightmares. You may also develop anxiety symptoms and mood changes in the day-time (see later). You should therefore reduce the nightly dose very slowly over several weeks to months. In this way the withdrawal symptoms will not be so severe, and gradually your general feeling of well-being will improve. For example, if you are taking nitrazepam (Mogadon) every night in a dose of two 5 mg tablets, you should break the tablets in half (2.5 mg) and then quarters (1.25 mg). You should reduce the nightly dose by half a tablet every month for 2 months; you will then be down to one tablet (5 mg) a night. Then reduce the nightly dose by a quarter of a tablet (1.25 mg) once a month until you are taking only one-quarter of a tablet every night. After a month on this dose you can stop it or try breaking it in half and taking one-eighth of a tablet every night for another month before stopping.

There is no hard and fast rule about how to stop sleeping drugs except to reduce your nightly dose very slowly over several months until you are completely off them. It is worth taking your time and being patient and not feeling guilty about taking sleeping drugs. As you slowly reduce the dose you should try non-drug treatments to help you to sleep (see earlier). If you find it difficult, see your doctor or a clinical psychologist or join a local self-help group. You will need support and counselling and to be taught how to relax.

What about elderly people who have developed the habit of taking sleeping drugs every night? Many of these individuals are widows, often living alone. Even if they are dependent upon them, I think it would be wrong to make them feel guilty about taking sleeping drugs. Nevertheless they should be weaned off them if they are depressed, anxious or tense; if they drink alcohol regularly; if they have increased the dose; if they are incontinent; or if they show signs of intoxication or have impaired kidney, heart or liver function. In any of these situations they should slowly be weaned off their sleeping drug. As for others in this situation, their general well-being would improve if they were to be slowly weaned off their sleeping drugs. In future 'new' elderly patients should never be prescribed a regular nightly dose of a sleeping drug.

Table 38.1 Sleeping drugs – harmful effects and warnings

Barbiturates

Barbiturates should no longer be used as sleeping drugs because of their harmful effects, in particular their potential for producing addiction and the danger to life associated with their intentional or accidental overdosage, especially when taken with alcohol.

Harmful effects include drowsiness, sedation, skin rashes, allergic reactions (particularly affecting the skin), incoordination of voluntary movement, hangover, impaired judgement and depression of breathing. Some patients can become paradoxically excited, restless and confused, particularly the elderly and people in pain. Children may become irritable and over-excited. Long-term use of phenobarbitone to treat epilepsy may cause folic acid deficiency anaemia, and defects of the blood clotting mechanisms may occur in newborn babies if their mothers took phenobarbitone during pregnancy. Rarely, barbiturates may cause liver damage. Long-term use of barbiturates in high doses produces symptoms like those produced by alcohol – disorientation, mental confusion, incoordination of voluntary movements (ataxia), dizziness, depression, skin rashes, difficulty in speaking and poor judgement.

Warnings Barbiturates must not be used in people who are allergic to them or who have severe kidney or liver disease or porphyria, nor in over-active children. They should be used with caution in individuals with mild to moderately impaired kidney or liver function or chronic chest disease (e.g. asthma, bronchitis). In the presence of severe pain, barbiturates may fail to produce sedation or sleep and may cause wakefulness, excitement and delirium unless they are given with an effective pain reliever.

Risks in elderly people Harmful effects may be more frequent and severe; therefore use with caution and in reduced dosage.

Risks in driving Barbiturates may affect your ability to drive; therefore do not drive until you know that it is safe to do so.

Risks with alcohol Barbiturates increase the effects of alcohol and may be dangerous. Do not drink alcohol when taking a barbiturate.

Tolerance to and dependence on barbiturates Barbiturates and all sleeping drugs produce *tolerance*, which is a lessened response to the effects of a drug over time so that a larger dose of the drug has to be taken in order to produce the same intensity of effect that was produced by the lower doses at the start of treatment. Barbiturates produce *dependence* similar to that produced by alcohol, which is why this type of dependence is often referred to as the barbiturate/alcohol type. *All other sleeping drugs produce a similar type of dependence.* The dependence takes the form of a strong need to go on taking the drug, a tendency to increase the dose, a reliance on the drug in order to cope (psychological dependence), and a serious physical dependence in which individuals cannot cope without it because of unpleasant symptoms if they try to reduce the dose, and serious, characteristic, symptoms if the drug is stopped suddenly. These *withdrawal symptoms* come on after a few hours and include weakness,

Table 38.1 Sleeping drugs – harmful effects and warnings (*cont.*)

anxiety, headaches, dizziness, tremors, vomiting, nausea, stomach cramps, insomnia and rapid beating of the heart. After a day or two the blood pressure on standing up after sitting or lying down may fall and produce dizziness, light-headedness, and fainting; convulsions may occur and hallucinations, and delirium tremens may develop after several days, followed by deep sleep. NOTE For definitions of the terms 'dependence' and 'addiction', see under 'Benzodiazepines' in Chapter 40.

Delirium tremens (the DTs)
The DTs produced by the sudden withdrawal of a barbiturate is similar to that produced by the sudden withdrawal of alcohol from a chronic alcohol abuser. People so affected become disorientated, confused and agitated; they see things that are not there (visual hallucinations), tremble and sweat, and develop a rapid pulse, rapid breathing and a high temperature.

Benzodiazepines
See Chapter 40.

chloral betaine
Chloral betaine is a complex of chloral hydrate and trimethyl glycine which dissolves in the stomach to release chloral hydrate. Welldorm previously contained dichloralphenazone but this was stopped because of unacceptable risks of harmful effects. For harmful effects and warnings, see 'chloral hydrate', below.

chloral hydrate
Harmful effects Chloral hydrate is corrosive to the skin and lining of the mouth unless well diluted. It may irritate the stomach, producing gastritis, nausea and vomiting, especially if it is taken on an empty stomach. Allergic skin rashes may occur within hours and up to 10 days after a single dose. It may produce hallucinations, agitation, confusion, hangover, unsteadiness, drowsiness, dizziness and light-headedness. High doses produce acute intoxication (like being drunk with alcohol), nausea and vomiting. Chronic high doses produce symptoms like chronic alcoholism but the gastritis is more severe and skin rashes may develop. Kidney damage may occur in people who become addicted to chloral hydrate.

Dependence Chloral hydrate produces dependence of the barbiturate/alcohol type (see above under Barbiturates).

Warnings Chloral hydrate should not be used to treat anyone who has impaired kidney or liver function, severe heart disease or a history of gastritis or peptic ulcers.

Risks in elderly people Harmful effects are likely to be more frequent and severe in elderly people, particularly hangover effects. Use with caution and use smaller doses.

Risks in driving Do not drive if you are taking this drug until you know how it affects you.

Risks with alcohol Chloral hydrate increases the effects of alcohol.

chlormethiazole
Harmful effects include drowsiness, indigestion, nausea, vomiting, sneezing, congestion of the nose (this may occur 15–20 minutes after taking the drug), increased production of phlegm and irritation of the conjunctivae of the eyes. These symptoms may be severe and associated with a severe headache and stomach upset. A transient fall in blood pressure may cause faintness and dizziness. It may trigger depression in someone suffering from manic–depressive illness, and it may, rarely, cause severe allergic reactions and depressed breathing. It may cause thrombophlebitis at the site of injection into a vein, and occasionally produce a paradoxical reaction of excitement and confusion instead of drowsiness.

Dependence Chormethiazole produces intoxication and dependence similar to those produced by the barbiturates and alcohol (see earlier, under 'Barbiturates').

Warnings Chlormethiazole should not be used in individuals who are allergic to it,

Table 38.1 Sleeping drugs – harmful effects and warnings (*cont.*)

or who have acute impairment of their breathing, or a history of drug and/or alcohol abuse. *It must not be prescribed to alcoholics who continue to drink alcohol.* It should be used with caution in people suffering from chronic chest diseases, or impaired liver or kidneys function. Chlormethiazole should be used with great caution in anyone with a history of drug abuse, alcoholism or a serious behavioural disorder. In overdose the drug causes coma, depressed breathing, a fall in body temperature (hypothermia) and a high risk of pneumonia. These dangers are particularly serious if the drug is taken with alcohol, a sedative or an anti-anxiety drug.

Risks in elderly people Harmful effects are likely to be more frequent and severe in elderly people, particularly if they drink alcohol. It may produce hangover effects and excessive drowsiness in the day-time. Use with caution and use smaller doses. Its routine use in elderly people is not recommended.

Risks in driving Chlormethiazole may affect your driving ability; therefore do not drive until you know that it is safe to do so.

Risks with alcohol You should not drink alcohol when you are taking this drug – it dangerously increases its effects.

chlormezanone
See Table 40.2.

cyclopyrrolones
Some of the actions produced in the body by cyclopyrrolones are similar to those produced by benzodiazepines. However, they produce different effects on patterns of sleep and are claimed to cause fewer hangover effects.

zopiclone is a cyclopyrrolone marketed for the short-term treatment of insomnia and other sleep difficulties. Although it is claimed that tolerance and withdrawal symptoms are not a problem with this drug, it is early days and its use should be very carefully monitored for such problems and for any addiction potential.

Harmful effects include a bitter metallic taste in the mouth after taking the drug, mild stomach and bowel upsets, allergic reactions, drowsiness, hallucinations and visual disturbances.

Warnings The dose should be reduced in anyone with impaired liver function, and individuals should be monitored for withdrawal symptoms.

Risks in elderly people Harmful effects may be more frequent and severe; therefore reduce dose by half.

Risks with alcohol It increases effect of alcohol, so do not drink alcohol while taking this drug.

Risks with driving It may interfere with your ability to drive and operate moving machinery.

methyprylone
Harmful effects include morning drowsiness, hangover, headache, dizziness, vertigo, unsteadiness, nausea, vomiting, diarrhoea, constipation and, rarely, raised temperature, hallucinations, convulsions, confusion, excitability, anxiety, depression and nightmares. Very rarely, it may cause low blood pressure, fainting, double vision, blurred vision, blood disorders, allergic reactions, skin rashes and itching.

Dependence Methyprylone produces intoxication and dependence similar to those produced by barbiturate drugs and alcohol (see earlier, under 'Barbiturates').

Warnings Methyprylone should not be used in people who are allergic to it. It should be used with caution in anyone suffering from impaired function of their kidneys or liver.

Risks in elderly people Harmful effects of methyprylone may be more frequent and severe in elderly people, particularly drowsiness, hangover and confusion. Use with caution and in smaller doses.

Risks in driving Methyprylone may affect your ability to drive, particularly when taken with alcohol or certain other drugs (see Chapter 89).

Risks with alcohol Methyprylone increases the effects of alcohol; so do not drink alcohol while taking this drug.

Table 38.1 Sleeping drugs – harmful effects and warnings (*cont.*)

promethazine
Harmful effects include drowsiness, dizziness and disorientation. For other potential harmful effects see antihistamines (Chapter 10).

Warnings Promethazine should not be used in people who are allergic to it or to phenothiazine anti-psychotic drugs nor in anyone suffering from asthma, bronchitis or other chest trouble. It should be used with caution in individuals with narrow-angle glaucoma or narrowing of the outlet from the stomach, and in people who have difficulty passing urine due, for example, to an enlarged prostate gland.

Risks in elderly people Harmful effects may be more frequent and severe, particularly drowsiness and abnormal movements (tardive dyskinesia). Use with caution and in smaller doses.

Risks in driving Promethazine may affect your ability to drive; therefore do not drive until you know that it is safe to do so.

Risks with alcohol It increases the effects of alcohol, so do not drink alcohol while taking this drug.

triclofos sodium
Harmful effects are similar to those described above under chloral hydrate, except that it does not irritate the skin or lining of the mouth and is less likely to cause irritation of the stomach.

Warnings The warnings given above under chloral hydrate apply to the use of triclofos. NOTE Chloral betaine, chloral hydrate, dichloralphenazone and triclofos produce intoxication and dependence similar to those produced by barbiturate drugs and alcohol (see earlier, under 'Barbiturates').

Table 38.2 Suggestions to doctors on when to prescribe sleeping drugs

Sleep disorders	*Treatment*
Due to a physical disorder – e.g. pain, itching, breathlessness	Treat the physical disorder; e.g. give a pain reliever, anti-itching drug or a bronchodilator
Due to an emotional disorder – e. g. anxiety, depression	Insomnia is a symptom; treat the whole patient. Provide counselling, advice and support. If tense and anxious, an anti-anxiety drug at night will help but only for 1–2 weeks and not regularly every night, only when needed. If the patient has symptoms of depression, an anti-depressant drug that produces drowsiness at night may help sleep. Anti-anxiety drugs and anti-depressant drugs should be used provided they are part of overall treatment and not just treating the symptom of insomnia in isolation
Transient sleep disturbance – e.g. jet lag, noisy environment	Avoid the use of sleeping drugs if possible. Very occasionally it may be helpful to prescribe a short-acting sleeping drug with minimal hangover effects, but only for a night or two (e.g. triazolam). This produces less hangover effect than longer acting ones

Table 38.2 Suggestions to doctors on when to prescribe sleeping drugs (*cont.*)

Sleep disorders	*Treatment*
Shift worker who needs to stay asleep	Drug use should preferably be avoided. Very occasionally it may be necessary to prescribe a quick acting sleeping drug with a short duration of action (e.g. temazepam). Advise patient to avoid regular daily use for more than a few days at a time
Short-term sleep disturbances – e. g. bereavement, family upset, divorce, etc.	Provide advice, support and counselling; if inability to sleep becomes a real problem, prescribe a small dose of a sleeping drug (e.g. temazepam) but for only 2 or 3 nights. Advise patients not to use it on consecutive nights, but to try to sleep without the drug if possible
Long-standing sleep disturbances (chronic insomnia)	Look for and treat any underlying physical disorders (e.g. pain, itching, breathlessness) or emotional disorder (e.g. anxiety, depression). Drug and alcohol misuse are common causes, as is cat-napping during the day. Advise patient to avoid tea, coffee, cola or alcohol in the evenings. Advise on non-drug treatments. Refer to clinical psychologist. Only prescribe a small dose of a sleeping drug for use occasionally, i.e. for the odd night or two. Avoid prescribing a sleeping drug for use every night. Give no more than one week's supply and then review the situation with the patient.

NOTES No 'new' patient should ever be prescribed more than 1 week's supply of a sleeping drug at any one time.

Attempts should be made to wean most regular users off their sleeping drug by following the sort of regimen described earlier.

No repeat prescription for a sleeping drug should ever be issued without the doctor seeing the patient.

Obviously, there are exceptions such as people suffering from a serious illness (e.g. cancer or AIDS), but in these patients the regular nightly use of a sleeping drug must only be part of an overall comprehensive treatment programme that has been tailored to the individual's needs.

Table 38.3 Sleeping drug preparations

Preparation	*Drug*	*Drug group*	*Dosage form*
Amytal	amylobarbitone	Barbiturate	Tablets
chloral hydrate	chloral hydrate	Sedative	Mixture
Dalmane	flurazepam	Long-acting benzodiazepine	Capsules
Dormonoct	loprazolam	Intermediate-acting benzodiazepine	Tablets
Halcion	triazolam	Short-acting benzodiazepine	Tablets
Heminevrin	chlormethiazole	Sedative	Capsules, sugar-free syrup

Table 38.3 Sleeping drug preparations (*cont.*)

Preparation	*Drug*	*Drug group*	*Dosage form*
loprazolam	loprazolam	Intermediate-acting benzodiazepine	Tablets
lormetazepam	lormetazepam	Intermediate-acting benzodiazepine	Tablets
Mogadon	nitrazepam	Long-acting bezodiazepine	Capsules, tablets
Nitrados	nitrazepam	Long-acting benzodiazepine	Tablets
nitrazepam	nitrazepam	Long-acting benzodiazepine	Tablets, mixture
Noctec	chloral hydrate	Sedative	Capsules
Normison	temazepam	Intermediate-acting benzodiazepine	Capsules
Remnos	nitrazepam	Long-acting benzodiazepine	Tablets
Rohypnol	flunitrazepam	Intermediate-acting benzodiazepine	Tablets
Seconal Sodium	quinalbarbitone sodium	Barbiturate	Capsules
Sodium Amytal	amylobarbitone sodium	Barbiturate	Capsules, tablets
Sominex	promethazine	Antihistamine	Tablets
Somnite	nitrazepam	Long-acting benzodiazepine	Suspension
Soneryl	butobarbitone	Barbiturate	Tablets
Surem	nitrazepam	Long-acting benzodiazepine	Capsules
temazepam	temazepam	Intermediate-acting benzodiazepine	Capsules, elixir, tablets
temazepam Gelthix	temazepam	Intermediate-acting benzodiazepine	Gel-filled capsules
temazepam Planpak	temazepam	Intermediate-acting benzodiazepine	Soft gelatin capsules of 10 mg, 5 mg and 2 mg strengths
triclofos	triclofos	Sedative-hypnotic	Elixir
Tuinal	amylobarbitone sodium	Barbiturate	Capsules
	quinalbarbitone sodium	Barbiturate	
Unisomnia	nitrazepam	Long-acting benzodiazepine	Tablets
Welldorm	chloral betaine	Sedative-hypnotic	Tablets, elixir
Zimovane	zopiclone	Cyclopyrrolone	Tablets

39

Depression

There is a continuum from feeling blue to feeling severely depressed and suicidal, and from feeling tired and fed up to possessing symptoms that totally interfere with your capacity to cope with your everyday life. If you feel sad and miserable for long periods, this is not just 'feeling blue'; doctors would call it 'depression'. There are many factors that may trigger an attack of depression in a susceptible person. These include social factors such as unemployment; family factors such as bereavement or divorce; or physical factors, such as a virus infection (e.g. influenza), surgery or a heart attack. Depression may be triggered by certain drugs; for example, reserpine given for raised blood pressure and some sulphonamide drugs. You may feel severely depressed after childbirth, during the menopause, just before a period or if you have vitamin deficiencies; but you may also be severely depressed for no obvious reason.

When you have a depressive illness, in addition to feelings of depression (feeling sad, miserable, weepy, suicidal) you may develop changes in behaviour. You may stop wanting to mix socially and start staying at home in the evenings. You may develop physiological changes such as alterations in sleep rhythm (particularly difficulty in getting off to sleep or early morning wakening), alteration in appetite, weight and/or sex drive, and loss of energy. You may develop physical symptoms; for example, headaches, dizziness, chest pains, palpitations, indigestion, diarrhoea and backache. These symptoms may make you worry about physical disease and so you may become hypochondriacal and think you have a cancer or heart disease. You may develop mental symptoms and feel unreal, divorced from yourself, as if you were looking from outside at yourself; you may have difficulty in concentrating and making decisions; your memory may be affected and you may keep thinking morbid thoughts about death, dying and suicide. You may become very tense and anxious (as if something dreadful is going to happen all the time). You may develop fears (e.g. fear of seeing people, fear of going out). You may become very agitated and irritable or very withdrawn and quiet, and you may become suspicious of other people and what they are doing. You may become obsessive, having to do things over and over again, and you may feel guilty, unworthy and blame yourself. You may recall all sorts of things from your past life and keep brooding on some event from the past which caused you anxiety or sadness.

Some depressive episodes are labelled as 'endogenous depression' (or psychotic depression) by doctors. Endogenous depression means it comes from 'inside' and there is often no obvious 'outside' cause why you should be depressed. On the other hand, you may become depressed because of an obvious 'outside' cause – for example, the death of a relative, the loss of a job. Doctors call this 'exogenous' or 'reactive' depression. Your depression is due to your reaction to the outside event. However, these are only labels and quite often there is no clear distinction between 'outside' and 'inside' events. They just cannot be separated that easily.

Mood changes where there is only depression may be referred to as *unipolar*, and *bipolar* where there is a swing from depression to elation (e.g. manic depression). The later is probably genetic ('blue genes') whereas the former may be an inherited tendency to bring the world down upon oneself.

This has been a very sketchy description of what doctors label depression. Patients may experience a few or many of these symptoms. Some symptoms may be mild and some intense, and, according to all sorts of factors in your upbringing, your culture, your personality and your environment, you will react in different ways. Certainly in Western society the puritan ethic of 'being firm and standing on one's own two feet' may produce awful feelings of guilt and unworthiness in which suicide appears to be the only way out. The problem is too complex to be simply labelled 'depression'.

The trouble is that doctors often label you as depressed and prescribe anti-depressant drugs when they really should label as 'depressing' those outside factors that are affecting you; prescribing drugs will not alter these, only how you react to them. This is why it is important for doctors to treat you as a whole person by discussing with you the various factors in your life that may be causing you to feel depressed. It does not help you if all the doctor does is to respond to a few of your symptoms with a prescription for anti-depressant drugs. I do not mean that the symptoms of depression should not be relieved by drugs, but that such treatment ought only to be a part of your overall treatment.

Drug treatment of depression

There is normally a balance between the amount of brain stimulants and depressants acting on the brain, and there are mechanisms for ensuring that too much stimulant or depressant does not accumulate in brain cells to produce an excessive response. Any disturbance in the balance between the amount of brain stimulants and depressants may affect our alertness and our mood and there is evidence that some patients who are depressed suffer from an under-production of brain stimulants. To combat this effect we have anti-depressant drugs which raise the level of stimulant chemicals in the brain, resulting in an elevation of mood and a reduction in the symptoms produced by depression.

Clearly, these anti-depressants are no solution for life's ills, nor are they necessary in mild depression, but in people with moderate or severe depression such drugs may relieve incapacitating symptoms and enable them to cope more easily. However, these drugs provide only relief from symptoms, they do not cure depression. There is no cure, but effective anti-depressant drug treatment will help individuals through the bad spells of their depression and make life tolerable until the underlying depression lifts, which it will sooner or later.

Tricyclic anti-depressants

Tricyclic anti-depressants are the main group of drugs used to treat depression. Given to people who are not depressed, these drugs make them feel sleepy and light-headed. Their movements become clumsy and they have difficulty in thinking and concentrating, but the drugs do not affect their mood. However, if tricyclic anti-depressants are given to patients who are depressed, after a period of 2–3 weeks their mood lifts and they begin to feel better physically and mentally. This clearly tells us that there is something different about the chemical response in the brain of patients who are depressed from those who are not.

It is not fully understood how tricyclic anti-depressants lift the mood and relieve the symptoms of depression. One effect may be to block the mopping up of stimulant brain chemicals (e.g. noradrenaline and serotonin) by nerve cells and therefore prolong their effects. Slowly the brain adapts to this increased stimulation and over a period of 2–3 weeks other changes occur that cause the mood of the depressed patients to lift and stay lifted as long as they continue to take an appropriate daily dose of the anti-depressant or until the underlying depression clears up on its own (which is usually the case).

In addition to increasing the effects of stimulant neurotransmitters in the brain, tricyclic anti-depressant drugs also affect chemical messengers in nerves that oppose these stimulant effects. These are in the parasympathetic nervous system, where tricyclic anti-depressant drugs block the neurotransmitter acetylcholine. This blocking produces what are called anticholinergic effects. These include blurred vision, dry mouth, dizziness, rapid beating of the heart, constipation, tremor and difficulty in passing urine. When you take tricyclic anti-depressant drugs these unwanted effects begin straight away whereas it takes 2–3 weeks for the depressive symptoms to start to improve. As the drug is continued in adequate daily doses, the body begins to tolerate the anticholinergic effects and they usually become progressively less troublesome, during which time the anti-depressant effects begin to take over.

There is marked variation in type and frequency of harmful effects from tricyclic anti-depressants between individuals and between different drugs. In other words, what is good for one patient may not be good for another. In children, tricyclic anti-depressants may produce alarming effects (see later) and they should be used with utmost caution.

Effects on the heart and circulation

Tricyclic anti-depressant drugs (particularly amitriptyline) may occasionally affect the nerves controlling the heart and arteries, producing a fall in blood pressure on standing up after sitting or lying down (postural hypotension), rapid beating of the heart (tachycardia) and changes on electrical tracings of the heart. Very rarely, high doses may depress the heart and produce heart block or serious disorders of heart rhythm, particularly, in patients with heart disease. Children are more vulnerable than adults to harmful effects on the heart. In people who have coronary artery disease or disease of the arteries supplying the brain, the fall in blood pressure produced by tricyclic anti-depressants may, rarely, trigger a heart attack or a stroke, respectively. They should therefore be used with utmost caution in these patients.

Dangers of using tricyclic anti-depressants in elderly people

Elderly people are more likely to suffer from harmful effects than are younger people. They are particularly likely to suffer from dizziness, a fall in blood pressure on standing up after sitting or lying down (postural hypotension), constipation, difficulty in passing urine, tremors and ankle swelling. They may become confused and delirious. Elderly people with glaucoma, heart disease, raised blood pressure or an enlarged prostate gland are at particular risk from the anticholinergic effects of tricyclic anti-depressants.

Anyone who is demented may become depressed but the use of tricyclic anti-depressants in these people may make the dementia much worse. Equally, some depressed elderly individuals may run the risk of being labelled 'demented' when in actual fact they are depressed and would improve dramatically if they were given anti-depressant treatment.

Dangers of taking tricyclic drugs with other drugs

The interactions of other drugs with tricyclic anti-depressants are listed in Chapter 89. The combined use of a tricyclic anti-depressant drug with a monoamine oxidase inhibitor (MAOI) anti-depressant drug is dangerous (see later). It may cause sweating, flushing, high temperature, restlessness, excitement, tremor, twitching, muscle rigidity, convulsions and coma. Therefore, tricyclic anti-depressant drugs should not be given to patients taking MAOI drugs or for 14 days after stopping an MAOI drug. There is no convincing evidence to suggest that this combination works any better than either drug used on its own. The combination of tranylcypromine and clomipramine is particularly dangerous.

Tricyclic anti-depressant drugs may increase the effects of sympathomimetic drugs on the heart. They may therefore produce harmful effects when given with sympathomimetic drugs present in decongestant cold and cough remedies and in asthma drugs.

Withdrawal effects

People may take tricyclic anti-depressant drugs regularly every day for years without feeling a need to increase the dose, and although the body becomes tolerant to the anticholinergic effects (blurred vision, constipation, etc.) it does not seem to become tolerant to the beneficial effects of relieving the symptoms of depression.

There are reports of patients experiencing withdrawal symptoms to tricyclic drugs such as anxiety and difficulties with sleeping when they are stopped suddenly, and of course symptoms of any underlying depression may surface. There are also very occasional reports that stopping imipramine suddenly may cause chills and cold-like symptoms.

No anti-depressant drug should ever be stopped suddenly – daily treatment should always be tapered off very slowly over weeks or months. This is in order to check whether the underlying depression has cleared or whether it is going to return. If it does return, the drug treatment should continue for another 3 months before trying again to reduce the daily dose.

Other anti-depressants

Mianserin (Bolvidon, Norval) and *maprotiline* (Ludiomil) are structurally different from tricyclic anti-depressants because they contain a four (tetra) ring nucleus instead of a three (tri) ring nucleus; they are referred to as tetracylic anti-depressants. It is not fully understood how they relieve depression but they appear to increase the availability of stimulant neurotransmitters in the brain. They produce fewer anticholinergic effects than the tricyclics (e.g. dry mouth, blurred vision, constipation, difficulty passing urine) and fewer effects on the heart and circulation. However mianserin may, rarely, cause serious blood disorders and liver damage, painful joints and flu-like symptoms, and maprotiline may, rarely, cause skin rashes and convulsions. For other harmful effects and warnings on the use of mianserin and maprotiline, see Table 39.1.

Trazodone (Molipaxin) is an anti-depressant that is not related to the tricyclic or tetracyclic anti-depressants. Its mode of action in relieving depression is not known but it may increase the effects of stimulant neurotransmitters in the brain. It also produces sedation and may help to relieve anxiety associated with depression. It causes fewer anticholinergic effects than the tricyclic anti-depressants (see earlier) and is less likely to cause harmful effects on the heart and convulsions when an overdose is taken. It may cause chronic erection of the penis (priapism).

Viloxazine (Vivalan) is an anti-depressant drug not related to the tricyclic or tetracyclic anti-depressants; it belongs to a group of drugs called oxazines. It blocks the mopping up of the stimulant neurotransmitter, noradrenaline, by nerve cells, and makes it more available to produce stimulation of the brain. It produces fewer anticholinergic effects than the tricyclic anti-depressants (see earlier), fewer harmful effects on the heart and circulation and less sedative effects.

Fluoxetine (Prozac) and *fluvoxamine* (Faverin) are anti-depressant drugs that block the mopping up, and therefore prolong the action, of the stimulant neurotransmitter, 5-hydroxytryptamine (5HT, serotonin). They have virtually no anticholinergic effects and produce fewer effects on the heart and circulation than the tricyclics. However, they cause more nausea and vomiting. (U)

Table 39.1 Anti-depressant drugs – harmful effects and warnings

Tricyclic anti-depressants

Harmful effects Harmful effects of tricyclic anti-depressant drugs vary between different drugs and between different individuals. They also vary in frequency and in type. Some harmful effects are directly related to the dose and some are related to how a particular individual reacts. Some harmful effects may be more likely to occur, or to occur with greater intensity according to what other disorders the person is suffering from. It is important, therefore, that treatment is tailored to each individual's particular needs and responses.

Not all of the following harmful effects have been reported with every tricyclic anti-depressant drug but they have been reported with one or more of them and should always be borne in mind whenever these drugs are used. They include dry mouth, blurred vision, constipation, difficulty in passing urine, lassitude, weakness, fatigue, lack of energy, confusion, inability to concentrate, disorientation, dizziness, restlessness, drowsiness, nervousness, insomnia, nightmares, numbness and pins and needles in the hands and feet, tremors, noises in the ears, parkinsonism-like effects, changes in weight, sweating, fall in blood pressure on standing up after lying or sitting down (may produce dizziness and faintness), rapid beating of the heart, palpitations, disorders of heart rhythm, heart attacks, convulsions, strokes, allergic skin rashes (e.g. nettle

Table 39.1 Anti-depressant drugs – harmful effects and warnings (*cont.*)

rash), sensitivity of the skin to sunlight, angioedema, nausea, stomach upsets, vomiting, loss of appetite, peculiar taste in the mouth, diarrhoea and black tongue.

Very rarely, tricyclic anti-depressant drugs may damage the bone marrow, producing blood disorders; damage to the liver, producing jaundice; swelling of the testicles and breasts in men; breast enlargement and leakage of milk in women; increased or decreased sexual drive (libido), impotence, changes to blood sugar levels; loss of hair (alopecia) and changes in weight. Some patients may become manic, and symptoms of schizophrenia may be triggered – especially in elderly people.

Tricyclic anti-depressants that produce *sedation* include amitriptyline, dothiepin, doxepin and trimipramine; those that produce *little sedation* include amoxapine, butriptyline, clomipramine, desipramine, imipramine, iprindole, lofepramine and nortriptyline. The ones that produce *stimulation* include protriptyline.

All tricyclic anti-depressants cause some anticholinergic effects (e.g. dry mouth, difficulty passing urine, blurred vision, constipation) and harmful effects on the heart; however, lofepramine appears to produce fewer of these effects than the others.

Some of the tricyclic anti-depressants are particularly associated with certain harmful effects although some occur only rarely. For example, *amitriptyline* is associated with serious disorders of heart rhythm; *iprindole* with liver damage and jaundice (usually in the first 14 days); *protriptyline* with heart disorders, aggravation of anxiety, tension and insomnia and with sensitivity of the skin to sunlight; and *trimipramine* with anticholinergic effects (dry mouth, blurred vision, constipation) and numbness and pins and needles in the hands and feet.

Warnings Tricyclic anti-depressants should not be used to treat anyone who is allergic to them, nor in individuals who suffer or have suffered in the past from convulsions, have difficulty in passing urine (e.g. enlarged prostate gland), who have closed-angle glaucoma or raised blood pressure, heart disease (they may trigger an attack of abnormal heart rhythm or rate) or over-active thyroid gland, or who are taking thyroid drugs. They should not be used with or within 14 days of taking a monoamine oxidase drug (a high temperature, convulsions and deaths have occurred from some such combinations), nor during the recovery stage of a heart attack (myocardial infarction). They should be used with caution in people with mild or moderate impairment of liver function, diabetes, serious mental illness (e.g. schizophrenia), or in anyone at risk of committing suicide.

People with any of the above conditions should be monitored closely and have a regular medical check-up every 2–3 months. Individuals with heart disorders should have an electric tracing of their heart (ECG) every 2–3 months.

Risks in elderly people Harmful effects of tricyclic anti-depressants may be more frequent and severe in elderly people, particularly their effects upon the heart and circulation, difficulty with passing urine, risks of producing glaucoma and effects on the brain producing, for example, confusion, restlessness and drowsiness. Their effects on lowering the blood pressure may be harmful in elderly people, causing faintness and light-headedness on standing up after lying or sitting down. They should therefore be used with caution and in lower doses than normal. *Protriptyline* is more likely to cause heart problems, and *mianserin* to damage the bone marrow, in elderly people than in younger people.

Risks in driving Tricyclic anti-depressants affect the function of the brain; therefore do not drive or operate machinery until you know that it is safe to do so. These effects can be made much worse by alcohol, sleeping drugs, sedatives or tranquillizers.

Table 39.1 Anti-depressant drugs – harmful effects and warnings (*cont.*)

Risks with alcohol Tricyclic anti-depressants may increase the effects of alcohol so it is advisable not to drink while you are taking any of these drugs.

Risks of suicide Tricyclic anti-depressant drugs take several weeks to work, during which time a severely depressed individual may feel suicidal. Therefore, it is advisable that the doctor prescribe only a small quantity of these drugs at any one time, because they can be dangerous in overdose.

Risks in schizophrenia People suffering from schizophrenia may develop a severe flare-up of their symptoms and become more paranoid and/or manic if they take tricyclic anti-depressants.

Other anti-depressants

fluoxetine (Prozac)
Harmful effects include nausea, headaches, diarrhoea, nervousness, tremor, drowsiness, fever, loss of appetite and weight, sweating, sexual dysfunction, weakness, anxiety, insomnia, dizziness and, rarely, skin rashes, convulsions and over-excitement (hypomania).

Warnings Fluoxetine must not be used in anyone who is allergic to it or who has severely impaired kidney function. It should be used with caution in people with epilepsy (particularly if it is unstable), heart disease, slight or moderate impairment of kidney function or impaired liver function or with diabetes.

Risks with driving It may affect your ability to drive, so do not drive until you know that it is safe to do so.

Risks with alcohol It may increase the effects of alcohol.

fluvoxamine (Faverin)
Harmful effects Nausea and vomiting are the commonest. Other symptoms include diarrhoea, headache, anxiety, agitation, loss of appetite, tremor and, rarely, convulsions and decreased heart rate and changes in electrical tracings of the heart (ECG).

Warnings It must not be used in anyone with epilepsy. Anxiety may worsen in the first few weeks of treatment. It should be used with caution in people with impaired kidney or liver function (treatment should start with low doses. Liver function tests should be carried out before treatment and at regular intervals during treatment).

Risks with alcohol It may increase the effects of alcohol, so do not drink alcohol when you are taking this drug.

Risks with driving It may affect your ability to drive, so do not drive until you know that it is safe to do so.

Risks with other drugs Note that there is the risk of convulsions and high temperature if given with an MAOI or with lithium.

maprotiline (Ludiomil)
Harmful effects Convulsions may occur, particularly in anyone with a history of epilepsy. Anticholinergic effects (dry mouth, difficulty passing urine, blurred vision, rapid heart beat, constipation) occur less frequently than with the tricyclic anti-depressants. Other possible harmful effects from maprotiline include drowsiness, dizziness, sweating, drop in blood pressure on standing up after sitting or lying down (this may produce faintness and light-headedness), tremor, pins and needles in the hands and feet, vivid dreams, skin rashes and impaired sexual functions. Serious harmful effects are very rare, but include damage to the bone marrow, producing blood disorders; liver damage, producing jaundice; and extreme excitement (hypomania). Mania and paranoid delusions may be made worse. Suddenly stopping the drug may produce insomnia, irritability and excessive sweating. Withdrawal symptoms in newborn babies may occur if the mother took the drug regularly during the last 3 months of pregnancy.

Warnings Maprotiline must not be used in anyone who suffers from mania, severe liver or kidney disease, narrow-angle glaucoma, retention of urine or recent myocardial infarction or who has

Table 39.1 Anti-depressant drugs – harmful effects and warnings (*cont.*)

a history of epilepsy. It should be used with caution in people with heart disease.

Risks in elderly people Harmful effects may be more frequent and severe, particularly agitation, confusion and a drop in blood pressure on standing up after sitting or lying down – this may produce faintness and light-headedness and cause an elderly person to fall. Smaller doses should be used and any increase in dosage should be carried out with utmost caution.

Risks with driving It may affect your ability to drive, so do not drive until you know that it is safe to do so.

Risks with alcohol It may increase the effects of alcohol, so do not drink alcohol if you are taking this drug.

mianserin (Bolvidon, Norval)

Harmful effects Drowsiness at the start of treatment is the most commonly occurring harmful effect. Occasionally, it may cause breast disorders (swelling, nipple tenderness, milk production), dizziness, fall in blood pressure on standing up after sitting or lying down (may produce faintness and light-headedness, especially in elderly people), swelling of the ankles, skin rash, sweating, tremor, painful joints and flu-like symptoms. Rarely, it may damage the bone marrow, resulting in serious blood disorders. This may occur after about 4–6 weeks of treatment and is reversible if the drug is stopped immediately. Liver damage with jaundice, excitement (hypomania) and convulsions may occur very rarely. Mania and paranoid delusions may be made worse.

Warnings It should not be used in people who suffer from mania or severe liver disease. It should be used with caution in anyone who has had a recent heart attack (myocardial infarction). It should, preferably, not be used in someone with a history of epilepsy, and it should be used with caution in people with diabetes, impaired liver or kidney function, narrow-angle glaucoma or enlarged prostate glands. Because of the (rare) risk of bone marrow damage producing serious blood disorders all patients should have a full blood count carried out *before* treatment and every 4 weeks during the first 3 months of treatment. Patients should report any sore throat, fever or sore mouth immediately and have a blood count carried out. The drug should be stopped immediately if jaundice, hypomania or convulsions occur, or if infection develops because of a reduced resistance caused by a fall in white blood cells due to bone marrow disease.

Risks in elderly people Harmful effects may be more frequent and severe; therefore it should be used with utmost caution and only small doses used to start treatment. Elderly people are more likely to suffer from damage to the bone marrow, causing serious blood disorders (see warnings above).

Risks with driving It may affect your ability to drive, so do not drive until you know that it is safe to do so.

Risks with alcohol It increases the effects of alcohol, so do not drink alcohol if you are taking this drug.

trazodone (Molipaxin)

Harmful effects It may cause drowsiness, and the following harmful effects occur occasionally: headache, nausea and vomiting, weakness, weight loss, tremor, dry mouth, changes in pulse rate (slow or fast), drop in blood pressure on standing up after sitting or lying down (may produce dizziness and light-headedness), constipation, blurred vision, restlessness, confusion, insomnia, skin rash and chronic erection of the penis (priapism). (If priapism occurs, the drug should be stopped immediately. The erection can be so severe as to require surgery, and occasionally it may cause lasting problems such as impaired erection or impotence.)

Warnings Trazodone should be used

Table 39.1 Anti-depressant drugs – harmful effects and warnings (*cont.*)

with caution in anyone who suffers from epilepsy (do not stop the drug suddenly), severe kidney disease or severe liver disease.

Risks in elderly people Harmful effects may be more frequent and severe; therefore use with caution.

Risks with driving It may affect your ability to drive, so do not drive until you know that it is safe to do so.

Risks with alcohol It may increase the effects of alcohol, so do not drink alcohol if you are taking this drug.

viloxazine (Vivalan)
Harmful effects It may cause nausea, headache, drowsiness and, occasionally, confusion, incoordination of movement (ataxia), dizziness, insomnia, tremor, pins and needles in the hands or feet, sweating, muscle and joint pains, mild rise in blood pressure and skin rashes. Anticholinergic effects (blurred vision, dry mouth, constipation, difficulty passing urine) occur less frequently than with the tricyclics. High doses are also less likely to cause a fall in blood pressure and harmful effects on the heart. Hypomania and aggression may be made worse. Very rarely, it may cause convulsions and liver damage, producing jaundice. Withdrawal symptoms may occur and include malaise, headache and vomiting.

Warnings It must not be used in anyone with mania, severe liver disease, a history of peptic ulcer or a recent heart attack (myocardial infarction). It should be used with caution in people with coronary heart disease (angina), congestive heart failure, heart block or epilepsy or in individuals who are at risk of committing suicide.

Risks in elderly people Harmful effects may be more frequent and severe; therefore use with caution. Use smaller doses and increase the dose only under strict medical supervision.

Risks with driving It may affect your ability to drive, so do not drive until you know that it is safe to do so.

Risks with alcohol It increases the effect of alcohol, so do not drink alcohol if you are taking this drug.

Monoamine oxidase inhibitor (MAOI) anti-depressant drugs

Monoamine oxidase is an enzyme present in the intestine, liver and brain, and it breaks down a group of stimulant neurotransmitters known as catecholamines (e.g. adrenaline and noradrenaline). Monoamine oxidase inhibitors (MAOIs) block this enzyme and therefore prolong the action of stimulant neurotransmitters. This action has a beneficial effect on the symptoms of depression in some people. However, their use has two major drawbacks – they also block the breakdown of other stimulant drugs and they can block the breakdown of stimulant chemicals in certain foods, to produce serious harmful effects.

The dangers of MAOIs blocking the breakdown of stimulant drugs

When monoamine oxidase is blocked, the body cannot break down naturally occurring stimulants such as adrenaline and noradrenaline; neither can it break down stimulant chemicals in medicines. MAOIs therefore increase the effects and dangers of stimulants such as sympathomimetic bronchodilator drugs used to treat asthma (e.g. isoprenaline, ephedrine); sympathomimetic drugs used as decongestants in cough and cold remedies (e.g. ephedrine, pseudoephedrine, phenylpropanolamine); amphetamine drugs used as stimulants; and amphetamine-related drugs used to suppress the appetite (e.g. fenfluramine) and as stimulants (e.g. methylphenidate). MAOIs also block the breakdown of dopamine, another stimulant nerve messenger, and if they are given with levodopa (a drug that is converted into dopamine by nerve cells and is used to treat parkinsonism), an excess level of dopamine may occur in the brain.

If someone who is on MAOI treatment takes one of the above drugs, a hypertensive crisis may occur: the blood pressure shoots up and the individual develops a severe headache, sweating, flushing, nausea, vomiting and palpitations. The rise in blood pressure may cause an artery in the brain to bleed which may cause death.

Severe reactions may also occur if an MAOI is taken with a tricyclic anti-depressant, especially amitriptyline or imipramine. A combination of the MAOI tranylcypromine and tricyclic clomipramine is particularly dangerous. Morphine and narcotic pain relievers may interact with MAOIs to produce a serious reaction, especially pethidine which may produce alarming effects, which include flushing, sweating, restlessness, muscle rigidity, depression of breathing, a fall in blood pressure and coma.

MAOI's may also prolong and intensify the effects of general anaesthetics, antihistamines, anticholinegic drugs, barbiturates and possibly other sleeping drugs, insulin and oral anti-diabetic drugs, and blood pressure-lowering drugs such as methyldopa, reserpine and guanethidine.

The dangers of MAOIs blocking the breakdown of stimulant chemicals in food

A most serious risk of MAOIs is that they can block the breakdown of stimulant chemicals in food and drink (e.g. tyramine in cheese and Chianti) and other stimulants in food (e.g. caffeine in chocolate and beverages, and levodopa in broad bean pods). In someone who is receiving treatment with MAOIs these stimulants are not broken down in the intestine and liver, and excessive amounts enter the main bloodstream and cause stimulation of the nervous system. This can produce a *hypertensive crisis*, see above.

The amount of tyramine in foods varies, depending upon their manufacture and storage, and the amount of tyramine taken into the body will depend upon the amount of tyramine-containing foods that are eaten. Protein foods that have been fermented, pickled, smoked or have gone off contain an increased amount of tyramine. Foods high in stimulant chemicals are listed later.

Warning *Stimulant drugs (see above) and foods and drinks containing stimulant chemicals (see below) should not be taken while on treatment with an MAOI and for 2 weeks after stopping such treatment.*

MAOIs should be used with caution

MAOIs are potentially dangerous drugs because of the harmful effects they may produce when taken with certain other drugs and foods. However, they can produce improvement in some people who are severely incapacitated by their depressive symptoms and in whom no other drug treatments work. In particular, individuals with atypical depression, in which anxiety and physical symptoms are dominant, and people who have severe phobias (e.g. agoraphobia) may be greatly helped by these drugs.

Table 39.2 Monoamine oxidase inhibitor anti-depressants (MAOIs) – harmful effects and warnings

Harmful effects These include dizziness, dry mouth, constipation, drop in blood pressure on standing after sitting or lying down, ankle swelling, drowsiness, weakness, fatigue, insomnia, stomach upsets, weight gain, tremor, twitching, agitation, blurred vision, difficulty in passing urine and, rarely, liver damage with jaundice, skin rashes, blood disorders, symptoms of mental illness and sexual disturbances. They may trigger mania and confusion. *Iproniazid* is more toxic than *phenelzine*, and in additon to those harmful effects listed above it may, rarely, cause inflammation of blood vessels (vasculitis) producing bleeding and bruising; and nerve damage producing numbness and pins and needles in the arms and legs. *Isocarboxazid* may, rarely, cause blood disorders, liver damage (hepatitis) and skin rashes.

Warnings MAOIs should not be given to anyone who is allergic to them, or who has a phaeochromocytoma, congestive heart failure, a history of liver disease or abnormal liver function tests, blood disorders, stroke or over-active thyroid gland. They should be used with caution in individuals with epilepsy.

Risks with certain other drugs and foods The most important risk when MAOIs are taken with certain other drugs and foods is the development of what is called a 'hypertensive crisis'. This crisis is produced by a sudden rise in blood pressure – the individual develops a severe headache starting at the back and spreading forward, palpitations, neck stiffness and soreness, nausea, vomiting, sweating (sometimes with fever and a cold, clammy skin), dilated pupils and discomfort on looking into the light. Either a fast or a slow heart beat may develop and be associated with a tight pain in the chest.

Bleeding into the brain may occur during one of these crises and deaths have occurred. The following foods and drugs should be avoided by anyone taking MAOIs and for 2 weeks after stopping them.

Foods and drinks high in stimulants: pickled herring, liver, dry sausages (salami, pepperoni), game, broad bean pods (fava bean pods), flavoured textured vegetable proteins, cheese (cottage cheese and cream cheese are allowed), yoghurt, banana skins. *Beers, lagers and wines* – it is best to avoid all alcoholic drinks, including low or alcohol free. *Yeast extracts* (e.g. Marmite), meat extracts (e.g. Bovril, Oxo). *Large amounts of chocolate* and drinks containing *caffeine* (tea, coffee, cola). Any foods that have undergone protein changes due to ageing, pickling, fermentation or smoking to improve flavour, particularly fish, meat, poultry and offal.

Over-the-counter medicines: cough and cold medicines, nasal decongestants, hayfever remedies, sinus remedies, asthma inhalant remedies, slimming remedies and 'pep' pills.

Prescription medicines: amphetamines, and amphetamine (e.g. diethylpropion) or amphetamine-related (e.g. fenfluramine) slimming drugs; cocaine; methylphenidate and pemoline used as stimulants; dopamine and dopamine precursors (e.g. levodopa used to treat parkinsonism); adrenaline, ephedrine and related bronchodilator sympathomimetic drugs used to treat asthma; phenylpropanolamine and other sympathomimetic drugs used in nasal decongestants, cold and cough remedies and hayfever preparations; methyldopa used to treat raised blood pressure; tyrosine, an amino acid used as a dietary supplement; phenylalanine, an amino acid that is an essential constituent of the diet and is used as a dietary supplement.

Risks with other drugs If you are on treatment with an MAOI, consult your pharmacist or doctor before taking any medicine (tablets, capsules, eye drops, nose drops, mouth sprays, suppositories, inhalants, etc.) whether prescribed by a doctor, dispensed by a pharmacist or bought from a pharmacy, drug store, supermarket, health food shop or herbalist.

Risks in elderly people MAOIs should, preferably, not be used in elderly people because of their potentially harmful effects.

Risk in driving MAOIs may produce dizziness and other symptoms that could interfere with your driving ability, so do not drive until you know that it is safe to do so.

Risks with alcohol Do not drink alcohol if you are taking an MAOI drug.

Lithium salts

Lithium salts are used to treat people suffering from severe states of excitement (manic illness) and to prevent relapse in patients suffering from manic–depressive illness in which periods of excitement alternate with periods of depression. Lithium calms patients down but we do not know how it works.

Balancing the benefits and risks of lithium

Lithium is short acting, and the margin between the dose that produces beneficial effects and the one that causes harmful effects is very narrow. It replaces sodium in the body, and its effects are very much determined by the level of sodium in the body. Loss of sodium from the body by restriction of fluids or the use of diuretics (water tablets) will increase the toxicity of lithium.

Harmful effects of lithium are related to dosage and vary according to the concentration of lithium in the blood. Toxic effects can also occur if the level of lithium in the blood rises too quickly, so it is important to divide the daily dose and take it at fixed intervals throughout the day.

Estimations of blood levels of lithium must be carried out every week at the start of the treatment in order to make sure that the concentration is within safe and effective limits (0.6–1.2 millimoles/litre). When levels remain steady, the frequency of blood tests may be reduced to once every month and then to every 2 months. Signs of toxicity include loss of control over voluntary movements (ataxia), rhythmic involuntary movements of the arms and legs (tremor), rhythmic movements of the eyes (nystagmus) and fits (convulsive siezures). Overdose may produce kidney damage. Different preparations of lithium may be absorbed into the bloodstream at different rates, and so the individual should always be kept on the same preparation when possible.

The effective use of lithium

Lithium treatment should be considered only for people with no heart or kidney disease and who take in a 'normal' amount of salt in their diets. It may be used to treat an acute attack of mania, to prevent recurrence of manic episodes in patients suffering from manic–depressive illness and to treat severe recurrent depression that does not respond to other treatment.

There is no doubt that lithium regulates mood and may benefit some people. However, it is a dangerous drug and should be used only by experts who are fully knowledgeable about the effects it may produce in the body. Regular estimations of the level of lithium in the blood are essential for its safe use and it should not be used where laboratory facilities for such measurements are not available.

Other drugs used to treat depression

Tryptophan

Tryptophan is an amino acid, and an essential constituent of the diet. It is a chemical forerunner (precursor) of a stimulant nerve messenger in the body called serotonin (or 5-hydroxytryptamine: 5HT), a deficiency of which is considered to be associated with a depressed mood. Two vitamins (pyridoxine and vitamin C) are involved in the conversion of tryptophan to serotonin. For this reason, they have been included in preparations of tryptophan used to treat depression.

Warning *Tryptophan preparations (e.g. Pacitron and Optimax) have been voluntarily withdrawn from the market because of reports that products containing tryptophan may cause a serious disorder called oesinophilia–myalgia, which results in fever, skin rashes, painful muscles, fluid retention and disorders of the lungs and nerves.*

Vitamin B_6 (pyridoxine)

In people deficient in pyridoxine (e.g. some women taking an oral contraceptive drug) the metabolism of tryptophan may be abnormal unless additional vitamin B_6 is taken. However, there is disagreement as to whether the use of vitamin B_6 prevents depression in some women on the pill.

Carbamazepine (*Tegretol*)

This drug is normally used to treat epilepsy, but it is also helpful in treating some patients suffering from manic–depression and in whom lithium does not work. It helps to reduce mood swings.

Flupenthixol

This is an anti-psychotic drug used to treat serious mental illness such as schizophrenia. However, it may also be useful in some people with depression. If given in low doses, it may help to reduce the withdrawn apathy and lack of response that may affect some depressed patients.

Table 39.3 Anti-depressant drugs

Preparation	*Drug*	*Drug group*	*Dosage form*
Allegron	nortriptyline	Tricyclic anti-depressant	Tablets
amitriptyline	amitriptyline	Tricyclic anti-depressant	Tablets
Anafranil	clomipramine	Tricyclic anti-depressant	Capsules, syrup, injection
Anafranil SR	clomipramine	Tricyclic anti-depressant	Tablets (sustained-release)
Asendis	amoxapine	Tricyclic anti-depressant	Tablets

Table 39.3 Anti-depressant drugs (*cont.*)

Preparation	*Drug*	*Drug group*	*Dosage form*
Aventyl	nortriptyline	Tricyclic anti-depressant	Capsules
Bolvidon	mianserin	Tetracyclic anti-depressant	Tablets
Camcolit	lithium carbonate	Lithium salt	Tablets (sustained-release)
Concordin	protriptyline	Tricyclic anti-depressant	Tablets
Domical	amitriptyline	Tricyclic anti-depressant	Tablets
Elavil	amitriptyline	Tricyclic anti-depressant	Tablets
Evadyne	butriptyline	Tricyclic anti-depressant	Tablets
Faverin	fluvoxamine	5HT re-uptake blocker	Enteric coated tablets
Fluanxol	flupenthixol	Anti-psychotic	Tablets
Gamanil	lofepramine	Tricyclic anti-depressant	Tablets
imipramine	imipramine	Tricyclic anti-depressant	Tablets
Lentizol	amitriptyline	Tricyclic anti-depressant	Capsules (sustained-release)
Liskonum	lithium carbonate	Lithium salt	Tablets (sustained-release)
Litarex	lithium citrate	Lithium salt	Tablets (sustained-release)
Ludiomil	maprotiline	Tetracyclic anti-depressant	Tablets
Marplan	isocarboxazid	MAOI	Tablets
mianserin	mianserin	Tetracyclic anti-depressant	Tablets
Molipaxin	trazodone	Triazolopyridine	Capsules, tablets, liquid
Nardil	phenelzine	MAOI	Tablets
Norval	mianserin	Tetracyclic anti-depressant	Tablets
Parnate	tranylcypromine	MAOI	Tablets
Parstelin	tranylcypromine	MAOI	Tablets
Pertofran	desipramine	Tricyclic anti-depressant	Tablets
Phasal	lithium carbonate	Lithium salt	Tablets (sustained-release)
Priadel	lithium carbonate	Lithium salt	Tablets (sustained-release), sugar-free liquid

Table 39.3 Anti-depressant drugs (*cont.*)

Preparation	*Drug*	*Drug group*	*Dosage form*
Prondol	iprindole	Tricyclic anti-depressant	Tablets
Prothiaden	dothiepin	Tricyclic anti-depressant	Capsules, tablets
Prozac	fluoxetine	5HT re-uptake blocker	Capsules
Sinequan	doxepin	Tricyclic anti-depressant	Capsules
Surmontil	trimipramine	Tricyclic anti-depressant	Tablets, capsules
Tegretol	carbamazepine	Anti-epileptic	Tablets, liquid
Tofranil	imipramine	Tricyclic anti-depressant	Tablets, syrup
Tryptizol	amitriptyline	Tricyclic anti-depressant	Capsules, tablets, syrup, injection
Vivalan	viloxazine	Oxazine anti-depressant	Tablets

Table 39.4 Combined anti-depressant drug preparations

Preparation	*Drug*	*Drug group*	*Dosage form*
Limbitrol 5 + 10	amitriptyline	Tricyclic anti-depressant	Capsules
	chlordiazepoxide	Benzodiazepine	
Motipress	nortriptyline	Tricyclic anti-depressant	Tablets
	fluphenazine	Phenothiazine anti-psychotic	
Motival	fluphenazine	Phenothiazine anti-psychotic	Tablets
	nortriptyline	Tricyclic anti-depressant	
Parstelin	tranylcypromine	MAOI	Tablets
	trifluoperazine	Phenothiazine anti-psychotic	
Triptafen and Triptafen M	amitriptyline	Tricyclic anti-depressant	Tablets
	perphenazine	Anti-psychotic	

Overview of the drug treatment of depression

Anti-depressant drugs are very effective at relieving the symptoms of depression. Although they do not cure the depression, they enable you to cope more effectively. In addition to relieving mental symptoms and lifting mood, anti-depressant drugs relieve many of the physical problems associated with depression such as difficulty with sleeping, loss of appetite, lack of energy, aches and pains, loss of weight and loss of interest in sex.

Choice of anti-depressant drugs

The tricyclic anti-depressants are the drugs of choice for treating moderate to severe depressive illness unless it is so severe that immediate electric shock treatment is indicated. They are most effective for treating endogenous depression (see earlier) associated with physical symptoms such as loss of appetite, loss of weight, loss of libido, lack of energy and disturbed sleep.

Controlled studies of the tricyclic anti-depressants have shown that they are roughly equal in their effectiveness when treating groups of patients. However, between individuals there may be a variation in response and some people do better on one tricyclic drug than another. It is important, therefore that the treatment for depression is tailored to each individual's needs.

The tricyclic anti-depressants differ mainly in the amount of sedation they produce and these differences can be usefully exploited. If sleep is disturbed, it may help to use a tricyclic drug that produces sedation (e.g. amitriptyline) in a single daily dose at bed-time; however, someone who is quiet and withdrawn may benefit from a tricyclic drug that stimulates (e.g. protriptyline) given in divided doses throughout the day.

Because of the time-lag between starting treatment and the lifting of the depression, it may occasionally be necessary for someone suffering from severe depression to be given electroconvulsive therapy (ECT), particularly if there is a serious risk of suicide. Some tricyclics such as amoxapine (Asendis) appear to act more quickly than others and may be worth trying. Sufferers should be advised that initial harmful effects such as dry mouth, blurred vision and constipation wear off within a week or two and that they should persist with treatment. It will help if they start on small daily doses that are then gradually increased every few days.

Failure of an individual to benefit from a tricyclic anti-depressant drug may mean that the blood level of the drug is too low to be effective, which may be caused by the patient failing to take the drug as directed or because the prescribed dose is too low.

Maprotiline, mianserin, trazodone or *viloxazine* have not been shown to be more effective in relieving symptoms of depression than the tricyclic anti-depressants despite claims of faster onset of action and less drowsiness. They produce fewer anticholinergic effects and fewer harmful effects on the heart and circulation but convulsions, damage to the bone marrow and liver changes, although very rare, occur more frequently than with the tricyclic drugs. They offer an alternative to the tricyclic drugs, as do *fluoxetine* and *fluroxamine*

The *monoamine oxidase inhibitors* may work when tricyclic and other anti-depressants fail. They are particularly useful in people with atypical depression (see earlier) especially in those with panic attacks and phobias (e.g. agoraphobia).

Lithium may be used to treat acute attacks of mania, to prevent recurrence of manic episodes in people suffering from manic–depressive illness and to treat severe recurrent depression that does not respond to other treatment. It reduces the number and severity of subsequent episodes. Treatment has to be continued for an indefinite period but it usually involves just one dose a day. Stopping treatment with lithium should be considered only if the individual remains well over several months with a minimum of symptoms. Initial treatment of an acute episode may have to include the use of an anti-psychotic drug (see Chapter 40) in high doses because it takes a few days before lithium starts to work. However, see risks of drug interactions – Chapter 89.

Carbamazepine (Tegretol) is an anti-epileptic drug that may be effective in patients with manic–depressive illness or who suffer from multiple mood swings and do not respond to lithium. It may be added to lithium treatment or substituted for it.

Flupenthixol (Fluanxol) is a phenothiazine anti-psychotic drug that may be beneficial in patients who are withdrawn, despondent and apathetic.

Treatment with anti-depressants must be individualized

In addition to the selection of a particular anti-depressant drug, its daily dosage must be tailored to an individual's response, particularly the balance between relief of symptoms of depression and harmful effects produced by the treatment.

During intial treatment, harmful effects such as drowsiness, dry mouth and constipation may be dominant and it takes a few weeks for the beneficial effects to develop. Treatment should be continued for 6 weeks and if there is no improvement the dose should be increased or the drug changed. Once improvement occurs it is important for the dose to be adjusted to achieve maximum relief of depressive symptoms and then to keep treatment at this effective level for a further 2–3 months before attempting to reduce the dose slowly over several weeks. If the depressive symptoms recur on reducing the dose, the treatment should be continued for a further few months and another attempt made to reduce the dose, and so on. Some patients may need long-term treatment for many months or even years. Sometimes in severe depression an individual may initially be very anxious and agitated and it may then be necessary to give a phenothiazine anti-psychotic drug, or an anti-anxiety drug with an anti-depressant drug at the start of treatment. However, such a combination should be used with caution and only for a short period of time until the anti-depressant has started to work and the anxiety and agitation have passed.

Comment

About 10–20 per cent of sufferers do not respond to anti-depressant drugs. This high rate of failure may be due to several factors. A person treated with an anti-depressant drug may not respond to treatment because the diagnosis was not correct, or the dose was inadequate, or the most appropriate anti-depressant drug for the individual's particular needs was not used. Treatment may also fail if he or she cannot tolerate the harmful effects or does not take the drug as directed. Many failed treatments are due to under-treatment, and it may help if the doctor carries out estimations of the concentration of the drug in the blood in order to monitor the patient's progress. The blood level of an anti-depressant drug should be high enough to be effective and low enough not to cause harmful effects.

40

Anxiety

Anxiety is an unpleasant feeling of tension and apprehension. It produces the same feelings as fear. We can all feel anxious in response to a threat or danger, some more than others; but when feelings of anxiety become severe and continuous, particularly without any obvious cause, you have a problem. When you are this anxious you may also develop incapacitating fears about simple everyday activities such as going out of the house alone. You may develop sheer panic attacks for no obvious reason. These may occur, for example, while you are travelling on a bus, sitting in the hairdressers or shopping in a supermarket.

Long-standing anxiety gives you a feeling of hopelessness as if you cannot cope any more. You find it difficult to think straight, you cannot make decisions and you develop all sorts of physical symptoms such as headache, giddiness, breathlessness, palpitations, stomach upsets, backache, restlessness and, above all, fatigue. You may worry that you have a physical disease or are going out of your mind.

The symptoms you feel are telling you that there is something very seriously wrong in your life. It may be obvious and totally devastating such as the death of a loved one, a divorce or being made redundant. Or you may have long-standing conflicts, for example with your marriage, with your children or parents, about your role in life, about your job and so on. Many experiences come together to cause anxiety, not only present day ones but ones from your past life. Some conflicts in your life sort themselves out but others can go on for years. Some of these conflicts may require tough decisions and there is no doubt that inability to make a decision produces further anxiety, particularly if you have no one to listen to you or to help you discuss your problems.

If you become so anxious and tense that it is affecting your ability to cope with everyday living, you need help to recognize and to try to understand why you are anxious and tense. You will need advice and help on how to cope. You will need to be taught how to relax both physically and mentally in order not to become totally exhausted by your tensions. You will also need help to regain your self-confidence. Clearly, none of these can be achieved by the use of anti-anxiety drugs.

The group of physical and mental symptoms labelled anxiety and depression cannot easily be separated; therefore I suggest that you read the introduction to Chapter 39 on depression as well as reading this chapter.

Anti-anxiety drugs

Up to the mid-sixties the most commonly used drugs to calm you down were the barbiturates. They were also used as sleeping drugs. They were prescribed extensively and indiscriminately by the million every year despite warnings about the dangers of addiction and overdosage. As a consequence, many patients became dependent on them and/or died as a result of intentional or accidental poisoning, particularly when they were taken with alcohol.

When barbiturates are used to calm you down (as sedatives) the gap between making you calm and making you drowsy is very narrow, which means you can easily become drowsy. That is why they were also used extensively as sleeping drugs.

In the fifties and sixties several new groups of drugs were introduced which were supposed to calm you down without producing drowsiness. Some only lasted a few years before they were withdrawn because they produced more dependence than the barbiturates; others are still around – for example, the meprobamates and the benzodiazepines. The former are no longer fashionable and so these days when we talk about anti-anxiety drugs we are really talking about the *benzodiazepines* – the 'downers' of the seventies and eighties.

Benzodiazepines

When used in 'calming' doses rather than 'sleeping' doses to relieve the symptoms of anxiety, the gap between calming you down and making you drowsy is much greater with some of the benzodiazepines than with the barbiturates. They are also much safer when an overdose is taken. Therefore, when they were introduced in the fifties and sixties they clearly needed a new image. The old term 'sedative' (a drug that calms you down) was obviously not suitable for the late fifties and 'swinging' sixties, and so they were marketed as 'tranquillizers' and advertisements to doctors carried tranquil scenes of sandy beaches, calm seas and swaying palm trees.

Benzodiazepines were not the first mood-altering drugs to be called tranquillizers. Meprobamate and related drugs had already been marketed as tranquillizers, and a decade earlier drugs used to treat schizophrenia and related serious mental disorders had also been marketed as tranquillizers; so to differentiate between them, the ones used to treat serious mental illness were referred to as *major tranquillizers*, and the benzodiazepines and other drugs used to treat mild symptoms of anxiety were called *minor tranquillizers*. This also differentiated them from the barbiturates, which were still referred to as sedatives. However, some barbiturates and some benzodiazepines were also marketed as sleeping drugs (see Chapter 38).

The terms minor and major tranquillizers are now obsolete, and we should talk about *anti-psychotic drugs* instead of major tranquillizers and *anti-anxiety drugs* instead of minor tranquillizers. Nevertheless, the term 'tranquillizers' is now part of our language. Today, the term tranquillizer usually refers to the benzodiazepines but some people still apply it to anti-psychotic drugs used to treat serious mental illness. However, there are dangers in using the term to describe all drugs that calm you down because those people who are against their use sometimes do not seem to understand that anti-psychotic drugs (the so-called 'major' tranquillizers) are an important and valuable part of treatment for patients suffering from schizophrenia and other serious mental illnesses, whereas anti-anxiety drugs (the 'minor' tranquillizers) are usually used to treat minor self-limiting symptoms caused by everyday problems of living. These differences should be recognized. Furthermore, patients can become dependent on the benzodiazepines and other anti-anxiety drugs, whereas they can not become dependent on the anti-psychotic drugs.

The start of the benzodiazepine bonanza

When various benzodiazepines were introduced on to the market in the sixties and early seventies, millions of pounds were spent world wide by the manufacturers to 'inform' doctors that anxiety and stress associated with ordinary everyday problems of living could be relieved by taking anti-anxiety drugs. Doctors were encouraged to respond to a patient's everyday problems of living as 'medical' problems needing drug treatment. Doctors were soon persuaded and within a few years of the first benzodiazepines being launched they issued millions of prescriptions for them annually. Benzodiazepines rapidly became among the top five drugs prescribed in most countries in the Western world. Despite this massive use of anti-anxiety drugs, the doctors knew no more about how to treat patients suffering from emotional problems than previously. They merely resorted to treating all kinds of physical and mental symptoms with anti-anxiety drugs. They successfully defined for their patients a method of coping with stress (i.e. pop a 'downer') and made sure that their patients had an endless supply by allowing them to pick up a repeat prescription every month from their receptionist without ever having to be bothered to see a doctor.

History repeats itself

The recent media interest in the misuse and dangers of benzodiazepines is like history repeating itself. A similar attack against the barbiturates occurred in the media in the late sixties, and doctors ran their own campaign to restrict the prescribing of those drugs. This was successful in so far as the prescribing of barbiturates decreased significantly. But patients were not provided with alternatives to drug treatment, they were merely given unlimited access to another group of downers – the benzodiazepines. In fact, the use of these drugs soon outstripped the excessive use of the barbiturates in the fifties and sixties. It was like having an air bed full of downers – you dented one part of it only to see another part bulging right up, and what is more the bed itself was getting bigger because more and more downers were being pumped into it by doctors!

The use of benzodiazepines by doctors

Throughout the seventies and into the eighties millions of prescriptions for benzodiazepine tablets and capsules were issued to patients. Some doctors applied little or no control over their supply, and many patients were kept on benzodiazepine anti-anxiety drugs for years on end, often for a disorder that did not need treating with such drugs in the first place. Unfortunately, some of these patients became dependent on their benzodiazepines.

The benzodiazepines were used by doctors to treat all kinds of physical and mental symptoms, often because they did not know what else to do. Twice as many women as men were prescribed benzodiazepines, probably because some doctors tended to see women as being less able to cope than men. This view of women was strengthened by advertisements for anti-anxiety drugs in doctors' journals in the late sixties and early seventies. These often carried pictures of harassed housewives with the clear message that the only way they would be able to cope was to pop a benzodiazepine!

As we move into the early nineties the situation is changing. The use of benzodiazepines is being repeatedly appraised in medical journals and their prescription is falling; but we are left with many thousands of people who are still dependent on them.

Effects produced by benzodiazepine

Benzodiazepines (e.g. Valium) are the most commonly used drugs to treat anxiety. They are referred to as anti-anxiety drugs, anxiolytics, anxiolytic sedatives, minor tranquillizers or tranquillizers.

All benzodiazepine drugs produce similar effects on the body. They calm you down if you are tense (anxiolytic effect), they may make you drowsy and send you to sleep (sedative–hypnotic effect), they relax muscles (muscle relaxant effect) and they can stop fits (anti-convulsant effect).

They act on the brain and spinal cord and, as the dose is increased, they produce drowsiness, sleep and then stupor. In high doses, they do not act on the brain like an anaesthetic but you feel as if you have had an anaesthetic because you lose your memory for events just after taking the drug, even though you were aware at the time of what was happening to you. This is why some dentists use these drugs and why you may be given them before surgery.

Benzodiazepines are 'downers' because they work like the 'dampening down' chemicals in the brain that are released naturally to block receptors in the nerve pathways excited by fear and tension. The benzodiazepines attach themselves to these receptors and block the pathways, reducing the feelings of fear and tension and therefore calming you down. In fact, these receptors are called 'benzodiazepine receptors' and it appears that the body produces its own 'benzodiazepines' to calm you down. This is one of the many interesting discoveries to come out of research into the effects of benzodiazepines on the brain.

Benzodiazepines also reduce the 'electrical' excitation of brain cells which occurs during a convulsion, and some of them are used to treat people suffering from epilepsy (see Chapter 37).

In high doses all benzodiazepines cause drowsiness and sleep, but some do this more than others at lower doses. This is why some of the benzodiazepines are marketed as sleeping drugs and some as anti-anxiety drugs. It is also why those used to treat anxiety should be taken in divided doses throughout the day in order to avoid a concentration in the brain high enough to produce drowsiness and sleep. This latter danger is particularly important in elderly people because the drugs last much longer in their bodies and so it is easy for a high concentration to accumulate in their brains.

Duration of action and risks of harmful effects

Benzodiazepines vary in how quickly they work and in the duration of their effects. This is related to the capacity of the body to get rid of them. They are broken down in the liver and passed out by the kidneys in the urine. Therefore, disorders of the liver and kidneys may produce a delay in getting rid of them and lead to toxic levels in the body. This may happen in elderly people, whose kidneys may not work as efficiently as when they were younger.

Intermediate-acting benzodiazepines (see Table 40.3) produce earlier and more intense withdrawal symptoms if they are stopped suddenly (see later) but there is a reduced risk of their accumulating in the body to produce harmful effects.

Long-acting benzodiazepines (see Table 40.3) usually cause less of a problem with regard to withdrawal symptoms (see later), but when taken regularly every day they and/or their breakdown products accumulate in the body, which may cause serious problems in individuals with impaired liver or kidney function who are not able to break them down or excrete them efficiently. The same risk applies to elderly people, who may also have some impaired functioning of their kidneys.

Harmful effects of benzodiazepines

The harmful effects produced by the benzodiazepines are listed in Table 40.1. Common harmful effects include drowsiness, light-headedness, fatigue, loss of control over voluntary movements (ataxia) and slurred speech. These effects may occur after a single dose as well as after repeated doses, and they may persist into the following day. They may be particularly harmful to elderly people.

Paradoxical effects

Occasionally, benzodiazepines may produce opposite effects (paradoxical effects) in some people. Instead of acting as 'downers' they act as 'uppers' and the indivudual becomes excited, aggressive and anxious. In a susceptible person an underlying depression may be triggered and the individual might become suicidal.

Tolerance, dependence and addiction to benzodiazepines

Tolerance

Tolerance to benzodiazepines may develop whether they are used to relieve anxiety or to promote sleep. This means that, after repeated doses, the drug may not work as effectively as it did at first and so, in order to obtain the same effects, it may be necessary to increase the dose.

Tolerance is a general phenomenon which may occur with many drugs. It may come on rapidly after only a few doses (this is called tachyphylaxis) or it may take days or weeks of regular daily use before it develops. Tolerance to a drug may be due to changes in how the body deals with it over time; for example, an increase in the rate of breakdown of the drug by the liver will reduce its concentration in the blood and at its sites of action, resulting in a reduction of its effectiveness.

Tolerance may also occur due to changes in the body caused by cells *adapting* to the actions of the drug. After repeated doses, physico-chemical changes occur, particularly in the cells of the brain and nervous system, which result in a reduced response by those cells to the same concentration of the drug. These effects may lead the user to increase the dose in order to produce the same level of response that was experienced with the original doses. Increasing the dose will increase the concentration of the drug at its sites of action and temporarily override the adaption of the cells. This type of tolerance occurs with the benzodiazepines.

Compared with non-tolerant individuals, those who become tolerant to the effects of a drug may experience not only a reduction in desired effects but also a reduction of undesired effects. However, as the dose increases there is progressively less difference between the harmful effects experienced by non-tolerant and by tolerant individuals, so the dangers of overdose become similar.

Because of tolerance to undesired effects, individuals who have increased their daily dose of a drug to compensate for tolerance to the desired effects, may not experience symptoms or show signs that they are taking an increased dose each day. In other words, it may not be obvious to a prescribing doctor that a patient is taking a higher daily dose than was prescribed at the start of treatment. This highlights the importance of checking the quantities of such a drug issued on repeat prescriptions over a fixed time. However, if people take doses in excess of what their bodies have adapted to, they may show signs of intoxication which, in the case of benzodiazepines, will be similar to those displayed by people intoxicated by alcohol.

Tolerance to a drug such as a benzodiazepine does not directly increase the probability that individuals may need to go on taking that drug, but the fact that they become involved with taking an increased dose may reinforce their perceived needs and a pattern of use may develop which might ultimately become compulsive (see below).

Psychological dependence

An important risk with taking benzodiazepines or similar drugs is that some individuals will eventually come to rely (or depend) on them. The intensity of this dependence may vary from a mild feeling that they cannot cope without the drug to a feeling of panic if they run out of a supply and a preoccupation with ensuring that they never do.

Some individuals may develop a craving for the drug and a compulsion to go on taking it, and the actual act of taking it then re-enforces their compulsion, which continues regardless of the severity and nature of the initial disorder being treated. In these people the drug produces a compulsion both by relieving unpleasant feelings and by producing pleasurable ones, and the facts that the drug is self-administered and that the desired effects are self-induced also contribute to its compulsive use.

Some regular users of a drug such as a benzodiazepine will become compulsive in their use; others may become reliant (dependent) upon it but not compulsive in their behaviour; yet others will become neither reliant nor compulsive. Clearly, different individuals will respond differently to the same drug. Moreover, different individuals respond differently to emotional upsets that may produce different physical and/or mental symptoms of varying degrees of intensity. Some people will be more sensitive to these symptoms than others, and may be less able to tolerate such symptoms without seeking relief; of these, some may find greater relief than others from a prescribed drug which may effectively suppress their symptoms. They may also be less able to tolerate any unpleasant symptoms that develop if the dose of the drug is reduced or the drug is stopped, and this may contribute to their reliance upon the drug.

The benefits that individuals experience from taking a mood-altering drug such as a benzodiazepine will depend on many factors. These include the drug and its dosage, the social situation in which the individuals find themselves, their personality and their ability to cope with the strains of everyday living. These complex factors interact and so it is almost impossible to predict which individuals may be vulnerable to the dependence-producing properties of a drug. Clearly someone who has previously been dependent on a mood-altering drug such as alcohol may be more vulnerable than others.

Physical dependence

Physical dependence refers to a physical state caused by the repeated use of a mood-altering drug. This physical state, which may affect many cells in the body but particularly those in the brain and nervous system, is an attempt by these cells to adapt to the changes which the drug produces – it is sometimes referred to as neuro-adaptation. Once this changed physicochemical state has developed, the drug must be taken at regular intervals or else the adaptation fails and the affected cells will react in such a way that the individual develops unpleasant and unwanted symptoms. These are referred to as *withdrawal symptoms* and they can be very severe if the drug is stopped abruptly. The complex of symptoms that occurs when a drug is stopped abruptly is sometimes referred to as an *abstinence syndrome*.

Some withdrawal symptoms are a flare-up of the symptoms that the drug had damped down; for example, anxiety may return when an anti-anxiety drug is stopped, and sleep may be disturbed when a sleeping drug is stopped. This rebound effect may cause the symptoms to be much worse than they were before the drug was started. Other withdrawal symptoms are an exaggeration of the opposite effects produced by the drug; for example, if a drug calms the individual by depressing the function of the brain and nervous system, its sudden withdrawal may trigger the opposite effects – excitation of the brain and nervous system which may result in severe anxiety, restlessness and even convulsions if the drug is stopped abruptly. Withdrawal symptoms when a benzodiazepine is stopped abruptly include excitement, restlessness, agitation, confusion, delusions, hallucinations and convulsions. They are similar to those that occur if barbiturates or alcohol are stopped abruptly. Because of these similarities, benzodiazepines are described as producing physical dependence of the barbiturate/alcohol type.

The appearance of withdrawal symptoms will depend upon the degree of alteration of function that cells in the brain and nervous system have undergone in order to adapt to the actions of the drug. The severity of withdrawal symptoms will be determined by the dose of the drug and the duration of its use, and the speed of appearance and the intensity of symptoms will depend on how fast the drug is removed from its sites of action in the body.

Short-acting drugs that are rapidly broken down and excreted by the body will produce a rapid onset of withdrawal symptoms if they are stopped suddenly, and the symptoms will last for a shorter period of time than those produced by long-acting drugs that are broken down and excreted more slowly. A long-acting drug will produce a more gradual onset of withdrawal symptoms and they will be more protracted because it may take several days for the drug to be completely cleared from its sites of action.

Withdrawal symptoms may be severe and develop very rapidly if a drug is given to block (antagonize) the effects of the drug at its sites of action. Such antagonists are used to treat overdosage with certain drugs; for example, a morphine antagonist may be used to treat morphine overdose and a benzodiazepine antagonist may be used to treat benzodiazepine overdose.

Cells in the brain and nervous system that are affected by the actions of a mood-altering drug start to adapt to its effects *from the very first dose*; depending upon the drug, the dose and the frequency of dosage, it may be a matter of hours, days or weeks before an individual develops a physical dependence sufficient to produce withdrawal symptoms if the drug is stopped abruptly.

With short- to intermediate-acting drugs the desired effects may wear off between doses and the individuals may experience a rebound of unpleasant symptoms until the next dose is taken. This may reinforce the need to go on taking the drug, and craving between doses may develop, resulting in compulsive use. An example of withdrawal effects is the day-time anxiety that may follow the nightly use of a short-acting sleeping drug.

Cross-dependence

The ability of one drug to relieve the symptoms caused by the withdrawal of another drug and its ability to maintain physical dependence is referred to as cross-dependence. This ability is related more to the similar effects the drugs produce in the body than to any chemical similarity. Cross-dependence may be partial or complete. Most anti-anxiety drugs, sedatives, sleeping drugs and alcohol can produce cross-dependence. A drug's ability to produce cross-dependence with another dependence-producing drug may therefore serve as a warning that the drug might have a potential for producing dependence.

Addiction

'Addiction' is a commonly used term although it is often misused and misunderstood. It is a useful term if its use is restricted to the description of dependence associated with a type of behaviour that includes compulsive use, an overwhelming desire to go on taking the drug even though harmful consequences of such actions are recognized, and a preoccupation with obtaining a supply of the drug. Addiction therefore refers to the drug-related *behaviour* of a dependent drug user, and it is important to note that an individual may be physically dependent on a drug but not addicted to it in so far as he or she does not display an addictive pattern of behaviour.

Benzodiazepine withdrawal symptoms

Many statements are made about the extent of dependence and addiction to benzodiazepines but these have usually come from studies of small numbers of patients and it is difficult to apply such findings to the millions of patients throughout the world who take benzodiazepines. Therefore it is not possible to make even a reasonable guess as to how many patients are physically dependent on them.

However, a substantial number of individuals who have taken a benzodiazepine regularly every day for more than 2–3 weeks will experience some withdrawal effects if they stop the drug abruptly, particularly if they have been using higher than average doses. They may experience a few or many of the following symptoms: increased anxiety, tension and panic; depression and feelings of suicide; irritability and outbursts of rage; overactivity and poor concentration; poor sleep and unpleasant and sometimes terrifying dreams; headaches, nausea and loss of appetite; a metallic taste in the mouth; palpitations, trembling, faintness, dizziness and sweating, flu-like symptoms, tight chest and pains in the stomach; and pain and stiffness in the jaw, face, head, neck and shoulders. They may become aware of sensations in their body – for example, creeping sensations in the skin – and they may become very sensitive to light, noise, touch and smell. They may get strange feelings of movement; feel depersonalized as if they are not themselves; feel unreal as if they are in a dream; and develop a fear of going out. Their arms and legs may feel heavy and wobbly, and they may develop pins and needles in them.

These symptoms may occur 2–3 days after stopping an intermediate-acting benzodiazepine. With long-acting ones these withdrawal symptoms occur in about 7 days after stopping the drug. In either case, symptoms usually last from 1 to 3 weeks but may go on for months.

Anxiety on stopping benzodiazepines

Anxiety (see earlier) may be a serious problem after stopping benzodiazepines, and may be worse than the symptoms individuals experienced before they ever started taking the drugs. It is like lifting a fire blanket off a smouldering anxiety that has been damped down by the drugs: it suddenly bursts into flames when the drug is stopped. These symptoms are both physical and mental but they will slowly burn themselves out over a few weeks to months. However, this burning out can be very painful. Some people may develop panic attacks which are so severe that they may become housebound and never want to go out for fear of developing an attack. During an attack, breathing may become rapid, the heart may beat quickly, and there may be light-headedness and dizziness. Sweating and trembling may occur and the legs may 'turn to jelly'. A feeling of total panic may develop as if something totally catastrophic is going to happen. These attacks last for only a few seconds and nothing does happen but the sufferer is left feeling totally exhausted. Some of these symptoms may be caused by rapid breathing, and there is no doubt that controlled breathing (from the abdomen) may stop some of them from developing.

How to withdraw benzodiazepines

If you have been taking a benzodiazepine regularly, whether for weeks, months or years, and wish to stop the drug with a minimum of withdrawal symptoms, it is important to reduce the daily dose of your drug slowly and to be prepared to experience a few or many symptoms in varying degrees of intensity. In addition to reducing the daily dose of the drug, you may need advice and counselling from your doctor or other health care worker, particularly a clinical psychologist. You will certainly need help from your closest relatives and friends, and you may find it useful to attend a self-help group. Relaxation tapes from your doctor or clinical psychologist may help you. These tapes contain instructions on how to relax to pleasant relaxing music. However, it is beyond the scope of this book to go into further detail and I will concentrate on how to withdraw the drugs.

Guidelines on withdrawing benzodiazepines

1. Change from an intermediate- to a long-acting benzodiazepine

When intermediate-acting benzodiazepines (see Table 40.3) are stopped, withdrawal symptoms come on more quickly and are more intense than if a long-acting drug is stopped. Therefore, if you are taking an intermediate-acting benzodiazepine it helps to replace it slowly, one dose at a time, with an equivalent dose of a long-acting one (e.g. diazepam).

2. Slowly and in gradual steps reduce the daily dose of the long-acting benzodiazepine

Once you have switched over from an intermediate-acting benzodiazepine to a long-acting one, or if you were on a long-acting drug in the first place, you need to withdraw the long-acting benzodiazepine gradually over several weeks or months, according to how you feel.

Different people will react differently to withdrawal, and the important point is to reduce the daily dose of your drug according to how you are feeling and not according to this schedule or that schedule. The trouble is that 'withdrawal' of benzodiazepines has been taken over by competing professional groups and all manner of schedules and guidelines keep appearing. These are often very subjective and based on experience with a relatively few individuals compared with the thousands of people who are dependent on benzodiazepines.

There is no magic to withdrawal and what is necessary is a gradual stepwise reduction in your daily intake of drugs. The trouble is that the doses of these drugs vary, and this can make it difficult to reduce the daily dose slowly. However, most are available in 2 mg tablets that can be broken in half and then quarters. For example, if you are taking diazepam (Valium) you should ask your doctor to switch your strength of tablets from whatever they are (e.g. 5 mg, 10 mg) to 2 mg tablets. This means that if you had been on one 10 mg tablet three times a day you should now be on five 2 mg tablets three times a day – i.e. 15 tablets daily.

A suitable withdrawal schedule would then be to reduce your daily dose by half a tablet (1 mg) or a whole tablet (2 mg) every 1 or 2 weeks, according to how you feel. As I said earlier, if you are taking an intermediate-acting benzodiazepine, it will help if you switch to a long-acting one and then slowly reduce the dose step by step over several weeks or months.

Rapid withdrawal

You can undergo *rapid* withdrawal, if you wish, by a stepwise reduction in daily dosage over a period of 5–6 weeks – it really is up to you and how you feel. However, withdrawal symptoms may be more intense, particularly if you have been taking high daily doses for many months or years.

Blood sugar

A low blood sugar may produce symptoms of anxiety in some people and aggravate withdrawal symptoms. It is important, therefore, to cut down on sweets, chocolates, cakes, biscuits, pastries, etc. Initially these help because they push up your blood sugar, but then the pancreas produces large amounts of insulin in response to the high blood sugar and this drives your blood sugar right down – what is called rebound hypoglycaemia (low blood sugar). To prevent these excess fluctuations in your blood sugar levels it is sensible to eat at regular intervals, particularly in the mornings and to eat a well balanced diet that contains adequate protein and fibre (wholemeal bread, cereals, vegetables). *Alcohol* and *caffeine* can stimulate insulin production and cause a fall in your blood sugar, so your intake of these should be reduced. Avoid alcohol if possible or take it only with or after a main meal, and use decaffeinated coffee or weak tea, particularly in the mornings. Do not forget that alcohol may depress your mood, and caffeine is a stimulant which may make you feel more nervous. It is also wise to stop smoking.

A beta blocker may help you over the worst period

Beta blockers are discussed in detail in Chapter 20. Because they block the effects of adrenaline, which is produced in excess in fear and tension, they may be useful in preventing some of the distressful symptoms when benzodiazepines are stopped. Such symptoms as trembling, sweating and rapid beating of the heart may be helped by taking a beta blocker. It may therefore be worth taking a beta blocker for 3–4 weeks during the period that you are withdrawing the benzodiazepine but read carefully about beta blockers in Chapter 20. Do not use the ones that affect the brain (see page 263).

When to use benzodiazepine to treat anxiety

Benzodiazepines do not cure your anxiety, they only relieve some of the symptoms. They can 'block' your mind so that you may not be able to work out, adapt to or learn from the situation in which you find yourself. They may actually blank out your emotions and therefore delay your emotional reactions to a situation so that years later when you try to stop their regular daily use, you may feel very much more distressed about the situation than you would have felt at the time without drugs.

Benzodiazepine drugs should only be prescribed to relieve severe anxiety that is disabling and interfering with the individual's ability to cope (but read Chapter 39 on depression). They should only be used very occasionally for *no more than 2–4 weeks* at a time. The smallest possible dose that controls symptoms should be used, and the individual's progress should be reviewed regularly and the treatment stopped as soon as possible. Prescriptions for benzodiazepines should *not* be issued without the patient seeing a doctor and no more than 1 week's supply should be given at any one time.

Alternatives to benzodiazepines

Non-drug treatments for anxiety should be available to all patients. These should include advice and support from a general practitioner and/or community psychiatrist, clinical psychologist, community psychiatric nurse and/or social worker; instruction and the provision of relaxation tapes and other aids to help relaxation; psychotherapy, behaviour therapy; and/or access to group therapy or a self-help group. These treatments should also be made available to any patient who wishes to come off anti-anxiety drugs or sleeping drugs.

Table 40.1 Benzodiazepines – harmful effects and warnings

Harmful effects of benzodiazepines vary between different drugs and between different individuals. They vary in frequency, severity and type. Most harmful effects produced by benzodiazepines are mild and are usually related to the doses used. They can easily be controlled by reducing the dose. More serious harmful effects are rare and are usually caused by high doses and/or by how a particular individual reacts. Not all of the following harmful effects have been reported with every benzodiazepine, but they have been reported with one or more of them and should be borne in mind whenever a benzodiazepine is used.

Harmful effects include drowsiness, light-headedness, fatigue, loss of control over voluntary movements (ataxia), confusion, constipation, depression, double vision or blurred vision, headache, low blood pressure, incontinence of urine or difficulty in passing urine, jaundice due to liver damage, changes in libido (sexual drive), altered salivation, nausea, skin rashes, slurred speech, forgetfulness, tremor, vertigo, blood disorders, depression of breathing and, with injectable preparations, thrombophlebitis at the site of injection.

Paradoxical reactions may occur, which include excitement, anxiety, hallucinations, spasm of muscles, rage and disturbed sleep. In a susceptible person, benzodiazepines can trigger underlying depression and the patient may become suicidal.

Warnings Benzodiazepines should not be used in people who are allergic to them, in children under the age of 6 months and in people with acute (narrow-angle) glaucoma. They should be used with caution in anyone who suffers from impaired kidney or liver function.

Risks in elderly people Harmful effects of benzodiazepines may be more frequent and severe in the elderly, the smallest dose possible should be used for the shortest duration of time possible. Elderly people run the risk of developing incoordination of movement, drowsiness and agitation. They may wet themselves in the night or have difficulty in passing urine, and they may become confused and forgetful.

Risks in driving Benzodiazepines may affect your ability to drive so do not drive until you know that it is safe to do so.

Risks with alcohol Benzodiazepines increase the effects of alcohol; so do not drink if you are taking a benzodiazepine.

Risks with other drugs Benzodiazepines should be used with caution with anti-epileptic drugs, morphine-related pain relievers, anti-psychotic drugs, barbiturates, MAOIs and other anti-depressants (see Chapter 89).

Miscellaneous anti-anxiety drugs

Barbiturates

Before the introduction of the benzodiazepines, millions of tablets and capsules of barbiturates were prescribed for the relief of anxiety and tension, and to produce sleep. These drugs are no longer in fashion. They are very dangerous in overdosage, and produced many deaths, particularly when taken with alcohol. They should not be used to treat anxiety and insomnia.

Meprobamate (Equanil)

This drug is less effective than the benzodiazepines. It carries a risk of and is more dangerous in overdose dependence, than the benzodiazepines.

Chlormezanone (Trancopal)

Chlormezanone is used as a sleeping drug and as an anti-anxiety drug when muscle tension is prominent. It is also used to treat muscle spasm. It has no advantage over the benzodiazepines.

Anti-psychotic drugs

Anti-psychotic drugs (previously known as major tranquillizers) should not be used to treat mild anxiety and tension. However, patients with psychotic illnesses may develop severe anxiety, which can be treated specifically with anti-psychotic drugs for short periods of time.

Antihistamines

The antihistamine hydroxyzine (Atarax) is occasionally useful for relieving tension in patients with itching skin rashes.

Beta blockers

These drugs are discussed in detail in Chapter 20. They are used to treat angina, raised blood pressure and disorders of heart rhythm, to relieve the symptoms caused by over-active thyroid gland and to prevent migraine attacks. Because they block the effects of adrenaline produced in excess in fear and tension, they are quite effective in relieving some of the physical symptoms of anxiety; for example, rapid beating of the heart, tremor and sweating, stomach symptoms (e.g. nervous indigestion) and bowel symptoms (e.g. nervous diarrhoea).

Buspirone (Buspar)

This is an anti-anxiety drug that is not related to the benzodiazepines. Although it is claimed to produce less risk of dependence than the benzodiazepines, it is in its early days and only time will tell. There is no cross-tolerance to the benzodiazepines, so if a patient is changed from a benzodiazepine to buspirone the same guidelines (see earlier) for slowly reducing the daily dosage of a benzodiazepine will have to be followed. Beneficial effects may take 2–4 weeks to develop.

General warnings on the use of sleeping drugs, sedatives and anti-anxiety drugs

All sleeping drugs, sedatives and anti-anxiety drugs depress brain function and can produce intoxication, psychological dependence, tolerance, physical dependence and addiction, increase the effects of alcohol and impair ability to drive motor vehicles and operate moving machinery.

Intoxication

Like alcohol, these drugs cause acute intoxication if taken regularly in a dosage above that normally recommended. Elderly and debilitated patients and people with impaired heart, kidney or liver function may develop intoxication at 'normal' dosage. Signs of intoxication are similar to those of alcohol intoxication – confusion, difficulty in speaking, unsteadiness on the feet, poor memory, faulty judgement, irritability, over-emotion, hostility, suspiciousness and suicidal tendencies.

Psychological dependence

These drugs are habit forming. When taken regularly every day for more than 2 weeks you may come to rely upon them – i.e. be psychologically dependent on them. You may soon feel as if you are unable to cope without them and you may panic if you think your supply is going to run out before you can get some more. You may come to depend on them in your everyday life.

Tolerance, dependence and addiction

Tolerance, dependence and addiction are discussed in detail early in this chapter, under 'Benzodiazepines'. They may develop to sleeping drugs, sedatives and anti-anxiety drugs.

Physical dependence to these drugs is referred to as 'physical dependence of the barbiturate/alcohol type' because they may produce withdrawal symptoms similar to those that occur when a barbiturate or alcohol is stopped abruptly. Classic barbiturate withdrawal symptoms due to physical dependence may develop within a few hours or a few days, and include weakness, anxiety, headache, dizziness, tremors, vomiting, nausea, stomach cramps, insomnia and rapid beating of the heart. After a day or two the blood pressure may drop upon standing up after sitting or lying down and produce dizziness, light-headedness and fainting; convulsions may occur and hallucinations and delirium tremens may develop after several days, followed by a deep sleep.

Dangers with alcohol

If you drink alcohol regularly you should not take these drugs. They all increase the effects of alcohol and the combination may be dangerous. Although you may be able to tolerate an increased dose of alcohol, sleeping drug, sedative or anti-anxiety drug, the lethal dose of these drugs remains unaltered, so their combination in high dosages could kill you. Another important point to remember is that, if taken regularly over several months, sleeping drugs, sedatives and anti-anxiety drugs may actually make you anxious, irritable and depressed. As your doctor probably prescribed these drugs in the first place in order to control such symptoms, you or he may be tempted to increase the dose in order to control these symptoms further. Yet the increased dose may actually make you worse. This also applies to alcohol, so remember: if you are getting anxious and miserable despite taking more alcohol and/or sleeping drugs, sedatives or anti-anxiety drugs, it is probably the drugs that are producing the effects. Individuals have become trapped on this downward course which may end in suicide.

Accidental overdose

Deliberately taking an overdose of a sleeping drug, sedative or anti-anxiety drug with suicidal intent accounts for most cases of overdose, but accidentally self-administered overdose may also occur. For example, if you take a dose of sleeping drug and fail to fall asleep, you may reach out and take another dose. The effects of this increased dose may make you confused and you may take further doses without knowing (or remember subsequently). Therefore, never keep sleeping drugs by your bedside; keep them locked in a drug cupboard. Take only the recommended dose and leave the bottle in the locked cupboard. If you are responsible for, or live with, someone who is elderly, debilitated or depressed, and taking sleeping drugs, supervise their administration.

Risks with driving

These drugs impair learned behaviour and interfere with your power to concentrate. They can also impair your ability to drive motor vehicles and operate moving machinery, to fly aeroplanes or to carry out hazardous work (e.g. working at heights) or hazardous sports (e.g. rock climbing). They depress a wide range of functions in many vital organs, particularly nerves, muscles, respiration, and the heart and circulation. They may produce any state from mild sedation to confusion and unconsciousness. Like alcohol, they may produce different effects according to the situation in which they are taken. At a discotheque they may produce excitement whereas if taken on retiring to bed they may produce sleep. The combination of a strange environment (e.g. admission to a hospital ward) and a dose of a sleeping drug may make elderly patients very confused and disorientated. This is a warning against the habit of giving patients sleeping drugs as a routine just because they are in hospital; although very convenient for the night staff, it is usually not necessary and may lead to the development of the sleeping-drug habit when the patient returns home.

Paradoxical effects

All sleeping drugs, sedatives and anti-anxiety drugs may produce paradoxical effects in some people. Instead of calming them down they make them hostile and aggressive. These effects vary from just becoming more talkative and excited, to becoming really aggressive and antisocial. They may also increase anxiety and tenseness and make you more sensitive to sounds, sight and touch.

Table 40.2 Other anti-anxiety drugs – harmful effects and warnings

buspirone (Buspar)
Harmful effects include dizziness, headache, nervousness, light-headedness, excitement, nausea. Rarely, there may be rapid beating of the heart, chest pain, drowsiness, confusion, dry mouth, fatigue and sweating.

Warnings Buspirone should not be used in people with epilepsy or who suffer from severe kidney or liver disease. It should be used with caution in individuals who have suffered from kidney or liver disease in the past. In order to prevent benzodiazepine withdrawal symptoms, reduce slowly any benzodiazepine the patient is taking before switching a patient to buspirone.

Risks in elderly people Harmful effects may be more frequent and severe; therefore use with caution.

Risks with driving It may affect your ability to drive, so use with caution and do not drive until you know that it is safe to do so.

Risks with alcohol It may increase the effects of alcohol, so do not drink alcohol when you are taking this drug.

Table 40.2 Other anti-anxiety drugs – harmful effects and warnings (*cont.*)

chlormezanone (Trancopal)
Harmful effects include drowsiness, weakness, dizziness, nausea, light-headedness, headache, lethargy, flushing, excitement, depression, dryness of the mouth and difficulty passing urine. Rarely, jaundice and skin rashes may develop.

Warnings Chlormezanone should not be used in anyone allergic to the drug, and used with caution in people with impaired kidney or liver function.

Dependence may develop (see earlier). The drug should not be stopped suddenly but should be withrawn slowly. It is long acting and may accumulate in the body, so the daily dosage should be reduced in patients with impaired kidney or liver function.

Risks in elderly Harmful effects may be more frequent and severe; therefore use with caution and in smaller doses.

Risks in driving May affect your ability to drive and operate moving machinery, so do not engage in these activities until you know that it is safe to do so.

Risks with alcohol It increases effects of alcohol, so do not drink alcohol if you are taking this drug.

meprobamate (Equanil)
Harmful effects Drowsiness is the most common harmful effect. Less common ones include incoordination of voluntary movements, dizziness, slurred speech, headache, vertigo, weakness, numbness and pins and needles in the hands and feet, blurred vision, feeling of extreme well-being (euphoria) and over-excitement. Rarely, there may be nausea, vomiting and diarrhoea; palpitations, rapid heart beat; fainting, fall in blood pressure; allergic reactions – skin rashes, itching, blood disorders, bruising, fever, swollen glands, chills, wheezing and dermatitis.

Warnings Meprobamate should not be used in individuals who are allergic to it. It should be used with caution in people with impaired kidney or liver function or who suffer from epilepsy.

Dependence Meprobamate may cause psychological and physical dependence similar to those described at the beginning of this chapter. Sudden withdrawal after regular daily use may cause recurrence of anxiety symptoms, and withdrawal symptoms which include vomiting, incoordination of voluntary movements, tremors, twitching, confusion, hallucinations and, rarely, convulsions. The onset of withdrawal symptoms occurs usually within 12–48 hours after stopping the drug, and clears up within a further 12–48 hours. After regular daily use, meprobamate should always be stopped slowly.

Risks in elderly people Do not use.

Risks with driving It affects your ability to drive, so do not drive until you know that it is safe to do so.

Risks with alcohol Meprobamate increases the effects of alcohol, so do not drink alcohol if you are taking this drug.

Table 40.3 Drugs used to treat anxiety

Preparation	*Drug*	*Drug group*	*Dosage form*
Almazine	lorazepam	Intermediate-acting benzodiazepine	Tablets
Alupram	diazepam	Long-acting benzodiazepine	Tablets
Atarax	hydroxyzine	Antihistamine	Tablets, syrup

Table 40.3 Drugs used to treat anxiety (*cont.*)

Preparation	*Drug*	*Drug group*	*Dosage form*
Atensine	diazepam	Long-acting benzodiazepine	Tablets
Ativan	lorazepam	Intermediate-acting benzodiazepine	Tablets, injection
Berkolol	propranolol	Non-selective beta blocker	Tablets
Buspar	buspirone	Anti-anxiety	Tablets
chlordiazepoxide	chlordiazepoxide	Long-acting benzodiazepine	Capsules, tablets
clobazam	clobazam	Long-acting benzodiazepine	Capsules
Diazemuls	diazepam	Long-acting benzodiazepine	Injection (emulsion); for injection or infusion
diazepam	diazepam	Long-acting benzodiazepine	Capsules, tablets, elixir
Equanil	meprobamate	carbamate	Tablets
Frisium	clobazam	Long-acting benzodiazepine	Capsules
Half-Inderal LA	propranolol	Non-selective beta blocker	Sustained-release capsules
Inderal	propranolol	Non-selective beta blocker	Tablets, injection
Inderal LA	propranolol	Non-selective beta blocker	Sustained-release capsules
Lexotan	bromazepam	Intermediate-acting benzodiazepine	Tablets
Librium	chlordiazepoxide	Long-acting benzodiazepine	Capsules, tablets
lorazepam	lorazepam	Intermediate-acting benzodiazepine	Tablets
meprobamate	meprobamate	carbamate	Tablets
Nobrium	medazepam	Long-acting benzodiazepine	Capsules
Oxanid	oxazepam	Intermediate-acting benzodiazepine	Tablets
oxazepam	oxazepam	Intermediate-acting benzodiazepine	Tablets, capsules
oxprenolol	oxprenolol	Non-selective beta blocker	Tablets
propranolol	propranolol	Non-selective beta blocker	Tablets
Solis	diazepam	Long-acting benzodiazepine	Capsules
Stesolid	diazepam	Long-acting benzodiazepine	Injection, rectal solution

Table 40.3 Drugs used to treat anxiety (*cont.*)

Preparation	*Drug*	*Drug group*	*Dosage form*
Tensium	diazepam	Long-acting benzodiazepine	Tablets
Trancopal	chlormezanone	Anti-anxiety	Tablets
Tranxene	clorazepate dipotassium	Long-acting benzodiazepine	Capsules
Trasicor	oxprenolol	Non-selective beta blocker	Tablets
Tropium	chlordiazepoxide	Long-acting benzodiazepine	Capsules, tablets
Valium	diazepam	Long-acting benzodiazepine	Tablets, sugar-free syrup, injection, suppositories
Xanax	alprazolam	Long-acting benzodiazepine	Tablets

41

Schizophrenia and other serious mental illnesses

Definitions

The term *psychosis* is a label applied generally to any kind of mental disorder, especially the more serious types in which there is a lack of insight by the individual about his or her condition.

The term *psychoneurosis* refers to a group of symptoms caused by a faulty emotional response to the stresses and strains of everyday life – for example, anxiety, tension, hysteria, reactive depression and obsessional and compulsive neurosis.

The term *neurosis* refers to a personality trait that makes an individual prone to develop emotional disturbances. A neurosis is less serious than a psychosis, and the individual has insight into his or her problems. We are all more or less neurotic, dependent upon the stresses and strains of our everyday lives.

Affective psychosis is a label applied to serious mental disorders associated with a disturbance of mood, especially *manic depression* in which the mood can swing from extreme excitement (mania) to the depths of depression (manic–depressive psychosis). In manic–depressive psychosis the individual may develop delusions (false beliefs) and feel suicidal.

Another serious mental disorder (or psychosis) is *schizophrenia*, in which individuals suffer from a breakdown of personality, which affects their thoughts and emotions. They may lose touch with reality and develop false beliefs (delusions) and see, hear, feel or smell things that do not exist in the 'real' world (hallucinations).

Drugs used to treat psychoses – anti-psychotic drugs

Drugs used to treat psychoses such as schizophrenia or mania are called anti-psychotic drugs. Because they calm people down, these drugs were previously referred to as major tranquillizers. The prefix 'major' was used to distinguish them from 'minor' tranquillizers or anti-anxiety drugs, used to treat mild mental symptoms. In recent years the term 'tranquillizer' usually has been used to refer to anti-anxiety drugs, especially the benzodiazepines (see Chapter 40), but it may still be used by some people to refer to anti-psychotic drugs as well.

The terms major and minor tranquillizers and even the term 'tranquillizer' should no longer be used (see discussion in Chapter 40). It is more helpful to use terms that give an indication of the type of disorder for which the drugs are used – for example, anti-psychotic drugs and anti-anxiety drugs. This helps to draw an important distinction between the anti-psychotic drugs, which are effective in treating *serious* symptoms of mental illness, and anti-anxiety drugs (e.g. benzodiazepines), which are often used inappropriately to treat *mild* physical and mental symptoms, caused by everyday problems of living.

In 'calming' people down, anti-psychotic drugs may produce a state of emotional quietness and indifference (see later). This state is referred to as a 'neuroleptic state' and these drugs were previously referred to as neuroleptics. This term should also be dropped in favour of the term anti-psychotic.

Harmful effects produced by anti-psychotic drugs

Anti-psychotic drugs calm people (tranquillize them) without affecting consciousness and without producing the paradoxical excitement sometimes caused by sedatives and anti-anxiety drugs. In addition, they produce other beneficial effects – particularly in individuals suffering from schizophrenia. They relieve distressing symptoms; severely disturbed schizophrenic people become less agitated and restless, and withdrawn individuals become more responsive and co-operative. After several days of treatment with these drugs, hallucinations and delusions disappear and thinking becomes more organized and coherent.

Effects on the brain

Anti-psychotic drugs affect nerve receptors at all levels of the nervous system, and one of their principal effects is to block a stimulant nerve transmitter (neurotransmitter) in the brain and nervous system, called dopamine. This blocking of dopamine may account for their effects in relieving symptoms of psychotic illness and the serious harmful effects that they may produce on those parts of the brain that control posture and involuntary aspects of movement and which rely on dopamine as a nerve transmitter. These processes are also affected in Parkinson's disease, which in part is due to a deficiency of dopamine (see Chapter 36).

Harmful effects on movement

Anti-psychotic drugs block dopamine in parts of the brain that are responsible for co-ordination of movement; this may produce a state like parkinsonism. The muscles become rigid, and movements become slow and can freeze. Rhythmic involuntary shaking movements may develop, affecting the tongue, face, mouth and jaw (e.g. puffing of the cheeks, puckering of the mouth, protrusion of the tongue, chewing movements). Sometimes these movements are associated with other abnormal involuntary movements of the arms and legs. These include:

- Restless movements: inability to keep still, jitteriness, agitation, difficulty with sleeping
- Dystonias: spasm of muscles, producing abnormal involuntary movements of the face, neck, back, arms and hands; difficulty in swallowing, protrusion of the tongue and abnormal movements of the eyes
- Parkinsonism: mask-like face, drooling, shaking (tremors), rigid muscles and shuffling walk
- Tardive dyskinesia: rhythmical involuntary movements of the tongue, face, mouth and jaw (e.g. puffing of the cheeks, puckering of the mouth, protrusion of the tongue, chewing movements); sometimes these movements are associated with abnormal involuntary movements of the arms and legs

Neurolepsis

In high doses, anti-psychotic drugs may reduce people's initiative and interest in their surroundings, spontaneous movement and displays of emotion. They just sit motionless and stare into space like zombies but can be roused and give sensible answers to direct questions. This state is called a 'neuroleptic state' and although it may be convenient for ward staff to have a 'quiet' patient this may not always help the patient; yet psychiatrists believed for years that to produce this state was a test of effectiveness of anti-psychotic drugs.

The neuroleptic state literally places the patient in a 'chemical straitjacket' – an emotional imprisonment which may be produced by any of the anti-psychotic drugs if used in high enough dosage. Fortunately, these days there is much less tendency to use anti-psychotic drugs in doses high enough to produce a neuroleptic state. However, it may occasionally be necessary to give a very violent and severely disturbed patient an injection of an anti-psychotic drug to calm them down and make them manageable. Although such injections are referred to as 'liquid coshes' they may well be preferable to applying a physical straitjacket or putting the patient in a padded cell. Nevertheless, there are risks and they should be used with caution (see later).

Harmful effects on the breasts

Another anti-dopamine effect of anti-psychotic drugs is on the pituitary gland (the master gland), which produces the hormone prolactin. This hormone is responsible for milk production in breast-feeding mothers. By their action in blocking dopamine, anti-psychotic drugs block the controlling effects the hypothalamus has on the production of prolactin by the pituitary gland, with the result that, in people receiving treatment with these drugs, prolactin is over-produced and the breasts may enlarge (gynaecomastia) and milk may be produced (galactorrhea) even in male patients.

Harmful effects on the blood pressure

Anti-psychotic drugs may affect the heart and circulation, particularly the blood pressure and the body's temperature. A drop in blood pressure on standing up after lying down or sitting down (postural or orthostatic hypotension) may be a serious problem with some anti-psychotic drugs, causing dizziness and faintness, particularly in elderly people.

Harmful effects on the temperature

A mild rise in temperature may occur in the first few days of treatment, particularly if an anti-psychotic drug is given by injection. However, a fall in temperature (hypothermia) is more common and is due to the effects of the drugs on the temperature control centre in the brain and on the blood vessels supplying the skin. This is important to remember in cold climates, because people taking this treatment, particularly the elderly, may develop hypothermia; but also note that the effects of anti-psychotic drugs on the body's temperature control can cause heat stroke in people who live in a hot climate.

Neuroleptic malignant syndrome

Very rarely, a patient treated with an anti-psychotic drug may develop a high body temperature (hyperthermia), varying levels of unconsciousness, rigidity of the muscles, paleness (pallor), rapid beating of the heart, changes in blood pressure and sweating, and the individual may be incontinent of urine. This group of signs and symptoms is known as the 'neuroleptic malignant syndrome', and it may be fatal. It has been reported with haloperidol, chlorpromazine, and flupenthixol. Any anti-psychotic drug being taken should be stopped at the earliest sign of this syndrome. There is no effective treatment and it usually lasts for about 5–10 days after stopping the drug. The symptoms may be very prolonged if the patient has been receiving a depot injection of an anti-psychotic drug.

Other harmful effects produced by anti-psychotic drugs

Other harmful effects of anti-psychotic drugs vary between different drugs and between different patients; they also vary in frequency and type. Some harmful effects are directly related to the dose and some are related to how a particular individual reacts. Some harmful effects may be more likely to occur, or occur with greater intensity according to what other disorders the patient is suffering from. It is important, therefore, that treatment always be tailored to the individual's needs and responses.

Not all of the following harmful effects have been reported with every anti-psychotic drug, but they have been reported with one or more of them, and should be borne in mind whenever these drugs are used: dry mouth, blocked nose, blurred vision, headache, nausea, constipation, drowsiness, apathy, pallor, depression, agitation, painful erection of the penis (priapism), inhibition of ejaculation, difficulty passing urine, flare-up of mental illness, fall in blood pressure (sometimes fatal), disorders of heart rhythm, abnormalities on electrical tracings of the heart (ECG) and blood disorders; rarely, there may be liver damage including jaundice, irregular menstrual periods, sensitivity of the skin to sunlight, allergic reactions (skin rashes, asthma, angioedema), mild fever, increased appetite and increase in weight.

Prolonged use of high doses may cause opacities in the lens and cornea of the eyes, and purplish pigmentation of the skin, cornea, conjunctiva and retina. Injections may cause pain and local swelling (nodules), a sudden fall in blood pressure and rapid beating of the heart.

Variations in response to anti-psychotic drugs

Different people may react differently to the same anti-psychotic drug given by mouth because absorption of the drug into the bloodstream from the intestine may vary and therefore its effects may be unpredictable.

Unborn babies, babies, infants and elderly people have a diminished ability to break down and get rid of these drugs from the body, so they are more prone to develop harmful effects. Children actually break them down more quickly than adults.

Doctors can cause some serious problems in their patients if they suddenly change them from one anti-psychotic drug to another. This is because patients may become tolerant to the effects of one of these drugs but not necessarily tolerant to the effects of another – which means that if high doses of one drug are stopped suddenly and replaced by another, severe effects (e.g. fall in blood pressure) may occur with the new drug.

Anti-psychotic drugs should not be stopped suddenly

People become tolerant to the sedative effects of anti-psychotic drugs over a few days to a few weeks and will progressively experience less sedation. However, anti-psychotic drugs do not produce dependence although if they are stopped suddenly some individuals experience muscle aching and difficulty with sleep. Because anti-psychotic drugs block dopamine, stopping them suddenly after prolonged daily use in high doses may make nerve receptors in the brain supersensitive to dopamine (what is called disuse supersensitivity). This may produce alarming attacks of severe uncontrollable movement of the limbs and face.

The use of anti-psychotic drugs in relieving the symptoms of schizophrenia

Anti-psychotic drugs are very effective in relieving some disturbing symptoms of schizophrenia. They are particularly useful for relieving tension, over-activity, hallucinations and delusions, insomnia, loss of appetite and self-neglect. They may have a dramatic effect in some withdrawn people but not in others. They are less likely to improve judgement, memory and a person's insight into his or her condition. They are more effective in treating acute symptoms than chronic symptoms.

Anti-psychotic drugs should be withdrawn very slowly over months because of the risks of triggering a breakdown. Individuals should be well supervised at this time because it may be 1–2 months after stopping all treatment before symptoms of a breakdown appear.

A large proportion of patients suffering from schizophrenia who improve on anti-psychotic drugs will be able to come off them after about a year or two without relapse. For the few individuals who are always prone to relapse, regular, well supervised maintenance doses of anti-psychotic drugs can help to prevent relapse and re-admission to hospital; however, the long-term benefits and risks must be balanced carefully for each individual, particularly the risk of tardive dyskinesia.

The relief and prevention of symptoms produced by anti-psychotic drug treatment may be very beneficial to patients and also to their carers, but it should be only part of an overall treatment strategy. This strategy should include a full and *continuing* range of professional support services both in hospital and in the community. It should be tailored to the individual's needs, and response over time and it should be flexible enough to provide the right kind of help whenever it is needed and attentive enough to spot and treat any early signs of trouble in order to *prevent* a breakdown.

Care for someone who suffers from schizophrenia should be comprehensive, continuing and tailored to that person's needs. It should offer various choices according to the individual's condition. In the past, too many of these unfortunate people were filled with drugs and nothing else was done for them. They were turned into institutionalized beings who caused no trouble, which was fine for the staff but degrading for them. We are still trying to cope with this legacy of the past 30 years as 'burned-out' patients walk aimlessly around the corridors and grounds of some of our mental hospitals, or just wander round the streets because it has been decided that they should be discharged into the community.

Comment

Anti-psychotic drugs are more effective in relieving the symptoms of schizophrenia than are other forms of treatment, both in acute episodes and in preventing breakdown. However, their benefits outweigh their risks *only* if they are used properly.

Choice of anti-psychotic drug

Different anti-psychotic drugs vary in the nature and extent of the harmful effects they produce, and the choice of drug is usually determined by how much sedation it causes and the degree of parkinsonism effects it may produce. In addition, different people react differently to any one of the anti-psychotic drugs; therefore, treatment should always be tailored to an individual's needs and response.

There is no point in using more than one anti-psychotic drug for the same person; there is no evidence that this practice reduces the risks of harmful effects.

Chlorpromazine, methotrimeprazine and promazine produce marked sedation and moderate parkinsonism effects. Pericyazine, pipothiazine and thioridazine produce moderate sedation and fewer parkinsonism effects. All the other anti-psychotic drugs produce less sedation but marked parkinsonism effects.

A recently introduced anti-psychotic drug, clozapine (Clozaril), produces anti-psychotic effects and also rapid sedation. It blocks the action of the several neurotransmitters in the brain but has less effect in blocking the effects of dopamine than the other anti-psychotic drugs and therefore is likely to cause less risk of involuntary movements. Claims for its use in improving tardive dyskinesia need further study. Its main disadvantage is that it may knock out the production of white blood cells by the bone marrow, leading to a serious and life-threatening reduction in the body's resistance to infection. Its use should therefore be restricted to treating individuals who have not improved on any other treatment, provided that white blood counts are carried out weekly for the first 18 weeks of treatment and every 2 weeks after that, and provided that patients report immediately if they develop symptoms of an infection (e.g. sore throat, fever). The drug must be stopped immediately if the white cell count drops below $3000/mm^3$.

Treatment of abnormal movements

Restless movements often disappear on their own. The dose of anti-psychotic drug should not be increased until these symptoms have cleared up. If they do not clear up, the dose should be reduced.

Dystonias usually clear up within 48 hours of stopping the drug. If moderately severe, the anti-psychotic drug should be stopped and a barbiturate given instead; this will usually stop them. If very severe, an anticholinergic anti-parkinsonism drug may help.

Parkinsonism effects are usually helped by giving an anticholinergic anti-parkinsonism drug, but only when necessary and only for a few weeks or months. These drugs may unmask tardive dyskinesia or make it worse (see later) and patients may come to 'rely' on them because of their effects on mood. If the symptoms are severe, it may be necessary to lower the dose or stop the drug.

Tardive dyskinesia may appear after long-term treatment or even after the drug treatment has stopped. It may develop with relatively small doses and after only short periods of treatment. It occurs more often in elderly people, especially elderly women; but in general there is no way of telling who may develop it, at what dose and after what duration of treatment. There is no known effective treatment for tardive dyskinesia.

Any anti-psychotic drug being used should be stopped at the earliest sign of the patient developing tardive dyskinesia. This may be nothing more than just a fine worm-like movement of the tongue.

Anticholinergic drugs used to relieve parkinsonism symptoms may unmask or make tardive dyskinesia worse.

Warning *Anticholinergic drugs should not be used as a routine in order to prevent parkinsonism. They are unnecessary because not every patient taking anti-psychotic drugs develops parkinsonism, and they may be harmful because anticholinergics may unmask or worsen tardive dyskinesia.*

The use of anti-psychotic drugs in controlling behaviour

A high dose of anti-psychotic drug by injection or by mouth may be very effective in an emergency for quietening a very severely mentally disturbed patient, whether the cause is due to brain damage, a behavioural disorder or a serious mental illness producing mania or agitation. However, the use of anti-psychotic drugs for these purposes has recently come in for much criticism, and not without grounds because in the past they were often used routinely to make patients quiet and more manageable. Nevertheless, if used with caution, they may benefit patients and tide them over particularly difficult episodes. High doses should be used only to control behaviour under strict medical supervision, and with the consent of the nearest relative or guardian.

Use in children

There is no convincing evidence that anti-psychotic drugs are beneficial in treating children with psychotic mental illness or with hyperactivity (attention-deficit disorder).

Depot injections of anti-psychotic drugs

Injections of anti-psychotic drugs are available which, when given into a muscle, form a 'depot' from which the active drug is slowly released over several weeks. These depot injections are given deep into a muscle at intervals of about 1–4 weeks. They are used to treat patients who should benefit from the long-term use of an anti-psychotic drug but who can not be relied on to take tablets by mouth regularly every day. Also, some patients may find it more convenient to have an injection just once every month than to take tablets every day. However, these injections produce an increased risk of parkinsonism effects and movement disorders; moreover, because they are depot injections, they go on working for several weeks. The selection of a particular drug to be given by depot injection should be made with great caution, and the dose and interval of dose worked out very carefully according to the individual's needs and response. Furthermore, no depot injection should be given to anyone without that patient's full consent (or that of his or her guardian); this demands that the patient (or guardian) should have the benefits and risks of such treatment explained to them in detail, particularly the risk of tardive dyskinesia.

The choice of depot injections will depend upon whether the patient is agitated and aggressive or apathetic and withdrawn (see earlier). The risk of harmful effects is about the same with all available preparations. Patients on regular depot injections appear to do better than patients given anti-psychotic drugs by mouth at the earliest sign of a flare-up of their disorder.

In addition to the harmful effects that anti-psychotic drugs produce when given by mouth, depot injections may also cause pain, redness and swelling at the site of injection.

Because of the risk of parkinsonism effects and movement disorders (particularly tardive dyskinesia), patients receiving depot injections should be seen and examined carefully at regular intervals (every 2–4 weeks). Also, any change from treatment by mouth to treatment by depot injection should be carried out with utmost caution and the dose by mouth should be reduced *gradually* over several days after the first depot injection.

Warnings on the use of anti-psychotic drugs

Low blood pressure (hypotension) produced by anti-psychotic drugs is related to the dose of the drug used. It may be dangerous in elderly people, who may develop dizziness and light-headedness, and they may fall and injure themselves.

Low body temperature (hypothermia) is also related to the dose of anti-psychotic drug used. This harmful effect may be especially dangerous in elderly people particularly in winter when treatment with anti-psychotic drugs may contribute to the risk of their developing hypothermia. In very hot climates they may contribute to the development of heat stroke.

The risk of developing *tardive dyskinesia* and the likelihood that it will become permanent are believed to increase as the duration of treatment increases and the total 'overall' dose of the drug increases. It is not possible to predict who will develop tardive dyskinesia and it is not known whether anti-psychotic drugs differ in their potential for causing it. There is no known treatment. There is no evidence that stopping anti-psychotic drugs intermittently (drug holidays) is of any benefit in preventing tardive dyskinesia, and it may make the patient's condition worse.

The continued long-term use of anti-psychotic drugs may actually mask the progression of underlying tardive dyskinesia, and it is not known what effect this has upon the outcome of the disease.

Because of the occasional risk of tardive dyskinesia, anti-psychotic drugs should be used with utmost caution. The smallest effective dose for the shortest duration of time should be used to treat acute episodes, and they should be used only for long-term treatment of chronic disorders that are definitely known to benefit from these drugs (e.g. schizophrenia) and for whom no other, equally effective and potentially less harmful, treatment is available.

Anti-psychotic drugs may produce *allergic reactions* in some people, who should not be given them if they have suffered from an allergic reaction to one of them in the past.

Because of the rare risk of *blood disorders*, patients should report any sore throat or other sign of infection immediately. If a blood test shows a *reduced white cell count*, the drug should be stopped and an antibiotic started.

There is a rare risk of *liver damage*; if fever and/or flu-like symptoms develop, tests of liver function should be carried out immediately, and if they show any abnormality the drug should be stopped.

Patients who suffer from *angina* should be observed carefully because the increase in activity produced by these drugs may make the angina worse. If this happens, the drug should be stopped.

Anti-psychotic drugs should be used with caution in patients suffering from *glaucoma*.

Table 41.1 Anti-psychotic drugs

Preparation	*Drug*	*Dosage form*
Anquil	benperidol	Tablets
chlorpromazine	chlorpromazine	Tablets, elixir
Clopixol	zuclopenthixol	Tablets, depot injection
Clopixol-Conc.	zuclopenthixol	Depot injection
Clopixol Acuphase	zuclopenthixol	Oily injection
Clozaril	clozapine	Tablets
Depixol	flupenthixol	Tablets, depot injection
Depixol-Conc.	flupenthixol	Depot injection
Dolmatil	sulpiride	Tablets
Dozic	haloperidol	Sugar-free oral liquid
Droleptan	droperidol	Tablets, sugar-free oral liquid, injection
Fentazin	perphenazine	Tablets
Fortunan	haloperidol	Tablets
Haldol	haloperidol	Tablets, sugar-free liquid, injection
Haldol Deconoate	haloperidol deconoate	Depot injection
Integrin	oxypertine	Capsules, tablets

Table 41.1 Anti-psychotic drugs (*cont.*)

Preparation	*Drug*	*Dosage form*
Largactil	chlorpromazine	Tablets, syrup, forte suspension, injection
Loxapac	loxapine	Capsules
Melleril	thioridazine	Tablets, suspension, syrup
Modecate and Modecate Concentrate	fluphenazine	Depot injection
Moditen	fluphenazine	Tablets
Moditen Enanthate	fluphenazine enanthate	Depot injection
Neulactil	pericyazine	Tablets, syrup forte
Nozinan	methotrimeprazine	Tablets, injection
Orap	pimozide	Tablets
Piportil Depot	pipothiazine palmitate	Depot injection
Redeptin	fluspirilene	Injection
Serenace	haloperidol	Capsules, tablets, sugar-free oral liquid, injection
Sparine	promazine	Suspension, injection
Stelazine	trifluoperazine	Tablets, spansules (sustained-release), sugar-free syrup, liquid concentrate, injection
Stemetil	prochlorperazine	Tablets, syrup, granules, injection, suppositories
Sulpitil	sulpiride	Tablets
Triperidol	trifluperidol	Tablets

42

Stimulants

Our state of mental alertness, which varies throughout the day, is under the control of chemical nerve transmitters (neurotransmitters) in the brain. Some of these transmitters depress the activity of brain cells and produce drowsiness and sleep, whereas others stimulate brain cells and produce wakefulness.

The balance between our degree of wakefulness and sleepiness is under the control of part of the brain called the reticular activating system (RAS). This system is stimulated by adrenaline and related nerve stimulants, and damped down by depressant nerve transmitters such as gamma-amino-butyric acid, or GABA for short. Drugs that cause a release of stimulant neurotransmitters such as adrenaline or mimic their actions (see Chapter 2) will produce increased alertness. They are referred to as *stimulants*, and include amphetamines, methylphenidate, pemoline, prolintane, caffeine and cocaine. In addition to increasing alertness, they also lift the mood and may produce a state of extreme well-being (euphoria).

Amphetamines ('speed')

Amphetamines are manufactured stimulants. In the brain and nervous system they cause the level of the body's own stimulants to increase. They cause a release of noradrenaline and dopamine from storage by displacing them and they also block their clearance back into storage. Amphetamines also stimulate receptors that are triggered by dopamine and serotonin (another stimulant nerve transmitter).

Amphetamines produce wakefulness, alertness, lifting of the mood (they are 'uppers'), and they give an increase in self-confidence. They produce elation, an exaggerated feeling of well-being (euphoria) and an increase in general activity. They also improve physical and mental performance.

Amphetamines prevent fatigue and also partly reverse it. In the Second World War they were widely used among the armed forces to combat fatigue. After the war their use spread to musicians, students, night-shift workers and long-distance lorry drivers who found that amphetamines kept them awake and more alert.

In the late fifties and early sixties doctors prescribed amphetamines by the millions each year to lift mood, give energy, as tonics and also as slimming pills because they reduce the appetite. Patients would ask for 'pep pills' and say they wanted 'pepping up'. Doctors would respond (or, more accurately, started the craze) by telling their patients 'I'm going to give you something to pep you up'. Amphetamines became freely available on prescription, and on the streets amphetamine misuse became a major social problem. Amphetamine misuse was widespread – from suburban housewives who took them for slimming but enjoyed the way they could 'whistle through their housework' to widespread use by 'mods and rockers' and multi-drug users. Some misusers took to 'main-lining' amphetamines into a vein in order to get a more rapid and intense response.

Harmful effects of amphetamines

Prolonged use and/or the use of high doses of amphetamines can produce restlessness, sleeplessness, nervousness and anxiety, and serious mental symptoms such as delirium, paranoid hallucinations and delusions, and panic states; suicidal or homicidal tendencies may develop. Some of these serious mental symptoms may be mistaken for schizophrenia; even though recovery is rapid if the drug is stopped, some people suffer permanent mental breakdown. Long-term use may also cause physical symptoms that include shaking, sweating, palpitations, chest and abdominal pains, fainting, sores and ulcers, liver damage, raised blood pressure and bleeding into the brain.

'Speed kills'

In the sixties 'abusers' who developed bad experiences (trips) became known among other drug takers as 'speed freaks' and in the end the drug underworld turned against amphetamines with the slogan that 'speed kills'. Not surprisingly against such a social menace, legal controls were eventually applied to their supply and use, and the news media influenced both public and medical opinion. In the seventies there was a dramatic reduction in the social and especially medical use of amphetamines.

However, they are still around as street drugs, and their illicit manufacture and use have increased significantly in recent years. Furthermore, a few doctors occasionally use amphetamine-related drugs to suppress the appetite of overweight patients despite the fact that there is no place for such treatment (see Chapter 43).

Tolerance and dependence

The brain soon becomes *tolerant* to amphetamines, so an individual will need to go on increasing the dose of the drug in order to produce the effects experienced initially. Furthermore, they reduce the level of natural stimulants in the brain, so after regular daily use over a period of a few weeks an individual will come to 'depend' upon the drug and feel let down if he stops it.

If amphetamines are suddenly stopped after regular daily use, the balance between natural stimulant nerve transmitters and depressant nerve transmitters will be disturbed – there will be a deficiency of natural stimulants and an excess of depressants. This imbalance produces unpleasant withdrawal symptoms that include tiredness, depression and an increased appetite.

Regular users can become dependent and addicted to amphetamines; not only do they need to go on taking the drug in ever-bigger doses to obtain the same 'high' but they also need to go on taking them in order to combat the depression and fatigue that develop when they try to stop the drug. Some users may become preoccupied with obtaining and taking the drug, and they may enter a downward spiral that includes main-lining the drug in order to get a better 'buzz' (effect), which carries with it the risk of getting infected with hepatitis and/or AIDS from contaminated blood on shared needles.

Medical use of amphetamines

As often happens in medicine, widespread prescribing by doctors slowly gives way to a realization that the risks from using a particular group of drugs far outweigh any benefit. This happened with the amphetamines and they are now recommended only for treating narcolepsy, a disorder in which there is a tendency to fall asleep during the day-time for no obvious reason and is probably due to an excess of depressant nerve transmitters in the brain. They may also be used to treat certain behaviour disorders in children (see later). Available preparations include Dexedrine (dexamphetamine).

Other stimulants

Methylphenidate is a mild stimulant that produces effects similar to those of the amphetamines. It is used in some countries to treat hyperactive children. It may cause insomnia, loss of appetite, instability, headache and increased heart rate.

Pemoline (Volital) is a stimulant that has been used to treat tiredness and depression, and also to treat hyperactive children. It may produce insomnia, loss of appetite, nausea, dizziness, headache, drowsiness and mild depression. Large doses may cause nervousness, rapid beating of the heart and hallucinations.

Prolintane is a mild stimulant that is combined with vitamins C and B in Villescon, which is marketed as a general tonic.

The use of stimulants to treat hyperactive children

Methylphenidate, dexamphetamine and pemoline have been shown to produce improvement in hyperactive children suffering from what is now called ADD – attention-deficit disorders. However, there is every possibility that any improvement that has been observed in children who have received treatment was probably due to the extra attention they received rather than to the drug treatment. (U)

NOTE The long-term use of stimulants in children may retard their growth.

Caffeine

Effects on the nervous system

Caffeine is present in some pain-relieving preparations and in 'pick-me-ups' that can be bought over the counter in chemists and drug stores. It is the most widely used stimulant. It is present in tea, coffee, cocoa and cola. It is a powerful stimulant of the brain and nervous system. It reduces drowsiness, delays or reduces fatigue, and helps clear thinking. As the dose is increased it produces nervousness, restlessness, insomnia and tremors. In still higher doses it can produce convulsions.

Caffeine stimulates the breathing centre in the brain, and can be used to treat newborn babies whose breathing has been depressed by drugs used during childbirth (e.g. morphine-related drugs).

Effects on the heart

In moderate to high doses caffeine increases the heart rate and may produce disorders of heart rhythm in some sensitive individuals. It increases the output of blood from the heart and dilates small arteries, producing a transient increase in blood flow to the hands and feet. However, in the brain it has an opposite effect and actually constricts the arteries supplying the brain. Caffeine improves the blood supply to the heart by causing dilatation of the coronary arteries.

Stomach acid

Caffeine causes an increase in the production of acid and pepsin in the stomach. It is therefore important for people with peptic ulcers to be cautious about how much coffee, tea, cola and cocoa they drink. They also need to control the amount of decaffeinated coffee that they drink, because, despite the absence of caffeine, this may stimulate acid production in the stomach and irritate its lining.

Other effects

In addition to relaxing muscles in the walls of arteries, caffeine also relaxes muscles of the bronchial tubes – a caffeine-related drug, theophylline, is used to treat asthma. Caffeine increases the capacity to do muscular work, and increases the production of urine (diuretic effect).

Risks of overdose

The average caffeine contained in a cup of tea is 40–100 mg, in brewed coffee about 100–150 mg and in instant coffee about 80–100 mg. Cocoa contains about 250 mg of theobromine and 5 mg of caffeine. A 12 oz bottle of a cola drink contains about 50 mg of caffeine. The average daily intake of caffeine may therefore be sufficient to cause problems in some people, although there is a significant variation between individuals as to how they respond to caffeine. Some people can drink cup after cup of coffee without much effect, yet some rare individuals may develop toxic effects with just one cup of coffee.

High use of coffee and/or tea or cola, resulting in an intake of caffeine of more than about 600 mg per day will, in some people, produce chronic caffeine poisoning – restlessness, anxiety, disturbed sleep, tremor, rapid beating of the heart and palpitations. The tannin in tea may constipate while the oils in coffee (whether decaffeinated or not) may irritate the lining of the stomach and intestine, producing indigestion and diarrhoea.

Dependence on caffeine

Most people are psychologically dependent on caffeine drinks (e.g. tea, coffee) and cannot start or get through the day without repeated 'fixes' of the drug. Tolerance develops to the effects of caffeine and sudden withdrawal may produce headaches.

Intoxication with caffeine is not that uncommon. Therefore, people who feel nervous, restless and have disturbed sleep should reduce the amount and/or strength of tea and/or coffee they drink each day. It may help to drink decaffeinated tea and/or coffee for most of the time.

Other risks from caffeine-containing beverages

There is a lack of convincing evidence from adequate and well controlled studies to demonstrate an association between drinking caffeine-containing beverages and cancer of the breast in women, coronary artery disease, raised blood pressure, cancer of the pancreas, kidney or bladder, risk in pregnancy and risk of spontaneous abortion.

Cocaine

Virtually the only medical use of cocaine is as a local anaesthetic and sometimes as additional treatment to morphine or a related drug in patients dying and in severe pain.

Cocaine is obtained from the leaves of the coca plant. It is a stimulant with high potential for abuse. Its effects are similar to those produced by amphetamines. It is known as 'coke', 'snow', 'gold dust', 'bernice', 'lady', 'she', 'Dama Blanca', 'crack', etc.

The taking of cocaine is surrounded by rituals of how and where it is taken. Whether it is taken at home, at work or at a party will influence how an individual responds to cocaine. It is therefore difficult to describe how it will affect someone because any drug experience will be complicated by these influences and by that individual's expectations and emotional make-up as well as how he or she responds directly to the effects of the drug. The dose taken may vary significantly between takers and so may the harmful effects – which are dependent upon the dose, frequency of dosage and the way it is taken. Also, the sensitivity of individuals to the harmful effects of cocaine may vary widely. These harmful effects include depression, anxiety and symptoms of serious mental illness, such as hallucinations, delusions and paranoia, which are often difficult to differentiate from schizophrenia.

Cocaine may be taken by mouth (Andean Indians chew coca leaves as a social ritual and as a mild stimulant). It may be snorted up the nose, where it is rapidly absorbed through the nasal lining to produce stimulation. The individual becomes talkative and full of energy and self-confidence. Snorting produces effects that last for about 20–40 minutes. Repeated snorting (every 20–30 minutes) leads to agitation, suspiciousness and paranoia. Regular use causes the lining membrane of the nose to shrink (cocaine rhinitis or cocaine sniffles). The nose may shrink, and occasionally the central panel of the nose (the septum) which separates the nostrils may perforate.

Other ways of taking cocaine include smoking and injection into a vein which produces an immediate effect. Repeated and regular use of cocaine can lead to intense anxiety, severe paranoia and hallucinations.

Crack is the free base of cocaine, which is cocaine separated from its hydrochloride salt. It vaporizes when heated and can be smoked and/or inhaled. This produces an instant 'high' just like injecting cocaine into a vein. The maximum effect is reached within half a minute and lasts about half an hour whereas snorting cocaine powder up the nose takes about half an hour to reach peak effect. Smoking or inhaling crack is more likely to produce addiction than snorting cocaine powder up the nose (see later). Inhalation may damage the throat and lungs due to the high temperature and corrosiveness.

During a 'high' from inhaling or injecting cocaine, users may develop acute cocaine psychosis and become severely anxious and paranoid, and develop hallucinations; as the concentration of the drug in the blood falls they may become violent. Jitters and anxiety may develop after the effects have worn off.

Addiction

Users may rapidly become tolerant to cocaine, so they have to keep on increasing the dose in order to achieve the same effects. In addition, they develop an overwhelming craving for the drug and become totally preoccupied with obtaining a supply of the drug and taking it. They become totally dependent on the drug emotionally, and if they stop the drug suddenly they go down into the depths of depression. The degree of this depression is directly related to the dose they were using. Overdose causes fits and breathing to stop. Death may occur.

Dangers with alcohol

Taking cocaine with alcohol may produce alarming behaviour because cocaine produces excitement and increases the energy while alcohol and related drugs produces poor judgement.

Harmful physical effects

Cocaine damps down the appetite, produces disturbed sleep and, although initially it may produce sexual arousal and delayed orgasm, its continued use may lead to loss of interest in sex. The appeal of cocaine as an aphrodisiac owes more to imagination than to its effects on the body.

As the dose of cocaine is increased, shaking develops and, later, convulsions. It increases the heart rate and initially can cause a rapid rise in blood pressure. A large intravenous dose of cocaine can cause heart failure and death due to its direct toxic effects on the heart. Cocaine increases the body's temperature and in high doses it causes chills followed by fever (cocaine fever).

43

Slimming

Slimming – a multi-million-pound industry

Slimming is a multi-million-pound business which uses all the persuasive powers of modern advertising, and tied closely to it are the fashion and beauty industries. We cannot escape the continuous brain-washing that to be slim is to be beautiful. New diets and new books on slimming seem to come out every week – not surprisingly, since the publishing industry also makes millions of pounds each year from persuading people that they need to lose weight.

These industries have created a need by telling us what weights we should be and how we should look. Because of this, millions of us strive each year to reach unnecessary, unrealistic and unachievable weight loss. We know this full well, because every year we try; yet we know that nine out of ten of us will regain the weight we have taken off within about 3 months of stopping any slimming programme.

Some people have big noses, others have little ones, some take size 10 shoes, others take size 6, yet when it comes to weight, everybody is supposed to slot into a narrow range of weights defined for us by the fashion industry and those who make money out of us losing weight.

Research findings do not help. We are told about enzymes, about white fat and brown fat and about environmental factors such as social class (the rich are slimmer than the poor). We know that fat children aged 7–11 years grow into fat adults. We know that most of us eat too much food for our requirements. We know we eat the wrong sorts of fattening foods and we know that we take too little exercise. We also know that if we are really overweight we run the risk of getting all kinds of horrible things such as heart disease, high blood pressure, diabetes, arthritis, chest disorders, gall stones and raised blood fats. (U)

Being overweight is a life-long problem

The trouble is that being overweight is a life-long problem. If we do not wish to be 'overweight', we must take life-long action. This is why the slimming industry is so lucrative; we are always ready to try something new. From the point of view of our general fitness we know what we should eat and what we should not eat. We know we should take more exercise. We know these facts, but it doesn't help us, and here is the real crunch. It is really all in our minds. Our desire to eat and our interest in food override our knowledge or wishes. We have been conditioned since childhood to associate eating with pleasure and the eating of certain foods with reward (be a good boy and you may have some sweeties, chips, ice-cream or whatever).

Slimming diets strengthen our preoccupation with food

I believe that dieting can strengthen our conditioning because we consciously or subconsciously associate slimming diets with 'punishment' for our being fat. In fact slimming diets, I would suggest, actually strengthen our preoccupation with food, so it is not surprising that most of us put weight back on when we stop a diet. We just cannot wait to start eating fattening foods again as a reward for the punishment we have just gone through.

How do we motivate ourselves to lose weight?

Many of us, particularly those with weight problems, are addicted to food and there are many psychological, social and cultural factors that influence the amounts and types of foods that we eat. Eating is pleasurable and satisfying. It can also be a method of coping – some of us eat more when we are anxious, tense or depressed. It is behavioural, it is an addiction; so to lose weight we have to change our behaviour, not just for a month or two but for life. Therefore, special slimming diets have very little part to play in the problem – we can't stay on a slimming diet for life! Such diets earn millions of pounds for the people who write about them or who sell them but they only change your behaviour temporarily.

'Going on' and 'coming off' diets does not help us. It can often make us feel a failure. What we have to do is slowly condition ourselves to take moderate exercise and to eat less over time while making sure that we eat sensible and nutritious food. We need to control our eating and it is a life-long problem. Unfortunately, to do this is very difficult for most of us and almost impossible for some of us. Some of us can motivate ourselves. Some people may be motivated if a medical examination shows them to be in great danger if they do not lose weight. Others will benefit from going to group therapy sessions where they recommend sensible eating and provide counselling and support, but many of these people regain weight once they stop group therapy.

In the end it all comes down to motivation – it is something 'inside your head' that not only tells you that you want to lose weight but also makes you determined to lose weight and to maintain that 'new' weight for the rest of your life. This is not helped by slimming drugs or diet – it is your motivation that helps you to stick to a diet!

Slimming drugs

In the fifties and sixties, amphetamines were frequently prescribed as 'pep pills' because they give you energy. In addition to being 'uppers' they also reduce your appetite; as a result, millions of prescriptions were issued every year for slimming, particularly to women. However, the reduction of appetite only lasts for a few weeks and then wears off, yet some doctors allowed patients to pick up repeat prescriptions for months and years on end without ever seeing them. As a consequence, thousands of women became addicted to them and some even had mental breakdowns because of the harmful effects that these drugs produce on the mind.

Amphetamine-related drugs used as slimming drugs

Diethylpropion (Apisate and Tenuate Dospan) and *phentermine* (Duromine and Ionamin) are prescribed by some doctors for slimming. These drugs are stimulants ('uppers') and, like the amphetamines ('speed'), they reduce your appetite for a few weeks which is supposed to help you to lose weight. The trouble is that they also give you a 'lift' when you are taking them and you may feel 'let down' when you stop them. Because of this stimulant effect, you may easily start to 'rely' on them and some people may actually become dependent and addicted to them. Because they give a lift, they are also used for 'kicks' by drug abusers.

Phenylpropranolamine is another amphetamine-related drug, which causes a transient reduction of appetite. It is a sympathomimetic drug (see Chapter 2) and in high doses may produce similar harmful effects to the amphetamines. It is present in some cold and cough remedies.

Fenfluramine (Ponderax) increases the concentration of a stimulant chemical in the brain known as serotonin, which helps to reduce the appetite. Fenfluramine is related to the amphetamines but it does not produce stimulation. Very rarely, some people may become tolerant to its effects and they may start to increase the dose to obtain the same effects; if they try to stop the drug suddenly they may develop severe depression – they have become dependent on the drug. Patients should be weaned off the drug slowly because of the risk of a severe depression of mood if the drug is stopped suddenly. Dexfenfluramine (Adifax) produces similar effects but is more specific in its actions on serotonin.

Mazindol (Teronac) is not related to the amphetamines. It stimulates the brain, and if taken daily it reduces your appetite for a few weeks, after which the effect wears off. It may produce mood changes and, although rare, cases of dependence have been reported.

Water tablets (diuretics)

Diuretics act on the kidneys to make them pass more salt and water in the urine. This causes a fall in the volume of the blood, which results in water being drawn out of the body tissues into the blood stream in order to restore the volume of blood to normal. As a result, your body weight goes down because it now contains less water than before. In other words, if you take water tablets for slimming, all you are doing is dehydrating your body. This is why jockeys take them before a race if they are overweight. It is also why boxers do vigorous exercise in order to sweat their weight down just before a fight; it reduces the amount of water in their bodies and reduces their weight. The weight of jockeys and boxers who do this will return to what it was, once they start drinking normally again after the race or the fight.

By taking water tablets you, too, will lose weight because you lose water; but once you stop them your body stops the kidneys passing urine until your body water is back to what it should be and your weight will be back to what it was.

These drugs do not make you lose fat – only water – and yet they may produce unpleasant harmful effects (see Chapter 22). They may cause serious disturbances to your body's water and salt levels.

Slimming remedies that contain bulk laxatives

These slimming remedies usually contain non-digestible plant substances and other agents to increase the bulk of your motions. They absorb water from the bowel contents. They include agar, bassorin (from tragacanth), cellulose derivatives (e.g. methylcellulose), ispaghula (*Plantago ovata*), karaya (sterculia) and psyllium. They act like bulk laxatives. You lose weight because they absorb water from the bowel and make you pass more water in your motions. This water is drawn from the bloodstream into the bowel and then, in order to keep the volume of the blood steady, water is drawn from the tissues into the bloodstream. This produces loss of weight by dehydration. As soon as you stop them, the body restores its water level by reducing the amount of urine you pass until your body water is back to normal – and of course your weight is back to what it was. The loss of water and salts can cause dehydration and muscle weakness. Bulk laxatives may cause obstruction to the intestine and should always be taken with plenty of fluids.

Drugs that increase the bulk of food and are supposed to reduce your appetite

These also act principally as bulk laxatives. They include Celevac (methylcellulose), Cellucon (methylcellulose), Guarem (guar gum), Nilstim (methylcellulose and cellulose), Prefil (sterculia). They attract and absorb water (hydrophilic) and swell. When used to reduce your appetite the idea is that they swell inside the stomach and make you feel full. They are therefore taken before expected meal-times in order to stop you feeling hungry. They can also be taken as meal replacements; for example, as special biscuits.

There is no convincing evidence that these preparations are any more effective than eating raw carrot, apples, celery or salads. Furthermore, their use before meals has not been shown to reduce hunger, because they move out of the stomach and into the intestine within half an hour of swallowing them; nor has it been shown that, although you may have to chew these preparations more than ordinary foods, this has the slightest effect on reducing your desire to eat. They do not help to produce a change in eating behaviour, which is what is needed in the long-term treatment of obesity.

Guar gum

In addition to guar gum acting as a bulk food and bulk laxative and taking fluids out of the bowel there is some evidence that it may reduce the rise in blood sugar that occurs after a meal. This may be because it reduces the absorption of carbohydrates. It is being tried in diabetic patients in an attempt to control the blood glucose level after meals, but there is no convincing evidence from adequate and well controlled studies that it helps you to lose weight. It may cause wind and a distended abdomen.

Herbal remedies

Herbal remedies usually contain drugs that are supposed to make you feel full and eat less, or drugs that make your kidneys pass more water and/or 'laxatives' that make you lose water in your motions. With many herbal preparations you will lose weight because you are losing water from your body. This dehydration may be harmful. As soon as you stop these drugs the body adjusts its water level back to normal by reducing the amount of urine you pass and your weight will go back to what it was before you started such treatment. They do not produce any loss of fat. Herbal remedies should not be used to aid slimming.

Thyroid drugs

Thyroid drugs affect the rate at which you burn up energy (metabolism). They may produce a loss of weight because fat is burned up as a source of energy. However, thyroid drugs make the body act as if the thyroid gland is overworking and they may seriously affect the whole body, particularly the heart. Harmful effects include rapid beating of the heart, restlessness, insomnia, excitability, angina, disorders of heart rhythm, headaches, sweating, fever, vomiting and excessive loss of weight. These effects are very dangerous in people with raised blood pressure or heart disease and in the elderly. Thyroid drugs should never be used to aid slimming.

Local anaesthetics by mouth

The Andean Indians chew coca leaf and this stops them from feeling hungry. Coca contains cocaine, which is a local anaesthetic but produces many other effects – which is probably why the Indians chew the leaf. Benzocaine is a local anaesthetic which is claimed to reduce the appetite if taken in gum or lozenges just before meal-times. It has only short-term effects and may produce harmful effects which include severe allergic reactions (see Chapter 28).

Drugs that are supposed to reduce the absorption of sugar in the diet

These are called *starch blockers* because they are supposed to prevent the digestion of starch in food. They are made up of a protein called phaseolansin, which is obtained from red kidney beans. This substance is said to block the conversion of starch to sugar in the intestine, thus preventing the absorption of sugar from starches in the food. In recent years many of these preparations were marketed in the USA but often they just contained ground-up kidney beans, which caused harmful effects in some people; they were withdrawn from the market for this reason.

Conclusion on the use of slimming drugs

Any benefit that may be produced by slimming drugs is very short lasting in what is, after all, a life-long problem. The risks of using them far outweigh any possible benefit and they should not be used. Remember that herbal remedies are drugs.

Table 43.1 Slimming drugs – harmful effects and warnings

diethylpropion
Harmful effects include headache, allergic and other types of skin rash and, occasionally, sleeplessness, nervousness, hallucinations, restlessness, tremor, constipation, agitation, nervousness, insomnia, anxiety, depression, rapid beating of the heart, raised blood pressure; rarely, there may be mental breakdown in susceptible individuals and enlargement of the breasts (gynaecomastia). *Tolerance* and *dependence* may occur.

Warnings Diethylpropion should not be used in anyone who is emotionally unstable, who has a serious mental illness or a history of drug or alcohol abuse, or who suffers from advanced hardening of the arteries (arteriosclerosis), over-active thyroid gland, high blood pressure, glaucoma, or allergy or sensitivity to amphetamines. It should be used with caution in people with mild or moderate raised blood pressure, angina, irregular heart beats, peptic ulcers, epilepsy, anxiety, tension or depression.

Risks in elderly people Harmful effects may be more frequent and severe.

fenfluramine (U)
Harmful effects Diarrhoea, drowsiness, dry mouth, dizziness and lethargy are the most common harmful effects. Occasionally, there may be headache, stomach upsets, blurred vision, sleep disturbances, retention of fluid in the tissues (e.g. ankle swelling), frequency of passing urine, constipation, shivering, palpitations and low blood pressure. Very rarely, it may cause skin rashes, impotence, loss of hair and haemolytic anaemia. Rebound mental depression may occur if the drug is stopped suddenly. *Tolerance* may occur and, rarely, *dependence*.

Warnings Fenfluramine should be used with caution in anyone with a history of mental depression. It should not be used in people with a history of drug and/or alcohol abuse, nor in someone with glaucoma or who is allergic or sensitive to amphetamines.

Risks in elderly people Harmful effects may be more frequent and severe.

Risks with driving It may affect your ability to drive, so do not drive when you are taking this drug.

Risks with alcohol It increases the effects of alcohol, so do not drink alcohol when you are taking this drug.

mazindol
Harmful effects include dry mouth, sweating and insomnia. Occasionally it

Table 43.1 Slimming drugs – harmful effects and warnings (*cont.*)

may cause constipation, nervousness, palpitations, restlessness, dizziness, tremor, mood changes, headache, depression, drowsiness, weakness, an unpleasant taste, nausea, skin rashes, sweating, clamminess of the skin, difficulty passing urine, impotence and changes in libido.

Warnings Mazindol should not be used in anyone with glaucoma or who is allergic to mazindol, who is agitated or who has a history of serious mental illness, drug or alcohol abuse or who has peptic ulcers, severe impairment of kidney, liver or heart function, severe blood pressure or disorders of heart rhythm.

Risks of dependence Mazindol is related to the amphetamines, which can produce dependence; therefore it should be used with caution.

Risks in elderly people Harmful effects may be more frequent and severe. Do not use.

Risks with driving It may impair your ability to drive so do not drive until you know that it is safe to do so.

phentermine

Harmful effects include restlessness, nausea, vomiting, dry mouth, swelling of the face, skin rashes, headache, constipation, frequency of passing urine, dizziness, nervousness, depression, insomnia, palpitations, rapid heart beat, high blood pressure, and rarely hallucinations and severe mental symptoms. *Tolerance and dependence* may occur.

Warnings Phentermine should not be used in people who are emotionally unstable, who have serious mental illness, who have a history of drug and/or alcohol abuse, or who suffer from advanced hardening of the arteries (arteriosclerosis), over-active thyroid glands, high blood pressure, glaucoma or allergy or sensitivity to amphetamines. It should be used with caution in anyone with mild or moderate raised blood pressure, angina, diabetes, irregular heart beats, peptic ulcers, epilepsy, anxiety, tension or depression.

Risks in elderly people Harmful effects may be more frequent and severe.

Table 43.2 Slimming drugs

Preparation	*Drug*	*Dosage form*
Adifax*	dexenfluramine	Capsules
Apisate	diethylpropion plus B vitamins (thiamine, pyridoxine, riboflavine, nicotinamide)	Sustained-release tablets
Duromine	phentermine	Sustained-release capsules
Ionamin	phentermine	Sustained-release capsules
Ponderax	fenfluramine	Sustained-release capsules
Tenuate Dospan	diethylpropion	Sustained-release tablets
Teronac	mazindol	Tablets

* For Adifax (dexfenfluramine) see Update.

44

Tonics

What is a tonic?

A tonic is anything that improves our feeling of well-being. Any activity that makes us feel better is a 'tonic', whether it is yoga or a game of tennis, a walk in the country or going to a concert, having a few days at home or going away for a holiday. Whatever we do, so long as it improves our feeling of well-being we can say that it has been a 'tonic' – it has done us good! However, the term 'tonic' is also used to describe any substance that we take in order to improve our feelings of well-being. We take such substances (which are mostly drugs or foods) as 'pick-me-ups'. We take them because we believe or have been led to believe that they will give us more vitality, and/or make us feel and look younger.

Placebo effects

Our expectations of the benefits of tonics are influenced by recommendations from relatives and friends and particularly by the powerful influence of advertisements in newspapers, magazines, books and on television. For a tonic to be effective we have to believe that it will benefit us. In other words, the beneficial effects that we experience from taking a tonic are mostly in our minds. They are what doctors call 'placebos'. The word placebo comes from a latin verb meaning 'to please' and placebos usually 'please us'.

In medicine, placebos are used for two purposes. One is as a control when testing the effectiveness of an active drug and the other is 'to please' the patient.

When testing the effectiveness of an active drug, it is important to know whether the effects produced were due to the drug or whether they were in the mind of the patient. To get over this problem, dummy tablets containing an inert substance are made to look just like the tablets of the active drug. These are called placebos. The effects produced by the dummy tablets and by the active tablets are then compared between different groups of patients and also in the same group of patients over time. This is called a blind trial because the patients do not know whether they are taking the dummy tablets or the active tablets. However, doctors may influence the results because they may believe in the active drug and may pass this belief on to their patients. To control for this it is necessary also to 'blind' the doctors so that they do not know whether they are prescribing the dummy tablets or the active tablets. It is only when the trial is finished that the doctors are told which were the active drugs. This is called a double-blind trial, and during the trial the dummy tablets and active tablets carry a secret code, usually known only to the pharmacist who dispenses them (see Chapter 1).

Doctors also use placebos to please their patients. Any treatment can produce what is called a 'placebo effect' – a beneficial effect that comes principally from the mind of the patient rather than being a direct effect of the drug. Any treatment from 'healers', whether they are doctors, surgeons, physiotherapists, psychiatrists, osteopaths or any other health care workers, can produce a placebo effect, and of course witchdoctors produce important placebo effects. The degree of response is determined by the patient's belief in the healer and the treatment and by the reassurance and belief that the healer imparts to the patient.

It is all a matter of believing

The more that patients believe in their healer, the more likely they are to benefit. In addition, different treatments may produce different responses. For example, the colour, shape and taste of drug preparations can influence response. Individuals report more pain relief from red capsules than from yellow ones, more drowsiness from blue capsules than red ones. A bitter taste appears to work better than a sweet one, and the less that tablets and capsules look like those in everyday use the more effective they will probably be.

Obviously some people are more susceptible to suggestion than others, but at least one in three of us will respond to a placebo given for the relief of pain, to calm us down or to make us sleep.

Tonics work because we believe – but there are dangers

All tonics produce a placebo effect (we feel better because we believe in them) but there are dangers to using tonics as general pick-me-ups, because feeling 'run-down' may be a useful warning of an underlying physical and/or mental disorder.

If we have no energy because we are anaemic then we need a blood test and appropriate treatment, not a tonic. If we have no energy because we are anxious and depressed then we need psychological treatment, not a tonic. If we have any physical disorder (e.g. diabetes) that makes us feel 'run-down' then we need specific treatment – we do not need a tonic. In other words, we need treating as a whole person, not just for the symptoms of 'run-downness', yet we spend millions of pounds every year on tonics whose beneficial effects are all in our minds.

The suggestion in advertisements that a particular tonic can help anybody who feels run-down is untrue, misleading and potentially harmful. There is no such substance as a 'general' tonic.

The misuse of iron as a tonic

Iron salts are often included in tonics because many individuals believe and have been led to believe that anaemia is a common cause of feeling run-down. You may develop iron-deficiency anaemia because you are losing blood regularly through, for example, heavy periods or a bleeding peptic ulcer. However, iron deficiency is only one cause of anaemia and the type of anaemia cannot be recognized without carrying out a blood test. Therefore, never treat yourself with iron without having a blood test, and do not let your doctor treat you for anaemia without sending you for a blood test. Remember that blood loss is the commonest cause of iron-deficiency anaemia and that iron is a specific treatment for iron-deficiency anaemia; it is not a tonic. If you do not need iron, you can over-treat with iron and cause problems related to excess iron in the body.

The misuse of vitamins as a tonic

There are optimal daily requirements for vitamins to prevent vitamin-deficiency disorders, and there are recommended doses for treating vitamin-deficiency disorders (see Chapter 45). There is no evidence that the regular daily use of doses above recommended requirements does the slightest bit of good. It may actually cause harm. The belief that, if taking 50 mg of a vitamin daily keeps you healthy, 500 mg will make you even more healthy is just not true.

Nerve tonics

Many decades ago it was found that nerve cells contain glycerophosphates; because of this the manufacture and sale of nerve tonics containing glycerophosphates and hypophosphates has proved an extremely lucrative business. This has happened despite the fact that the use of these drugs has never been shown to produce any physical benefit at all. However, they are harmless and have a psychological effect. Unfortunately, they are mixed with all sorts of bitters (appetite stimulants), laxatives and stimulants, some of which may produce harmful effects if taken regularly over time.

Some *tonic wines* contain hypophosphates and vitamins, but people who take them should realize that it is the alcohol in the wine that makes them feel better and which they miss if they stop taking it.

Appetite stimulants

Bitters, which appear in many tonics, are supposed to stimulate your appetite. They stimulate salivation and the production of gastric juice by taste and smell. They often contain various vitamins and iron salts. Certain alcoholic drinks are also used for this purpose (aperitifs). However, persistent loss of appetite is not the sort of symptom you should treat yourself without first having a complete medical check-up.

Yeast

Yeast is the basis of many tonics. It supplies you with a few vitamins and is often combined with caffeine to stimulate you. Some yeast preparations may contain obsolete drugs, which can be harmful.

Digestive tonics

Over-the-counter remedies containing digestive enzymes such as pepsin and pancreatin, liver salts and bile salts are valueless. Some contain small quantities of obsolete laxatives.

Health foods

The beneficial effects produced by this wide range of usually very expensive products are principally in the mind. They work because we believe they work, and the more expensive they are the more they seem to work. There is no harm in this provided we are not physically or mentally ill and require more specific treatments and provided that the products do not contain harmful ingredients.

Herbal remedies

Herbal remedies contain extracts of drugs from herbs. They often contain several drugs, some of which may be ineffective or present in ineffective doses, and some may be obsolete. They clearly have a strong placebo effect (see earlier) in those people who believe in them. Some of their principal effects appear to be concerned with increasing the volume of the urine (diuretic effect), increasing the volume of the motions (laxative effect) and depressing the brain (sedative effect).

45

Vitamins

Vitamins are constituents of the diet that are essential in small amounts for the maintenance of normal growth and function of the body, but they are not made within the body. They are present in the tissues of plants and animals, and a well balanced diet consisting of meats, dairy produce, fish, grains, vegetables and fruit will provide an adult with his daily requirements. These daily requirements have been worked out over the past 50 years and are listed in Table 45.1.

A deficiency of food produces a deficiency of vitamins, and so there is a significant difference between the number of people who develop vitamin deficiencies in the developing countries compared with the number in the well fed West. Western countries suffer from over-production and over-storage of food and their people suffer mainly from diseases related to over-eating. This contrasts with developing countries who suffer from under-production and shortage of food and whose people suffer from diseases caused by under-feeding – malnutrition. It is in these countries that we see the ravages of starvation and the many dreadful diseases produced by a deficiency of vitamins. For example, deficiency of vitamin A is a major cause of blindness in thousands of people in south-east Asia.

Although starvation is the main cause of severe vitamin deficiency in some areas of the world, mild vitamin deficiency can occur in prosperous countries – not because of food shortage but because of food manufacturing techniques, food fads and dieting. In prosperous countries poverty can also lead to a diet low in vitamins, particularly among elderly people. It may also occur because of self-neglect and poor diets in drug addicts and alcoholics.

Failure to effectively absorb vitamins from food is a physical cause of vitamin deficiency. This can result from disease of the liver, gall bladder, stomach or intestine; surgical removal of parts of the stomach or intestine is also an important cause of vitamin deficiency. The body may develop an increased requirement for vitamins (e.g. in pregnancy) or it may not be able to use vitamins properly because of a genetic defect in the body's biochemistry.

The rate at which the body's stores of vitamins become used up varies greatly. Stores of vitamins that are soluble in water (B and C) can quickly become used up, but if you take in more than the body can store, these vitamins are just passed out in the urine. Those vitamins that are soluble in fat (e.g. A, D, E, K) are stored in the body, and a deficient intake may take months to become apparent.

Specific vitamin-deficiency disorders are very rare, and what we usually see are multi-vitamin deficiencies caused by a generally poor diet. The development of disorders caused by deficiencies of vitamins is slow and symptoms are mixed, so we rarely see the classic pictures of specific vitamin deficiency described later.

The use of vitamins

Vitamins are used to treat diseases caused by vitamin deficiencies (see later) and also to prevent vitamin-deficiency disorders developing by giving them as supplements to an individual's diet.

The doses of vitamins used to treat established vitamin-deficiency disorders are much higher than those used to prevent deficiencies. The latter need only be at a level to supplement a diet that is deficient in vitamins in order to bring the daily intake up to recommended levels. Beyond this, there is *no merit in taking more.* Unfortunately, the manufacturing and selling of vitamin preparations is a multi-million-pound business and millions of people are persuaded to take vitamins every day which they do not need and in doses that are potentially harmful.

There is no convincing evidence of the benefits of megavitamin treatment (massive doses of vitamins) despite its current fashion. The body requires an optimal amount of vitamins each day and the amounts required for normal body activities are very small indeed.

When vitamins are taken, not as part of a well-balanced diet but in highly concentrated forms, they must be regarded as *drugs* and as such they may produce harmful effects. Those vitamins that are soluble in water (the B vitamins and vitamin C), if taken in excess of the body's requirements, are quickly excreted. High-dose preparations may occasionally cause harm and their use is often unnecessary and wasteful. Fat-soluble vitamins such as A, D and E, if taken in excess of daily requirements, may accumulate in the body until toxic concentrations are reached.

People who need to take multi-vitamin preparations

Multi-vitamin preparations may be of benefit to people whose diet is inadequate; for example, those who are poor, frail and/or elderly; those who are faddy about their food or who are on strict slimming or vegetarian diets; and alcoholics and drug addicts who take in too little food.

Some disorders of the stomach and intestine may result in an inadequate absorption of vitamins, and people with such disorders will require supplementary vitamins. Babies and toddlers may need multi-vitamins, as may patients during a long debilitating illness. Also, children on special diets to treat errors of metabolism, food intolerances or allergies should be given a multi-vitamin preparation each day.

Comment Taking multi-vitamins is no substitute for a good nutritious diet. Yet, paradoxically, it is often those individuals who can best afford a good diet and who should not need extra vitamins who actually take supplementary vitamins.

Injections of high potency preparations of water-soluble vitamins (B and C) should be reserved for serious disorders such as acute illness with a high fever, alcoholism, confusion following an illness or surgery, and neuritis of the nerves supplying the arms and legs (peripheral neuritis). They should be used with caution because there is a risk of producing a serious allergic reaction (anaphylaxis). Intravenous use should be by slow infusion.

Vitamin A

Sources

Vitamin A is formed in the liver from carotene, which is a pigment responsible for the yellow and orange colour of certain fruits and vegetables (e.g. carrots). Those high in carotene include dark green vegetables (e.g. spinach or broccoli), carrots, apricots, melons and pumpkins. Animal and fish foods provide a major source of already formed vitamin A, particularly liver and kidneys, fish liver oils and dairy produce (milk, eggs, cheese).

Vitamin A deficiency diseases

Deficiency of vitamin A rarely occurs in people who have the opportunity to eat a normal diet. If deficiencies in the diet occur, it takes many months before symptoms develop because the body stores of vitamin A have to be used up first.

Vitamin A deficiency may be caused by malnutrition, and serious diseases such as tuberculosis and cancer may cause an increased excretion of vitamin A. Any disorder that affects the absorption of fat from the intestine will cause vitamin A deficiency (e.g. cystic fibrosis, coelic disease). Drugs such as cholestyramine, used to lower blood fat levels, may cause defective absorption of vitamin A and other fat-soluble vitamins (D, E, K) from the intestine.

Lack of vitamin A is a common cause of eye damage in children suffering from malnutrition in parts of the world where famine occurs. Of course, it is also associated with other vitamin and food deficiencies.

Deficiency of vitamin A affects surface cells throughout the body – the skin becomes dry and scaly, sweat and tear glands become blocked, the eyes become dry and itching and may ulcerate, and the cornea may be damaged, affecting vision. Deficiency may also cause night-blindness due to defective formation of the pigment at the back of the eye.

Risks of overdosing with vitamin A

Excessive doses of vitamin A may cause vitamin A intoxication, resulting in fatigue, loss of weight, loss of appetite, irritability, vomiting and stomach upsets, fever, itching and loss of hair. Anaemia, headaches, difficulty with vision and enlargement of the liver may occur. The skin looks yellow, goes dry and cracks. The bones and joints become swollen and painful, and in children growth may become stunted. The pressure inside the skull may increase and produce symptoms that may be mistaken for a brain tumour; this usually occurs in children.

Acute overdose of vitamin A causes drowsiness, irritability, headaches and peeling of the skin. The use of large doses of vitamin A or eating liver rich in Vitamin A in the first 3 months of pregnancy may damage the baby.

Derivatives of vitamin A are being used to treat some skin disorders (see Chapter 75). They are also being tested for their possible effects in preventing certain types of cancer, but we still need more convincing evidence of these alleged benefits.

B vitamins

These include:

vitamin B_1 – thiamine, aneurine
vitamin B_2 – riboflavine
vitamin B_6 – pyridoxine
niacin – nicotinic acid, nicotinamide, nicotinic acid amide, niacinamide (vitamin B_3)
folic acid – pteroylglutamic acid
pantothenic acid – vitamin B_5
biotin – vitamin H
vitamin B_{12} – cyanocobalamin

Vitamin B_1 (thiamine)

Sources

Foods rich in vitamin B_1 include brown rice, wheat germ, whole wheat, eggs, liver, pork, beef, peas, beans and nuts, yeast and oatmeal.

Vitamin B_1 deficiency disease

Deficiency of vitamin B_1 causes inflammation of the nerves, producing numbness, pins and needles, weakness of muscles and difficulty in walking. It also causes heart failure and oedema (fluid in the tissues). Nausea and vomiting may occur. This group of disorders is known as beri-beri. The swollen tissue type is known as wet beri-beri and the nerve type as dry beri-beri but people usually suffer from both together. Vitamin B_1 deficiency may also damage the brain (Wernicke's encephalopathy) and cause mental confusion and psychotic illness (Korsakoff's syndrome). These disorders may occur in alcoholics on poor diets deficient in vitamins, in people on hunger strike and in patients with severe and persistent vomiting (e.g. of pregnancy). The amount of vitamin B_1 required goes up with the amount of carbohydrate in the diet, and people given large amounts of glucose solution need added vitamin B_1 (thiamine).

Riboflavine (vitamin B_2)

Sources

Foods rich in riboflavine include yeast, milk, eggs, cheese, liver and kidneys, wheat germ and wheat bran, soya flour, yoghurt, green vegetables and beans.

Riboflavine deficiency usually occurs along with other vitamin deficiencies and is due to a poor diet. The need for riboflavine increases during periods of increased cell growth, such as during pregnancy and wound healing. Deficiency may occur in alcoholics, and low levels of riboflavine have been noted in women on the contraceptive pill. Some vegetarians may develop a deficiency and so may people who take very little milk in their diet.

Riboflavine (vitamin B_2) deficiency disease

Deficiency of riboflavine produces sore lips (angular stomatitis), ulcers of the mouth, a sore magenta-coloured tongue, skin rashes (seborrhoeic dermatitis) and blood vessels on the cornea of the eye (vascularization of the cornea). The patient may go on to develop seborrhoeic dermatitis of the face, a generalized dermatitis, and itching and burning eyes.

Pyridoxine (vitamin B_6)

Sources

Foods rich in pyridoxine include yeast, eggs, meat, fatty fish, potatoes, bananas, fruits and vegetables, peanuts, yeasts, soya flour, whole grain cereals and brown rice.

Pyridoxine deficiency disease

Deficiency of pyridoxine in infants produces irritability and convulsions. Deficiency in adults causes dermatitis, dry skin on the face, sore lips and tongue, sores in the mouth, and damage to nerves, producing numbness and pins and needles in the hands and feet, and muscle weakness. Depression, mental dullness and anaemia may also occur.

Hydralazine, penicillamine and oestrogens interfere with the body's use of pyridoxine and may cause a deficiency. Isoniazid used to treat tuberculosis may also affect the body's use of pyridoxine. Patients on a poor diet may develop signs of nerve damage when taking these drugs, due to their interference with the use of pyridoxine. These symptoms are cured by taking pyridoxine. It may also relieve the fits and mental symptoms caused by cycloserine, also used to treat tuberculosis.

Opinion is divided as to whether pyridoxine should be given routinely to patients receiving treatment with isoniazid or cycloserine for tuberculosis. It seems a sensible thing to do but of course it is equally, if not more important, to try to ensure that the patient takes an adequate diet.

Pyridoxine reduces the effects of levodopa used to treat parkinsonism. The combined oral contraceptive (the 'pill') may interfere with the use of pyridoxine in some women and cause depression, which may respond to pyridoxine. There is no convincing evidence from adequate and well controlled studies of the benefit of pyridoxine in preventing pregnancy sickness. For its use in premenstrual syndrome, see Chapter 68.

Pyridoxine dependency

In addition to pyridoxine deficiency disease caused by poor diet or drugs, there is a group of disorders in which an individual does not show signs of deficiency of pyridoxine and yet seems to require high amounts of the vitamin. These disorders are rare and include a type of anaemia that responds to pyridoxine and which can easily be mis-diagnosed as due to iron deficiency.

Risks of overdosing with pyridoxine

In doses above 500 mg per day pyridoxine may cause nerve damage to the sensory nerves. This has been noted in women taking large doses of pyridoxine to relieve premenstrual syndrome. High doses of pyridoxine also block the production of the milk-producing hormone, prolactin, and affect various processes in the body. Do not take more than 50 mg daily without medical advice.

Niacin (*nicotinamide*)

Sources

Foods rich in niacin include liver, kidney, fish, poultry, meats, yeast, milk, yoghurt, cheese, eggs, wheat germ, wheat bran, nuts, vegetables and brown rice.

Humans can make niacin from tryptophan (an essential amino acid from protein in food) which is a precursor of serotonin, a nerve messenger, and has been used to treat depression. Requirements for niacin are increased during vigorous exercise when large amounts of calories are burned up, during acute illness or infection and following injury or burns. A diet high in calories requires additional niacin, and so does a diet low in protein or a diet consisting mainly of maize.

Niacin deficiency disease

Deficiency affects the skin, producing dermatitis; the intestine, producing diarrhoea; and the brain, producing dementia – what are called the three Ds. The mouth is sore (stomatitis), the tongue becomes red and swollen, and nausea, vomiting and diarrhoea are common. Damage to the brain produces headache, dizziness, insomnia, and, if severe, delusions, hallucinations and dementia. Damage to the spinal cord and nerves produces disorders of sensation (numbness and pins and needles) and weakness and paralysis of movement. These signs and symptoms caused by niacin deficiency are known as *pellagra*.

Risks of overdosing with niacin

Overdose may cause flushing, irritation of the stomach lining, a rise in blood uric acid, interference with glucose levels in the blood and, occasionally, liver damage, producing jaundice. High doses should not be used by mouth in people with peptic ulcers and, because niacin can cause a release of histamine, it should be used with caution in anyone with asthma.

Folic acid

Sources

Foods rich in folic acid (pteroylglutamic acid) as folates include fresh green vegetables, wheat germ, wheat bran, eggs, yeast, liver, kidneys, peanuts, soya flour, oranges, bananas, avocados, beans, beetroot and brown rice. Canning, long exposure to heat and refining can reduce the folic acid content of food significantly. Fresh green vegetables are the best source of folic acid.

Folic acid deficiency disease

Deficiency produces anaemia and may be caused by poor diet, by disorders that interfere with the absorption of folic acid from the small intestine and by pregnancy. In alcoholism the diet is usually poor in folic acid; also, alcohol is toxic to liver cells and interferes with the use of folic acid. Anticonvulsant drugs (e.g. phenytoin, primidone, phenobarbitone), methotrexate, trimethoprim and oral contraceptives reduce the blood level of folic acid and may produce anaemia, which responds to folic acid. Anti-malarial drugs and nitrofurantoin may also cause anaemia by interfering with folic acid metabolism.

Pantothenic acid (vitamin B_5)

Sources

Foods rich in pantothenic acid include yeast, liver and kidneys, wheat bran, soya flour, egg yolks, poultry, meat, whole grains, pulses and vegetables.

Pantothenic acid deficiency disease

A deficiency disease has not been recognized in humans but a deficiency syndrome has been produced under experimental conditions, causing abdominal pains, cramps, vomiting, muscle tenderness, weakness, nerve damage (pins and needles in the hands and feet) and insomnia.

Biotin (vitamin H)

Sources

Rich food sources include yeast, eggs, liver and kidneys, peanuts, wheat bran, wholemeal bread, corn, fish, meats, rice and vegetables. It is made by bacteria in the intestine.

Biotin deficiency disease

Deficiency can be caused by eating a large amount of raw egg white. A protein in egg white, avidin, binds to biotin to prevent its absorption. Cooking eggs destroys the avidin and releases the biotin. Deficiency may also follow long-term tube-feeding lacking biotin. It produces dermatitis and loss of hair (alopecia).

Vitamin B_{12}

Sources

Foods rich in vitamin B_{12} (cyanocobalamin) include meat, milk, cheese and eggs.

Vitamin B_{12} deficiency disease

Vitamin B_{12} deficiency disease is discussed in detail in Chapter 47. To be absorbed into the blood stream, vitamin B_{12} has to combine with a substance secreted by the stomach, known as the intrinsic factor. Vitamin B_{12} is known as the extrinsic factor, and the combination of intrinsic and extrinsic factors is absorbed through the small intestine. Vitamin B_{12} is stored in the liver. One of its many actions is upon blood formation by the bone marrow. Deficiency produces a special type of anaemia called megaloblastic anaemia, which is usually due to lack of the intrinsic factor in the stomach (as in pernicious anaemia); to disorders of the small intestine, affecting absorption of extrinsic/intrinsic complex; and, rarely, to dietary deficiency of vitamin B_{12} in strict vegetarians or in those living in the tropics.

Vitamin C (ascorbic acid)

Sources

Foods rich in vitamin C include citrus fruits, rose hips and green vegetables. Cooking reduces the vitamin C content of food.

Vitamin C deficiency disease

Deficiency of vitamin C is rare in Western countries but may occur among alcoholics and drug addicts, in patients with serious mental illness who do not eat an adequate diet, in elderly, poor and neglected people, and in patients with disorders of their stomach and intestine which interfere with the absorption of vitamin C from food.

A deficiency causes delay in wound healing. Early signs of deficiency include loss of appetite, weakness, and joint and muscle pains. Prominent hair roots may develop in the skin, particularly on the thighs and buttocks. The hairs become coiled and the hair root openings blocked. In severe deficiency, bleeding abnormalities develop and there is bleeding into the skin (bruising), joints, muscles and other organs, the lining of the stomach and intestine, liver, kidneys and other organs. The gums become swollen and they bleed and become infected. If left untreated the teeth will fall out. In infants, vitamin C deficiency causes bleeding into the gums and skin, retarded physical growth, anaemia and impaired growth of bones. The syndrome of symptoms and signs of severe vitamin C deficiency is called scurvy.

Other uses of vitamin C

Vitamin C helps the absorption of iron from food. Lack of evidence of the benefits of vitamin C in treating colds is discussed in Chapter 3.

Because vitamin C promotes healing, large doses have been used to promote healing after surgery, injury or fractures, to treat cold sores and rectal polyps or to stimulate the immune system. However, there is no convincing evidence from adequate and well controlled studies of the benefits of vitamin C in these disorders.

Mega doses of vitamin C are also claimed to lower cholesterol and blood fat levels and to prolong life in patients dying from cancer, but there is no convincing evidence of such benefits from adequate and well controlled studies.

Risks of high doses of vitamin C

The risks of high doses of vitamin C include indigestion, diarrhoea and kidney stones. A rebound deficiency of vitamin C in the blood can occur if high daily doses are suddenly stopped. Rebound scurvy has been reported in newborn babies whose mothers took high daily doses of vitamin C throughout their pregnancies.

Vitamin C in high doses makes the urine acid, and this may cause drugs such as the tricyclic anti-depressants to be excreted more rapidly and therefore to be less effective. High concentrations of vitamin C in the urine may give a false positive test for glucose in the urine.

Vitamin D

Vitamin D is the name of a group of similarly structured chemicals which includes vitamin D_3 (cholecalciferol) and vitamin D_2 (ergocalciferol).

Sources

Foods rich in vitamin D include fish oils and oily fish, margarine, eggs and milk. It is also produced by the body after exposure of the skin to sunshine. The average diet of babies and some children may not provide sufficient vitamin D, particularly if they are not exposed to an adequate amount of sunshine.

Vitamin D_3 is the natural form of vitamin D; it is produced from cholesterol in the skin after exposure to sunlight. If sun exposure is not sufficient to stimulate production by the skin, the body has to rely on vitamin D from the diet (e.g. fish oil, eggs, milk).

Vitamin D_2 is obtained from ultraviolet radiation of ergosterol, a steroid found in plants and some fungi.

Vitamin D from the skin and from food is concentrated and made active by the liver. It is then made into a more active form by the kidneys under stimulation from the parathyroid glands and depending on the levels of calcium and phosphorus in the blood. This explains why signs and symptoms of vitamin D deficiency may develop in people with kidney or liver disease – they are unable to make the active forms of vitamin D. In the body, vitamin D acts as both a vitamin and a hormone (see Chapter 68, under 'Osteoporosis').

Anti-epileptic drugs such as phenytoin and phenobarbitone can increase the breakdown of vitamin D in the liver and cause bone disease (see later).

Bones, the intestine and the kidneys are primary targets for the active forms of vitamin D but many other tissues also possess vitamin D receptors. Vitamin D controls the absorption of calcium and phosphorus by the intestine, and, with parathyroid hormone and calcitonin, it controls the movement of calcium in and out of bone. It also regulates the excretion of calcium and phosphorus in the urine (see Chapter 68, under 'Osteoporosis').

Vitamin D deficiency may occur because of lack of sunshine, poor diet (e.g. vegetarian diets) or poor absorption from the intestine because of disease of the intestine. Signs and symptoms of vitamin D deficiency may also occur in liver and kidney disease and in disorders of the parathyroid gland. Phosphates in laxatives, if they are used regularly over a prolonged period of time, may contribute to vitamin D deficiency.

Vitamin D deficiency diseases

Rickets is a bone disorder caused by defective calcium and phosphorus absorption and metabolism which occurs when infants and children are short of vitamin D. This is caused by a diet poor in vitamin D and lack of sunshine. Soft patches develop in the skull, the forehead sticks out (frontal bossing), the rib joints are swollen (rickety rosary), and the legs are bowed.

The adult counterpart of rickets is called *osteomalacia* (bone softening). In the past, women who kept indoors, had poor diets and multiple pregnancies were prone to develop osteomalacia. Vegetarian Asians, particularly women who cover themselves in clothing, may need to take a vitamin D preparation each day, especially during the winter months. Vitamin D deficiency may follow surgical removal of parts of the small intestine, which can cause defective vitamin D absorption. Kidney disease and certain anti-epileptic drugs (see Chapter 37) may cause osteomalacia. Symptoms include bone pain and tenderness, backache, muscle weakness and spontaneous fractures.

The treatment of rickets and osteomalacia is to give vitamin D daily by mouth. The recovery is dramatic but patients need to be followed up carefully in order to prevent overdosing with vitamin D. During treatment, the level of calcium in the blood and urine should be checked regularly. High blood calcium levels should be avoided. These may result from an increased absorption of calcium from the intestine and an increased movement of calcium in and out of bone. The phosphate level should also be checked because phosphate binds to calcium and may be deposited in kidneys, eyes, brains and heart.

Risks of overdosing with vitamin D

Excessive vitamin D in the body (hypervitaminosis) may occur due to overdosing with vitamin D, abnormal conversion of vitamin D to its active forms in certain diseases (e.g. sarcoidosis) and a change in the sensitivity of some tissues in the body to vitamin D.

Initial signs and symptoms of vitamin D intoxication include weakness, tiredness, headache, nausea and passing large volumes of urine. These are caused by a rise in calcium levels in the blood and urine. As a result of the high levels of calcium in the blood, calcium is deposited in the kidneys (producing stones), in blood vessels, the heart, lungs and skin. This can be serious in infants, who seem to be very sensitive to vitamin D intoxication. The disorder is treated by stopping vitamin D and, if the blood calcium is high, by giving a diet low in calcium, corticosteroids (e.g. prednisolone) and plenty of fluids.

Vitamin K

Sources

There are two main types of vitamin K – K_1 and K_2. Foods rich in vitamin K_1 include green vegetables and liver. Vitamin K_2 is produced by bacteria in the intestine. Synthetic vitamin K preparations include menadiol (Synkavit).

Vitamin K deficiency diseases

Vitamin K is necessary for the production of various blood-clotting factors by the liver (see Chapter 26) and proteins for bone formation. Deficiency of vitamin K causes a reduction in blood-clotting factors resulting in bleeding and delayed blood clotting.

Vitamin K is soluble in fat and requires bile salts for its absorption from the intestine. Deficiency may be caused by disorders of the intestine that interfere with fat absorption, by obstruction to the production of bile (e.g. obstructive jaundice); and by some drugs (e.g. sulphonamides, tetracyclines and, particularly, some of the cyclosporins; see Chapter 50). These drugs kill the bacteria in the intestine that produce vitamin K_2.

Anti-clotting drugs by mouth (see Chapter 26), which block the use of vitamin K to make blood-clotting factors, are the main cause of bleeding disorders due to vitamin K deficiency.

Vitamin K_1 (phytomenadione; Konakion) is given routinely by intramuscular injection to newborn babies to prevent bleeding; this is necessary because it will take time for bacteria in the bowel to start producing vitamin K. Synthetic vitamin K (menadiol) should not be used in newborn babies because there is a risk of damaging the red blood cells (haemolytic anaemia), causing jaundice and kernicterus (see Chapter 26).

Deficiency of vitamin K in adults is treated with synthetic vitamin K (menadiol; Synkavit) because it is soluble in water and therefore does not need fats for its absorption.

Risks of overdose with vitamin K

Vitamin K_1 injected into a vein has been reported to cause flushing, chest pain, breathlessness and death, but whether this was caused directly by the vitamin K_1 or the solution in which it was suspended is not certain.

Vitamin E

Sources

Vitamin E (tocopherols) is present in various forms in vegetable oils, margarine, nuts, seeds, dried fruits, soya bean, wheat germ, maize, rice germ, cotton seed and green leaves (e.g. lettuce).

Opinions about the need for vitamin E in our diet are sharply divided. Those who promote and sell vitamin E preparations make many claims for its benefits, and so much magic and mystique have been built up about its uses that it is often difficult to separate fact from fiction.

Vitamin E deficiency diseases

Deficiency of vitamin E in the diet is very rare but, because it is soluble in fat and requires bile for its absorption from the intestine, vitamin E deficiency may occur in serious disorders of the intestine that affect fat absorption (such as surgical removal of parts of the intestine). Low levels of vitamin E have also been found in young children with a congenital blockage of the bile duct. These children develop muscle weakness, which responds to vitamin E by injection. Vitamin E deficiency may also occur in children with cystic fibrosis and in adults with gall bladder disease, which causes a reduction in the amount of bile in the intestine. Vitamin E deficiency has occurred in the past in premature babies who were tube-fed with a formula that did not contain vitamin E.

Vitamin E acts as an anti-oxidant and has been found of some use in preventing eye damage in premature babies who are given oxygen by a ventilator. However, a number of premature infants in the USA died when they were given vitamin E by intravenous injection. Whether these deaths were due to the vitamin E or to the formulation is not known.

A specific group of signs and symptoms caused by a deficiency of vitamin E has not been described. Anaemia may occur due to the life of red blood cells being shortened, and some symptoms of nerve damage have been associated with vitamin E deficiency. In premature infants (who have inadequate stores of vitamin E), a deficiency is associated with the breaking up of red blood cells (haemolytic anaemia), an increase in blood platelets and a collection of fluid in the tissues (oedema).

The myths about vitamin E

Some of the myths about vitamin E have come from experiments on animals in which vitamin E deficiency produces numerous disorders. These include damage to the nervous tissue, muscles of the skeleton and heart muscle, and to the blood-forming tissues in bone marrow. As a consequence, vitamin E has been tried in patients suffering from disorders that can be related to such damaged tissues. To date it has not been convincingly proved that a deficiency of vitamin E is the cause of such disorders in humans or that vitamin E improves them.

Vitamin E is promoted as an anti-ageing vitamin, yet there is no evidence for such a claim; nor is there any evidence that it has any effect

Table 45.1 Vitamins – daily requirements for healthy adults

Vitamin	*Amount*
Vitamin A	1 mg
Vitamin B complex	
Thiamine	1 mg
Riboflavine	1.5 mg
Niacin	15–20 mg
Pyridoxine	3 mg
Pantothenic acid	5 mg
Biotin	100 micrograms
Folate (folic acid)	200 micrograms
Vitamin B_{12}	3 micrograms
Vitamin C	30–60 mg
Vitamin D	3 micrograms (none if adequate sunshine)
Vitamin E	10 mg
Vitamin K	100 micrograms

on sterility or virility in humans. The latter idea has come out of animal studies that have shown that vitamin E deficiency produces irreversible sterility in male rats. In female rats a deficiency of vitamin E causes death of the fetus and a premature end to pregnancy but there is no evidence of its benefits in preventing abortion in humans. Nor is there any evidence of its benefits in people suffering from disorders of menstruation or menopausal symptoms.

There is no convincing evidence from adequate and well controlled studies of the benefit of vitamin E in preventing cancer, in treating circulatory disorders or in preventing or treating coronary artery diseases, particularly the symptom of angina. There is also no convincing evidence that vitamin E improves athletic performance, improves your sex life, benefits fibrocystic disease of the breast or prevents caratacts.

Vitamin E seems to protect the fatty surfaces of cells. Diets high in polyunsaturated fatty acids increase an animal's requirements for vitamin E but this has not been shown in humans, probably because such diets also contain high levels of vitamin E anyway (e.g. sunflower oil). Selenium is a trace element that is involved with vitamin E in the body. It can prevent or reverse some of the symptoms of vitamin E deficiency in animals. Vitamin E also protects animals against various drugs and metals but no such action has been shown in humans.

There is a relationship between vitamin A and vitamin E. Vitamin E seems to 'protect' vitamin A, and vitamin A absorption from food is increased by the presence of vitamin E. High doses of vitamin E may cause bowel upsets.

Other vitamins

Aminobenzoic acid

This has sometimes been included in the vitamin B group. It is involved in the production of folic acid by micro-organisms. It is not a true vitamin for humans. It is also known as para-aminobenzoic acid or PABA. It is a growth factor for bacteria, which is blocked by sulphonamide drugs (Chapter 54) and certain anti-cancer drugs that block folic acid (Chapter 76). It is used in sunscreen preparations (see Chapter 75); it may cause contact dermatitis and make the skin allergic to the sun's rays.

Bioflavoids

These were previously called vitamin P but there is no evidence that they function as vitamins. They are usually found along with vitamin C in, for example, citrus fruits (skin and pulp), tomatoes, grapes, apricots and green peppers. They are also called flavones, and all kinds of unsubstantiated claims have been made for their benefits in the treatment of heavy periods, varicose veins, bruising, haemorrhoids, nose bleeds and bleeding gums. There is no evidence that deficiency causes bleeding under the skin and easy bruising.

Choline

This is a precursor in the production of acetylcholine, an important nerve messenger in the body (see Chapter 2). It can be manufactured in the body and it is therefore not strictly a vitamin. No deficiency disease has been reported. Despite the claims, there is no convincing evidence from adequate and well controlled studies of its benefits in treating angina, atherosclerosis, stroke, thrombosis, Alzheimer's disease or senile dementia.

Inositol

This is found in muscle and brain. It is not a true vitamin because the body can make it. It is present in cereals and vegetables as phytic acid (a combination of inositol and phosphorus), and is a major constituent of lecithin. Despite the claims, there is no convincing evidence from adequate and well controlled studies of its benefits in treating anxiety or schizophrenia, or in restoring hair growth.

Laetrile

Laetrile is present in vitamin B complex, and the richest sources of it are peach kernels and apple pips. It provides a source of cyanide in the body which is claimed to destroy cancer cells.

No deficiency disease has been reported and no dietary requirements are known. Overdose produces cyanide poisoning – cold sweats, headaches, nausea, lethargy, low blood pressure, breathlessness and blueness of the lips. There is no convincing evidence of its benefit in treating cancer.

Lecithins

Lecithins are complex mixtures of choline, inositol, fatty acids and phosphorus. They are present in animal and vegetable cells. Rich sources include wheat, soya beans, peanuts, liver, meats, fish, eggs, corn, oats and rice. Despite the claims, there is no convincing evidence from adequate and well controlled studies of their benefits in treating raised blood pressure, angina, strokes, senile dementia or Alzheimer's disease, in reducing cholesterol and other blood fats or in dissolving gall stones.

Oil of evening primrose

Fats are natural organic compounds that act as structural and storage materials in plants and animals. They are mixtures of glycerol esters and can be split by water into glycerol and fatty acids. Fats differ from oils because they are solid at 20°C whereas oils are liquid.

Saturated fats contain fatty acids that cannot absorb any more hydrogen, whereas *unsaturated fats* can absorb additional hydrogen. The role of saturated fats and unsaturated fats in causing fatty deposit in arteries is discussed in Chapter 25.

Linoleic, linolenic and arachidonic acids are unsaturated fatty acids. They are essential for the normal functioning of all membranes and are involved in cell growth. They are therefore also known as *essential fatty acids*.

Oil from the seeds of the evening primrose contains large amounts of unsaturated fatty acids and of gamma-linolenic acid (GLA), which is usually produced in humans from linoleic acid.

Claims are frequently made for the benefits of essential fatty acids in human disorders ranging from skin diseases to multiple sclerosis; yet there is no convincing evidence from adequate and well controlled studies of their benefit in these conditions.

The major claim for oil of evening primrose is that not only does it contain essential fatty acids but it also contains gamma-linolenic acid (GLA), which is a precursor (a forerunner) for the development of an anti-inflammatory chemical (a prostaglandin) (see Chapter 30). However, the body makes its own GLA from linoleic acid in food; therefore any benefit claimed for oil of evening primrose must be backed by evidence that the body is failing to make prostaglandins because of a shortage of gamma-linolenic acid and that this deficiency and/or any other defect in the manufacture of prostaglandins in the body is corrected by taking oil of evening primrose. As yet there is no convincing evidence of such abnormalities in the numerous diseases that oil of evening primrose is claimed to benefit. Furthermore, we lack convincing evidence, from adequate and well controlled studies, of the benefits of oil of evening primrose in any disorder other than atopic eczema (but see Chapter 75). (U)

Comment Any deficiencies of essential fatty acids and other fatty acids are best corrected by eating a. well balanced and adequate diet, because deficiencies of such micro-nutrients seldom occur singly. A poor diet is much more likely to produce a *general* deficiency of vitamins and micro-nutrients rather than specific ones.

Are there any benefits from taking extra vitamins and/or minerals?

Taking extra vitamins and/or minerals over and above the normal recommended requirements has become a way of life for many over-fed people of the West. People who can afford an adequate and well balanced diet, which should supply all their needs, seek relief from numerous real and/or imaginary symptoms by taking extra vitamins and minerals. They seek perpetual 'youth' and 'zest' and hope to slow down the natural progression of ageing by 'popping' handfuls of vitamins and mineral pills every day. They are aided and abetted by the slick advertising used by the manufacturers and suppliers of vitamins, minerals and so-called health products. Yet most of the benefits claimed for these products are unsubstantiated. Their principal effects are in the mind (see Chapter 44), and there is something very sickening about the millions of pounds spent on extra vitamins, minerals and health products by people in parts of the world where there is too much food available compared with parts of the world where people are starving because of a shortage of food and in whom diseases (not imaginary symptoms) are caused by a deficiency of vitamins.

Current fashions

Fashions for taking various extra vitamins, minerals and health products come and go. At present pyridoxine, vitamin C, vitamin E, oil of evening primrose, calcium, chromium magnesium, zinc and selenium are in fashion. These days it is almost impossible to pick up a women's magazine or a health magazine that does not go on about pyridoxine, vitamin E or oil of evening primrose. Zinc is now supposed to cure all kinds of things from acne to anorexia nervosa, and selenium is recommended for treating disorders as diverse as arthritis, angina, cataracts and cancer.

Treatment claims

Below are listed some symptoms and disorders that are supposed to benefit from treatment with extra vitamins and/or minerals. But these claims are not based on findings from adequate and well controlled studies – in other words, there is no convincing evidence of such benefits.

Acne No convincing evidence that extra pyridoxine helps to prevent premenstrual flare-up of acne.

Ageing No convincing evidence that taking vitamin supplements helps, unless used to augment a diet deficient in the recommended requirements; for example, an elderly person living alone on a poor diet may benefit from vitamin supplements, but the best treatment is to ensure an adequate and balanced diet.

No convincing evidence that vitamin B complex, vitamin C or vitamin E are of special benefit in preventing ageing despite popular claims.

Alcoholism Alcoholics may benefit from the B complex of vitamins and folic acid but there is uncertainty as to whether their condition is due to an inadequate diet lacking in vitamins or whether drinking alcohol to excess increases the body's need for the B complex group of vitamins. There is no convincing evidence that oil of evening primrose is of benefit.

Alopecia (loss of hair) No convincing evidence that taking extra vitamins, particularly B vitamins and oil of evening primrose, is of the slightest benefit. No convincing evidence that zinc is of any benefit.

Alzheimer's disease No convincing evidence of the benefits of taking extra vitamins nor of a direct association between excessive intake of aluminium and Alzheimer's disease.

Angina No convincing evidence that extra vitamin E is of benefit in treating angina.

Anorexia nervosa No convincing evidence that taking extra zinc is of benefit.

Aphthous ulcers (mouth ulcers) No convincing evidence of the benefits of taking extra zinc (by mouth and/or cream) in preventing or treating aphthous ulcers.

Arteriosclerosis (hardening of the arteries) No convincing evidence that taking extra vitamin E, C or A is of benefit in preventing or treating arteriosclerosis.

Arthritis No convincing evidence of the benefits of taking extra B vitamins, vitamin C or calcium in the treatment of rheumatoid arthritis and osteoarthritis. No convincing evidence of the benefits of taking extra copper by mouth or of wearing a copper bangle or of taking oil of evening primrose or fish oils.

Asthma No convincing evidence of the benefits of taking extra B vitamins and vitamin C in treating or preventing asthma.

Atherosclerosis (fatty deposits in arteries) No convincing evidence of the benefits of taking extra pyridoxine, vitamin C or vitamin E in the treatment of atherosclerosis.

Autism No convincing evidence that taking massive doses of B vitamins or vitamin C is of benefit.

Backache No convincing evidence that taking large doses of vitamin C is of benefit in disc injuries.

Bedsores No convincing evidence that taking high doses of vitamin C is of benefit. No convincing evidence that taking extra zinc by mouth is of benefit.

Blindness No convincing evidence that taking extra vitamin A improves night vision, *unless* the individual has vitamin A deficiency.

Body odour No convincing evidence of the benefits of taking extra pyridoxine, magnesium, zinc or para-aminobenzoic acid in reducing body odour.

Boils No convincing evidence of the benefits of taking extra zinc by mouth in preventing or treating boils.

Bronchitis No convincing evidence of the benefits of taking high doses of vitamins A and C in preventing or treating bronchitis.

Bruises No convincing evidence that taking extra vitamin C helps to reduce the risk of bruising in people engaged in body contact sports.

Burns No convincing evidence of the benefits of taking high doses of vitamins C and E in treating burns.

Cancer No convincing evidence of the benefits of taking high doses of carotene or vitamin A, C and/or E in treating or preventing cancers. No convincing evidence of the benefits of taking laetrile despite repeated claims to this effect.

Cataracts No convincing evidence of the benefits of taking extra vitamin B_1, vitamin C, vitamin E and/or calcium in preventing cataracts.

Chilblains No convincing evidence of the benefits of taking extra B vitamins or vitamin D in treating or preventing chilblains.

Cigarette smoking No convincing evidence that taking extra vitamin B_1 or vitamin C reduces the harmful effects of cigarette smoking.

Colds No convincing evidence of the benefits of taking extra vitamin A or C in preventing or treating colds.

Cold sores No convincing evidence of the benefits of taking extra vitamin C or zinc in treating or preventing cold sores.

Constipation No convincing evidence of the benefits of taking extra vitamin B_1 in treating or preventing constipation.

Contraceptives No convincing evidence that women on the combined oral contraceptive pill require supplementary pyridoxine, vitamin B_{12}, vitamin E or vitamin C. There is some evidence that pyridoxine may help to reduce depression in certain women who take the pill.

Convalescence No convincing evidence that taking extra vitamin C accelerates recovery.

Deafness No convincing evidence that taking extra vitamin A will help to prevent deafness.

Dental decay No convincing evidence that taking extra pyridoxine or vitamin C helps to prevent tooth decay.

Depression No convincing evidence of the benefits of taking extra pyridoxine in preventing or treating depression.

Dermatitis No convincing evidence of the benefits of taking high doses of B complex vitamins or vitamin A.

Diabetes mellitus No convincing evidence that diabetic patients require additional pyridoxine, vitamins C, E or A, or that they require additional zinc, magnesium or chromium.

Dry skin No convincing evidence that taking high doses of vitamin A is of benefit in helping to prevent dry skin. There is no convincing evidence of the benefits of using vitamin E skin applications to prevent or to treat dry and/or ageing skin.

Eczema No convincing evidence of the benefits of taking extra vitamin A, extra B vitamins, extra vitamin C or zinc in treating or preventing attacks of eczema. The possible benefits of evening primrose oil are discussed under eczema, page 1021.

Eyes No convincing evidence that taking extra vitamin B_2 helps to prevent or relieve blood-shot eyes, particularly after eye surgery.

Fatigue There is no evidence that fatigue with or without changes in mood is due to early deficiency of B vitamins, vitamin C or vitamin E, magnesium or potassium.

Fertility No convincing evidence that taking extra vitamin E will help fertility.

Gall stones No convincing evidence that taking high doses of vitamin C will help to prevent cholesterol gall stones.

Gangrene No convincing evidence that high doses of vitamin E help to prevent gangrene in diabetic patients.

Glandular fever No convincing evidence that taking high doses of B vitamins or vitamin C speeds recovery.

Glaucoma No convincing evidence of the benefits of taking high doses of vitamin C in preventing or treating glaucoma.

Haemorrhoids No convincing evidence of the benefits of taking high doses of vitamin C in preventing or treating haemorrhoids.

Hayfever No convincing evidence of the benefits of taking high doses of B vitamins, vitamin C or vitamin E in preventing or treating hayfever.

Heart disease No convincing evidence of the benefits of taking high doses of B vitamin complex, vitamin E, vitamin C or pyridoxine or evening primrose oil in preventing or treating coronary artery disease. People living in hard water areas seem to develop less heart disease than those in a soft water area; this may be due to the calcium and magnesium in hard water.

It has also been observed that people living in areas with a low level of selenium in the soil may be at greater risk of developing coronary heart disease than are those in areas where the level of selenium is high, and that selenium may protect against coronary heart disease.

There is no convincing evidence that taking additional potassium, chromium or manganese in the diet reduces the risk of coronary heart disease.

Hepatitis No convincing evidence that taking high doses of vitamin C is of benefit in treating viral hepatitis.

Hyperactivity in children No convincing evidence of the benefits of taking high doses of B vitamins, vitamin C or vitamin E in treating hyperactive children.

Impotence No convincing evidence of the benefits of taking extra vitamin A in preventing or treating impotence.

Kidney stones No convincing evidence of the benefits of taking extra pyridoxine or magnesium in preventing calcium stones. Magnesium may suppress stone formation in people prone to develop them.

Learning disabilities There is no convincing evidence that taking extra vitamin C or vitamin E improves mental ability. There is no convincing evidence that taking vitamin supplements improves performances in non-verbal tests of reasoning.

Leg ulcers No convincing evidence of the benefits of taking extra zinc by mouth and/or applied directly to the ulcer in speeding up the healing of leg ulcers.

Loss of sense of smell No convincing evidence that taking high doses of vitamin A or zinc helps to restore the sense of smell in someone who has lost it.

Lumbago No convincing evidence of the benefits of taking extra thiamine (a B vitamin) or calcium in relieving lumbago.

Memory loss No convincing evidence of the benefits of taking extra B vitamins in improving memory in elderly people.

Menopause No convincing evidence of the benefits of taking extra B vitamins in helping mood nor of vitamin E in helping hot flushes. See, however, the use of calcium in preventing osteoporosis (Chapter 68).

Migraine No convincing evidence of the benefits of taking high doses of vitamins in preventing or treating migraine, nor of the benefits of magnesium supplements.

Mosquito bites No convincing evidence that taking thiamine (a B vitamin) by mouth acts as an insect repellent and keeps mosquitoes away.

Muscle cramps No convincing evidence of the benefits of taking additional calcium or potassium in treating night cramps, or other muscle cramps. Nor is there any evidence of the benefit of taking vitamins C or E.

Osteoporosis See discussion on the treatment of osteoporosis (Chapter 68).

Painful menstrual periods No convincing evidence of the benefits of taking extra calcium in reducing painful periods.

Pins and needles (paraesthesia) Pyridoxine may relieve the symptoms of nerve damage caused by certain drugs (e.g. isoniazid) but it is unwise to take pyridoxine to treat symptoms of nerve damage (numbness, pins and needles in the hands and feet, etc.) without a proper diagnosis. No convincing evidence that taking pyridoxine relieves the symptoms of nerve damage in multiple sclerosis.

Parkinson's disease No convincing evidence that taking extra vitamin C helps to reduce the harmful effects of levodopa. Pyridoxine blocks the effects of levodopa (see Chapter 36).

Pregnancy No convincing evidence that a deficiency of B vitamins damages the unborn baby. A pregnant woman should take iron and small doses of folic acid daily throughout pregnancy. Opinion is divided on the need to take other vitamins daily during pregnancy. High doses of vitamins, particularly high doses of vitamin A and pyridoxine, should not be taken in pregnancy.

Pregnancy sickness No convincing evidence of the benefits of taking extra pyridoxine in preventing or relieving pregnancy sickness.

Premenstrual syndrome (PMS) For the use of pyridoxine in PMS, see Chapter 68.

Prickly heat No convincing evidence that taking high doses of vitamin C is of benefit in preventing or treating prickly heat.

Prostate problems No convincing evidence of the benefits of taking oil of evening primrose or extra zinc in reducing inflammation or enlargement of the prostate gland.

Psoriasis No convincing evidence of the benefits of taking extra zinc in treating the skin lesions or in preventing or treating the arthritis that can occur in psoriasis.

Resistance to disease No convincing evidence of the benefits of taking extra vitamin A, B vitamins and vitamin C in improving resistance to infection.

Restless legs No convincing evidence of the benefits of taking high doses of vitamin E in preventing or treating restless legs.

Retention of fluids with periods No convincing evidence of the benefits of taking high doses of vitamins C and E or pyridoxine in reducing fluid retention at period times (the bloated feeling).

Schizophrenia No convincing evidence of the benefits of taking high doses of B complex, folic acid, vitamin C or vitamin B_{12} in preventing or treating schizophrenia.

Seborrhoeic dermatitis No convincing evidence of the benefits of taking extra B vitamins, extra biotin in children, or extra pyridoxine in adults in treating or preventing seborrhoeic dermatitis.

Shingles No convincing evidence of the benefits of taking high doses of B complex, vitamin C or vitamin B_{12} in the treatment of shingles or in preventing the neuralgia that may follow an attack.

Stomach ulcers No convincing evidence of the benefits of taking high doses of vitamin A, C or E in treating or preventing stomach ulcers.

No convincing evidence that vitamin C taken with aspirin can reduce the risk of bleeding from the stomach caused by aspirin.

Sunburn No convincing evidence of the benefits of taking high doses of vitamins E or C or of extra zinc in preventing or treating sunburn.

Thrombophlebitis No convincing evidence of the benefits of taking high doses of vitamin E in preventing or treating thrombophlebitis.

Toxaemia of pregnancy No convincing evidence that toxaemia of pregnancy is related to a deficiency of folic acid or pyridoxine.

Travel sickness No convincing evidence of the benefits of taking pyridoxine in preventing travel sickness.

Varicose veins No convincing evidence of the benefits of taking high doses of vitamins C or E in preventing or treating varicose veins.

Warts No convincing evidence of the benefits of taking extra vitamin E by mouth and/or applied locally in treating warts.

Wound healing No convincing evidence of the benefits of taking extra vitamins A, C or E or zinc in speeding up the healing of wounds.

46

Minerals

Calcium, iodine, iron, magnesium, phosphorus, potassium, sodium and sulphur are essential elements of importance to human nutrition. In addition to these important elements the body also requires very small traces of other elements to function effectively; these are called trace elements and include chromium, cobalt, copper, manganese, molybdenum, nickel, selenium, tin, vanadium and zinc. Fluoride is also considered to be essential (see later).

The mineral content of plants varies according to the composition of the soil in which they grow and, in turn, this affects the mineral content of livestock that feed on the plants. The mineral content of our food therefore varies according to the origin of our food. The mineral content of the water we drink also varies by regions, so our total intake of minerals will vary from region to region. In addition, our total intake may be affected by how much processed food we eat because highly refined foods are low in minerals (but see 'Sodium', below).

We only have ideas on optimal requirements for some minerals (e.g. calcium, copper, iodine, magnesium, manganese, phosphorus and zinc). Estimates are made for the rest, based on 'average' diets. Furthermore, we have little information about the harmful effects of overdosing with most of these minerals.

We know much more about the effects of the main elements than the trace elements, and very much more about some trace elements than others. However, the current fashion for tube-feeding (parenteral feeding) has brought to light the problems that may occur if patients become deficient in any of the trace elements. They are involved in controlling chemical reactions in cells and in organizing the molecular structure both within cells and in the surface membrane of cells. The body's requirement for trace elements is very carefully balanced and any excess may damage cells, whilst a shortage may interfere with normal functions.

Sodium

Sodium is necessary to maintain the proper fluid volume of the body. Most of the sodium is in the blood inside blood vessels (intravascular fluids) and in the fluid that bathes the cells (extravascular or extracellular fluid). The remainder is in the cells of the body (intracellular).

The amount of sodium in the diet of individuals varies widely. Sodium in food is present mainly as salt (sodium chloride), but natural foods are not high in salts and we increase our salt intake by adding salt in cooking and at the table. Processed food is particularly high in salt. Bacon, processed meats and tinned foods are all high in salt. Bread contains salt, and sodium monoglutamate used as a flavouring agent adds to the amount of sodium that we take in every day. Foods from animals and fish are high in salt, and many medicines, from penicillin antibiotics to vitamins, are high in sodium.

Sodium and chloride are easily absorbed from the intestine and are excreted by the kidneys. Excessive sweating can produce a significant loss of salt (sodium chloride) from the body, which is why people doing any kind of physical work in tropical climates require added salt. It is also why furnace workers in the past would drink salted beer. Athletes indulging in heavy physical training in tropical climates should take salt solutions after training, but it makes sense for these to be well balanced solutions of water and several salts because other salts may also be lost after excessive sweating.

Sodium is the principal mineral in the body fluid, where it is complemented by chloride. It is mainly responsible for regulating the distribution of fluids between the blood and the tissues by the process known as osmosis (the diffusion of a solvent from a weaker to a stronger solution through a semi-permeable membrane). The body can adapt to large variations in sodium (salt) intake by adjusting the output of sodium in the urine, and there is a close relationship between the amount of sodium and the amount of water in the body. Loss of water from, for example, sweating, passing large volumes of urine or vomiting and diarrhoea causes a loss of both sodium (as salt: sodium chloride) and water.

Sodium is also essential for normal functioning of nerves and muscles, including the heart, and is involved in chemical reactions inside cells and in the transport of nutrients into cells.

Low blood sodium (hyponatraemia)

There are two forms of sodium deficit. One form is a decrease in body sodium due to an excess of water relative to the concentration of sodium. It may occur if sodium loss is in excess of water loss or if sodium and water loss is treated with water alone; for example, taking water or water and glucose to treat salt and water loss due to excessive sweating and exercise or due to vomiting and diarrhoea. This can be dangerous because the water dilutes the body fluids and the kidneys excrete the dilute urine without affecting the salt concentration of the blood. Treatment should consist of water containing balanced amounts of electrolytes (e.g. sodium and potassium) – see 'Treatment of acute diarrhoea', Chapter 16.

The other form of sodium deficit is when both sodium and water are lost from the body. A loss of sodium and water may be caused by excessive sweating and dehydration as in heat exhaustion brought on, for example, by hard exercise in a high temperature. Vomiting and diarrhoea produce a loss of salt and water, which may be particularly dangerous in babies and infants.

The kidneys exert efficient control over the body's sodium and water and keep them at a steady level. Loss of sodium and water may therefore occur if the kidneys do not function effectively because of disease. However, a common cause of loss of sodium and water in the urine is the use of diuretics (water tablets) by doctors to treat heart failure and raised blood pressure. These drugs cause loss of water and sodium from the body. Several diseases that affect the glands (e.g. pituitary gland), liver or heart may also cause a loss of sodium and water.

Symptoms of a low level of sodium in the body include loss of appetite, headache, nausea, vomiting, fatigue and muscle weakness, confusion and delirium. When there is a sudden and severe loss of both salt and water, as for example in severe vomiting and diarrhoea, the blood volume, blood pressure and output of urine fall and the patient may have fits and go into a state of shock.

Loss of sodium with loss of water, resulting in a low blood volume, may be due to overdosing with diuretics. In some of these patients (usually elderly) swelling of the tissues (e.g. ankle swelling) may still be present but the worst thing is to continue treatment with the water tablets. These must be stopped and the patient given additional salt and adequate fluids by mouth.

Treatment of sodium loss involves giving salt and water solution by mouth or by infusion into a vein. The solution for infusion must be of equal concentration to body fluids; this is called 'isotonic' or 'normal' saline. Adults suffering from a severe loss of salt and water may require up to 8 litres of solution before they improve and their blood pressure and pulse return to normal.

Severe sodium loss is usually associated with water loss and a disturbance in the acidity of the blood. In addition, there is often loss of potassium and magnesium; therefore once the blood pressure is back to normal, any other deficiency should be corrected.

High blood sodium (hypernatraemia)

Excess of sodium in the body may be caused by excessive loss of water from the body due to sweating without adequate water intake, by fever, by excessive amounts of sodium in the food as when infants are over-fed with processed food or when patients are tube-fed. It may also occur in diabetes insipidus (see Chapter 60).

Symptoms of excess sodium in the body include nausea, vomiting, diarrhoea, cramps, restlessness, weakness, thirst, flushing of the skin, fever, rapid heart rate, dizziness, headache, a fall in blood pressure, twitching, rigidity, convulsions and coma.

Excessive salt combined with excess water in the body causes swelling of the tissues (oedema). It may occur in heart failure, kidney failure and liver failure. It may also be the result of over-treatment with intravenous salt solution, or be caused by drugs; for example, corticosteroids, male sex hormones, oral contraceptives because of their oestrogen content, phenylbutazone and carbenoxolone.

Treatment involves treating the underlying causes, the restriction of salt and water intake and the use of diuretics (water tablets).

Warnings *Sodium chloride solutions should not be given to patients who suffer from congestive heart failure or severe impairment of kidney function or when the tissues are swollen (oedema) with excess of sodium in the body. They should be used with caution in people taking corticosteroids and drugs that cause sodium to be retained in the body (e.g. carbenoxolone, phenylbutazone).*

Potassium

Potassium is the principal mineral in the fluid inside cells and is closely involved in the function of cells. It is an essential component in the body's use of carbohydrates, storage of sugars and the production of body proteins. It is involved in the transmission of electrical activity through muscles, including the heart. The turnover of potassium in the body depends upon the turnover of sodium; if the kidneys conserve sodium, potassium is lost in its place; if the diet contains low amounts of sodium and potassium, the kidneys conserve sodium and lose potassium.

Potassium is present in many foodstuffs. Foods containing high amounts of potassium include dried fruits, soya flour, molasses, wheat bran, fresh fruit, salads, vegetables, meat and poultry, wholemeal bread and fish. Tea, coffee and cocoa are high in potassium.

Low blood potassium (hypokalaemia)

A low potassium may be caused by a decreased intake of potassium in the diet (malnutrition, starvation, alcoholism and patients being tube-fed and receiving no food and fluids by mouth) or by an increased loss due to vomiting or diarrhoea or the regular use of laxatives, or in disturbances that affect the acidity of the blood such as diabetes. Surgical removal of parts of the intestine (e.g. ileostomy, colostomy), Cushing's syndrome, diabetes insipidus, ulcerative colitis and/or Crohn's disease may cause a low blood potassium. Loss of potassium may also occur in kidney disease, after severe burns or injury and during surgery.

A common cause of potassium loss is the use of diuretic drugs (water tablets) prescribed by doctors to treat heart failure and raised blood pressure. They cause a loss of both sodium and potassium. Corticosteroids also cause an increased loss of potassium in the urine.

A low level of potassium in the body can cause muscle weakness, thirst, drowsiness, pins and needles in the hands and feet, mental confusion, distension of the bowel, breathlessness, a fall in blood pressure, irregularities of the heart beat, kidney damage and paralysis.

A low blood potassium increases the toxicity of digoxin and related drugs on the heart. Since a low blood potassium may be produced by diuretic drugs, these drugs should be used with utmost caution in any patient who is also taking digoxin.

NOTE The level of potassium in the blood does not necessarily indicate the level of potassium in the body, and it is important to be medically examined as well as having a blood test.

Treatment with potassium salts may be given by mouth or intravenously. The blood potassium level should be checked before treatment and each day during treatment. When given into a vein to treat severe potassium loss, it must be done with utmost caution and continuous electric tracings of the heart (ECGs) should be carried out in order to spot any harmful effects on the heart. It should also be used with utmost caution in patients with impaired kidney function, excessive vomiting and/or diarrhoea. Leakages of potassium solution from the site of intravenous injections may damage local tissues and cause phlebitis and spasm of the vein.

A glucose solution containing a potassium salt and sodium chloride (salt) should be given by mouth to treat fluid loss caused by vomiting and diarrhoea (see Chapter 16).

The need to give potassium salts to patients who take diuretic drugs on a regular basis is discussed in Chapter 22.

High blood potassium (hyperkalaemia)

A high blood potassium may occur after excessive intake of potassium by mouth or by infusion into a vein. It may be produced by excessive transfusion of whole blood. Diuretics (water tablets) that conserve potassium (see Chapter 22) may cause a rise in blood potassium levels and it may also occur in kidney failure and adrenal failure or if the blood becomes too acid or after an injury. A high blood potassium causes pins and needles in the face, hands and feet, muscle weakness, paralysis, and mental confusion. It produces harmful effects on the heart (e.g. disorders of heart rhythm) and causes a fall in blood pressure.

Small doses of potassium given directly into a vein may produce serious harmful effects and death if the kidneys are not functioning efficiently and are not able to excrete potassium effectively in the urine.

Treatment Foods that contain potassium (see earlier) should be stopped, and if the patient is on a potassium-retaining diuretic (see Chapter 22) this too must be stopped. If the high potassium has produced harmful effects on the heart, a calcium gluconate injection should be given into a vein slowly over about 5 minutes using continuous electrical tracings of the heart to monitor for harmful effects. High blood potassium levels can be reduced by an infusion of dextrose solution containing insulin or by an infusion of sodium bicarbonate solution. A mild rise in blood potassium can be treated with sodium polystyrene sulphonate. It is a resin that will exchange sodium for potassium, and may be taken by mouth or as an enema. Alternatively, a calcium resin may be used.

Magnesium

Magnesium is a very important mineral in the body. It is essential for the structure of bone and is involved in the use of carbohydrates and proteins by the body and in chemical processes that affect nerves and muscles. It is closely dependent on calcium (it can mimic calcium) and it is not possible to correct a disorder caused by calcium deficiency without correcting any magnesium deficiency.

Foods containing magnesium include soya beans, nuts, yeast, wholewheat flour, rye flour, brown rice, dried fruit, seafoods, vegetables and meats.

Low blood magnesium (hypomagnesaemia)

A low blood magnesium is often associated with a low blood calcium and potassium. Prolonged diarrhoea (including abuse of laxatives) and vomiting is the commonest cause of magnesium loss. Deficiency may also occur as a result of reduced intake from a poor diet, malnutrition or a high-fibre diet. It may occur because of failure to absorb magnesium from food as well as in several diseases, which include under-active parathyroid glands, diabetes, alcoholism and acute kidney failure. Diuretic drugs (water tablets) may produce a loss of magnesium.

Deficiency affects the nervous system, skeletal muscle, stomach and intestine, and the heart and circulation. It may produce nausea, vomiting, dizziness, muscle weakness and cramps, tremors and jerking movements and ataxia. A serious deficiency may cause mental depression, apathy, confusion, agitation, convulsions, delirium, and harmful effects on the heart (disorders of rhythm).

Treatment is by infusion into a vein of magnesium chloride in a glucose solution.

High blood magnesium (hypermagnesaemia)

A high blood level of magnesium may occur in kidney failure. It may also occur after kidney dialysis, after the intravenous use of magnesium sulphate in the treatment of toxaemia of pregnancy, after the regular use of magnesium sulphate as a laxative, and after the regular daily use of indigestion mixtures containing magnesium, particularly in patients with impaired kidney function.

Symptoms include drowsiness, flushing, thirst, depression, low blood pressure, weakness, harmful effects on breathing, disorders of heart rhythm, coma and stoppage of the heart.

Treatment involves the intravenous injection of calcium gluconate. Dialysis of the blood may be necessary as well as intravenous fluids.

Calcium

Calcium is a major component of teeth and bone and is necessary for the clotting of blood. It is also essential for normal functioning of the muscles and nerves, and for normal functioning the heart. About 99 per cent of the body's calcium is held in bones. All this calcium comes from food, particularly from milk and cheese but also from vegetables, beans, cereal grains and from drinking water.

There is a close balance between calcium in the blood and calcium in the skeleton, which is regulated by hormones produced by the parathyroid and thyroid glands. Vitamin D is also essential for this balance. There is an inverse relationship between calcium and phosphorous in the blood (see discussion in Chapter 68, under 'Osteoporosis').

Low blood calcium (hypocalcaemia)

A low blood calcium may be caused by a deficiency of vitamin D (Chapter 45). It may also occur in malnutrition and any condition of the intestine that interferes with its absorption into the bloodstream (e.g. Crohn's disease). Any disorder in which there is defective absorption of fat from the food will interfere with calcium absorption because the calcium will form insoluble soaps with the fats. Chronic kidney failure, under-active parathyroid glands and diabetes may reduce absorption of calcium from the intestine, and certain substances in food may interfere with calcium absorption. These include foods rich in oxalic acid (e.g. soya beans, rhubarb, spinach) and foods rich in phytic acid (the outer layers of cereal grains – for example, wholemeal bread contains more phytic acid than white bread). A low blood magnesium may be associated with a low blood calcium, and so may an excessive intake of fluoride.

A decreased intake of calcium in the diet during pregnancy or breast feeding may cause a fall in blood calcium levels. Calcium absorption from the intestine decreases with advancing age and at the menopause (see Chapter 68). Several drugs may lower the blood calcium; for example, corticosteroids, anti-epileptic drugs and oestrogens (e.g. in oral contraceptives).

Rich sources of calcium are to be found in milk and cheese, and the fashion now for eating less milk and dairy products may possibly cause problems in later life (see 'Osteoporosis' in Chapter 68). Foods rich in protein, vitamin D and lactose improve the absorption of calcium from food, as does acid in the stomach and magnesium.

A low blood calcium level may cause diarrhoea, pins and needles, wheezing, mood changes, muscle cramps, convulsions, changes on electrocardiograph tracings (ECGs), dermatitis and tetany (see next).

Tetany

A low blood calcium increases the excitation of nerves. In children, acute symptoms start with numbness and tingling around the mouth, tips of the fingers and toes. The muscles of the wrists and hands then go into spasm and the thumb becomes pressed on to the fingers (carpopedal spasm). The muscles in the voicebox go into spasm and produce a high-pitched noise on breathing in and out (stridor), and convulsions can develop. Adults develop the numbness and pins and needles around the mouth and in the hands and feet but spasms of the wrist and fingers and stridor occur less often than in children and convulsions are rare.

Treatment to control tetany involves the slow injection into a vein of a solution of calcium gluconate. Treatment of the low blood calcium will vary according to the underlying disorder that caused it.

High blood calcium (hypercalcaemia)

The principal causes of high blood calcium levels are malignant cancers, over-active parathyroid glands and excessive intake of vitamin D. It may also result from the use of thiazide diuretics and the over-use of calcium-containing indigestion mixtures plus milk in the treatment of stomach and duodenal ulcers.

Symptoms of a high blood calcium include loss of appetite, nausea, vomiting, abdominal pain, constipation, passing large volumes of urine, muscle weakness, mental symptoms, drowsiness, confusion, coma, bone pains, kidney stones and kidney damage due to deposits of calcium, harmful effects on the heart (disorders of rhythm), and stoppages of the heart (cardiac arrest).

Treatment involves reducing calcium intake by mouth, drinking large volumes of water and the use of sodium phosphate and other salts by mouth or by injection according to the severity of the hypercalcaemia and according to kidney function. Calcitonin and corticosteroids may be used; mithramycin (see Chapter 76) has been used in cancers of the bone that cause an increase in the blood calcium levels. See sodium clodronate in Update.

Phosphorus (phosphate)

Foods high in phosphorus (as phosphates) include yeast, dried skimmed milk, wheat germ, soya flour, hard cheese, seeds, nuts, eggs, meat, fish and high-protein foods. Phosphate is essential for the chemical processes that go on inside cells. It is also closely involved with calcium, and 85 per cent of phosphate in the body is present in bones combined with calcium.

Low blood phosphate (hypophosphataemia)

Phosphate depends on vitamin D for its absorption from food and its take-

Table 46.1 Calcium supplements

Preparation	*Dosage form*
Cacit (calcium carbonate)	Effervescent tablets
Calcichew (calcium carbonate)	Chewable tablets
Calcimax (calcium laevulinate and calcium chloride plus calciferol, thiamine, riboflavine, pyridoxine, cyanocobalamin, ascorbic acid, nicotinamide and calcium pantothenate)	Syrup
calcium gluconate	Tablets, effervescent tablets, injection
calcium lactate	Tablets
Calcium Sandoz (calcium glubionate and calcium lactobionate)	Syrup, injection
Chocovite (calcium gluconate plus vitamin D_2) (calciferol)	Tablets
Citrical (calcium carbonate)	Granules
Ossopan 800 (hydroxyapatite: provides calcium and phosphorus)	Tablets, granules
Sandocal 400 and 1000 (calcium lactate gluconate, calcium carbonate, citric acid)	Effervescent tablets
Titralac (calcium carbonate and glycine)	Tablets

NOTE Requirements for calcium vary with age – these are discussed under osteoporosis (Chapter 68).

up by bone from the blood. Reduction in the phosphate absorbed from food can be caused by indigestion mixtures that contain aluminium hydroxide. This binds to the phosphate in the intestine and prevents its absorption. Moderate deficiency may occur in patients with over-active parathyroid glands, in rickets and osteomalacia, and in vitamin D deficiency. Severe deficiency may occur in chronic alcoholism, diabetic coma and as a result of tube-feeding.

The symptoms of phosphate deficiency include debility, loss of appetite, bone softening and pains, weakness and pins and needles. Severe deficiency causes blood disorders, slows down the heart and can affect the brain and nerves, producing tremor, confusion, fits and coma.

Treatment depends upon the cause and the severity of the deficiency. Moderate deficiency will respond to milk or a balanced solution of sodium and potassium phosphate salts by mouth. Rarely, even in severe cases, is it necessary to give solutions by injection into a vein.

High blood phosphate (hyperphosphataemia)

A raised blood phosphate may occur in patients with over-active parathyroid glands and with a low blood calcium and a raised blood magnesium level in acute kidney failure.

Excessive intake by mouth may cause diarrhoea and prevent the absorption of iron, calcium, magnesium and zinc from the intestine. High levels of blood phosphate cause a low level of blood calcium. Symptoms of a high blood phosphate level include pins and needles in the hands and feet, listlessness, mental confusion, weakness, raised blood pressure and disorders of heart rhythm.

An acute severe rise in blood phosphate may occur if too much phosphate solution is given into a vein. It causes a marked fall in blood calcium, producing tetany (see earlier) and convulsions which may be fatal. In patients who have low blood calcium levels due to kidney disease or other disorder, a rise in phosphorus may cause a further fall in blood calcium and trigger tetany (see earlier).

Treatment Reduction of blood phosphate levels is achieved by dietary restriction of foods containing high amounts of phosphate and the use of calcium carbonate by mouth. This binds to phosphates to prevent absorption from the intestine. The use of aluminium compounds to bind phosphates in patients with kidney failure (e.g. on dialysis) is controversial because of the risk of aluminium poisoning leading to aluminium-related dementia and softening of the bones (osteomalacia).

Iodine

Iodine is essential for the manufacture of thyroid hormones by the thyroid gland. Deficiency of iodine produces enlargement of the thyroid gland, which is called a goitre. Iodine is widely distributed in living matter. Fish and other seafoods are a good source of iodine whilst vegetables and milk contain some iodine. In mountainous regions well away from the sea, iodine may be so deficient in the diet and the soil that goitre is fairly common. In these areas the addition of iodine to table salt (iodization) is recommended.

Goitre has now almost disappeared from developed industrialized countries because most of the table salt in those areas at risk is now iodized. However, in many remote mountainous areas of the world it remains a problem and millions of people suffer from iodine deficiency.

Certain foods can interfere with the take-up of iodine by the thyroid gland; these include brassica (e.g. cabbage), cassava, kale, soya beans, groundnuts and mustard seeds. Certain drugs may interfere with the take-up of iodine by the thyroid gland (see Chapter 63) and some medicines contain iodine (e.g. cough and cold remedies).

Fluoride

There is now sufficient evidence to show that traces of fluoride in bones and teeth help to prevent tooth decay (caries). The main source of fluoride is drinking water but only hard water. There is very little, if any, fluoride in soft water. Fluoride is also present in seafish and tea.

The use of fluoride to prevent dental caries

It has now been convincingly demonstrated that in those parts of the world where the natural water contains 1 part or more per million of fluoride the incidence of dental caries is lower than in comparable areas whose natural water contains less fluoride than this. Fluoride increases the resistance of tooth enamel to acid, it improves the laying down of minerals in teeth and it interferes with bacterial growth. It is more effective if it is taken when the enamel is being laid down on the teeth before they erupt – that is, in childhood. If fluoride becomes deposited in these teeth they will be more resistant to dental caries than teeth that have not had fluoride deposited in them. Fluoride is not deposited in fully developed teeth, so it is obviously of much more benefit in children than in adults.

Harmful effects of fluoride

In parts of the world where there is a high concentration of fluoride in the drinking water the teeth may become mottled, the enamel looks dull and becomes pitted. This is called fluorosis. There is no risk to health and the teeth are resistant to caries. Where the drinking water contains very high amounts of fluoride (over 10 parts per million) the bones may become hardened (sclerosed) and calcium may be laid down in tendons and ligaments.

Comment

In those countries where the fluoride in drinking water was previously low and it is now added to the drinking water, there has been a fall in the extent of dental decay among children. However, this has coincided with an increased interest in dental decay in children in these countries, and much more dental health education and other activities, as well as the use of fluoride in toothpastes and other dental preparations. Nevertheless, there is convincing evidence that fluoride reduces tooth decay, and this is not in question. What is in question is how to supply an appropriate amount of fluoride to children while, at the same time, not exposing them and everyone else to a source of fluoride for the rest of their lives, the long-term effects of which we do not know.

The decision to use fluoride preparations in children should depend upon whether their drinking water is fluoridized and upon the amount they drink. It may be difficult to ensure a safe dose range in some children because fluoride is present in some toothpastes and even available as tablets to give to children.

Warning *Fluoride tablets should be kept out of the reach of children. The dose causing acute toxicity in adults is 5 g but deaths have occurred with 2 g. In children a fatal dose may be as low as 0.5 g of sodium fluoride.*

Chromium

Chromium is essential for the maintenance of normal blood glucose levels. It links up with a B vitamin (nicotinamide) to form what is called the glucose tolerance factor (GTF). This factor helps insulin to attach itself to receptors at its site of action.

GTF is involved in controlling blood glucose and cholesterol and it stimulates the production of proteins. However, claims for its benefits in slimming (reducing fat and building muscle) have not been subjected to adequately controlled trials.

The richest source of glucose tolerance factor is Brewer's yeast. Foods that contain small amounts of chromium include liver, egg yolk, molasses, beef, hard cheeses, fruit juices, bran, wholegrains and milk.

Chromium deficiency may occur in patients being tube-fed, in people on a diet high in refined and processed food or on prolonged slimming diets, and in starvation and alcoholism. It causes disorders of blood glucose levels and nervous disorders that include loss of control over voluntary movements and confusion. Symptoms include those of a low blood glucose level (weakness, sweating, palpitations, faintness, dizziness), alcohol intolerance, nervousness and symptoms like early diabetes (frequent passing of urine, thirst, hunger, weight loss).

Excess chromium intake by mouth causes nausea, vomiting, ulceration of the stomach and intestine, liver damage, kidney damage and disordered functioning of the nerves and brain.

Cobalt

Cobalt is present in vitamin B_{12} which has been discussed in detail earlier (see Chapter 45). There is a link between cobalt, iodine and thyroid hormone production which is not fully understood. Deficiency of the mineral cobalt is unknown but vitamin B_{12} deficiency is well documented. Cobalt used to be added to beer to improve the 'head' when it was poured out, but it was found to produce toxic effects on the heart and deaths occurred among heavy beer drinkers.

Copper

Foods high in copper include liver, shellfish, yeast, olives and nuts, but much of the copper we take in comes from copper pipes and food containers and from food processing. Some cough and cold remedies contain copper, and anti-fungal solutions used to clean swimming pools also contain copper.

Copper is essential for blood formation. It helps to form the red pigment, haemoglobin, in red blood cells. In addition, it is part of many enzymes in the brain, nerves and supportive tissues of the body. It is necessary for skin and hair pigmentation. Copper is excreted through the bile, urine and saliva.

Deficiency of copper occurs in several inherited nerve and brain disorders, and it may develop in patients being tube-fed (parenteral nutrition). Poor absorption from the intestine may occur in cystic fibrosis and other disorders that affect the absorption of food, and in certain kidney diseases.

Despite claims in 'health' magazines that a deficiency of copper produces failure to thrive in infants, and loss of pigmentation of hair and skin, brittle bones and loss of the sense of taste in adults, there is no convincing evidence from adequate and well controlled studies of its benefits in treating these disorders. No beneficial effect produced by copper has been reported in the medical literature apart from that in anaemia. However, because copper deficiency is usually present with other nutritional deficiencies, it is not even certain whether a deficiency causes anaemia (see Chapter 47).

A raised blood level of copper may occur in response to inflammation (e.g. rheumatoid arthritis). Excess intake of copper may cause nausea, vomiting, painful muscles and dissolving of red blood cells (haemolysis). In Wilson's disease, a rare inherited disease of copper storage, there is an inability to excrete copper and it becomes deposited in the liver, causing liver damage; in the brain, producing abnormal involuntary movements; and in the cornea of the eyes, producing a greenish-brown discoloration. Treatment involves the use of penicillamine, which binds the copper and removes it from the deposits.

Copper has a contraceptive effect when present in the womb. It is added to intra-uterine contraceptive devices (IUDs).

Copper bracelets are worn as a folk remedy for rheumatic conditions, but despite claims that some copper is absorbed through the skin to produce a beneficial effect, there is no convincing evidence from adequate and well controlled studies of such a benefit.

Manganese

Manganese is essential for the normal functioning of many enzyme systems in the body, and for the formation of the red pigment, haemoglobin, in the red blood cells. Sources in food include cereals, wholemeal bread, nuts, beans, fruit, green leafy vegetables and tea.

Deficiency in laboratory animals has been associated with impaired growth, abnormalities of bones, ataxia, convulsions and disorders of fat metabolism.

Manganese poisoning produces a Parkinson-like syndrome.

Low blood levels of manganese have been noted in diabetes, schizophrenia, rheumatoid arthritis and several other disorders but the significance is not known. Claims that manganese may help tardive dyskinesia (see Chapter 41) have not been substantiated.

Molybdenum

Molybdenum is a component of many enzymes in the body. The effects of molybdenum deficiency in humans are not known, although dental decay and sexual impotence have been suggested without any convincing evidence. There may be an association between a high intake of molybdenum and gout. Foods that contain molybdenum include buckwheat, beans, wheat germ, liver, soya beans, wholegrain and cereals. Deficiency may occur through eating foodstuffs grown in soil low in molybdenum or by eating large amounts of refined and processed foods.

Nickel

Nickel deficiency has been reported in animals and birds. Its effect in humans is not known. In animals deficiency of nickel impairs iron absorption from the intestine, producing iron-deficiency anaemia. Low blood levels may occur in cirrhosis of the liver, and chronic kidney failure and high blood levels may occur after a heart attack or stroke, severe burns and in toxaemia of pregnancy and cancer of the womb or lung.

Selenium

Selenium is essential for the formation of an enzyme that protects the constituents of cell membranes from damage from oxidizing chemicals. The daily requirement of selenium is not known. It is probably dependent on the presence of other trace minerals such as zinc, copper, manganese and a supply of vitamin C and E, and iron. Foods that contain selenium include liver, fish, shellfish, wholegrains, cereals, dairy produce, fat and vegetables.

Selenium deficiency may occur in patients being tube-fed, and in people whose diet is high in processed and refined foods. It may also occur in areas where the concentration of selenium in the soil is low (e.g. parts of China).

Deficiency of selenium causes a type of heart disease called Keshan disease. Symptoms are relieved by giving selenium as sodium selenite by mouth. The relationship between a low blood selenium level and coronary artery disease requires further investigation.

Selenium deficiency has been reported in patients with alcoholic cirrhosis of the liver. This may be due to a reduced intake coupled with an increased excretion. There appears to be a relationship between selenium deficiency and protein starvation (Kwashiorkor disease). There also appears to be a possible relationship between selenium and cancer. People who live in areas with low selenium levels in the soil may be at a greater risk of developing cancer. Vitamin E may be involved with selenium in 'protecting' against cancer. However, none of the evidence is totally convincing and we need more research in this interesting field.

Excessive intake of selenium retards growth and produces muscular weakness, infertility, damage to the liver, difficulty in swallowing and talking, and depression of breathing.

Selenium is another trace element that is now in fashion with health writers, and it is claimed to help all kinds of disorders from arthritis, high blood pressure and angina, to hair and nail problems and cataracts. However, there is no convincing evidence from adequate and well controlled studies to support any of these claims.

Warning *Do not mistake selenium, a trace element essential to humans, with selenium* ***sulphide****, which is used in shampoos and is highly dangerous if taken accidentally by mouth.*

Silicon

Silicon is found in high concentrations in tendons and eye tissues and also in the wall of the main artery from the heart, the aorta. It is necessary for mammalian bone growth and the laying down of calcium in bone (calcification).

Sulphur

Sulphur is mainly supplied by sulphur-containing amino acids from proteins in the food. Therefore, deficiency may occur if there is a deficiency of protein in the diet.

Tin

The effects of tin in humans are not known. Deficiency has been found to produce retarded growth in rats. Food sources of tin are unknown because of the difficulty in measuring it. Tinned foods contain more than fresh foods.

Tin preparations have been used to treat boils, carbuncles and acne, and also tapeworm. Its use by mouth may cause severe headache and vomiting, disorders of balance, double vision, retention of urine and colic, unconsciousness, paralysis in the arms and legs, and death. It should not be used to treat such disorders.

Vanadium

Deficiency disorders have been reported in animals and birds. Little is known about its effects in humans. Deficiency in animals causes a reduction in red blood cell production, resulting in anaemia, a raised blood fat level and lack of growth of bone and teeth.

Excess of vanadium may be associated with manic–depression.

Food sources of vanadium include parsley, lobster, radishes, lettuce and fish bone. Processed foods may contain more vanadium than fresh food because of contamination during manufacturing.

Zinc

Zinc is essential for the development and function of cells in the body. It is a constituent of many enzyme systems. It is present in liver, yeast, shellfish, meats, wholegrain cereals and green vegetables. Oysters are rich in zinc.

A high-fibre diet may interfere with the absorption of zinc from the intestine. However, there is much disagreement about the signs and symptoms of zinc deficiency in adults. Chronic zinc deficiency in children has occasionally been associated with poor growth, poor appetite and impaired sense of taste. A zinc deficiency syndrome of dwarfism and under-development of the sexual organs has been reported in the Middle East but these children also suffered from protein deficiency.

A rare inherited disorder of zinc metabolism causes a skin rash, loss of hair, mental irritability, muscle wasting and depression.

Acute zinc deficiency has been described in patients being tube-fed (parenteral nutrition). They develop diarrhoea, irritability, depression, a skin rash, loss of hair, loss of taste and defects in their immune system (resistance to infection). Zinc deficiency may occur in protein-losing disorders (e.g. some kidney diseases), poor absorption from the intestine as in inflammatory bowel disorders (e.g. ulcerative colitis), cirrhosis of the liver, chronic alcoholism, diabetes, loss from injuries or burns, and in patients on kidney dialysis. Zinc loss in the urine may be increased by diuretics (water tablets), cisplatin, penicillamine and alcohol. According to the disorder being treated, it may be necessary to give zinc on a short- or long-term basis.

Zinc taken in excess may cause nausea and vomiting.

Zinc is fashionable at the moment with health magazine writers and all sorts of claims are made for its benefits in treating disorders from anorexia nervosa and acne to the common cold, osteoporosis and even schizophrenia. It is also claimed that it accelerates wound healing and helps bedsores to heal. Unfortunately, there is no convincing evidence that zinc deficiency occurs in these disorders and, similarly, there is no convincing evidence from adequate and well controlled studies of its benefits in treating them.

NOTE A test for zinc deficiency is to taste zinc sulphate solution (0.1%). People with a severe deficiency of zinc cannot distinguish between the taste of the zinc solution and plain water.

47

Anaemias

Anaemia is one of the world's great health problems. It can be defined as a reduction in the number of red blood cells (erythrocytes) in the blood or a reduction in the haemoglobin level in a sample of blood to below a normal range that takes account of age and sex.

Haemoglobin is the red pigment in red blood cells which carries oxygen from the lungs to the tissues and carbon dioxide back from the tissues to the lungs. Men have more haemoglobin than women.

Causes of anaemia

Anaemia due to loss of blood

Anaemia can be caused by a loss of blood which may be sudden and acute, such as haemorrhage due to an injury, or it may be slow and prolonged (chronic), for example due to heavy menstrual periods or slight bleeding each day from a stomach ulcer.

Sudden, acute loss of blood causes a sudden drop in the volume of the whole blood and can produce shock. The body attempts to restore the volume of lost blood by drawing fluids from the tissues into the blood stream. This results in dilution of the blood and the appearance of anaemia some 24–36 hours later. If there is no further bleeding, increased red cell production will correct the anaemia in a few weeks provided the body's stores of iron are adequate. However, if the acute loss of blood is severe, these mechanisms do not have time to work and the patient will die unless a blood transfusion or a plasma substitute is given to push up the blood volume near to normal.

Chronic blood loss (e.g. bleeding peptic ulcer, heavy periods) does not produce a fall in blood volume because the body has time to compensate. However, the loss of red blood cells causes a loss of iron, which uses up the body's stores of iron and leads, over time, to the development of iron deficiency (see later).

Anaemia due to inadequate production of red blood cells

These anaemias may be due to:

- A deficiency of iron, vitamin B_{12} or folic acid
- Toxic effects from some inflammatory disease which may be infectious (e.g. tuberculosis) or not infectious (e.g. rheumatoid arthritis), from liver disease or kidney disease, or from drug treatments
- Glandular disorders, such as under-active pituitary gland, thyroid gland, adrenal gland or gonads (testes and ovaries)
- Disorders of development of red blood cells or of haemoglobin (e.g. thalassaemia; see later)
- Damage to those cells in the bone marrow that are responsible for manufacturing red blood cells; this may be due to drugs, radiation or some other toxic agent
- Replacement of the bone marrow by invading cells – for example, leukaemic cells in a patient suffering from leukaemia or due to invasion by cancer cells from a cancer elsewhere (cancer secondaries or metastases); scar tissue (fibrosis) may also reduce the bone marrow's ability to make red blood cells

NOTE *Erythropoietin* is secreted by the kidneys in response to a decreased oxygen supply and it stimulates red cell production by the bone marrow (see Update).

Anaemia due to deficiency of iron

Iron-deficiency anaemia occurs because of a loss of blood (e.g. heavy periods in women), a lack of iron in the diet, failure to absorb iron from the food due to some disorder of the intestine, or a defective ability to absorb iron.

Anaemia due to a deficiency of iron in the diet is common throughout the world. It affects millions of people, particularly the poor and under-fed. In developing countries a large proportion of infants and pregnant mothers are anaemic due to poor nutrition. It occurs much less frequently in Western countries but, nevertheless, it is surprisingly high considering how rich in foods these countries are.

How the body uses iron

The total iron content of the healthy body is maintained between narrow limits. Any loss of iron is precisely balanced by absorption of iron from food. Every day we lose iron in cells that normally slough off the skin, the lining of the stomach and intestine and the lining of the bladder. Iron is also lost in the hair and nails and in the sweat. In this way we lose 'naturally' about 1 mg of iron every day. In women, additional iron is lost in the blood when menstruating, to the baby when pregnant and in the milk when breast feeding.

Most of the body's iron is used over and over again because red blood cells last for only about 120 days, after which they are taken by big white cells (macrophages) to the spleen where they are broken down and the iron is extracted. A small proportion of the iron is stored and the rest is used to make haemoglobin.

Only about 5–10 per cent of iron from the average Western diet is absorbed from the intestine in order to maintain the proper balance of iron. This absorption increases significantly if the body stores of iron are reduced or if red cell manufacture is speeded up (e.g. due to a loss of blood).

Lack of iron in the diet, loss of iron from bleeding or not being able to absorb iron from food lead to iron being used up from the body stores. This is a most important point to remember because red cell production is not affected until the body stores of iron have been used up. This means that the signs and symptoms of anaemia come on late – after several months of iron deficiency.

Iron from food comes from digestion of haemoglobin in animal foods and/or from iron salts in the food. The absorption of iron salts from the food can be affected by many factors. Acidity of the stomach contents and acids in the diet can increase absorption whereas chemicals in cereals and nuts can interfere with the absorption of iron. Vitamin C (ascorbic acid) can counter this effect.

The absorption of iron from food by the intestine is under a very complex regulatory system which responds according to the body's needs. The absorption of iron from the duodenum is increased if your body's iron is low, but once your body's stores are back to normal this absorption will decrease. Some of the iron is stored as ferritin in the cells of the lining of the intestine, and much of this is lost when the cells slough off because they are replaced every 3–4 days. The rest is attached to a protein for transfer in the bloodstream. This 'shuttle' protein is called transferrin and an estimate of the amount of iron attached to available transferrin is a measure of the degree of anaemia. It is referred to as the iron-binding capacity of the blood. Normally only about one-third of the binding sites on the transferrin are occupied by iron. The iron is transferred to receptors on cells, particularly those cells in the bone marrow that develop haemoglobin and those that store iron as ferritin.

It is not difficult to understand why loss of blood produces iron-deficiency anaemia: 95 per cent of iron in the body has been recycled from broken down red blood cells and if red blood cells are lost through bleeding their iron is not available for recycling. In this recycling the 'haem' is separated from its protein 'globin'. The haem is then broken down to iron and bilirubin. The latter is a red pigment that is taken to the liver and then excreted through the bile into the intestine where it is converted into a brown pigment, which accounts for the colour of the faeces.

The release of iron from its stores is reduced by infections, cancer and chronic inflammatory disorders (e.g. rheumatoid arthritis), which may explain why people with chronic diseases develop anaemia.

There is more to the diagnosis than anaemia

In its fully developed form, iron-deficiency anaemia can be diagnosed in the laboratory because the red cells become smaller than normal (microcytosis) and paler than normal (hypochromia – low colour), and the concentration of iron in blood plasma is reduced. Tests will also show a reduction in iron storage and usage.

However, iron-deficiency anaemia is not a disease; it is a sign that something is going wrong – too little iron in the diet, inability to absorb iron, loss of iron through loss of blood, or some underlying chronic disease. In women of child-bearing age menstruation, pregnancy and breast feeding are the common causes of iron-deficiency anaemia. In men and in women after the menopause, iron-deficiency anaemia should be regarded as due to the loss of blood unless proved otherwise. Patients should be checked for blood in their motions from a bleeding peptic ulcer, for bleeding piles and for any other disorder that may cause chronic bleeding.

Because iron is drawn from the body's stores, the onset of iron-deficiency anaemia is slow and people cope well before they slowly develop the symptoms of anaemia – tiredness, dizziness, palpitations and breathlessness.

Drug treatment of anaemia due to iron deficiency

Preventing iron-deficiency anaemia

The regular daily use of iron in order to prevent iron-deficiency anaemia developing is necessary in premature babies, twins and infants after caesarean delivery, in pregnancy and in people who have undergone surgical removal of parts of their stomach or small intestine. It may also be necessary in breast-feeding mothers depending upon their diet and in women with heavy periods. Also, female blood donors may need to take iron regularly every day. It is not necessary and it can be harmful to take iron regularly every day if you are not suffering from iron-deficiency anaemia (see criticisms of the use of iron as a 'tonic', in Chapter 44).

Treating iron-deficiency anaemia

Because iron-deficiency anaemia is a sign of disease, every effort must be made to identify and treat any underlying cause. Iron is very effective for treating iron-deficiency anaemia but is of no benefit in anaemias not caused by a deficiency of iron.

The response of a patient with iron-deficiency anaemia to iron treatment depends upon the cause and the severity of the anaemia, the presence or absence of any underlying illness, and that individual's ability to take and to absorb iron from the various types of iron preparations that are available.

The degree of improvement will depend upon the severity of the anaemia and the amount of iron made available to the bone marrow. When adequate doses of iron are taken regularly every day there should be a rapid improvement in symptoms, with a reduction in tiredness and fatigue. This response occurs within a few days of starting treatment, before evidence of any change in the haemoglobin and red blood cells. As the iron treatment is continued, the haemoglobin should rise by 100–200 mg/100 ml each day and the red blood cells should gradually return to normal. It takes 1–3 months of regular daily treatment with iron to reach normal values. After this, iron treatment should be continued for at least 3 months in order to allow the iron stores in the body to build up to normal.

Preparations and dosage

Despite the many preparations of iron that are available and their heavy sales promotion by drug companies, simple iron salts are best (e.g. ferrous sulphate, ferrous gluconate and ferrous fumarate). Of these, ferrous sulphate is the cheapest and the drug of choice. Ferric salts are not as well absorbed as ferrous salts and are not recommended.

The response to iron treatment is related to the amount of iron that becomes available in the body rather than the type of iron salt used. The dose of iron by mouth should be between 100 and 200 mg daily to treat iron deficiency anaemia and about 60 mg daily to prevent it. The content of ferrous iron in commonly used preparations is as follows:

Preparation	*Amount*	*Amount of iron available*
Ferrous fumarate	200 mg	65 mg
Ferrous gluconate	300 mg	35 mg
Ferrous glycine sulphate	225 mg	40 mg
Ferrous succinate	100 mg	35 mg
Ferrous sulphate	300 mg	60 mg
Ferrous sulphate (dried)	200 mg	65 mg

Iron is best absorbed on an empty stomach but iron preparations may irritate the stomach and produce nausea and pain. This harmful effect may be reduced if they are taken with or just after food. This will reduce the amount of iron absorbed but this has to be balanced by the fact that people are more likely to stick to the prescribed dosage if they do not experience stomach upsets.

Slow-release preparation of iron (once a day dosage)

These preparations are designed to resist the acid in the stomach, thus avoiding irritation of the stomach lining by delaying the release of iron salts until they are in the intestine. They release iron slowly as the preparation moves along the intestine. This avoids high concentrations in any one part and reduces the risk of irritation, but absorption of iron from these once-a-day preparations may mot be as efficient as with ordinary iron preparations. They are often referred to as *sustained release* preparations.

Combined iron preparations

Vitamin C in iron preparations

A common additive to iron preparations is vitamin C, which, if given in a dose of 200 mg or more, increases the absorption of iron by up to 30 per cent. However, the benefits of increased absorption are counter-balanced by an increased risk of irritation of the stomach and therefore it offers no advantage over simply increasing the dose of the iron salts.

B vitamins in iron preparations

There is no evidence that including B vitamins in iron preparations is of the slightest benefit; it merely increases the cost.

Folic acid in iron preparations

The only indication for using an iron preparation containing folic acid is in the prevention of folic acid-deficiency anaemia in pregnancy.

Minerals in iron preparations

There is no evidence that including other minerals in iron preparations is of the slightest value; they merely increase the cost. In particular, there is no evidence that adding small doses of copper and/or magnesium to iron preparations improves the formation of haemoglobin.

Risks of iron treatment

Some patients taking iron preparations by mouth complain of nausea and stomach pains. These symptoms may be reduced by taking the iron with or just after meals (see earlier). The symptoms may also be related to dose and may be reduced by starting on a small dose (120 mg ferrous sulphate three times daily) and gradually building up the daily dose during the first week of treatment. Regular daily use of iron preparations may cause diarrhoea or constipation. These harmful effects do not necessarily respond to a reduction in the dosage. Constipation can be a real problem in elderly people who may develop an obstruction of the bowel.

Reducing the daily dosage in order to reduce harmful effects is sensible but it means that improvement will take a little longer.

Warnings on the use of iron preparations

Liquid iron preparations stain the teeth black. It therefore helps if it is sucked through a straw. Iron salts colour the motions black.

Iron preparations should not be given to patients who are having repeated blood transfusions. This may lead to an overload of iron in the body.

Failure to respond to iron treatment by mouth may mean that the iron tablets are not being taken regularly every day as directed. This may be because the iron is causing stomach upsets or because the individual just forgets to take them; whatever the reason, it is usually an indication of poor communication between doctor and patient. However, failure may be due to the fact that more iron is being lost from bleeding than the iron tablets are replacing, or that the patient has some other illness that affects his response to iron. It may also be due to an inability of the patient to absorb the iron. And of course the diagnosis may be wrong – iron treatment is only of use in treating and preventing anaemia due to iron deficiency!

Acute iron poisoning occurs particularly in young children. As few as ten tablets of iron may kill a young child; therefore keep all tablets in cupboards out of reach of children. The iron irritates the lining of the stomach, killing the cells and producing pain and bloody diarrhoea, shock and breathlessness. The child may then appear to improve but, as the acidity of the blood changes, he may become unconscious and die.

Overload of iron in the body (iron overload) results in iron being deposited in the heart, liver, pancreas and other organs of the body. These deposits cause the affected organ to malfunction, and death may occur.

Iron overload occurs most often in people who suffer from an inherited disorder, haemochromatosis, in which their mechanisms for controlling the absorption of iron do not work efficiently and they absorb excessive amounts of iron into their bodies. It may also occur in patients who are given frequent blood transfusions.

Iron overload may also occur in some individuals who take iron regularly every day when they are not suffering from iron-deficieny anaemia and have adequate body stores of iron. In these people the mechanism for controlling iron absorption from the intestine may be marginally defective, so they take in more iron than they need.

Haemosiderosis is a disorder in which there is iron overload in the body as the result of excessive and rapid breakdown of red blood cells in certain blood disorders (see haemolytic anaemia, earlier).

Iron by injection

Iron may be given by injection in the form of Imferon (iron dextran) or Jectofer (iron sorbitol). These preparations offer an alternative to taking iron preparations by mouth but it is important to remember that the rate of improvement of the anaemia is similar to that which follows iron treatment by mouth. Some doctors think, quite wrongly, that by giving iron by injection they will provide a more rapid cure for their patient's iron-deficiency anaemia. Although giving iron by injection does not speed up the response to iron treatment, it does increase the storage of iron in the body much more quickly than iron taken by mouth.

Indications for using iron injections

Injections of iron should be used only if patients are unable to take iron by mouth because of stomach upsets, because they will not take their iron as directed, if they are unable to absorb iron from their intestine because of some disease, because of severe chronic blood loss, or because they have a disorder such as ulcerative colitis in which their symptoms are made worse by oral iron.

Imferon (*iron dextran injection*)

Harmful effects Severe allergic reactions to Imferon injections are very rare. They occur usually within the first few minutes after an injection. Breathing difficulties develop and/or the blood pressure falls rapidly and the heart stops. Other allergic symptoms include nettle rash (urticaria), skin rashes, itching, nausea and shivering. An injection of Imferon must be stopped immediately at the first sign of any allergic reaction.

Other harmful effects include soreness and inflammation at the site of injection, brown discoloration of the skin following an intramuscular injection, phlebitis at the site of an intravenous injection, flushing and a drop in blood pressure following an intravenous injection, and swollen glands and an increase of pain in the joints of patients suffering from rheumatoid arthritis.

Delayed reactions to Imferon injections may occur, particularly when large doses are injected into a vein (intravenously). The individual develops fever and painful joints and muscles. The onset of these reactions varies from several hours to several days after the injection. They last for a few days and then clear up completely.

Warnings *It should not be used in anyone who is allergic to it or who has heart disease (e.g. angina, disorders of heart rhythm) or severe liver disease or are in the acute stages of kidney disease, nor should it be given intravenously to individuals with asthma.*

Because of the rare risk of severe allergic reactions, Imferon should not be used unless full resuscitation facilities and drugs are immediately to hand.

Patients should be kept under careful observation during and for 1 hour after injection.

It should be used with extreme caution in anyone with impaired kidney function, acute or chronic infections, or a history of allergies (hayfever, eczema, asthma). These individuals should be given intramuscular injections in gradually increasing doses. People who suffer from allergies should be given a test dose before injection, and an antihistamine if the drug is given by intravenous injection.

A high incidence of painful joints has been reported among patients with rheumatoid arthritis who have been given intravenous injections. Therefore, intravenous injections should be used with utmost caution and only when really necessary in these individuals.

Risk of cancer Cancer of the tissues (sarcoma) has been produced in rats, mice and rabbits when very high doses have been used. However, it is difficult to estimate the risks of cancer in humans because of the long time between the exposure to a cancer-producing agent and the subsequent development of a cancer. Such a risk is considered to be very rare indeed.

The manufacturer's guidelines on giving Imferon injections should be followed precisely.

Jectofer (*iron sorbitol injection*)

Harmful effects About one-third of the dose is excreted in the urine within 24 hours of the injection. This causes the urine to turn black at the peak of its excretion. Very rarely, it may cause serious disorders of heart rhythm.

Warnings *Jectofer should not be used to treat patients suffering from liver or kidney disease or who have an acute infection of their urine because it increases the excretion of white blood cells and therefore could interfere with the body's resistance to infection. It is important to use correct recommended doses according to body weight, especially in underweight patients. Iron by mouth should be stopped 24 hours before Jectofer is given.*

Anaemia due to chronic disease

A mild to moderate anaemia frequently occurs with long-standing infections (e.g. tuberculosis), inflammatory disorders (e.g. rheumatoid arthritis) and cancers. In these conditions there is a fault in the transport of iron around the body, the red blood cells have a shorter life and bone marrow production of haemoglobin and red blood cells is defective. This anaemia does not benefit from iron treatment and any improvement relies on the treatment of the underlying disorder.

One principal cause of anaemia in chronic kidney failure is a failure of the kidneys to produce a factor that stimulates the production of red blood cells by the bone marrow. (Red blood cell production is referred to as erythropoiesis and the factor is referred to as erythropoietin.) Other causes of anaemia include an increased rate of destruction of red blood cells and bleeding from the stomach and/or intestine and other sites.

Table 47.1 Iron preparations by mouth – harmful effects and warnings

Harmful effects Discomfort in the stomach and intestine, diarrhoea and vomiting occur in about one in five people. These harmful effects are related to the amount of iron in each preparation rather than to the type of preparation used. Iron absorbtion is better between meals but stomach upsets can be reduced by taking iron preparations with or just after food. Regular daily use of iron may cause constipation in some people. Large doses of iron preparations may irritate the lining of the stomach and intestine and cause diarrhoea, vomiting and bleeding from the lining.

Warnings Iron should not be used in anyone having repeated blood transfusions or in individuals suffering from anaemia *not* due to iron deficiency. It should be used with caution in people with a disorder of iron storage, abnormal haemoglobins, or disorders of the stomach and intestine that may increase the absorption of iron into the blood. Mixtures containing iron salts should be well diluted and sucked through a straw in order to prevent discoloration of the teeth. The absorption of iron salts and tetracycline antibiotics is diminished when they are taken together; therefore iron salts should be taken at least 3 hours before or 2 hours after taking a tetracycline antibiotic.

Table 47.2 Iron preparations by mouth

Preparation	*Drug*	*Dosage form*
Fe-cap	ferrous glycine sulphate	Capsules
Feospan	ferrous sulphate	Sustained-release capsules
Fergon	ferrous gluconate	Tablets
Ferrocap	ferrous fumarate	Sustained-release capsules
Ferrocontin Continus	ferrous glycine sulphate	Sustained-release tablets
Ferrograd	ferrous sulphate	Sustained-release tablets
Ferromyn	ferrous succinate	Elixir
ferrous gluconate	ferrous gluconate	Tablets
ferrous succinate	ferrous succinate	Tablets
ferrous sulphate	ferrous sulphate	Tablets
Fersaday	ferrous fumarate	Tablets
Fersamal	ferrous fumarate	Tablets, syrup
Galfer	ferrous fumarate	Capsules
Ironorm	ferrous sulphate	Capsules, oral drops
Niferex	polysaccharide-iron complex	Tablets, elixir
Niferex-150	polysaccharide-iron complex	Capsules
Plesmet	ferrous glycine sulphate	Syrup (elixir)
Slow-Fe	ferrous sulphate	Sustained-release tablets
Sytron	Sodium irondetate	Sugar-free elixir

Table 47.3 Iron and folic acid preparations used to prevent anaemia in pregnancy

Preparation	*Drug*	*Dosage form*
Fefol	ferrous sulphate, folic acid	Spansules (sustained-release capsules)
Ferfolic SV	ferrous gluconate, folic acid	Tablets
Ferrocap-F 350	ferrous fumarate, folic acid	Sustained-release capsules
Ferrocontin Folic Continus	ferrous glycine sulphate, folic acid	Sustained-release tablets
Ferrograd Folic	ferrous sulphate, folic acid	Sustained-release tablets
Folex-350	ferrous fumarate, folic acid	Tablets
Galfer FA	ferrous fumarate, folic acid	Capsules
Lexpec with Iron	ferric ammonium citrate, folic acid	Sugar-free syrup
Lexpec with Iron-M	ferric ammonium citrate, folic acid	Sugar-free syrup
Meterfolic	ferrous fumarate, folic acid	Tablets
Pregaday	ferrous fumarate, folic acid	Tablets
Slow-Fe Folic	ferrous sulphate, folic acid	Sustained-release tablets

Erythropoietin (U)

The availability of a preparation of erythropoietin has revolutionized the treatment of anaemia in chronic kidney failure. It successfully corrects the anaemia by stimulating the bone marrow to produce red blood cells.

NOTE Erythropoietin is now being misused by some athletes in order to improve their stamina. It increases the production of red blood cells and thus increases the oxygen-carrying capacity of the blood. A similar effect is produced when athletes train at high altitudes. The lack of oxygen in the atmosphere stimulates red cell production, and so when the athletes return to lower altitudes they have an increased red cell count and their blood has a greater oxygen-carrying capacity.

Anaemia due to deficiency of vitamin B_{12}

Vitamin B_{12} and folic acid (a B vitamin) are essential for cell growth. Vitamin B_{12} deficiency affects all cell growth, particularly those cells which undergo a rapid turnover – for example, cells of the skin, cells lining the mouth, stomach and intestine, and cells in the bone marrow that form red blood cells.

The effects of vitamin B_{12} deficiency on bone marrow cells cause a special type of anaemia called megaloblastic anaemia. 'Megalo' means large and 'blastic' means immature, so megaloblastic anaemia is diagnosed by the appearance of 'large immature' red blood cells in the bone marrow and blood. Pernicious anaemia (see later) is an example of this type of anaemia.

In addition to affecting the formation of red blood cells and producing anaemia, a deficiency of vitamin B_{12} may produce damage to nerve cells in the spinal cord, causing pins and needles in the hands and feet, numbness and difficulty in walking. It may also damage brain cells – producing irritability, sleepiness and disorders of behaviour (megaloblastic madness). Nerve damage can also affect smell, taste and vision (particularly in tobacco smokers). In addition, a deficiency of vitamin B_{12} may damage the cells on the surface of the tongue, producing a smooth red tongue, and the cells lining the stomach and intestine, producing defective absorption of food.

Pernicious anaemia is the commonest anaemia caused by a defective absorption of vitamin B_{12}. Other disorders that produce defective B_{12} absorption include surgical removal of the stomach (gastrectomy) and myxoedema. Ulcerative inflammation of the small intestine (e.g. Crohn's disease) and surgical removal of parts of the small intestine may also result in defective B_{12} absorption.

A serious lack of vitamin B_{12} in the diet (e.g. in vegans) may result in a deficiency of vitamin B_{12}, and some drugs may cause it (e.g. calcium adsorbing drugs by mouth, aminosalicylic acid and biguanide oral anti-diabetic drugs). Prolonged use of nitrous oxide anaesthetic may cause a megaloblastic anaemia because it inactivates vitamin B_{12}. The treatment is to give vitamin B_{12} by injection.

Sources of vitamin B_{12}

Vitamin B_{12} is manufactured only by certain micro-organisms present in soil and sewage and in the intestine. Humans therefore depend entirely on micro-organisms to produce vitamin B_{12} for them. Foods that contain vitamin B_{12} come mainly from animals – meat, liver, fish, eggs and milk. Vegetable products contain no vitamin B_{12} unless contaminated with vitamin B_{12}-producing micro-organisms from soil. The liver holds a large store of vitamin B_{12}, so anaemia due to vitamin B_{12} deficiency will not develop for several years after stopping vitamin B_{12} in food or developing a disorder that prevents its absorption from the intestine into the bloodstream (see later).

Pernicious anaemia

Vitamin B_{12} in food is liberated by the acid and juices in the stomach. It then attaches itself to a protein in the stomach juice, called 'intrinsic factor', which is essential for vitamin B_{12} to be absorbed further down the intestine. Some patients lack intrinsic factor and are not able to absorb vitamin B_{12}; they develop a megaloblastic anaemia called pernicious anaemia or Addisonian pernicious anaemia. It is an autoimmune disorder, see page 80.

Vitamin B_{12} stores

About 90 per cent of the body's store of vitamin B_{12} is in the liver. Every day some is excreted into the bile and reabsorbed through the intestine. This explains why patients who have had surgery to the small intestine can develop vitamin B_{12} deficiency despite the small amount needed each day from food.

Diagnosis

The diagnosis of vitamin B_{12} deficiency is made by determining the concentration of vitamin B_{12} in the blood and by tests of acid production by the stomach. The latter is necessary because, in addition to a reduced vitamin B_{12} level in the blood, there is also a lack of acid production (achlorhydria) in the stomach in patients suffering from pernicious anaemia.

Vitamin B_{12} treatment

Vitamin B_{12} by injection into a muscle must be given to individuals suffering from pernicious anaemia or who have had part or all of their stomach removed surgically. Vitamin B_{12} injections should also be given to individuals who have been shown to have vitamin B_{12} deficiency due to disorders of their small intestine. Once vitamin B_{12} is started by injection, the treatment is for life and a dose of 1 mg of vitamin B_{12} (as hydroxocobalamin) by intramuscular injection every 3 months should be adequate maintenance treatment. Strict vegetarians (vegans) should take vitamin B_{12} by mouth.

Vitamin B_{12} preparations

Two vitamin B_{12} preparations for injection are used – hydroxocobalamin and cyanocobalamin. The latter has been used for decades but hydroxocobalamin is now recommended because its effects last longer (up to 3 months).

Dangers of using folic acid in vitamin B_{12} deficiency

Folic acid deficiency may also cause a megaloblastic anaemia; if a patient diagnosed as vitamin B_{12} deficient fails to respond to vitamin B_{12} injections, tests for folic acid deficiency (see later) should be carried out because the use of vitamin B_{12} may mask an underlying deficiency of folic acid. However, the reverse situation is much more serious. If folic acid is given to patients with vitamin B_{12} deficiency, the bone marrow and blood improve just as if vitamin B_{12} were given. This is because vitamin B_{12} is essential to the use of folic acid by growing and dividing cells. Clearly, if you give folic acid, this has beneficial effects; but folic acid does not affect the damage to the cells in the brain, spinal cord and nerves produced by vitamin B_{12} deficiency. This means that if someone with vitamin B_{12} deficiency is given folic acid, the blood improves and the individual feels better but the nerve damage will progress unless treatment with vitamin B_{12} is given.

Despite the popular use in the past of vitamin B_{12} injections as a general tonic and to treat all manner of disorders, there is no evidence that it is of the slightest benefit to anyone except those people suffering from vitamin B_{12} deficiency.

Warning *Megaloblastic anaemia occurring in pregnancy should not be treated with vitamin B_{12} (see later).*

Anaemia due to deficiency of folic acid

Folic acid (pteroylglutamic acid) belongs to the B group of vitamins. It is present as folate polyglutamates (folates) in fresh green vegetables, meat, liver, wholemeal bread, and fruit. The digestive juices in the upper small intestine break them down to folates, which are absorbed and enter the blood stream where they are transported by proteins to the cells of the body. They are stored as folate polyglutamates in cells and the supply is maintained by absorption from food and by recycling through the liver into the bile and then back into the bloodstream from the upper part of the small intestine. The body stores can last for a few months.

Folic acid (from folates) is converted in the body to an enzyme that is essential for cell growth and division. Deficiency of folic acid causes megaloblastic anaemia. 'Megalo' means large and 'blastic' means immature, so megaloblastic anaemia is diagnosed by the appearance of 'large immature' blood cells in the bone marrow and blood. The deficiency causes a defective step in cell division. Vitamin B_{12} deficiency also causes this defective step, which is why megaloblastic anaemia caused by vitamin B_{12} deficiency can be reversed by giving folic acid. However, this is dangerous as stated earlier because the folic acid does not prevent the progressive brain and nerve damage caused by vitamin B_{12} deficiency.

Deficiency of folates (folic acid)

Folate deficiency produces a megaloblastic anaemia (large, immature red cells). A sore tongue (glossitis) is not as common as with vitamin B_{12} deficiency, and brain and nerve damage is very rare. The *diagnosis* of folate deficiency is made by measuring the concentration in the blood. The changes in red blood cells in the bone marrow and blood are similar to those seen in vitamin B_{12} deficiency.

A deficiency of folates can occur because of inadequate intake due to poor diet or overcooking of foods (particularly by boiling in water). Alcohol may damage the liver and interfere with the recycling of folates which, along with the poor diet eaten by alcoholics, may lead to the development of folic acid deficiency. Diseases of the intestine also may interfere with the absorption of folates (e.g. coeliac disease and tropical sprue), as may surgical removal of part of the upper small intestine.

Over-activity of the bone marrow due to cancer, leukaemia and certain types of anaemia (e.g. haemolytic) may cause folate deficiency. Certain anti-cancer drugs may interfere with the use of folates in the cells, and folic acid deficiency may occur in patients on renal dialysis.

The anti-epileptic drugs phenytoin and primidone cause folate deficiency by interfering with folate absorption from the intestine and the storage of folates.

Pregnancy increases the requirements for folates because the baby takes in folates at the expense of the mother. Breast feeding also increases the requirements for folates.

Oral contraceptive drugs may block steps in the use of folates in some women.

Treatment of folic acid deficiency

Folic acid deficiency responds rapidly to folic acid by mouth. For people suffering from severe folic acid deficiency or who cannot take folic acid by mouth, an injection is available.

Folic acid by mouth is usually adequate for most individuals. Even in the presence of poor absorption due to an intestinal disorder the dose used by mouth is usually high enough to ensure that sufficient of the vitamin is absorbed. Treatment for 4–5 weeks usually corrects the deficiency and replaces the body store. Treatment should be continued daily until the underlying problems in the diet are corrected. Some patients may need daily treatment on a continuing basis.

Folic acid in small doses (200–500 micrograms) should be given regularly every day to pregnant mothers and, depending upon their diet, patients on renal dialysis. People with chronic haemolytic anaemia may require 5 milligrams (mg) of folic acid daily, every other day, or just one dose weekly to keep them supplied with an adequate amount of folic acid.

Patients suffering from diseases where there is rapid turnover of cells (e.g. haemolytic anaemia) should be treated with folic acid. Daily folic acid should also be given to individuals who develop a folic acid deficiency because of a drug treatment they are receiving.

Haemolytic anaemias

A healthy red blood cell has an active life of about 120 days. This life span may be shortened if the red cell structure is defective due to some inherited disorder or if the haemoglobin is defective.

In haemolytic anaemias the red blood cells burst open in the blood stream and release haemoglobin, which is taken to the liver to be broken down.

Anaemia develops if destruction of red blood cells occurs faster than the bone marrow can produce new ones. An indication of the degree of anaemia is the appearance in the blood of immature red blood cells, which means that the bone marrow is pushing them out so fast that they have no time to mature. In addition, because of the high number of red cells being broken down, there is excessive pressure on the bile system (see Chapter 83) which excretes the red pigment, bilirubin. This pigment is a breakdown product from the haem in haemoglobin after the iron has been extracted for recycling. The increase in bilirubin production may result in mild jaundice (see Chapter 83).

Haemolytic anaemias due to non-hereditary causes

Haemolytic anaemias may be due to the body reacting against its own cells (autoimmune disease; see later), to infections e.g. (malaria), toxic reaction in some cancers, inflammatory disorders (e.g. rheumatoid arthritis), metabolic disorders and drugs (see Chapter 78), blood transfusion reaction (see later) and in the newborn. In these cases the red blood cells are broken down in the spleen, liver and bone marrow and other organs.

Autoimmune haemolytic disease

Autoimmune diseases are discussed in Chapter 9. In autoimmune haemolytic anaemia the body forms antibodies against its own red blood cells, which destroy them. The majority of the antibodies work at body temperature and are called 'warm' antibodies. However, some work at low temperatures and are called 'cold' antibodies.

Warm antibodies may occur in certain leukaemias, and in people taking methyldopa used to treat raised blood pressure. The destruction of red blood cells may produce anaemia, fever, vomiting and prostration. The disorder is diagnosed by the Coombe's test – a special protein (anti-human globulin) is added to a sample of the patient's blood which has the antibodies on the surface of the red blood cells. The test is positive if the red cells clump together (agglutinate).

Treatment of this type of autoimmune haemolytic anaemia involves the use of a corticosteroid drug (e.g. prednisolone) starting with a high daily dose and slowly reducing the dose over several weeks. If there is failure to improve, the patient's spleen is removed.

Cold antibodies occur mainly in the elderly. The antibody reaction causes the red cells to clump together to produce a sludge that blocks the small arteries. The patients may develop cold 'dead' fingers and toes (Raynaud's phenomenon) and anaemia. The condition is worse in cold weather. The only effective treatment is to keep warm.

Blood transfusion reaction

Different people have different blood groups, and the groups are classified according to the presence or absence of certain proteins on the surface of the red blood cells. When blood is transfused from one person to another these proteins act as antigens (foreign proteins) and trigger the production of antibodies.

Blood-group antigens that have been recognized include A, B, O, M, N, S and Rh (rhesus). They are very important in matching a patient's blood for blood transfusions. If the blood is not of the same group as that of the patient, antibodies will develop to the antigens on the transfused red blood cells. This antibody–antigen reaction, or 'immune reaction', will destroy the transfused red blood cells. Symptoms usually start after only a few millilitres of blood have been given, and if the transfusion is stopped immediately there should be no serious problems. If it is not, the patient may develop a severe blood transfusion reaction: shivering and restlessness; nausea, vomiting and pain in the chest and back; the skin will become cold, clammy and blue; the temperature, pulse and breathing will increase; and the blood pressure will fall. The red pigment released from the red blood cells may produce jaundice and also damage the kidneys. Symptoms begin to subside over the next 24–48 hours but some patients may die.

The best treatment is obviously preventative, which demands meticulous matching of the patient's blood. Any blood transfusion should be run in slowly at first (up to about 100 ml) and stopped if there is the slightest sign of a reaction. Unconscious patients receiving a blood transfusion should be kept under continuous observation. An important safety measure in matching the blood is to cross-match – test a sample of the recipient's serum against the donor's red blood cells.

Haemolytic disease of the newborn

An important blood group is called the rhesus factor. The majority (85 per cent) of people have red blood cells that contain a rhesus factor on their surface. The factor is known as Rh antigen D. These people are called rhesus positive. The 15 per cent of people who do not have this antigen on their red blood cells are called rhesus negative. The factor is inherited and is a dominant factor. This means that some children of a rhesus positive father and a rhesus negative mother will be rhesus positive. They will have the rhesus factor on their red blood cells but their mother will not. If this happens the mother may develop antibodies to the rhesus factor (the antigen) on the red blood cells of her unborn baby. Usually with the first pregnancy nothing happens unless the mother has previously been made sensitive to the rhesus factor because of a previous blood transfusion. If she has been made sensitive or if she has other babies, there is a risk that she will make antibodies which will then pass across into the baby and destroy its red blood cells.

The most common cause of the mother developing antibodies to her baby's red blood cells is during delivery of the baby when some of the baby's blood may 'leak' into her bloodstream from the placenta (afterbirth). The degree of sensitization of the mother will depend upon the number of red blood cells from the baby that enter her bloodstream just after delivery. As a consequence of being sensitized the mother may produce antibodies against her baby's red blood cells in a subsequent pregnancy.

If the mother's antibodies enter the baby's bloodstream they will destroy the baby's red blood cells (haemolytic anaemia). The baby will then develop swelling of the tissues due to accumulation of fluids (oedema) and enlargement of the liver and spleen. After 24 hours a deep jaundice develops due to excessive amount of bile pigment in the baby's blood. Normally, this red pigment (bilirubin) from destroyed red blood cells passes through the liver where it undergoes a chemical change and is excreted into the bile. In babies, the liver is not mature enough to carry out this chemical change on the large amount of bilirubin being produced. As a result, the blood level of unchanged (or 'free') bilirubin rises. This free bilirubin, unlike bilirubin that has undergone a chemical change in the liver, can cross from the baby's blood into the baby's brain through the natural protective barrier (the blood/brain barrier) where it damages nerve cells. This condition is known as *kernicterus*, and free bile pigment in the brain causes serious brain damage, which includes convulsions, coma and rigidity of the muscles. There is a risk of death. If the child survives, subsequent problems caused by the damage to nerve cells include athetosis (slow involuntary movements, particularly of the arms and legs), spasticity (rigid spasm of muscles), deafness and mental impairment.

Prematurity is another cause of kernicterus because the premature baby's liver is so underdeveloped that it cannot get rid of even 'normal' amounts of bilirubin pigment into the bile.

The treatment of haemolytic disease of the newborn is to carry out a complete exchange transfusion of the baby's blood as soon as the disorder is suspected. The baby's blood is drawn off from one point while a blood transfusion is given through another point.

Preventing rhesus problems

If the mother is rhesus negative (Rh-negative) and the father is rhesus positive (Rh-positive) the mother's blood should always be tested for antibodies between the 32nd and 36th week of each pregnancy. If no antibodies are present, everything should be all right but the baby's blood (from its umbilical cord) should be tested for antibodies immediately after delivery. If these are present the baby should have an exchange blood transfusion.

If there is evidence that any of the baby's red blood cells have entered the mother's bloodstream, she should be given an injection of gamma-globulin containing anti-D immunoglobulin within 72 hours of delivery. This will destroy any of the baby's red blood cells that have leaked into her bloodstream. This will stop the mother developing antibodies to the rhesus factor on the baby's red blood cells and therefore prevent the risk of haemolytic anaemia developing in future babies.

Haemolytic anaemias due to hereditary factors

Haemolytic anaemia may be due to some hereditary abnormality of the red blood cells or of the haemoglobin pigment in red blood cells, and the following are some examples.

Hereditary spherocytosis

In this condition the walls of the red blood cells are abnormal and the cells look thick and round (spherocytes). Their life span is reduced and their destruction is sufficient to cause anaemia and episodes of jaundice. Treatment involves blood transfusions, and removal of the spleen in severe cases. The disorder is most common in African black people.

Enzyme abnormality (glucose-6-phosphate dehydrogenase (G6PD) deficiency)

This disorder is most common in African blacks (West and East Africa). It is a hereditary disorder in which there is an enzyme deficiency in red blood cells which renders the cells liable to damage from certain drugs (e.g. anti-malaria drugs and sulphonamide drugs). In addition, infections may make the red blood cells more sensitive to the damaging effects of drugs such as aspirin, chloramphenicol and chloroquine. These drugs may easily trigger an attack of haemolytic anaemia. The damage to the red blood cells (haemolysis) produced by drugs is related to the dose given. Treatment is to stop the drug, and give a blood transfusion if necessary.

Abnormal haemoglobins

Sickle cell anaemia is an inherited transmission of an abnormal haemoglobin known as haemoglobin S, which makes the red cells crescent or sickle shaped. It is found mainly in African blacks living near the equator. Factors for the development of haemoglobin are transmitted from both parents, so some children may be affected and carry the trait but not have the disease whilst others may have the disease. The abnormal haemoglobin causes haemolytic anaemia, which begins at about the age of 4 months. The anaemia is associated with an increased risk of infections and, later, with enlargement of the heart, leg ulcers, gall stones, delayed growth and delayed puberty. Over-growth of the bone marrow in the first year of life causes the shape of the skull to be deformed. Dehydration and infections may trigger fever, jaundice and severe pains in bones and other tissues. This is caused by small blood vessels being blocked by damaged red blood cells that cut off the blood supply to the tissues supplied by these vessels. Pregnancy can be particularly hazardous in patients with sickle cell anaemia because damage to the bone marrow may cause pieces to come loose and enter the blood stream, to block off an artery elsewhere (embolism).

Treatment of sickle cell anaemia involves general medical care. Patients are at particular risk from malaria and other infections. They should take life-long anti-malarial treatment if they live in a malaria area. In Africa it is unlikely for children with sickle cell anaemia to live to adult life.

Thalassaemia (Cooley's anaemia) is an inherited abnormality of haemoglobin affecting people who live in the Mediterranean, Middle East and Far East. According to whether one or both parents carry the 'trait', their offspring may develop a mild form of the disease which can seem, initially, to be just like iron-deficiency anaemia but which does not improve with iron treatment. This is called *thalassaemia minor*. If both parents carry the trait, an offspring can develop the full-blown disease, called thalassaemia major.

Thalassaemia major is a very serious disease which requires blood transfusions. In addition to severe anaemia, there is over-growth of the bone marrow, producing an abnormal shaped skull which gives the patient a mongoloid appearance. Growth is retarded, and the spleen and liver become enlarged.

48

Anti-bacterial drugs – antibiotics

An infectious disease is caused by the invasion of the body by harmful or potentially harmful micro-organisms and their subsequent multiplication in the body. Infectious diseases are caused by bacteria, viruses, fungi, worms and protozoa. Drugs used to treat these infections are called anti-bacterial, anti-viral, anti-fungal, anti-helminthic and anti-protozoal drugs, respectively.

Anti-bacterial drugs

The term anti-bacterial refers to any substance that destroys bacteria or blocks (inhibits) their growth. Those drugs that kill bacteria may be called bactericidal and those that inhibit their growth may be called bacteriostatic. The most important group of anti-bacterial drugs used to treat infections is the antibiotics Some groups of antibiotics are also used to treat fungal infections (see Chapter 56).

Antibiotics

An antibiotic is a chemical substance produced by certain bacteria or fungi that stops the growth of, and may eventually kill other groups of bacteria and/or fungi. The important point in this definition is that antibiotics are produced by one group of micro-organism (e.g. penicillin comes from a certain type of fungus) and they kill another group of micro-organism (e.g. penicillin kills certain types of bacteria).

Antibiotics differ in their origin (produced by bacteria or fungi), in their chemical structure and in their action and effects on the range of bacteria or fungi that they are active against. Some may only be active against a specific micro-organism; they are then said to have a narrow spectrum of activity. Others may be active against a wide range of bacteria or fungi, in which case they are called broad-spectrum antibiotics. Antibiotics that are active against bacteria are called anti-bacterial antibiotics, and those that are active against fungi are called anti-fungal antibiotics.

Many antibiotics are now manufactured synthetically without having to rely entirely on bacteria or fungi to produce them. Those that are partially produced by micro-organisms and then modified by adding chemicals are often referred to as semi-synthetic antibiotics. Whatever their origin, the blanket term antibiotic is used to describe them.

Anti-bacterial antibiotics vary in the ways in which they act on bacteria in order to inhibit their growth (bacteriostatic) or kill them (bactericidal). But these actions are often a matter of degree, and a bacteriostatic in high doses will become bactericidal.

The body's natural resistance to infection and the effectiveness of antibiotics

The effectiveness of an antibiotic in treating an infection is determined by the 'natural resistance' of the individual to infection. This resistance is determined by the body's own defence system, which attacks any infecting micro-organisms. This defence system is called the immune system and is described in detail in Chapter 9. If the body's immune system is working efficiently, antibiotic treatment will be much more effective than if the immune system is not working well. Failure of the immune system can be caused by drugs (such as those used to prevent rejection in transplant patients) or due to diseases that severely impair the immune system (e.g. AIDS). When the immune system is not working effectively the patient not only has more chance of catching an infection but also has less chance of improving from antibiotic and other treatments for that infection. It is therefore important to remember that antibiotics cannot cure bacterial or fungal infections alone; they require an effective and efficient defence system in the body. They are also useless against viral infections.

Anti-bacterial antibiotics

Other factors can also influence the body's response to antibiotic treatment. Local factors at the site of infection may lessen the effectiveness of an antibiotic (e.g. the presence of pus or blood, the acidity of the tissues and the blood supply and oxygen supply to the site). For example, bacteria are much harder to kill if they are inside an abscess that is full of pus and has a hard wall of inflamed tissue around it; in these cases it is necessary to open the abscess and drain the pus before the antibiotic can really get to work.

The presence of some foreign material can affect the body's immune system and thus lessen the effectiveness of antibiotics. For example, in patients who have had a replacement hip joint put in, the body's white cells start trying to 'fight' the synthetic joint. This activity weakens their natural ability to fight infections, and if a patient develops an infection at the site, any antibiotic treatment given may be less effective than it would be otherwise.

Harmful blood levels of antibiotics

Most antibiotics are broken down in the liver and excreted by the kidneys in the urine. Any disorder of function of the liver or kidneys may cause an increase in the harmful effects produced by antibiotics because their concentration in the blood will reach toxic levels. This applies particularly to unborn babies and premature and newborn infants whose kidneys and livers have not fully developed. It also applies to elderly people whose liver and kidney functions may often be slowed down. 'Normal' doses of antibiotics in such elderly people may produce harmful effects.

Bacterial resistance to antibiotics

As stated earlier, some antibiotics are active against a specific group of bacteria and some are active against several groups of bacteria. However, if bacteria come into a lot of contact with a particular antibiotic, they can develop a resistance to that antibiotic and other chemically similar antibiotics. This stops the antibiotics from being active against that group of bacteria.

A group of bacteria can become resistant to an antibiotic because some of the group have a natural resistance to that antibiotic. In this case, the antibiotic will knock out the sensitive ones and leave the resistant ones to multiply. These then become dominant and spread to infect other patients.

In addition to the emergence of naturally resistant bacteria within any group of bacteria being attacked by an antibiotic, a number of bacteria will develop genetic changes and mutate. Some of these genetic changes may result in the bacteria being resistant to the antibiotic, and if this happens they will multiply while their 'colleagues' will be killed off. In this way a strain of 'new' bacteria resistant to that particular antibiotic will emerge.

Transfer of antibiotic resistance

A genetic element in bacteria, called plasmid, makes copies of itself when bacterial cells multiply. It is responsible for transmitting special codings that make future bacteria resistant to certain antibiotics. It is sometimes known as the resistance factor or R factor.

Some of these codes may be within viruses that infect bacteria. These viruses are called bacteriophages and they can infect only bacteria. When they multiply inside the bacteria they cause the bacteria to dissolve, which releases more viruses. These viruses then spread into other bacteria where they become part of the organism's nucleus, and not only make it resistant to the virus but also transfer the codes that give it resistance to a particular antibiotic or group of antibiotics.

Misuse of antibiotics

From this very simple description of bacterial resistance to antibiotics you will realize what a real problem it has been, is and will be in the future. Yet much of the problem is caused by unnecessary use and over-use of antibiotics. This has encouraged the development of bacterial resistance to antibiotics and has created an ever-increasing demand for more and more antibiotics to replace those to which bacteria have become resistant. This has contributed significantly to the ever-increasing drug bill.

Antibiotic misuse covers the whole spectrum of medical practice – from the unnecessary use of antibiotics to treat virus infections (e.g. viral sore throats) by some family doctors (see later) to the blunderbuss use of antibiotics by some surgeons in the hope of preventing post-operation infections.

Antibiotic treatment needs tailoring to an individual's needs

The risk of using standard doses of antibiotics is that whether a patient is small or big, is male or female, is young or old, has healthy or unhealthy livers and/or kidneys and has a mild, moderate or severe infection, that person may be given the *same* daily dosage of an antibiotic as all other patients. Unfortunately, this may sometimes result in failure of treatment in some patients and the appearance of harmful drug effects in others. Too high a dose of an antibiotic may produce serious harmful effects in someone whose kidneys or liver are not working effectively (see earlier) whereas too low a dose may be inadequate to control the infection but sufficient to encourage the emergence of bacteria resistant to the antibiotic being used.

The same criticism applies to the route of administration (by mouth or by injection), the times between dosages and the duration of treatment. These should be varied according to the antibiotic being used, the severity of the infection and the potential harmful effects of the antibiotics in the particular individual being treated.

Every drug treatment is always a balance of benefits and risks for the person being treated. In antibiotic treatment, a sufficient amount of the antibiotic has to be given to kill the infecting micro-organism without damaging the patient. The balance of potential benefits to potential risks varies according to the condition of the patient, the antibiotic being used, the infecting micro-organism and the dose needed to be effective. This requires knowledge of the patient, the disease, the benefits and risks of using available antibiotics and also of laboratory reports on the type of infecting micro-organism and its sensitivity to various antibiotics.

Doctors' actions determine patients' expectations

Patients are sometimes as much to blame as doctors for the misuse of antibiotics because they often expect antibiotic treatment for a minor infection whether it is bacterial or not; but of course what a patient expects may well be what he has been led to expect by the doctor's previous prescribing. For example, a doctor who looks at little Johnnie's throat and says 'Yes, it is inflamed; I will give him some penicillin', has done two things that will affect the behaviour of Johnnie's parents in the future, the next time Johnnie gets a sore throat. By the mere act of prescribing penicillin, available only on prescription, the doctor has said 'Yes, this is a medical problem which needs to be seen by a doctor', and has defined a treatment for little Johnnie's sore throat in the future – that it should be treated with penicillin.

Doctors often talk about demanding patients but they may create a demand by defining patients' problems as medical and then responding by prescribing drugs.

Patients may also be responsible for failed antibiotic treatments by not taking the dose as directed for the stated number of days. They feel better after a day or two and then fail to complete the course of antibiotics. This can lead to the development of resistance by the infecting bacteria and the flare-up of the disorder after a day or two because not all the infecting bacteria were killed. Of course, if the sore throat (or whatever) was due to a virus infection, they may well feel better in two or three days, but that's not because of the antibiotic – it is in spite of it!

The importance of identifying the infecting bacteria and testing their sensitivity to various antibiotics

Different bacteria respond differently to any one antibiotic, so it is important to know which antibiotic will be most effective in treating a specific infection. Tests are available that identify the infecting bacteria; further tests using various antibiotics are then carried out to determine which of them are most effective at killing the bacteria (sensitivity tests). These tests give the doctor a guide to the selection of the most effective antibiotic.

It is obviously good practice for a sample of infecting micro-organism (e.g. a throat swab) to be sent to the laboratory for identification and for antibiotic sensitivity testing in order to decide on the most appropriate antibiotic. This should preferably be done before any treatment is started. Initial treatment may then be 'blind' until the results of the laboratory tests are back. This is standard practice in the treatment of tuberculosis. Unfortunately, too many antibiotic treatments are started blindly and then samples sent off to the laboratory for testing. Obviously, this causes problems in testing for antibiotic sensitivities, and certain techniques have to be used to 'remove' the antibiotics from the bacteria.

In reporting on which antibiotics are the most effective the laboratory staff have to be careful in how they report their findings. This is because doctors may go for their 'favourite' one, even though it is much more expensive than the others that are listed and which are equally effective. Doctors may also prescribe the first one on the list even though it may be the most expensive and no more effective than the others. Sometimes, having sent off a sample for testing, the results may be either forgotten or ignored, which is a waste of laboratory time.

I do not wish to imply that no antibiotic should be used blindly (before the results of laboratory tests on the bacteria are available). In some situations this is clearly impractical and could be harmful to the patient. However, I do wish to warn against the blind use of antibiotics to treat conditions such as sore throats and mild fevers. These are usually due to virus infections and such treatments do not benefit the patient. What is more, they are potentially harmful because of the risk of making the patient allergic to that particular antibiotic, which could cause serious problems if the drug were needed to treat a much more serious disorder in future. Also, such blind use encourages the development of bacterial resistance (see earlier).

Combining antibiotics

Different antibiotics act differently, and by using two or more together it is possible to obtain increased antibiotic effects if one drug increases (enhances) the effects of the other. On the other hand, one drug may block (inhibit) the action of another antibiotic, in which case there will be a decrease in the effectiveness of the antibiotic treatment. Also, the harmful effects of one antibiotic may be increased by giving it with another antibiotic drug. The combination of two or more antibiotics may be used if the infection is caused by two or more types of bacteria. Some antibiotics supplement the action of other antibiotics, and this can result in a combined action that is greater than the sum of the effects of the two drugs given separately. This is called synergism, and there are some useful examples – such as the use of penicillin and streptomycin against certain streptococcal infections.

Sometimes the combined use of antibiotics may reduce the development of resistant bacteria during treatment. This method is used in treating tuberculosis, in which the development of resistant bacteria may be a problem.

The use and misuse of antibiotics to prevent infections

A staggering amount of antibiotics are used to 'prevent' infections. Yet some of these attempts to prevent infections may be useless and/or harmful. They are always very expensive.

Prevention may work if an effective antibiotic is given for a specific infection: for example, the use of penicillin to prevent a type of streptococcal infection of the throat in patients with rheumatic fever; the prevention of gonorrhoea or syphilis immediately after sexual contact with an infected partner; or the use of rifampicin to prevent meningococcal meningitis in people who have been in direct contact with someone suffering from meningococcal meningitis. Another example is in dentistry; during certain dental procedures bacteria may enter the blood stream, and in patients with disease of their heart valves the bacteria may settle on the valves and produce an infection of the lining of the heart (endocarditis). In these individuals, antibiotics should be given just before the dental procedures in order to try to prevent such a serious complication.

Huge quantities of antibiotics are routinely pumped into patients every day before, during and after surgical operations. This is in order to prevent infection developing in the wounds. These practices increase the risk of producing resistant bacteria, which then spread to other patients to infect their wounds – which is why a large number of bacterial infections in patients in surgical wards are resistant to the commonly used antibiotics. Antibiotics are no substitute for 'clean' surgery using sterile techniques. The use of antibiotics in surgical operations should be very selective; for example, in operations on the bowel there is a risk of infection getting into a wound, or operations where a synthetic product is inserted (e.g. an artificial hip joint or heart valve).

Superinfection

The normal balance of micro-organisms living in the body (e.g. in the lungs, bladder, gut) may be disturbed by any antibiotic that kills some

Table 48.1 Suggested anti-bacterial drugs for some commonly occurring infections

Disorder	*Anti-bacterial drugs*
Acne	tetracycline by mouth
Bronchitis (flare-up)	ampicillin or amoxycillin or co-trimoxazole or trimethoprim or erythromycin or tetracycline
Conjunctivitis (purulent)	chloramphenicol or gentamicin eye drops
Dental abscess	amoxycillin or metronidazole
Gall-bladder infections	gentamicin or a cephalosporin
Gonorrhoea	ampicillin with probenecid, or ciprofloxacin or spectinomycin or cefuroxime
Impetigo	topical chlortetracycline and/or flucloxacillin by mouth
Middle ear infection	penicillin G or penicillin V
Non-gonococcal urethritis	tetracycline
Sinusitis	erythromycin or co-trimoxazole
Syphilis	procaine penicillin, or tetracycline or erythromycin
Tonsillitis	penicillin G or penicillin V or erythromycin
Typhoid fever	chloramphenicol or co-trimoxazole or amoxycillin

Table 48.2 Suggested anti-bacterial drugs for preventing some commonly occurring disorders

Prevention of a recurrence of rheumatic fever	penicillin V or sulphadimidine daily
Prevention of meningococcal meningitis in contacts	rifampicin
Prevention of heart valve infections in patients having dental treatment under a local anaesthetic	amoxycillin or erythromycin or amoxycillin plus gentamicin
Prevention of tuberculosis in susceptible contacts	isoniazid
Prevention of infection after surgery on the stomach or gall bladder	gentamicin or cephalosporin
Prevention of infection after surgery of bowel	gentamicin plus metronidazole
Prevention of infection after hysterectomy	metronidazole

bacteria and not others. This may lead to an over-growth of one group of micro-organisms (e.g. bacteria or fungi). This over-growth is called a superinfection and may be defined as the development of a new infection while being treated with an antibiotic for another infection.

Superinfections may cause serious problems because the 'new' infection may not be sensitive to the commonly used antibiotics and may prove very difficult to treat. The risk is greatest with broad-spectrum antibiotics, which kill a wide range of bacteria. This allows one organism to become dominant; for example, when antibiotics are taken by mouth a thrush infection of the mouth, intestine and anus may develop. Also, certain antibiotics taken by mouth may cause a severe form of colitis (semi-membranous colitis) due to an over-growth of a very toxic bacterium (*Clostridium difficile*). The prolonged use of antibiotics when they are not necessary increases the risks of superinfection after, for example, surgery.

Antibiotic policies

Because of the great use of antibiotics in hospitals, the emergence of antibiotic-resistant bacteria and the costs of these drugs, some health authorities have introduced limits to the use of antibiotics. These are usually referred to as 'antibiotic policies' and are aimed at encouraging a more rational use of antibiotics, cutting down the cost of antibiotic usage and, hopefully, reducing the emergence of antibiotic-resistant bacteria. There is an urgent need for something similar in general practice.

49

Penicillins

Penicillin obtained from a mould became available for use in 1941. The original crude extracts of the fermentation of the mould contained several penicillins and, by adding various chemicals to the fermentation, a number of naturally produced penicillins have since been developed. These include benethamine penicillin, benzathine penicillin, benzylpenicillin (penicillin G) and phenoxymethylpenicillin (penicillin V). In addition, the chemical structure of the penicillin may be altered to produce what are called semi-synthetic penicillins. They are not wholly synthetic because the basic penicillin structure is still obtained from moulds by fermentation.

These products are all known as penicillins, and penicillin G is often taken as the main example. The semi-synthetic penicillins have advantages over penicillin G because most of them are more resistant to the acid in the stomach and are more effective by mouth, some of them are active against many more types of bacteria (they are broad-spectrum antibiotics) and some are effective against bacteria that have developed a resistance to penicillin G. However, it is important to remember that when bacteria are sensitive to penicillin G or penicillin V, the other penicillins are not usually as effective.

Penicillins damage the developing cell walls of multiplying bacteria, making them burst. They therefore kill bacteria (they are bactericidal), but only when the bacteria are multiplying.

Penicillin resistance

Bacteria may become resistant to the effects of penicillins in two ways. In one, they may produce enzymes that inactivate some of the penicillins by disrupting the chemical ring structure (the beta-lactam ring) of the penicillin nucleus. They are therefore known as beta-lactamases or penicillinases. In the second way, some bacteria develop a tolerance, or resistance, to penicillin and they just go on multiplying in the presence of doses that would previously have killed them.

Dosage forms of penicillins

The dosage varies according to the penicillin used, the route of administration, the disorder being treated and the patient. Benzylpenicillin is best given by injection; procaine penicillin, which is long acting, is given by intramuscular injection; and penicillin V is effective by mouth. Methicillin, cloxacillin and flucloxacillin are active against penicillinase-producing resistant bacteria; they may be given by injection, and cloxacillin and flucloxacillin may be given by mouth but should be strictly reserved for treating such infections.

Ampicillin is usually taken by mouth, except in serious infections, when it is given intravenously. It has become widely prescribed for upper and lower respiratory infections, urinary infections (e.g. cystitis) and other infections.

Amoxycillin is very effective and need only be given every 8 hours by mouth. It has the same spectrum of activity as ampicillin but is better absorbed.

Classification of penicillins

The basic structure of the penicillins consists of two rings and a side chain. Modifications of this side chain structure have enabled the development of very effective semi-synthetic penicillins. One of the rings in the penicillin nucleus is called a beta-lactam ring and that is why penicillins are called beta-lactam antibiotics. Cephalosporin antibiotics (see later) contain this ring and are also beta-lactam antibiotics.

Penicillins are classified according to the range and type of bacteria that they are active against and according to whether they are resistant or sensitive to the enzyme penicillinase, which some bacteria produce to destroy the penicillin nucleus. Penicillins are therefore grouped into:

- Penicillinase-sensitive penicillins – sensitive to penicillinase
- Penicillinase-resistant penicillins – resistant to penicillinase
- Broad-spectrum penicillins – active against a wide range of bacteria
- Anti-pseudomonal penicillins – active against a group of bacteria (pseudomonas)* which cause serious infections
- Mecillinams – active against a range of Gram-negative bacteria

* Pseudomonas bacteria may infect wounds, the eyes and the urinary tract, and are associated with the production of thick bluish-yellow pus. They belong to a main group of bacteria that are known as *Gram-negative* bacteria because in the laboratory they do not colour with a special violet stain called Gram's stain. They are responsible for many commonly occurring infections. *Gram-positive* bacteria hold the violet stain.

Penicillinase-sensitive penicillins

Penicillin G (benzylpenicillin) was the first penicillin to be used in patients, and still is a very important antibiotic. The antibiotic of first choice when treating a whole range of infectious diseases, it is active against specific bacteria (e.g. streptococcus, pneumococcus, meningococcus). It is important that its use be supported by laboratory tests both to identify the infecting bacteria and to test the sensitivity of the bacteria to penicillin G because some have developed resistance to it.

Penicillin G is not well absorbed when given by mouth, and acid in the stomach makes it inactive. It is therefore given by injection.

After absorption into the blood stream, it spreads throughout all fluids in the body but only a small amount enters the brain fluid. It is rapidly excreted by the kidneys and that is why attempts have been made to try to prolong its duration of action. These include combining it with probencid, which blocks its excretion by the kidneys, or making it into salts that do not dissolve easily – for example, procaine penicillin, benzathine penicillin and benethamine penicillin. These salts dissolve slowly, and so, when given by deep intramuscular injection, they form a depot from which the penicillin G is slowly released for up to 24 hours.

Penicillin V (phenoxymethylpenicillin) is actually less active than penicillin G but, because it is not destroyed by the acid in the stomach, it can be given by mouth. However, despite its very widespread use by mouth, its absorption from the gut is not reliable and tests have shown that blood levels of penicillin V can vary significantly. It is also less active than penicillin G against certain bacteria. It should not therefore be used for serious infections. There are many much more effective and reliable antibiotics. In any case, with serious infections, laboratory tests should always be carried out to determine the most effective antibiotics. It is frequently used to treat tonsillitis and ear infections in children. It is also used to prevent streptococcal infections occurring in children who have had rheumatic fever.

Phenethicillin has a similar range of actions against bacteria but it is no more effective than penicillin V.

Penicillinase-resistant penicillins

When penicillin G was first introduced, it was active against a range of micro-organisms – especially staphylococci that cause wound infections, boils and abscesses. However, its indiscriminate over-use, particularly in hospitals, soon resulted in a group of bacteria that produce a beta-lactamase enzyme (penicillinase) that destroys a central ring (the beta-lactam ring) of the penicillin nucleus, making the antibiotic inactive. This caused many problems until the introduction of penicillins that are actually resistant to penicillinase. Three such penicillins are available – *cloxacillin, flucloxacillin* and *methicillin.* These three drugs are active against penicillin-resistant staphylococci and they should be used only to treat infections by these bacteria. They are less active than benzylpenicillin against bacteria that are not resistant to it.

They are not a substitute for penicillin G in non-resistant infections. Also, that they can be given by mouth does not mean that they are a better alternative treatment for infections. Against non-resistant infections, penicillin G by injection remains a very effective and cheap drug.

Flucloxacillin is not destroyed by the acid in the stomach and can therefore be taken by mouth. It may also be given by injection. Cloxacillin may also be taken by mouth but it is less well absorbed than flucloxacillin; it is also given by injection. Methicillin is made inactive by the acid in the stomach and is given only by injection.

The same old story of over-use

These penicillinase-resistant penicillins have now been so over-used in hospitals that strains of staphylococcal bacteria have now emerged that are resistant even to methicillin and cloxacillin. To treat staphylococcal penicillin-resistant wound infections and abscesses in hospitals, doctors are now left with a restricted choice; for example, the use of vancomycin (see later).

Broad-spectrum penicillins

Ampicillin was the first broad-spectrum penicillin introduced for the treatment of infections. It was a revolution. It is active against a whole range of bacteria and is very effective. *Amoxycillin* represented an improvement on ampicillin in so far as it is better absorbed when taken by mouth, even when taken with food, and it produces less diarrhoea. It reaches higher blood levels and a higher concentration at the sites of infection. Other ampicillin-related antibiotics include bacampicillin, ciclacillin, mezlocillin, and pivampicillin and talampicillin (see Table 49.1). Co-fluampicil (Magnapen) contains flucloxacillin (see earlier) and ampicillin.

Skin rashes in glandular fever

Although allergic reactions to ampicillin, amoxycillin and related penicillins are rare, they often produce a measles-like rash if taken by patients suffering from glandular fever. As glandular fever is caused by a virus infection that is not affected by antibiotics, it is clearly an unnecessary hazard to treat it, or any other virus infection, with antibiotics.

An attempt to overcome the problem of bacterial resistance

Research to overcome the problem of penicillinase-producing bacteria resistant to ampicillin, amoxycillin and related antibiotics came up with a product called *clavulanic acid*. This is not an antibiotic but it blocks the penicillinase that is produced by resistant bacteria and that inactivates these antibiotics. A combined preparation containing amoxycillin and clavulanic acid is available. This preparation (co-amoxiclav: Augmentin) is active against penicillinase-producing bacteria that are resistant to ampicillin, amoxycillin and related drugs. Sulbactam also blocks penicillinase, it is combined with ampicillin in Dicapen.

Anti-pseudomonal penicillins

Carbenicillin and ticarcillin and their close relatives azlocillin, carfecillin and piperacillin are active against pseudomonal infections and certain proteus infections that are resistant to ampicillin and related drugs. Timentin contains ticarcillin and clavulanic acid, and is active against penicillinase-producing bacteria that are resistant to ticarcillin.

Pseudomonal infections are very serious infections which cause a bluish-yellow pus. They have increased significantly in hospitals over the past 40 years as a result of the widespread use of antibiotics in hospitals. Patients with diminished resistance to infections because they are receiving treatment with drugs that depress the immune system, e.g. corticosteroids or who are suffering from a disease which causes an immune deficiency such as leukaemia or AIDS, are at risk of severe infections with these bacteria.

Mecillinams (amidino penicillins)

This is a group of penicillin antibiotics effective against a range of Gram-negative bacteria (e.g. salmonella, which causes dysentery).

Mecillinam has a wide spectrum of activity. It has to be given by injection. Pivmecillinam is a special preparation of mecillinam, which is called a pro-drug. The preparation is taken by mouth and is absorbed into the blood stream, taken to the liver where the mecillinam part of the preparation is split off and enters the blood stream.

Harmful effects of penicillins

Allergic reactions

Allergic reactions to penicillins occur occasionally; when a penicillin is given to someone who has become allergic, a reaction may occur, producing skin rashes, swellings of the skin, face and throat (angioedema), fever and swollen joints. A severe allergic shock (anaphylactic shock) may, very rarely, occur and may cause death. It is more common after injections and in people who have previously had an allergic reaction to penicillin or who are allergic to cephalosporins.

In addition to allergy from penicillins taken into the body, penicillin may also produce allergic reactions if it is included in skin ointments, ear drops, eye drops, or throat lozenges. Penicillin allergy may also follow the handling of penicillin (e.g. nurses drawing up injections), breathing it in or drinking milk from cows treated with penicillin for mastitis. For these reasons, penicillin should not be used in local applications and throat lozenges. The latter may produce a sore tongue, mouth and lips and cause a black furring of the tongue.

Cross-allergy to penicillins occurs because the allergy is to the basic penicillin structure. If you are allergic to one (say, penicillin V) you will probably be allergic to another (e.g. ampicillin).

Diarrhoea

All penicillins given by mouth may cause diarrhoea, nausea, heartburn and itching of the anus (pruritus ani). Diarrhoea is commonest with ampicillin, which may occasionally cause severe colitis. Contaminants from the manufacturing process may also account for some cases of diarrhoea.

Damage to the brain

A very rare harmful effect of the penicillins is irritation of the brain, producing disorders of brain function. This occurs when very high doses are used intravenously or intramuscularly or when normal doses are used in people with impaired kidney function. Injection of high doses of penicillin into the spinal fluid may cause convulsions and should be avoided.

Raised blood salts

A problem with penicillin preparations is that they contain sodium or potassium as penicillin salts. In patients with impaired kidney function, high doses of penicillins may produce high blood levels of sodium and potassium – which may be harmful.

Rash in glandular fever

Ampicillin, amoxycillin, bacampicillin, ciclacillin, pivampicillin and talampicillin may produce a measles-like skin rash in patients suffering from glandular fever or chronic lymphatic leukaemia. This is different from the usual penicillin rash and is specific to these penicillins. It is not an allergic reaction, so penicillins may be used in future in these individuals.

Other harmful effects

Penicillins by mouth may occasionally cause a black tongue due to a fungal infection, and, very rarely, they may cause blood disorders, severe colitis (pseudo-membranous colitis) and superinfection.

Warnings on the use of penicillins

Penicillins should not be used in patients who are known to be allergic to one of the penicillins. People who suffer from nettle rash, asthma or hayfever or who are allergic to a cephalosporin are more prone to allergic reactions to penicillins than are people who do not.

The dosage of some penicillins should be reduced in patients who suffer from impaired kidney function; for example, the dose should be reduced and a longer time should be allowed between doses when using amoxycillin, ampicillin, azlocillin, mezlocillin and piperacillin.

Bacampicillin, pivampicillin and talampicillin should not be used in patients who suffer from severe impairment of their kidney or liver function.

Procaine penicillin should not be injected into a vein, it is only for injection into a muscle (intramuscular).

If, in order to save life, penicillin has to be given to an individual who has had a previous severe allergic reaction to penicillin, it is possible to check for the intensity of the allergy by testing patches of penicillin and its breakdown products on the skin. If the test is positive, the individual may be desensitized to penicillin by giving gradually increasing doses at regular intervals, first by mouth and then by intravenous injection. Full resuscitative equipment and drugs should be immediately at hand and a catheter should be placed in a vein ready to give adrenaline at the earliest sign of a reaction.

Table 49.1 Penicillin preparations

Preparation	*Drug*	*Drug group*	*Dosage form*
Ambaxin	bacampicillin	Broad-spectrum penicillin	Tablets
Amfipen	ampicillin	Broad-spectrum penicillin	Capsules, syrup, powder for injection
Amoxil	amoxycillin	Broad-spectrum penicillin	Capsules, dispersible tablets, syrup, sugar-free syrup (Amoxil Syrup SF), sachets of sugar-free powder (Amoxil 3g Sachet SF), injection powder for reconstitution, paediatric suspension
amoxycillin	amoxycillin	Broad-spectrum penicillin	Capsules, syrup, injection
ampicillin	ampicillin	Broad-spectrum penicillin	Capsules, syrup
Apsin VK	penicillin V potassium (penicillin VK)	Penicillinase-sensitive penicillin	Tablets, syrup
Baypen	mezlocillin	Broad-spectrum penicillin	Injection (powder in vial)
Celbenin	methicillin	Penicillinase-resistant penicillin	Injection (powder in vial)
Crystapen	benzylpenicillin (penicillin G)	Penicillinase-sensitive penicillin	Injection (unbuffered powder in vial)
Depocillin	procaine penicillin	Penicillinase-sensitive penicillin	Injection (powder for reconsititution)
Distaquaine V-K	penicillin V potassium (penicillin VK)	Penicillinase-sensitive penicillin	Tablets, syrup
Econocil VK	penicillin V potassium (penicillin VK)	Penicillinase-sensitive penicillin	Capsules, tablets

Table 49.1 Penicillin preparations (*cont.*)

Preparation	*Drug*	*Drug group*	*Dosage form*
Floxapen	flucloxacillin (sodium in capsules and injection; magnesium in syrup)	Penicillinase-resistant penicillin	Capsules, syrup and syrup forte, injection (powder in vials)
flucloxacillin	flucloxacillin	Penicillinase-resistant penicillin	Capsules, syrup
Ladropen	flucloxacillin	Penicillinase-resistant penicillin	Capsules, injection (powder in vials)
Orbenin	cloxacillin	Penicillinase-resistant penicillin	Capsules, syrup, injection (powder in vials)
Penbritin	ampicillin	Broad-spectrum penicillin	Capsules, syrup and syrup forte, paediatric suspension, injection (powder in vials)
penicillin VK	penicillin V potassium	Penicillinase-sensitive penicillin	Capsules, elixir, tablets
Penidural	benzathine penicillin	Penicillinase-sensitive penicillin	Suspension, oral drops
phenoxymethyl-penicillin	penicillin V potassium (penicillin VK)	Penicillinase-sensitive penicillin	Capsules, tablets, elixir
Pipril	piperacillin	Broad-spectrum penicillin	Injection (powder in vials), infusion (powder in bottles)
Pondocillin	pivampicillin	Broad-spectrum penicillin	Tablets, suspension, sachets (granules); also Pondocillin Plus tablets
Pyopen	carbenicillin	Anti-pseudomonal penicillin	Injection (powder)
Securopen	azlocillin	Anti-pseudomonal penicillin	Injection (powder in vials and in infusion bag)
Selexid	pivmecillinam	Amidino penicillin; active against Gram-negative bacteria	Tablets, suspension (granules in sachets)
Selexidin	mecillinam	Amidino penicillin; active against Gram-negative bacteria	Injection (powder in vials)
Stabillin V-K	penicillin V potassium (penicillin VK)	Penicillinase-sensitive penicillin	Tablets, elixir

Table 49.1 Penicillin preparations (*cont.*)

Preparation	*Drug*	*Drug group*	*Dosage form*
Stafoxil	flucloxacillin	Penicillinase-resistant penicillin	Capsules
Talpen	talampicillin	Broad-spectrum penicillin	Tablets, syrup
Temopen	temocillin	Penicillinase-resistant penicillin	Injection (powder in vials)
Ticar	ticarcillin	Anti-pseudomonal penicillin	Infusion bottle, injection (powder in vial)
V-Cil-K	penicillin V potassium (penicillin VK)	Penicillinase-sensitive penicillin	Tablets, capsules, syrup, paediatric syrup
Vidopen	ampicillin	Broad-spectrum penicillin	Capsules, syrup

Table 49.2 Combined penicillin preparations

Preparation	*Drug*	*Drug group*	*Dosage form*
Ampiclox	ampicillin	Broad-spectrum penicillin	Injection (powder in vial); also neonatal injection (powder in vial)
	cloxacillin	Penicillinase-resistant penicillin	
Augmentin	clavulanic acid	Beta-lactamase inhibitor	Tablets, dispersible tablets, Augmentin Junior and Paediatric (sugar-free powders for suspension), intravenous injection (powder in vial)
	amoxycillin	Broad-spectrum penicillin	
Bicillin	procaine penicillin, penicillin G	Penicillinase-sensitive penicillins	Injection (powder for reconstitution)
co-amoxyclav	amoxycillin	Broad-spectrum penicillin	see under Augmentin
	clavulinic acid	Beta-lactamase inhibitor	
co-fluampicil	flucloxacillin	Penicillinase-resistant penicillin	see under Magnapen
	ampicillin	Broad-spectrum penicillin	

Table 49.2 Combined penicillin preparations (*cont.*)

Preparation	*Drug*	*Drug group*	*Dosage form*
Dicapen	sulbactam	Beta-lactamase inhibitor	Injection (powder in vial)
	ampicillin	Broad-spectrum penicillin	
Magnapen	ampicillin	Broad-spectrum penicillin	Capsules, syrup, injection
	flucloxacillin	Penicillinase-resistant penicillin	
Miraxid	pivampicillin	Broad-spectrum penicillin	Tablets, paediatric suspension
	pivmecillinam	Amidino penicillin; active against Gram-negative bacteria	
Timentin	clavulanic acid	Beta-lactamase inhibitor	Injection (powder in vial)
	ticarcillin	Anti-pseudomonal penicillin	
Triplopen	benethamine penicillin, procaine penicillin, penicillin G	Penicillinase-sensitive penicillins	Injection (powder in vial)

NOTE Beta-lactamases are penicillinases.

50

Cephalosporins

The cephalosporins are a group of semi-synthetic beta-lactamase antibiotics active against a wide range of bacteria (i.e. they are broad-spectrum antibiotics). They are related to a natural mould antibiotic called cephalosporin C. They are active against much the same groups of bacteria as the penicillins and they act in a similar way by damaging the walls of the bacteria.

Over the past decade so many cephalosporins have been introduced on to the market that it is difficult to categorize them. They are sometimes referred to as first, second and third generation cephalosporins according to their range of activity on various groups of bacteria but this does not really help. However, there are differences between cephalosporins in whether they are active if taken by mouth or whether they can only be given by injection, in how they are excreted by the kidneys, in whether they enter the brain fluids or not and which bacteria they are most active against.

Cephalosporins that can be taken by mouth are cefaclor, cefadroxil, cefuroxime, cephalexin and cephradine. The other cephalosporins must be given by injection.

Cephalosporins share a similar chemical structure with penicillins in so far as the nucleus of their structure also contains what is called a beta-lactam ring and, as with the penicillins, this ring can be damaged by certain bacteria that produce beta-lactamase enzymes (or cephalosporinases) which break open the ring and make the antibiotics inactive.

With the extensive use of cephalosporins by doctors we are now seeing more and more bacteria resistant to cephalosporins emerging each year. This is because some bacteria develop beta-lactamases and others mutate so that resistant strains are produced. Cross-resistance to cephalosporins may be shown by bacteria resistant to the penicillinase-resistant penicillins, methicillin and cloxacillin.

Harmful effects of cephalosporins

Allergy to cephalosporins

The most common harmful effects produced by the cephalosporins are allergic reactions. Any one of the cephalosporins is likely to cause allergic reactions, which are similar to those produced by the penicillins. This may be because they share a similar chemical structure.

Immediate allergic reactions may rarely occur, causing a severe allergic emergency (anaphylaxis), wheezing and nettle rash (urticaria). A delayed allergic reaction comes on after several days and produces a measles-like rash with fever. Swollen glands and fever may occur on their own without a rash.

About 10 per cent of patients allergic to penicillins will be allergic to the cephalosporins. But there is no skin test to predict this cross-allergy. About 5 per cent of patients will be allergic to cephalosporins.

Risk of kidney damage

Cephaloridine (a first generation cephalosporin) may occasionally cause kidney damage, particularly when given in a high dose and when given along with a loop diuretic drug such as frusemide or ethacrynic acid. Other cephalosporins have caused kidney damage in patients whose kidney function is already impaired. The risk of kidney damage is increased in elderly people if a cephalosporin is given with other antibiotics that may cause kidney damage (e.g. gentamicin or tobramycin).

Risk of bleeding

Several of the cephalosporins interfere with blood-clotting factors and may occasionally cause bleeding, particularly in elderly and debilitated patients. Latamoxef may, rarely, produce severe bleeding.

Other harmful effects

Cephalosporins may occasionally cause nausea, vomiting and diarrhoea and, very rarely, blood disorders, severe colitis (pseudo-membranous colitis) and superinfection. Injections of cephalothin may be painful.

If alcohol is taken with latamoxef, it may produce flushing of the face, throbbing headache, palpitations, rapid beating of the heart, nausea, vomiting, fall in blood pressure and collapse if taken with large amounts of alcohol. This is called a disulfiram (Antabuse) reaction.

Warnings on the use of cephalosporins

Cephalosporins should not be used in an individual who has had an allergic reaction to any of the cephalosporins. They should not be used in people who suffer from porphyria.

Cephalosporins should be used with caution in anyone allergic to penicillins or who have impaired kidney function (see Chapter 84).

Cephalosporins may give a false positive test for sugar in the urine and a false positive test for haemolytic anaemia (see Coombe's test in haemolytic anaemia, Chapter 26).

Harmful effects from cephalosporins may be more frequent and severe in elderly people because they may have impaired kidney function.

Other beta-lactam antibiotics

Imipenem is a carbapenem; it is a derivative of the beta-lactam antibiotic thienamycin. It is formulated with cilastatin in the preparation Primaxin (powder in vial for intravenous infusion). Cilastatin is structurally related to imipenem but has no anti-bacterial activity; however, it blocks an enzyme in the kidneys that breaks down imipenem and thus keeps a high concentration in the blood. This is very important in treating infections, particularly those of the urinary tract.

Harmful effects include nausea, vomiting, diarrhoea and, rarely, colitis, blood disorders and convulsions. It may, very rarely, cause disturbed kidney and liver function tests.

Warnings *Imipenem must not be used in patients who are allergic to penicillin or who have impaired kidney function, epilepsy, colitis or other chronic inflammatory disorders of the intestine.*

Aztreonam is a monocyclic beta-lactam (monobactam) available as Azactam (powder in vial for injection). It is active only against Gram-negative bacteria.

Harmful effects are similar to those of other beta-lactam antibiotics; they include nausea, vomiting, diarrhoea, abdominal cramps, altered taste and mouth ulcers. Rarely, it may cause allergic reactions, skin rashes, damage to the liver (producing jaundice) and blood disorders. The injection site may be painful.

Table 50.1 Cephalosporin preparations

Preparation	*Drug*	*Dosage form*
Baxan	cefadroxil	Capsules, suspension
Cefizox	ceftizoxime	Injection (powder in vials)
cephalexin	cephalexin	Capsules, tablets
Ceporex	cephalexin	Capsules, tablets, suspension, syrup, paediatric drops
Claforan	cefotaxime	Injection (powder in vials)
Distaclor	cefaclor	Capsules, suspension
Fortum	ceftazidime	Injection (powder in vials)
Kefadol	cephamandole	Injection (powder in vials)
Keflex	cephalexin	Capsules, tablets, suspension
Keflin	cephalothin	Injection (powder in vials)
Kefzol	cephazolin	Injection (powder in vials)
Mefoxin	cefoxitin	Injection (powder in vials)
Monaspor	cefsulodin	Injection (powder in vials)
Suprax	cefixime	Tablets
Velosef	cephradine	Capsules, syrup, powder for suspension, injection (powder in vials)
Zinacef	cefuroxime	Injection (powder in vials)
Zinnat	cefuroxime	Tablets

Warnings *Aztreonam should not be used in people who are allergic to it or during pregnancy. It should be used with caution in individuals with impaired liver or kidney function, with penicillin and/or cephalosporin allergy or in breast-feeding mothers.*

51

Tetracyclines

The first tetracycline to be discovered was aureomycin, in 1948; it was grown from moulds. Another one, called terramycin, was discovered in 1950. Two years later, their chemical structure was determined and it was found to consist of a basic structure of four rings. The antibiotics were therefore called tetracyclines and the generic name of chlortetracycline was given to aureomycin, and oxytetracycline to terramycin. The names Aureomycin and Terramycin remained as brand names. Oxytetracycline (Terramycin) is also available under other brand names (see Table 51.1).

Since the fifties, numerous other tetracyclines have been produced and tested but only a few have proved to be of value. These include clomocycline, demeclocycline, doxycycline, lymecycline, a lysine complex of a tetracyline called methacycline, minocycline and tetracycline.

Harmful effects of tetracyclines

Harmful effects on the bowel

One of the problems with the tetracyclines is that they are only partially absorbed from the intestine and enough reaches the lower intestine to kill off some of the bacteria that live there. This may alter the balance between bacteria and fungi and lead to a superinfection with thrush (*Candida*), which may infect the mouth, bowel, anus and vagina, producing soreness and irritation. This may occur whether the tetracyclines are taken by mouth or by injection because some of the tetracycline in the blood is passed through the liver into the bile and out into the intestine.

The disturbance of bacteria in the intestine caused by tetracyclines may also result in diarrhoea, and sometimes in a serious form of colitis – pseudo-membranous colitis. This is an ulcerating colitis caused by toxins from an over-growth of a certain bacteria called *Clostridium difficile*.

Another serious risk with tetracyclines is the development of additional infections (superinfections) with resistant bacteria such as *Pseudomonas* or *Proteus*, which may cause severe enteritis and, very rarely, death. This is more likely to follow the use of tetracyclines for abdominal operations. These superinfections may also affect the lungs.

Demeclocyline (demethylchlortetracycline), doxycycline and minocycline are better absorbed than the other tetracyclines, and so less gets to the lower intestine to produce intestinal problems.

Tetracyclines are excreted in the urine and in the bile. Doxycycline is excreted principally through the bile and hence is the safest tetracycline to use in patients suffering from kidney failure. Because its breakdown products, which are excreted into the intestine, are largely inactive, it has less effect on natural bowel bacteria than other tetracyclines, and therefore it carries a lower risk of superinfections.

Harmful effects on teeth, bone and nails

Tetracyclines are deposited in growing teeth, producing discoloration and staining of the teeth in young children. It is not only the first set of teeth that is affected – the adult teeth may also be stained for life and there is an added risk of tooth decay. Tetracyclines are also deposited in bone, and they may cause bone growth to slow down in young infants and in unborn babies during the last few months of pregnancy.

The effects of tetracyclines on teeth and bone may occur before the baby is born (during the last 6 months of pregnancy), through infancy and into childhood. Therefore they should not be given to children under the age of 12 years.

Tetracyclines may discolour nails and make them sensitive to sunlight at any age if taken over a long period. Doxycycline is said to cause less staining than other tetracyclines, and demeclocycline is the worst.

Risks of harmful effects in patients with impaired kidney function

Tetracyclines may affect protein production in the body and also kidney function. These may be indicated by a rise in the blood level of breakdown products of proteins (as estimated by blood urea levels, for example). Urea and other waste products are excreted by the kidneys and this may have no consequences if the kidneys are healthy. However, if their function is impaired because of disease or ageing, the amount of these waste products may rise in the blood, producing loss of appetite, vomiting and weakness. This is kidney failure, and it may occur unexpectedly in elderly patients who are given tetracyclines, usually for a chest infection. Doxycycline and minocycline may be used to treat patients with impaired kidney function.

Other harmful effects

These include loss of appetite, nausea, vomiting, sore tongue, difficulty in swallowing, black or discoloured tongue and itching and/or thrush of the genitals and anus. Skin rashes may occur and the skin may become sensitive to sunlight and artificial ultraviolet light (this is more common with demeclocycline than the others).

Tetracyclines may occasionally cause allergic reactions and, very rarely, these may be severe. They may also, rarely, cause blood disorders.

Warnings on the use of tetracyclines

Tetracyclines must not be used in patients who are allergic to them or who have kidney failure. Nor should they be used in the last half of pregnancy or in breast-feeding mothers or in babies, infants and children under the age of 12 years when tooth development is taking place. Tetracyclines damage the teeth, producing a permanent yellow–grey–brown discoloration and poor enamel production (see earlier).

Doxycycline and minocycline may be used in patients with impaired kidney function, but the dose of other tetracyclines should be reduced in patients suffering from mild to moderate impairment of kidney function. Tetracyclines should not be given by intravenous injection to patients with impaired kidney function.

The use of out-of-date tetracycline products has caused damage to the kidneys and changes in the acidity of the blood, producing nausea, vomiting and protein and sugar in the urine. These damaging effects are thought to be due to the product degrading on exposure to moisture, heat or acid.

Sensitivity to sunlight caused by tetracyclines may result in severe sunburn.

Table 51.1 Tetracycline preparations

Preparation	*Drug*	*Dosage form*
Achromycin	tetracycline	Capsules, tablets, syrup, injection (powder in vial)
Achromycin V	tetracycline	Capsules
Aureomycin	chlortetracycline	Capsules
Berkmycen	oxytetracycline	Tablets
Deteclo	tetracycline, chlortetracycline, demeclocycline	Tablets
Imperacin	oxytetracycline	Tablets

Table 51.1 Tetracycline preparations (*cont.*)

Preparation	*Drug*	*Dosage form*
Ledermycin	demeclocycline	Capsules, tablets
Megaclor	clomocycline	Capsules
Minocin	minocycline	Tablets
Mysteclin	tetracycline plus nystatin (an anti-fungal)	Tablets
Nordox	doxycycline	Capsules
Oxymycin	oxytetracycline	Tablets
oxytetracycline	oxytetracycline	Capsules, tablets, mixture
Sustamycin	tetracycline	Sustained-release capsules
Terramycin	oxytetracycline	Capsules, tablets
Tetrabid	tetracycline	Sustained-release capsules
Tetrachel	tetracycline	Capsules, tablets
tetracycline	tetracycline	Capsules, tablets, mixture
Tetralysal	lymecycline	Capsules
Vibramycin	doxycycline	Capsules, syrup
Vibramycin-D	doxycycline	Dispersible tablets

Doxycycline preparations may occasionally cause ulcers of the oesophagus (gullet). They should therefore be taken with at least half a glass of water whilst standing or sitting up straight, and at least one hour before going to bed.

52

Aminoglycosides

Aminoglycosides include amikacin, framycetin, gentamicin, kanamycin, neomycin, netilmicin, streptomycin and tobramycin. They all have a similar chemical structure. They are not absorbed into the bloodstream when taken by mouth, but there is a risk of absorption in patients suffering from inflamed bowel disease and liver failure. They are given by injection and some are used in local applications to treat infections of the skin, eyes and ears.

Aminoglycosides are broad-spectrum antibiotics which kill bacteria (bactericidal). They are given by injection to treat serious infections. Bacteria can develop resistance to these antibiotics, and resistance to one of the group may be associated with resistance to others.

Amikacin, gentamicin, kanamycin, netilmicin, streptomycin and tobramycin are not absorbed from the intestine and have to be given by injection. Framycetin and neomycin are too toxic to be given by injection and are principally used in anti-infective skin applications and in eye and ear drops. They may be given by mouth to sterilize the bowel before surgery on it. Streptomycin is used to treat tuberculosis (see Chapter 55).

Harmful effects of aminoglycosides

Most harmful effects are related to the dose and duration of treatment. They occur more commonly in the elderly and in people with impaired kidney function. They should, preferably, not be used for more than 7 days.

High doses and/or prolonged use, particularly in patients with a low blood potassium, may occasionally cause damage to the kidneys and damage to the nerves in the ears, producing dizziness, vertigo, noises in the ears and deafness (which may be irreversible). Other harmful effects produced by nerve damage include numbness, tingling of the skin, muscle twitching, convulsions, lethargy and confusion.

Aminoglycosides may, rarely, cause loss of appetite, loss of weight, skin rashes, itching, generalized burning, fever, headache, nausea, vomiting, allergic reactions, joint pains, loss of hair and sore mouth.

Prolonged use may cause a fall in level of magnesium in the blood; rarely, a severe colitis (pseudo-membranous colitis) may occur.

Local applications may cause allergic rashes; if applied extensively to the skin or to burns, some of the antibiotic may be absorbed and may, rarely, produce nerve damage in the ear, resulting in deafness and vertigo.

Warnings on the use of aminoglycosides

Aminoglycosides must not be used in patients with hearing loss, disorders of balance (e.g. vertigo) or in the blind, nor in someone who is allergic to any one of them.

Anyone receiving treatment with aminoglycosides should be kept under close observation. The risk of harmful effects is increased if the patient becomes dehydrated, therefore plenty of fluids should be given during treatment. IV diuretics may be dangerous because they increase the concentration in the blood.

Harmful effects may be more frequent and severe in elderly people; therefore use smaller doses and/or increase the time between doses. Kidney function and hearing function should be checked regularly, and blood levels of the drug monitored (see below).

Aminoglycosides are excreted principally by the kidneys, so they must be used with utmost caution in anyone with impaired kidney function; impaired excretion will cause a rise in the concentration of the drug in the blood, increasing the risks of toxic effects, which are mainly damage to the ears (affecting hearing and balance) and damage to the kidneys.

The risk of damage to the nerves in the ears, affecting hearing and balance, is greater in people with impaired kidney function and in individuals with normal kidney function treated with high doses and/or for longer periods of time than recommended. Warnings of damage include dizziness, vertigo, noises in the ears and hearing loss.

Tests of kidney function and hearing function should be carried out before treatment and at regular intervals during treatment.

No other drug that may produce harmful effects on the nerves in the ears or kidney damage should be used at the same time as an aminoglycoside, whether by injection, by mouth or applied to skin or elsewhere. They include cisplatin; the anti-bacterial drugs cephaloridine, polymyxin B, colistin, streptomycin and vancomycin; and the loop diuretics bumetanide, ethacrynic acid and frusemide (see Chapter 89).

Diuretics given intravenously may reduce the volume of fluid in the body and increase the risks of harmful effects from the aminoglycosides. Aminoglycosides may be absorbed in sufficient amount from the bladder (e.g. if they are used in bladder wash-outs) to cause damage to the kidneys and to the nerves in the ears.

Allergic reactions may occasionally occur, particularly with streptomycin, which may also cause severe allergic skin rashes in those who handle the drug (e.g. nurses).

Aminoglycosides affect nerves that supply muscles, and they may produce serious muscle fatigue and difficulty with breathing in people who have myasthenia gravis. Large doses given during surgical operations may produce a temporary disorder like myasthenia gravis in which the muscles are totally fatigued. This effect may also occur if an aminoglycoside is given to someone who has been given neuromuscular blocking drugs or a large volume of blood that has been treated with citrate to prevent it from clotting.

Need to monitor blood levels

Harmful effects to aminoglycosides are more likely to occur if they are given in high doses for prolonged periods of time. This is why it is very important to monitor blood levels in all patients and to keep the dose so adjusted as to avoid toxic levels. Blood levels should be measured one hour after an injection and just before the next dose.

Use of aminoglycosides

Because of the risk of deafness and disorders of balance, streptomycin is now used only to treat tuberculosis.

Gentamicin is the most frequently used aminoglycoside. It is active against a broad spectrum of bacteria and, like all antibiotics, it should preferably be used only when laboratory tests have identified the infecting bacteria and antibiotic sensitivity tests have been carried out on them.

Amikacin, kanamycin, netilmicin and tobramycin have similar uses and produce effects and harmful effects similar to those of gentamicin.

Neomycin is too toxic to be given by injection. Because it is not well absorbed, it can be given by mouth to 'sterilize' the bowel before surgery of the bowel. Its main use is in topical applications to the skin, eyes and ears. Patients may become allergic to neomycin applications, and when used on large areas of skin (e.g. in the treatment of burns) enough may be absorbed into the blood stream to produce harmful effects (e.g. deafness and disorders of balance). Framycetin is similar to neomycin and is used only in topical applications. If absorbed, it is very toxic to hearing and balance and to the kidneys.

Table 52.1 Aminoglycoside preparations

Preparation	*Drug*	*Dosage form*
Amikin	amikacin	Injection, paediatric injection
Cidomycin	gentamicin	Injection, paediatric injection
Genticin	gentamicin	Injection (powder in vial)
Kannasyn	kanamycin	Injection (powder in vial)
Nebcin	tobramycin	Injection
neomycin	neomycin	Elixir
Netillin	netilmicin	Injection
Nivemycin	neomycin	Tablets, elixir
Soframycin	framycetin	Tablets

53

Other anti-bacterial drugs

Other groups of anti-bacterial drugs include:

aminoglycoside-like – spectinomycin
chloramphenicol – chloramphenicol
fusidic acid and its salts – sodium fusidate
glycopeptides – teicoplanin, vancomycin
lincosamides – clindamycin, lincomycin
macrolides – erythromycin
polymyxins – colistin
quinolones – acrosoxacin, ciprofloxacin, enoxacin, nalidixic acid, ofloxacin (U)
rifampicin – rifampicin

Harmful effects and warnings

Acrosoxacin is a quinolone antibiotic. It is used to treat acute gonorrhoea in both sexes.

Harmful effects include dizziness, drowsiness, headache and stomach upsets.

Warnings Acrosoxacin should be used with caution in people who suffer from impaired liver or kidney function. Repeated courses of treatment in anyone under 18 years of age should be avoided because of risk of damage to joints. Because it may produce drowsiness and dizziness, do not drive until you know that it is safe to do so.

Chloramphenicol is a chloramphenicol antibiotic. It is restricted to hospital use, for the treatment of such disorders as typhoid fever and meningitis caused by *Haemophilus influenzae* infection.

Harmful effects include allergic reactions, nausea, vomiting, sore tongue, sore gums, diarrhoea, colitis and superinfection. Occasionally, long-term use may damage the nerves, producing numbness and pins and needles in the arms and legs, and damage to the main nerve in the eyes, producing impaired vision. In premature and newborn babies it may, rarely, produce Grey syndrome – distension of the abdomen with or without vomiting, progressive paleness and blueness of the skin, collapse of the circulation, irregular breathing and death. Stopping the drug early may reverse the process.

It may, very rarely, damage the bone marrow, knocking out blood cell production and thus causing aplastic anaemia. This may develop during treatment and is irreversible even if the drug is stopped. It may also occur weeks or months after treatment, causing blood cell production to be completely knocked out. Just over half the patients recover; the remainder die.

Warnings Chloramphenicol must not be used in people who are allergic to it. Repeated courses and prolonged treatment should be avoided. The dose should be reduced in patients suffering from impaired kidney or liver function. Blood counts before and at regular intervals during treatment should be carried out. Blood levels should be monitored in newborn babies and children under 4 years of age.

Cinoxacin is a quinolone antibiotic used to treat infections of the urinary tract (see Chapter 33).

Ciprofloxacin is a quinolone antibiotic used to treat infections of the chest, urinary tract, stomach and intestine, and gonorrhoea.

Harmful effects include nausea, diarrhoea, vomiting, abdominal pain, headache, restlessness, tiredness, dizziness, itching and, rarely, skin rashes, painful joints and muscles. Vary rarely, it may produce sensitivity of the skin to sunlight, severe allergic reactions, confusion, hallucinations and convulsions, blurred vision, liver damage, kidney damage, blood disorders, pseudo-membranous colitis and Stevens–Johnson syndrome. It may cause pain and soreness at site of injection.

Warnings Ciprofloxacin may cause haemolysis in patients with a glucose-6-phosphate dehydrogenase defect; therefore use with caution. It must not be used in anyone who is allergic to quinolone antibiotics, nor in growing adolescents unless absolutely necessary. It should be used with caution in people with epilepsy or severe impairment of kidney function. Anyone taking this drug should drink plenty of fluids, to prevent crystals forming in the urine. It may impair your ability to drive and operate moving machinery, particularly if it is taken with alcohol.

Clindamycin is a lincosamide antibiotic. Its use is restricted to treating selected infections affecting the bone, the skin and the abdomen (peritonitis) by organisms that are sensitive to clindamycin.

Harmful effects include nausea and vomiting, and it frequently causes diarrhoea. Occasionally it may cause a severe form of colitis called pseudo-membranous colitis. Diarrhoea and colitis may occur up to several weeks *after* treatment has ceased. Allergic skin rashes and other allergic reactions may also occur.

Warnings Clindamycin should not be used in patients suffering from a chronic diarrhoeal disorder (e.g. ulcerative colitis), nor in people who are allergic to it or to lincomycin. It should be used with caution in anyone who suffers from allergies or from impaired liver or kidney function. Stop the drug immediately if diarrhoea occurs.

Colistin is a polymyxin antibiotic active against Gram-negative bacteria. It is not absorbed when given by mouth. It is used in topical applications to treat other skin infections, burns and wounds; to treat ear infections; and to 'sterilize' the bowel before surgery and to wash out the bladder.

Harmful effects include tingling around the mouth, dizziness and, occasionally, muscle weakness which, rarely, may cause difficulty with breathing.

Warnings Colistin must not be used in people who are allergic to the drug or who suffer from myasthenia gravis. The dose should be reduced in patients suffering from impaired kidney function; tests of kidney function should be carried out before treatment starts.

Enoxacin is a quinolone used to treat infections of the urinary tract, gonorrhoea, infections of the skin and shigella gastroenteritis.

Harmful effects include nausea, vomiting, dizziness, altered taste, indigestion, headache, stomach pains, occasionally skin rashes and, rarely, fatigue, rapid beating of the heart, insomnia, tremor and, very rarely, convulsions.

Warnings Enoxacin must not be used in people who are allergic to quinolone antibiotics. It should be used with caution in the elderly and in people with a low blood potassium level, epilepsy or narrowing of the arteries to the brain (cerebral arteriosclerosis).

Erythromycin belongs to a group of antibiotics called macrolides. It is active against almost the same groups of bacteria that are sensitive to the natural penicillins. According to the dose used and the infecting bacteria, it may inhibit their growth (bacteriostatic) or kill them (bactericidal). It is used as an alternative to penicillin in people who are allergic to penicillin. It is the treatment of choice in Legionnaire's disease, and is used to treat whooping cough, chest infections in children and some penicillin-resistant infections.

Bacteria quickly become resistant to erythromycin, especially if it is given for more than one week.

Harmful effects include abdominal cramps and, rarely, nausea, vomiting and diarrhoea. Mild allergic reactions may occur, which include nettle rash and other skin rashes, and, very rarely, disorders of the heart rhythm. Long-term treatment may lead to superinfection. Rarely, liver damage, with or without jaundice, may occur.

Warnings Erythromycin must not be given to people who are allergic to the drug or who have impaired liver function.

Lincomycin is a lincosamide antibiotic. It is related to clindamycin but it is less well absorbed from the intestine and there is a greater risk of diarrhoea. Its use is restricted to treating serious infections caused by bacteria sensitive to lincomycin.

Harmful effects include nausea and vomiting, and frequently it causes diarrhoea. It may occasionally cause a severe form of colitis called pseudo-membranous colitis, which is more common in middle-aged and elderly females, particularly following surgery.

Warnings Lincomycin must not be used in patients suffering from a diarrhoeal disorder (e.g. ulcerative colitis), nor in anyone who is allergic to the drug. It should be used with caution in patients who suffer from allergies, impaired liver or kidney function. Stop the drug immediately if diarrhoea occurs.

Nalidixic acid is a quinolone used to treat Gram-negative infections of the intestine and urinary tract. It is discussed in Chapter 33.

Ofloxacin is a quinolone drug used to treat infections of the urinary and genital tract and chest infections.

Harmful effects include stomach and bowel upsets, skin rashes, allergic reactions and pseudo-membranous colitis. It may occasionally cause transient changes in tests of liver function; rarely, it may cause joint and muscle pains and damage to the bone marrow, producing blood disorders.

Warnings It should not be used in anyone with epilepsy, or in growing adolescents. It should be used with caution in people with serious mental illness or impaired kidney function (the dose should be reduced). Exposure to strong sunlight or ultraviolet rays should be avoided.

Risks with driving: because it may cause dizziness and visual disturbances, it may affect your ability to drive or operate moving machinery.

Polymyxin B is a polymyxin antibiotic, which may be used to treat Gram-negative infections of the intestine, general infections, certain types of meningitis and infections of the eyes.

Harmful effects Occasionally it may cause drowsiness, irritability and damage to nerves, producing incoordination of movement (ataxia), pins and needles and numbness in the arms and legs and around the mouth, and blurred vision. Rarely, it may cause kidney damage, damage to the nerves of hearing and balance, producing deafness and vertigo, and damage to nerve endings in muscles, which may cause weakness and paralysis that can result in difficulty with breathing. Allergic reactions are rare with topical applications. It may cause pain at injection sites.

Warnings Polymyxin B must not be used in people allergic to polymyxin, nor in patients with impaired kidney function or myasthenia gravis. Kidney function should be tested before treatment starts and at frequent intervals during treatment.

Rifampicin is a rifampicin antibiotic. It is used to prevent meningococcal meningitis in close contacts and to treat tuberculosis. It is discussed in detail in Chapter 55.

Sodium fusidate is a salt of fucidic acid. It is active against a narrow spectrum of bacteria. It may be used to treat infections caused by penicillin-resistant staphylococci, especially of bone (osteomyelitis).

Harmful effects include nausea, vomiting, occasionally skin rashes and, rarely, jaundice with reversible changes in liver function.

Warnings Regular tests of liver function should be carried out.

Spectinomycin is an aminoglycoside-like antibiotic. It is used to treat gonorrhoea caused by a penicillin-resistant organism or in patients allergic to penicillins.

Harmful effects include soreness at the site of injection, nettle rash, nausea, vomiting, chills, fever and insomnia.

Warnings Spectinomycin is not effective in the treatment of syphilis. All patients with gonorrhoea should have a test for syphilis at the time of diagnosis and after 3 months treatment with spectinomycin. This is because there is a risk of getting both infections and the treatment of gonorrhoea may mask the progression of the underlying syphilis which, if present, will need specific and prolonged treatment.

Teicoplanin is a glycopeptide antibiotic related to vancomycin but has a long duration of action and may be given once daily. It is used to treat serious infections.

Harmful effects include nausea, vomiting and diarrhoea, allergic reactions (e.g. skin rash, fever, wheezing), headache and dizziness. Rarely, it may cause blood disorders, disturbances of kidney and liver function, tinnitus and hearing loss, and vertigo. Pain, redness and thrombophlebitis may occur at the site of injection.

Warnings The dose should be reduced if kidney function is impaired; blood counts and tests of liver function should be carried out before and at regular intervals during treatment. If treatment is prolonged, hearing tests should be carried out, and if other drugs are used that are known to damage the kidneys, tests of kidney function should be carried out.

Vancomycin is a glycopeptide antibiotic. It is used to treat pseudo-membranous colitis caused by antibiotics.

Harmful effects It may occasionally cause nausea, chills, fever, allergic reactions, throbbing pains in the muscles of the back of the neck, raised blood pressure, flushing of the skin over the neck and shoulders with a red rash and nettle rash during rapid administration of the drug (red man syndrome); very rarely, it may cause blood disorders; damage to the nerves in the ear, causing deafness and vertigo; and kidney damage.

Warnings Vancomycin must not be used in people who are allergic to it. The drug should be used with caution in patients with impaired kidney function. When injected into a vein the drug may irritate and cause thrombophlebitis; it should therefore be diluted in 200 ml of glucose or saline solution and injected slowly. If possible, patients with impaired kidney function or impaired hearing should not be given the drug by injection. Regular tests of liver and kidney function should be carried out as well as regular blood counts. Patients should also have regular measurements of the level of the drug in the blood.

Risks in elderly people: harmful effects, particularly damage to hearing, may be more frequent and serious in the elderly. Patients over 60 years of age should have regular kidney and liver function tests and blood tests; the level of the drug in their blood should be measured regularly.

Table 53.1 Other anti-bacterial preparations

Preparation	*Drug*	*Dosage form*
Aerosporin	Polymyxin B (polymyxin)	Injection (powder in vial)
Arpimycin	erythromycin succinate (macrolide)	Granules for suspension
Chloromycetin	chlorampenicol (chloramphenicol)	Capsules, suspension
Cinobac	cinoxacin (quinolone)	Capsules
Ciproxin	ciprofloxacin (quinolone)	Tablets, solution for infusion
Colomycin	colistin (polymyxin)	Tablets, syrup, injection (powder in vial)
Comprecin	enoxacin (quinolone)	Tablets
Dalacin C	clindamycin (lincosamide)	Capsules, paediatric liquid, injection
Eradacin	acrosoxacin (quinolone)	Capsules
Erycen	erythromycin (macrolide)	Enteric-coated tablets, suspension
Erymax	erythromycin (macrolide)	Capsules containing tasteless enteric-coated pellets
Erythrocin	erythromycin stearate (macrolide)	Tablets
Erythromid	erythromycin (macrolide)	Enteric-coated tablets
Erythromid DS	erythromycin (macrolide)	Enteric-coated tablets (double strength)

Table 53.1 Other anti-bacterial preparations (*cont.*)

Preparation	*Drug*	*Dosage form*
erythromycin	erythromycin (macrolide)	Enteric coated tablets, mixture (as succinate)
erythromycin stearate	erythromycin stearate (macrolide)	Tablets
Erythroped	erythromycin ethyl succinate (macrolide)	Granules in sachets, granules in sachet (forte and paediatric)
Erythroped A	erythromycin succinate (macrolide)	Tablets, granules in sachets
Fucidin	sodium fusidate (salt of fusidic acid)	Tablets, suspension, intravenous infusion (powder in vial with separate ampoule of buffer)
Ilosone	erythromycin estolate (macrolide)	Capsules, tablet, suspension, forte suspension
Kemicetine	chloramphenicol (chloramphenicol)	Injection (powder in vial)
Lincocin	lincomycin (lincosamide)	Capsules, injection, syrup
Rifadin	rifampicin (rifampicin)	Capsules, syrup, injection
Rimactane	rifampicin (rifampicin)	Capsules, syrup, injection
Targocid	teicoplanin (glycopeptide)	Injection (powder in vial)
Tarivid	ofloxacin (quinolone)	Tablets
Trobicin	spectinomycin (aminoglycoside-like)	Injection (powder in vial)
Uriben	nalidixic acid (quinolone)	Suspension
Vancocin	vancomycin (glycopeptide)	Infusion (powder in vial)
Vancocin Matrigel	vancomycin (glycopeptide)	Capsules

Metronidazole and tinidazole

These drugs belong to a group of drugs known as the nitroimidazoles, because of their chemical structure. In addition to metronidazole and tinidazole, which are used to treat *bacterial* infections (see later) and *protozoal* infections (see Chapter 59) the group include: clotrimazole, econazole, ketoconazole and miconazole, which are used to treat fungal infections (see Chapter 56) and mebendazole and thiabendazole used to treat worm infections (see Chapter 59).

Metronidazole and tinidazole are effective drugs against parasitic infections (e.g. amoebic dysentery, giardiasis, trichomonas infections of the vagina). They are also very effective against anaerobic bacteria (bacteria that do not require oxygen to survive and multiply). These anaerobic bacteria can cause and/or complicate many infections; for example, brain abscess, severe pneumonia, infection of bone (osteomyelitis), infection following childbirth, deep-seated abscesses, wound infections following surgery, acute ulcerative disorders of the mouth, tooth abscesses, bedsores and leg ulcers.

The discovery of the importance of anaerobic bacteria in causing these often severe and unpleasant infections and the effectiveness of metronidazole and tinidazole in treating them has been revolutionary. The effects of metronidazole and tinidazole can be dramatic. Unfortunately, it is the old story: they are now being over-used, not only to treat infections but also to prevent infections. They are also used to treat colitis caused by antibiotics (pseudomembranous colitis). Tinidazole has a longer duration of effect.

Table 53.2 Metronidazole and tinidazole – harmful effects and warnings

Harmful effects Serious harmful effects occur very rarely with recommended doses; they are more likely to occur when high doses are used for prolonged periods of time. Reported harmful effects include nausea, loss of appetite, vomiting, diarrhoea, stomach upsets, abdominal cramps, constipation, metallic taste in the mouth, furred tongue, sore mouth and thrush of the mouth. Very rarely, there may develop blood disorders (affecting white blood cells), drowsiness, dizziness, vertigo, confusion, ataxia, weakness, insomnia, allergic reactions, dry mouth, dry vagina or vulva, fever, blocked nose, difficulty passing urine and dark urine. High doses and/or prolonged treatment may, very rarely, cause convulsions and nerve damage, producing numbness or pins and needles in the arms and legs.

Warnings Metronidazole and tinidazole must not be used in people who are allergic to them. They should be used with caution in patients with disorders of the nervous system or with impaired kidney function. If either is used for more than 10 days, patients should have regular medical check-ups to test for harmful effects.

Risks in elderly people Harmful effects may be more frequent and severe; therefore use with caution.

Risks with driving Some harmful effects (e.g. dizziness) may affect your ability to drive; do not drive if you develop these symptoms.

Risks with alcohol Do not drink alcohol when taking either of these drugs; they may produce unpleasant reactions. (See disulfiram reaction under alcohol, in Chapter 87.)

Table 53.3 Metronidazole and tinidazole preparations

Preparation	*Drug*	*Dosage form*
Elyzol	metronidazole	Suppositories
Fasigyn	tinidazole	Tablets
Flagyl	metronidazole	Tablets, capsules, suppositories, injection
Flagyl S	metronidazole	Suspension
Flagyl Compak	metronidazole, nystatin	Tablets (with yellow pessaries of nystatin 100,000 units)
Metrolyl	metronidazole	Tablets, suppositories
metronidazole	metronidazole	Tablets, intravenous infusion, suppositories
Zadstat	metronidazole	Tablets, intravenous infusion, suppositories

54

Sulphonamides and trimethoprim

Sulphonamides

In 1935 it was found that the red dye prontosil rubra protected mice from streptococcal infection and that the active anti-bacterial drug in the body of the mice was a breakdown product of the red dye, called sulphanilamide. Following this discovery hundreds of similar drugs have been produced and tested for anti-bacterial activity. They belong to the sulphonamide group and they stop bacteria from multiplying (they are bacteriostatic) by interfering with the use of folic acid in the bacterial cells.

From their introduction, the sulphonamides were prescribed extensively by doctors, which led to the appearance of resistant bacteria and a high incidence of harmful effects (see later). However, as penicillin and other antibiotics were introduced, the popularity of the sulphonamides decreased and their use is now limited to the treatment of certain disorders such as infections of the urinary tract (see later).

Harmful effects of sulphonamides

Harmful effects from sulphonamide drugs are relatively common, and vary according to the particular sulphonamide used and the susceptibility of the individual. Patients who break down certain drugs slowly in their livers may be more at risk. Generally, harmful effects are mild and often related to the length of treatment and not always to the dose. Serious harmful effects are rare.

The harmful effects that have been reported include the following.

Allergic reactions and skin rashes Allergic reactions to sulphonamides may occur occasionally. They include serious skin rashes, conjunctivitis, sensitivity of the skin to sunlight, nettle rash, itching; drug fever and chills, severe allergic reactions; serum sickness-like symptoms (fever, swollen glands, painful joints); bruising and bleeding into the skin (purpura); inflammation of arteries (periarteritis nodosa); systemic lupus erythematosus (an immune disorder producing inflammation of the skin, blood vessels, heart, lungs, nerves and joints); severe dermatitis; and a skin rash with conjunctivitis and ulcers of the eyes, mouth and urethra (Stevens–Johnson syndrome).

Blood disorders Sulphonamides may occasionally damage the bone marrow and thus affect red blood cell production, causing anaemia, and white blood cell production, causing reduced resistance to infection. They may damage red blood cells, causing haemolytic anaemia, and interfere with the body's use of folic acid, producing folic acid deficiency anaemia. Destruction of red blood cells (haemolytic anaemia) may occur in patients who suffer from an abnormality of red blood cells: glucose-6-phosphate dehydrogenase deficiency.

NOTE sulphonamides may, rarely, knock out red cell and/or white cell production completely.

Mouth, stomach and intestinal disorders Sulphonamides may occasionally produce sore gums, sore tongue, loss of appetite, nausea, vomiting, abdominal pains, diarrhoea, colitis (pseudo-membranous colitis).

Liver disorders Sulphonamides may occasionally damage the liver, producing hepatitis and jaundice – which may be very severe.

Kidney disorders Sulphonamides may occasionally cause crystals in the urine and severe kidney damage, leading to kidney failure. Crystals in the urine are more common with the less soluble sulphonamides (e.g. sulfamerazine, sulphadiazine and sulphapyridine).

Disorders of the brain and nerves Sulphonamides may occasionally cause headache, drowsiness, dizziness, noises in the ears (tinnitus), vertigo, numbness and pins and needles in the arms and legs, incoordination of movements (ataxia), convulsions and meningitis.

Mental disorders Sulphonamides may occasionally cause hallucinations, depression, apathy and nervousness.

Other harmful effects Other occasional harmful effects produced by sulphonamides include painful joints, painful muscles, weakness, fatigue, insomnia, bad dreams and confusion.

Calcium sulphaloxate and sulphaguanidine produce fewer harmful effects because they are poorly absorbed from the intestine. They were previously used to treat infections of the intestine but should no longer be used for this purpose; nor should they be used to prepare the intestine for intestinal surgery.

Sulfametopyrazine and other long-acting sulphonamides accumulate in the body and are more likely to produce harmful effects. Sulphonamide drugs should not be used towards the end of pregnancy (see Chapter 79).

Sulphaguanidine frequently causes skin rashes.

Warnings on the use of sulphonamides

Sulphonamides should not be given to premature babies, babies under 2 months of age, nor to women just before childbirth because of the risk of producing kernicterus in the baby.

They should not be given to people with kidney or liver failure, jaundice or folic acid deficiency anaemia, nor to anyone who is allergic to sulphonamides or trimethoprim. In individuals suffering from impaired kidney function the dose should be reduced or the interval of time between doses should be increased. Sulphadiazine should not be used at all in anyone with severe kidney impairment.

Individuals on long-term treatment with sulphonamides should have regular blood tests to check their white and red cell counts and also to check for other blood disorders. Anyone taking sulphonamides should drink plenty of fluids in order to prevent crystals forming in the urine.

Sulphonamides should be given with caution to people with severe allergies or asthma, and with great caution to people who are deficient in folic acid (see page 719) or who are sensitive to sunlight.

Present-day use of sulphonamides

The use of sulphonamide drugs alone should be limited to treating urinary infections. Because of bacterial resistance and the availability of more effective and less harmful antibiotics they should no longer be used to treat or prevent infections of the throat and chest, bacillary dysentery and meningococcal meningitis. Rifampicin is now the drug of choice for preventing meningococcal meningitis in people who have been in contact with someone suffering from that disease.

Although the use of sulphonamide drugs alone has gone out of fashion, the combination of a sulphonamide drug (sulphamethoxazole) with trimethoprim is in fashion. This combination, known as co-trimoxazole, is widely used, and it is important to be aware that it contains a sulphonamide and that all the warnings on the use of sulphonamides also apply to co-trimoxazole.

Combinations of a sulphonamide with trimethoprim (co-trimoxazole)

Trimethoprim is a broad-spectrum anti-bacterial drug that blocks the use of folic acid inside bacterial cells at a stage just after the one that sulphonamides block. Therefore, the use of trimethoprim and a sulphonamide together successfully blocks vital processes in the cellular development of bacteria. This is an example of one drug potentiating the action of another by acting 'synergistically'. Whereas sulphonamides alone are bacteriostatic (they stop bacteria from multiplying), this combination is bactericidal (it kills the bacteria).

There is an optimal ratio of concentrations for the two drugs if they are to act together; because trimethoprim is twenty times stronger than sulphamethoxazole, the most effective ratio is 20 parts of sulphamethoxazole to 1 part of trimethoprim. The aim of a preparation of the combined drugs is therefore to get this 20 to 1 concentration ratio to the site of infection in the body (i.e. the target site). This is difficult because their rates of absorption through the intestine vary, as do their rates of excretion from the kidneys.

The most effective combination is one containing 5 parts of sulphamethoxazole to 1 part of trimethoprim: co-trimoxazole. The development of bacterial resistance is lower with this combination than with each drug used separately. The combination reaches satisfactory blood levels in about 1 hour after absorption, reaching a peak in 2–4 hours, which lasts for up to 7–8 hours and then tapers off by about 24 hours.

Harmful effects of co-trimoxazole and trimethoprim

Because co-trimoxazole interferes with the use of folic acid in bacteria, it may have this effect on the cells of the body, particularly in people who are deficient in folic acid; for example, the elderly and people who have a chronic illness. This harmful effect may result in the development of folic acid deficiency anaemia in these individuals.

The harmful effects produced by co-trimoxazole are a combination of those produced by a sulphonamide drug (see earlier) and those produced by trimethoprim (see later), and here is the real problem. Trimethoprim produces harmful effects similar to those produced by sulphonamides, and the combination causes many more skin rashes than either drug used alone. Some of these, although very rare, may be serious and occur more commonly in elderly people.

Co-trimoxazole may, rarely, produce kidney and liver damage; very rarely, fatal blood disorders have occurred in elderly people, in whom it should no longer be used. In patients suffering from AIDS it may produce a severe reaction, including fever, malaise, skin rash and blood disorders. People who have had a kidney transplant may develop blood disorders because of this drug.

Because co-trimoxazole contains two drugs, bacterial sensitivity to each drug should be tested. It should be used only if the infecting bacteria are sensitive to both drugs, when it will obviously be more effective than a sulphonamide alone. Co-trimoxazole is used to treat infections of the respiratory, urinary and intestinal tracts and of the skin.

Trimethoprim may be used alone for the treatment of urinary tract infections and chest infections. Harmful effects are less than with the combination.

Harmful effects include nausea, vomiting, sore tongue, itching, skin rashes and blood disorders (e.g. anaemia due to folic acid deficiency).

Warnings Trimethoprim must not be used in people who are allergic to it or who have anaemia due to folic acid deficiency, nor in patients suffering from severe liver disorders or blood disorders or in newborn babies. The dose should be reduced in patients with moderate impairment of kidney function and in anyone who may become deficient in folic acid. Monthly blood tests for anaemia should be carried out on patients taking long-term treatment.

Table 54.1 Sulphonamide and trimethoprim preparations

Preparation	*Drug*	*Drug group*	*Dosage form*
Bactrim	co-trimoxazole	Sulphonamide/folic acid inhibitor	Tablets, double-strength tablets, dispersible tablets, adult suspension, paediatric syrup, paediatric tablets, intramuscular injection, intravenous infusion
Chemotrim Paed	co-trimoxazole	Sulphonamide/folic acid inhibitor	Paediatric suspension
Comox	co-trimoxazole	Sulphonamide/folic acid inhibitor	Tablets, dispersible tablets, forte tablets, paediatric suspension
co-trimoxazole	co-trimoxazole	Sulphonamide/folic acid inhibitor	Tablets, dispersible tablets, mixture, intramuscular injection, solution
Enteromide	calcium sulphaloxate	Sulphonamide	Tablets

Table 54.1 Sulphonamide and trimethoprim preparations (*cont.*)

Preparation	*Drug*	*Drug group*	*Dosage form*
Fectrim Forte	co-trimoxazole	Sulphonamide/folic acid inhibitor	Dispersible tablets, tablets (Fectrim Standard), paediatric tablets (Fectrim Paediatric)
Ipral	trimethoprim	Folic acid inhibitor	Tablets, paediatric suspension
Kelfizine W	sulfametopyrazine	Sulphonamide	Tablets
Laratrim Forte	co-trimoxazole	Sulphonamide/folic acid inhibitor	Tablets (Laratrim Forte), adult suspension, paediatric suspension
Monotrim	trimethoprim	Folic acid inhibitor	Tablets, sugar-free suspension, injection
Septrin	co-trimoxazole	Sulphonamide/folic acid inhibitor	Tablets, dispersible tablets, forte tablets, paediatric tablets, adult suspension, paediatric suspension, intramuscular injection, intravenous infusion
sulphadiazine	sulphadiazine	Sulphonamide	Tablets, injection
sulphadimidine	sulphadimidine	Sulphonamide	Tablets, paediatric oral suspension
sulphaguanidine	sulphaguanidine	Sulphonamide	Tablets
Sulphamezathine	sulphadimidine	Sulphonamide	Injection
Syraprim	trimethoprim	Folic acid inhibitor	Tablets, injection
trimethoprim	trimethoprim	Folic acid inhibitor	Tablets, mixture, sugar-free injection
Trimopan	trimethoprim	Folic acid inhibitor	Tablets, sugar-free, paediatric suspension
Uromide	sulphaurea phenazopyradine	Sulphonamide Anaesthetic	Tablets

55

Tuberculosis

The infecting organisms that cause tuberculosis enter the body through the lungs and the intestines. However, illness does not always follow infection, and whether a person develops an illness or not depends on many factors such as the individual's age, sex, natural resistance to infections, standards of living and nutrition, and general physical condition.

The initial, or primary, tuberculosis infection usually affects the lungs but can affect the tonsils or the bowel where it produces enlarged glands in the abdomen. In 90–95 per cent of people the body's immune system controls the infection and these primary sites of infection heal over and scar; but if this healing is not complete because of the general health of the individual, some bacteria may survive and may enter the blood to spread the infection to other parts of the body – bones, joints, kidneys. This may happen months or even years after the primary infection – *reactivation infection* – and it comes on gradually, causing loss of appetite and weight, debility and fever.

In 5–10 per cent of patients the primary infection does not heal and progresses to produce complications at the site of infection such as collapse of a lung or an abscess. The infection may also spread through lymph glands to infect the lining covers of the lungs, producing pleurisy, or the lining covers of the heart, producing inflammation (pericarditis). It may also spread into the blood stream to infect many organs (miliary tuberculosis) and even cause an infection of the lining covers of the brain (meningitis). A similar type of disease may develop in someone who has a dormant primary infection and who becomes re-infected with tuberculosis bacteria – reinfection tuberculosis.

Progressive tuberculosis of the lungs may develop directly from a primary infection, it may follow the reactivation of an apparently healed primary infection, or the infection may spread to the lungs via the blood stream from an infected lymph gland (post-primary pulmonary tuberculosis).

Drug treatment of tuberculosis

The availability of effective anti-tuberculosis drugs (anti-tuberculous drugs) has had a dramatic effect in reducing complications and deaths from tuberculosis. Problems and failure of treatment are now due to the serious risk of the bacteria developing resistance to the drugs used, lack of education of doctors and poor education of patients.

Attempting to reduce the risks of bacterial resistance

Because of the very real problem that the bacteria which cause tuberculosis can easily become resistant to anti-tuberculous drugs, treatment is now always planned in two phases – an *initial phase* and a *continuing phase*. This approach attempts to control the risk of resistant bacteria developing.

Bacterial resistance develops to all anti-tuberculous drugs if they are given singly; they are therefore always used in combination. Before any drug treatment is started, a sample of sputum or infected tissue is sent off to the laboratory to confirm the diagnosis and to test available drugs against the infecting tuberculous bacteria in order to determine which drugs are most effective and to identify those drugs to which the bacteria have developed a resistance. However, it may take 3 months to obtain the results of these tests so, rather than delay initial treatment, it is given blind.

The *initial phase* of treatment always involves the use of at least three different drugs given together. The aim of such high powered treatment is to try to knock out the infection as quickly and as effectively as possible, just in case the infecting bacteria are resistant to one or more of the drugs being used. It usually involves the daily use of the following three drugs given together – isoniazid, rifampicin and pyrazinamide. Ethambutol or streptomycin may be added to the initial phase treatment. These drugs should be continued for at least 8 weeks, and preferably until the results of the drug-sensitivity tests are available.

Continuation phase treatment should directly follow the initial phase of treatment and includes isoniazid and rifampicin. Ethambutol may be used with either isoniazid or rifampicin. Streptomycin should be used only when absolutely necessary. Alternative drugs include capreomycin, cycloserine or pyrazinamide.

The duration of total treatment varies from 6 to 18 months, according to the drugs used and the patient's response.

With effective initial phase treatment it should be possible to knock out the tuberculosis infection completely. This clearly depends on the selection of an effective combination of drugs and the continuation of treatment for at least 8 weeks and, preferably, until the sensitivity tests are back from the laboratory. Equally, effective continuation treatment depends upon the doctor selecting the right combination of drugs and continuing treatment for an adequate duration of time.

Patients who are not able to take daily treatment by mouth and who are not very good at sticking to their treatment regimens (see below) may be put on to treatment that involves much more supervision. This usually includes twice-weekly treatment with high doses of isoniazid and rifampicin.

Failure of treatment

Most failures of treatment are due to patients who do not take their prescribed drugs as directed. Another important cause of failure is inappropriate prescribing by doctors, who may use the wrong combination of drugs, use too high or too low dosages, or stop treatment too early.

Prevention of tuberculosis

Tuberculin skin test for tuberculosis (the Mantoux test)

The Mantoux test is performed by injecting tuberculin into the skin (intradermally). Tuberculin is a purified protein derivative (PPD) of the active material in the liquid medium after growth of the tuberculosis organism. The individual who has tuberculosis will be 'sensitive' to the material in the Mantoux test and will develop a red, hard swelling at the site of injection. This will develop in about 6 hours, to reach a maximum in 36–60 hours and then fade over the next few days. A positive Mantoux test is defined as 10 mm or more of red hardness (induration) at 48 hours. A negative test is no reaction or an immediate reaction which disappears in 48 hours.

The reaction to the Mantoux test may be 'reduced' if the individual has a virus infection, has received immunization against a virus infection, has an immune deficiency caused by disease (e.g. AIDS) or by drugs (e.g. corticosteroids, anti-cancer drugs), or is suffering from malnutrition, old age or an overwhelming infection.

Tuberculin testing of people who have been in close contact with someone with active tuberculosis (contacts) is essential because not only does the Mantoux test identify those contacts who have the disease but it also helps to identify those close contacts who have not picked up the disease and who may benefit from BCG vaccination. The *Heaf test* was a multi-puncture method of injecting tuberculin into the skin. The apparatus was called a Heaf gun and the result was read in 3 days.

Warning *Because of the risk of transmitting hepatitis and AIDS, the Heaf gun should no longer be used. It has been replaced by a disposable* ***tine test unit*** *– a* *disc with four prongs 2 mm long coated with Old Tuberculin. A new disc is used for each individual.*

An uninfected person in close daily contact with someone with active tuberculosis (e.g. live bacteria present in the sputum) may be at risk of contracting the disease. To prevent this risk it may be necessary to give the uninfected person the anti-tuberculous drug isoniazid daily for 12 months (see Table 55.1 for harmful effects and warnings on use). Similar treatment is necessary for contacts who have evidence of a primary infection and for contacts who are immune deficient because of disease (e.g. AIDS) or drug treatment (e.g. someone taking corticosteroids or immunosuppressive drugs).

BCG vaccination

For comments on the use of BCG vaccination, see Chapter 11.

Table 55.1 Drugs used to treat tuberculosis – harmful effects and warnings

capreomycin
Harmful effects include allergic skin rashes (e.g. nettle rash) sometimes with fever; kidney damage, liver damage; damage to the nerves of the ear, causing hearing loss, noises in the ears and vertigo; blood disorders; pain and hardness of the skin at injection sites.

Warnings Capreomycin must be used with utmost caution in individuals with impaired hearing and/or balance, or with impaired function of their kidney or liver. It must not be given with other drugs that may damage the nerve in the ears that is responsible for hearing and balance, nor to anyone who is allergic to it. Tests of kidney and liver function should be carried out before and at regular intervals during treatment, as should tests of hearing and balance.

Risks in elderly people Harmful effects may be more frequent and severe; therefore use with caution.

cycloserine
Harmful effects occasionally affect the brain and nervous system, and appear to be related to the use of high doses (more than 500 mg daily). They include headache, dizziness, vertigo, drowsiness and, rarely, convulsions, confusion, disorientation with loss of memory, serious mental symptoms, sometimes with suicidal tendencies, severe irritability and aggression, weakness, numbness and pins and needles in the arms and legs and coma. Very rarely it may cause megaloblastic anaemia and, occasionally, allergic skin rashes.

Warnings Cycloserine should not be used in anyone who is allergic to it, or who suffers from epilepsy, depression, anxiety, severe kidney impairment or excessive alcohol use. The dose should be reduced in individuals with impaired kidney function. The toxicity of cycloserine is closely related to dose; therefore, blood levels of the drug should be checked regularly, at least every week in people with impaired kidney function, those receiving high doses (500 mg or more daily) and those showing signs of harmful effects. The value of pyridoxine (vitamin B_6) in preventing damage to nerves has not been proved.

Risks in elderly people Harmful effects

Table 55.1 Drugs used to treat tuberculosis – harmful effects and warnings (*cont.*)

may be more frequent and severe; therefore use reduced dosage.

ethambutol
Harmful effects include a decrease in vision due to damage to the optic nerve (the main nerve to eye); this is related to dosage and duration of treatment, and may affect one or both eyes. Vision usually recovers when the drug is stopped but, very rarely, the damage may be permanent. Red/green colour-blindness may also occur. Ethambutol may damage other nerves, producing numbness and pins and needles in the arms and legs. There are very rare reports of it causing allergic rashes, transient abnormalities of liver function tests, jaundice and nerve damage.

Warnings Ethambutol must not be used in people who are allergic to it or who suffer from optic neuritis. It should be used with caution in anyone with impaired kidney function; the dosage should be reduced, and regular estimates should be carried out of the level of the drug in the blood. Tests of kidney and liver function and tests of the blood should be carried out at regular intervals during treatment. Patients should have regular and complete eye examinations by an optometrist (opthalmic optician). You should report immediately if you notice any deterioration in your vision.

Risks in elderly people Harmful effects may be more frequent and severe; therefore use with caution, checking kidney function and using reduced dosage.

isoniazid
Harmful effects The drug is generally well tolerated and harmful effects occur mainly when high doses are used in people who break the drug down slowly. They include nausea, vomiting, allergic reactions, skin rashes, insomnia, damage to nerves; producing numbness and pins and needles in the arms and legs; nerve damage is preventable by giving pyridoxine. It may cause pain and swelling of the hand (shoulder-hand syndrome). Rarely, there may be restlessness, muscle twitching, convulsions, impairment of memory, serious mental symptoms, reduced white blood cells (agranulocytosis) liver damage (hepatitis) and disorders such as systemic lupus erythematosus and rheumatoid arthritis. The risk of getting hepatitis is related to age and is highest among people aged 50–64 years. It may occur after many months of treatment. The risk is increased by the daily consumption of alcohol. Occasionally, deaths from hepatitis caused by isoniazid have occurred.

Warnings Isoniazid must not be used in individuals who are allergic to it or who have liver disease caused by drugs. It should be used with caution in people who drink excessively, who have epilepsy or have impaired liver or kidney function. Because of the risk of liver damage, patients should be checked every month during treatment: regular tests of liver function should be carried out and you should report any symptoms that may suggest liver damage (e.g. fatigue, weakness, malaise, loss of appetite, nausea and vomiting). If there is any suggestion of liver damage the drug should be stopped immediately.

Risks in elderly people Harmful effects may be more frequent and severe; therefore use with caution.

pyrazinamide
Harmful effects Liver damage is the most common harmful effect and may vary from abnormal liver function tests with no symptoms, through mild damage with loss of appetite, fever, malaise and a tender enlarged liver, to more serious liver damage and jaundice. The risk of liver damage is reduced by keeping the dose at the manufacturer's recommended level. It may also cause loss of appetite, nausea, vomiting, painful joints, active

Table 55.1 Drugs used to treat tuberculosis – harmful effects and warnings (*cont.*)

gout, blood disorders, allergic reactions, nettle rash, difficulty in passing urine, malaise, fever and flare-up of peptic ulcers.

Warnings Pyrazinamide must not be used in people who are allergic to it, or who have liver disease, raised blood uric acid levels and/or gouty arthritis. It should be used with caution in anyone with impaired kidney function or diabetes. Liver function tests should be carried out before and at regular intervals during treatment. At the earliest sign of liver damage the drug should be stopped.

Risks in elderly people Harmful effects may be more frequent and severe; therefore use with caution.

rifampicin

Harmful effects include loss of appetite, nausea, vomiting, diarrhoea; influenza-like symptoms (chills, fever, bone pains, shortness of breath); kidney damage, flushing, itching, liver damage with jaundice and/or a shock-like state; skin rashes, headache, drowsiness, fatigue, irregular menstrual periods, dizziness, incoordination of movements, inability to concentrate, confusion and blurred vision. It may give urine, faeces, saliva and other body secretions a red–orange colour. It may affect the tears and discolour soft contact lenses. Rarely, it may cause blood disorders such as thrombocytopenic purpura, haemolytic anaemia and disorders of white blood cells. Harmful effects that occur following intermittent treatment are probably due to an immune response.

Warnings Rifampicin must not be used in patients with porphyria or who are allergic to it. The dose should be reduced in individuals with impaired liver function and in alcoholics. Tests of liver function should be carried out before and at regular intervals during treatment. Treatment should not be stopped and re-started, as this increases the risk of kidney damage.

Risks in elderly people Harmful effects may be more frequent and severe; therefore use with caution.

streptomycin

Harmful effects It may occasionally cause pins and needles in and around the mouth, vertigo, lassitude, headache and allergic reactions, damage to the nerves of the ear producing deafness (which may be permanent), noises in the ears and vertigo. Rarely, large doses may cause kidney damage, and very rarely, blood disorders and lupus erythematosus may occur. For other harmful effects of aminoglycosides, see Chapter 52.

Warnings Streptomycin should not be used in people who are allergic to it, who have hearing loss or vertigo or who are blind or who suffer from myasthenia gravis. The risk of damage to the nerves supplying the organ of balance is directly related to the dose and duration of treatment. Advanced age and impaired kidney function increase the risk of such damage. Recovery is usually complete after stopping the drug. Hearing loss may, rarely, occur with prolonged treatment and is usually permanent. Tests of kidney function should be carried out before and at regular intervals during treatment. If kidney function is impaired the dose should be reduced and the blood levels of streptomycin measured and kept within a safe range. The use of other drugs that damage nerves and/or the kidneys should be avoided. The damage to nerves may occasionally cause paralysis of breathing, especially during surgery if the streptomycin is given soon after a general anaesthetic and a muscle relaxant drug (e.g. tubocurarine). Tests of hearing and balance should be carried out before and at regular intervals during treatment. Noises in the ears requires immediate tests of hearing and balance or the drug to be stopped, or both. Contact with the skin may cause an allergic reaction; therefore

Table 55.1 Drugs used to treat tuberculosis – harmful effects and warnings (*cont.*)

nurses and others handling the drug should be cautious and wear plastic gloves. The drug should be injected deep into large muscles (e.g. the buttock) and injection sites should be alternated. Concentrations of greater than 500 mg/ml are not recommended. It should be given with caution to patients with impaired kidney function. Reducing the acidity of the urine may help to reduce the irritating effects on the kidneys. High doses in infants may produce a floppy child associated with stupor, coma and depressed breathing.

Risks in elderly people Harmful effects may be more frequent and severe; therefore use with caution. Blood levels should be checked at regular intervals during the first few weeks of treatment. In patients over 60 years of age the blood level of streptomycin 24 hours after injection should not exceed 1 microgram/ml.

Table 55.2 Preparations used to treat tuberculosis

Preparation	*Drug*	*Dosage form*
Capastat	capreomycin	Injection (powder in vial)
cycloserine	cycloserine	Capsules
isoniazid	isoniazid	Tablets, elixir
Myambutol	ethambutol	Tablets
Mynah	ethambutol and isoniazid	Tablets of varying strengths of ethambutol
Rifadin	rifampicin	Capsules, syrup, intravenous infusion (powder in vial)
Rifater	isoniazid, pyrazinamide and rifampicin	Tablets
Rifinah	rifampicin and isoniazid	Tablets, of varying strengths of rifampicin
Rimactane	rifampicin	Capsules, syrup, intravenous infusion (powder in vial)
Rimactazid	rifampicin and isoniazid	Tablets
streptomycin	streptomycin	Injection (powder for reconstitution)
Zinamide	pyrazinamide	Tablets

56

Fungal infections

The term 'mycosis' refers to a disease caused by fungi. The extent and nature of diseases caused by fungi (mycoses) vary a great deal between different areas of the world. In some areas, fungal diseases are regularly present in the community whereas in other areas they occur only under certain circumstances – for example, in individuals who have immune deficiency and in whom resistance to infection is reduced because of drug treatments or disease.

Immune deficiency caused by drugs

Treatments that cause immune deficiency and weaken the body's defence system against infection include corticosteroids, radiotherapy and drugs used to treat cancer.

Sometimes drugs are used with the specific aim of suppressing the immune system. They suppress part of, or the whole of, the body's immune system and are used in order to reduce the tendency of the body to reject a tissue or organ transplanted from another person.

Immune deficiency caused by disease

Any disease that damages the immune system will weaken the body's defence system and make the individual open to the risk of severe widespread infections from all kinds of micro-organisms (e.g. bacteria, fungi, viruses) that normally would not cause problems in healthy people. AIDS is an example of a disease that lowers the body's resistance to infection by damaging the immune system.

Fungal diseases

Fungal infections are spread by spores or hyphae. Normally they are breathed in or land on the skin to cause an infection. From the skin and lungs the fungus may spread to other parts of the body. Fungal infections last a long time (they are chronic infections) and usually any drug treatment has to be prolonged in order to obtain a cure.

Most fungi are harmless to humans; however, if the body's resistance to infection is lowered, fungi can cause local infections (e.g. of the skin and lungs) which may then spread throughout the body to infect virtually any organ.

Local fungal infections of the skin, mouth, vagina or anus are usually associated with some local damage to the surface or to treatment with antibiotics. The latter disturbs the local balance of bacteria and fungi, and makes it easier for fungus to start to grow. A common example of this is vaginal thrush in someone given antibiotics by mouth.

Some patients may be allergic to fungi and develop asthma and other respiratory disorders.

Anti-fungal drugs

Because fungi particularly attack people who are immune deficient (see earlier), it is important to treat the whole patient in order to correct, if possible, any predisposing factors. Any anaemia, infection or other underlying disorder should be treated and the patient should be given vitamins, minerals and a nutritious diet. Also, it is important to remove any contact with an infected animal, whether it is a dog, farm animal, pigeon or even bats in a cave.

Anti-fungal drugs include the following.

Amphotericin is an antibiotic that either kills fungi (fungicidal) or interferes with their multiplication (fungistatic), according to the dose used and the fungus being treated. It is active against a wide range of fungi and yeasts. Its activity may be increased by giving it with certain anti-bacterial drugs and other anti-fungal drugs (e.g. flucytosine). It is an effective drug which may be given by mouth or infusion into a vein but it may produce serious harmful effects (see later), so expected benefits need to be balanced against the risks.

As with the treatment of all fungal infections, the use of amphotericin has to be prolonged – usually about 6–10 weeks but sometimes as long as 16 weeks.

Clotrimazole is used only in local applications to treat vaginal thrush and ringworm and other forms of infection of the skin.

Econazole is used only in local applications to treat vaginal thrush (see later).

Fluconazole is active by mouth and is used to treat general thrush infections and thrush infections of the vagina, mouth and throat, and intestine. It need only be given in a single dose each day. It has less effect than ketoconazole on the breakdown of other drugs by the liver. It may also be given by intravenous infusion.

Flucytosine is effective in the treatment of generalized (systemic) fungal infections caused by certain yeasts (e.g. thrush). It may be given by mouth or by infusion into a vein. Fungi may become resistant to flucytosine, so its use as a single drug should be restricted. However, it increases the effects of amphotericin and the two are often used together to treat severe generalized infections.

Griseofulvin is given by mouth for the treatment of fungus infections of the nails and hair. It is used to treat infections of the skin only if applications of anti-fungal preparations have failed and/or if the disease is widespread over the body. It concentrates in keratin, which is a protein on the surface layer of the skin which forms a major component of nails and hair. The drug is deposited in developing keratin-producing cells and makes them resistant to fungal infection. Therefore, any new growth of hair, nails or skin is free from the infection. The keratin containing the fungus is got rid of through the loss of scales from the skin, cutting the nails and cutting the hair. The infected keratin gradually becomes replaced by uninfected keratin.

As with all anti-fungal drug treatment, griseofulvin should be continued for weeks or even months.

Itraconazole is used to treat thrush of the vagina and vulva, and fungal skin infections. It can remain in tissues (e.g. the skin) for up to 4 weeks. It enters infected cells in the base of the skin, and as the cells work their way to the surface the infected cells are shed.

Ketoconazole is taken by mouth. It requires acid in the stomach if it is to dissolve and be absorbed into the blood stream; therefore drugs that block acid production (see Chapter 15) reduce its absorption. It may, rarely, produce serious liver damage (see later), so expected benefits from using it should be carefully balanced against such risks. It is useful in treating histoplasmosis and a range of other serious fungal infections. It is better for long-term treatment. In acute infections it is less useful because its absorption from the intestine is erratic and it is slow to work. It may antagonize the effects of amphotericin. Ketoconazole affects the metabolism of several other drugs and may also affect the body's manufacture of steroids.

Miconazole is used in local applications, by mouth and by intravenous infusion. Because of its harmful effects (see later) the intravenous use of miconazole should be strictly limited to the treatment of severe, generalized fungal infections that have not responded to other treatments. An important use of meconazole is in local applications for the treatment of vaginal thrush and ringworm and other infections of the skin.

Natamycin is an anti-fungal antibiotic used in local applications to treat yeast infections (e.g. thrush) of the genitals, anus, skin, nails and mouth. It is also used in an inhalation for treating fungal and yeast infections of the lungs.

Nystatin is an antibiotic with a structure similar to amphotericin. It both kills fungi (fungicidal) and prevents their multiplying (fungistatic). It is available in ointments, creams, mouth-washes, tablets, pastilles and suspensions. It is too toxic to be given by intravenous injection but it is safe by mouth for treating fungal infections of the intestine because it is not absorbed into the bloodstream and is passed out in the motions. It is active against a number of yeasts and fungi but its main use is in treating yeast infections, particularly thrush of the mouth, skin, genitals and anus and of the oesophagus, stomach and intestine.

There is no evidence that nystatin combined with an antibiotic (e.g. tetracycline) reduces the incidence of thrush of the mouth caused by antibiotics in patients who are prone to develop thrush because of their general condition (see earlier).

Tioconazole (Trosyl nail solution) is used to treat fungal infections of the nails. It may cause local irritation and rarely an allergic reaction.

Drug treatment of fungal infections of the skin

A goup of fungi called dermatophytes can infect the skin and scalp, producing 'ringworm'. They can also infect the hair and nails, and also the groin (dhobie's itch) and feet (athlete's foot). Favus is a fungus infection of the scalp which produces a white smelly growth.

Anti-fungal drug treatment of skin infections should be carried out only after the tissue has been scraped and the scraping examined under the microscope to confirm the diagnosis of a fungus infection. Most ringworm infections of the skin can be treated successfully with anti-fungal drugs applied locally (e.g. miconazole or a related drug). Other preparations are less effective in treating these disorders.

If the fungal skin infection is widespread or resistant to topical treatment, griseofulvin is given by mouth. This drug concentrates in keratin, which is a protein in the surface layer of the skin, and forms a major component of hair and nails (see earlier). Griseofulvin by mouth is the anti-fungal treatment of choice for fungal infections of the hair and nails. (U)

Yeast infections of the skin may also occur. A common yeast infection is caused by *Candida*, which produces thrush (candidiasis or moniliasis). It may affect the skin, nails, mouth, anus and vagina, and infect nappy rash in babies. Thrush affecting the mouth, genitals and anus may follow treatment with antibiotics and/or may be a sign that the individual has diabetes. Anyone who develops thrush should have the urine tested for sugar. Thrush may be transmitted by skin contact and by sexual intercourse. Severe and extensive thrush may develop in patients who have an immune deficiency (e.g. AIDS).

Thrush infections of the skin are treated effectively by local applications of nystatin, amphotericin or miconazole or a related drug.

Genital thrush

Yeast infections (e.g. thrush) can affect the vagina, producing vaginitis, and the vulva, producing vulvitis. Usually they are infected together so the disease is called vulvo-vaginitis. It produces soreness, itching and a whitish discharge. On the tip of the penis it may produce redness and soreness (balanitis) and it may infect the anus. Direct sexual contact can spread the disease. Vaginal thrush may occur in pregnancy, in women taking the pill and in women who have taken a course of antibiotics. Genital thrush may occur in people suffering from diabetes.

The treatment of vaginal thrush involves the use of an anti-fungal cream and/or pessaries which must be applied well up the vagina. Vulvitis is treated with anti-fungal creams. Vaginal thrush easily recurs if it is not treated properly, and doctors may miss diagnosing it in patients with diabetes, in pregnant women, in women taking the pill and in those who have been or are on antibiotics. Thrush producing inflammation of the end of the penis (balanitis) is treated with local applications of clotrimazole, an anti-fungal drug.

Genital thrush may come from a sexual partner, who should be treated at the same time, or from a focus of infection around the anus, around the nails or in the navel. These areas should be treated with local applications of an anti-fungal drug at the same time if the infection recurs. Also, it always makes good sense to check for diabetes by having your urine tested for sugar.

If vaginal thrush is really resistant to treatment, local treatment should be continued at the same time as anti-fungal treatment by mouth. Some local abnormality in the vaginal wall may predispose to recurrent thrush and other infections, as may any change in the balance of bacteria that normally live there. This may be caused by taking antibiotics by mouth for some other disorder (e.g. tonsillitis). The balance may also be disturbed by certain chemical disorders of the vaginal wall; for example, if there is an increase in the amount of sugar in the cells as in diabetes (see earlier) or if the cells lose their acidity. In the latter case, preparations such as Aci-gel (acetic acid) may help to restore the normal vaginal acidity and prevent recurrence of the infection.

Anal thrush should be treated with local applications of an anti-fungal drug, and if appropriate the sexual partner should also be treated.

General fungal infections of the body (systemic infections)

Histoplasmosis is an example of a general fungal infection; it affects humans in its yeast state but infects soil as a fungus at other times, where its spores can lie dormant for years. It should always be suspected in any obscure infection of the lungs associated with enlarged lymph glands with or without enlargement of the liver and/or spleen. Infection is caused by inhaling the spores in infected dust. The disease attacks dogs, rats, mice and humans. The fungus grows within soil that is covered in chicken, bat or pigeon droppings. Birds carry the yeast on their feathers and bats in their bowels. People can get 'cave disease' from exploring bat-infested caves. Amphotericin is used to treat severe infections.

Lung diseases caused by fungi

Aspergillosis is a common fungal infection of the lungs. The spores are inhaled into the lungs, where they lodge and then germinate. The infection may just remain local in a small patch, but in someone who has immune deficiency (e.g. AIDS) it may spread throughout the lungs and cause serious problems. Thrush and other fungal infections may also produce serious lung disorders in these patients.

The treatment of fungal infections of the lungs is difficult and not always successful. Drugs used include amphotericin, nystatin, natamycin, flucytosine and miconazole or a related drug. The dose and the way the drug is given (e.g. by mouth or injection) will depend upon the disorder being treated and the general condition of the individual.

Table 56.1 Anti-fungal drugs – harmful effects and warnings

amphotericin
Harmful effects When given by mouth there is negligible absorption into the blood stream and harmful effects do not occur at recommended doses. Prolonged treatment with high doses may occasionally cause stomach upsets. *When given by intravenous infusion* harmful effects are fairly common at recommended doses and some may be serious; they include chills, fever, headache, loss of appetite, nausea, vomiting, anaemia, low blood potassium, kidney damage, kidney stones, noises in the ears (tinnitus), malaise, diarrhoea, muscle pains, pain and thrombophlebitis at injection sites and, rarely, disorders of heart rhythm, high or low blood pressure, bleeding gastroenteritis, blood disorders, hearing loss, blurred vision, convulsions, nerve damage, itching, flushing, liver damage and allergic reactions. *Topical applications* may produce itching, irritation and skin rash.

Warnings Amphotericin must not be used in people who are allergic to it. Amphotericin infusions should be given only under strict hospital supervision. Risks of intravenous therapy must be balanced against benefits in potentially fatal fungal infections. Tests of liver and kidney function should be carried out before and at regular intervals during treatment. Blood counts and tests of the chemistry of the blood (e.g. potassium) should be carried out at weekly intervals. Other drugs should be used with great caution. Harmful effects may be reduced by giving aspirin, an antihistamine or an anti-vomiting drug. A small dose of corticosteroid intravenously may reduce fever, and an injection of heparin may reduce the risk of thrombophlebitis at the injection site. The site of injection should be changed frequently.

fluconazole*
Harmful effects include nausea, allergic reactions, headache and stomach upsets.

Warnings Fluconazole must not be used in people who are allergic to it or related drugs. It should be used with caution in individuals with impaired kidney function. Do not continue treatment for more than 14 days except in immune deficiency disorders.

flucytosine
Harmful effects At the recommended dose, harmful effects are infrequent, and usually mild and transient. They include nausea, vomiting, diarrhoea and skin rashes. Very rarely, blood disorders may occur.

Warnings Flucytosine should be used with caution in people suffering from impaired kidney or liver function, anaemia or other blood disorders. Blood counts and tests of kidney and liver function should be carried out before treatment starts and at frequent intervals during treatment. It should be used with extreme caution in anyone with a low blood potassium level; blood potassium levels should be measured before treatment. The level of the drug in the blood should be monitored regularly in individuals with impaired kidney function.

griseofulvin
Harmful effects Transient drowsiness, headache, nausea, vomiting, diarrhoea and stomach pains may occur. High doses and/or prolonged treatment may, very occasionally, cause skin rashes, sensitivity of the skin to sunlight, allergic reactions, systemic lupus erythematosus, thrush of the mouth, fatigue, mental confusion, insomnia, numbness and pins and needles in the hands and feet. Very rarely, it may cause kidney and liver damage, disturbed menstrual periods and bleeding from the stomach and/or intestine.

Warnings Griseofulvin must not be used in people who suffer from liver failure or porphyria, nor to prevent fungal infections. Regular tests of kidney and liver function and blood counts should be carried out in patients on prolonged treatment. There is a possibility that an individual allergic to penicillins may also be allergic to griseofulvin. Avoid exposure to intensive natural or artificial sunlight.

Table 56.1 Anti-fungal drugs – harmful effects and warnings (*cont.*)

Risks in elderly people Harmful effects may be more frequent and severe; therefore use with caution.

itraconazole*
Harmful effects include nausea, abdominal pain, indigestion and headache.

Warnings When appropriate, women of child-bearing age should avoid intercourse or use a contraceptive during treatment and for 1 month after treatment has stopped. It should be used with caution in patients with impaired liver function, and should not be used in pregnancy or when breast feeding.

ketoconazole*
Harmful effects The most commonly occurring harmful effects are nausea, vomiting, abdominal pain, itching and headache. Rarely, a reduced platelet count (thrombocytotopenia), changes in liver function tests and liver damage (hepatitis) may occur. A severe allergic reaction (anaphylaxis) may, rarely, follow the first dose. Other allergic reactions include nettle rash and angioedema. Very rarely, it may cause the breasts to enlarge.

Warnings Ketoconazole must not be used in anyone who is allergic to it or to a related drug or who has impaired liver function. The risk of developing liver damage (hepatitis) is greater in individuals on long-term treatment (more than 14 days), therefore tests of their liver function should be carried out before treatment, after the first 10 days and twice monthly during treatment.

miconazole*
Harmful effects By mouth it may cause mild stomach upsets. *Intravenous infusion* may cause nausea, vomiting, diarrhoea, loss of appetite, fever, flushing, drowsiness and a transient fall in blood sodium. Thrombocytopenia (reduced blood platelets) may occur very rarely. Itching, skin rashes, pain and thrombophlebitis at injection sites may occur occasionally. Rapid injection may cause rapid heart beat. *When used on the skin* it may cause irritation and allergy.

Warnings Miconazole should not be used in people who are allergic to it. When administered by intravenous infusion, it should be given slowly over 30 minutes, especially in individuals with heart or circulatory disorders. Frequent blood counts should be carried out during treatment, and the site of injection should be changed frequently in order to reduce risk of developing thrombophlebitis.

Risks in elderly people Harmful effects of intravenous use may be more frequent and severe; therefore use with caution.

natamycin
Harmful effects include mild irritation when applied to the skin or to the lining of the vagina.

nystatin
Harmful effects When used in high doses by mouth it may, rarely, cause nausea, vomiting and diarrhoea.

Warning Nystatin should not be used in people who are allergic to any one of the components in nystatin preparations.

tioconazole*
Harmful effects Application may cause mild irritation and rarely an allergic reaction.

Warning It should not be used in pregnancy or when breast feeding.

* *Warning* Cross-allergy may occur to these drugs.

Table 56.2 Anti-fungal preparations

Preparation	*Drug*	*Dosage form*
Alcoban	flucytosine	Tablets
Daktarin	miconazole	Tablets, oral gel, injection
Diflucan	fluconazole	Capsules, intravenous infusion
Fulcin	griseofulvin	Tablets, suspension
Fungilin	amphotericin	Tablets, suspension, lozenges
Fungizone	amphotericin	Intravenous infusion; powder in vial
griseofulvin	griseofulvin	Tablets
Grisovin	griseofulvin	Tablets
Nizoral	ketoconazole	Tablets, suspension
Nystan	nystatin	Tablets, pastilles, oral suspension granules (sugar-, lactose- and corn-starch free powder for suspension)
nystatin	nystatin	Mixture
Pimafucin	natamycin	Cream, vaginal tablets, suspension for inhalation
Sporanox	itraconazole	Capsules containing coated pellets

57

Viral infections

Fortunately most of us recover from most viral infections, but some can be very serious and even fatal, particularly in individuals who are immune deficient because of drug treatments or because of diseases such as AIDS.

Anti-viral drugs

There are a number of anti-viral drugs available that are of benefit in treating various virus infections, but their benefits and risks have to be balanced in each individual being treated. Anti-viral drugs include the following.

Acyclovir is used to treat herpes simplex infections of the skin, lips and mouth, genital herpes and herpes zoster (shingles). It may be taken by mouth (Zovirax tablets and suspension), applied locally (Zovirax cream) or given by intravenous infusion (Zovirax infusion). It is also available as Zovirax eye ointment.

Amantadine is used to treat and prevent influenza in individuals at risk of complications; for example, elderly people with serious chest or heart disorders. It is taken by mouth (Symmetrel capsules and syrup). Its benefits in treating herpes infections have not been demonstrated convincingly.

Foscarnet is used to treat cytomegalovirus (CMV) infections of the eyes in patients with AIDS in whom ganciclovir should not be used. It is given by intravenous infusion (Foscavir infusion).

Ganciclovir is used to treat life- or sight-threatening CMV infections in immune deficient patients (e.g. patients with AIDS). It is given by injection (Cymevene powder in vial).

Idoxuridine is a topical anti-viral drug. It is too toxic to take by mouth or injection. It may be used to treat cold sores (herpes simplex), herpes simplex of the genitals and shingles (herpes zoster). Local applications include Herpid solution, Iduridin solution and Virudox solution. Idoxuridine is included in Idoxene eye ointment and Kerecid eye drops to treat herpes simplex infections of the eyes.

Inosine pranobex may be used to treat herpes simplex infections of the skin and lips, although its benefits have not been demonstrated convincingly. It is taken by mouth (Imunovir tablets).

Tribavirin is used to treat severe virus infections of the lungs (respiratory syncytial virus (RSV) bronchiolitis). It is given by nebulization (Virazid powder for nebulization).

Vidarabine is used to treat chickenpox and shingles (herpes zoster) in individuals who are immune deficient (e.g. due to AIDS).

Zidovudine (Retrovir) is used to treat AIDS and AIDS-related complex. It is taken by mouth (Retrovir capsules).

The use of anti-viral drugs

Herpes simplex infections

Most people infected for the first time with a herpes simplex virus develop only a mild flu-like illness. However, in patients with immune deficiency whose defence system against infection is not functioning effectively, because of drug treatment for some other disorder (e.g. anti-cancer drugs) or because of an illness that affects the immune system (e.g. AIDS), herpes infections can be serious and life threatening.

There are two strains of herpes – types 1 and 2. The type 1 virus causes non-genital infections (e.g. cold sores; see later). Type 2 affects mainly the genitals, and infection is transmitted by sexual intercourse.

In addition to a mild flu-like illness, the very first infection (primary infection) with herpes simplex (type 1) may cause ulcers on the gums and mouth (commonest in infants), inflammation and ulcers on the throat and ulcers in the eyes. Type 2 causes ulcers and sores on the genitals and/or the anus.

A primary infection may also affect the skin (e.g. of the fingers) and, rarely, can produce inflammation of the brain (encephalitis). A newborn baby may develop a general herpes infection picked up from its mother during childbirth if she suffers from genital herpes; because a newborn baby's immune system is not fully developed, the infection may be very serious and life threatening.

Warnings *Genital herpes in a mother is an indication for a caesarian delivery in order to ensure that the baby does not come into direct contact with the herpes ulcers on her genitals.*

A serious problem with herpes simplex infections is that they keep recurring, often over many years. These recurrent infections occur because, in between attacks, the viruses lie dormant in the roots of the nerves that supply the infected part of the skin and re-infection may occur because something irritates the skin in that area. For example, a common site for re-infection is the lips (cold sores) and exposure to strong sunlight, another infection (e.g. a cold), general debility, or a menstrual period may trigger another cold sore. The genitals are also a common site for recurrent herpes infections.

Anti-viral drug treatment of herpes simplex infections

Anti-viral drugs help to reduce spreading of the viruses from herpes ulcers and help healing. They also give some relief from pain and soreness.

Herpes of the lips (cold sores) and the skin may benefit from acyclovir by mouth or from the application of idoxuridine solution. Acyclovir by mouth may also be used over the long term to help prevent herpes simplex in an individual who is immune deficient (e.g. suffering from AIDS).

Herpes ulcers of the eyes respond to preparations of acyclovir, idoxuridine or vidarabine applied locally.

Herpes of the mouth may benefit from local treatment with a tetracycline mouth-wash and acyclovir or inosine pranobex by mouth if the ulcers are persistent.

Inflammation of the brain (herpes encephalitis) is serious; 80 per cent of infected patients die. Acyclovir or ganciclovir by infusion into a vein may be of benefit.

Genital herpes An attack of genital herpes may benefit from treatment with acyclovir applied locally and also given by mouth or injection. Acyclovir may also be taken by mouth to suppress genital herpes over the long term, especially in immune deficiency disease (e.g. AIDS). Subsequent attacks do not respond to acyclovir as well as the first attack. Inosine pranobex by mouth may also be used to treat an initial attack of genital herpes.

Herpes infection of the newborn is dangerous and may be fatal. Acyclovir or vidarabine should be given by infusion into a vein. This may be of benefit but the death rate is high.

Chickenpox and shingles

Chickenpox (varicella) and shingles (herpes zoster) are caused by the same virus (varicella-zoster virus), which spreads by droplets from the nose and mouth and from contact with the sores.

Chickenpox is highly infectious and mainly affects children under the age of 10 years. Second attacks are very rare. In patients with immune deficiency whose resistance to infection is impaired by drug treatment or disease (e.g. AIDS), chickenpox can be very serious and even fatal.

Shingles is caused by an invasion of the roots of nerves by the virus. It causes pain, blisters and sores in the area of skin supplied by the nerve. An attack of shingles results from a reactivation of the chickenpox/shingles virus that has lain dormant for months or years. The frequency and severity of shingles increases with age. It can be very severe in people with immune deficiency whose resistance to infection is impaired by drug treatment or disease (e.g. AIDS).

Treatment of chickenpox

In chickenpox no drug treatment is necessary in the majority of individuals. If the spots become infected, an antiseptic ointment may be used. Children with immune deficiency whose resistance to infection is impaired because of drugs or disease (e.g. anti-cancer drugs or AIDS) should be given human immunoglobulin (see Chapter 11). Acyclovir or vidarabine by injection may reduce the development of complications in these children.

In some countries a vaccine against chickenpox is undergoing trials in children with immune deficiency. However, because it involves the use of a live virus that has been weakened (attenuated), there is always the risk that the virus may enter nerve cells and lie dormant for years, to produce an infection at some later date. This risk must clearly be balanced against the benefits of using the vaccine in children with an immune deficiency in whom chickenpox may be a very serious illness. Because chickenpox is usualy a mild disease the general use of a vaccine is not indicated.

Treatment of shingles

There is no specific treatment for the rash of shingles but calamine lotion may soothe it. The pain may be relieved by a mild pain reliever such as paracetamol, but sometimes it can be very severe and persistent and needs a stronger pain reliever. The use of a corticosteroid (e.g. prednisolone) by mouth to relieve the pain has now gone out of fashion. A tricyclic anti-depressant (e.g. amitriptyline) may occasionally relieve the pain. Idoxuri-dine applied to the rash may possibly help and acyclovir by mouth may reduce the duration of the pain and the risk of continuing pain in the nerve after the rash has cleared up (post-herpetic neuralgia).

Shingles may be very severe in people with an immune deficiency because of drug treatment or disease (e.g. anti-cancer drugs or AIDS). In these individuals it is worth trying acyclovir by mouth or intravenous infusion or vidarabine by intravenous infusion.

Shingles affecting the eye

When shingles affects the nerve that supplies the surface of the eye, it may cause ulcers on the cornea. These produce scarring, blurring of vision and other problems if they are not treated. They should always be treated urgently by an eye specialist. Anti-viral preparations used to treat shingles affecting the eye include idoxuridine eye drops and vidarabine ointment.

Influenza

Influenza is caused by three types of viruses – A, B and C. Influenza A usually causes a worldwide spread of the disease (a pandemic). When it spreads rapidly through a particular community, it is called an epidemic. The B virus is associated with smaller outbreaks at local level (endemic). Influenza C is rare. The time from catching the infection to getting the first symptoms (the incubation period) is 24–48 hours. The illness causes headaches, aches and pains and fever, and there may be a cough. Recovery takes place over about 5 days. Sometimes a secondary bacterial infection may develop and produce complications (e.g. bronchitis). In general, there is no specific treatment for influenza apart from rest, fluids and mild pain relievers (see Chapter 3 for treatment of the common cold).

The anti-viral drug amantadine has been shown to be effective in preventing an attack of influenza A in people who have been in contact with infected persons. In an influenza A epidemic, amantadine may be of use in treating people who run the risk of developing serious complications; for example, patients with severe heart and lung disease, the elderly and patients debilitated by illness. When used to prevent an attack of influenza, it should be continued for as long as the epidemic lasts – which is usually about 6–8 weeks. Because amantadine does not interfere with the body's defence response to the influenza A virus, it may be given with an anti-influenza A vaccine, when it should be continued for 2 weeks after the injection.

The use of amantadine in preventing attacks of influenza A in vulnerable people has not caught on; perhaps there is some confusion because it is also used to treat parkinsonism. The latter use was discovered accidentally while testing the drug to prevent influenza infections.

The use of amantadine in people who have developed influenza A is a subject of controversy. Some claim that if it is given within the first 48 hours of an attack it may be of benefit, but convincing evidence to support such an observation is not available.

Influenza vaccines

Resistance to influenza (immunity) is absolutely specific for a particular influenza virus; therefore, if a new strain (from an epidemic or pandemic) can be identified, specific vaccines can be prepared that will give about 75 per cent protection against the infection. Obviously, they can be prepared only when a pandemic or epidemic has developed and the virus identified. (See also the discussion on the use of vaccines in Chapter 11.)

Table 57.1 Anti-viral drugs – harmful effects and warnings

acyclovir
Harmful effects from short-term use by mouth or intravenous infusion include nausea, vomiting, headache, diarrhoea, loss of appetite, fatigue, swelling of ankles, skin rash, leg pains, taste of medicine in mouth and sore throat. *Long-term use* may cause diarrhoea, nausea, vomiting, vertigo, painful joints, headache, numbness and pins and needles in hands and feet, skin rashes, fever, insomnia, fatigue, changes in liver or kidney function tests, palpitations, sore throat, muscle cramps, irregular menstrual periods, acne, irritability, hair loss and depression.

Warnings These preparations of acyclovir should not be used in people who are allergic to it. Drink plenty of fluids. The dose should be reduced in anyone suffering from impaired kidney function.

Risks in elderly people Harmful effects may be more frequent and severe; therefore use with caution, and in reduced doses.

Topical applications (e.g. creams)
Harmful effects These may produce transient burning or stinging of the skin and, occasionally, redness and dryness of the skin.

Warnings Topical applications should not be used in the eyes, mouth or vagina, and not at all in anyone known to be allergic to it.

Harmful effects from eye ointments include transient mild stinging, soreness of the eyelids (blepharitis) and superficial damage to the cornea (superficial punctate keratopathy).

Warning It must not be used in people known to be allergic to acyclovir.

amantadine
Harmful effects when taken by mouth include nervousness, inability to concentrate, insomnia, dizziness, stomach upsets, dry mouth, ankle swelling and, rarely, blood disorders, discoloration of the skin, convulsions, hallucinations and feelings of detachment.

Warnings Amantadine must not be used in people who suffer from epilepsy, peptic ulcers or severe impairment of kidney function. It should be used with caution in anyone with heart disease, raised blood pressure, kidney disease, recurrent eczema,

Table 57.1 Anti-viral drugs – harmful effects and warnings (*cont.*)

liver disease or serious mental illness (psychoses).

Risks in elderly people Harmful effects may be more frequent and severe; therefore use with caution.

foscarnet
Harmful effects include headache, nausea, vomiting, fatigue and skin rashes. It may cause a drop in blood calcium levels sufficient to produce symptoms, a drop in blood sugar levels, impaired kidney function and epileptic seizures. Undiluted solutions may cause thrombophlebitis at the site of injection.

Warnings Foscarnet should not be used during pregnancy or in breast-feeding mothers. It should be used with caution in individuals with impaired kidney function and low blood calcium levels prior to treatment. Blood calcium levels and kidney function tests must be carried out every other day during treatment. The individual on treatment must drink plenty of fluids.

ganciclovir
Harmful effects when given by intravenous infusion include fever, blood disorders, impaired liver and kidney function, sore throat, nose bleeds, swelling of the face, stomach and bowel upsets and skin rashes. It may cause pain and damage to the tissues at the site of injection.

Warnings Ganciclovir should not be used in pregnancy, and women of child-bearing potential should avoid sexual intercourse or practise contraception during treatment. Men should avoid sexual intercourse or use a condom during and for 90 days after treatment. Mothers should not breast feed during treatment or for 72 hours after treatment has stopped. It should not be used in patients who are allergic to it or to acyclovir, or who have a very low white blood count. Blood tests should be carried out before treatment and every 1–2 days during the first 14 days of treatment. It should be used with caution in patients with impaired kidney function or who are receiving radiation treatment and/or drugs that may damage the bone marrow. Patients should take plenty of fluids during treatment.

idoxuridine
Harmful effects It may sting when applied to the skin, cause changes in taste, and overdose may maserate the skin.

Warnings Skin solutions should not be used in people who are allergic to idoxuridine or dimethylsulphoxide (present in Herpid or Virudox preparations). Avoid contact with eyes, do not use in the mouth or vagina and avoid contact with clothes. Eye applications may cause local pain, irritation and swelling in the eye.

Warnings They should be used with caution in pregnancy.

inosine pranobex
Harmful effects when taken by mouth include an increase in the level of uric acid in the blood and urine.

Warnings It should not be used in patients who suffer from gout, raised blood uric acid levels or impaired kidney function.

tribavirin
Harmful effects of powder nebulization include worsening of chest condition, bacterial pneumonia, and an increase in red blood cells.

Warnings Tribavirin should not be used in women who are pregnant or who are of child-bearing potential.

vidarabine
Harmful effects of injections include loss of appetite, nausea, vomiting, diarrhoea, tremor and, occasionally, dizziness, hallucinations, confusion, serious mental symptoms, incoordination of movements, weight loss, malaise, itching skin rashes and decreased white and red blood cell counts. It may cause pain at the site of injection.

Warnings The treatment must be stopped if the patient becomes intolerant to the drug. It should be used with

Table 57.1 Anti-viral drugs – harmful effects and warnings (*cont.*)

caution in anyone with impaired kidney function (the dosages must be reduced). Regular tests of the blood should be carried out during treatment in order to check whether there is any reduction in the number of white and/or red blood cells and platelets.

Harmful effects of eye applications include watering of the eyes, redness of the eyes, pain, discomfort on looking into the light, burning sensation, irritation, allergy and, rarely, damage to the cornea.

Warning It should not be used in patients who become intolerant to it – if there is no response after 7 days of treatment, the drug should be stopped.

zidovudine

Harmful effects It may occasionally damage the bone marrow – knocking out red cell production, causing anaemia, and white cell production, increasing the risk of infections. Rarely, the anaemia may be so severe as to require a blood transfusion. The anaemia develops in about 2–4 weeks, and the reduced white cell count in about 4–6 weeks. Blood counts should be carried out every 2 weeks for the first 3 months of treatment and then every month after that. When treatment is stopped the bone marrow recovers rapidly and another course of treatment can be started in about 2 weeks. Only a very few patients have had to come off the drug because of harmful effects. Other harmful effects include nausea, headache, abdominal pain, fever, painful muscles, numbness and pins and needles in the arms and legs, vomiting, insomnia and loss of appetite.

Warnings Zidovudine must not be used in patients known to be allergic to it or who have a low white cell count or a low red cell count. It should be used with caution in anyone with impaired kidney or liver function. It should not be used in breast-feeding mothers.

Risks in elderly people Harmful effects may be more frequent and severe; therefore use with caution.

Risks with other drugs Regular, daily use of paracetamol may increase the damaging effect of zidovudine on the bone marrow. Any drug that impairs the function of the liver, kidneys or bone marrow may increase the risks of using zidovudine (see Chapter 89).

58

Malaria

Human malaria results from infection by a parasite, a single-cell protozoa called *Plasmodium*. There are four common species of plasmodium – *P. falciparum*, *P. malariae*, *P. ovale* and *P. vivax*. Malaria is prevalent throughout most of the tropical and sub-tropical countries of the world below an altitude of about 1500 metres, excluding the Mediterranean countries, the USA and Australia. Millions of people are attacked and many people, particularly children, die each year from malaria.

Malaria is transmitted from an infected human to an uninfected human by infected female mosquitoes that feed on human blood. It may also be transmitted by the transfusion or inoculation of infected blood, and, very rarely, it may pass from an infected pregnant mother into her unborn baby.

The female mosquito picks up the infection by drinking blood from an infected person which contains sexual forms of parasite (gametocytes). These mature and the females are fertilized in the mosquito's stomach. The products of this bisexual fertilization then make their way into the salivary glands of the mosquito, where they multiply. When the mosquito 'bites' a person, these developing 'spores' are transferred into the blood stream of the person who has been 'bitten'. They are carried to the liver where they multiply asexually and grow. After a period of 5–16 days (but sometimes after months or years), hundreds of new parasites are released from the liver into the blood stream where they enter red blood cells and start to multiply and so the cycle keeps repeating itself.

Some of the parasites released from the red blood cells develop sexual forms, both male and female, and these circulate in the blood stream. When a mosquito bites that person, the blood containing these sexual forms enters the mosquito's stomach where they mature and the females are fertilized, and so the whole cycle starts over again.

Symptoms

After infection from a mosquito bite, the individual feels no symptoms while the parasites are multiplying in the liver. However, as they enter and are then released from the red blood cells (the so-called 'blood stage') the patient develops severe shivering, fever, headache and nausea. In *P. ovale* and *P. vivax* infections each cycle in the red blood cells takes 48 hours and the fever recurs every 48 hours. This is called benign tertian malaria. With *P. falciparum*, the cycle is less than 48 hours and the fever and symptoms are more or less continuous; it is the most dangerous type, which is why it is called malignant tertian malaria. With *P. malariae* infections the fever recurs every 72 hours and is called benign quartian malaria. Between the fevers, the patient often feels well except for weakness.

The parasites *P. ovale* and *P. vivax* may lie dormant in liver cells for months and even years and then suddenly flare up. This is why the first attack of malaria with these infections may occur long after the individual has returned from the infected area. It also explains why people infected with these parasites may relapse after treatment of the 'blood stage' of the infection. *P. falciparum* and *P. malariae* do not lie dormant in the liver; however, a flare-up of symptoms may develop if the parasites have not been completely cleared from the red blood cells by treatment or if the body's immune response is deficient.

Complications

Because the parasites damage red blood cells, malaria may cause anaemia. Young red blood cells are particularly affected, and red blood cells that are not infected may be damaged by the body's own defence system which may not easily differentiate between infected and non-infected red blood cells. The destruction of the red blood cells (haemolytic anaemia) causes the spleen to enlarge because it acts as a graveyard of dead red cells. This increased activity can also lead to an early death for some non-infected red cells.

In *P. falciparum* malaria the infected red cells may stick in small blood vessels and block the flow of blood, producing ischaemia – a lack of oxygen supply to the affected organ. This may happen, for example, in the brain, kidneys, liver and intestine. The rupture of these red blood cells and the release of more parasites in the already congested organs may lead to more damage. These complications may cause fever and unconsciousness (cerebral malaria), kidney failure, liver failure and severe vomiting and diarrhoea respectively.

Blackwater fever is fever associated with the passing of dark red, almost black, urine. The dark red, black colour of the urine is caused by the presence of a red pigment (haemoglobin) which has been released into the blood stream from bursting red blood cells. It occurs most often with the dangerous *P. falciparum* infections and in patients who have been forgetful about their drug treatment. It also occurs in people who have a genetic weakness in the functioning of their red blood cells (a deficiency of glucose-6-phosphate dehydrogenase). An attack of haemolysis may be triggered by taking quinine or by fatigue.

Treatment of an acute attack of malaria

Benign malaria

Chloroquine by mouth is the treatment of choice for an acute attack (blood stage) of benign tertian malaria caused by *P. ovale* and *P. vivax* and benign quartian malaria caused by *P. malariae*. Amodiaquine may also be used.

Radical cure of benign malaria caused by P. ovale *and* P. vivax

A radical cure in *P. ovale* and *P. vivax* infections aims at killing the parasites in the liver and preventing a relapse. Following treatment with chloroquine for the blood stage, primaquine is used to achieve a radical cure – but only when the individual has left the area and is free from the risk of re-infection. The patient must be under medical supervision because of the risk of haemolytic anaemia due to primaquine in patients who have a genetic defect in their red cell function, called glucose-6-phosphate dehydrogenase deficiency. This must be tested for in all patients *before* treatment is started; if it is present, a smaller daily dose of primaquine should be used over a longer period of time.

Malignant tertian malaria (falciparum malaria)

Malignant tertian malaria, caused by *P. falciparum* infection, is dangerous and requires early diagnosis and early treatment. The drug of choice is chloroquine but drug treatment has been made more difficult because of the emergence of chloroquine-resistant parasites. Therefore, treatment will depend upon whether or not the infection was caught in an area of the world where chloroquine-resistant parasites are known to be present. However, because treatment may fail with any of the anti-malarial drugs due to the development of resistant parasites, it is important that blood tests are carried out every 12 hours in order to measure the degree of infection and its response to treatment.

If the parasites are sensitive to chloroquine, patients should be given a course by mouth or, if seriously ill, by continuous intravenous infusion, changing later to chloroquine by mouth. An intravenous infusion of quinine and tetracycline by mouth should be given if there is any doubt about the sensitivity of the parasite to chloroquine or if the individual has been taking chloroquine for prevention and still suffers an acute attack of malaria (what is referred to as breakthrough attacks). If the strains are resistant to chloroquine, an alternative is to give a course of quinine by mouth (or, if seriously ill, by intravenous infusion) plus a single high dose of Fansidar by mouth. If the parasites are also resistant to Fansidar, a course of tetracycline or mefloquine should be given with the quinine. Sensitivity of the parasites to the drug should be checked and daily counts of the numbers of parasites in the blood should be carried out. If these remain high and complications develop, consideration should be given to an exchange transfusion – drawing the blood from a vein on one arm and giving fresh blood into a vein in the other arm.

Preventing malaria

The aim of prevention is to use drugs to attack the parasites during the blood stage; this will keep the individual free from fever and chills. The choice of drug depends upon the extent and type of malaria, the risk of exposure and a balance of the expected benefits and risks of the drug to be used in a particular individual. This approach may be called suppression, suppressive prophylaxis, prophylaxis or chemoprophylaxis.

Preventive treatment does not stop an individual from getting infected and therefore other sensible precautions should be taken (see later). Anti-malarial drugs should be taken 1 week before exposure, during the period of exposure and for at least 4 weeks afterwards. The drugs most commonly used are chloroquine or proguanil but up-to-the-minute advice should always be obtained from a specialist medical adviser.

Preventive treatment suppresses symptoms but does not necessarily eradicate the infection. It is important to note that chloroquine eliminates only the first (primary) attack of fever in patients suffering from *P. vivax* or *P. ovale* malaria but has no effect on future relapses that may occur months and years later. This is because it does not kill the parasites when they are in the liver. Therefore, fever occurring during or after a visit to an infected area may still be malaria despite the fact that the individual took anti-malarial drugs.

The prophylaxis of malaria is complicated because of parasites that are resistant to chloroquine and other anti-malarial drugs and because of rare but serious harmful effects from Fansidar (pyrimethamine plus sulfadoxine), Maloprim (pyrimethamine and dapsone) and amodiaquine. In addition, some countries now have low risks of malaria and some have high risks. Prophylaxis will also depend upon whether an individual is visiting an area of risk for a short or a long time.

No single drug or combination of drugs can provide absolute protection against malaria. Drugs most commonly used include chloroquine, mefloquine, proguanil and Maloprim. Because of the risks of harmful effects, Fansidar and amodiaquine should no longer be used.

Because they have no liver stage, *P. falciparum* and *P. malariae* respond well to preventative treatment but infection with chloroquine-resistant *P. falciparum* parasites in various parts of the world makes blanket prevention with chloroquine not possible and advice should always be sought from specialist medical advisers.

Take sensible precautions

Because drug prevention is not totally safe against malaria, travellers should take common sense precautions against being bitten by mosquitoes – particularly at night. They should wear a hat, buttoned-up long-sleeved shirt or blouse and trousers, and avoid dark colours. In their bedroom they should use a mosquito net over their beds at night and make sure there are no holes in it and tuck it well under the mattress early in the evening. (Protection afforded by the net may be improved by impregnating with permethrin every 6 months.) They should use insecticidal sprays to kill any mosquitoes that enter the room during the day-time and apply a mosquito repellent such as diethyltoluamide if they go outside, particularly in the evenings. They should also use a vaporizing device in their bedrooms during the night.

People who visit a risk area should report immediately to a hospital if they develop a fever, whether or not they are taking preventative drug treatment. If they develop a fever within 12 months of returning from a risk area, they should report to a hospital to be checked for malaria. Individuals who develop a fever within 2 months of returning from a *P. falciparum* risk area should seek medical advice immediately because this can be a life-threatening disorder. If there is the slightest doubt, treatment with quinine should be started immediately (by mouth or intravenous infusion) and a tetracycline by mouth. Mefloquine or Fansidar by mouth are alternatives, according to results of tests of the sensitivity of the parasites to the drugs. Daily parasite counts should be made; if they are high and complications develop, an exchange blood transfusion may be necessary.

Preventing and treating malaria in pregnancy

If possible, pregnant women should not travel to high-risk zones.

Prevention

Chloroquine and proguanil may be used in anti-malarial doses during pregnancy, but up-to-date advice should always be sought from an expert medical adviser. Pregnant women taking proguanil should be given folic acid supplements.

Treatment

Acute malaria is dangerous in pregnancy and should be treated with drugs described earlier under 'Treatment of an acute attack of malaria'.

Table 58.1 Drugs used to treat malaria – harmful effects and warnings

amodiaquine
Harmful effects include nausea, vomiting, diarrhoea, insomnia, vertigo and lethargy. Prolonged use may cause deposits in the cornea of the eyes, bluish-grey pigmentation of the finger nails, skin and roof of the mouth. Rarely, liver damage and blood disorders may occur, and nerve damage, producing numbness and pins and needles in the arms and legs.

Warnings An eye examination should be carried out before treatment and at regular intervals during treatment (3–6 months) in any individual receiving treatment for a prolonged period of time (6 months or more). Amodiaquine should not be used in people with an eye disease or any visual defect or in anyone allergic to this group of drugs. It should be used with caution in patients with impaired kidney or liver function. Harmful effects are more likely to occur in alcoholics; therefore use with caution. Anyone on prolonged treatment should have regular complete medical examinations to test for any symptoms or signs of harmful effects, and regular blood counts should be carried out. It may cause a flare-up of symptoms in people suffering from psoriasis or porphyria.

Risks in elderly people Harmful effects may be more frequent and severe; therefore use with caution.

Risks with driving Damage caused by the drug to the eyes may make you unfit to drive.

chloroquine (Avloclor, Nivaquine)
Harmful effects include nausea, vomiting and headache. *Doses used to treat malaria are usually well tolerated, but the high doses used to treat rheumatoid arthritis may cause harmful effects, some of which are occasionally serious.* They include itching, skin rashes, severe mental symptoms, convulsions, fall in blood pressure, changes in electric tracings of the heart (ECG), double vision and difficulty in focusing. Prolonged use of high doses may cause deposits in the cornea of the eyes and damage to the retina. These changes may occur long after the drug has been stopped. Pigmented deposits and opacities in the cornea are often reversible if the drug is stopped at the earliest possible sign of any

Table 58.1 Drugs used to treat malaria – harmful effects and warnings (*cont.*)

eye trouble. However, damage to the retina at the back of the eye, which causes defective vision, loss of colour vision and blind spots, is often not reversible after the drug has been stopped. This damage to the retina appears to be due to the overall dose taken in a course of treatment. If this exceeds 100 g, damage occurs. Rare harmful effects include loss of hair, sensitivity of the skin to sunlight, skin rashes, noises in the ears (tinnitus), reduced hearing due to damage to the nerve supply to the ears, muscle weakness, bleaching of the hair, bluish-black pigmentation of the skin and lining of the mouth, and blood disorders.

Warnings An eye examination should be carried out before treatment and at regular intervals during treatment (3–6 months) in anyone receiving treatment for a prolonged period of time (6 months or more). Chloroquine should not be used by people with eye disease or any visual defect or who are allergic to this group of drugs. It should be used with caution in individuals with impaired kidney or liver function. Harmful effects are more likely to occur in alcoholics, therefore use with caution. Everyone on prolonged treatment should have regular complete medical examinations to test for any symptoms or signs of harmful effects, and regular blood counts should be carried out. The drug may cause a flare-up of symptoms in patients suffering from porphyria and a severe flare-up of psoriasis.

Risks in elderly people Harmful effects may be more frequent and severe; therefore use with caution.

Risks with driving Damage to the eyes caused by the drug may make you unfit to drive.

Fansidar
(Contains pyrimethamine (see below) and sulfadoxine, a sulphonamide)

Harmful effects include drug rashes (stop immediately), itching and slight hair loss. Rarely, it may cause allergic reactions, including Stevens–Johnson syndrome, headache, feelings of fullness, nausea, vomiting, sore mouth and fever, blood disorders and nerve damage.

Warnings Fansidar should not be used in people allergic to sulphonamides, neither should it be used in daily treatment (for prevention) in anyone with severe kidney or liver disease or blood disorders. Excessive exposure to the sun should be avoided. Regular blood counts should be carried out if treatment is prolonged (more than 6 months).

Maloprim
(Contains pyrimethamine (see below) and dapsone, a sulphone drug)

Harmful effects are rare; they include blood disorders, haemolysis and skin rashes. High doses (of dapsone) may cause muscle and joint pains, cough, nettle rash and swollen glands.

Warnings Maloprim should not be used in people allergic to sulphonamides, sulphones or pyrimethamine. It should be used with caution in anyone with severe impairment of kidney or liver function, and in individuals who may develop folic acid deficiency (e.g. pregnant women); the latter group should be given additional folic acid.

mefloquine
Harmful effects Occasionally, it may cause nausea, vomiting and diarrhoea, abdominal pain, headache and dizziness. Rarely, it may cause mood changes, rashes, itching and slowing of the heart rate, weakness and changes in test results of liver function.

Warnings Should not be used for prevention in individuals with impaired kidney or liver function, history of mental disorders or convulsions. May affect ability to drive or operate moving machinery.

primaquine
Harmful effects At recommended doses harmful effects are infrequent in lightly pigmented people. However, in darkly pigmented people it may damage red blood cells, producing haemolytic anaemia and also in patients with glucose-6-phosphate dehydrogenase deficiency. It

Table 58.1 Drugs used to treat malaria – harmful effects and warnings (*cont.*)

may damage haemoglobin in red blood cells, producing blueness, abdominal pains and weakness (methaemoglobinaemia).

Warnings Primaquine should be used with caution in non-caucasians because 5–10 per cent have a genetic abnormality that makes them liable to develop haemolytic anaemia and methaemoglobinaemia (glucose-6-phosphate dehydrogenase deficiency). A small test dose should be used to start treatment and then the daily dose slowly increased and repeated blood counts should be carried out to monitor for blood disorders.

Risks in elderly people As in adults, but monitor carefully.

proguanil (Paludrine)
Harmful effects include mild stomach upsets, skin rashes and hair loss.

Warning Proguanil should be used with caution in anyone with severe kidney failure.

Risks in elderly people As in adults, but monitor carefully.

pyrimethamine (Daraprim; in Fansidar and Maloprim)
Harmful effects Large doses and prolonged treatment may cause loss of appetite and vomiting, a sore tongue and blood disorders.

Warning Pyrimethamine should be used with caution in anyone with impaired liver or kidney function. It may cause folic acid deficiency, so additional folic acid should be given when the drug is used in high doses. Regular blood tests should be carried out in individuals on high doses.

quinine
Harmful effects Long-term daily use may cause cinchonism, which is characterized by blurred vision, nausea and tinnitus when mild but includes vertigo, fever, vomiting, abdominal pain, skin rash and itching when severe. In addition to cinchonism, quinine may cause severe allergic reactions in sensitive people; for example, allergic skin rashes, wheezing and angioedema. Very rarely, it may cause blood disorders and kidney damage.

Warnings Quinine should not be used in people who are allergic to it or who have tinnitus or a damaged nerve to the eyes (optic neuritis). It should be used with caution in anyone with myasthenia gravis – it may make the condition worse – or with heart disease or disorders of heart rhythm (atrial fibrillation). Individuals deficient in glucose-6-phosphate-dehydrogenase are at risk of developing haemolysis and blackwater fever (see earlier in this chapter).

Table 58.2 Drugs used to treat malaria

Preparation	*Drug*	*Dosage form*
Avloclor	chloroquine (as phosphate)	Tablets
Daraprim	pyrimethamine	Tablets
Fansidar	pyrimethamine and sulfadoxine	Tablets
Lariam	mefloquine	Tablets
Maloprim	pyrimethamine and dapsone	Tablets
Nivaquine	chloroquine (as sulphate)	Tablets, syrup, injection
Paludrine	proguanil	Tablets
primaquine	primaquine	Tablets
quinine	quinine	Tablets, injection

59

Some parasitic infections (including worms)

Amoebic dysentery

The amoeba that cause amoebic dysentery live in the intestine of humans and spread from human to human in the form of cysts in contaminated faeces, which infect drinking water and food. Lettuce is a common vehicle for infection. The time from contact to the appearance of the disease (the incubation period) may vary from 2 weeks to a few years. Amoebic dysentery is a chronic disease causing grumbling stomach pains and two or more rather loose motions each day. Intermittent diarrhoea and constipation are common, and the stools may be slimy and bloody and smell awful.

Amoeba may spread from the intestine to the liver, to produce an abscess that causes fever, sweating and malaise.

Drugs used to treat amoebic infections

Metronidazole and *tinidazole* are very effective drugs for treating acute amoebic dysentery and amoebic infections of the liver.

Chloroquine is also used to treat amoebic infections of the liver but is slower to work and less reliable than metronidazole.

Diloxanide is the drug of choice for treating chronic amoebic dysentery in which cysts are passed in the motions. A course of diloxanide should always be given following treatment of acute amoebic dysentery with metronidazole or tinidazole, or following a course of chloroquine for an amoebic infection of the liver.

Emetine is the old-fashioned treatment of amoebic infections. It is no longer used because of its serious harmful effects, particularly damage to the heart.

Giardiasis

Giardiasis is a parasitic infection of the small intestine caused by a protozoa

(*Giardia intestinalis, G. lamblia*). Infection is world wide, particularly in the tropics. The protozoa, which are whip shaped and therefore called flagellates, attach themselves to the lining of the small intestine and cause inflammation and wasting of the lining. The infection causes attacks of urgent diarrhoea, discomfort in the abdomen and loose pale motions. It may be associated with distension of the abdomen, pain and nausea. The damage to the lining of the small intestine may interfere with the absorption of nutrients and vitamins, and lead to malnutrition.

Drug treatment

Tinidazole or *metronidazole* by mouth produce a dramatic cure. Tinidazole is long acting and can be given as a single dose.

Mepacrine by mouth is an alternative to tinidazole or metronidazole.

Leishmaniasis

This is a group of diseases caused by a protozoon (*Leishmania*) that is transmitted to humans by female sand flies. The disease may take several forms, discussed below.

Visceral leishmaniasis (kala-azar)

This type of leishmaniasis is caused by *Leishmania donovani*. It is widespread throughout parts of the Middle and Far East, East Africa, China, Russia, India and South America. Humans appear to be the main source of the infection (the host) but in some areas, such as the Mediterranean basin, dogs and foxes are the hosts. The disease mainly affects children and young adults; tourists are particularly susceptible.

The protozoa invade the blood system and are spread to many tissues. The disease affects the lining of the small intestine and can interfere with the absorption of nutrients, resulting in malnutrition. It may also spread to the liver, spleen and bone marrow where it interferes with white cell production to cause immune deficiency; damage to red cell production, causing anaemia; and damage to platelet production, causing bleeding.

Treatment

The best treatment is prevention – insecticides, insect repellents, protective clothing and mosquito nets. Drug treatment involves the use of antimony drugs (e.g. sodium stibogluconate).

Oriental sore

In the Middle and Far East (the Old World) certain types of *Leishmania* protozoa cause ulcers of the skin (Oriental sores). The source (hosts) are gerbils and other desert rodents. The skin ulcers may respond to antimony compounds but the diffuse ulcerating type of lesion has to be treated with pentamidine. A lasting immunity can be achieved by injecting a culture of protozoa (*L. major*) into the upper arm; this produces a single sore but protects against further trouble.

Skin lesions can also be caused in South and Central America by a *Leishmania* protozoon transmitted by sand flies from a variety of rodents which act as the source (hosts). The nose and mouth can be attacked by the ulcers and produce serious disfigurement. Treatment is with antimony compounds. Amphotericin may help the nose and mouth ulcers.

Toxoplasmosis

Toxoplasmosis is caused by the protozoal parasite *Toxoplasma gondii*. It occurs naturally in mice, guinea-pigs, cats, rabbits and several other small animals and also in birds. Humans become infected from cysts in the faeces of such animals.

The most serious form of the disease affects newborn babies. The parasite is found all over the baby's body – in the eyes, brain, heart, lungs and adrenal glands. This 'congenital' type of toxoplasmosis causes abnormal development of the brain (water on the brain: hydrocephalus; or a small shrunken brain: microcephaly). It also causes convulsions, tremors and paralysis, and the baby may develop a large infected liver with jaundice. Infected babies usually die, but if they survive they are usually severely handicapped.

Toxoplasmosis infection is spread from the mother to the baby in the womb. The mother catches the infection from cysts passed in a cat's faeces or from eating under-cooked beef or lamb.

In adults the disease may produce no symptoms in some people but in others it may produce acute problems causing aches and pains, fever, skin rashes, pneumonia, jaundice and inflammation of the heart. It may cause enlarged lymph glands and changes in the white blood cells. It may also cause a chronic inflammation inside the eye.

Treatment

People who are immune deficient (e.g. with AIDS) or who have eye damage from toxoplasmosis should be treated with a combination of a sulphonamide and pyrimethamine. An alternative treatment is a tetracycline antibiotic. Individuals with eye disorders may require corticosteroid eye drops.

Diseases caused by worms

Threadworms

Threadworm (*Enterobius vermicularis*) infections are widespread throughout the world. The worm affects children particularly. Its life follows a cycle – eggs are swallowed and, as they pass into the intestine, they develop and mate. The pregnant females move down into the bowel and make their way into the anus where they lay their eggs. This causes severe itching, particularly in bed at night. Children scratch their itching anuses, infect their fingers with ova and then put their fingers in their food and mouth and re-infect themselves. Children also touch each other's hands and this is how the infection is easily spread in nursery school.

Adult worms can easily be seen moving out of the anus and over the skin to the genitals; they can also be seen in the motions (the male worm is 2–5 mm long and the female is 8–12 mm long). In girls the worms may spread up from the anus into the vagina where they can cause severe irritation and ascending infection up into the womb and fallopian tubes.

Treatment

The important part of treatment is strict hygiene in the family and in nursery schools. Infected children must wash their hands and scrub their nails after going to the toilet and before meals. They should also take a bath or shower every morning to wash the worms and eggs from the anus and genitals. They should try not to scratch themselves and put their fingers in their mouths. The whole family should practise good hygiene and be treated.

Drug treatment includes:

- *mebendazole* – a single dose by mouth; it should not be used in children under the age of 2 years
- *piperazine* – one dose by mouth daily for 7 days (the dose varies according to age); it may be repeated after 1 week if no improvement
- *pyrantel* – a single dose by mouth

Roundworm

The roundworm *Ascaris lumbricoides* causes a disease known as ascariasis. It is a large worm; adult females may measure 20–45 cm in length. The worms live for about 18 months in the body before they die. The intestine may contain any number of worms from one to hundreds. The female produces 200,000 eggs per day; they are passed in the faeces and after about 10 days in soil they become infective and contaminate water and food.

The eggs enter humans from food contaminated with human faeces. The eggs hatch in the duodenum and the larvae penetrate the wall of the intestine into the blood stream where they are carried to the lungs. In the lungs they move out of the blood stream and climb up the bronchial tubes into the throat. They are then swallowed into the intestine where they mature, to start producing eggs after about 2 months. A large proportion of the world's population is infected with roundworms.

In the lungs they may produce fever, pain, cough, malaise and breathlessness, and in the intestine they may cause pain, diarrhoea, vomiting and loss of appetite. They may also interfere with the absorption of nutrients and vitamins, producing malnutrition, especially in children. A bunch of worms may block the intestine and cause a serious obstruction.

Drug treatment

Levamisole (not available in the UK), mebendazole, piperazine and pyrantel are all effective. Containment of the infection must rely on better education and sanitation.

Tapeworms

There are many types of tapeworm. Humans are the source (the host) of tapeworms where they live in the intestine attached by suckers in their heads. They have no gut and absorb nutrients through their surface. Tapeworms consist of segments and cross-fertilization takes place between segments. Eggs are produced, which are passed in the faeces. These infected faeces contaminate foods that are eaten by animals (e.g. cattle and pigs) and by fish. These animals are intermediate hosts in the development of the tapeworm. Humans get infected by eating these infected animals (e.g. uncooked or under-cooked beef, pork and fish), and this allows the next stage of development in the life cycle of the tapeworm.

In the intermediate hosts the surfaces of the eggs are dissolved in the stomach juice and they hatch to release larvae into the intestine. These pass through the intestine wall and circulate round the body where they settle in various tissues, particularly muscles where they form cysts around themselves. These cysts (or cysticerci) are the cause of 'measly' beef and pork.

Beef tapeworm (Taenia saginata)

Humans normally get infected from eating uncooked or under-cooked beef (rare steaks and kebabs) containing cysts (cysticerci). The cysts are dissolved by the stomach juices and the baby worm attaches itself to the wall of the intestine.

Usually only one tapeworm develops; it hangs on to the intestinal wall by its suckers and reaches a length of 4–8 metres. Tapeworms are usually in the upper part of the small intestine and cause no symptoms, but occasionally they cause irritation, producing wind, cramps or diarrhoea. Segments (proglottides) appear in the stools. Eggs may also appear in the stools and can be obtained from the anus by applying sticky tape. These eggs contaminate animal food and are eaten by intermediate hosts (cattle) and so the cycle continues.

Pork tapeworm (Taenia solium)

Humans normally get infected from eating uncooked or under-cooked pork containing cysts (cysticerci). The cysts are dissolved by the stomach juice and the baby worm attaches itself to the wall of the small intestine.

Usually only one tapeworm develops; it hangs on by its suckers and reaches a length of 2–4 metres. There are usually no symptoms, and eggs and segments are passed in the faeces. These eggs may contaminate animal food and be eaten by intermediate hosts (e.g. pigs, sheep, camels), and so the cycle continues.

The development of pork tapeworm cysts in humans

Humans may develop pork tapeworm cysts (cysticercosis) by eating food or water contaminated with human faeces infected with eggs of the pork tapeworm. Also, eggs may be transferred from the anus to the mouth by the fingers, and sometimes eggs may enter the stomach from the intestine during a severe bout of vomiting.

Once in the stomach, the pork tapeworm's eggs are dissolved in the stomach juice. This allows them to hatch and to release their larvae, which work their way through the wall of the intestine to circulate all around the body, and wherever they settle they make cysts around themselves. The cysts may develop in any organ or tissue of the body. Inside the cysts the larvae mature over a few months but eventually they die, leaving a hard cyst. These cysts may cause no problems in the skin or muscles except for some aches and pains and fever in the early stages. However, if they develop in the brain, they may cause problems such as water on the brain (hydrocephalus) by blocking the drainage of brain fluid. They may also cause pressure and inflammation in the brain, resulting in epilepsy, paralysis and personality changes. The cysts may lodge in the eyes and cause inflammation, blurred vision and blindness, and in the heart to produce heart failure.

Fish tapeworm (Diphyllobothrium latum)

These are the largest tapeworm and can reach 10 metres in length. They attach themselves to the wall of the small intestine. Segments and eggs pass out in the faeces and these can infect freshwater areas where copepods (a group of crustaceae) breed. The larvae develop in the copepods, which are then eaten by pike, perch or salmon. Humans become infected by eating these fish raw or under-cooked. Poor sewage disposal allows infected human faeces to enter freshwater lakes and so the cycle continues.

The most harmful effect of fish tapeworm is that it can interfere with the absorption of vitamin B_{12}, causing anaemia.

Drug treatment of tapeworms

One dose of *niclosamide* or *praziquantel* after a light breakfast, followed by a purgative after 2 hours.

Hydatid disease (echinococcosis)

The dog and certain wild canines are the source (host) of a small tapeworm (*Echinococcus granulosus*). These animals pass the eggs in their faeces, which contaminate the ground. The eggs may be taken in by other animals (e.g. sheep, cattle and camels) during feeding, and hatch in the intestines of these animals. The larvae then enter the blood stream and are spread round the body, to form cysts (hydatid cysts) in various tissues.

The eggs may also be taken in by humans directly from dogs' faeces or by drinking water contaminated with the eggs. The eggs hatch in the small intestine and the larvae work their way through the wall of the intestine into the blood stream, to be taken to the liver, where they form a cyst. The cyst may enlarge and become hardened, or it may rupture, causing the release of many cysts. Occasionally larvae travel to the lungs or brain, where they form cysts. Symptoms will depend on the size and location of the cysts. A rare form has a cycle between foxes and voles; it may affect humans and invade the liver.

Treatment

Treatment consists of surgical removal of the cyst, avoiding spillage of its contents. Mebendazole may be of some value, particularly in people who cannot have surgery or whose lungs are affected.

Improved hygiene, worming of dogs and inspection of meat should help to reduce the spread.

Hookworms

Hookworms are roundworms with conspicuous teeth. They are about 1 cm in length and attach themselves to the lining of the small intestine and drink blood. This can lead to anaemia and a low blood protein in the infected person (the host). The females produce thousands of eggs, which contaminate the faeces and hatch in soil within 48 hours. The larvae can survive for several months in soil. Upon coming into contact with the skin of humans, the larvae penetrate it, enter the blood in the veins and are carried to the lungs. They then climb through the lung tissue and up the breathing tubes into the throat where they are swallowed into the stomach and then reach the small intestine where they hook on and start sucking blood – the cycle is completed.

Light infections produce few symptoms but heavy infections (thousands of worms) may cause hookworm disease – abdominal pain and diarrhoea, chronic blood loss, causing anaemia, and low blood proteins which may result in weakness, fatigue and retarded growth in children. The severe anaemia may cause heart failure.

Treatment

Drugs used include bephenium, levamisole, mebendazole, pyrantel and thiabendazole. Tetrachloroethylene is also used in some countries.

Schistosomiasis (or bilharziasis)

This is a chronic worm infection, which is estimated to affect over 200 million people in the world. It is one of the most important public health problems facing tropical and sub-tropical countries. The schistosomes are worms that live in the body of humans as parasites. They are transmitted by freshwater snails.

Humans may be infected by three species of schistosomes – *Schistosoma haematobium, S. japonicum* and *S. mansoni*. Each species is particular to a certain area of the world and causes a specific illness resulting in a substantial amount of suffering and many deaths.

The schistosome worms live and mate in the venous blood – *S. haematobium* live in the veins around the ureters and bladder; *S. mansoni* live in the main veins that drain the intestine (the inferior mesenteric veins) and *S. japonicum* live in other main veins that drain the intestine (the superior mesenteric veins).

The female worms lay their eggs in the blood stream and, according to their location, the eggs then break their way out of the body by entering the bladder or intestine to be passed in the urine or faeces. Those eggs that do not escape get trapped in the wall of the bladder or intestine and cause areas of inflammation. They may also spread to the liver and cause inflammation in the liver.

The eggs are present in the urine and faeces of infected humans, so passing urine or emptying the bowels into freshwater lakes contaminates the water with eggs, where they hatch in a few hours. The baby worms swim near the surface of the water and are capable of infecting snails for up to 8 hours. Once they enter the snail they multiply by the hundreds and schistosome worms develop in about 4–6 weeks. Under certain conditions of light and temperature they mature enough to infect humans. They emerge from the snails into the water and remain infective to humans for about 72 hours. If a human paddles or swims in the infected water, the worms attach themselves to the skin by suckers. Within minutes they have burrowed deep into the skin, helped by a special chemical they produce from a gland on their heads that penetrates the skin and by a vibratory movement of their bodies. During the few minutes while they are penetrating the skin, they shake off their tails and change into a different shape so that they can easily lie in tunnels burrowed under the skin. At this stage they no longer need oxygen and would die if they re-entered the water. They remain in the skin for 1–3 days before entering and migrating along veins to the lungs and then to the liver in about 4–6 weeks. In the liver they undergo a further development and finally they migrate to the areas where they mate (see above).

Eggs can be seen in the urine and faeces within about 5–9 weeks of first being infected. The worms live in the body for 3–10 years and continue to produce eggs at regular intervals.

The infection is more common in the young and in males and is probably related to the frequency with which they enter and swim in infected waters. Three distinct disease syndromes are caused by schistosomiasis and are related to three distinct stages in the development of the worms: swimmer's itch, and acute and chronic schistosomiasis.

Swimmer's itch is an allergic dermatitis caused when the young worms enter the skin from infected water. The disease may go no further than this.

Acute schistosomiasis (Katayama fever) is a serum-sickness-like syndrome (see Chapter 11) which occurs 3–9 weeks after infection. There is fever, headache, pains in the abdomen and an enlarged spleen and liver. It is an acute allergic reaction that coincides with the production of eggs in the body (see earlier).

Chronic schistosomiasis is caused by eggs that fail to be excreted in the urine and faeces. They remain in the bladder or intestine and, along with the chemicals they produce to help their escape through the wall of the bladder or of the intestine, they trigger severe immune reactions. This causes immune cells and chemicals to move in on the eggs, which results in the production of what are called schistosome egg granulomas. A granuloma is a tumour containing granulomatous tissue which is the 'debris' left after a severe immune/inflammatory reaction. These tumours then increase in size because scar tissue is laid down on them. They may become large enough to cause all kinds of problems; for example, blockage to the flow of urine through a ureter, which causes a back-pressure into the kidney, resulting in kidney damage or blockage to the flow of blood in the liver and spleen. These lesions may occur in any tissue or organ of the body.

NOTE Several schistosome species use migratory birds as their definitive hosts and fresh- and salt-water molluscs as their intermediate hosts. Swimming in infected waters can cause the swimmer's itch stage of the disease only.

Drug treatment

Praziquantel is effective against all types of human schistosomes. Oxamniquine is active only against *S. mansoni*, and metriphonate is effective against *S. haematobium*.

If treatment is given early enough during the course of the disease, it may be possible to not only kill the worms but also to reverse some of the damage. In the later stages, treatment will kill the worms and prevent them from causing further damage.

Control

The most cost-effective approach to the control of schistosomiasis at present is the mass treatment of communities, using a single dose of praziquantel combined with an all-out attack on snails using chemicals (molluscicides).

The drug treatment causes a low egg count in the urine and faeces for years. However, at the same time there is need for health education programmes as well as a need to dramatically improve living standards, to provide toilets, to improve agricultural practices of irrigating fields and to discourage washing, swimming and playing in infected waters.

Filariasis

Filaria are a genus of parasitic worm that infect tissues under the skin and in the lymphatics. There are eight types that commonly affect humans and three of them are responsible for most diseases caused by filariae. They are transmitted by biting insects (mosquitoes, black fly, horse fly and midges) and they go through complex life cycles in the body. The adults are thin worms about 2–50 cm long.

The type that live under the skin cause severe skin rashes and can affect the eyes. The type that live in the lymphatic system cause allergic and inflammatory reactions that block the flow of lymph producing back-pressure of fluid into the tissues, causing the affected area to swell up. The blockage may affect the drainage from the breasts, scrotum, legs or arms. These areas can swell up to a tremendous size. The leg can be so swollen that it looks like an elephant's leg, which is why it is called elephantiasis. The scrotum can become so enormous that it has been known for one affected individual to push his scrotum round in a wheel-barrow!

Drug treatment

Diethylcarbamazine is effective against most types of infections. It kills the worms but triggers a severe allergic reaction. If the infection persists, suramin is used; it kills adult worms but may also damage the kidneys. Ivermectin is another effective drug.

Dracontiasis

Dracontiasis is caused by the female guinea-worm, which lives under the skin in humans. It is transmitted from a small crustacean (cyclops) that lives in wells and ponds. When the cyclops is eaten by humans the larvae penetrate the intestine wall and spread to settle down in tissue under the skin and elsewhere. The mature female worms work their way through the surface of the skin to the surface, to release their eggs; this causes acute allergic symptoms, severe blisters and inflammation of the skin and joints.

Drug treatment

Metronidazole and niridazole are both effective at killing the worms. The worms should be removed from the skin and sterile dressings applied.

Table 59.1 Drugs used to treat amoebic, worm and other parasitic infections – harmful effects and warnings

bephenium (Alcopar)
Harmful effects include nausea, diarrhoea, vomiting, headache and vertigo.
Warning It must not be used in anyone with persistent vomiting.

diethylcarbamazine (Banocide)
Harmful effects include allergic reactions (caused by death of the worms), which may be severe; generalized itching and congestion of the conjunctivae may occur. These reactions may be modified by giving treatment with a corticosteroid and an antihistamine by mouth. Damage to eyes may occur during treatment for onchocerciasis.
Warnings *Risks in elderly people* Harmful effects of treatment may be more frequent and severe; therefore use with caution, particularly if the individual suffers from loiasis, lymphatic filariasis or, especially, onchocerciasis. Patients should have an eye examination before and at regular intervals during treatment.

diloxanide furoate (Entamizole [with metronidazole])
Harmful effects include wind and belching, vomiting, itching, nettle rash and transient protein in the urine.

emetine hydrochloride
Harmful effects include pain and abscess at the site of injection; nausea, vomiting and diarrhoea; dizziness, headache; muscle weakness; skin rashes; heart symptoms (pain in chest, breathlessness), rapid heart beat, fall in blood pressure and changes on the electrocardiograph. Large doses and prolonged use may cause damage to the heart (resulting in heart failure), kidneys, stomach and intestine and skeletal muscle.
Warnings Emetine hydrochloride should not be used in people with heart or kidney disease. The heart should be carefully monitored during treatment.
Risks in elderly people Harmful effects may be more frequent and severe; therefore use with caution.

levamisole
Harmful effects include nausea, vomiting, abdominal pain, taste disturbances, headache, fatigue, confusion, insomnia, dizziness, fever, flu-like symptoms, painful joints and muscles, inflammation of blood vessels, fall in blood pressure, skin rashes, blood disorders and protein in the urine.
Warnings Levamisole must not be used in patients with serious liver, kidney or blood disorders.
Risks in elderly people Harmful effects may be more frequent and severe; use with caution.

mebendazole (Vermox)
Harmful effects Abdominal pain and diarrhoea may occur rarely in cases of massive infestation and expulsion of worms.

mepacrine
Harmful effects include dizziness, headache, nausea and yellow colour of the skin; large doses may cause vomiting and mental disturbances. Prolonged use may

Table 59.1 Drugs used to treat amoebic, worm and other parasitic infections – harmful effects and warnings (*cont.*)

cause dermatitis (sometimes very severe) and, rarely, liver damage and damage to the bone marrow, producing blood disorders.

metronidazole
See Chapter 53.

metriphonate (Bilarcil)
Harmful effects may cause nausea, vomiting, abdominal pain, headache and vertigo.

niclosamide (Yomesan)
Harmful effects include nausea, vomiting, abdominal discomfort, loss of appetite, diarrhoea or constipation, drowsiness, dizziness, headache, skin rash, itching anus, irritation in the mouth, bad taste in the mouth, sweating, palpitations, loss of hair, backache, irritability, allergic reactions.

Warnings Niclosamide should not be used in people who are allergic to the drug. It kills worms in the intestine only; it is without effect on cysticercosis.

nimorazole (Naxogin 500)
Harmful effects include nausea, vomiting, rashes, vertigo, drowsiness, incoordination of movements and intolerance to alcohol. For other potential harmful effects, see metronidazole (Chapter 53).

Warnings Nimorazole should not be used in patients with active disorders of the brain or nervous system. Treatment should be stopped if incoordination of movements develops.

Risks in elderly people Harmful effects may be more frequent and severe; therefore use with caution.

Risks with alcohol Do not drink alcohol when you are taking this drug.

niridazole
Harmful effects include loss of appetite, nausea, vomiting, diarrhoea, dizziness, headache and abdominal pain. Occasionally, insomnia, disorders of heart rhythm, anxiety, confusion and hallucinations may occur and, rarely, convulsions, allergic reactions, numbness and pins and needles in arms and legs and haemolytic anaemia in people with a glucose-6-phosphate dehydrogenase deficiency. It may colour the urine deep brown.

Warnings Niridazole should not be used in people with epilepsy, severe heart disease or a history of mental illness. Do not use it with isoniazid. It should be used with great caution in patients with impaired liver function due to heavy infection.

Risks in elderly people Harmful effects may be more frequent and severe; therefore use with caution.

oxamniquine (Mansil, Vansil)
Harmful effects include pain at the site of injection, which may be associated with hardness of the skin at the site, and fever. This occurs within about 48 hours of the injection and lasts for 2–7 days. Muscle pains, headache, dizziness, sleepiness, insomnia, diarrhoea, skin rashes, red discoloration of the urine, minor abnormalities of electrical tracings of the heart (ECG) and abnormalities of liver function tests have been reported.

piperazine (Antepar, Ascalix, Pripsen)
Harmful effects Occasionally it may cause nausea, vomiting, diarrhoea, headache, nettle rash, numbness and pins and needles in the hands and feet. High doses and prolonged daily use (over 14 days) may, very rarely, cause severe nerve damage which includes sleepiness, vertigo, incoordination of movements, weakness, tremor and convulsions. Rarely, it may cause cataracts and allergic reactions (e.g. nettle rash, fever, painful joints).

Warnings Piperazine must not be used in people with liver disease, epilepsy or severe kidney disease or in anyone who is allergic to it. It should be used with caution in people with impaired kidney function or who are suffering from severe

Table 59.1 Drugs used to treat amoebic, worm and other parasitic infections – harmful effects and warnings (*cont.*)

malnutrition or anaemia, who may develop epilepsy or who have evidence of brain or nerve disorders. Because of its potential to produce nerve damage, especially in children, prolonged and repeated use in excess of the recommended dose should be avoided.

praziquantel (Biltricide)
Harmful effects are usually mild and transient; they include malaise, headache, dizziness, abdominal discomfort with or without nausea, rise in temperature, nettle rash and allergic reactions.

Warnings Praziquantel must not be used in people who are allergic to it, nor to treat cysticercosis of the eyes.

Risks with driving Do not drive on the day of treatment or on the following day.

pyrantel (Combantrin)
Harmful effects are usually mild and transient; they include loss of appetite, abdominal cramps, nausea, vomiting, diarrhoea, headache, dizziness, drowsiness, insomnia and skin rashes.

Warning Pyrantel should be used with caution in patients with liver disease.

sodium stibogluconate (Pentostam)
Harmful effects include loss of appetite, chest and abdominal pain, coughing, nausea, vomiting, weakness, diarrhoea, rash, bleeding from the nose and gums, fever, rigors, vertigo, flushing of the face, painful muscles, jaundice, abnormalities on electrical tracings of the heart (ECG) and allergic reactions (which may be severe).

Warnings Sodium stibogluconate should not be used in patients with pneumonia or inflammation of the liver (hepatitis), kidneys (nephritis) or heart (myocarditis). Because of the risk of severe allergic reactions, full resuscitative facilities should be immediately to hand when it is administered. It should be used with caution in patients with heart disease: antimony accumulates in the electrical pathways of the heart and may cause disorders of heart rhythm.

Risks in elderly people Harmful effects may be more frequent and severe; therefore use with caution.

suramin
Harmful effects include nausea, vomiting, abdominal pain, diarrhoea, nettle rash, collapse, increased sensitivity, and numbness and pins and needles in the hands and feet due to nerve damage, fever, skin rash, dermatitis, discomfort on looking into the light, watery eyes, blurred vision, and protein and blood cells in the urine. Very rarely, it may cause a reduced white cell count and damage to red blood cells (haemolytic anaemia).

Warning Suramin must not be used in patients with kidney disease or disease of the adrenal glands.

Risks in elderly people Harmful effects may be more frequent and severe; therefore use with caution.

tetrachloroethylene
Harmful effects include drowsiness, confusion, giddiness, headache, nausea and vomiting; very rarely, severe symptoms may follow use – these include kidney and liver damage, nerve damage and convulsions. Harmful effects are more likely to occur in alcoholics.

Warnings Treatment for roundworms should *precede* the use of tetrachloroethylene. It should not be used in alcoholics or in patients with impaired liver function, severe debility or anaemia, or with any inflammatory or ulcerative disorders of the intestine.

Risks in elderly people Harmful effects may be more frequent and severe; therefore use with caution.

thiabendazole (Mintezol)
Harmful effects include loss of appetite, nausea, vomiting and dizziness. Less frequently, stomach upsets, itching, diarrhoea and drowsiness may occur.

Table 59.1 Drugs used to treat amoebic, worm and other parasitic infections – harmful effects and warnings (*cont.*)

Rarely, there may be collapse, noises in the ears (tinnitus), irritability, eye disturbances, blurred vision, yellow vision, numbness, bedwetting, raised blood sugar, low blood pressure, itching around the anus, blood in the urine, liver damage and jaundice. Allergic reactions may occur and include fever, flushing of the face, dry eyes, swelling of the lips, mouth and skin (angio-oedema), skin rashes, swollen glands, Stevens–Johnson syndrome and, rarely, anaphylaxis. The urine may smell as it does after eating asparagus. Live ascaris may appear in the mouth and nose.

Warnings Treatment of anaemia, dehydration and malnutrition should be given *before* treatment with thiabendazole is started. Thiabendazole should not be used in people who are allergic to it, nor to treat mixed infections of ascaris because it may cause these worms to migrate. It should be used with caution in patients with impaired kidney or liver function, and their progress should be monitored. It should be used only to treat worm infection and *not* to prevent infection. It competes with theophylline and related drugs for metabolism in the liver; this reduces the breakdown of these drugs, so their blood level may increase to toxic levels. The blood levels of theophylline and related drugs should be carefully monitored and, if necessary, their dose reduced.

Risks with driving It may interfere with your ability to drive, so do not drive while on treatment.

tinidazole (Fasigyn)
See Chapter 53.

The pituitary gland

The pituitary gland is located in the base of the brain. It has two lobes – one at the front, the anterior lobe, and one at the back, the posterior lobe. It is connected by a stalk to a part of the brain called the hypothalamus. The hypothalamus contains nuclei which produce substances that control the secretions of the anterior lobe. It also has nerve fibres which run into the posterior lobe in order to control its functions.

Hormones produced by the anterior lobe of the pituitary gland

The anterior lobe produces seven hormones, four of which act on other glands (called target glands) and three of which act on specific tissues in the body. Secretion of each hormone is under the control of the hypothalamus, which responds to the level of hormones in the blood produced by the target glands. For example, if the thyroid hormone level is high the hypothalamus will send out a message to the pituitary to make it reduce its production of thyroid-stimulating hormone, and vice versa. A similar response will occur to the various levels of hormones produced by the adrenal glands and the gonads (testes in males, and ovaries in females). The hypothalamus also responds to nervous stimulation, physical activity and various metabolic activities in the body.

Hormones produced by the posterior lobe of the pituitary gland

The posterior lobe is under nervous control from the hypothalamus. It secretes two hormones, vasopressin and oxytocin.

Vasopressin is responsible for increasing the absorption of water from the urine back into the blood stream. It is therefore known as an anti-diuretic hormone (a diuretic is any substance that increases the volume of the urine). Vasopressin reduces the volume of the urine by reducing the volume of water in the urine. The secretion of vasopressin responds to the concentration of the blood: a rise stimulates the kidneys to absorb more water from the urine in order to dilute the blood back to its normal concentration. A fall in the volume of the blood produces a similar effect and the increased water that is absorbed from the urine by the kidneys helps to push up the volume of the blood. Nervous stimulation (e.g. pain) also triggers an increased secretion of vasopressin.

Oxytocin in the female stimulates the expression of breast milk, and it causes the womb to contract during childbirth.

Disorders produced by over-secretion of hormones from the anterior lobe of the pituitary gland

Gigantism

This is a condition of excessive tallness that is produced by over-secretion of growth hormone (GH) in young people before puberty and before the bones have stopped growing.

Acromegaly

This is a chronic disease that is characterized by gradual enlargement of the soft tissues of the hands and feet and the bones of the face and chest. The skin becomes thick and coarse, and the nose, lips, tongue and ears increase in size, as do internal organs such as the heart and liver. About one-third of sufferers develop diabetes and, as the disease progresses, they may also develop arthritis and a raised blood pressure. It is due to over-secretion of growth hormone in adult life.

Treatment

Bromocriptine stimulates dopamine receptors in the brain, one effect of which is to stimulate those nerves running from the hypothalamus to the pituitary gland that cause the pituitary gland to reduce its production of growth hormone and prolactin (the milk-producing hormone). It is used to treat over-secretion of growth hormone in addition to the surgical removal of the gland or its destruction by irradiation.

Cushing's disease

Cushing's disease is caused by an over-secretion of corticosteroids from the adrenal glands as a result of over-stimulation of the glands by ACTH (adrenocorticotrophic hormone) secreted by an over-active anterior lobe of the pituitary gland. This over-activity may be due to a tumour of the anterior lobe or to over-stimulation by the hypothalamus.

Cushing's syndrome

Cushing's syndrome refers to a group of signs and symptoms similar to those produced by Cushing's disease. It is caused by over-secretion of corticosteroid hormones due to a tumour of an adrenal gland which over-secretes independently of ACTH. Over-secretion of corticosteroids may also be caused by certain cancers that produce ACTH (e.g. cancer of the lung). However, by far the commonest cause is the over-use of corticosteroids (see Chapter 62). Cushing's syndrome is discussed in Chapter 61.

Over-production of the milk-producing hormone (prolactin)

Over-secretion of prolactin (the milk-producing hormone), which is produced in both men and women, may be due to a tumour of the anterior lobe of the pituitary gland. It may also be caused by drugs that block the effects of dopamine, a nerve transmitter in the brain which stimulates the nerves that run from the hypothalamus to the anterior lobe of the pituitary gland and which are responsible for causing a reduction in the gland's production of prolactin. Drugs that block dopamine and remove this control include drugs used to treat serious mental illness (anti-psychotic drugs), certain drugs used to treat vomiting (e.g. metoclopramide), and methyldopa used to treat raised blood pressure. The female sex hormones (oestrogens) also stimulate prolactin secretion during pregnancy. Decreased function of the ovaries and testes may be associated with a raised secretion of prolactin.

Over-production of prolactin causing a raised blood level of prolactin may cause spontaneous enlargement of the breasts (gynaecomastia) and flow of milk from the breast (galactorrhoea) in both men and women. It may cause loss of menstrual periods (amenorrhoea) in women and infertility in both men and women.

Treatment

Bromocriptine which stimulates dopamine nerve receptors in the brain (see earlier) reduces prolactin secretion and helps to restore the function of the ovaries or the testes – provided, of course, that the secretion of gonadotrophins is not affected.

Under-activity of the anterior lobe of the pituitary gland (hypopituitarism)

Hypopituitarism is most commonly caused by a tumour of the gland. There are other rare causes, including damage to the gland following haemorrhage after childbirth (known as Sheehan's syndrome).

Under-activity of the anterior lobe of the pituitary gland leads to under-activity of the thyroid gland and to under-activity of the ovaries or testes, producing loss of sexual drive (libido) and impotence. Growth of hair becomes scanty, the skin becomes pale, milk flow from the breasts can occur in both men and women, and signs and symptoms of under-activity of the adrenal glands develop (Chapter 61). Treatment involves giving adrenal hormones, thyroid hormones and sex hormones.

Disorders produced by under-secretion of growth hormone and gonadotrophin

Under-secretion of growth hormone (GH) in children results in failure to grow and a short stature, and under-secretion of gonadotrophin results in sexual under-development (pituitary infantilism). The commonest cause is a genetic inability of the hypothalamus to secrete growth hormone-releasing factor. Treatment was previously with growth hormone obtained from the pituitary glands of dead people. This has now been replaced by human growth hormone preparations produced in the laboratory by genetic engineering (e.g. somatropin).

Under-activity of the posterior lobe of the pituitary gland

Diabetes insipidus

Lack of secretion of vasopressin by the posterior lobe of the pituitary gland produces excessive thirst and the passing of large volumes of dilute urine. This is called diabetes insipidus. It is fairly rare and may be due to several causes, including a tumour of the gland.

Treatment

Treatment of diabetes insipidus due to failure of the posterior lobe or the hypothalamus involves the use of vasopressin (Pitressin) or terlipressin (Glypressin) by injection or desmopressin (DDAVP injection or nasal drops,

Desmospray nasal spray) or lypressin (Syntopressin) nasal spray. The treatment should be tailored to the needs of each individual and adjusted to produce a mild increase in the volume of urine over each 24-hour period in order to avoid the harmful effects of too much water being retained in the body (water intoxication). Desmopressin has the longest duration of action and, unlike vasopressin and lypressin, it produces no constricting effects upon arteries.

An anti-diabetic drug chlorpropamide, carbamazepine (an anti-epileptic drug) and the blood fat-lowering drug clofibrate may also help to reduce the large volume of urine being passed in people with partial diabetes insipidus. They appear to make the kidneys more sensitive to any vasopressin that is still being produced. They are only of use in mild cases. The great danger of using chlorpropamide is that it may cause a serious fall in the blood sugar level.

Diabetes insipidus may be due to kidney disease that causes the kidneys not to respond to vasopressin. This may be produced by poisoning with heavy metals such as lead and by lithium used to treat depression. The treatment of this type of diabetes insipidus is to use a thiazide diuretic (e.g. chlorthalidone) which, instead of increasing the volume of the urine, may produce an opposite, or paradoxical, effect and reduce the volume of the urine. A thiazide diuretic may also help patients with partial diabetes insipidus caused by a disorder of the posterior lobe of the pituitary gland or of the hypothalamus and who are still capable of producing some vasopressin.

Table 60.1 Drugs used to treat diabetes insipidus – harmful effects and warnings

vasopressin
Harmful effects include tremors, sweating, vertigo, pallor around the mouth, 'pounding' in the head, abdominal cramps, wind, nausea, vomiting, nettle rash and wheezing. Allergic reactions may be mild and local at the site of injection or occasionally general and, very rarely, severe. It may cause overloading of the body with water (water intoxication) producing drowsiness, listlessness and headache, leading, very rarely, to coma and convulsions. Constriction of the coronary arteries may, occasionally, cause angina pain.

Warnings Vasopressin must not be used in anyone with disorders of the circulation, especially coronary artery disease (e.g. angina). In such individuals even small doses of vasopressin may trigger an attack of angina, and large doses may cause a heart attack. The early signs of water intoxication should be looked for and the drug stopped or the dose reduced – they include drowsiness, listlessness and headache. If these early signs are spotted and treatment is adjusted the serious consequences of water intoxication should be prevented. It should not be used in individuals with chronic kidney disease (chronic nephritis) until there is evidence of a fall in waste

Table 60.1 Drugs used to treat diabetes insipidus – harmful effects and warnings (*cont.*)

products in the blood (e.g. blood urea and other nitrogenous compounds).
Vasopressin should be used with caution in people with epilepsy, migraine, asthma, heart failure or any disorder where water retention may trigger problems.

desmopressin
It should be used with caution in people with impaired kidney function or disorders of the heart or circulation. Fluid overloading should be avoided after testing.

lypressin
It may cause nausea, abdominal pain and an urge to have the bowels opened. Nasal drops may occasionally cause congestion of the nose and ulceration of its lining.
It should not be used in people with disorders of the circulation and used with caution in asthma, epilepsy and heart failure.

terlipressin
It may cause headache, raised blood pressure and abdominal cramps. It should be used with caution in people with disorders of the heart and circulation.
Fluid balance, blood pressure and blood chemistry should be monitored.

Table 60.2 Hypothalamic and anterior pituitary hormone preparations

Preparation	*Drug*	*Drug group*	*Dosage form*
Acthar Gel	corticotrophin in hydrolized gelatin	Adrenal-stimulating hormone	Injection
ACTH/CMC	corticotrophin	Adrenal-stimulating hormone	Injection
Fertiral	gonadorelin	Gonadotrophin-releasing hormone (LHRH)	Injection
Genotropin	somatropin	Biosynthetic human growth hormone	Injection (powder in vial)
Gonadotraphon LH	human chorionic gonadotrophin	Gonadotrophin	Injection (powder in vial)
HRF	gonadorelin	Gonadotrophin-releasing hormone (LHRH)	Injection (powder in vial); used to assess pituitary function
Humatrope	somatropin	Biosynthetic human growth hormone	Injection (powder in vial)
Metopirone	metyrapone	Blocks corticosteroid production by adrenals and increases ACTH production by pituitary	Capsules; used to assess function of anterior pituitary
Metrodin	urofollitrophin	Gonadotrophin (FSH) (from human menopausal urine)	Injection (powder in vial)

Table 60.2 Hypothalamic and anterior pituitary hormone preparations (*cont.*)

Preparation	*Drug*	*Drug group*	*Dosage form*
Norditropin	somatropin	Biosynthetic human growth hormone	Injection (powder in vial)
Pergonal	menotrophin	Gonadotrophin (FSH and LH) from human post menopausal urine	Injection (powder in vial)
Profasi	human chorionic gonadotrophin	Gonadotrophin	Injection (powder in vial)
Saizen	somatropin	Biosynthetic human growth hormone	Injection (powder in vial)
Synacthen	tetracosactrin	Adrenal stimulating hormone (to test adrenal function)	Injection (suspension with zinc phosphate complex)
Synacthen Depot	tetracosactrin	Adrenal stimulating hormone	Injection (aqueous suspension with zinc phosphate complex)

Table 60.3 Preparations used to treat diabetes insipidus

Preparation	*Drug*	*Dosage form*
DDAVP	desmopressin	Nasal drops, injection
Desmospray	desmopressin	Nasal spray
Glypressin	terlipressin	Injection (powder in vial)
Pitressin	vasopressin	Injection
Syntopressin	lypressin	Nasal spray solution

Table 60.4 Hypothalamic and anterior pituitary hormone preparations – uses, harmful effects and warnings

corticotrophin (ACTH, Acthar) See pages 840–41

gonadorelin (Fertiral, HRF) See page 945

human chorionic gonadotrophin See page 944

metyrapone (Metopirone)
It blocks aldosterone production (see page 829). It is used to treat individuals suffering from Cushing's syndrome who develop severe fluid retention due to too much aldosterone production. It is also used to diagnose whether the Cushing's syndrome is dependent upon ACTH or not (see pages 828–9).

Harmful effects include nausea, vomiting, a fall in blood pressure and allergic reactions.

Warning It should not be used in pregnancy and breast feeding mothers and it should be used with caution in individuals suffering from an underactive pituitary gland (hypopituitarism).

Table 60.4 Hypothalamic and anterior pituitary hormone preparations – uses, harmful effects and warnings (*cont.*)

menotrophin (Pergonal)
It is a gonadotrophin used to stimulate the ovaries in women suffering from infertility (see chapter 69) and to stimulate the ovaries to produce several eggs in women undergoing in-vitro (IVF) or in-vivo fertilization. It is also used to treat males whose testicles may not have developed due to failure of their pituitary gland to produce gonadotrophin (hypogonadotrophic hypogonadism).

Harmful effects include pain at injection site and rarely fever and joint pain, allergic reactions, overstimulation of the ovaries (see under Humegon, page 1266–7) and multiple pregnancy.

Warnings It should not be used in pregnancy. Any hormonal disorder should be treated first (e.g. underactive thyroid or adrenal glands).

somatropin (Genotropin, Humatrope, Norditropin, Saizen)
It is a bio-engineered synthetic human growth hormone. Its structure is identical to that of the natural growth hormone produced in humans. It is used to treat children who fail to grow because their pituitary glands are not producing sufficient growth hormone for their needs. It may also be used to treat poor development of the ovaries or testes and to treat Turner's syndrome (failure of the ovaries or testes to develop properly associated with webbing of the neck, short stature and other abnormalities).

Harmful effects include fluid retention, pain and wasting of fat at site of injections and underactivity of the thyroid gland. The body may produce antibodies against the growth hormone but the long term effects of treatment are not known.

Warnings Should not be used in individuals whose bones have stopped growing, who have any type of active tumour, in pregnancy or in breast-feeding mothers. It should be used with caution in individuals with brain tumours causing failure to grow, with ACTH deficiency or in diabetics. It should only be used by doctors experienced in treating individuals with growth hormones and provided full laboratory X-ray services are available to monitor the child's progress. Thyroid function must be carefully monitored.

tetracosactrin (Synacthen)
It is a depot adrenal stimulating hormone (see corticotrophin, pages 840–41). It is used to treat disorders such as Crohn's disease, ulcerative colitis and rheumatoid arthritis. It is also used to test the function of the adrenal glands.

Harmful effects and Warnings See chapter 62.

urofollitrophin (Medtrodin)
It is a gonadotrophin extracted from the urine of menopausal women. It possesses both FSH and LH activity. It is used to treat absent or scanty menstrual periods due to underactivity of the pituitary gland. It is also used to stimulate egg production in women undergoing in-vitro (IVF) and in-vivo fertilization.

Harmful effects include pain at site of injection, allergic reactions, overstimulation of the ovaries (see under Humegon, pages 1266–7) and multiple pregnancy.

Warnings Women should be carefully monitored for signs of overstimulation of the ovaries.

61

The adrenal glands

We have two adrenal glands which are situated at the top of each kidney – they are therefore often referred to as suprarenal glands (above the kidneys). Each gland has an inner central part called the medulla and an outer part called the cortex.

NOTE In this book the term 'adrenal glands' refers only to the cortex of the adrenal glands. When referring to the medulla the term 'adrenal medulla' (and not 'adrenal glands') is used.

The *adrenal medulla* secretes adrenaline and noradrenaline, and the *cortex* secretes many steroid compounds which belong to four main groups – glucocorticosteroids (e.g. hydrocortisone [cortisol]), mineralocorticosteroids (e.g. aldosterone), male sex hormones (e.g. androsterone) and also small amounts of female sex hormones (oestrogen and progesterone).

The production and secretion of glucocorticosteroids and sex hormones are under the control of ACTH (adrenocorticotrophic hormone) from the anterior lobe of the pituitary gland, whereas production of the mineralocorticosteroid aldosterone is under the control of the renin–angiotensin system (see page 282).

ACTH secretion responds to the level of corticosteroids in the blood; if this is high, ACTH secretion falls, and if it is low, ACTH production is increased. This sort of response is often called a negative feedback system, and it serves to keep the production of corticosteroids steady. There is also an in-built daily rhythm in the production of ACTH, which peaks early in the morning. This is controlled by our biological clocks. In addition, any factor that puts stress on the body (e.g. injury or infection) causes an increased production of ACTH. This is part of our survival system against stress, whatever the cause.

The glucocorticosteroids produce many effects, which are discussed in detail in Chapter 62. The mineralocorticosteroid aldosterone is discussed in Chapter 21. The sex hormones produced by the adrenal glands are discussed in Chapter 66 (female sex hormones) and Chapter 72 (male sex hormones).

Over-activity of the adrenal glands

Over-activity of the adrenal glands may be caused by some disorder of the pituitary gland, resulting in an over-production of adrenocortical-stimulating hormone (adrenocorticotrophin, ACTH). This causes an over-production of corticosteroids by the adrenal glands and the development of *Cushing's disease.* The most striking picture of people with Cushing's disease is a fat face (moon face), increased deposits of fat around the lower part of the back of the neck (buffalo hump) and a redistribution of fat so that the individuals develop a fat abdomen and thin arms and legs. They will have a raised blood pressure due to salt and water retention in the body, and muscle weakness due to loss of potassium in the urine. The over-production of male sex hormones causes hair to grow (hirsutism), acne and disorders of menstruation.

The treatment of Cushing's disease is to surgically remove both adrenal glands, which may be preceded by metyrapone treatment and followed by corticosteroid maintenance treatment. However, in some patients the removal of both adrenal glands may cause severe pigmentation of the skin and a tumour in the anterior lobe of the pituitary gland (Nelson's syndrome). This may be prevented by irradiating the pituitary gland when removing the adrenal glands or after the operation if the ACTH blood level starts to rise excessively. An alternative to removing the adrenal glands is to irradiate the pituitary gland or selectively remove the tumour by microsurgery.

An excess of corticosteroids in the body may also be produced by other disorders. This excess will result in signs and symptoms identical to those in Cushing's disease – these signs and symptoms are therefore referred to as *Cushing's syndrome.* The causes of Cushing's syndrome may be divided into two groups, discussed below.

Cushing's syndrome dependent on ACTH stimulation of the adrenal glands

Too much stimulation of the adrenal glands may be caused by doctors giving too big a dose and too frequent doses of ACTH in the treatment of various disorders, and by certain cancers (e.g. cancer of the lung) that produce their own ACTH which over-stimulates the adrenal glands (the ectopic ACTH syndrome).

Cushing's syndrome not dependent on ACTH stimulation of the adrenal glands

This may, rarely, be due to a cancer of the adrenal glands but the most common cause of this type of Cushing's syndrome is the over-use of corticosteroid drugs (see Chapter 62). High and regular doses of corticosteroid drugs produce all the signs and symptoms of Cushing's syndrome but, because they produce high blood levels of corticosteroids, they stop the production of ACTH by the pituitary gland – which causes the adrenal glands to shrink from under-use. This is why it is very dangerous to stop corticosteroid drugs suddenly and why it takes many months to years before the pituitary and adrenal glands recover from such treatment.

Treatment

This will depend upon the cause but, because many cases are now caused by the over-use of corticosteroid drugs, the most common treatment is the gradual reduction and withdrawal of these drugs. The treatment of a tumour of an adrenal gland is to remove it surgically. For a cancer elsewhere that is producing ACTH (e.g. in the lungs), improvement may be obtained with metyrapone, aminoglutethimide or trilostane, which interfere with the production of corticosteroids by the adrenal glands and correct the patient's potassium deficiency.

Over-production of aldosterone

Primary over-production of aldosterone (primary hyperaldosteronism) may be due to a tumour of an adrenal medulla, causing Conn's syndrome which is characterized by drinking a lot of water and passing frequent large volumes of urine due to impaired control of salt and water balance, episodes of muscular weakness due to potassium loss, and a raised blood pressure.

Over-production of aldosterone (aldosteronism) may occur in cirrhosis of the liver (scarring and shrinking of the liver) associated with an abnormal accumulation of fluid in the abdominal cavity (ascites), and it is sometimes associated with severe heart failure. Treatment is with spironolactone, which blocks the effects of aldosterone in the kidneys, causing a reduction in potassium loss.

Aldosteronism may also be caused by a defective blood supply to a kidney (renal ischaemia), produced by a narrowing of the main artery to the kidney (renal artery stenosis). This may be amenable to surgical removal of the narrowing.

Under-activity of the adrenal glands

An insufficient secretion of adrenal hormones may occur because of shrinkage of the adrenal glands (Addison's disease) due to some chronic infection such as tuberculosis; because of an autoimmune reaction in which the body produces antibodies to its own tissues, in this case the adrenal glands; or it may be due to a failure to develop the enzymes required to produce the hormones. Under-activity of the adrenal glands may also result from a failure of the pituitary gland to produce ACTH (see earlier) but a common cause these days is the *over-use of corticosteroid drugs.* These suppress ACTH production and cause the adrenal glands to shrink.

Under-activity of the adrenal glands produces weakness and loss of weight; increased pigmentation to areas of the skin exposed to sunlight or subject to pressure or friction in skin creases; patches of loss of pigmentation (vitiligo); low blood pressure; loss of appetite, nausea, vomiting and diarrhoea alternating with constipation; low blood sugar levels in response to carbohydrate meals, which produce tiredness and lack of energy; irregular or loss of menstrual periods; and occasionally loss of hair.

Women with autoimmune Addison's disease suffer from early shrinking of their ovaries because their ovaries are attacked by the same antibodies that attack the adrenal glands.

Insufficient production of adrenal hormones due to under-activity of the pituitary gland often causes additional problems such as a deficiency of growth hormone and/or gonadotrophins. There is usually loss of hair and the skin is pale, as opposed to the pigmentation that occurs in Addison's disease. The blood pressure is not affected because the production of aldosterone is independent of hormones from the pituitary gland.

Treatment of under-activity of the adrenal glands

Treatment of primary under-activity of the adrenal glands depends upon the cause, but all patients require hormonal replacement treatment with glucocorticosteroids (e.g. hydrocortisone) and a synthetic mineralocorticosteroid such as fludrocortisone. People with secondary under-activity of the adrenal glands usually do not require fludrocortisone because they continue to produce aldosterone.

Treatment during periods of stress Patients whose adrenal glands are under-active will require additional corticosteroids during periods of stress (injury, infection, surgery). These problems are discussed in detail in Chapter 62.

Acute adrenal failure (acute adrenal crisis, Addisonian crisis) is a medical emergency requiring intravenous hydrocortisone and intravenous fluids (5% glucose in isotonic saline) followed by large, and then gradually reducing, daily doses of hydrocortisone by mouth. It may follow the sudden stoppage of corticosteroid drugs in a patient who has been on regular daily dosage with them.

Defective production of adrenocortical hormones

Defective production of 'normal' adrenocortical hormones due to some enzyme deficiency in the adrenal gland from birth or developing in infancy may cause an over-production of ACTH by the pituitary gland. This results in over-stimulation of the adrenal gland and the formation of adrenal hormones to the point where the production can go no further because of a deficiency of the appropriate enzymes. This may cause all kinds of problems because various hormones are affected at various stages in their production. This may result in an over-production of sex hormones, resulting in masculinized female babies with cliteral enlargement and fusion of the labia of the vagina so that they look like little boys. If the affected babies grow into early childhood they may develop early puberty (precocious puberty). However, their growth becomes stunted because their precocious puberty causes the long bones to stop growing. Mild cases may develop in very early puberty, with the result that the children grow very tall and develop early sexual drive (libido).

Corticosteroids

The cortex part of the adrenal glands (which lie on either side of the body just above the kidneys) produces a number of hormones, which belong to a large group of chemicals called *steroids*. The steroids produced by the adrenal cortex are referred to as *adrenocortical steroids* because they are made by the adrenal cortex. They are divided into three groups according to their principal effects upon the body: glucocorticosteroids, mineralocorticosteroids and sex hormones.

Glucocorticosteroids

Those adrenocortical steroids that principally affect the use of sugar, protein and calcium in the body are called glucocorticosteroids. They are very important because they also help to combat the effects of injury and stress. They are frequently used in medical treatment to reduce the immune response, to relieve inflammation and to relieve allergic symptoms. They include hydrocortisone and cortisone (which is broken down in the liver to hydrocortisone). The shortened term *corticosteroids* (or even 'steroids') is often used to refer to these adrenocortical steroids.

Mineralocorticosteroids

Another group of adrenocortical steroids principally affect water and salt in the body, and these are called mineralocorticosteroids. They include deoxycortone and aldosterone.

Sex hormones

The third group of adrenocortical steroids affect sexual development and are called sex hormones. They are produced by the adrenal cortex and are in addition to those produced by the sex glands (testes and ovaries). Although some female sex hormones (oestrogens) are produced by the adrenals, the principal ones are male sex hormones (androgens). This is why women with over-active adrenal glands may develop beards and a deep voice in addition to other problems.

The use of corticosteroids to relieve inflammation

In the late 1940s the anti-inflammatory effects of the adrenocortical hormone cortisone were discovered, and it was introduced onto the market as a 'wonder drug' for the treatment of rheumatoid arthritis. Also introduced was adrenocorticotrophic hormone (ACTH), which is produced by the pituitary gland and stimulates the adrenal glands to produce cortisone.

For the first time, drugs were available that had a dramatic effect in relieving inflammation of joints in rheumatoid arthritis. Their use was quickly extended to the treatment of other inflammatory and allergic diseases. The media coverage was extensive and they soon became widely used and over-used, which led to many patients developing serious problems due to the harmful effects of these drugs. This was because cortisone (and ACTH) not only reduce inflammation but they also produce many other effects on various chemical processes in the body, particularly those involved with sugar, protein, salt and calcium metabolism. These 'other' effects on the body resulted in many patients suffering from unwanted effects as a result of being given too large a daily dose for too long. Serious harmful effects also occurred if treatments were stopped suddenly because this can have disastrous consequences (see later).

The harmful effects of cortisone and its dramatic effects in reducing inflammation led drug companies to search for synthetic corticosteroids that would have reduced effects upon the chemical processes of the body (metabolic effects) and, hopefully, be more specific in their effects upon inflammation. In this search they have been successful and there are corticosteroid drugs now available whose anti-inflammatory effects are greater than their metabolic effects when used in recommended doses. However, the message is clear: in the doses used to relieve inflammation, corticosteroids are potentially *harmful* drugs; if used over prolonged periods of time, they may produce slow and increasing damage to many tissues and organs in the body and may result in *serious harm* to the patient.

Corticosteroids – risk of high dosage and/or prolonged treatment

High doses and/or prolonged treatment may produce an exaggeration of some of the normal actions of corticosteroids.

The prolonged use of high daily doses of corticosteroids produces Cushing's syndrome, see page 828.

Effects on water and salts

Corticosteroids cause an increase in salt (sodium chloride) retention by the kidneys, which leads to an increase in the fluid volume of the body because, if salt is retained by the kidneys, water is retained. This leads to a rise in blood pressure, and a gain in weight, which may trigger heart failure in a susceptible person. In addition, they result in a loss of potassium by the kidneys which causes a low blood potassium (hypokalaemia), which may in turn produce apathy, muscular weakness and mental confusion.

Effects on glucose

Corticosteroids increase the production of glucose by the liver but decrease its use by the body for energy. This causes an increase in the blood glucose level (hyperglycaemia) and glucose appears in the urine (glycosuria). In people prone to develop diabetes, corticosteroids may trigger the disease. In diabetic patients, corticosteroids may increase their daily requirements for insulin or oral anti-diabetic drugs.

Effects on protein and muscles

The normal use of protein in the body is reduced by corticosteroids and their breakdown is increased. This produces protein loss from the body, leading to muscle weakness and wasting. In addition, the protein framework of bone is weakened through protein loss, and bones become soft (see effects on bone, later).

High doses of corticosteroids may occasionally produce marked weakness of muscles, particularly those in the upper arms and legs, shoulders and pelvis. This is known as steroid myopathy and may be associated with a reduction in the size of the affected muscles (loss of muscle mass).

Effects on the skin

Because of protein loss, the skin wastes (skin atrophy), producing stretch-like marks (striae) in the skin rather like stretch marks seen after pregnancy. Protein loss also weakens the walls of small blood vessels, which become fragile and burst easily, producing bruising (ecchymosis). The skin becomes fragile, and corticosteroids interfere with healing. They may increase sweating and flushing of the face and an increase or decrease in skin pigmentation. Acne may develop.

NOTE Even the small doses of corticosteroids used in inhalations may, over time, cause thinning of the skin and purpura.

Effects on fat

Fat deposits in the body become redistributed away from the arms and legs into deposits on the face (producing a 'moon' face), on the back of the neck and around the neck (producing a 'buffalo hump') and on the abdomen.

Effects on inflammation

Corticosteroids suppress inflammation by preventing the release of inflammation-producing chemicals. They relieve the redness, swelling, local heat and tenderness of inflammation. They stop the processes of inflammation whatever the cause, whether mechanical, chemical, immunological, infectious or allergic. In other words, and this is important to understand, they stop or suppress inflammation but they do *not* cure the underlying cause. The inflammatory symptoms of the underlying disease may disappear but the disease itself is not affected. However, this suppression of the symptoms of inflammation can be life saving in some patients even though it may produce problems in others.

Warnings *Normally, we have to rely on the signs and symptoms of inflammation (e.g. swelling, pain) to know that something is wrong; likewise the doctor has to rely on the signs and symptoms of inflammation to make a diagnosis. If these are absent because they have been suppressed by corticosteroids, the underlying disease may be masked and this may have serious consequences. For example, in a patient who is taking corticosteroids, an underlying infection (e.g. tuberculosis) may actually progress without producing symptoms and this may be very dangerous.*

Corticosteroids may interfere with skin tests for allergies by reducing the response. They may also interfere with the body's response to immunization and vaccinations.

Effects on bone

Because of protein loss the protein framework of bone is weakened. In addition, corticosteroids reduce the absorption of calcium from the intestine and this leads to a reduction in the concentration of calcium in the body. This stimulates the parathyroid glands to produce a hormone that takes calcium from bone in order to maintain the blood calcium level. This hormone stimulates those cells in bone that actually dissolve bone (osteoclasts). This produces softening of the bones, which is made worse by the fact that corticosteroids also block the action of bone-forming cells (osteoblasts). They produce two actions that soften bones – decreased bone formation and increased bone loss (resorption). The softening of the bones is called osteoporosis. It particularly affects the vertebrae of the spine, which may collapse and cause pain and arching of the back. The softening may also affect the ribs, producing pain and predisposing to fractures of the ribs. The long bones of the arms and legs are more prone to fracture, and the hip and shoulder joints may be damaged due to crumbling of the head of the bones – the femur and humerus respectively. For a further discussion of osteoporosis, see Chapter 68.

Effects on growth

Corticosteroids slow down cell division and may arrest bone growth in children. Relatively small doses in children may produce stunted growth (see later).

Effects on mental state

Corticosteroids may affect behaviour, leading to nervousness, insomnia and mood changes. Serious mental illness may occasionally develop, including, in some patients, symptoms of schizophrenia or manic–depression. A patient's mood may be so affected by corticosteroids that he or she may attempt suicide. On the other hand, some patients may develop a feeling of extreme well-being (euphoria).

Effects on the eyes

High doses of corticosteroids over prolonged periods of time may occasionally lead to the development of cataracts in adults. These have also been reported in children. They may also increase the pressure inside the eyes and cause glaucoma. Occasionally, they may cause the eye to protrude (exophthalmos).

Effects on menstrual periods

Corticosteroids may cause the periods to become scanty and/or irregular.

Effects on sex life

Corticosteroids may reduce libido and produce impotence.

Effects on the brain

Corticosteroids may increase the pressure of the fluid inside the brain, producing symptoms that could be mistaken for a tumour. Rarely, they produce headaches, vertigo and convulsions.

Allergy

Rarely, corticosteroid injections may produce allergic skin rashes (e.g. nettle rash) and severe allergic reactions (anaphylactic reactions).

Effects on the body's response to stress

The production of corticosteroids by the adrenal glands is under the control of the anterior lobe of the pituitary gland in the brain. This is the master gland and if the blood level of corticosteroids falls, the pituitary gland produces a hormone – adrenocorticotrophin (ACTH) – that stimulates the adrenal glands to produce more. If the blood level of corticosteroids is high, the pituitary gland reduces its production of the ACTH so that the adrenal glands reduce their production of corticosteroids. In this way, a careful balance is always maintained. In addition to responding to the blood level of corticosteroids produced by the adrenal glands, ACTH is also released in response to stress (e.g. injury, infection, surgery). This is because the body requires more corticosteroids at times of stress in order to gear up the body ready to cope.

If an individual is taking high doses of corticosteroids for a prolonged period of time, the pituitary gland stops producing ACTH in response to the very high blood levels of these drugs. The adrenal glands then shrink from disuse. This means that such people are not able to produce corticosteroids in response to stress, and when exposed to injury, infections or surgery they may occasionally collapse. To avoid such dangers, these individuals will need increased doses of corticosteroid drugs if they are injured, develop an infection or undergo a surgical operation.

Warning *It may take up to 2 years for the pituitary and adrenal glands to return to normal functioning after just 1 month's treatment with a corticosteroid. Therefore the same dangers and warnings discussed above apply equally to anyone who has taken a corticosteroid by mouth regularly every day for 1 month or more at any time in the previous 2 years. In the event of accident or surgery, their response to stress will need boosting with extra hydrocortisone. People who have received a corticosteroid daily for 1 month or more should carry their steroid warning card with them at all times for 2 years after they stopped such treatment.*

Effects on the stomach

Most doctors consider that corticosteroids increase the risk of developing peptic ulcers and increase the risk of bleeding and perforation in patients who suffer from peptic ulcer. Unfortunately, information from adequate and well controlled studies of these dangers is lacking, but what information is available suggests that corticosteroids may cause ulcer problems – particularly in people who have a peptic ulcer or have had one in the past. The danger appears to be related to the daily dose and length of treatment – the higher the daily dose and the longer the treatment, the greater the risk. Special coated tablets (enteric coated) which release the corticosteroid in the intestine rather than in the stomach do not appear to help reduce the dangers. Another way of trying to prevent ulceration of the stomach is to give, in addition, a drug that is used to treat peptic ulcers. However, we need more evidence on whether giving such a drug (e.g. an H_2 blocker) with a corticosteroid helps to prevent an ulcer from developing or recurring.

There is no convincing evidence that peptic ulcers caused by corticosteroids heal more slowly or bleed or perforate more easily than other peptic ulcers.

Withdrawal effects

Because corticosteroid drugs suppress the production of naturally occurring corticosteroids, any withdrawal of these drugs leaves the individual without any corticosteroids. This may produce fever, painful muscles, painful joints, runny nose, conjunctivitis, loss of weight and malaise. Rarely, there may be raised pressure in the brain and swelling of the back of the eyes (papilloedema).

The *sudden* stopping of corticosteroids in someone who has been taking them daily for months to years may trigger a major crisis similar to that produced when the adrenal glands are damaged (adrenal crisis). The individual suddenly develops nausea, vomiting and abdominal pain and becomes cold, pale, restless and sweating; the blood pressure falls and the pulse becomes feeble and rapid – in other words the patient is in a state of collapse or clinical shock and requires *urgent* treatment.

Warnings on the use of corticosteroids

Corticosteroid drugs should not be used, or should be used with utmost caution, in patients suffering from an infection, unless specific anti-infective treatment is given. They should not be given to people who have been immunized with a live virus (e.g. poliomyelitis). Corticosteroids may impair ability to resist infection and they may mask the signs and symptoms of underlying infections (see earlier).

Prolonged treatment with corticosteroids reduces the body's ability to respond to stress (e.g. injury, infection, surgery) and an increased dose should always be given at these times (see earlier).

Corticosteroids may trigger diabetes in a susceptible person, and they increase requirements for insulin or oral anti-diabetic drugs in diabetic people receiving treatment.

Corticosteroids by mouth or by injection should be avoided in anyone suffering from psoriasis because, if the drug is stopped or the dose reduced, the condition may flare up and become very much worse and very much more difficult to treat.

Corticosteroids should be withdrawn gradually (see earlier).

Corticosteroids should be used with caution in people with peptic ulcers, osteoporosis, raised blood pressure, glaucoma, epilepsy, under-active thyroid, serious mental illness, serious kidney disorders (e.g. chronic nephritis), secondary cancer, cirrhosis of the liver, thrombophlebitis or skin rashes caused by infectious diseases (e.g. measles), and in pregnancy.

Risks in elderly people

Harmful effects from corticosteroids may be more frequent and severe in elderly people, particularly the risks of fluid retention (oedema), effects on the stomach (see earlier), risks of producing cataracts and the risks of bone softening (osteoporosis).

Risks with anaesthetics

In addition to the risks of surgery in a patient on long-term treatment with corticosteroids, there is an additional risk that an anaesthetic may cause a serious fall in blood pressure during and just after the operation. Anaesthetists should always check whether a patient is taking corticosteroids. Always carry your steroid treatment card with you at all times.

Risks in children

Prolonged use of corticosteroids in children causes stunting of growth and should be avoided if possible. The harmful effect on growth may be reduced by using ACTH or by giving the corticosteroid as a single dose in the mornings on alternate days. Treatment with growth hormone has no effect on this stunting because corticosteroids affect the metabolism of cartilage.

NOTE High doses of corticosteroids by inhalation (to treat asthma) may stunt growth.

Risks with immunizations and vaccinations

Corticosteroid drugs may interfere with the body's response to immunizations and vaccinations.

Adrenocorticotrophic hormone (ACTH, corticotrophin)

This is a very complex chemical produced by the anterior lobe of the pituitary gland. The pure substance was isolated from the pituitary glands of slaughtered animals in the 1940s and it was first synthesized 20 years later. The synthetic preparations are less likely to cause allergic reactions because they are not contaminated with animal protein. ACTH stimulates the adrenal glands to produce corticosteroids (the most important of which is hydrocortisone) and, to a lesser extent, male sex hormones (androgens).

The principal effects of ACTH are those of corticosteroids. Therefore, it should not be used with the idea that it will have selective anti-inflammatory effects – it will always cause disturbances of salt and water balance. ACTH is inactive when given by mouth and has to be given by injection. When given by intravenous injection it produces rapid effects which quickly wear off. Its effects may be prolonged by giving the injection under the skin or into a muscle, but even then they last for only about 6 hours.

ACTH is occasionally used to treat adrenal deficiency disorders (e.g. Addison's disease) and disorders that respond to corticosteroids. Because it does not produce disuse changes in the adrenals, it is easier to withdraw ACTH than corticosteroids and therefore it may be of use in short-term treatment. However, in the long term it is not as useful because it is not as selective and it has to be given by injection.

ACTH may produce the harmful effects described under corticosteroids; in particular, diabetes may be made worse and insulin dosage may have to be increased. High blood pressure occurs more often but stomach troubles are less frequent. It may produce allergic reactions and increase skin pigmentation, and long-term use may cause the adrenal glands to undergo changes of 'over-use' and the pituitary changes of 'under-use'. Therefore, it should always be withdrawn slowly after long-term use. ACTH on alternate days is sometimes used in children to try to reduce the possibility of growth retardation, which may occur on regular daily use of corticosteroids.

A long-acting ACTH injection is available (Acthar Gel injection). Tetracosactrin (Synacthen and Synacthen Depot), a synthetic polypeptide resembling ACTH, is used for diagnosis and treatment.

Different corticosteroid preparations produce different degrees of effect on the body's chemistry

Fludrocortisone and deoxycortone produce the most harmful effects on the body's chemistry. Cortisone, hydrocortisone, ACTH and tetracosactrin are less harmful, and betamethasone, dexamethasone, methylprednisolone and triamcinolone produce the least harmful effects on the body's chemistry. The commonly used prednisolone produces only slight effects on the body's chemistry. However, in the end it is how safely these drugs are prescribed that increases the benefits and reduces the risks.

Replacement treatment with corticosteroids

Replacement treatment with corticosteroids is necessary in people who are not able to make adequate amounts themselves because of some disorder of their adrenal glands. These individuals will require corticosteroids in doses sufficient to meet their normal requirements – what is called physiological replacement dosages. They will require both a glucocorticosteroid (e.g. hydrocortisone) and a mineralocorticosteroid (e.g. fludrocortisone) by mouth every day. Patients will also require corticosteroid replacement treatment if they have undergone surgical removal of their adrenal glands.

In acute insufficiency (e.g. stopping corticosteroids abruptly) hydrocortisone should be given intravenously.

People suffering from adrenal insufficiency due to inactivity of the pituitary gland will need hydrocortisone maintenance treatment but may not need a mineralocorticosteroid because the production of aldosterone is under the control of the renin–angiotensin system (see Chapter 21). They may also require thyroid hormone and sex hormones.

Use of corticosteroids in stress

Early in this chapter I gave attention to the problems that may occur in patients who have been on long-term treatment (1 month or more) with corticosteroids. 'Normal' people who develop a serious infection or injury or who have a surgical operation produce an extra amount of corticosteroids daily in order to protect themselves during this period. Usually they produce about 300 mg of hydrocortisone in a 24 hour period during the time of the stress. Once the stress is over they revert to producing normal amounts of hydrocortisone, which averages about 20 mg every 24 hours. To compensate for this loss in production at the time of stress, patients taking corticosteroid drugs should be given an injection of hydrocortisone (100 mg) into a muscle just before a surgical operation or if they are injured or develop an infection. This dose should be repeated 8-hourly (by mouth if possible) for 24 hours and then halved every 24 hours until the normal maintenance dose is reached on about the fifth day after the operation – this is usually 25 mg daily of hydrocortisone in patients receiving replacement treatment because of some disease of their adrenal glands, and about 7.5 mg of prednisolone or its equivalent in patients on long-term anti-inflammatory or anti-allergic treatment with corticosteroids.

Suppressive treatment with corticosteroids

The major uses of corticosteroids are to suppress inflammation, to suppress allergic responses and to suppress immune responses. As stated earlier, corticosteroids are available whose anti-inflammatory and other suppressive effects are greater than their effects on salt and water balance and other chemical processes in the body (see earlier). However, these unwanted effects may easily occur if they are used in too high a dose and too regularly.

Equivalent anti-inflammatory doses of those corticosteroids commonly used are:

betamethasone	0.75 mg
cortisone	25.00 mg
dexamethasone	0.75 mg
hydrocortisone	20.00 mg
methylprednisolone	4.00 mg
prednisolone	5.00 mg
prednisone*	5.00 mg
triamcinolone	4.00 mg

* Prednisone is converted to prednisolone in the liver.

In emergencies hydrocortisone is injected into a vein; for example, to treat severe allergic reactions and in severe attacks of asthma – but it does not work immediately.

The corticosteroids most commonly used by mouth to continue treatment are prednisolone, betamethasone and dexamethasone. These are equally effective but prednisolone is the most commonly used.

Corticosteroids suppress inflammation and allergic reactions, and are used to relieve symptoms in disorders such as rheumatoid arthritis, ulcerative colitis and Crohn's disease, certain types of asthma and chronic chest disorders, skin diseases, aphthous ulcers in the mouth, various immune diseases and some cancers.

Balancing the benefits and risks of corticosteroids

Corticosteroid treatments are always a balance of benefits to risks for the particular individual being treated; they should not be used in high doses over prolonged periods of time. The dangers of long-term regular daily use of corticosteroids by mouth should always be carefully considered. The optimal daily dose of prednisolone is 7.5 mg and the dose should not exceed 10 mg daily (or the equivalent dose of one of the other corticosteroids). A single (higher) dose on alternate days, rather than daily may help to prevent the adrenal glands from shrinking. Because the adrenal glands are most active at night, it will also help if daily doses (or doses on alternate days) are given in the mornings. They should be used in the minimum dose possible to achieve maximum benefit. This can often be better achieved by targeting the drug locally – for example, using an inhaler to treat asthma, using an enema to treat ulcerative colitis, or using topical applications to treat skin disorders.

Corticosteroids can be life saving in some serious conditions but more often they are used to relieve symptoms. They do not cure or stop the progression of disorders such as rheumatoid arthritis, and some patients have suffered more from the over-use of corticosteroids than from their underlying disease.

Table 62.1 Corticosteroid preparations (by mouth and injection)

Preparation	*Drug*	*Dosage form*
Betnelan	betamethasone (glucocorticoid)	Tablets
Betnesol	betamethasone (glucocorticoid)	Soluble tablets, injection
Cortisone	cortisone (glucocorticoid–mineralocorticoid)	Tablets
Cortistab	cortisone (glucocorticoid–mineralocorticoid)	Tablets
Cortisyl	cortisone (glucocorticoid–mineralocorticoid)	Tablets
Decadron	dexamethasone (glucocorticoid)	Tablets, injection
Decadron Shock-Pak	dexamethasone (glucocorticoid)	Injection (intravenous)
Decortisyl	prednisone (glucocorticoid)	Tablets
Deltacortril	prednisolone (glucocorticoid)	Enteric-coated tablets
Deltastab	prednisolone (glucocorticoid)	Tablets, injection
Depo-Medrone	methylprednisolone (glucocorticoid)	Injection
dexamethasone	dexamethasone (glucocorticoid)	Tablets
Efcortelan Soluble	hydrocortisone (glucocorticoid–mineralocorticoid)	Injection (powder in vial)
Efcortesol	hydrocortisone (glucocorticoid–mineralocorticoid)	Injection
Florinef	fludrocortisone (mineralocorticoid)	Tablets
hydrocortisone	hydrocortisone (glucocorticoid–mineralocorticoid)	Tablets, injection (powder in vial)
Hydrocortistab	hydrocortisone (glucocorticoid–mineralocorticoid)	Tablets, injection
Hydrocortone	hydrocortisone (glucocorticoid–mineralocorticoid)	Tablets
Kenalog	triamcinolone (glucocorticoid)	Injection
Ledercort	triamcinolone (glucocorticoid)	Tablets
Medrone	methylprednisolone (glucocorticoid)	Tablets

Table 62.1 Corticosteroid preparations (by mouth and injection) (*cont.*)

Preparation	*Drug*	*Dosage form*
Precortisyl	prednisolone (glucocorticoid)	Tablets
Precortisyl Forte	prednisolone (glucocorticoid)	Tablets
Prednesol	prednisolone (glucocorticoid)	Tablets
prednisolone	prednisolone (glucocorticoid)	Tablets, enteric-coated tablets (prednisolone EC)
prednisone	prednisone (glucocorticoid)	Tablets
Sintisone	prednisolone (glucocorticoid)	Tablets
Solu-Cortef	hydrocortisone (glucocorticoid–mineralocorticoid)	Injection (powder in vial)
Solu-Medrone	methylprednisolone (glucocorticoid)	Injection (powder in vial)

NOTE For corticosteroid preparations injected directly into joints, see Chapter 30.

63

Thyroid disorders

Functions of the thyroid gland

The thyroid gland is in the neck, in front and on both sides of the windpipe (the trachea) below the voicebox (the larynx). It produces two hormones, called thyroxine and triiodothyronine, which determine the rate of chemical processes that occur in the body (metabolism) and exert control over the burning up of oxygen by cells to release energy. In babies, infants and children these hormones are also essential for physical and mental growth and development through their control of the body's use of proteins and their effects on the brain and nervous system.

The thyroid gland also produces another hormone, calcitonin, which is involved in the control of calcium levels in the blood and bone formation.

The role of iodine

Iodine is essential for the production of thyroid hormones. The thyroid gland takes up iodine from the blood stream and concentrates it before using it to produce hormones. This is why radioactive iodine is useful in the treatment of an over-active thyroid gland (see later).

Control of the thyroid gland

Thyroid function is under the control of the anterior lobe of the pituitary gland, which produces a thyroid-stimulating hormone called thyrotrophin, or TSH for short. The release of TSH by the pituitary is governed by a part of the brain, called the hypothalamus, which produces thyrotrophin-releasing hormone (TRH). There is a feedback mechanism produced by the levels of thyroid hormones in the blood stream: if they are high TSH production is decreased; and if they are low, it is increased. TSH works directly on the thyroid gland and controls the release of thyroid hormones into the blood stream. It also controls the uptake of iodine by the gland.

Over-active thyroid gland

Over-activity of the thyroid gland is called *thyrotoxicosis* or *hyperthyroidism*. There are two main types of thyrotoxicosis. One is a diffuse enlargement of the thyroid gland that occurs early in adult life, particularly in women, and is often called Graves' disease. The other type occurs in older adults and is associated with a lumpy (nodular) enlargement of the thyroid gland.

Graves' disease is due to an abnormal defence response (immune response) by the body. In this disease, antibodies are produced that stimulate the receptors in the thyroid gland normally stimulated by TSH. This makes the gland over-work even though blood tests show the levels of TSH to be reduced or not detectable. People who develop this disease appear to be predisposed to it because of some genetic factor.

Thyrotoxicosis which develops due to nodular swellings of the thyroid is probably due to repeated stimulation of a nodular goitre (see later) – it is usually called *thyrotoxic nodular goitre* or *toxic nodular goitre*.

Symptoms

The symptoms of thyrotoxicosis include loss of weight despite a good appetite. This is due to an increase in the burning up of the body's stores of energy sources. Thyroid hormones also increase the actions of adrenaline-like substances in the body and produce rapid beating of the heart, palpitations, trembling, sweating, diarrhoea and nervousness.

People with Graves' disease may develop protrusion of their eyeballs (exophthalmos). This complication is much less common in those suffering from a toxic nodular goitre. Exophthalmos may be an autoimmune response, and some individuals with severe exophthalmos improve with corticosteroid therapy (e.g. intravenous methylprednisolone).

Treatment

There are two stages to the treatment of over-active thyroid gland. The first is to use drugs to reduce the over-activity and to relieve the symptoms. The second stage is long term and involves a choice from three types of treatment – the continued use of anti-thyroid drugs, the use of radioactive iodine to destroy the gland or surgical removal of part of the gland.

First stage of treatment

The first stage of treatment involves the use of anti-thyroid drugs and beta blocker drugs.

Anti-thyroid drugs (carbimazole (Neo-Mercazole) and propylthiouracil)

Two drugs are currently in fashion for treating thyrotoxicosis: carbimazole and propylthiouracil. They interfere with the use of iodine by the thyroid gland and block the production of thyroid hormones. Unfortunately, they may, rarely, damage the blood-forming tissues in the bone marrow and cause a serious reduction in white blood cells (agranulocytosis), which lowers the patient's resistance to infection and may result in recurrent fevers and sore throats. It occurs more frequently in the first few months of treatment. This serious complication may develop rapidly and routine blood tests do not pick it up quickly enough. It is therefore best for the patient to rely on early warning symptoms of a sore throat and fever and to stop the drug immediately these symptoms develop. Full recovery usually follows and alternative treatments should then be given.

Initial treatment with anti-thyroid drugs Improvement with anti-thyroid drug treatment occurs over a period of about 8 weeks and is judged by the relief of symptoms, a fall in pulse rate, and the loss of weight stops. In addition, it is helpful to measure the levels of thyroid hormone, thyroid-stimulating hormone or thyroid-stimulating hormone receptor antibodies in the blood in order to assess progress. Starting doses are usually high in order to achieve a speedy response, and then the daily dose is slowly reduced depending upon the response of the patient.

Once the patient settles down, the aim of treatment is to maintain the thyroid gland in a fairly 'normal' state of activity (euthyroid state) for the smallest daily dosage of drug as possible. Some people recover completely after one course of treatment whereas others may need further treatment. *Protruding eyes* (exophthalmos) is not improved by anti-thyroid drugs but they may prevent it from getting worse.

Need for patient education Improvement depends particularly upon whether the patient takes the treatment as directed. Good compliance with treatment requires that a patient has a good understanding of the disorder and of the benefits and risks of taking anti-thyroid drugs. This means that there must be good communication between the doctor and the patient.

Beta blockers

These drugs (e.g. propranolol) are discussed in detail in Chapter 20. In severe thyrotoxicosis they relieve the symptoms of anxiety, palpitations, increased bowel activity and tremor. They are useful for treating severe symptoms of thyrotoxicosis, particularly at the start of treatment while waiting for anti-thyroid drugs to produce their benefits. However, it is important to note that, although they relieve these symptoms, they have no effect on the thyroid gland and thyroid hormone production. Furthermore, they have no effect on the increased activity of cells throughout the body, which continue to burn up oxygen at an increased rate despite the reduced blood supply to tissues created by the beta blockers. In mild to moderate thyrotoxicosis they make it difficult to assess the underlying response to anti-thyroid drugs, which relies on an improvement in the symptoms that beta blockers relieve.

Long-term treatment with anti-thyroid drugs

Patients improve significantly during the first few months of treatment with anti-thyroid drugs. However, after this initial phase, opinion is divided about the benefits of the long-term use of anti-thyroid drugs. These drugs do not cure the disease. They decrease thyroid hormone production and relieve symptoms, which will help those people in whom the underlying thyrotoxicosis is going to burn out of its own accord (i.e. undergo a natural remission). Such a remission can be predicted if the individual shows good improvement despite a reduction in dosage and if the gland gets smaller.

If thyroid hormone levels increase when the dose is decreased, it is unlikely that the individual is going to develop a remission, and will therefore require surgery. Unfortunately, there is no way of predicting before treatment is started which patients are going to go into a natural remission. However, 'natural remission' may represent a progressive change from over-activity of the thyroid gland to under-activity. In other words, if left alone would some people with over-active thyroid glands slowly develop under-active glands? It is doubtful if we will ever know because sufferers from thyrotoxicosis usually need treatment to relieve their distressing symptoms and because virtually all of them receive some sort of treatment from their doctors.

Anti-thyroid drug treatment in adults should not be continued for more than 1–2 years, after which time alternative treatment (surgery or radioactive iodine) should be considered.

Potassium perchlorate should not be used Potassium perchlorate and related drugs interfere with the concentration of iodine in the thyroid gland and have been used over the past few decades to treat over-active thyroid gland. Fortunately, they have now gone out of fashion because they damage the blood-forming tissues in the bone marrow and produce severe blood disorders. They should not be used.

Iodine

Iodine is the oldest treatment for thyroid disorders. In an over-active gland it produces a rapid improvement (within 24 hours) and after 10–15 days of daily treatment the individual is greatly improved. Unfortunately, this improvement does not continue and the over-activity returns and is sometimes much worse. Iodine is therefore useful only for preparing patients for surgical removal of part of the thyroid gland and in a thyroid emergency – what is called a thyroid crisis or thyroid storm (see later).

Harmful effects of iodine Occasionally, patients may develop an acute allergy to iodine if it is injected into a vein. They develop a swelling of the throat and run a risk of suffocating. They may also develop bleeding into the skin, painful joints, fever and enlarged lymph glands. Regular daily use of iodine by mouth over a prolonged period of time may cause iodine intoxication (iodism) with symptoms like a severe cold, sore mouth and gums and a sore throat. The symptoms disappear within a few days of stopping the drug.

Radioactive iodine

Radioactive iodine is treated by the body like ordinary iodine. It is taken up and concentrated in the thyroid gland where its radiation destroys the thyroid tissues. With a carefully selected dose of radioactive iodine (iodine$_{131}$) it is possible to knock out the thyroid gland completely without damaging the surrounding tissues. This is because 90 per cent of the rays are beta rays which penetrate only as far as half a millimetre.

Anti-thyroid drugs are usually given for a month or two before radioactive iodine treatment in order to relieve symptoms. They are stopped during the week of treatment and, according to the individual's symptoms, they are sometimes re-started for a further month or two.

In about 80 per cent of patients an appropriate dose of radioactive iodine will stop the thyroid gland from over-working within about 6 months. The remaining 20 per cent will need a second course of treatment with radioactive iodine. At least 6 months should be allowed from the first treatment with radioactive iodine before a second dose is considered.

Harmful effects of radioactive iodine The principal complication of radioactive iodine treatment is that it results in under-activity of the gland (hypothyroidism, see later). This occurs in about 10 per cent of patients in the first year and increases by 5 per cent per year up to about 20 years.

Despite fears, the use of radioactive iodine since the 1940s has produced no increased risk of developing cancer of the thyroid gland or leukaemia.

Wider use of radioactive iodine For years it was agreed that radioactive iodine should be reserved for patients over the age of 45 years and should not be used for anyone under this age, particularly in women of child-bearing age. However, it is now considered safe in women under the age of 45 years if they are not pregnant and take precautions not to get pregnant for at least 6 months after treatment. These precautions are to prevent any possible damage to eggs in the ovaries, which may affect the baby if a woman does get pregnant.

The radiation risk to the ovaries from radioactive iodine treatment of the thyroid gland is no greater than from a special X-ray of the stomach (a barium meal). Radioactive iodine treatment is dangerous to the unborn baby because it crosses the placenta and enters the baby's blood stream; it is picked up and concentrated in the baby's thyroid gland and destroys it.

Patient education Patients should fully understand that radioactive iodine destroys thyroid tissue and that between 80 and 100 per cent of them will eventually develop signs and symptoms of under-active thyroid gland (hypothyroidism). They should understand the benefits and risks of treatment, why treatment is needed and the early signs of under-active thyroid gland. They must also understand that they will need to be checked up at regular intervals (about every 6 months) until hypothyroidism appears and is then treated with thyroid hormones. (For symptoms of hypothyroidism, see later.)

This advice requires good communication between the doctor and the patient, which should be both oral and written. Unfortunately, this sometimes does not happen and patients slip into hypothyroidism and develop all kinds of problems for themselves and their relatives which could easily have been prevented by the appropriate use of thyroid hormones in the right dose, at the right time for each particular patient.

Over-active thyroid gland in pregnancy

The peak incidence of Graves' disease is in women of child-bearing age, so it is not that uncommon for a woman suffering from the disease to become pregnant. Depending on the severity of the disease, there is a risk of abortion and of a thyroid crisis (storm) during labour. These risks have to be balanced against the benefits and risks of using available treatment to control the over-active thyroid gland.

Obviously, radioactive iodine is out of the question because it will destroy the unborn baby's thyroid gland; and here it is well to remember that thyroid hormones are essential for growth and development, particularly of the brain and nervous system. Anti-thyroid drugs offer the treatment of choice but their risks must be balanced with any expected benefits, bearing in mind that they enter the baby's blood stream and block the production of thyroid hormones by the baby's thyroid, which may result in a goitre (see later). This must be balanced against the fact that excess thyroid hormones being produced by the mother's thyroid gland do not enter the baby's blood stream and do not harm the baby.

Of the two anti-thyroid drugs available, carbimazole and propylthiouracil, the latter is safer because in some newly born babies carbimazole has been found to cause a circular patch of baldness and skin damage on the baby's head (aplasia cutis). Clearly, propylthiouracil should be given in the lowest dose possible to bring the thyroid down to 'normal' functioning. Preferably, it should be stopped in the last 3 weeks of the pregnancy in order to stop the baby being born with a goitre. If anti-thyroid drugs are continued after the pregnancy, the baby must not be breast fed because the drugs enter the milk and can affect the baby's thyroid gland.

If a pregnant woman does not respond well to anti-thyroid drugs, part of the gland should be removed surgically sometime during the middle 3 months of the pregnancy, the patient having first had a course of anti-thyroid drugs and iodine (see later).

Over-active thyroid gland in children

Radioactive iodine should not be given to children and young adults, and surgical removal of part of the gland is often not as successful in relieving symptoms as it is in adults. The only treatment that is left is the anti-thyroid drugs – carbimazole or propylthiouracil. These may have to be continued for as many years as is necessary until they are not needed or until surgery or radioactive iodine can be given.

Thyroid crisis (or storm)

Some patients may suffer very severe symptoms of thyrotoxicosis, triggered by some stress or infection. They develop a high temperature, abdominal pain, exhaustion, delirium, delusions, mania, dehydration and heart failure.

This is called a thyroid crisis or storm. It may also occur after thyroid surgery if the pre-surgery treatment was not adequate, or after any surgical procedure if the over-activity of the thyroid gland was not recognized and treated.

Treatment involves the use of intravenous fluids and glucose, hydrocortisone and iodine (as potassium iodide), propylthiouracil by mouth, external cooling, paracetamol or chlorpromazine to help to bring the temperature down, and propranolol and digoxin if heart failure is present. Any precipitating cause such as an infection should be treated. However, the best treatment is prevention, or at least early recognition, because the condition may be fatal.

Surgery

Surgical removal of part of the thyroid gland is very effective treatment. Over-activity of the gland (thyrotoxicosis) rarely recurs but about half of the patients ultimately develop under-activity (hypothyroidism) and will need thyroid hormone treatment for the rest of their lives.

Anti-thyroid drugs should be used for about 1–2 months before surgery until the thyroid is working at a 'normal' level (euthyroid); then iodine is given every day for about 7–10 days in order to reduce the blood supply in the gland which is very high when the gland is over-working. If patients cannot take anti-thyroid drugs because they are allergic to them or have developed some other harmful effect, iodine alone may be used before surgery. Alternatively, iodine may be combined with a beta blocker (e.g. propranolol) for 1–2 weeks.

Table 63.1 Drugs used to treat over-active thyroid gland – harmful effects and warnings

carbimazole (Neo-Mercazole)
Harmful effects usually occur in the first 8 weeks of treatment. They are usually mild and transient, and include nausea, headache, stomach upsets, joint pains, skin rashes and itching. Occasionally, hair loss may occur. Rarely, damage to the bone marrow may produce a reduction in white blood cells.

Warnings Carbimazole must not be used in anyone who has previously had harmful effects from the drug, or whose thyroid gland is pressing on the windpipe because treatment may worsen this pressure.

Risks in pregnancy Benefits of using carbimazole in pregnancy must be balanced against any potential risks to the baby. Mothers should be carefully monitored; if their condition is satisfactory, treatment should be stopped 3–4 weeks before delivery. The smallest possible effective dose should be used which, preferably, should not exceed 15 mg daily. After childbirth the baby's progress should be carefully monitored for

Table 63.1 Drugs used to treat over-active thyroid gland – harmful effects and warnings (*cont.*)

any evidence of under-activity of the thyroid gland and its effects on development.

iodine (aqueous iodine oral solution, potassium iodide tablets)
Harmful effects include symptoms like a common cold, headache, runny eyes, conjunctivitis, pain in the cheeks (salivary glands), laryngitis, bronchitis and skin rashes. On prolonged treatment, harmful effects include depression, insomnia and impotence.

propylthiouracil
Harmful effects usually occur in the first 8 weeks of treatment. They are usually mild and transient, and include nausea, headache, stomach upsets, joint pains, skin rashes and itching. Occasionally, hair loss may occur. Rarely, there may develop a tendency to bleed easily, and damage to the bone marrow may produce a reduction in white blood cells.

Warnings Propylthiouracil should not be used in people whose thyroid gland is pressing on the windpipe, as the treatment may worsen this pressure. The dose should be reduced in anyone with impaired kidney function.

Risks in pregnancy Benefits of using propylthiouracil in pregnancy must be balanced against any potential risks to the baby. Mothers should be carefully monitored; if the condition is satisfactory, treatment should be stopped 3–4 weeks before delivery. The smallest possible effective dose should be used. After childbirth the baby's progress should be carefully monitored for any evidence of under-activity of the thyroid gland and its effects on development.

Under-active thyroid gland

The term 'hypothyroidism' refers to a condition caused by under-activity of the thyroid gland, whereas the term 'myxoedema' refers to hypothyroidism that is complicated by thickening of the skin. This thickening of the skin is caused by deposits of a protein substance (mucoid) under the skin. Some doctors call severe hypothyroidism 'myxoedema' and so both terms are often used to mean the same disorder; however, 'myxoedema' should not be used unless the individual has the skin changes.

Causes of hypothyroidism

Under-activity of the thyroid gland is almost always due to a disorder of the thyroid gland itself. Very occasionally, it may be due to an under-active pituitary gland (the master gland) or the hypothalamus (the part of the brain that controls the pituitary gland). If the pituitary gland is not working properly, the production of thyroid-stimulating hormone (TSH) is decreased and the thyroid starts to under-work.

A common cause of under-working of the thyroid gland is treatment for over-activity of the gland – for example, anti-thyroid drugs, radioactive iodine and surgical removal of part of the gland.

The thyroid gland may spontaneously start under-working in middle age. This affects women more frequently than men. It may be associated with enlargement of the gland (a goitre) or the gland may shrink (atrophy). The commonest cause of hypothyroidism occurring in someone who has a goitre is Hashimoto's disease. This occurs mainly in adult women and is an abnormal defence (immune) response by the body to its own thyroid tissue. The body produces antibodies that attack its own thyroid tissue as if it were some foreign tissue. This may also occur as a 'natural' outcome of Graves' disease (see earlier), which may end up with the gland shrinking (atrophy) and under-working (hypothyroidism). This may mean that Graves' disease, Hashimoto's disease and atrophy of the gland are all stages in one over-all immune disease affecting the thyroid gland; but why the body should turn on its own thyroid gland and damage it in this way is not understood. However, there does seem to be a genetic factor which predisposes an individual to such an attack.

Symptoms

Hypothyroidism in adults produces effects that are the reverse of hyperthyroidism (over-working). Instead of being hot and sweating the patients are cold and the skin is dry. Instead of being over-active and anxious they become slow both physically and mentally. They gain weight, feel cold, become tired and forgetful. They may become constipated, menstrual periods may become heavy or prolonged, and they may develop aches and pains all over and loss of hair. If they develop myxoedema the skin becomes thickened and puffy, particularly on the face and around the eyes. The thyroid gland may be enlarged (goitre). Hypothyroidism may be difficult to recognize in elderly people.

In children it may be difficult to diagnose hypothyroidism, which may present as a deterioration in school work, lack of interest in physical activities and a slowing down of growth. Babies develop what is called cretinism: there is a marked reduction in physical and mental development, the face is pasty, the forehead wrinkled, the lips are thick and the tongue is enlarged and sticks out. Cretinism may be inherited or develop in areas where there is a deficiency of iodine (endemic goitre; see later).

Drug treatment of hypothyroidism

Hypothyroidism is usually permanent and requires life-long treatment with a thyroid hormone. Response to treatment is both dramatic and effective. It should be started with a small daily dose (usually by mouth), slowly building up to a dose that fully meets the patient's needs. The daily dosage will vary according to the individual's response and general condition, and the presence or absence of heart disease.

Replacement of thyroid hormone should be gradual because of the risk of over-stimulating the heart and circulation, particularly in the elderly and in people with heart disease or raised blood pressure. To prevent this a beta blocker may be added at the start of treatment.

Babies should be routinely checked at birth for thyroid hormone deficiency because low levels will produce cretinism (see earlier). If the level of thyroid hormone is low, treatment should be started immediately with injections of a thyroid hormone and repeated at intervals in order to prevent abnormal physical and mental development.

Liothyronine (Tertroxin tablets, Triiodothyronine injections) and thyroxine (Eltroxin tablets) are used to treat hypothyroidism. Liothyronine acts more quickly than thyroxine and is used when a speedy response is required, as in treating hypothyroid coma (or myxoedema coma), which is a state of collapse that may develop in someone with severe hypothyroidism.

Goitre

The term 'goitre' is used to describe an enlargement of the thyroid gland. This may be a simple enlargement which is smooth and diffuse (simple goitre) or it may be lumpy in which case it is called nodular goitre. Goitre may be associated with over-activity of the thyroid gland (thyrotoxicosis, see earlier) or with under-activity (hypothyroidism).

Goitre may occur in a small number of people in a population, and can be due to several causes. This is usually referred to as a *sporadic goitre.* On the other hand, goitre may affect a whole group of people in a population, when it is usually caused by some factor in the environment. It is then called *endemic goitre,* and its commonest cause is a deficiency of iodine in the diet. This occurs particularly in populations living inland in mountainous areas well away from the sea. When endemic goitre affects most women in an area some babies will be born with cretinism. This may principally affect brain and nerve development, producing mental deficiency, deafness, mutism, spasticity and loss of control over voluntary movements (ataxia), or it may produce stunted growth and myxoedema, in which the skin is pale and puffy.

Less common environmental factors include a high level of calcium in the water, which interferes with the absorption into the body of iodine from food; and certain substances in food called goitrogens (goitre-making), which prevent the thyroid gland from concentrating iodine sufficiently to manufacture thyroid hormones. Goitrogens are present in brassicas, cassava and soya beans.

In goitre the gland gets larger because there is defective production of thyroid hormones. This stimulates the pituitary gland to produce more thyroid-stimulating hormone (TSH), which causes the gland to get bigger but it still cannot produce thyroid hormones because either there is a lack of iodine or some other factor is present that interferes with their production. This effect may be continuous and produce a diffuse smooth enlargement of the gland; or the iodine supply may be sporadic and work in stops and starts, affecting different parts of the gland and thus producing a lumpy or nodular goitre.

A long-standing simple smooth goitre may become nodular over the years and grow very large so that it presses on the windpipe and causes difficulty with breathing. Some nodules may start to over-work and produce thyroid hormones in excess. This is called toxic nodular goitre (see earlier). However, the nodules usually do not function.

Drugs may cause goitre

Anti-thyroid drugs may produce goitres; so may prolonged treatment for depression using the drug lithium and sulphonamides used to treat infections. Goitre may result from the prolonged use of cough medicines that contain iodine.

Treatment of goitre

If the thyroid gland is under-active, the treatment is to give thyroid hormone (e.g. thyroxine) in order to reduce the production of thyroid-stimulating hormone (TSH) by the pituitary gland. In addition, the patient should take an adequate diet containing iodine. The treatment is suitable for both simple and nodular goitre. Surgery may be necessary in nodular goitre. The treatment of goitre associated with over-activity of the gland is discussed earlier in this chapter.

Endemic goitre should be prevented by ensuring an adequate intake of iodine in the diet by, for example, including iodine in table salt.

Table 63.2 Drugs used to treat under-activity of the thyroid gland – harmful effects and warnings

liothyronine sodium (Tertroxin, Triiodothyronine Injection)
Harmful effects include fast beating of the heart, irregular heart rate, angina, muscle cramps, headache, restlessness, excitability, flushing, sweating, diarrhoea, excessive weight loss and menstrual irregularities.

Warnings Liothyronine should not be used in people who suffer from angina or from disorders of the heart or circulation. Individuals with under-active adrenal glands will require treatment with corticosteroids before they start taking liothyronine. Diabetics may need to have their dose of anti-diabetic drug adjusted; it accumulates in the body and has a delayed effect.

thyroxine sodium (thyroxine, Eltroxin)
Harmful effects include fast beating of the heart, irregular heart rate, angina, muscle cramps, headache, restlessness, excitability, flushing, sweating, diarrhoea, excessive weight loss and menstrual irregularities.

Warnings Thyroxine should not be used in people who suffer from angina or from disorders of the heart or circulation. Individuals with under-active adrenal glands will require treatment with corticosteroids before they start taking thyroxine. Diabetics may need to have their dose of anti-diabetic drug adjusted; it accumulates in the body and has a delayed effect.

64

Disorders of the parathyroid glands

The parathyroid glands lie behind the thyroid gland, which is in the neck, in front of the main windpipe (the trachea) and just below the voicebox (the larynx). There are usually four parathyroid glands, an upper pair and a lower pair. They are reddish discs about 5 mm in diameter. They secrete two hormones – parathyroid hormone (PTH) and calcitonin. These hormones control the levels of calcium and phosphorus in the blood and are closely involved with the body's use of calcium and phosphorus in bone formation and with the excretion of phosphorus in the urine. Also closely involved with them is vitamin D (see 'Osteoporosis', in Chapter 68).

Over-active parathyroid glands

Over-activity may be due to a tumour of one of the glands or it may occur secondarily to a long-standing disease of the kidneys, which causes a reduced production of active vitamin D by the kidneys, a loss of calcium in the urine and a fall in the blood calcium level. The parathyroid glands respond to this fall by increasing the secretion of parathyroid hormone. This draws calcium from bone and results in an increased level of calcium in the blood. A similar response may result in the bone softening that occurs in osteomalacia and in rickets caused by vitamin D deficiency (vitamin D is essential for the absorption of calcium from the intestine). Similar bone softening may also occur in disorders of the intestine that interfere with the absorption of calcium and vitamins from the food.

The high levels of calcium in the blood may cause weakness, loss of appetite, nausea, vomiting, constipation, drowsiness and confusion; if the bones are involved, bone softening may cause backache and other bone pains. The excess calcium in the urine may cause kidney stones, and deposits of calcium in the kidney may produce kidney disease.

Treatment

If one gland is over-active because of a tumour it is removed surgically. If other glands are over-active they are removed surgically and a small piece of parathyroid tissue transplanted under the skin in the forearm. If the blood calcium increases again, the size of this transplant can be easily adjusted by cutting some of it away under local anaesthetic.

Under-active parathyroid glands

If the parathyroid glands are under-active, there is a fall in the blood calcium and a rise in blood phosphate levels. This produces tetany (see Chapter 46), mental illness, cataracts, calcium deposits in various organs and thrush infections, particularly of the finger nails. The condition is very rare. It may follow partial or total surgical removal of the thyroid gland in which the parathyroid glands are accidentally removed along with the thyroid tissue. It may also develop as a consequence of an autoimmune disease in which the body produces antibodies against its own parathyroid tissues.

Treatment

Treatment is difficult; it involves the use of calciferol (vitamin D_2), which promotes the absorption of calcium and phosphorus from the intestine.

65

Diabetes

Diabetes (diabetes mellitus) is a complex disorder that affects how the body deals with carbohydrates. It has many causes, which result in a deficiency of insulin production by the pancreas, or a block to its actions in the tissues of the body, or both. Whatever the cause, the result is a high concentration of glucose in the blood (hyperglycaemia), and a variety of complications, which can affect the blood vessels, the nerves, the eyes and the kidneys.

Insulin and glucose

Insulin is a hormone secreted by the pancreas. It controls the use of carbohydrates, fats and proteins from food. Its secretion is controlled by many factors, the most important of which is the concentration of glucose in the blood. If the concentration of glucose increases, the production of insulin increases; if the concentration of glucose in the blood falls, the production of insulin falls.

The body obtains most of its energy from *glucose*, which is a simple sugar broken down in the intestine from more complex sugars (or carbohydrates) and absorbed into the blood stream. Insulin enables cells to take up glucose to burn it for energy or to store it for future use. In diabetes not enough insulin is produced and therefore cells are unable to take up glucose from the blood and it accumulates in the blood, to reach a high concentration (hyperglycaemia). In addition, the production of glucose from proteins in the liver (gluconeogenesis) is increased (see later).

Controlling the production of insulin

Insulin's role is to organize the use and storage of all substances from food that the body uses for fuel. Its secretion is therefore stimulated not only by the concentration in the blood of glucose from carbohydrates but also by the concentration of amino acids from proteins and fatty acids from fats.

The stomach and intestine also play a part in controlling insulin production. There is a close interplay between insulin production, the presence or absence of food in the stomach and intestine, hormones produced by the stomach, and nervous stimulation of the pancreas, stomach and intestine. For example, glucose taken by mouth stimulates insulin production more than if it is given by injection into a vein. This is because hormones released by the stomach and intestine when food is present send 'early' messages to the pancreas to produce more insulin in anticipation of the food products that will shortly be absorbed into the bloodstream. These hormones that give anticipatory signals are called incretins. Therefore, when we talk about the regulation of insulin secretion we must also include the parts played by hormones from the stomach and intestine. In other words, the pancreas, stomach and intestines are not only involved in the digestion of food, they are also directly involved in how that food is used by the body.

There is a fine balance between the activities of nerves that stimulate the secretion of insulin and those that stop its secretion. This balance is controlled by a centre in the brain (the hypothalamus), which also controls the appetite and regulates feeding behaviour. The nervous control of insulin secretion is therefore complex and can be affected by physical stress, mental stress, hunger and even thinking about food.

Problems caused by a lack of insulin

Lack of glucose for energy

In the absence of insulin, the passage of glucose through the walls of all cells in the body is defective and not enough glucose gets into the cells to produce energy for their everyday activities.

Muscle protein is broken down and the muscles waste

In the absence of insulin, the normal protein breakdown in the body is unopposed with the result that, in diabetes, protein breakdown proceeds faster than protein build-up – which is one of the reasons why diabetic patients lose weight.

In addition, in the absence of insulin the conversion of stored carbohydrates (glycogen) into glucose is reduced in the liver and muscles. This process, which is called glycogenolysis, normally provides a ready source of energy during exercise etc. If it does not occur, the body starts to break down muscle protein into glucose instead. This is called gluconeogenesis, and it leads to the accumulation of protein breakdown waste products (urea and ammonia) in the blood and urine.

Fats are broken down

When needed for energy, fatty acids are released from fat deposits in the body and enter the bloodstream where they are taken to cells in the muscles and other tissues to be burned. The enzyme that breaks fats down to fatty acids is lipase, and its actions are normally blocked by insulin, by adrenaline and related chemicals and by glucagon (see below). In the absence of insulin, the release of fatty acids into the blood stream is unchecked and this causes problems. The excess fatty acids are not broken down properly in the liver, resulting in an accumulation of organic compounds (ketone bodies) and acids which enter the bloodstream. Some of the ketone bodies are used by the cells for energy but the acids increase the acidity of the blood and alter the acidity of the urine, which causes a loss of potassium in the urine – which may be dangerous. The increased acidity of the urine also causes some loss of sodium.

Over-production of glucose

In the absence of insulin, the production of glucose from proteins in the liver (gluconeogenesis) is increased (see earlier) and leads to an over-production of glucose.

Anti-insulins (e.g. glucagon)

There are a number of anti-insulin (or counter-regulatory) hormones that keep the concentration and production of insulin under control. They include glucagon, growth hormone, corticosteroids, and adrenaline and related chemicals. From the point of view of diabetes, glucagon is the most important. It is produced by alpha cells in the pancreas in response to a low blood sugar, stress and other factors. Its main action is in the liver where it binds itself to certain receptors and stimulates a series of chemical processes that result in the production of glucose.

Diabetes

Diabetes may be separated into two general disease syndromes (a syndrome being a group of signs and symptoms caused by a disease).

Type I or *insulin-dependent diabetes mellitus* (IDDM) occurs in people with little or no ability to produce insulin. These individuals develop high blood glucose levels and other chemical changes that produce severe symptoms unless they are treated with insulin. They are absolutely dependent on insulin treatment for their survival. This most severe form of the disease usually appears in people under 35 years of age, particularly between childhood and adulthood (10–16 years of age). Older terms for this disorder were juvenile-onset diabetes and ketosis-prone diabetes. It develops rapidly.

Type II or *non-insulin-dependent diabetes mellitus* (NIDDM) occurs mostly in people over 40 years of age whose pancreas still has the ability to make insulin, but they appear to be resistant to insulin and they have a reduced ability to burn off calories, which predisposes them to become overweight. Insulin treatment is not essential for their survival and they do not develop the serious chemical changes which develop in insulin-dependent patients. Previous terms for this form of diabetes were maturity-onset diabetes, adult diabetes, non-ketotic diabetes and stable diabetes.

Sometimes a patient does not fit neatly into one category or the other; for example, some non-insulin-dependent patients may require insulin in order to keep well and some non-insulin-dependent diabetics will become insulin dependent over time as the ability of their pancreas to produce insulin becomes exhausted.

Resistance to the effects of insulin

Insulin production by the pancreas does not appear to decrease with age but older people develop a resistance to the actions of insulin, which may be due to a reduction in the number of insulin receptors in the body. Poor diet, physical inactivity and increasing weight also increase resistance to the actions of insulin.

Symptoms of diabetes

People with *insulin-dependent diabetes* pass a lot of urine (polyuria), drink a lot of fluids (polydipsia) and eat a lot (polyphagia). They lose weight and feel tired, and are susceptible to infections. They may develop serious chemical disturbances such as an increase in the acidity of the blood (acidosis) and an excessive amount of organic compounds (ketones) in the blood. The latter is referred to as ketosis. The combined effects are usually referred to as ketoacidosis.

Non-insulin dependent diabetic individuals are usually older than 40 years of age, most are overweight and they may develop polydipsia (drink a lot of fluids), polyuria (pass a lot of urine), loss of weight, weakness, fatigue, dizziness, headaches and blurred vision. Many adult people do not know they have diabetes until sugar in the urine is detected at a routine medical. Others may present with serious complications of the disease affecting their eyes, nervous system and/or arteries.

Diagnosis of diabetes

The diagnosis of diabetes is suggested by the appearance of sugar (glucose) in the urine, and it is confirmed by measuring the concentration of glucose in the blood – blood glucose levels after fasting and at other times in the day are measured. In general, glucose appears in the urine only when the blood glucose levels are high.

Another test for diabetes is the glucose tolerance test (GTT) which measures an individual's response to a dose of glucose by mouth after a period of fasting. In diabetes the fasting blood glucose level is above normal. After taking the glucose by mouth it rises to a level higher than normal, and after 2 hours the level remains above normal. Glucose also appears in the urine.

Causes of diabetes

Diabetes clearly runs in families but whether it is genetically inherited is difficult to determine because of complicating factors such as diet, stress and other factors in the environment which can markedly influence whether or not an individual develops the disease.

Non-insulin-dependent diabetes

Abnormalities of insulin (and, to a lesser extent, glucagon) secretion may contribute to the development of non-insulin-dependent diabetes. There is evidence that it may, rarely, be caused by genetic abnormalities that affect the manufacture of insulin in the pancreas but whilst in some patients insulin secretion by the pancreas is reduced, in others it is not. It therefore appears that in the latter group of patients it is the target tissues that are resistant to the effects of insulin. This may be due to a reduction in the number of insulin receptors in the body with ageing. However, studies of insulin production in response to glucose given by mouth or by injection suggest that in non-insulin-dependent diabetics the B cells in the pancreas may not be able to 'recognize' glucose in the blood as well as they should, and they fail to respond by producing insulin. Therefore, insulin deficiency and insulin resistance may both contribute to the high blood glucose levels in people suffering from non-insulin-dependent diabetes. In addition, increased production of glucose by the liver may also contribute to the high blood sugar level. This may be due to a resistance of the liver cells to the restraint that insulin normally applies to the liver's production of glucose. Also, excess production of glucagon (anti-insulin hormone) may contribute to the high blood sugar level.

Non-insulin-dependent diabetes is common in overweight people who eat lots of sugary foods. Rarely, it may be caused by a chronic inflammation of the pancreas, producing scarring (chronic pancreatitis) and occasionally triggered by some drugs; for example, diuretics, corticosteroids and oral contraceptive drugs.

Insulin-dependent diabetes

In insulin-dependent diabetes there must be a strong inherited (genetic) abnormality but, in addition, there is evidence that individuals who develop the disease have often had a virus illness in the preceding few months. There is also evidence that the disease may be an abnormal defence response in the body, because 90 per cent of patients with newly diagnosed insulin-dependent diabetes have circulating antibodies to cells of the pancreas. This means that the body's natural defence system is reacting against its own tissues (in this case the pancreas) as if the pancreatic cells were foreign invaders (see Chapter 9).

Strong arguments are made for the role of genetic abnormalities, virus infections and abnormal immune responses as the causes of insulin-dependent diabetes. However, it is probable that each may contribute to the development of insulin-dependent diabetes in a particular individual.

Early complications of diabetes

Ketoacidosis

A lack of insulin may lead to a rapid change in the chemistry of the body, called ketoacidosis. This may develop suddenly in someone who has unrecognized insulin-dependent diabetes. It may also occur when an insulin-dependent diabetic develops any form of stress (e.g. an acute infection) and fails to increase the dose of insulin. The signs and symptoms of ketoacidosis include intense thirst and passing large volumes of urine, constipation, cramps, altered vision, abdominal pain (with or without vomiting) especially in children, weakness, drowsiness, dehydration and over-breathing. There may be a smell of acetone in the breath (a smell like nail varnish remover); sometimes the blood pressure and the temperature fall, and the individual may go into a coma. The diagnosis and treatment of ketoacidosis are discussed later, under 'Diabetic emergencies'.

Late complications of diabetes

Late complications of diabetes include damage to the eyes, nerves, kidneys and arteries.

Eyes

Diabetes may damage the small arteries of the retina, causing bleeding and scarring. This may cause blindness by damaging the seeing part of the retina. Diabetes may also cause glaucoma and affect the lenses, producing cataracts.

Nerves

Diabetes may damage nerves. It is usually the sensory nerves (touch, pain, etc.) that are affected although nerves responsible for movement may also be involved. The feet and legs are affected the most and, because pain sensation is reduced, patients do not notice when they injure the skin. As a result, painless ulcers (e.g. on the feet) may develop which can become infected and turn into abscesses.

Diabetes may sometimes damage the nerves supplying the hands, producing clumsiness and numbness of the fingers. It may also damage the big nerves which supply the legs, producing pain, burning sensations and pins and needles in the legs and feet.

Rarely, diabetes may damage nerves in the autonomic nervous system, producing disorders of sweating, blood pressure, pulse rate, breathing, sexual function, bladder function and disorders of the stomach and bowel.

Kidneys

Diabetes may damage the small arteries in the kidneys, leading to scarring and failure of the kidneys to function efficiently. It is one of the most important causes of kidney failure. It is associated with a rise in blood pressure (hypertension), which should be treated as early as possible with an ACE inhibitor (see Chapter 21).

Arteries

A major cause of death in diabetes is damage to the arteries. It causes atherosclerosis which is more prevalent than in non-diabetic patients, its onset is earlier and it develops more rapidly. Atherosclerosis is discussed in detail in Chapter 25. The principal damage is the laying down of cholesterol and fat in the lining walls of the arteries. These deposits become scarred and may break (ulcerate), which causes the development of a blood clot (thrombosis) on its surface. This process is related to the increased levels of cholesterol and fats in the blood in diabetes.

Atherosclerosis associated with diabetes may affect the coronary arteries and increase the risk of angina and coronary thrombosis. It may affect the arteries in the limbs, resulting in poor circulation to the hands and feet. Not only can this complicate any nerve damage but it may also lead to a poor supply of oxygen to the tissues, resulting in gangrene of the toes or fingers.

The risks from diabetes are increased if the individual's cholesterol and blood fats are high, if he or she smokes cigarettes and/or has untreated hypertension (raised blood pressure).

Treatment of diabetes

The severity of the disease varies from person to person, and treatment varies according to whether or not the individual is insulin dependent.

The aims of treatment are:

- To try to keep blood glucose levels as near normal as possible
- To try to prevent serious long-term damage to the eyes, kidneys, nerves, heart and circulation
- To interfere with normal life-style as little as possible

Dietary treatment

Diet is an integral part of treatment of diabetes, and in some non-insulin-dependent diabetics it should be the main treatment. Dietary treatment is different for non-insulin-dependent and for insulin-dependent patients. The former are often overweight and have some insulin production whereas the latter are not usually overweight and have no insulin production. Diabetic diets are concerned with reducing the overall intake of calories while maintaining a nutritious and well balanced diet.

Drugs used to treat diabetes

Drugs that can be taken by mouth

Two principal groups of drugs are available which, when taken by mouth, cause a fall in the concentration of glucose in the blood. They are the sulphonylureas and the biguanides.

The sulphonylureas These drugs actually stimulate the pancreatic cells to secrete insulin. They are therefore of no use in insulin-dependent diabetics who are not capable of secreting insulin but they may be of use in non-insulin-dependent people who retain a capacity to secrete insulin. However, after several months' treatment, insulin levels may fall to previous levels while the blood glucose level remains improved – which indicates some other effects.

There is some evidence that sulphonylureas may increase the number of insulin receptors and may help to 'increase' the effects of available insulin on fat cells and on cells in the liver and muscles, but it is not understood how they produce these effects.

Harmful effects of sulphonylureas Harmful effects are generally mild and infrequent. They include headache, hunger, and stomach and bowel upsets – nausea, vomiting, loss of appetite and diarrhoea. Allergic reactions may occur (usually in the first 6–8 weeks of treatment) and include itching, nettle rash, other rashes; rarely, dermatitis, fever and jaundice may occur. Sensitivity of the skin to sunlight (photosensitivity) has been reported with chlorpropamide, which may also cause flushing of the face when alcohol is drunk. Very rarely, there may be damage to the bone marrow, producing blood disorders.

Any of the sulphonylureas may cause a fall in blood glucose level (hypoglycaemia) which may continue for several days such that prolonged and repeated treatment with glucose may be necessary. Individuals may develop hypoglycaemia after just one dose, or after several days, weeks or months of regular daily treatment. Most hypoglycaemic reactions to the sulphonylureas occur in people over 50 years of age and are more likely to occur in anyone who has liver or kidney disease. Overdose or inadequate and irregular meals may trigger an attack. Other drugs may also interact with the sulphonylureas, producing hypoglycaemia (see Chapter 89). Sulphonylureas should not be used in elderly people.

Warnings on the use of sulphonylureas Chlorpropamide causes nausea, flushing and palpitations if it is taken with alcohol. The attack comes on within 20 minutes of taking alcohol and lasts up to 1 hour. The individual may also feel light-headed and breathless. It is rare in insulin-dependent diabetics and in people without diabetes. It seems to be associated with non-insulin-dependent diabetes and may be an inherited characteristic. *Tolbutamide* may rarely cause such an attack.

Some individuals may become allergic to sulphonylurea drugs; if this happens a sulphonylurea drug should not be used in future.

A sulphonylurea drug should not be used in patients suffering from diabetic ketoacidosis (see earlier) whether they are in coma or not. This condition should be treated with insulin.

There appears to be a possible relationship between the use of the sulphonylurea tolbutamide and an increased risk of death from heart disease, compared with patients treated with diet alone or diet and insulin. Because sulphonylurea drugs are chemically similar and produce similar actions and effects, it seems sensible to bear this warning in mind when using any one of these drugs.

The short-acting tolbutamide may be used in patients with impaired kidney function, as may gliclazide and gliquidone which are principally broken down in the liver.

Insulin should be used temporarily in patients who develop an infection, injury, undergo surgery or who have a heart attack.

It is important to stick to your prescribed diet and regular exercise programme and to test your urine and/or blood for glucose at regular intervals.

The biguanides Drugs in this group do not have an effect on insulin secretion. They reduce the absorption of carbohydrates from the stomach and intestine, increase the use of glucose by the tissues and decrease the production of glucose from protein (gluconeogenesis, see earlier). They do not cause a marked fall in blood glucose concentration in normal individuals. The two main drugs in this group are phenformin and metformin.

Phenformin has been taken off the market because it occasionally produced a serious chemical disorder of the blood called lactic acidosis. This is due to an accumulation of organic acids in the blood which interfere with the use of oxygen by the tissues. Lactic acidosis may cause nausea, vomiting, abdominal pains, rapid over-breathing (hyperventilation), heart failure, drowsiness and death. Individuals who break down phenformin slowly may be at greater risk.

Metformin (Glucophage) is the only biguanide available for use in the UK. It must not be used in anyone allergic to the drug or who is suffering from diabetic coma or ketoacidosis, severe impairment of kidney function, chronic liver disease, heart failure or recent heart attack (myocardial infarction), severe infection, injury, dehydration, alcoholism (use insulin instead), or who is prone to develop lactic acidosis. It should be used with caution in people with mild to moderate impairment of kidney function.

Stop 2–3 days before surgery and switch to insulin. Kidney function tests should be carried out before and at regular intervals during treatment and patients should have a vitamin B_{12} test of their blood every 12 months.

Metformin may, rarely, produce lactic acidosis in people with kidney disease who do not excrete the drug efficiently; this causes the level of metformin in the blood to rise to toxic levels. Lactic acidosis may rarely occur in alcoholics.

Harmful effects produced by metaformin are usually mild and transient, and include loss of appetite, nausea, vomiting and diarrhoea. Prolonged treatment may cause a decreased absorption of vitamin B_{12} from food.

Overview of the benefits and risks of anti-diabetic drugs by mouth

A major study in the USA was set up in 1961 to establish whether control of blood glucose concentrations helps to prevent or delay damage to blood vessels in people suffering from non-insulin-dependent diabetes. The researchers reported that the over-all death rate was higher in those patients who were treated with anti-diabetic drugs by mouth than in the group who were not. However, this study has been criticized because of deficiencies in the selection of patients and absence of information on whether the patients took all the prescribed drugs as directed. Nevertheless, subsequent studies have still not produced convincing evidence about the benefits of anti-diabetic drugs by mouth in preventing long-term complications of diabetes.

The present consensus is that anti-diabetic drugs by mouth should be used only in patients suffering from non-insulin-dependent diabetes in whom weight reduction, dietary control and education have failed, who are unwilling or unable to take insulin and in whom blood glucose levels are only mildly increased. These drugs may then control blood glucose levels under ordinary circumstances. However, they are not adequate in someone undergoing surgery, in a severely injured person or in someone with a fever due to an infection. These people will require insulin.

About 10–20 per cent of patients do not respond to anti-diabetic drugs by mouth. This is called 'primary' failure. In other patients, their blood glucose concentrations become well controlled by sulphonylureas for several months on end and then suddenly go out of control. This is called 'secondary failure' and it happens quite frequently. In such patients in Great Britain it is suggested that metformin should be added to the treatment because it works differently from the sulphonylureas. However, this practice is questionable.

Warning *Anti-diabetic drugs by mouth should not be used in sufferers from insulin-dependent diabetes. Deaths have occurred from acidosis and dehydration in such patients who have been treated with sulphonylureas.*

Failure to improve on oral anti-diabetic drugs may be due to failure of the pancreas and not the treatment. These patients should be treated with insulin rather than increasing the use of oral anti-diabetic drugs.

In people over 60 years of age, oral anti-diabetic drugs should be used only when diet has failed. Short-acting drugs (e.g. tolbutamide) should be used in order to prevent the risk of hypoglycaemia in the night, and regular medical check-ups should be carried out with particular attention to the heart, kidney function and liver function.

The need to treat the patient as an individual

The effective treatment of someone suffering from non-insulin-dependent diabetes takes time and patience. Different people burn up energy at different rates and their daily activities vary, so they may react differently to treatment. Successful treatment therefore needs tailoring to the individual's needs and response to treatment.

Diabetes is a life-long disease which may produce serious complications. It is very important that patients understand fully about the disease and its treatment, in particular about the long-term benefits and risks of drug treatment compared with no drug treatment.

Insulin

Insulin is the main drug for treating anyone suffering from insulin-dependent diabetes. It is also used to treat many individuals who suffer from non-insulin-dependent diabetes.

Insulin is destroyed in the stomach if it is taken by mouth so it has to be given by injection, usually under the skin (subcutaneous). It is usually injected into the upper arms, thighs, buttocks or abdomen using a syringe and needle but various injection devices are available which hold one or more insulin preparations in a cartridge pen which has a meter and allows fixed doses to be released at intervals. Insulin can also be given under the skin by continuous infusion using a pump (infusion pump). This allows a continuous supply of insulin and boosts the supply when needed (e.g. after meals); it thus prevents serious falls in blood glucose (hypoglycaemia). However, these pumps are bulky, and can go wrong. They are not convenient for vigorous physical activities and there is a risk of skin infection. Patients using such pumps may easily slip into ketoacidosis. Pumps are also available that can deliver insulin directly into a vein or into

Table 65.1 Drugs used to treat diabetes: oral preparations

Preparation	*Drug*	*Drug group*	*Dosage form*
chlorpropamide	chlorpropamide	Sulphonylurea	Tablets
Daonil	glibenclamide	Sulphonylurea	Tablets
Diabinese	chlorpropamide	Sulphonylurea	Tablets
Diamicron	gliclazide	Sulphonylurea	Tablets
Dimelor	acetohexamide	Sulphonylurea	Tablets
Euglucon	glibenclamide	Sulphonylurea	Tablets
glibenclamide	glibenclamide	Sulphonylurea	Tablets
Glibenese	glipizide	Sulphonylurea	Tablets
Glucophage	metformin	Biguanide	Tablets
Glurenorm	gliquidone	Sulphonylurea	Tablets
metformin	metformin	Biguanide	Tablets
Minodiab	glipizide	Sulphonylurea	Tablets
Orabet	metformin	Biguanide	Tablets
Rastinon	tolbutamide	Sulphonylurea	Tablets
Semi-Daonil	glibenclamide	Sulphonylurea	Tablets
Tolanase	tolazamide	Sulphonylurea	Tablets
tolbutamide	tolbutamide	Sulphonylurea	Tablets

the abdominal cavity; pumps that are processed to respond to local glucose levels are under trial. There are implant devices that can be worked by remote control (programmed implantable medication systems, PIMS). A nasal aerosol of insulin is also under trial.

The daily doses of insulin and the types of insulin used will vary according to the blood glucose level and the calorie intake and level of daily activities of the individual being treated. Some doctors attempt tight control of the blood glucose level in the hope of preventing complications, particularly eye damage. Others are less rigid and try to prevent low blood glucose levels (hypoglycaemia), which may easily occur if too fine a control is kept on the blood glucose level.

Flexible control of blood glucose level may be best in the elderly and in people who are not highly motivated, but in younger patients it is considered by some experts that it is better to keep tight control on the blood glucose levels and, hopefully, reduce the risk of blindness than to worry about attacks of hypoglycaemia.

In general, it is quite easy to relieve obvious symptoms of a raised blood glucose but it is very difficult, if not impossible, to keep the blood glucose at desired levels throughout a 24-hour period without producing an attack of hypoglycaemia. How close you get to this depends on the types of insulin used and how they are used.

Insulin preparations

Pork and beef insulins

These insulins are obtained from the pancreas of slaughtered animals. Pork (porcine) insulin is chemically similar to human insulin and produces fewer allergic reactions than beef (bovine) insulin.

Soluble preparations for injection are available in both acid solution (Acid Insulin Injection) and neutral solution (Neutral Insulin Injection).

The neutral solution is absorbed more rapidly into the blood stream from the injection site and reduces the risk of pain and discomfort at the site of injection. Both Acid Insulin Injection and Neutral Insulin Injection are short acting (maximum 2–4 hours and last up to about 8 hours). They are the only forms of insulin that should be used to treat diabetic emergencies and during surgical operations.

NOTE Neutral Insulin Injection is dispensed if a doctor orders insulin injection or soluble insulin.

By altering the acidity and adding zinc to insulin suspensions the zinc combines with the insulin to produce larger particles which, after injection, act as a depot to produce a slow release of insulin. These preparations are called insulin zinc suspensions (IZS) or lente insulins (lente meaning 'slow'). The size of particles determines the speed of action. Amorphous IZS has a rapid onset of action and acts for a moderate duration of time (semilente). Crystalline IZS has a slower onset of action and a prolonged duration of action (ultralente). When the two types are mixed a preparation with an intermediate duration of action is produced.

Another method of making insulin act over a longer period is to add protamine (a protein obtained from fish sperm) to a suspension of insulin. The protamine and insulin form a complex that is much less soluble and from which insulin is released slowly after injection. The duration of action of this complex may be prolonged by adding zinc to form Protamine Zinc Insulin (PZI). However, its use is complicated by the hazard that, if the blood glucose is controlled through the day-time, it may fall too low during the night and early morning. Attempts to balance this effect resulted in the combined use of a smaller dose of the long-acting PZI with the short-acting soluble insulin. The combined effects provide sufficient cover during the day without too high a dose of PZI working on through the night. They should not be mixed in the same syringe because excess protamine in the PZI may attach itself to the soluble insulin. Such a combination is still needed in some severe cases of diabetes but its use has generally been replaced by the lente insulins.

Some patients may be allergic to protamine, and an alternative protein preparation is available – Globulin Zinc Suspension. However, this may also cause allergic reactions in some people. Isophane Insulin is an intermediate-acting insulin that contains less protamine and zinc than PZI.

Purity of pork and beef insulin preparations

By means of special biochemical procedures (chromatographical separation), impurities from the pancreas are removed from insulin preparations, thus reducing the risk of allergic reactions which has previously impaired their effectiveness. These are called highly purified insulins. They should be used especially when there is evidence of fat wasting at injection sites (fat atrophy) and also in patients who need very high doses of insulin because they are becoming tolerant to conventional insulins. It is also recommended that purified insulin be used in pregnancy and after surgery, in order to reduce the risks of allergy in later years when insulin may be required again. Children should also be treated with purified insulin.

When conventional insulins are replaced with purified insulins, the dose of the latter may need reducing. This should be done slowly over several days.

Human insulins

'Human insulins' are not obtained from humans, they are manufactured in laboratories by using enzymes to modify the protein structure of pork insulin (enzyme-modified pork insulins, emp); by genetic engineering using pork insulins (pork recombinant insulin, prb); and by genetic engineering using yeast cells and pork insulin (pyr). Like beef and pork insulins, human insulin preparations may be short acting (about 8 hours with a peak at 1–2 hours) and include both neutral and acid formulations. When formulated with zinc and/or protamine, preparations of human insulin may be intermediate or long acting (up to 35 hours with an onset of action in 1–4 hours). In addition, mixtures are available containing neutral human insulin and isophane insulins (see above) which gives a two-stage response (biphasic response).

It is important to note that all insulin preparations, whether pork, beef or human, can very occasionally produce allergic reactions, and human insulin appears to be no safer in this respect than pork insulins. The risk is greatest with beef insulins (see earlier).

Variations in the duration of action of insulin preparations

Commercial insulins come in concentrations of 100 units per millilitre (U100) and 500 units per millilitre (U500). They vary in their duration of action and they are usually grouped as short (rapid), intermediate (medium) and long acting. The duration of their effects varies considerably between different people, and what may be short acting in one person may be medium acting in another. The duration of action must therefore be worked out for each individual.

Variations in response may be caused by circulating anti-insulin antibodies because the body's defence system may regard the injected insulin as a foreign invader and neutralize it. Response may also vary with the rate of absorption of insulin into the blood stream following injection under the skin. Furthermore, there may be marked variations in absorption throughout a 24-hour period according to whether the individual exercises the injected arm or leg and whether he or she massages the site of injection. Differences in purity of the insulin preparation may also affect duration of response, although most preparations now available are purified or highly purified preparations (see earlier).

Using insulin – a partnership between patient and doctor

Control of blood glucose and its symptoms will depend upon the type of insulin used, the number of injections required each day and the methods of assessing control. The most suitable mixture of short-, intermediate- and long-acting insulin preparations has to be worked out for each individual in order to control the blood glucose levels, particularly after food and through the night. The right treatment is what is right for the particular individual. Treatment should not be standardized.

It is important that diabetics learn how to assess their own progress in terms of how they feel, what they eat, when they eat and what their urine and blood tests for glucose show. Self-testing of the urine for glucose gives only a rough indication of what is happening to the concentration of glucose in the blood. It should not be relied upon as a sole guide to insulin treatment, and, where appropriate, diabetics should also have equipment to test their blood glucose levels.

Where possible, diabetic patients should manage their own disease and should be well informed about diabetes, its complications and its treatments. This means that doctors, nurses and pharmacists should undergo continuing education on diabetes and its treatment in order to be able to provide diabetics with up-to-date advice.

Many insulin schedules have been proposed but no single method is better than any other, provided the doctor and the patient actually understand what they are doing. Also, no single schedule in an individual should be rigidly fixed because his or her needs will vary according to all kinds of factors such as growth, stress, infection and the development of insulin antibodies (see earlier). Dosages may need to be altered because of physical activity, changes in eating habits or changes in other drug treatments (e.g. corticosteroids, diuretics). In addition, absorption of the injected insulin into the blood stream may vary according to the site of injection, and because of other factors as discussed earlier. This means that the doctor and patient must regularly review treatment *together* and decide on changes *together*.

NOTE It is advisable to use insulin preparations from the same manufacturer because different manufacturers may use different additives (e.g. suspensions, buffers, preservatives). These may influence the individual's response.

Harmful effects of insulin

Allergy to insulin

A minority of people beginning treatment with insulin may develop local allergic reactions at the injection site. This involves redness and itching, and occasionally the site of injection may become hardened (indurated). These reactions usually clear up with continued use of insulin. An antihistamine may be used to provide relief of symptoms. These allergic reactions occur much less frequently these days because of the availability of highly purified insulins.

Occasionally a generalized allergic reaction to insulin may occur, causing nettle rash (urticaria) and, very rarely, an allergic emergency (anaphylactic shock). This usually occurs when a particular insulin preparation has been stopped and then re-started; it may be necessary to 'desensitize' the patient to that particular insulin preparation (see Chapter 10).

Highly purified beef insulins carry the greatest risk of allergic reactions whereas highly purified pork insulins have an insignificant risk. Human insulin preparations carry less risk but there is still a rare risk of allergic reactions because they contain various additives and the preparations may undergo a chemical change in the vial.

Fatty dents and lumps at insulin injection sites

Impurities in conventional insulin injections may cause wasting of fat (fat atrophy or lipoatrophy), producing dents at injection sites. This reaction may be reversed by substituting a highly purified pork insulin and injecting into the affected site. Overgrowth of fatty tissue (fat tumours, lipid hypertrophy) may also occur at the site of an insulin injection, which is probably directly due to the effects of the insulin on fat. This problem may be helped by rotating the sites of injection.

Blurring of vision and ankle swelling

Many patients develop blurring of vision after starting insulin, which makes reading difficult. This is because insulin has an effect on the lenses of the eyes and changes their shape slightly. The blurring goes off in a few weeks. Ankle swelling (oedema) due to fluid retention may also occur in the first few weeks of treatment with insulin.

Dangers of changing one insulin preparation for another

People respond differently to different preparations of insulin. Therefore any change from pork to beef or beef to pork insulins, or from conventional insulins to highly purified insulins or human insulins should be done knowingly and with great care because of the risks of producing allergies and changes in response to similar dosages.

Other drug treatments may affect the blood glucose-lowering effects of insulin

The fall in blood glucose that insulin produces may be temporarily reduced by adrenaline and related drugs. It may be increased by alcohol, monoamine oxidase inhibitor anti-depressant drugs and by propanolol and related beta blockers. Beta blockers may also reduce some of the symptoms of hypoglycaemia and so the patient may be developing hypoglycaemia and not realize it – this could be dangerous. Diuretics may increase blood glucose levels.

Hypoglycaemia (low blood glucose, 'hypo attacks', insulin reaction)

Hyoglycaemia (low blood sugar) is a major danger of insulin treatment. This is because blood glucose levels are normally maintained within narrow limits, in spite of meals, periods of fasting, resting or effort. There is a very fine balance between glucose production, storage and needs, which are under the control of insulin, glucagon, nervous control (adrenaline and related chemicals), corticosteroids and growth hormone. Even with insulin treatment, it is not possible to maintain this fine control of the blood glucose system.

Causes of hypoglycaemia

In every diabetic taking insulin the blood glucose level goes up and down throughout the day according to the timing of insulin injections and meals. Because hypoglycaemic symptoms occur when the blood glucose level is low it is important for all patients to know the times of day when their blood glucose falls and to be able to recognize the warning symptoms and the relief from symptoms that taking sugar or glucose produces. The commonest times are before lunch and during the night. Where possible it is therefore helpful for all patients to measure their own blood glucose levels at intervals throughout the day in order to determine the danger times for themselves.

Hypoglycaemia may be produced by overdosing with insulin, by not taking enough carbohydrates in the diet, by missing or delaying meals or by physical activity. It may occur when changes are made in the type of insulin (e.g. changing from beef to human insulin without adjusting the dose). Unexplained falls in blood glucose levels may be due to the development of other disorders affecting the thyroid or adrenal glands or the absorption of carbohydrates from the stomach and intestine.

At the beginning of insulin treatment in a new diabetic patient there is a 'honeymoon' period for a few days when everything seems fine. Then for no reason the patient becomes unstable and the insulin requirements decrease, sometimes considerably. To prevent the risk of hypoglycaemic attacks, the insulin dose should always be reduced and then the effective daily dosage worked out before the patient leaves hospital.

Symptoms of hypoglycaemia

About half the glucose produced in the body is used up in the brain. Early warning symptoms that someone is developing hypoglycaemia are shaking and trembling, feeling nervous, sweating, hunger, palpitations, pins and needles in the tongue and mouth, and, occasionally, headaches. As the blood sugar falls, it begins to affect the brain, starting with visual disturbance (double vision), difficulty in concentrating and thinking, and slurring of speech. As it gets lower the individual becomes confused, develops behaviour changes and may become truculent. Children may become 'naughty'. Eventually the individual becomes restless, sweats profusely, becomes unconscious and may have fits and die if glucose is not given.

Preventing hypoglycaemic attacks

All diabetic patients should:

- Carry glucose or sugar sweets with them at all times
- Carry a diabetic warning card with them at all times
- Take extra carbohydrates at times when they know their blood glucose goes down and before vigorous exercise
- Take glucose immediately they feel the early warning symptoms of hypoglycaemia

Glucagon injections

This drug rapidly increases the blood glucose level by blocking the effects of insulin. It may be given by injection into a muscle, into a vein or under the skin. It is an alternative to intravenous glucose (see below); for example, when it would be difficult to give an injection into a vein. A supply of glucagon is also useful for an emergency when a doctor is not available to give glucose intravenously. It should be available to nurses on wards where patients are being given insulin treatment and also to relatives of patients taking insulin.

Intravenous glucose

Unconscious patients should be given 20–50 ml of 50% glucose directly into a vein, by a doctor or a paramedic.

Changing from beef or pork to human insulins

When changing from beef insulin to human insulin the dose of the latter should be reduced. Most patients transferred in this way have little trouble but some experience changes in their symptoms of hypoglycaemia. The early warning symptoms produced by adrenaline stimulation (e.g. sweating, tremor, palpitation) may become less and the symptoms produced by the effects of a low blood sugar on the brain may become more obvious (e.g. inability to concentrate, visual disturbances, headache, slurring of speech). Some of these problems may be caused by too great a dose reduction when changing from beef to human insulin, by using tighter control of blood glucose levels which may itself reduce warning symptoms of hypoglycaemia, or by doctors changing preparations without adequate knowledge and understanding of the consequences.

When changing from pork insulin to human insulin the dose may work more quickly following injection under the skin, and very rarely some patients may experience unexpected hypoglycaemia. Doctors should be aware of the risks of changes in the symptoms of hypoglycaemia when switching someone from animal insulins and take the opportunity to advise their patients.

Treatment of diabetes in pregnancy

Diabetics who become pregnant

Before the 1950s about 1 in 4 diabetic pregnancies ended in the death of the baby. Now only about 1 in 100 babies from diabetic mothers are born dead. This is still two or three times greater than the 'normal' death rate for babies.

About half of the babies who die suffer from some abnormality, which highlights the importance of proper control of diabetes from the time of conception, particularly during the first 6–12 weeks of pregnancy. Control of the diabetes should be the optimum possible throughout the whole of the pregnancy (from conception to delivery). This calls for knowledge and understanding by the doctors, nurses and, above all, the patient. Pregnant diabetics should also act as their own doctors. They should test their blood and urine regularly and change their dose and frequency of insulin injections accordingly. Good self-care added to good obstetric and nursing care should prevent most problems.

Diabetes developing during pregnancy

Diabetes developing during pregnancy needs very careful handling even if it is mild because there is an added risk to the baby. Every pregnant woman should have her urine tested routinely for glucose. Mothers who have had diabetes in previous pregnancies should be watched carefully; so should mothers with a history of diabetes in their family and those who have previously had a big baby (more than 4500 g) or an unexplained death of a previous baby.

Breast feeding by mothers taking insulin causes no problems for the baby. The mother should take extra carbohydrates and fluids.

Diabetic emergencies (ketoacidosis)

As stated earlier, a lack of insulin results in serious disturbances in the levels of glucose, proteins and fats in the body. This causes chemical disturbances of the blood, called ketoacidosis. The blood glucose level is high and glucose is present in the urine, the acidity of the blood is increased, breakdown products of fats and proteins (ketone bodies) appear in the blood (and urine), the blood potassium level may be raised and the blood sodium may be reduced. The individual becomes seriously dehydrated and drowsy, and over-breathes. There is a smell of acetone (like nail varnish remover) in the breath. Vomiting may occur and cause further serious disturbances of the body's fluids and salts.

In an insulin-dependent diabetic, ketoacidosis will occur if insulin is stopped or the dose is reduced in error or deliberately, or during infections when the body actually requires more insulin. It may also develop in someone who has previously not been diagnosed as having insulin-dependent diabetes.

The onset of ketoacidosis is slow, over hours and days, and symptoms of diabetes are always present (e.g. excessive thirst, passing large volumes of urine). Therefore there is no excuse for a missed diagnosis. Most attacks of ketoacidosis occurring in patients could have been predicted and prevented.

All patients and doctors should know that, in any illness, injury, infection or surgical operation, the blood glucose level increases. This means that under such circumstances, diabetic patients will require more insulin than usual, and some who normally take anti-diabetic drugs by mouth will require insulin by injection during the illness or before, during or after surgery.

NOTE Ketoacidosis may not always be associated with a raised blood glucose level even though the ketoacidosis may be at a dangerous level. Likewise, patients with a raised blood glucose and severe dehydration may go into coma even though they do not have ketoacidosis. The latter disorder is referred to as hyperosmolar diabetic coma and usually occurs in elderly people.

Treatment

Treatment of ketoacidosis involves the intravenous (into a vein) administration of fluids (normal saline at first, changing to dextrose saline when the blood glucose has returned to normal) and insulin. A clear solution of insulin (neutral insulin injection) should be used for intravenous use. Sufficient insulin should be given to maintain the level of insulin in the blood at a safe level until the chemistry of the blood and the blood glucose are back to normal. Infusion rates of insulin should be steady and it is best to use a slow infusion pump if available; otherwise the insulin should be given by intramuscular injection, but absorption of the insulin may be impaired if the patient's blood pressure is low and the blood circulation is poor.

Potassium chloride is given if the potassium is low and sodium bicarbonate is given to correct the acidity of the blood if it is seriously disturbed. Any underlying infection should be treated.

NOTE In ketoacidosis, insulin must be given by injection into a vein or muscle, and not under the skin.

Treatment during surgery

During surgery on insulin-dependent diabetics, neutral insulin should be continued, preferably by slow infusion into a vein. This should be continued until the patient can eat and drink, at which stage the individual is switched to neutral insulin injected under the skin. The dose, frequency and type of insulin to keep the patient stable are then worked out. For minor surgery, neutral insulin may be administered slowly into a vein by a minipump and the dose varied according to the blood glucose levels, which should be monitored throughout the procedure.

According to their blood glucose levels, patients on anti-diabetic drugs by mouth may need a neutral insulin injection on the day of surgery.

Treatment of diabetes in elderly people

In elderly people who suffer from diabetes it is often more difficult to balance the benefits and risks of treatment than it is in younger people. Treatment must be tailored to the individual's needs according to whether that person is insulin-dependent or not and according to age and general physical and mental state.

Elderly diabetics need regular medical examinations to check on their general physical state and their blood glucose levels. They need careful care of their feet to make sure they are not developing ulcers, and their eyes need checking at intervals for signs of damage from the diabetes. Any drugs that cause a rise in blood glucose levels (e.g. thiazide diuretics and corticosteroids) should be used with caution; diabetics will also need watching carefully if they develp an infection (e.g. bronchitis) because their treatment may need changing during the time of infection.

Dietary treatment is safest in elderly diabetic patients. It is important to take time and patience to go through the diet that they have been taking and to advise them on the kind of diet that will keep their blood glucose down but which is easy to follow.

Anti-diabetic drugs by mouth should be used only if it is not possible to control the blood glucose level by diet alone. To prevent hypoglycaemia the minimum effective dose possible should be used. To prevent the risks of hypoglycaemia (particularly in the night) long-acting drugs should not be used; it is better to use a short-acting drug (see Table 65.2). Nevertheless, hypoglycaemia is always a risk. A sulphonylurea anti-diabetic drug should be used but occasionally metformin may help overweight patients who have not managed to reduce their weight.

Insulin should always be used if oral anti-diabetic drugs have not relieved the symptoms or not brought the blood glucose level under control, if the patient gets dehydrated and loses weight or if the patient develops an infection or needs surgery.

Hypoglycaemia can be a serious risk in elderly people.

Guar gum

Guar gum is obtained from the seeds of *Cyamopsis psoraloides*. It is soluble and high in fibre. If taken before meals it swells up and slows down the emptying of the stomach. This reduces the rate of absorption of carbohydrates from the intestines and helps to reduce the rise in blood glucose which normally occurs after a meal. It may be used *in addition* to diet, insulin or oral anti-diabetic drugs.

Guar gum is not very pleasant to take. It is available as granules to dissolve in water (e.g. Guarem and Guarina). It may cause nausea, wind and diarrhoea, particularly at the start of treatment. It may affect the absorption of other drugs and it should not be used in patients who have a narrowing of the oesophagus, stomach or intestine because it may cause an obstruction.

Table 65.2 Short-, intermediate- and long-acting insulin preparations

Preparation	*Drug*	*Duration of action*
Human Actrapid	neutral soluble insulin* (human)	Short-acting
Human Actrapid Penfill	neutral soluble insulin* (human)	Short-acting
Human Insulatard	isophane insulin* (human)	Intermediate-acting
Human Monotard	insulin zinc suspension* (human)	Intermediate-acting
Human Protaphane	isophane insulin* (human)	Intermediate-acting
Human Protaphane Penfill	isophane insulin* (human)	Intermediate-acting
Human Ultratard	crystalline insulin zinc suspension (human)	Long-acting

* Highly purified

Table 65.2 Short-, intermediate- and long-acting insulin preparations (*cont.*)

Preparation	*Drug*	*Duration of action*
Human Velosulin	neutral soluble insulin* (human)	Short-acting
Humulin I	isophane insulin (human)	Intermediate-acting
Humulin Lente	30% amorphous and 70% crystalline insulin zinc suspension (human)	Intermediate-acting
Humulin S	soluble insulin (human)	Short-acting
Humulin Zn	crystalline insulin, zinc suspension (human)	Intermediate-acting
Hypurin Isophane	isophane insulin* (beef)	Intermediate-acting
Hypurin Lente	insulin zinc suspension* (beef)	Long-acting
Hypurin Neutral	neutral soluble insulin* (beef)	Short-acting
Hypurin Protamine Zinc	protamine zinc insulin* (beef)	Long-acting
Insulatard	isophane insulin* (pork)	Intermediate-acting
Lentard MC	insulin zinc suspension* (beef and pork)	Intermediate-acting
neutral insulin	neutral soluble insulin* (beef)	Short-acting
Semitard MC	amorphous insulin zinc suspension* (pork)	Intermediate-acting
Velosulin	neutral soluble insulin* (pork)	Short-acting
Velosulin Cartridge	neutral soluble insulin* (pork)	Short-acting

* Highly purified

Table 65.3 Biphasic-acting combined insulin preparations

Preparation	*Drug*	*Duration of action*
Human Actraphane	isophane insulin* (human) 70%	Intermediate-acting
	neutral soluble insulin* (human) 30%	Short-acting
Human Initard (50/50)	isophane insulin* (human) 50%	Intermediate-acting
	neutral soluble insulin* (human) 50%	Short-acting
Human Mixtard 30/70	isophane insulin* (human) 70%	Intermediate-acting
	neutral soluble insulin* (human) 30%	Short-acting

Table 65.3 Biphasic-acting combined insulin preparations (*cont.*)

Preparation	*Drug*	*Duration of action*
Humulin M1	isophane insulin (human) 90%	Intermediate-acting
	neutral soluble insulin (human) 10%	Short-acting
Humulin M2	isophane insulin (human) 80%	Intermediate-acting
	neutral soluble insulin (human) 20%	Short-acting
Humulin M3	isophane insulin (human) 70%	Intermediate-acting
	neutral soluble insulin (human) 30%	Short-acting
Humulin M4	isophane insulin (human) 60%	Intermediate-acting
	neutral soluble insulin (human) 40%	Short-acting
Initard 50/50	isophane insulin* (pork) 50%	Intermediate-acting
	neutral soluble insulin* (pork) 50%	Short-acting
Mixtard 30/70	isophane insulin* (pork) 70%	Intermediate-acting
	neutral soluble insulin* (pork) 30%	Short-acting
Penmix 30/70	isophane insulin* (human) 70%	Intermediate-acting
	neutral soluble insulin* (human) 30%	Short-acting
Rapitard MC	biphasic preparation of beef and pork insulin*	Intermediate- and short-acting

* Highly purified

66

Female sex hormones

The newborn baby girl's ovaries contain thousands of eggs (ova). Each ovum is in a fluid-filled sac called a follicle. Before puberty, many of these follicles enlarge but then shrink.

Puberty

At puberty the ovaries begin to undergo cyclical changes under stimulation from hormones produced by the master gland (the pituitary). The uterus and vagina enlarge, the breasts develop, fat is laid down in certain areas giving the characteristic female figure, and hair starts to grow under the arms and on the pubis.

Menstruation

The pituitary gland produces two hormones that affect the growth of the ovaries. They are called gonadotrophins because they make the gonads (ovaries) grow. One is follicle-stimulating hormone (FSH), which stimulates the development of follicles around the ova in the ovaries. This makes the follicles grow, and as one of them starts to grow more than the others it starts to produce its own female sex hormones, called oestrogens. These oestrogens are released into the bloodstream to work on many tissues and organs in the body. One major effect is on the lining of the uterus, making it grow thicker. As the blood concentration of oestrogens increases, the pituitary's production of FSH decreases and the other gonadotrophic hormone takes over. This is called luteinizing hormone (LH) and it acts on the follicle, making it rupture and release the ovum. This process is known as ovulation. LH also ensures the continuing development of the follicle after it has released the ovum and converts it into a yellowish body (corpus luteum), producing a different female sex hormone, called progesterone, which belongs to the group of female sex hormones known as progestogens. Progesterone is released into the blood stream to work on many tissues and organs in the body. One major effect is to act on the lining of the uterus, making it ready to receive a fertilized ovum.

The first change in the uterus when its lining thickens under the influence of oestrogens is called the proliferative phase (phase of growth). The subsequent phase, after ovulation, when progesterone makes it undergo special changes in preparation for receiving a fertilized egg (ovum) is called the secretory phase. The description is used because cells develop that will be ready to secrete nutritious fluids if conception occurs and the fertilized egg settles on the lining of the uterus. Doctors, by taking a scraping (or biopsy) from the lining of the uterus, are able to tell whether the lining has undergone both changes – proliferative and secretory – and, therefore, whether the patient has ovulated. They are also able to determine whether oestrogens and progesterone have been made in sufficient quantities to produce the changes.

Progesterone inhibits the production of LH by the pituitary whereas oestrogens stimulate its production. There is thus a delicate balance between FSH and LH production by the pituitary gland and the production of oestrogens and progesterone by the developing follicle and the corpus luteum respectively.

Before puberty the production of FSH and LH by the pituitary is not enough to stimulate the development of a follicle around an ovum and only small quantities of oestrogens and progesterone are produced by the ovaries. Two or three years before the development of menstruation, pubertal changes are already taking place. This is thought to be due to the growth and development of the pituitary gland, and also the part of the brain (the hypothalamus) that exerts control over the pituitary gland. As the pituitary gland develops, it starts to increase its production of FSH and LH. These get to work on the ovaries and cause groups of follicles to develop. As they grow, they start to produce more and more oestrogens. These oestrogens work on various tissues in the body, producing the secondary sexual characteristics; in addition, the lining of the uterus starts to thicken and the first menstrual period develops (the menarche).

After the first menstrual period the pituitary and hypothalamus are also developing and at times produce too little gonadotrophic hormone to affect the production of oestrogens by the ovaries. Thus the lining of the uterus does not thicken and a young girl may go several months without a period or she may have irregular periods. As the pituitary settles down, the periods will become more regular and menstruation will start to occur approximately every 28 days.

During these first few months, ovulation does not usually occur because the pituitary does not produce sufficient LH hormone; but as the cycles without ovulation continue (usually known as anovulatory cycle), more and more oestrogens are produced by the follicles and LH production increases, eventually causing ovulation (release of the ovum).

At the time of ovulation, the lining of the uterus is ready to receive the ovum, which after ovulation leaves the ovary and passes down a fallopian tube into the cavity of the uterus. If the ovum is not fertilized by a male sperm (and this often takes place as the ovum passes down the tube), it slowly disintegrates as it passes down the cavity of the uterus.

If the ovum is not fertilized, LH production falls and the corpus luteum shrinks, resulting in a decreasing production of progesterone and oestrogens. As the level drops, the blood vessels supplying the lining of the uterus close, the lining disintegrates and menstrual bleeding starts. When progesterone production by the shrinking corpus luteum declines, the pituitary responds by producing more LH. In response to a decreased production of oestrogens the pituitary starts to produce more FSH and the cycle starts all over again. The increase of FSH and LH starts to work on the ovaries, a new group of follicles starts to develop and the whole sequence of changes is repeated.

Pregnancy

If the ovum is fertilized, it burrows into the lining of the uterus and becomes anchored. It develops a layer of cells around it (the trophoblast), which multiply and eventually form the placenta (afterbirth). At this early stage the trophoblast cells surrounding the developing fertilized ovum (now called an embryo) start to produce chorionic gonadotrophin hormone ('chorionic' because it is produced by the cells which go to form part of the placenta called the chorion, and 'gonadotrophin' because it works on the gonads, or ovaries). Chorionic gonadotrophin, like LH, works on the corpus luteum in the ovary and maintains its development. This results in an increased production of progesterone by the corpus luteum, despite the fall-off in LH production by the pituitary.

Under stimulation from progesterone, the lining of the uterus continues to provide nutrition for the developing embryo until the placenta is developed. This then takes over essential duties – supplying nutrients, carrying away unwanted products, supplying oxygen and other gases to the developing baby and carrying away carbon dioxide. In addition, the placenta (which links the baby's blood supply directly to the mother's) continues to produce chorionic gonadotrophin but also starts to produce its own oestrogens and progesterone.

This delicate and complex balance of hormones ensures that the pregnancy becomes established. After about 12 weeks the chorionic gonadotrophin production by the placenta starts to fall off, the corpus luteum shrinks at about 16–18 weeks, and production of chorionic gonadotrophin reaches a low level which lasts throughout the pregnancy. At the same time, production of oestrogens and progesterone by the placenta continues to increase throughout the pregnancy, falling abruptly after delivery. The fall in oestrogens then stimulates the pituitary to produce FSH, a group of follicles gradually starts to develop in an ovary and the menstrual cycle is set in motion again.

The high levels of oestrogen and progesterone in pregnancy are responsible for breast development. Some chorionic gonadotrophin hormone is excreted in the urine and gives a positive urine pregnancy test early in pregnancy.

After childbirth the sucking of the baby at the breast stimulates production of a milk-producing hormone (prolactin) by the pituitary gland. This stimulates further milk production (supply meets demand). At the same time, prolactin serves a useful purpose by stopping the production of FSH by the pituitary and thus preventing the development of follicles in the ovaries. This prevents the breast-feeding mother from menstruating for several months after delivery, depending, of course, on how long she breast feeds. However, it does not necessarily mean that a breast-feeding mother cannot get pregnant.

Menopause

As the ovaries get older, the follicles start responding less to FSH. This results in decreased production of oestrogens and, for a time, increased production of FSH. Also, LH production falls and ovulation fails to occur during some cycles. As ovarian function continues to decline, ovulation stops altogether. Oestrogen and progesterone production fall right off and eventually menstrual periods stop. Various menopausal changes may occur, which include increase in weight, hot flushes, bone changes and psychological symptoms. The lack of oestrogens produces shrinking of the secondary sex organs – the breasts become smaller, the vulva and vagina undergo changes and the ovaries and uterus shrink (see Chapter 68).

Female sex hormones

From this brief description of the hormonal control of puberty, menstruation, pregnancy and the menopause you will see that there are two groups of hormones that control numerous functions in the female body – oestrogens and progestogens. Many synthetic preparations of these hormones are available and they are used for a wide variety of disorders.

Female sex hormones – oestrogens

The main sources of oestrogens in the body are the ovaries, and the placenta in pregnant women. They are also produced in small amounts by the adrenal glands and by the testes in males. Over 20 different oestrogens have been isolated from the urine of pregnant women. There are three main oestrogens at work in the female body – oestradiol, oestriol and oestrone. Oestradiol is the most powerful and is produced mainly by the ovaries. In the liver, oestradiol is easily converted into oestrone, which is converted into oestriol. All three are excreted in the urine. During pregnancy, large quantities of oestrogens are made by the placenta, and urine from pregnant women contains a large amount of oestrogens.

Oestrogens are responsible for the development of secondary sexual characteristics in girls. By their direct actions on tissues they cause the growth and development of the vagina, uterus and fallopian tubes; they contribute to the development of the breasts and the female figure; they affect bone growth, and the growth of hair in the armpits and in the pubic region, and the pigmentation of the nipples and genitals. Oestrogens also contribute to the control of the menstrual cycle (see earlier).

The *naturally occurring oestrogens*, in order of potency, are oestriol, oestrone and oestradiol. *Semi-synthetic oestrogens* include derivatives of oestradiol – ethinyloestradiol and esters of oestradiol such as oestradiol valerate. Mestranol is converted to ethinyloestradiol in the body.

Completely synthetic oestrogens include dienoestrol, and stilboestrol and its derivatives (e.g. diethylstilboestrol).

Conjugated oestrogen is a mixture of oestrogens (oestrone and equilin) obtained wholly or partly from horses' urine or made synthetically from purified oestrone and equilin. *Esterified oestrogen* is made from a salt of oestrone and equilin.

All oestrogen preparations can cause the same spectrum of effects, including harmful effects, when taken in equally effective doses (therapeutic doses). The semi-synthetic oestrogen ethinyloestradiol is the most active oestrogen that can be taken by mouth and it is the one most commonly used (see 'Oral contraceptives', Chapter 67).

For further discussion of the benefits and risks of oestrogen preparations, see under 'The menopause' in Chapter 68.

The need in women for male sex hormones

In addition to the main oestrogen production by the ovaries and placenta in women, many other tissues in both men and women produce oestrogens; for example, the liver, muscles, hair follicles and fat tissues. These sources form a useful supply of oestrogens in males and in women after the menopause. An interesting point is that this production of oestrogen requires a source of male sex hormone (testosterone). In women it is provided by the ovaries and the adrenal glands. The male sex hormone testosterone and its active breakdown product androstenedione are needed in women not only for the manufacture of oestrogen in the body but also they make a contribution to female growth at puberty. They may contribute to the development of acne in female teenagers and they are mainly responsible for the libido (sex drive) of women.

Harmful effects of oestrogens

Oestrogens cause salt and water retention in the body and may account for the fluid retention that occurs in the latter half of the menstrual cycle. They can also reduce blood fat levels and may protect against coronary heart disease but this potentially beneficial effect may be reduced if they are taken with a progestogen as in hormone replacement therapy (HRT).

Reported harmful effects from oestrogens include break-through bleeding, spotting, changes with periods; loss of periods during or after treatment; painful periods or premenstrual syndrome (PMS); thrush of the vagina; symptoms similar to those produced by cystitis; tenderness and enlargement of the breasts with or without some milk production; nausea, vomiting, bloated feelings, headache, migraine, dizziness, depression, increase or decrease in weight, changes in libido. Rarely, they may cause jaundice; various types of skin lesion, including chloasma (pigmentation on the face); increased hair on the body, loss of hair from the scalp; and involuntary movements (chorea).

Warnings on the use of oestrogens

Oestrogens should not be used in women who suffer from cancer of the breast or a cancer dependent on oestrogens, known or suspected pregnancy, undiagnosed bleeding from the vagina, active thrombosis or a past history of thrombosis.

Long-term use of oestrogens in certain animals increases the frequency of cancer of the breast, cervix, vagina and liver.

The regular daily use of oestrogens for more than a year in women after the menopause may increase the risk of developing cancer of the womb. This risk is greater the longer the use and the higher the daily dose of oestrogens. The risk is reduced if the oestrogens are used in cycles (3 weeks on and 1 week off), if they are used in low doses and particularly if they are combined with a progestrogen – see hormone replacement therapy after the menopause (Chapter 68). Prolonged daily use of oestrogens may also increase the risk of getting cancer of the breast. (The risk with oestrogen and cancer of the breast in post-menopausal women is discussed in Chapter 68.)

Oestrogens used in the treatment of cancer of the prostate in males may, rarely, cause cancer of the breast – this risk is related to the dose and duration of treatment. The large doses of oestrogen used are also associated with an increased risk of thrombosis.

Oestrogen treatment in post-menopausal women increases the risk of them developing gall stones. A similar risk has been noted in women taking the combined oral contraceptive pill for 2 years or more.

There is an increased risk of thrombosis in women taking the combined oral contraceptive pill, which is related to the dose of oestrogen. This applies particularly after surgical operations in women taking the combined oral contraceptive pill. Therefore you should stop taking it 4 weeks before surgery or during prolonged periods of immobilization (e.g. being confined to bed for some injury). Advice to women receiving oestrogens after the menopause is not clear on this point but it is obviously better to be safe and stop treatment 4 weeks before surgery.

Oestrogens should be used with utmost caution in patients suffering from any disorder of the blood vessels supplying the brain (cerebrovascular disease) or the heart (coronary artery disease) because of the increased risk of a stroke or a heart attack, respectively.

An increase in blood pressure is not uncommon in women taking combined oral contraceptive pills. This may also occur in women taking oestrogens after the menopause.

Combined oral contraceptive pills may make diabetes worse, so women on the pill or taking oestrogens after the menopause should be checked for diabetes at regular intervals.

Oestrogen treatment may cause a severe rise in blood calcium levels in people suffering from cancer of the breast with secondaries in bone. If this occurs the drug should be stopped.

Oestrogens may cause fluid retention and aggravate epilepsy, migraine, heart disease or kidney disease. Patients with these disorders should be kept under careful observation.

There is an increased risk of developing mental depression in women taking the combined oral contraceptive pill. Although this is probably due to the progestogen, oestrogens should nevertheless be given with caution to post-menopausal women who have had an episode of serious mental depression in the past.

Fibroids of the womb may increase in size on oestrogen treatment.

Women who have had jaundice in pregnancy run a risk of developing jaundice on oestrogen treatment (including the pill). If jaundice occurs, oestrogen treatment (including the pill) should be stopped and the woman should have a full medical check-up, including tests of liver function.

Oestrogens should be given with caution to patients who suffer from impaired kidney function.

Because oestrogens affect the use of calcium and phosphorus in the body, they should be used with caution in people with disorders of bone metabolism that are associated with a high blood calcium or with impaired functioning of the kidneys.

Oestrogens should be used with utmost caution in young people who have not finished growing because they may stop growth prematurely – note the possible risks of oral contraceptive pills in young girls.

Oestrogen preparations are easily absorbed through the skin. When applied to the skin they may have a general effect on the body. Workers who handle these drugs may develop enlarged breasts and other harmful effects if they do not take protective precautions.

Risks in pregnancy

Oestrogens should not be taken during pregnancy. Their use in early pregnancy may be associated with an increased risk of damage to the unborn baby. Baby girls may, rarely, develop cancer of the vagina or cervix in later life if their mothers took high doses of the oestrogen diethylstilboestrol during pregnancy. The use of high doses of diethylstilboestrol (DES) in pregnancy has also been associated with an increased risk of abortion, ectopic pregnancies, premature delivery and death of newborn babies.

The possible risk from oestrogens during pregnancy, particularly early pregnancy, applies to the use of combined oral contraceptives (see warnings, earlier); of oestrogen-containing pills used to diagnose early pregnancy (these should no longer be used); and of oestrogens to prevent abortion (they should no longer be used for this purpose). Also, note the risks of the 'morning-after' pill (post-coital pill), although this is taken so soon after sexual intercourse that if an egg is fertilized it has hardly had time to start developing; nevertheless there is a slight risk.

If you become pregnant while taking a preparation containing oestrogen, you should be aware of the possible dangers.

Risk in breast feeding

Do not breast feed if you are taking an oestrogen-containing drug.

Before starting oestrogens

Doctors should take a complete family history and a personal medical history before starting a patient on treatment with oestrogens. This should be followed by a detailed medical examination with special emphasis on the blood pressure, breasts, abdomen, an internal examination and a cervical smear. This examination should be repeated every 12 months for as long as the individual is taking a preparation containing oestrogen (e.g. the oral contraceptive pill).

The use of oestrogens

Painful menstrual periods

The drug treatment of painful periods (dysmenorrhoea) is discussed in Chapter 68.

Heavy and/or irregular menstrual periods

The drug treatment of heavy and/or irregular periods is discussed in Chapter 68.

Oral contraceptives

The most common use of oestrogens is in combination with progestogens in oral contraceptives (see Chapter 67).

Stopping breast feeding

Oestrogens in high doses have been used for decades to stop the breasts filling up with milk in mothers who, after childbirth, did not wish to or could not breast feed their babies. However, this treatment is associated with a risk of developing thrombosis in the deep veins of the legs and pelvis and the life-threatening risk that a piece of the thrombus may come loose and travel in the blood stream to the lungs. Oestrogens should no longer be used for this purpose.

If drug treatment is needed it is now the fashion in the UK to use bromocriptine to suppress milk production. Bromocriptine stimulates certain nerve receptors in the brain (dopamine receptors) and is used to treat Parkinson's disease in which there is a deficiency of dopamine. It also blocks the release of the milk-producing hormone, prolactin, by the pituitary gland (see page 821) and that is why it is used to stop milk production.

Table 66.1 Oestrogen preparations

Preparation	*Drug*	*Dosage form*
Estraderm	oestradiol	Transparent transdermal patches
ethinyloestradiol	ethinyloestradiol	Tablets
Harmogen	oestrone (piperazine oestrone sulphate)	Tablets
Hormonin	oestradiol, oestriol and oestrone	Tablets
oestradiol	oestradiol	Implants
Ortho Dienoestrol	dienoestrol	Vaginal cream
Ortho-Gynest	oestriol	Pessaries, vaginal cream
Ovestin	oestriol	Tablets, cream
Premarin	conjugated oestrogens	Tablets, vaginal cream
Progynova	oestradiol	Tablets
Tampovagan Stilboestrol and Lactic Acid	stilboestrol with lactic acid	Pessaries

Treating menopausal symptoms

The use of oestrogens in the treatment of menopausal symptoms is discussed in Chapter 68.

Anti-oestrogens

Clomiphene, cyclofenil and tamoxifen block the actions of oestrogens at oestrogen receptor site; they are referred to as anti-oestrogens.

The important action of these drugs is their ability to stimulate the production of gonadotrophins (LH and FSH) by the master gland (the pituitary). They do this by blocking oestrogen receptors so that the pituitary thinks the level of oestrogens in the body is low and it stimulates the ovaries to produce more oestrogens. They are therefore used to treat infertility caused by a failure to ovulate and to treat people with absent periods or disorders of menstrual bleeding caused by failure to ovulate. Tamoxifen is also used to treat patients suffering from certain cancers that require oestrogens for their growth (see Chapter 76).

Preparations

clomiphene (Clomid tablets, Serophene tablets)
cyclofenil (Rehibin tablets)
tamoxifen (Emblon tablets, Noltam tablets, Nolvadex tablet preparations, Tamofen tablets)

Female sex hormones – progesterone and progestogens

Natural progesterone is a female sex hormone formed by the ovaries (first by a follicle and then by the corpus luteum). In pregnancy the placenta takes over production of progesterone. In both males and females the adrenal glands also produce some progesterone.

The production and actions of progesterone are discussed earlier in this chapter. Its chief function is to prepare the lining of the womb to receive a fertilized egg. If fertilization takes place, progesterone is then responsible for maintaining the pregnancy and for breast development.

Progesterone causes the body temperature to rise during the last 2 weeks of the menstrual cycle, and this rise in temperature is a sign that ovulation has occurred. This is why recording the daily temperature throughout the menstrual cycle is used as a test to determine whether you are ovulating.

The term 'progestogen' is used to describe any drug that produces actions and effects in the body similar to those produced by the naturally occurring progesterone.

There are two main groups of progestogens:

1. Progesterone and synthetic drugs chemically related to it; for example allyloestrenol, dydrogesterone, hydroxyprogesterone and medroxyprogesterone
2. Synthetic drugs related to the male sex hormone, testosterone; for example ethisterone, ethynodiol, lynoestrenol and norethisterone

Natural progesterone lasts only a few minutes in the body because it is rapidly broken down by the liver. For this reason progesterone by mouth is ineffective, so it is given via the vagina (as pessaries), via the rectum (as suppositories) or via an injection into a muscle. By these routes it does not enter the liver so quickly.

The *synthetic progestogens* are effective when taken by mouth and are much longer acting than the naturally occurring progesterone. Those related to testosterone produce some male hormone effects (masculinization).

Depot injections of progestogens (e.g. medroxyprogesterone (Depo-Provera) or norethisterone (Noristerat). These long-acting preparations given by depot injections into a muscle provide contraceptive cover for about 2 months (see Chapter 67). They may be useful for providing contraception after an injection against german measles but this should not be carried out routinely without the written consent of the woman. They are also frequently used to provide contraception for poor and under-privileged women, usually living in areas where medical services are scarce.

In addition to the harmful effects and warnings listed above these depot injections may cause heavy bleeding if given just after childbirth. They may occasionally cause episodes of infertility and irregular periods after treatment is stopped. Swelling, discoloration of the skin and abscess may occur at the site of injections.

Progestogens require oestrogens

For progestogens to work they require oestrogens either to have prepared the 'target' sites beforehand (e.g. the lining of the uterus) or to work simultaneously with them. In other words, progestogens act mainly on tissue that is 'sensitized' by oestrogens. This is why it is often better to give oestrogens and progestogens together when treating disorders of the menstrual cycle. Progestogens modify some of the effects of oestrogens but their actions are blocked if there is too much oestrogen.

Harmful effects of progestogens

Progestogens may occasionally cause breast tenderness and milk production, itching and skin rashes, depression, acne, break-through bleeding, spotting, changes in menstrual flow, loss of periods, fluid retention (e.g. ankle swelling), changes in weight, changes in libido, mental depression, rise in temperature, insomnia, nausea and sleepiness. Very rarely, they may cause changes in the neck of the womb, changes in liver function tests, jaundice, allergic reactions, hairiness, allergic skin rashes with and without itching, eye damage, ectopic pregnancy and cysts of the ovaries. For potential harmful effects of using an oestrogen/progestogen combination pill, see Chapter 67.

Warnings on the use of progestogens

Progestogens should not be used in anyone with thrombophlebitis or any type of thrombosis or a stroke, or who have a history of these disorders, nor in people with liver disease, cancer of the breasts or genitals, undiagnosed vaginal bleeding or missed abortion.

Be on the alert for the earliest sign of thrombosis. Stop the drug immediately if any impairment of vision develops, or if migraine develops.

Pre-treatment medical examinations and annual medical examinations should include a breast examination, an internal examination and a cervical smear.

Because progestogens may cause fluid retention, they should be used with caution in people with epilepsy, migraine and heart or kidney disorders.

Anyone with undiagnosed vaginal bleeding should have a full medical examination including internal examination and a cervical smear.

Individuals with a history of depressive illness should be treated with caution and the drug stopped if depression occurs.

Diabetic patients should be carefully monitored.

Risk in pregnancy

Progestogens should be used with utmost caution in pregnancy, particularly the use of high doses during the first 3 months of pregnancy (see later). Preparations containing a progestogen should no longer be used to test for pregnancy.

Risk in breast feeding

High doses of progestogens reduce milk production. They also enter the milk. The combined oral contraceptive pill should not be taken when breast feeding but a progestogen-only pill may be used because they contain only low doses of a progestogen.

Risks of cancer

Laboratory studies suggest that long-term use of high doses of progestogens may be associated with cancer of the breast in beagle dogs, and cancer of the womb in monkeys. The relevance of these findings to humans is not established.

Use of progestogens

Oral contraception

The most common use of progestogens is alone or in combination with oestrogens in oral contraceptives (see Chapter 67). The ones used in combined oral contraceptives (the 'pill') and progestogen-only contraceptives include desogestrel, ethynodiol, gestodene, levonorgestrel, lynoestrenol and norethisterone.

Miscarriages

Injections of various synthetic progestogens have been used for many years to try to prevent miscarriages, despite lack of evidence that these injections are of any use and despite the fact that, if used in the first 3–4 months of pregnancy, they may possibly cause damage to the unborn baby.

In the vast majority of women the cause of a miscarriage is a defective egg which she needs to get rid of, and progestogens are unlikely to affect the body's natural reactions. However, because of their effects on the muscle of the womb, they may actually delay a spontaneous miscarriage.

In a few pregnant women who have had a previous miscarriage it may be shown from laboratory tests that they are not producing sufficient amounts of progesterone to maintain their pregnancy and these individuals may benefit from a course of treatment with the naturally occurring progesterone.

Heavy and irregular menstrual periods

The use of progestogens to treat heavy and irregular periods is discussed in Chapter 68.

Premenstrual syndrome

The use of progestogens to treat premenstrual syndrome is discussed in Chapter 68.

Loss of menstrual periods (amenorrhoea)

The use of progestogens to treat amenorrhoea is discussed in Chapter 68.

Menopause

The use of progestogens and oestrogens in the treatment of menopausal symptoms is discussed in Chapter 68.

Table 66.2 Progestogen preparations

Preparation	*Drug*	*Dosage form*
Cyclogest	progesterone	Suppositories
Depo-Provera	medroxyprogesterone	Depot injection
Depostat	gestronol	Depot injection
Duphaston	dydrogesterone	Tablets
Gestanin	allyloestrenol	Tablets
Gestone	progesterone	Injection
Menzol	norethisterone	Tablets
Primolut N	norethisterone	Tablets
Proluton Depot	hydroxyprogesterone	Depot injection
Provera	medroxyprogesterone	Tablets
Utovlan	norethisterone	Tablets

Table 66.3 Progestogen/oestrogen preparations

Preparation	*Drug*	*Dosage form*
Cyclo-Progynova 1 mg and 2 mg	oestradiol (oestrogen) levonorgestrel (progestogen)	Tablets
Estrapak	oestradiol (oestrogen) norethisterone (progestogen)	Oestrogen skin patch and norethisterone tablets
Menophase	mestranol (oestrogen) norethisterone (progestogen)	Tablets (phased doses)
Prempak-C	conjugated oestrogens norgestrel (progesterone)	Tablets (phased doses)

67

Oral contraceptive drugs

To understand the use of oral contraceptives read Chapter 66, on female sex hormones. It is most important that you understand the hormonal control of the menstrual cycle and in particular the parts played by the female sex hormones, oestrogens and progestogens.

There are three types of oral contraceptives:

1. Combined oestrogen/progestogen preparations containing fixed doses (usually known as 'the pill')
2. Phasic preparations containing oestrogens and progestogens in varying doses
3. Progestogen-only preparations containing fixed doses

The 'pill' – the combined oestrogen/progestogen oral contraceptive

These oral contraceptives are the most widely used and have the lowest failure rate in terms of unwanted pregnancies. They contain varying doses and types of oestrogens and progestogens. The dose of oestrogen is usually below 50 micrograms. Many go as low as 30 micrograms. With low-dose oestrogen pills (30–35 micrograms) the degree of protection is reduced and it is very important not to miss one. Combined pills containing less than 30 micrograms of an oestrogen are even less reliable. The dose of progestogen in combined pills also varies but it is not as critical as the dose of the oestrogen.

How the combined oestrogen/progestogen pill works

The combination of an oestrogen and a progestogen in the 'pill' stops the ripening and release of an egg from the ovary (ovulation). It does this because the pituitary gland responds to the high blood level of oestrogen and progestogen produced by the pill by reducing its release of follicle-stimulating hormone (FSH) and luteinizing hormone (LH), which are necessary for the growth of the egg and its release. The combination of oestrogen and progestogen also causes the lining of the womb to become thin so that it would be difficult for a fertilized egg to bed down in its surface. In addition, the mucus in the neck of the womb becomes thick and sticky and forms a mucous plug that stops sperms from entering the womb (this is an effect produced principally by progestogens). The combination also slows down movement in the walls of the fallopian tubes and reduces secretion into the tubes, which makes it difficult for the egg to pass through the fallopian tubes into the womb.

The dose of oestrogen and safety

A principal effect of oestrogens in oral contraceptives is to stop the production of FSH and therefore a follicle does not develop and ovulation is prevented. However – and this is very important – the production of FSH is related to the circulating level of oestrogen, so a small dose of oestrogen may actually lead to increased FSH production and therefore stimulation of the follicle-producing ovulation. An equally important point to remember is that a medium dose of oestrogen may merely delay ovulation; but, as we shall see later, the principal risks of the pill are thought to be due to its oestrogen content and so the smallest effective dose has to be used, which may not be enough to stop some women ovulating. The safest dose to avoid serious harmful effects is 50 micrograms or less of ethinyloestradiol or mestranol – so take note. The names of the oestrogen and progestogen in your pills will be entered in small type on the packet – look for these.

The dose of progestogen and safety

If the dose of progestogen in the pill gets too low, you can get a 'show' in between periods (break-through bleeding); there is then an added risk that you may ovulate and could get pregnant. If you get break-through bleeding on a particular pill, you will need to change to a pill that contains a higher dose of progestogen (see Table 67.1). Also, a higher dose of progestogen in a pill gives you a wider margin of safety if you happen to forget to take one, but note the risks (see later).

How to take the combined pill (the pill)

Starting on the pill

The term 'the pill' usually refers to the most commonly used type of oral contraceptive – oestrogen/progestogen combinations. The first course of the pill is usually started on the fifth day of the menstrual period, taking the day that the period started as the first day. You then take a pill daily for 21 days, followed by an interval of 7 days without taking the pill, during which time you will have a period. This means that you will have a menstrual cycle of 28 days, because this is what most women are used to. After 7 days off the pill, you then start the next course so that in a 28-day cycle you take the pill for 3 weeks and stop it for 1 week. Alternatively, when you first go on the pill you may start it on the first day instead of the fifth day, if you wish. If you do this, you need not take the extra precautions that you should take for 14 days when you start the pill on the fifth day (see later).

The pill comes in pop-out calendar packets on which are marked the days of the week so that it is easy for you to remember when you stopped and need to re-start. If you do not have a good memory there are preparations available that contain seven dummy tablets. The dummy tablets are a different colour from the contraceptive pills but all you have to do, having started the first course, is to take one pill every day – you do not have to remember when to stop and when to start.

If you forget

If you forget a pill, take it as soon as you remember and then take your next pill at the normal time. If you forget to take a pill for 12 hours or more (particularly the first or last in the packet) you should take it as soon as you remember and then take that day's pill at your usual time and continue the course *but* you should avoid sexual intercourse or take extra precautions for the next 7 days. If the 7 days run beyond the end of the packet, open a new packet and continue taking one every day until you come to the end of the new packet. Do not leave a gap. Your period will now be delayed until you have finished the second packet of pills but this will do no harm. You may also get some bleeding on the days you are taking the tablets but again this will do no harm. If you are on an ED pill (see Table 67.2) do not take the seven dummy tablets but go straight on to the active pills.

If you forget to take the pill for 2 days (36 hours or more), ovulation may occur. Stop the course of pills, avoid sexual intercourse or use another method of contraception and wait until you have had a period before starting the next course. Start the next course on the fifth day but take extra precautions for 2 weeks because it will be like starting a new course.

If you think you have got pregnant

If you think you may have got pregnant during the days when you forgot to take the pill, or if you are scared or worried that you have got pregnant, stop the pill. If you have a 'normal' period, start the new course, but if you are at all suspicious and particularly if your period is scanty or does not begin, do not start a new month's course. Wait until 40 days from the first day of your previous period and have a urine pregnancy test done (you may get a false negative before this time). Advise your doctor or pharmacist of any other drugs your are taking, as some may interfere with the test. If the test is negative, use extra contraception for the first 14 days when starting your next course on the fifth day of your next period because this will be like starting a new course.

It is best to stop the pill at least 3 months before you want to try to get pregnant.

If you miss a period

If after the first month on the pill you do not have a period, carry on as normal. If you miss two periods, stop the pill and have a urine pregnancy test done.

If you get break-through bleeding

If you have been on the pill for some time and then get break-through bleeding between periods, stop the pill and consult your doctor. You will need an internal examination and a cervical smear to check that everything is all right.

If you get diarrhoea or vomiting

If you have an episode of diarrhoea or vomiting while on the pill, this may interfere with its absorption. You should avoid sexual intercourse or take extra precautions for the rest of the month.

If you take other drugs

Drugs that may interact with oral contraceptives are listed in Chapter 89. Some antibiotics (e.g. ampicillin) may interfere with the absorption of the pill and you should avoid sexual intercourse or take extra precautions during the course of treatment and for the rest of the month. Certain drugs (e.g. barbiturates, phenytoin and rifampicin) may increase the breakdown of the pill in the liver and reduce its effectiveness. Patients taking these drugs run a risk of getting pregnant even though they are on the pill.

After childbirth and when breast feeding

After childbirth, the pill should not be started for 3–4 weeks because of the risk of developing thrombosis. They may be taken while breast feeding but in some women they may reduce the supply of milk. Progestogen-only pills do not affect milk flow.

*Harmful effects and risks of using the pill**

Depression

The progestogen in the pill may occasionally cause a depressed mood in some women, but it is not the progestogen alone – it seems to require oestrogen as well to produce this unpleasant effect, and so it is the combination that causes the trouble. There is a suggestion that vitamin B_6 may help to control this depression and it is certainly worth trying.

Risk of thrombosis

The greatest risk from the pill is the development of thrombosis in a vein and the shooting off of part of this clot (thrombus) into the lungs, resulting in death. This process is called thrombo-embolism and the thrombus usually occurs in the deep veins of the legs or pelvis. It may also occur in the vessels supplying the brain (cerebral thrombosis), producing a stroke.

This *very rare* risk of thrombosis is not related to how long you have been on the pill, but it is thought to be roughly proportional to the dose of oestrogen in a preparation. It is safer to use a dose of oestrogen of 50 micrograms or less, and the majority of pills do not go above this. There is no difference whether the oestrogen is mestranol or ethinyloestradiol.

There is a greater risk of thrombosis if you are over 35 years of age, if you smoke and if you are overweight. The risk is also greater in women who suffer from diabetes, raised blood pressure and/or raised blood fat level.

Risk of a stroke

The very rare risk of suffering a stroke increases as the dose of oestrogen in the pill increases. It is also greater with the advancing age of the user, with cigarette smoking and with being overweight. Having diabetes, raised blood pressure and/or a raised blood fat level also increases the risks of having a stroke.

Risk of a heart attack

There appears to be a very rare risk between taking the pill and developing

* For risk of liver tumours, see under HRT, page 936.

a coronary thrombosis. People at high risk are those with raised blood pressure who are also heavy smokers, or those with high blood fat levels and a family history of a parent or brother or sister dying from a coronary thrombosis under the age of about 60.

Changes in the body's chemistry

The pill has many effects upon the body's metabolism. For example, blood sugar and fat levels may be raised.

Blood clotting

Blood clotting may be affected by high-dose oestrogen preparations, which may increase the very rare risk of thrombosis.

Itching vagina and thrush infections

The pill may predispose to infections of the cervix, particularly by thrush (candida). Itching vagina (pruritus vulvae) may occasionally be produced by the pill, and vaginal discharge and itching are more likely to occur if you are given a tetracycline or another such broad-spectrum antibiotic for some other infection.

Itching and skin rashes

Itching of the skin may rarely occur and some women get a brownish colour (chloasma) on their face which is also seen in pregnancy. A blistering skin rash (porphyria) on exposure to the sun may rarely occur, and some women's hair goes thin for a few months after stopping the pill.

Risk of eye disorders

Very rarely, the pill may damage the nerves in the eye and/or cause a thrombosis in a blood vessel, producing blurred vision or double vision. The pill may affect your ability to wear contact lenses.

Risks of gall bladder disease

There appears to be a rare but increased risk of gall bladder disease in women taking the pill.

Risks of raised blood pressure

The blood pressure may rise in some women taking the pill. This is related to the length of time on the pill.

Risks of headaches

Migraine may start or get worse on the pill, and persistent headache may occur. Mild headache and flushing may also occur.

Risk of the pill and surgery

Because of the risk of thrombosis following surgery the pill should be stopped 6 weeks before non-emergency operations unless they are minor. It may be started again 2 weeks after becoming fully mobile. If stopping is not possible, sub-cutaneous heparin should be given.

Risks of cancer

In women taking an oral contraceptive over a prolonged period of time the possible long-term risk of their developing cancer of the breast, uterus, cervix or vagina should always be considered, although at present there is no confirmed evidence of such risks. However, studies of these risks are difficult because of the prolonged delays in the development of cancer and the many other factors that are known to influence the incidence of cancers of this kind. It does mean, though, that women taking oral contraceptives should have annual medical examinations, including breast screening and cervical screening. Liver cancers have, very rarely, been reported in women taking the pill.

Some other symptoms

Other symptoms that may occasionally occur on the pill include loss of appetite, nausea and vomiting; cramps in the legs and abdomen; fluid retention (bloated feeling), tenderness of the breasts, white vaginal discharge, dry vagina, increase in weight, dizziness, swelling of the ankles, changes in libido (may be increased or decreased) and painful muscles and joints.

Changes in menstruation

Spotting, which is a very slight show of blood between periods, is usually of no significance. Carry on taking the pill, as it usually clears up. If it recurs the next month, consult your doctor.

Break-through bleeding, which is bleeding between periods like a small period, may be stopped by taking two pills a day for 2 or 3 days and then going back on the normal course. Alternatively, you may carry on the course and see how things are with the next month's course. If it recurs, consult your doctor. Another way is to stop the pill for 7 days and then start another course. Whichever you choose, if break-through bleeding occurs 2 months running, you must see your doctor and have a gynaecological examination, which will usually include a cervical smear test. Such an examination is also necessary if spotting or break-through bleeding occurs for the first time after prolonged use of the pill or if it recurs at irregular intervals. Decreased flow is nothing to worry about.

Reduced or absent periods

In some women the pill may make periods lighter and relatively painless. Women with a past history of scanty periods or irregular periods may miss periods altogether. This is not a matter for concern but it may make it difficult to decide whether you are pregnant if you missed taking the pill as directed. If you think you might be pregnant, follow the procedure described earlier.

Following childbirth

The pill should not be used during the first 3–4 weeks after childbirth because of the risk of thrombosis.

Breast feeding and the pill

The combined pill used immediately after childbirth may interfere with the production of breast milk. There may be a decrease in the quantity and quality. A progestogen-only pill does not affect breast feeding and should be used in preference to a combined pill. Use oral contraceptives.

Problems with periods after stopping the pill

Occasionally, after stopping the pill some women fail to have a period. This is more common in women with late puberty who previously had irregular periods. It is caused by failure of the pituitary gland to recover from its suppression by the high blood levels of oestrogens and progestogens while on the pill. The hypothalamus may also not recover its full function. The lining of the uterus in these women may not respond to oestrogens produced by their own ovaries because they have been under daily influence, for many months, of the oestrogen and progestogen in the pill they have been taking. Loss of periods does not appear to be harmful and if a women does not want to get pregnant there is no need to give a drug to stimulate ovulation.

Failure to get pregnant when off the pill

After being on the pill it may take some women months to years to get pregnant but this is not related to the length of time that they were taking the pill.

Warnings on the use of the pill

Do *not* take the pill:

- If you are pregnant or suspect that you may be pregnant
- If you suffer from undiagnosed vaginal bleeding
- If you have suffered or are suffering from a thrombosis in an artery or vein, angina, heart valve disease, or heart attack or stroke, or chorea
- If you have sickle cell anaemia
- If you are prone to develop thrombosis or circulation disorders
- If you have suffered from jaundice or severe itching in pregnancy
- If you have jaundice, any type of infectious hepatitis, porphyria or liver tumour (adenoma)
- If you suffer from otosclerosis in which the deafness is getting worse
- If you have cancer of the breast or womb dependent upon oestrogens for growth
- If you have attacks of severe migraine (e.g. associated with pins and needles in hands and/or feet); an increase in the frequency or severity of headaches indicates that a medical examination is required

Do not take the pill for 6 weeks before a surgical operation or for 2 weeks after.

Do not take the pill for 4 weeks after childbirth. A progestogen-only pill has fewer harmful effects if you are breast feeding and may be taken during this time.

Precautions on the pill

The pill may cause *fluid retention*, so use it with caution if you suffer from epilepsy, migraine, asthma, liver, kidney or heart disease. Use it with caution if you have multiple sclerosis or Raynaud's disease or if you are on kidney dialysis.

If you smoke, a progestogen-only pill may be safer, particularly if you are over 35 years of age.

If you are 35 and are taking the pill, you should not smoke.

To reduce the risk of thrombosis, it is better to use a pill that contains 50 micrograms or less of an oestrogen. If you have had a superficial thrombophlebitis you may take the pill, but regular medical supervision is necessary. It is best not to use the pill if you have a high blood fat level.

If you are at the menopause (and being on the pill will not affect your symptoms), stop the pill for 2 or 3 months to see if a period comes on; if it does, go back on the pill for another 2 or 3 months. If you do not have a period, do not go back on the pill but take alternative contraceptive precautions for 2 years if you are under 50 years of age or for 1 year if you are over 50.

If you have diabetes or a family history of diabetes, you should be cautious, although having diabetes does not stop you going on the pill. However, if you have signs of damaged arteries from your diabetes, you should not take the pill, nor if you smoke, have a raised blood fat level or if your blood pressure is raised.

If you are due to have thyroid tests, stop the pill for 2 months before – it interferes with tests for thyroid function.

Be cautious when using corticosteroids – they may send your blood pressure up.

Remember that, if you have a bout of diarrhoea or vomiting, you may not absorb sufficient of the drug to be effective, and you should use additional contraceptive precautions for the rest of the month.

Antibiotics such as ampicillin interfere with the absorption of the pill from the intestine, and you should take *extra* precautions during the course of treatment and for 14 days after or until the next period starts.

If you are ever in doubt, always continue to take the pill as directed but take additional precautions until the end of the month.

Varicose veins are not a reason for not taking the pill.

Piles (haemorrhoids) are not a reason for not taking the pill.

If you have raised blood pressure, you should be cautious about using the pill or other oral contraceptive. If you have a normal blood pressure and develop a rise in blood pressure on the pill, you should stop taking it.

If you suffer from epilepsy, use a pill with a high dose of oestrogen (e.g. ethinyloestradiol) but no greater than 50 micrograms. This is because anti-epileptic drugs increase the breakdown of the pill in the body and lessen its effectiveness.

It may be best not to take the pill if you have had previous episodes of severe mental depression. Remember that you may get depressed if you change from a high- to a low-dose oestrogen pill.

Remember that you need to avoid sexual intercourse or use additional contraceptive methods if you change pills (e.g. from high dose to low dose). Check with your doctor or pharmacist.

Young girls (under 16 years of age) should not start taking the pill until their periods are occurring regularly. Young girls taking the pill for more than 9 months should stop their pill for 1 month and be checked to see if they are ovulating. If they are, they can carry on with the pill. If they are not ovulating, they should not be taking the pill and should be referred to a gynaecologist.

Interaction with other drugs

Drugs that may interact with oral contraceptives and reduce their effectiveness are listed in Chapter 89.

Vitamin C and the pill

There is no evidence that high doses of vitamin C help to protect against the harmful effects of the pill. However, they can increase the risk of thrombosis and increase the absorption of oestrogen – this can convert a low-oestrogen pill into a high-oestrogen pill.

When to stop the pill immediately

- If you get pregnant
- If your blood pressure goes up
- Six weeks before a surgical operation or when confined to bed after an accident or an illness
- If you get jaundice
- At the first signs of a thrombosis (e.g. pain and swelling in the calf)
- If you get migraine and have never previously had an attack
- If you have had migraine before and develop a very severe attack
- Frequent severe or unusual headaches
- Any disturbance of vision

The choice of combined oestrogen/progestogen preparations

Progestogens act on the uterus, which has been made sensitive (primed) to the effects of oestrogens. Various preparations may therefore be compared by how long they can delay a menstrual period when given in equally effective doses. In this way oestrogens may also be compared, and from such studies we have learned that ethinyloestradiol is abut 20 times more potent than naturally occurring oestradiol and about twice as potent as mestranol. Similarly, the progestogens can be ranked in order of potency (from strongest to weakest) – for example, norgestrel, norethisterone, megestrol. What is more, different chemical structures of the same drug can vary in potency; for example, levonorgestrel is about twice as potent as norgestrel. It is also worth noting that about 90 per cent of norethisterone acetate, ethynodiol acetate and lynoestrenol are converted to norethisterone in the body.

In the body, the ratio of oestrogen to progestogen is delicately balanced to give optimum chances of getting pregnant. Some women may produce too much oestrogen and therefore have heavy, frequent periods, whereas others may produce too much progesterone and suffer from scanty and irregular periods. Both these groups of women do not produce the ideal balance of hormones to encourage conception and they may therefore be sub-fertile. It follows, therefore, that if an oestrogen is given to some

Table 67.1 Oral contraceptives: combined oestrogen and progestogen pills – fixed doses

Name	*Oestrogen: dose (micrograms)*	*Progestogen: dose (milligrams)*
Brevinor	ethinyloestradiol 35 mcg	norethisterone 0.5 mg
Conova 30	ethinyloestradiol 30 mcg	ethynodiol 2 mg
Eugynon 30	ethinyloestradiol 30 mcg	levonorgestrel 0.25 mg
Femodene*	ethinyloestradiol 30 mcg	gestodene 0.075 mg
Loestrin 20	ethinyloestradiol 20 mcg	norethisterone 1 mg
Loestrin 30	ethinyloestradiol 30 mcg	norethisterone 1.5 mg
Marvelon	ethinyloestradiol 30 mcg	desogestrel 0.15 mg
Mercilon	ethinyloestradiol 20 mcg	desogestrel 0.15 mg
Microgynon 30	ethinyloestradiol 30 mcg	levonorgestrel 0.15 mg
Minulet	ethinyloestradiol 30 mcg	gestodene 0.075 mg
Neocon 1/35	ethinyloestradiol 35 mcg	norethisterone 1 mg
Norimin	ethinyloestradiol 35 mcg	norethisterone 1 mg
Norinyl-1	mestranol 50 mcg	norethisterone 1 mg
Ortho-Novin 1/50	mestranol 50 mcg	norethisterone 1 mg
Ovran	ethinyloestradiol 50 mcg	levonorgestrel 0.25 mg
Ovran 30	ethinyloestradiol 30 mcg	levonorgestrel 0.25 mg
Ovranette	ethinyloestradiol 30 mcg	levonorgestrel 0.15 mg
Ovysmen	ethinyloestradiol 35 mcg	norethisterone 0.5 mg

*Femodene ED as for Femodene, 21 active tablets plus 7 dummy tablets – take 1 tablet each day for 28 days.

women it may produce scanty periods or even absent periods if given in sufficient dosage (the principle of preparations used to delay the onset of menstruation). When the drugs are stopped, withdrawal bleeding will occur.

The effects produced by oestrogens can be balanced by adding progestogens. As the doses of these increase, the risk of pregnancy gets less; but, unfortunately, harmful effects start to increase. High doses of oestrogens and progestogens will produce the harmful effects mentioned earlier. Clearly there is a spectrum of desired effects and harmful effects produced by the various combination oestrogen/progestogen pills. Therefore, a pill should be chosen for you which takes into account how regular and heavy your periods were and its potential for producing harmful effects in you.

Re-read this chapter and Chapter 66, on female sex hormones, and make a note of the facts that apply particularly to you; for example, whether you previously had scanty periods or heavy periods, whether you are overweight or smoke, whether you have a raised blood pressure or have had a previous thrombosis, whether you have previously had some episodes of depressed mood, what harmful effects you have felt on certain contraceptive preparations, and so on. Remember, you may be on the pill for many years; it is most important for you to choose the pill that suits you the best.

Table 67.2 Oral contraceptives: biphasic and triphasic combined oestrogen and progestogen pills

Name	*Oestrogen: dose (micrograms)*	*Progestogen: dose (milligrams)*
BiNovum	ethinyloestradiol 35 mcg daily for 21 days	norethisterone 0.5 mg daily for 7 days, then 1 mg daily for 14 days
Logynon*	ethinyloestradiol 30 mcg daily for 6 days, then 40 mcg daily for 5 days, then 30 mcg daily for 10 days	levonorgestrel 0.05 mg daily for 6 days, then 0.075 mg daily for 5 days, then 0.125 mg daily for 10 days
Synphase	ethinyloestradiol 35 mcg daily for 21 days	norethisterone 0.5 mg daily for 7 days, then 1 mg daily for 9 days, then 0.5 mg daily for 5 days
Trinordiol	ethinyloestradiol 30 mcg daily for 6 days, then 40 mcg daily for 5 days, then 30 mcg daily for 10 days	levonorgestrel 0.05 mg daily for 6 days, then 0.075 mg daily for 5 days, then 0.125 mg daily for 10 days
TriNovum†	ethinyloestradiol 35 mcg daily for 21 days	norethisterone 0.5 mg daily for 7 days, then 0.75 mg daily for 7 days, then 1 mg daily for 7 days

* Logynon ED as for Logynon: 21 active tablets plus 7 dummy tablets – take one tablet each day for 28 days.
† TriNovum ED as for TriNovum: 21 active tablets plus 7 dummy tablets – take one tablet each day for 28 days.

Biphasic and triphasic oral contraceptives

It makes sense to try to reduce the dose of both drugs in the pill and to try to mimic the pattern of oestrogen and progestogen production by the body. Biphasic and triphasic pills are an attempt to do this by varying the dose of oestrogen and progestogen through the cycle. However, they are more complex to take and there is a greater margin of error if you forget to take one. They may produce premenstrual syndrome, and painful periods and vaginal discharges are more common. They contain both oestrogens and progestogens, and the harmful effects and warnings discussed under the 'pill' also apply to phasic preparations.

Phasic pills should be considered for use by smokers in their early 30s, possibly by women over 45 years of age and by women with absent periods on the 'ordinary' pill.

Progestogen-only preparations

These pills contain only a progestogen and they are therefore useful in women who should not take or who cannot tolerate an oestrogen-containing pill. They are suitable for women over 35 years of age, especially if they smoke, and for women who suffer from diabetes, who have a past history of thrombosis or who develop a transient raised blood pressure on a combined pill. They may be used before the periods start after childbirth without affecting breast feeding.

Progestogen-only pills make the mucus in the neck of the womb thick and sticky so that sperm cannot easily swim through. They also affect the surface of the womb, which may prevent a fertilized egg from implanting, and they affect the fallopian tubes.

How to use progestogen-only pills

Progestogen-only pills are started on the first day of the cycle (without the need for extra precautions) and then taken every day without missing a day even through a period. They are slightly less reliable than the combined pills and the risks from missing a dose are greater. They should be taken *at the same time* in each 24 hours and preferably several hours before the usual time of sexual intercourse. If you delay taking a dose by 3 hours or more, you are at risk. If this happens, take the missed pill and complete the course but avoid sexual intercourse or take additional precautions for the next 48 hours. If you miss two consecutive daily doses, stop the course and avoid sexual intercourse or take extra precautions until your next period starts. If you swap over from a combined pill to a progestogen-only pill, you should take the first dose of your progestogen-only pill the very next day after taking the last dose of your combined pill. If you have vomiting or severe diarrhoea, the pill may not work – continue with the course but avoid sexual intercourse or take extra precautions for 48 hours.

Harmful effects of progestogen-only contraceptives

Reported harmful effects include tenderness and swelling of the breasts, nausea, break-through bleeding, spotting, changes in menstrual flow, loss of periods, fluid retention (e.g. ankle swelling), changes in weight, acne, skin rashes with and without itching, mental depression, changes in libido, insomnia, headache and sleepiness. Very rarely, jaundice, allergic reactions, ectopic pregnancy and cysts of the ovaries may occur.

Warnings on the use of progestogen-only contraceptives

Progestogen-only preparations should not be used in women with severe disease of the arteries, coronary heart disease, a stroke due to thrombosis, high blood fat levels, a liver tumour, sex hormone-dependent cancer of the breast or genitals, undiagnosed vaginal bleeding, as a diagnosis for pregnancy or in women who are allergic to a particular preparation or who have had a previous ectopic pregnancy or who are pregnant. They should be used with caution in women with heart disease, raised blood pressure, history of thrombosis, cancer dependent on hormones, impaired liver function, history of liver disease in pregnancy, ovarian cysts, focal migraine or depressive illness. Diabetic patients should be carefully monitored. Progestogen-only pills may mask the start of the menopause.

Because progestogen-only pills cause fluid retention they should be used with caution if you suffer from epilepsy, migraine, asthma or heart or kidney disorders.

Pre-treatment medical examinations and annual medical examinations should include a breast examination, an internal examination and a cervical smear.

The progestogen-only pill should be stopped at the first sign of thrombosis, if you become jaundiced, if you think you may be pregnant or if you develop severe migraine or any visual disturbances.

Progestogen-only pills need not be stopped before or following non-emergency surgery.

Long-lasting injections of a progestogen

Medroxyprogesterone acetate (Depo-Provera) is a long-acting progestogen preparation, which is given by intramuscular injection. One injection provides contraception for 3 months. It produces problems similar to those of oral preparations, particularly irregular and sometimes heavy periods during the first 2–3 months. It may cause back pain, fluid retention, increase in weight and transient infertility on long-term treatment (see also page 897).

Norethisterone enanthate (Noristerat) long-acting oily injections provide contraception for up to 8 weeks. It produces similar problems to oral progestogens which include irregular and sometimes heavy periods, headache, dizziness, nausea, change in weight, breast discomfort and bloated feelings.

Morning-after pills (post-coital contraception)

There are two methods of providing contraception after sexual intercourse if you have not taken any precautions: hormone pills or the use of an intra-uterine device.

Table 67.3 Oral contraceptives: progestogen-only preparations

Name	*Progestogen*	*Dose*
Femulen	ethynodiol	0.5 mg
Micronor	norethisterone	0.35 mg
Microval	levonorgestrel	0.03 mg
Neogest	norgestrel	0.075 mg
Norgeston	levonorgestrel	0.03 mg
Noriday	norethisterone	0.35 mg

Table 67.4 Depot progestogen contraceptives

Name	*Progestogen*	*Dose*
Depo-Provera	medroxyprogesterone	150 mg/ml injection
Noristerat	norethisterone	200 mg/ml injection

Hormone pills

Hormone pills can be given either as oestrogen only or as combined oestrogen/progestogen.

Oestrogen-only treatment

High doses of ethinyloestradiol should not be used The use of high doses of ethinyloestradiol (5 mg daily for 5 days) may produce severe nausea and vomiting in 20 per cent of patients, and there is a risk of a pregnancy developing outside the womb (e.g. in a tube). This is called ectopic pregnancy and may occur in 10 per cent of women in whom the method fails.

Stilboestrol should not be used The use of stilboestrol in the first 3 months of an established pregnancy may produce abnormalities in the baby, and has been associated with the production of vaginal cancer in girl offspring when they reach their teens.

Combined oestrogen/progestogen

The use of a combined oestrogen/progestogen pill that contains a high dose of oestrogen may be used for morning after contraception (e.g. Schering PC4). These post-coital contraceptive pills contain 50 micrograms of the oestrogen ethinyloestradiol so remember: do not take any type of contraceptive pill – it *must* be Schering PC4. It probably works by stopping the fertilized egg from implanting in the lining of the womb.

Only four pills are taken: the first two pills must be taken within 72 hours of unprotected intercourse and the next two exactly 12 hours later. The next period will often be delayed for up to 1 week, during which time sexual intercourse should be avoided.

The post-coital contraceptive pill causes nausea in 50–60 per cent of individuals and vomiting in 30 per cent but these symptoms are short-lived and rarely severe. Other harmful effects such as headaches, dizziness, breast tenderness and withdrawal bleeding may occur. Your doctor should prescribe an extra dose in case you vomit up the first dose. You should have a pregnancy test 3–4 weeks after taking the pill. If you do get pregnant there is a slight risk that the pill may have damaged the baby.

Post-coital intra-uterine device

An alternative to the morning-after pill (post-coital pill) is the insertion of an intra-uterine device within the first 72 hours. Pain and abnormal bleeding may occur and there is always a risk of infection. These devices should not be used in young women who have not had a baby and may want a baby in the future.

68

Menstrual problems, menopause, osteoporosis and hormone replacement therapy

Premenstrual syndrome

The label premenstrual syndrome (PMS) covers a wide variety of mental and physical symptoms which occur regularly in the same phase of each menstrual cycle and which are followed by a phase in the cycle that is free from symptoms. There are three common patterns to the cycle of PMS: just before a period; at ovulation for a few days and recurring just before a period; and starting at ovulation and getting progressively worse just before a period. PMS may also occur after pregnancy and at the menopause.

The symptoms appear to be related to fluctuations in the production of oestrogens and progesterone by the ovaries but other factors may also contribute to the syndrome; for example, changes in the control of water and salt balance in the body, low blood sugar levels (hypoglycaemia), high levels of the milk-producing hormone prolactin and psychological factors.

The label premenstrual tension (PMT) covers only the mental symptoms; for example, depression and irritability.

Drug treatment of PMS

Progesterone

The fact that the symptoms of PMS occur regularly in the last 2 weeks of the menstrual cycle suggests that there may be a deficient production of progesterone during this phase (the luteal phase). Such a deficiency may occur after pregnancy and also at the menopause.

However, several studies have failed to show that PMS sufferers actually have a deficient production of progesterone in the last 2 weeks of their menstrual cycle, and some studies of the use of the natural hormone progesterone given during this time as pessaries, suppositories or injections have not produced convincing evidence of its benefits. We need more evidence and we also need evidence that the natural hormone (progesterone) is more beneficial than the synthetic progestogen dydrogesterone.

None the less, provided that PMS has been properly diagnosed by keeping a daily calendar of all physical and mental symptoms and the cyclic nature of those symptoms clearly identified and principally located in the 2 weeks just before a period starts, it may be worth trying progesterone as pessaries or suppositories or dydrogesterone by mouth daily for the last 2 weeks of each cycle.

Oestrogens

Some of the symptoms of PMS that may follow childbirth in some women may be helped by oestrogens, particularly symptoms of depression. Oestrogens may also help to relieve some of the symptoms of PMS that appear at the menopause in some women. See the discussion of oestrogen preparations under 'Hormone replacement therapy'.

Stopping ovulation

Because PMS symptoms occur between ovulation and the beginning of a period, another approach to hormonal treatment is to stop ovulation. This can be achieved by taking a combined oestrogen and progestogen oral contraceptive (the 'pill'). However, in PMS sufferers this often makes the condition worse. Whether this is due to the progestogen in the oral contraceptive causing a reduction in the production of natural progesterone (see above) or whether it is due to the oestrogen in the pill is not certain, but the former seems more probable.

Blocking prostaglandin production

In painful periods (spasmodic dysmenorrhoea) certain chemicals called prostaglandins are released in the womb that cause it to go into painful spasms. These chemicals also enter the blood stream and are thought to be responsible for other symptoms such as headaches and stomach upsets which may accompany painful periods.

Prostaglandins are involved in many processes in the body, including inflammation. If their production is blocked by drugs, the symptoms of inflammation are reduced. Drugs that have this effect (e.g. aspirin, ibuprofen, mefanamic acid, see NSAIDs, page 440) are of use in treating painful periods and some of the associated symptoms. They may also relieve some PMS symptoms in those women whose symptoms continue during their periods and who also suffer from painful periods.

Pyridoxine (vitamin B_6)

Pyridoxine (vitamin B_6) acts as a co-enzyme, which is the non-protein part of certain enzymes that act as catalysts for various chemical reactions in the body. Our requirements for pyridoxine increase with the amount of protein in our diet and we generally require about 2.0 mg daily. No specific deficiency disorder has been recognized although biochemical tests show that about one-third of alcoholics are deficient in pyridoxine.

With regard to PMS, claims and counter-claims are frequently made for the benefits of pyridoxine but there is no convincing evidence from adequate and well controlled studies of its benefits in PMS. A daily dose of 50 mg by mouth may relieve some emotional symptoms in some women but it is not possible to relate PMS to a deficiency of pyridoxine. Regular use of high doses (200 mg daily) has been associated with severe nerve damage.

Magnesium

There is no convincing evidence from adequate and well controlled studies that taking additional magnesium is of benefit, nor is there any convincing evidence that women who suffer from PMS have a deficiency of magnesium.

Evening primrose oil

There is no convincing evidence from adequate and well controlled studies that evening primrose oil is of benefit in PMS. See the discussion on the effects and use of evening primrose oil in Chapter 45.

Diuretics (water tablets)

Retention of water in the body may occur during the last 2 weeks of the menstrual cycle; this may cause tension and other mental symptoms and a bloated feeling. Diuretics increase the volume of urine that is passed and this may help to reduce some premenstrual symptoms in some women. Diuretics are discussed in Chapter 22. A thiazide diuretic is suitable for this purpose. However, they are of little use in treating the whole premenstrual syndrome (PMS).

Tamoxifen

This drug is an anti-oestrogen: it blocks oestrogen receptors in the body. Its use to treat PMS is still experimental.

Heavy periods (menorrhagia)

One cause of heavy periods is an hormonal imbalance between oestrogen and progestogens which may occur in young girls when they are starting their periods (menarche) and particularly in menopausal women as their ovaries stop functioning. In these individuals there is usually a continuous action of oestrogens set against a defective production of progesterone. This continuous action of oestrogens on the lining of the uterus causes it to become much thickened, so when a period does occur, the bleeding is heavy. Also, the periods may be irregular because of a failure to ovulate regularly due to the defective production of progesterone.

When a period is heavy and continuous, a dose of a progestogen by mouth every 4–6 hours will stop the period within 24 hours. Periods may also be made less heavy and more regular by taking a progestogen daily from the 20th to the 25th day of the menstrual cycle. Treatment is often more effective if an oestrogen is also taken daily throughout the cycle. A combined oestrogen/progestogen combination oral contraceptive (the 'pill') may be used for this purpose.

Another drug that may be tried in the treatment of menorrhagia is danazol (Danol), a synthetic steroid drug that damps down the production of follicle-stimulating hormone (FSH) and luteinizing hormone (LH) by the pituitary gland. This reduces the production of oestrogens and progesterone by the ovaries, which may help to reduce heavy periods in some women.

Other drugs that may be beneficial in reducing heavy blood loss include: a non-steroidal anti-inflammatory drug (e.g. mefenamic acid [Ponstan]); tranexamic acid (Cyklokapron), a drug that stops blood clots from being dissolved (an anti-fibrinolytic); and ethamsylate (Dicynene), a drug that helps to stop bleeding (haemostatic).

Painful periods (dysmenorrhoea)

Dysmenorrhoea is pain associated with the periods. It may be primary (i.e. no obvious cause) or secondary due to some underlying disorder.

Primary dysmenorrhoea

This is the commonest – it is sometimes called functional or spasmodic dysmenorrhoea. The pain of primary dysmenorrhoea is thought to be caused by contractions of the womb and a reduced blood supply to the womb caused by the local release of prostaglandins which are produced during the last phase of the cycle (the secretory phase). For this phase to occur, a woman needs to have ovulated and therefore dysmenorrhoea does not occur if the woman does not ovulate (see hormone therapy, later). Factors that may make the periods more painful include the passage of blood clots through a narrow neck of womb, lack of physical exercise, a malpositioned womb and anxiety. Dysmenorrhoea is more common in adolescence and tends to decrease with age and following pregnancy.

In addition to crampy and colicky pains in the lower abdomen, there may be a dull ache in the back and down the legs; some women may develop headache, nausea, constipation or diarrhoea, frequency of passing urine and, occasionally, vomiting. The symptoms may start the day before a period, reach a peak during the first day and then taper off over the next 2 days. In addition, premenstrual symptoms may occur, such as irritability, nervousness, depression and a bloated feeling.

Treatment

There are two main approaches to the treatment of primary dysmenorrhoea: pain relief and hormonal therapy.

Pain relief A hot-water bottle on the lower abdomen may help to relieve some discomfort. Because the pain and other symptoms such as headaches and nausea are due to the release of prostaglandins, it will help to block their production by taking an anti-inflammatory drug such as aspirin, ibuprofen (e.g. Brufen), naproxen (e.g. Naprosyn) or mefenamic acid (Ponstan). Treatment should be taken at regular intervals, starting 2 days before the period is due and continuing during the first 2 days of the period. If the pain is still severe, codeine may be added to the treatment.

Hormonal treatment If dysmenorrhoea is not relieved by pain relievers, suppression of ovulation ought to be considered using a combined oestrogen/progestogen preparation (e.g. an oral contraceptive pill). Treatment should continue for 3 or 4 months and then be stopped to see how the periods are without treatment. However, if the woman is sexually active, she may continue to use the pill both as a contraceptive and to prevent her dysmenorrhoea.

Other hormonal treatments include the use of a progestogen from the

5th to the 25th day of a cycle; for example, dydrogesterone (Duphaston) or norethisterone (Primolut N, Utovlan). Treatment should be repeated for about 3 months and then stopped to see how the periods are without treatment.

Secondary dysmenorrhoea

Causes of secondary dysmenorrhoea include endometriosis, fibroids, and tightening of the neck of the womb which may follow cauterization treatment for an ulcer.

Endometriosis

Endometriosis is one of the most common causes of secondary dysmenorrhoea. It is a disorder in which endometrial tissue (i.e. tissue that lines the womb) develops in areas other than in the womb. It may occur because material shed from the womb during a period travels along the fallopian tubes and enters the abdominal cavity or because some tissues in the abdominal cavity may transform into endometrial tissue. Patches of endometrial tissue may also occur away from the abdominal cavity; for example, in the lungs, navel, vagina, vulva, or in surgical scars, which suggests spread via the blood and lymphatic systems.

Painful periods may develop after several years of pain-free periods and it may be associated with pain on intercourse (dyspareunia). The periods may be heavy and irregular, and there may be pain in the back passage. About 25–50 per cent of affected women are infertile. Treatment is difficult and should be tailored to each individual depending upon her symptoms, age, desire to have a baby and the extent of the disease. Treatment centres around suppressing the function of the ovaries combined with surgical removal of abnormally located patches of endometrium.

There are three forms of drug treatment aimed at suppressing the function of the ovaries:

1. The continuous use of oral contraceptives (without a 1-week break every month) for at least 6 months, followed by cyclical use as normal (e.g. 3 weeks on and 1 week off)
2. The use of a depot intramuscular injection of the progestogen medroxyprogesterone (Depo-Provera) every 2 weeks for 6 months or longer
3. The use of danazol (Danol), which blocks the release of pituitary hormones (LH and FSH) that stimulate the ovaries. The drug is taken daily for at least 6 months (U)

Danazol may frequently cause weight gain, fluid retention, fatigue, headache, nausea, dizziness, backache, flushing, decreased breast size, oily skin and acne, muscle cramps and emotional instability. Very rarely, it may cause jaundice and raised blood pressure in the brain. It should not be used in pregnancy, when breast feeding or in women who suffer from porphyria. It should be used with caution by women with severe impairment of liver, heart or kidney function, migraine, epilepsy or diabetes or in women who are prone to put on weight easily.

The menopause

The term 'menopause' refers to the stopping of the menstrual periods due to a declining function of the ovaries and a failure to ovulate. The menopause comes on between the ages of 40 and 50 years and, as the function of the ovaries declines, the periods become irregular due to a reduced production of oestrogens and progesterone. This is a gradual process which can last 1–2 years. The term 'climacteric' means a critical period of life but it is often used specifically to refer to the menopause.

Premature menopause refers to the menopause coming on before the age of 40 years due to early failure of the ovaries. Smoking may be associated with an early menopause.

Artificial menopause refers to menopausal changes that occur following surgical removal of the ovaries or irradiation of the lower abdomen including the ovaries.

Symptoms of the menopause

The decline in function of the ovaries is associated with numerous symptoms, which include hot flushes and sweating, particularly at night; painful muscles, bones and joints; dizziness, faintness and palpitations; fatigue, inability to concentrate; depression, anxiety, insomnia, tension and irritability. Nausea, wind, constipation or diarrhoea may occur. Osteoporosis may start (see later) and the menstrual periods may become heavy and/or irregular.

The lining of the vagina shrinks (vulvo-vaginal atrophy) and may cause pain on sexual intercourse, with occasional bleeding, and difficulty in passing urine.

Menopausal symptoms may vary in intensity and duration. In some women they last for only a few months whilst in others they may go on for a few years.

Treatment of menopausal symptoms

Hormone replacement therapy (HRT)

The benefits and risks of HRT are discussed later (see page 931).

Hot flushes

Oestrogens relieve the hot flushes and sweating associated with the menopause. They also relieve the shrinking of the vagina and the symptoms that it causes.

Natural oestrogens are used (e.g. oestradiol, oestriol, oestrone) because they may possibly produce fewer long-term harmful effects than the synthetic, more potent oestrogens used in higher doses in oral contraceptives. They may be taken by mouth, as a skin patch or as an implant (see later, under HRT).

Because continuous use of oestrogens may over-stimulate the lining of the womb and increase the risk of cancer, it is safer to take oestrogens on a cyclical basis (e.g. 3 weeks on and 1 week off). It also helps to reduce the risk of cancer if a progestogen is taken by mouth for all or part of the 3 weeks (see discussion under 'Hormone replacement therapy, HRT', later). Women who have had their wombs removed may take oestrogens on their own because there is no risk of their getting cancer of the womb.

Vaginal problems

An *oestrogen vaginal cream* or pessary may help to relieve painful intercourse and other symptoms caused by shrinking of the vagina. The preparation should be used daily for 1–3 weeks and then about twice weekly. A lubricant jelly should be used before sexual intercourse.

Warnings *Oestrogens from vaginal creams are absorbed and may cause bleeding from the womb. They should not be used in women with a history of breast cancer. Do not take oestrogens by mouth* **and** *apply oestrogen creams or pessaries to the vagina; you may overdose.*

Emotional problems

HRT is very effective treatment for hot flushes, vaginal problems and osteoporosis (see later). However, despite the often exaggerated claims for HRT there is no convincing evidence that HRT is any better than a placebo (dummy treatment) at relieving the emotional symptoms which may occur around the time of the menopause. However, it may relieve menopausal depression in some women.

Osteoporosis

This is a common disorder of bone in which the actual amount of bone in the skeleton is decreased to such a level that parts of the skeleton can no longer provide mechanical support. More bone is dissolved than new bone is laid down, and the bones themselves become thin, honeycombed and weakened. Osteoporosis is a major cause of fractures – particularly crush fractures of the vertebrae of the spine, producing a bent spine, and fractures of the hips and wrists from falls. It affects both men and women in old age (senile osteoporosis). In women it can also come on earlier than in men, in the years following the menopause, when it is called post-menopausal osteoporosis.

About four out of every ten women will fracture a bone before they are 70 years of age because of osteoporosis; these fractures, which usually affect the wrist, spine or hips, usually occur with minor accidents. It takes only a slight fall for an elderly woman with osteoporosis to fracture her hip bone and it takes only a few days of ice and snow for casualty departments to fill with elderly women with fractured wrists.

We are all familiar with the 'widow's hump', the bent spine caused by the vertebrae collapsing due to osteoporosis, but we must now recognize that a large number of other fractures in elderly women are also due to osteoporosis.

Fractures as a result of osteoporosis cause pain and disability, and there is an increased death rate during the year following a hip fracture in elderly people. The cost of medical and surgical services for elderly patients who have fractured a bone because of osteoporosis runs into many millions of pounds.

Factors that may contribute to osteoporosis

From middle age onwards we all lose bone progressively due to a failure to lay down new bone. Our genetic coding inherited from our parents, our sex, race, diet, the amount of physical activity we do and many other factors will all determine the amount of bone we develop as young adults. This will have implications when we get older; for example, people with 'light' skeletons will suffer from more bone problems as they get older than people with 'heavy' skeletons. Lightweight women in particular appear to be at greatest risk from developing osteoporosis in later life, especially white and Asian women.

The amount of calcium we take into our bodies from our food is very important because, if it is insufficient, calcium is taken from bone to make up the balance. What we take in depends upon the amount of calcium in our food and our ability to absorb it from our intestine into our bloodstream. As we get older we are less able to absorb calcium from our food. Therefore, some middle aged and elderly people may need to eat more calcium-containing foods, in order to ensure that they absorb sufficient amounts of calcium into their bodies.

Vitamin D is also important because calcium cannot be absorbed from the intestine in the absence of vitamin D. Most of us obtain a sufficient amount of vitamin D from the effects of the sun's rays on our skin but some of us (e.g. elderly housebound people) may need to rely on a supply of vitamins from foods rich in vitamin D (e.g. oily fish) or from tablets of vitamin D (see chapter 45).

Osteoporosis may develop because of the over-use of corticosteroid drugs, if the thyroid gland over-works, if the ovaries and testes stop working, if cancer of the bone marrow develops, if there is disease of the intestine which interferes with the absorption of calcium from food, if part of the stomach or intestine has been removed surgically, or if the liver stops functioning efficiently because of disease (e.g. cirrhosis).

High alcohol intake, smoking and, particularly, decreased physical activity may be factors that increase the risk of developing osteoporosis.

The menopause and osteoporosis

The menopause contributes to osteoporosis. It has been shown that, after removal of the ovaries, bone loss increases for several years. After natural menopause, bone loss is also greater than new bone formation. This appears to be related to a fall in the blood level of oestrogens which possibly makes bone more responsive to hormones from the parathyroid gland. These hormones increase if the blood calcium falls and they cause calcium to be drawn from the bones in order to push up the blood calcium.

The menopause may also decrease the production of another hormone, called calcitonin, which is produced by the parathyroid and thyroid glands. This hormone opposes the actions of parathyroid hormone and reduces blood calcium by decreasing the dissolving of bone.

However, it is important to note that not all post-menopausal women develop osteoporosis even though they are all deficient in oestrogen.

Preventing and treating osteoporosis

Hormone replacement therapy (*HRT*)

This is discussed later.

The use of calcium

Calcium is necessary for bone formation, and it appears that the amount of calcium we take in during childhood and early adult life affects our bone mass – which reaches a peak around about our early thirties. Because it is our bone mass that will help to prevent osteoporosis in later life, it is very important that we take in adequate amounts of calcium.

Pregnant women, breast-feeding mothers, elderly people and women at the menopause should also ensure that their calcium intake is adequate, and this may mean taking calcium tablets in addition to a well balanced diet. People who have developed osteoporosis should ensure that their total calcium intake is about 1500 mg daily. (A pint of low fat milk contains 750 mg of calcium.)

Weight

A reduced calorie intake and a weight that is less than normal for your age, height and build will predispose you to develop osteoporosis. Being overweight seems to help, possibly by putting more stress (tension) on the bones because of the weight that has to be carried around and because the increased number of fat cells allows more conversion of male sex hormones produced by the ovaries and adrenal glands to be converted into oestrogens.

Exercise

Exercise, posture and gait throughout life are very important in preventing osteoporosis. Weight-bearing exercises (e.g. walking, shopping, gardening, jogging, golf) appear to be most important because these exercises put tension on bones which increases new bone formation.

However, it is the old story: carry out weight-bearing exercises only in moderation. Excessive exercise leads to loss of periods and loss of bone, particularly if combined with a low-calorie diet (e.g. women athletes or ballet dancers).

Vitamin D

There is no evidence that vitamin D is of benefit in preventing or treating post-menopausal osteoporosis, except of course if there is evidence of vitamin D deficiency which will then interfere with the absorption of calcium from the intestine.

Fluoride

Fluoride may increase bone density but not reduce the risk of fractures. It must be given along with calcium supplements or the laying down of new bone will be poor or defective. An effective dose and duration of treatment have not been worked out.

Anabolic steroids

These are discussed in Chapter 73. They are of benefit in men who have been castrated or whose testes are not functioning. In women there is a risk of masculinization and a rise in blood fat levels.

Calcitonin

This hormone is produced by the parathyroid and thyroid glands and helps to regulate the blood calcium level. It reduces the dissolving of bone and it may prove useful for preventing and treating osteoporosis. It has to be given by injection or nasal spray. An alternative approach is to use intermittent treatments, first with calcitonin and then with a drug that stimulates the laying down of new bone e.g. parathyroid hormone, which is difficult to use on its own because it has to be given with careful blood monitoring.

Zinc, magnesium, boron, fish oils

There is no convincing evidence from adequate and well controlled studies that taking additional zinc, magnesium, boron or fish oils is beneficial in preventing or treating osteoporosis, nor is there evidence that people with osteoporosis have a deficiency of these elements.

Alcohol

The regular daily consumption of large amounts of alcohol reduces bone mass at any age; therefore heavy drinkers should cut down on their alcohol intake.

Diphosphonates

Etidronate (Didronel) prevents bone from dissolving and its long-term use stops osteoporosis from getting worse and may also cause some improvement.

Risks from other drug treatments

Prolonged use of *corticosteroid drugs* and *heparin*, particularly in high doses, may cause osteoporosis. Anti-epileptic drugs such as *phenytoin* and *phenobarbitone* may interfere with vitamin D in the body. *Indigestion mixtures* that contain magnesium and/or aluminium may bind phosphates in food, preventing their absorption.

Hormone replacement therapy (HRT)

Hormone replacement therapy (HRT) is treatment with the female sex hormone, oestrogen, in order to replace the deficiency that occurs following the menopause.

One major effect of taking oestrogens is that they make the lining of the womb thicker. If they are taken regularly every day the lining will overgrow and become sensitive to factors that trigger the development of cancer.

To prevent this continuous over-growth and reduce the risk of cancer, oestrogens are taken in cycles (3 weeks on and 1 week off) and a progestogen is added to the treatment for the last 10–14 days of each cycle. The effect of this approach is that, when the oestrogen and progestogen are stopped, the lining of the womb is shed (see discussion under 'Risks of using HRT', later). The bleeding is usually light and trouble free. A tampon or sanitary towel needs to be worn for about 3–5 days.

NOTE Women who have had a hysterectomy (surgical removal of the womb) have, of course, no risk of cancer of the womb and may be treated with an oestrogen alone.

Oestrogens used in HRT

All oestrogens can cause the same spectrum of harmful effects if given in equal effective doses (equitherapeutic doses) but the risk of developing these can be reduced in HRT because only *small* doses are required and less powerful oestrogens (e.g. natural oestrogens) can be used.

All oestrogens by mouth are broken down on their first pass through the liver. Furthermore, they may be poorly absorbed from the intestine which is why other routes may be more reliable; for example, implants or adhesive plasters.

Implants are wax-coated pellets of an oestrogen that is slowly released over a period of months. They are inserted into a fatty layer under the skin of the abdomen, thigh or buttocks under local anaesthetic. They may be useful for people who are forgetful but their beneficial effects may taper off at the end of the 6 months.

Adhesive plasters (transdermal preparations) are like a first aid dressing, and each patch has enough oestrogen to last for 3 days. The plasters are water-proof and transparent, and contain a measured amount of oestrogen. The patch may irritate the skin in some women and it may come loose in the bath or shower. They are suitable for treating hot flushes and vaginal symptoms but note that in women with a womb a progestogen will still have to be taken by mouth. Their use compared with oestrogens by mouth has not been fully evaluated in the prevention of osteoporosis.

Progestogens used in HRT

Many preparations of progestogens are available to be taken by mouth (see Table 66.2). No one particular progestogen can be recommended because accurate comparative information is not available. They are well absorbed from the intestine and they are reliable and effective. Their harmful effects are discussed in Chapter 66.

A typical HRT

A typical HRT for women who have not had their wombs removed includes an oestrogen skin patch applied to a clean, non-hairy area of skin below the waist and replaced with a new patch every 3–4 days using a different site. Such a patch will release about 50–100 micrograms of oestrogen every 24 hours. In addition, one progestogen tablet should be taken daily from day 15 to day 26 of each 28-day treatment with oestrogen. Eight patches and twelve tablets should be one month's treatment. The alternative by mouth is 1 oestrogen tablet daily for 11 days and then a combined oestrogen/progestogen tablet for 10 days and nothing for 7 days.

The benefits of HRT

To relieve hot flushes and other symptoms of the menopause

HRT will relieve hot flushes and vaginal problems (see page 926). To relieve these symptoms HRT should be taken for about 1–2 years.

To prevent osteoporosis

Only one woman in four develops post-menopausal osteoporosis; unfortunately, in those women who develop osteoporosis it is often not diagnosed until they present with symptoms such as a fractured wrist, by which time the condition is already well developed.

It is very difficult without bone scanning tests to predict those women who may develop osteoporosis but there are several risk factors that should be considered together. Women at risk of developing osteoporosis come into more than one of the following groups:

- Women who have undergone an early menopause or who have had their ovaries surgically removed
- White or Asian women who, at the menopause, are excessively thin
- Women who have a blood relative who suffers from or who suffered from osteoporosis
- Women who have sustained a fracture of the hip or forearm before the age of 65 years
- Women who are immobile due to disability or any other reason
- Women who are heavy drinkers
- Women who are on corticosteroid therapy or have recently taken corticosteroids
- Women who suffer from a glandular disorder that affects bone (e.g. over-active adrenal glands)

Women in the above groups stand a greater risk of having or developing osteoporosis and therefore if you come into more than one of these groups you should receive HRT for 5–10 years from the start of your menopause in addition to taking a well balanced diet and being physically active.

Women who do not come into more than one of these groups do not require HRT to prevent osteoporosis and should rely on a well balanced diet and physical activity.

If osteoporosis has developed, HRT will prevent further loss of bone and help to relieve pain but it may have no effect on the bone damage that has already occurred.

NOTE Pre-menopausal women who have had their womb and ovaries removed, their ovaries irradiated or who develop a premature menopause have a high risk of developing osteoporosis. They should take oestrogen-only HRT for at least 10 years. Pre-menopausal women who have had their womb removed but not their ovaries should also consider taking oestrogen-only HRT for at least 10 years.

To prevent heart attacks and strokes

The use of oestrogen-only HRT after the menopause reduces the risk of heart attacks and strokes. However, in women who have not had their womb removed the need to add progestogen to the treatment may lessen these benefits.

Risks of using HRT

For the purposes of this section, 'the pill' refers to a combined oestrogen/progestogen oral contraceptive and HRT refers to combined oestrogen and progestogen treatment.

Risk of cancer of the womb

There is an increased risk of cancer of the lining of the womb (endometrial cancer) in post-menopausal women who take oestrogens over a prolonged period of time. This rare risk is independent of other known risk factors associated with cancer of the womb. The risk from the use of oestrogens depends both on the duration of use and the dose used – the longer the use and/or the higher the dose, the greater the risk of cancer. In view of these findings the smallest effective dose of oestrogen should be used in HRT and treatment should be in cycles – 3 weeks on and 1 week off.

The risks of developing a cancer of the womb may be further reduced if a progestogen preparation is also taken daily in the last half of the cycle. The progestogen causes the lining of the womb to be shed at the end of each month with bleeding. This is not a normal menstrual period and, because it occurs when the drugs are stopped, it is called withdrawal bleeding. The shedding of the lining of the womb lowers the risk of cancer because it stops the continuous growth of the lining that occurs when oestrogens are taken alone.

HRT in women who have *not* had a hysterectomy (removal of their womb) therefore consists of combined treatment with an oestrogen and a progestogen preparation (see Table 68.1). Women who *have* had a hysterectomy are at no risk of cancer of the womb and may take oestrogen on its own.

Because of the rare risk of cancer of the lining of the womb, it is advisable to have an internal examination every 12–18 months. A woman on HRT who develops any sort of bleeding from her vagina (other than withdrawal bleeding during the 1 week when she is off treatment) should seek medical advice.

There is no increased risk of cervical cancer, and women should attend for routine screening every 4–5 years. However, any woman taking HRT who shows early changes on her cervical smear should be seen and examined at regular intervals (every 6 months).

Risk of cancer of the breast

In post-menopausal women there is a possibility that the prolonged use of HRT may be associated with cancer of the breast. At present there is no convincing evidence of this risk from well controlled studies but such a risk should always be borne in mind in women on HRT even though the dose of oestrogen used is low. While on treatment they should regularly examine their own breasts and have a mammogram every 2–3 years if they are aged 50 years or over.

HRT should be used with caution by women with a history of cancer of the breast in members of their family or if they have breast nodules, fibrocystic disease of the breast or abnormal mammograms. All women should have a mammogram before starting on HRT.

HRT should not be used by women who have a known or suspected cancer of the breast.

Risk of gall stones

This risk is rare but women taking HRT run a two to three times greater chance of developing gall stones than women not on HRT. This risk may be greater when a semi-synthetic oestrogen is taken by mouth, and may be less if a natural oestrogen is used as a skin patch or implant.

Risk of thrombosis

Because HRT consists of using an oestrogen and a progestogen preparation there is a rare possibility that it may cause thrombosis problems similar to those caused by the pill. However, as lower doses are used and natural oestrogens are less powerful than synthetic ones, such risks will be reduced; this may be why, so far, they have not been reported. Nevertheless, this does not rule out the possibility in certain women who may be prone to develop such complications. HRT should not, therefore, be used by women suffering from active thrombophlebitis or a related disorder or who have previously suffered thrombosis while taking the pill or while taking an oestrogen or progestogen preparation for some purpose other than contraception.

Risk of strokes

There is a very rare but increased risk of a stroke in women taking the pill over many years. It is therefore advisable that women should consider not using combined oestrogen/progesterone HRT if they are suffering from a stroke or have suffered from a stroke in the past or have evidence of disease affecting the arteries that supply the brain (cerebral arteries). Note that oestrogens on their own offer protection against a stroke (see earlier).

Risk of heart attack

There is evidence that the use of an oestrogen on its own may protect against artery disease and heart attacks but the addition of a progestogen to the treatment may negate this benefit. Therefore, because there is a very rare but increased risk of a heart attack in women who take the pill over a long period of time this should be kept in mind by women taking HRT that involves the use of both an oestrogen and a progestogen.

HRT should not be used by women who suffer from coronary artery disease (e.g. who suffer from angina and/or have had a previous heart attack).

Risk of liver tumours

Because there is a very rare risk that the pill may be associated with benign tumours of the liver, which may rupture and bleed into the abdomen, such a very rare possibility should be considered in any woman on HRT who develops a swelling in her abdomen with pain, tenderness and shock. HRT should not be used by women who developed a liver tumour while taking the pill or after taking an oestrogen-only preparation.

Risk of a raised blood pressure

A rise in blood pressure may occur in some women taking the pill. This rise in blood pressure is related to the progestogen in the oral contraceptive, the duration of treatment and the advancing age of the user. The high blood pressure may persist after the pill has been stopped. A similar rise in blood pressure may occasionally occur in women taking HRT. Therefore post-menopausal women who are taking HRT should have their blood pressure checked before treatment and at regular intervals during treatment (e.g. every 6–12 months). This applies particularly to women with a history of raised blood pressure (hypertension), kidney disease or a history of raised blood pressure during pregnancy (toxaemia).

Women with a history of raised blood pressure in members of their family and women who developed excessive weight gain or fluid retention with their periods are more likely to develop a raised blood pressure on HRT, and they too should have their blood pressure checked at frequent intervals.

Risk in diabetes

Because severe diabetes may damage the arteries (see Chapter 65), HRT should be used with caution.

Blood sugar levels may increase in some women who take the pill. This is due to the oestrogen content, and although low doses of natural oestrogens are used in HRT it is still advisable that women who suffer from diabetes and go on to HRT should have their blood sugar levels checked and their diabetic treatment reviewed at regular intervals, because it may be necessary to increase the dose of their insulin.

Risk of fluid retention

Both the oestrogen and progestogen in HRT may cause some retention of fluid, so HRT should be used with caution by women who suffer from any disorder that could be made worse by fluid retention; for example, epilepsy, heart disease, asthma or kidney disease. They will need to have regular medical check-ups.

Risk of depression

The pill may trigger mental depression in some women. It is not clear whether this is due to the oestrogen or to the progestogen. Therefore women on HRT who have a previous history of depression (whether on the pill or not) should watch out for any change in mood if they take HRT. However, HRT may relieve menopausal depression in some women.

Risk of headache

Some women may develop headache or migraine while taking the pill. Even though HRT contains lower doses of natural oestrogens, if a woman on HRT develops migraine or her migraine gets worse or if she develops headaches which are of a new type for her, or if they are recurrent, severe or persistent, she should consider stopping HRT.

Risk of an increase in size of fibroids

Tumours of the muscle of the womb are called fibroids, and some types of fibroids may rapidly increase in size if a woman takes oestrogens as in HRT.

Risk in women who have suffered from jaundice during pregnancy

Women who have suffered from jaundice during pregnancy have a slight risk of developing a recurrence of the jaundice if they take the pill. Because of this risk a woman on HRT who has previously suffered jaundice in pregnancy should stop her HRT if she becomes jaundiced (yellowness of the skin and eyes) and have the cause of her jaundice fully investigated.

Risk in women with impaired liver disease

Because oestrogens are broken down in the liver, any impairment of liver function may result in a reduced rate of breakdown and a rise in the blood level of the oestrogen. This may increase the risk of harmful effects. Therefore, HRT should not be used by women with severe liver disease.

Risk of increasing blood calcium levels

Oestrogens affect the body's use of calcium and may cause an excessive increase in blood calcium levels in women suffering from certain bone diseases or from kidney disease (which may cause a decreased excretion of calcium in the urine and a raised blood calcium level). Therefore, HRT (even though it includes low doses of natural oestrogens) should be used with caution by women who have a raised blood calcium level due to some bone disease or kidney disease.

Risk of raised blood fat levels

Raised blood fat levels may occur in some women taking the pill. Even though HRT includes low doses of natural oestrogens, it is advisable that women have their blood fat levels checked *before* they start HRT; if these are raised, they should not go on to HRT but rather they should have treatment for their raised blood fats.

NOTE Oestrogen-only treatment lowers blood fat levels.

Risk of vitamin B_6 (pyridoxine) and folic acid deficiency

Women who take the pill over a prolonged period of time may develop deficiency of vitamin B_6 (pyridoxine) and folic acid. The implications of these deficiencies are not known but if a woman is on HRT for many years it may be helpful if she takes a B complex vitamin tablet every day – one that contains vitamin B_6 (pyridoxine) and folic acid.

Risk of abnormal bleeding from the vagina

In some women the pill may cause spotting and bleeding in between periods (break-through bleeding). Similarly, in post-menopausal women taking HRT such bleeding could be due to the treatment. However, it could also be due to some underlying disorder (e.g. cancer of the womb). Therefore, if a woman taking HRT develops any bleeding from her vagina other than the withdrawal bleeding that occurs when each 3-week course of treatment is stopped, she should consult her doctor.

Risk of disturbances of vision

Progestogens may very rarely affect vision; therefore any woman on HRT who develops a disturbance of her vision should stop the treatment and consult her doctor.

Risk of abnormal laboratory tests

Both oestrogens and progestogens may alter laboratory tests on the blood; therefore the laboratory should be informed if a woman is taking HRT. Tests of liver function, thyroid function and blood clotting tests may be affected.

Risk during surgery

There is an increased risk of thrombosis following surgery in women taking the pill. Even though HRT involves the use of low doses of natural oestrogens, it is advisable that women taking HRT should stop their treatment 4–6 weeks before surgery or during any period of prolonged immobilization.

Risk of varicose veins

There is a rare but increased risk of developing superficial thrombophlebitis in varicose veins in women taking the pill. This risk appears to be related to the progestogen. Therefore, women on HRT who suffer from varicose veins should be aware of this possibility.

Risk in pregnancy

The use of the pill in early pregnancy may damage the unborn baby, so HRT should not be used if there is the slightest risk of being pregnant or becoming pregnant.

Risks of smoking

Cigarette smoking increases the risk of serious harmful effects on the heart and blood vessels from the pill. This risk increases with age (over 35 years) and with heavy smoking (15 or more per day). Even though HRT involves the use of low doses of natural oestrogens, it is none the less advisable that women taking HRT should not smoke.

Drug interaction

For interaction of oestrogens and progestogens with other drug treatment, see Chapter 89.

Harmful effects of HRT include swelling and tenderness of the breasts, lower abdominal cramps, backache, period pains, migraine-like headache, depression, anxiety, nausea and fluid retention. The progestogen supplement may cause premenstrual syndrome (PMS). To avoid fluid retention, PMS and vaginal bleeding, smaller amounts of progestogen should be used.

Table 68.1 HRT preparations

Preparation	*Drug*	*Drug group*	*Dosage form*
Cyclo-Progynova (1 mg)	oestradiol levonorgestrel	natural oestrogen progestogen	Tablets Tablets
Estraderm	oestradiol	natural oestrogen	Self-adhesive skin patches (release 25, 50 or 100 micrograms over 24 hours)
Estrapak	oestradiol	natural oestrogen	Self-adhesive skin patches (release 50 micrograms over 24 hours)
	norethisterone	progestogen	Tablets
Harmogen	piperazine oestrone	natural oestrogen	Tablets
Hormonin	oestriol and oestrone	natural oestrogens	Tablets
Menophase	mestranol	semi-synthetic oestrogen	Tablets
	norethisterone	progestogen	Tablets
Ovestin	oestriol	natural oestrogen	Tablets
Premarin	conjugated oestrogens	natural oestrogens	Tablets
Prempak-C	conjugated oestrogens	natural oestrogens	Tablets
	norgestrel	progesterone	Tablets
Progynova	oestradiol	natural oestrogen	Tablets
Trisequens	oestradiol and oestriol	natural oestrogens	Tablets
Trisequens Forte	norethisterone	progestogen	Tablets
Oestrogen vaginal applications			
Ortho Dienoestrol	dienoestrol	natural oestrogen	Cream
Ortho-Gynest	oestriol	natural oestrogen	Cream, pessaries
Ovestin	oestriol	natural oestrogen	Cream
Premarin	conjugated oestrogens	natural oestrogen	Cream
Tampovagan	stilboestrol lactic acid	synthetic oestrogen acid	Pessaries
Vagifem	oestradiol	natural oestrogen	Pessaries
Oestrogen-only implants			
Oestradiol implants (Organon)	oestradiol	natural oestrogen	Implants 25 mg lasts 36 weeks 50 mg lasts 44 weeks 100 mg lasts 57 weeks

69

Infertility

Fertility and infertility

For conception to occur and pregnancy to become established it is necessary for both partners to have a healthy and functioning reproductive system. The man must produce healthy sperm and the woman must produce a healthy egg (ovum). The egg must be able to pass freely down a fallopian tube into the uterus and sexual intercourse must occur at this time in order to ensure that the sperm have an egg to fertilize. At the same time, the lining of the womb must be in a suitable state to allow the fertilized egg to embed itself in its surface and start to divide.

The ability to conceive and for pregnancy to become established is referred to as *fertility*, and the inability to do this is referred to as *infertility*.

Infertility may be due to some abnormality in the male partner (male infertility) or in the female partner (female infertility).

The commonest causes of infertility include sexual intercourse taking place at the wrong time during the menstrual cycle of the woman (i.e. not during her time of ovulation); the man producing too few and/or unhealthy sperm; the woman failing to ovulate (produce an egg); the woman having a blockage in her fallopian tubes due to some previous infection; or the woman having some abnormality that interferes with the implantation of the fertilized egg in the lining of the womb.

Failure to ovulate and/or failure of a fertilized egg to implant in the lining of the womb may be due to some imbalance in the hormone control of these activities, which may be aggravated by stress or a physical illness.

Treatment of infertility

Obviously the first step is to exclude infertility in the male partner by checking the number and activity of sperm in his ejaculate.

If the male partner's sperm count is normal, the woman should have a gynaecological examination to identify any physical abnormality. She should also have tests of her hormone production, particularly to see if she is ovulating effectively and is producing adequate amounts of progesterone between ovulation and the start of her menstrual periods.

Drugs used to treat infertility (U)

Failure of the pituitary gland to produce adequate amounts of follicle-stimulating hormone (FSH) results in a failure to ovulate and infertility. Failure of the pituitary gland to produce luteinizing hormone (LH) leads to infertility despite ovulation because there is a deficient production of progesterone after ovulation. This results in a lack of preparation of the lining of the womb for pregnancy to occur or to be maintained.

If there is evidence of a lack of ovulation due to some hormonal defect, fertility drugs may be used. Such treatment has to continue for several months and may not always be successful.

Clomiphene (Clomid, Serophene) is usually the first drug of choice. It is an anti-oestrogen used to treat infertility in women in whom the pituitary gland is producing some FSH and LH but in whom there is evidence of failure to ovulate secondary to some other cause. Clomiphene stimulates the release of FSH by blocking the oestrogen receptor sites in the hypothalamus. The hypothalamus reacts as if the blood level of oestrogen were low and stimulates the pituitary gland to produce more FSH, which then stimulates the ovaries to produce an ovum and set the menstrual cycle going. One tablet of clomiphene (50 mg) is taken daily for 5 days starting on the fifth day of the menstrual cycle and ovulation occurs 5–10 days after the last dose. Couples are advised to have sexual intercourse during this phase.

Clomiphene may occasionally thicken the mucus at the neck of the womb and make it difficult for sperm to get through. This effect may be counteracted by giving an oestrogen drug before the clomiphene treatment.

An important risk of using clomiphene is that so much FSH is produced that the ovaries may produce more than one egg (ovum). This risk is exploited in artificial fertilization procedures. The surgeon aims at producing several eggs which can then be fertilized with the husband's sperm. This is done in the hope of ensuring that at least one egg becomes fertilized, but sometimes several do and that is why some women may have two, three, four or more babies following such procedures.

Other anti-oestrogens that may be used include *cyclofenil* (Rehibin) and *tamoxifen* (Emblon, Noltam, Nolvadex, Tamofen).

Follicle-stimulating hormone (FSH) (Metrodin, Pergonal) is used to treat infertility in women who have evidence of an under-active pituitary gland and who do not respond to clomiphene. It stimulates the ripening of the egg, and is usually given with *chorionic gonadotrophin* (HCG) (Gonadotraphon LH, Profasi) which acts like LH and promotes release of the egg and the production of progesterone. Treatment has to be carefully controlled in order to avoid the production of several eggs and the risk of a multiple pregnancy. The drugs are given by injection during the second week of the menstrual cycle, and courses may have to be repeated several times before pregnancy occurs.

Gonadorelin (Fertiral) is a gonadotrophin-releasing hormone (LHRH) which stimulates the pituitary gland to produce both FSH and LH. It may also be used to treat infertility associated with under-functioning of the ovaries caused by under-production of FSH and LH by the pituitary gland.

Bromocriptine (Parlodel) is used to treat infertility in women who are infertile because they do not ovulate due to over-production of the milk-producing hormone prolactin. Bromocriptine stimulates dopamine receptors in the pituitary gland, causing a reduction in the production of prolactin. It may also be beneficial in some women who are infertile but who do not over-produce prolactin.

Table 69.1 Drugs used to treat infertility – harmful effects and warnings

Chorionic gonadotrophin (HCG) (Gonadotraphon LH, Profasi)
Harmful effects include fluid retention (e.g. ankle swelling), headache, tiredness, sexual precocity (with high doses) and mood changes. Swelling and redness at the site of injection may occur, and it may cause over-stimulation of the ovaries in women who have received menotrophin (FSH).

Warnings HCG requires very careful monitoring in order to avoid multiple pregnancies and to avoid the hyperstimulation syndrome (see under Humegon in Update section).
It should be used
with caution in individuals with epilepsy, heart failure, migraine or kidney disorders.

Clomiphene (Clomid, Serophene)
Harmful effects are related to the dose used and the length of treatment. They include enlargement of the ovaries, over-stimulation of the ovaries, hot flushes, distension and bloated feeling in the abdomen; blurred vision and spots and flashes in front of the eyes (worse after being in the light), rarely cataracts; dermatitis and skin rashes, hair thinning, weight gain, breast tenderness; allergic reactions; dizziness, light-headedness, vertigo, nervous tension, insomnia, fatigue, depression, mood changes and jaundice.

Warnings Clomiphene should not be used in women with impaired liver function, undiagnosed bleeding between periods or ovarian cysts except polycystic disease. Use the smallest dose possible in order to prevent enlargement of the ovaries. NOTE Maximum enlargement of an ovary may occur several days *after* stopping the drug. You should report any discomfort in your abdomen immediately and be examined for a possible cyst of the ovary or other cause. Enlargement of an ovary or a cyst caused by the drug usually shrinks within a few days or weeks of stopping treatment. There is a risk of multiple pregnancies; there is also a risk of abnormalities in the unborn baby but so far this risk does not appear to be any higher than in the general population. About one woman in five loses her baby due to miscarriage or a similar cause. If you develop visual problems, you should not drive; the drug should be stopped and you should have your eyes examined by an eye specialist.

Risks in pregnancy The risk of taking the drug after conception has already occurred does not appear to increase the risk of birth defects in the baby.

Cyclofenil (Rehibin)
Harmful effects are infrequent. They

Table 69.1 Drugs used to treat infertility – harmful effects and warnings (*cont.*)

include hot flushes, abdominal discomfort, nausea and, rarely, jaundice.

Warnings – see under clomiphene, above.

Follicle-stimulating hormone (FSH)
Metrodin (urofollitrophin: from human menopausal urine); **Pergonal** (menotrophin: from human menopausal urine)
Harmful effects include fever, joint pain, irritation at the site of injection and over-stimulation of the ovaries.

Warnings There is a risk of multiple pregnancies, and a higher risk of miscarriage than in the general population. The risk of abnormalities in the unborn child does not appear to be increased.

Gonadorelin (Fertiral)
Harmful effects include rash at the site of injection. Rarely – with high doses – there may be abdominal pain, nausea, headaches or increased menstrual bleeding.

Warnings Gonadorelin should not be used in women with endometrial cysts or polycystic disease of the ovaries.

Bromocriptine (Parlodel)
Harmful effects include nausea, headache, vomiting, constipation, coldness of fingers and toes, and fall in blood pressure on standing after lying down (may produce dizziness, light-headedness and faintness).

Warnings For general warnings, see 'bromocriptine' in Chapter 36.

Risks in pregnancy If pregnancy occurs while on treatment it is advisable to stop the drug after the first missed period. When pregnancy is undesirable or unwanted, sexual intercourse should be avoided or a mechanical type of contraception should be used (e.g. a condom) but not an oral contraceptive pill. In women of child-bearing age being treated for conditions other than increased prolactin production, the lowest possible dose should be used in order to avoid suppression of LH function.

Risks with driving A fall in blood pressure in the first few days of treatment may produce symptoms that affect your ability to drive, so do not drive until you know that it is safe to do so.

Risks with alcohol Tolerance to the effects of bromocriptine may be reduced by alcohol.

Tamoxifen
See Chapter 76.

Drug treatment of male infertility

Hormonal treatment may help only if the sperm are normal but are being produced in a decreased number. This may be due to the pituitary gland producing too little FSH and LH to stimulate full sperm production. In these cases the drug treatment described above for female infertility may be tried but it may take several months of continuous treatment to produce an increased number of sperm.

Vaginal and vulval conditions

Applications to the vulva and vagina consist of creams, dusting powders, pessaries and medicated tampons.

Ointments are too 'solid' and do not dissolve. They interfere with evaporation from the surface of the vagina and vulva, and block the secretions.

Vaginal douches may be harmful because they alter the acidity of the lining of the vagina and also disturb the balance between bacteria and fungi that normally live in the vagina.

Dryness and shrinking of the vagina

Women at and after the menopause may develop shrinking of the vagina with dryness of its lining, which may make sexual intercourse painful. In these women a local application of an oestrogen preparation may be helpful but should not be used at the same time as hormone replacement treatment (HRT) by mouth; this is because oestrogens are absorbed into the blood stream from vaginal applications, and with combined use (by mouth and vagina) there is a risk of overdosing with oestrogens and the development of harmful effects.

Oestrogen applications are also used to treat other causes of dryness and shrinking of the vaginal surface – for example, kraurosis vulvae and vaginal prolapse. In the latter it is used to prepare the vaginal surface ready for surgery on a prolapse.

Because of the risks of absorption of the oestrogens into the blood stream, oestrogen vaginal applications should be used in as small an effective amount as possible and for the shortest duration of time possible.

Thrush of the vagina

Anti-fungal drugs such as nystatin or miconazole or a related drug are effective in treating thrush. Vaginal preparations include pessaries and medicated tampons. If the vulva is infected, an anti-fungal cream is applied to the vulva at the same time as the vaginal treatment. For severe and recurrent thrush infections of the vagina and vulva it may be necessary to take an anti-fungal drug by mouth (e.g. nystatin) as well as using a vaginal and vulval application.

Vaginal preparations that restore the acidity of the lining of the vagina (e.g. Aci-Jel) may help to discourage the growth of thrush and encourage the normal balance between bacteria and fungi.

Recurrence of thrush infections of the vagina and vulva is common, so a course of treatment should always be completed even if the thrush appears to have cleared up after a day or two.

Some drug treatments by mouth may cause vaginal thrush; for example, antibiotics and oral contraceptive pills. Vaginal thrush may occur in pregnancy. It may also occur in diabetes, so patients with vaginal thrush should always have their urine tested for sugar.

Re-infection of the vagina with thrush may occur if thrush is spread on the fingers from other areas (e.g. the umbilicus, nail beds and fingers, from the anus or from infected faeces). It may also spread from a thrush infection of the bladder and from an infected sexual partner. The latter source of infection is important, and in a regular sexual relationship both sexual partners should have a full course of anti-fungal drug treatment.

Treatment of other fungal infections

Anti-fungal applications used to treat fungal infection of the vagina or vulva include creams and pessaries (vaginal tablets) of amphotericin, clotrimazole, econazole, isoconazole, ketoconazole, miconazole or natamycin – see Table 56.2.

Trichomonal infections of the vagina

Trichomonas is a genus of protozoa, a parasite that lives in the vagina and causes a white discharge. They frequently infect the urethra as well but they do not infect the womb. The most effective drugs for treating trichomonal infections of the vagina are metronidazole, nimorazole or tinidazole by mouth. The sexual partner should also be treated at the same time.

Gynatren is a vaccine prepared from *Lactobacillus acidophilus* which is given at 2-weekly intervals for three doses. It stimulates antibody production against lactobacilli, which are associated with trichomonas protozoa in the vagina and also supposedly against the parasites themselves. It is claimed that it restores the normal acidity of the vagina and the normal balance between bacteria and fungi.

Harmful effects include local inflammation at the injection site and fever.

Warnings *Gynatren should not be used during a fever, or in patients with impaired heart or kidney function or blood disorders. Allergic reactions are possible, so full resuscitative facilities should be available at the time of injection.*

Bacterial infections of the vagina

The treatment of gonorrhoea and other sexually transmitted diseases is discussed in Chapter 34. Bacterial infections that are not sexually transmitted usually develop because of some local damage or injury to the vagina; for example, following surgery or some sexual activity.

Metronidazole or tinidazole are effective drugs for treating bacterial infections of the vagina. They are given by mouth. Local vaginal applications containing an anti-bacterial drug may also be used; for example, Sultrin (cream or pessaries) which contains three sulphonamide drugs.

Antiseptic vaginal applications

These include povidone-iodine (Betadine Vaginal Gel and pessaries and Betadine VC solution in an antiseptic vaginal cleansing kit). Because of the risk of absorption of iodine into the blood stream these preparations should not be used in pregnancy or in breast-feeding mothers. The absorbed iodine may interfere with tests of thyroid function, and the iodine may, rarely, cause local irritation and allergy.

Table 70.1 Preparations used to treat vaginal and vulval infections

Preparation	*Drug*	*Drug group*	*Dosage form*
Aci-Jel	acetic acid	Antiseptic	Jelly
Betadine	povidone-iodine	Antiseptic	Pessaries, vaginal gel, antiseptic vaginal cleansing kit (Betadine VC kit)
Canesten	clotrimazole	Anti-fungal	Topical cream, vaginal cream, vaginal tablets, vaginal tablets and topical cream (Duopak)
Canesten 1	clotrimazole	Anti-fungal	Vaginal tablets
Canesten 10% VC	clotrimazole	Anti-fungal	Vaginal cream
Diflucan	fluconazole	Anti-fungal	Capsules by mouth

Table 70.1 Preparations used to treat vaginal and vulval infections (*cont.*)

Preparation	*Drug*	*Drug group*	*Dosage form*
Ecostatin	econazole	Anti-fungal	Topical cream, pessaries, pessaries and topical cream (Twinpack)
Ecostatin-1	econazole	Anti-fungal	Long-acting pessaries
Fasigyn	tinidazole	Anti-protozal anti-bacterial	Tablets by mouth
Flagyl and Flagyl 400	metronidazole	Anti-protozoal/anti-bacterial	Tablets by mouth
Flagyl-S	metronidazole	Anti-protozoal/anti-bacterial	Suspension by mouth
Flagyl Compak	metronidazole and nystatin	Anti-protozoal/anti-bacterial	Tablets by mouth plus vaginal pessaries
Fungilin	amphotericin	Anti-fungal	Topical cream
Gynatren	inactivated lactobacilli	Vaccination against recurrent trichomoniasis	Intramuscular injection
Gyno-Daktarin	miconazole	Anti-fungal	Vaginal cream, pessaries, tampons, pessaries and vaginal cream (Combipack)
Gyno-Daktarin 1	miconazole	Anti-fungal	Vaginal capsules
Gyno-Pevaryl	econazole	Anti-fungal	Cream, pessaries, pessaries and topical cream (Combipack)
Gyno-Pevaryl 1	econazole	Anti-fungal	Pessaries, pessaries and topical cream (Gyno-Pevaril ICP: Combipack)
Imunovir	inosine pranobex	Anti-viral against genital herpes and warts	Tablets by mouth
Metrolyl	metronidazole	Anti-fungal	Tablets by mouth
Monistat	miconazole	Anti-fungal	Vaginal cream
Naxogin 500	nimorazole	Anti-protozoal	Tablets by mouth
Nizoral	ketoconazole	Anti-fungal	Topical cream, tablets or suspension by mouth
Nystan	nystatin	Anti-fungal	Vaginal cream, topical gel, pessaries, tablets by mouth; effervescent pessaries, topical gel and tablets by mouth (Triple Pack)
Pevaryl	econazole	Anti-fungal	Topical cream, lotion

Table 70.1 Preparations used to treat vaginal and vulval infections (*cont.*)

Preparation	*Drug*	*Drug group*	*Dosage form*
Pimafucin	natamycin	Anti-fungal	Topical cream, vaginal tablets
Sporanox	itraconazole	Anti-fungal	Capsules (with coated pellets inside) by mouth
Sultrin	sulphathiazole sulphacetamide sulphabenzamide	Sulphonamide Sulphonamide Sulphonamide	Vaginal cream, vaginal tablets
Travogyn	isoconazole	Anti-fungal	Topical cream, vaginal tablets
Zadstat	metronidazole	Anti-protozoal/ anti-bacterial	Tablets by mouth

NOTES Apply vaginal creams into the vagina as directed.
Apply topical creams to the surface of the anus or genitals.

71

Abortion, labour and childbirth

Inducing abortion

Prostaglandins

The prostaglandins *dinoprost* (Prostin F_2 alpha) and *dinoprostone* (Prostin E_2) are used to induce an abortion up to the 20th week of pregnancy. They are also used to empty the womb after death of the fetus. Up to the 14th week, a prostaglandin may be applied as a pessary to the neck of the womb in order to soften and dilate it before surgical removal of the fetus. After 14 weeks of pregnancy, labour can be induced by a prostaglandin applied as a pessary and/or given by injection into a vein (intravenously). A prostaglandin gel may also be applied to the neck of the womb to help it to become soft and to dilate. An injection of a prostaglandin through the wall of the womb and directly into the amniotic fluid (the fluid inside the baby's membrane) may also be used to induce labour after the 14th week of pregnancy.

Harmful effects of prostaglandins include nausea, vomiting and diarrhoea, when taken by mouth.

Warnings Prostaglandins should not be used if the woman is sensitive to them or when prolonged contraction of the womb could be harmful (e.g. previous caesarean section, six or more pregnancies). They should not be used with oxytocin. The intravenous route may produce harmful effects and is seldom used. Continuous administration for more than 2 days is not recommended.

Drugs used to induce and augment labour

It may be necessary to give drugs to induce (start off) labour if the mother's or the baby's health is at risk. They may also be used to help a woman in labour who is not making sufficient progress (i.e. to augment labour).

The use of drugs to induce or augment labour varies significantly between hospitals and between doctors. Some appear to use them all too readily whilst others may be too hesitant. However, their use over all has increased in the past three decades without good evidence from adequate and well controlled studies that the benefits of their *routine* use outweigh their risks.

Drugs used to induce and augment labour include prostaglandins and oxytocin.

Prostaglandins

The prostaglandin *dinoprost* (Prostin F_2 alpha) is used as a vaginal tablet (pessary) or gel to soften and dilate the neck of the womb to help a normal labour or to induce labour. For harmful effects and warnings, see above.

Oxytocin

Oxytocin (Syntocinon) stimulates the womb to contract and is given by slow intravenous infusion, preferably using an infusion pump. It is used to induce or assist labour, often along with rupture of the membranes. The contractions of the womb must be carefully monitored and the dose of oxytocin controlled so as to prevent over-stimulation.

Harmful effects When oxytocin is given in high doses with large volumes of electrolyte-free fluid, symptoms of water intoxication may develop. These include loss of appetite, headache, nausea, vomiting, abdominal pain, lethargy, drowsiness, unconsciousness and convulsions. The womb may be over-sensitive to oxytocin and go into spasm, and high doses may produce a violent contraction and rupture of the womb.

Warnings Oxytocin should not be used if the womb is not contracting effectively, if there is any mechanical obstruction to delivery, failed trial labour or severe toxaemia, if the baby is distressed or if the afterbirth is misplaced over the neck of the womb (placenta praevia). It should be used with caution in women with raised blood pressure, or who have had four or more pregnancies, a previous caesarian section or who are having more than one baby (e.g. twins).

Prevention and treatment of bleeding after abortion or delivery

Bleeding due to incomplete abortion can be controlled with a combination of *ergometrine* and *oxytocin* (*Syntometrine*) given by injection into a vein or into a muscle. The dose will vary according to the patient's condition and the amount of blood she has lost.

To prevent bleeding after childbirth *ergometrine, with or without oxytocin,* is commonly used by intramuscular injection *after* the baby's first shoulder has been delivered. Bleeding from the womb after childbirth when the womb is not contracting may be controlled by ergometrine intravenously or by oxytocin by intravenous infusion if the ergometrine does not work.

Harmful effects of ergometrine include headaches, dizziness, noises in the ears, abdominal pain, nausea, vomiting, raised blood pressure, chest pain, palpitations, breathlessness and slowing of the pulse rate.

Warnings Ergometrine should not be used in women with severe blood pressure, severe or persistent septic infection, disease of the circulation or severe kidney or liver disease. It should be used with caution in women with toxaemia or impaired liver or kidney function. It should not be used to induce labour; if used at delivery, this should be only when the baby's first shoulder has been delivered. Its effects on the womb are reduced by the general anaesthetic halothane.

Harmful effects of combined ergometrine and oxytocin (*Syntometrine*) include nausea, vomiting and abdominal pain.

Warnings The combination should not be used in women with a severe disorder of the liver or kidneys. It should be used with caution by intravenous route in women with mild or moderate impaired kidney or liver function, raised blood pressure or in the presence of a septic infection.

A prostaglandin (carboprost: Hemabate) may be given by intramuscular injection if combined ergometrine and oxytocin fail to stop the bleeding (see Update).

Premature labour

If the womb starts to contract before the 34th week, the mother may go into premature labour. To help to prevent this the mother is put to bed and given a sympathomimetic drug (see Chapter 2) to relax the muscle of the womb. Initially this is given by injection, and later by mouth.

Such treatment should be used only if the expected benefits of preventing labour outweigh the risks.

Sympathomimetic drugs used to prevent premature labour include isoxsuprine, ritodrine, salbutamol and terbutaline.

Harmful effects of sympathomimetics are discussed in Chapter 2. They include nausea, vomiting, flushing, sweating, tremor, rapid beating of the heart, fall in blood potassium and a fall in blood pressure with high doses.

Warnings Sympathomimetics should not be used in women who have had a recent haemorrhage, who have heart disease, premature separation of the placenta, severe anaemia, ruptured membranes, infection, raised blood pressure, pre-eclampsia (toxaemia), compression of the baby's cord or over-active thyroid gland.

Table 71.1 Drugs used to induce abortion, induce and augment labour, prevent and treat bleeding after abortion or childbirth and to treat premature labour

Preparation	*Drug*	*Drug group*	*Dosage form*
Bricanyl	terbutaline	beta-receptor stimulant	Injection
Cervagem	gemeprost	prostaglandin	Pessaries
Duvadilan	isoxsuprine	beta-receptor stimulant	Injection
ergometrine	ergometrine	uterotropic (causes uterus to contract)	Tablets, injection
Hemabate	carboprost	prostaglandin	Injection
Prepidil	dinoprostone	prostaglandin	Gel in single-use syringe
Prostin E_2	dinoprostone	prostaglandin	Tablets, solution for injection, plus diluent (extra-amniotic), vaginal gel, vaginal tablets
Prostin F_2 alpha	dinoprost	prostaglandin	Intravenous infusion, intra-amniotic injection
Syntocinon	oxytocin	uterotropic (causes uterus to contract)	Injection
Syntometrine	ergometrine, oxytocin	uterotropic (causes uterus to contract)	Injection
Ventolin	salbutamol	beta-receptor stimulant	Tablets, solution for intravenous infusion
Yutopar	ritodrine	beta-receptor stimulant	Tablets, injection

Abortion pill

This pill contains mifepristone which is an anti-progesterone. It blocks progesterone receptors in the uterus and elsewhere. If taken shortly after ovulation it stops the corpus luteum from being formed and causes a 'period' to come on. It should be taken no later than the 49th day after the first day of the last period and a prostaglandin is taken by injection or vaginally 48 hours later to stimulate the uterus to contract and expel its contents.

72

Male sex hormones

The development and maintenance of reproductive organs is under the control of chemicals known as steroid hormones. These hormones are produced by the male and female sex glands and by the adrenal glands. The hormones concerned with the development and maintenance of the male reproductive system are called androgens, and the most powerful of these is known as testosterone.

The function of male sex hormones

The master gland (the pituitary) produces hormones that stimulate the testes to make male sex hormones, the principal one being testosterone. At puberty, under this stimulation, testosterone is made in sufficient amounts to produce changes usually known as secondary sexual characteristics. The voicebox enlarges and the voice gets deeper, the genitals get bigger and hair begins to appear on various parts of the body. The skin thickens and becomes greasy, and acne may develop. There is also a spurt in growth as muscles develop and bones grow. These latter effects are called anabolic effects – 'anabolism' means making living tissue from nutrients in food.

Testosterone is also responsible for the growth and development of the testicles to produce sperm, and sufficient testosterone is also necessary for the development of normal sexual drive (libido) and fertility (the development of normal healthy sperm). In addition, in order to produce fertilization the sperm need to be in a special fluid – the seminal fluid. This is produced by secretions from the prostate gland and the seminal vesicles under stimulation from testosterone.

Male sex hormones are called androgens because they produce male characteristics. They have two principal effects: *androgenic* – they affect the development and maintenance of sexual organs and function; and *anabolic* – they affect growth and muscle bulk (body-building effects). Those male sex hormones that have predominantly sexual effects will also produce some anabolic effects, and those that principally produce anabolic effects will also have some effects on sexual function.

Testosterone is the natural male sex hormone produced by the testes, and in addition there are several synthetic preparations available with principally androgenic effects. There are also several synthetic male sex hormone with principally anabolic effects.

Male sex hormones that produce marked effects on sexual function (androgenic effects) and also some body building (anabolic effects) include mesterolone, methyltestosterone, testosterone and testosterone esters.

Male sex hormones that produce mainly body building (anabolic effects) and relatively weak effects on sexual function (androgenic effects) are discussed in Chapter 73.

Use of male sex hormones

To encourage sexual development

Male sex hormones that have principally sexual effects are used to treat disorders caused by failure of the testes to make these hormones. This failure may be primary, due to lack of development or under-development of the testes; or secondary, due to failure of the pituitary gland (the master gland) to produce sufficient hormones – luteinizing hormone (LH) and follicle-stimulating hormone (FSH) to stimulate the production and release of testosterone.

In under-development or if used in adolescent males with delayed puberty, male sex hormones produce development of the secondary sexual characteristics. They also stimulate growth, but may result in stunting of growth because they also cause the growing ends of the long bones in the arms and legs to close off early and stop growing.

In small doses they stimulate the production of sperm by the testes, but in high doses they cause the pituitary to stop the production of LH and FSH, which results in a stoppage of sperm production.

As replacement treatment

Male sex hormones are used to treat adult men who have been castrated.

To improve sexual function

Male sex hormones are of no use in treating male sterility (lack of sperm production) and they are of no use in treating impotence (inability to attain or maintain an erection) unless this is due to testicular failure causing a diminished production of testosterone. They may occasionally be used to increase sex drive (libido) in adult men with a low production of testosterone.

In failure of the testes due to lack of development, male sex hormones rarely reverse sterility because the pituitary gland produces insufficient gonadotrophins. Treatment is therefore given with injections of gonadotrophins – chorionic gonadotrophin (HCG) and menotropin (FSH). These will stimulate sperm production as well as male sex hormone production.

To counter the effects of oestrogens (female sex hormones)

Male sex hormones were previously used in women to treat abnormal menstruation and painful periods, and to suppress milk production after childbirth. But the harmful effects (e.g. growth of hair on the face) were often worse than the symptoms of the disorder being treated and they are not recommended. They may be used to treat certain patients with a type of breast cancer that depends on oestrogens. Small doses combined with a female sex hormone (oestrogen) have also been used to treat menopausal symptoms.

For a discussion of the normal interactions between androgens and oestrogens, see Chapter 66.

Harmful effects of male sex hormones

Male sex hormones (androgens) may cause nausea and loss of appetite, headache, anxiety, depression, nerve damage, numbness and pins and needles in the arms and legs; increase in the weight of the skeleton, prolonged erections (priapism), retention of salt and water in the body, producing swelling of tissues (e.g. ankle swelling); and they may cause a rise in blood sodium, chloride, potassium, calcium and phosphate. They may cause a rise in the blood fat levels (e.g. cholesterol) and increase the risks of developing fatty deposits in the arteries (atherosclerosis). Androgens can affect blood-clotting factors in the blood and increase the risk of bleeding in patients taking anti-blood-clotting drugs (anti-coagulants).

High doses, prolonged treatment and/or too frequent use may cause sexual changes, as follows.

In women – virilization, which includes enlargement of the clitoris, irregular periods, loss of periods, increased libido (sexual drive), enlargement of the breasts, hoarseness and deepening of the voice, hairiness (e.g. on the face), male-type baldness and acne. The voice changes and enlargement of the clitoris are usually irreversible even if the drug is stopped as soon as these develop. The use of a female sex hormone along with a male sex hormone will not stop virilization in females.

In pre-pubertal boys – enlargement of the penis, frequent erections, skin pigmentation, hairiness, acne and stunted growth.

In post-pubertal males – enlargement of the breasts, excessive frequency and duration of erections of the penis which may be persistent (priapism); reduced sperm count and reduced volume of seminal fluid may occur with high doses and/or prolonged treatment.

Danger to the liver

After 2–3 months of treatment, some male sex hormones (e.g. methyltestosterone, ethyloestrenol, stanozolol) may produce liver damage and jaundice at relatively small doses.

Prolonged use of high doses of male sex hormones may cause blood-filled cysts in the liver and spleen; these may be associated with liver failure and bleeding into the abdomen. Stopping the drug usually results in complete disappearance of the cysts.

Risks of liver cancer

There are rare reports of liver cancer developing in patients who have received methyltestosterone and possibly other related male sex hormones for prolonged periods of time.

Risks in elderly people

Male sex hormones may increase the risk of developing enlargement of the prostate gland and cancer of the prostate in elderly men.

Warnings on the use of male sex hormones

Male sex hormones should not be used in men who suffer from cancer of the prostate or breast, nephrosis, raised blood calcium, coronary heart disease or untreated heart failure. In women with breast cancer, male sex hormones may cause a rise in blood calcium level by stimulating the dissolving of bone (osteoporosis). They should be used with caution in people suffering from treated heart failure, impaired kidney or liver function, high blood pressure, diabetes, epilepsy, migraine or enlarged prostate glands.

Male sex hormones should be stopped immediately:

- In women – if they develop hoarseness of their voice, acne, more hair on their face or changes with their menstrual periods
- In men – if they develop acne or a worsening of acne, and/or if they develop frequent or persistent erections of the penis
- In anyone – if they develop nausea, vomiting, changes in skin colour or ankle swelling

Liver function tests should be carried out before and at regular intervals during treatment in anyone taking male sex hormones.

In pre-pubertal boys and girls, X-rays of the long bones should be carried out to determine whether the ends of the long bones have stopped growing.

Blood fat levels should be measured before and at regular intervals during treatment; if they are raised, treatment should not be started or it should be stopped.

Red blood cell counts and haemoglobin levels should be monitored at regular intervals in order to check for a rise in red blood cells (polycythaemia).

Anti-male sex hormone (chemical castration)

An anti-androgenic drug *cyproterone* (Androcur) is used to treat severe over-sexuality and sexual deviation in males. It inhibits sperm production and produces reversible infertility. It may also damage the sperm (see page 973). (U)

Table 72.1 Male sex hormone preparations

Preparation	*Drug*	*Dosage form*
methyltestosterone	methyltestosterone	Tablets
Primoteston Depot	testosterone	Oily injection
Pro-Viron	mesterolone	Tablets
Restandol	testosterone	Capsules
Sustanon 100	testosterone	Oily depot injection
Sustanon 250	testosterone	Oily depot injection
testosterone implants	testosterone	Implant
Virormone	testosterone	Injection

73

Anabolic steroids

As stated in Chapter 72, male sex hormones produce two main effects – *androgenic* (development and maintenance of sexual function) and *anabolic* (body-building function). The male sex hormones marketed as 'body builders' produce some effects on sexual function (androgenic) in males but when used in women they cause less masculinization than those male hormones that produce predominantly androgenic effects.

Masculinization means the development of male characteristics in women – deep voice, acne, male pattern of baldness and hair growth, shrinking of the breasts, increase in size of the clitoris and increase in libido (sexual drive).

Male sex hormones that are marketed as body builders are often referred to as anabolic steroids. 'Anabolism' means making living tissue from nutrients in food and 'steroid' refers to a group of organic chemicals related to cholesterol. All anabolic steroids are derivatives of testosterone, the principal male sex hormone made by the testes. They include nandrolone (Deca-Durabolin, Durabolin), oxymetholone (Anapolon 50) and stanozolol (Stromba).

When male sex hormones are given to men who have been castrated or whose testes have not developed, in addition to their effects on sexual development they produce an increase in anabolism (body-building effect) leading to an increase in muscle bulk and weight. However, in 'normal' men who have not been castrated, their effects in producing an increase in muscle bulk and weight are short lived. This is because treatment with male sex hormones has a *very limited* duration of effect in influencing muscle growth in men who have normal sexual function.

The idea that male sex hormones can be used *specifically* for body building is naive because the sexual effects and the body-building effects of male sex hormones are not due to different actions. They are due to the same actions but on different tissues. Clearly, the effects produced on the genitals and the muscles are different but the receptor sites at which male sex hormones work are exactly the same in every tissue of the body. In other words, you can not separate the effects and produce a 'pure' body-building steroid. Any anabolic steroid will always have some general effects on male sex hormone receptors throughout the body. Therefore, every anabolic steroid that is available produces some effects on sexual development and function. In other words, any one of them could be used to treat a patient who has a defective production of male sex hormones (e.g. a castrated male).

Medical use of anabolic steroids

In convalescence

The use of anabolic steroids to 'build up' patients recovering from injury, surgery and acute illnesses has not been shown to be of benefit. Neither have they been shown to be effective in chronically ill patients who have lost weight due to protein breakdown. These patients need a good nutritious diet

In osteoporosis

The use of anabolic steroids to treat osteoporosis is discussed in Chapter 68.

To treat aplastic anaemia

Anabolic steroids have the ability to stimulate blood cell production by the bone marrow. Oxymetholone and nandrolone may be used for this purpose as part of the treatment of patients suffering from aplastic anaemia, which is a severe anaemia caused by damage to the bone marrow from drugs, irradiation or some other toxic factor.

To treat hereditary angioedema

Stanozolol may be used to prevent reactions in people suffering from hereditary angioedema, which is an inherited predisposition to develop painful allergic-like swellings of the skin. Attacks may be triggered by injury, virus infections and emotional upsets. The swellings of the skin may be accompanied by nausea, vomiting and stomach pains. Occasionally, the linings of the air passages may become swollen and interfere with breathing.

To treat Behçet's syndrome

Behçet's syndrome is characterized by inflammation and ulcers of the skin, genitals, blood vessels, eyes, stomach, intestine and brain. The cause is not known. Treatment involves the use of corticosteroids and immunosuppressants. Occasionally, stanozolol may be of benefit to the damaged blood vessels.

To dissolve thrombi

The use of anabolic steroids to dissolve clots in blood vessels (thrombi) is discussed in Chapter 26.

To prevent itching due to chronic obstruction of the bile system

The use of anabolic steroids to prevent itching is discussed in Chapter 75.

Dangers of using anabolic steroids in children

The use of anabolic steroids to increase height in under-developed children may actually stunt growth because they stop the growth of long bones by prematurely closing the growing ends of the bones. They may produce masculinization in girls.

The misuse of anabolic steroids in sports

Anabolic steroids have been used for many years by weight lifters to increase their muscle bulk and, hopefully, their strength; by body builders to increase their muscle bulk; and by shot putters, javelin throwers and others to improve the strength of their throw. In more recent years some track and other athletes have used anabolic steroids to increase the duration and intensity of their training and, hopefully, to increase their competitive performances. The use of anabolic steroids for all these purposes is illegal within the sporting organizations concerned, and yet there is evidence that they are still being used despite stringent drug-testing at national and international levels.

The willingness of some athletes to use anabolic steroids illegally is a matter of concern; their willingness to risk serious harmful effects as well as the consequences of their illegal actions is of interest because we lack convincing evidence from adequate and well controlled studies that anabolic steroids actually improve competitive performance in, for example, track athletics. But they increase aggressiveness (and therefore competitiveness) and they increase muscle bulk. The mystique that surrounds their use adds to any perceived benefits and, even though some benefits may be just in the mind, the state of mind of some athletes is so central to their performance that steroids could actually influence that performance. In other words, if any athletes think that they are able to train harder and longer under the influence of anabolic steroids then they will, and if they think that they are going to perform exceptionally well then they probably will – particularly if their coaches have recommended their use because they believe in them, a belief that will 'rub off' on to the athletes.

If the claimed 'benefits' of anabolic steroids to athletes are to be unravelled we need careful scientific studies designed to compare the use of anabolic steroids with dummy compounds. Such studies will require that the athletes, athletics coaches and others involved do not know which athletes were taking the real drug and which were taking the dummy ('double-blind' studies). Furthermore, in order to be valid, these studies should be carried out in a competitive atmosphere on competitive athletes, and be controlled for the many factors that may influence both the training of athletes and their athletic performance in a competitive event. The latter would be very difficult and the former well nigh impossible because no top flight athlete would want to take dummy tablets and compete in competitive events against colleagues who might be taking the active drug. Furthermore, the doses used by athletes are much higher than those used for medical purposes, so such a trial would be quite unethical because of the risks from such high doses.

In the end the results would be academic, anyway: if it is shown that anabolic steroids improve performance, they should be banned; and if they don't, there is no point in using them.

Harmful effects of anabolic steroids

Harmful effects of anabolic steroids include nausea, fullness of the stomach, loss of appetite, vomiting and diarrhoea, excitation, insomnia, depression and psychological 'addiction'. They may also cause retention of salts and water in the body, producing swelling of tissues (e.g. ankle swelling), and a rise in blood sodium, chloride, potassium, phosphates and calcium. They may cause a rise in blood pressure and in blood glucose levels, so it may be necessary to change the dose of insulin or anti-diabetic drug by mouth in diabetic patients. Anabolic steroids increase blood fat levels (e.g. cholesterol) and increase the risk of developing fatty deposits in arteries (atherosclerosis), which increases the risk of premature death from coronary artery disease or stroke. Some anabolic steroids (e.g. oxymetholone) can reduce the uptake of iron from food and cause the blood level of iron to fall, producing anaemia. They can affect blood-clotting factors in the blood and increase the risk of bleeding in patients taking anti-blood-clotting drugs.

In women – anabolic steroids may produce masculinization (virilization), which includes enlargement of the clitoris, irregular periods or loss of periods, increased libido (sexual drive), enlargement of the breasts, hoarseness and deepening of the voice, hairiness (e.g. on the face), male-type baldness and acne. The voice changes and enlargement of the clitoris are usually irreversible even if the drug is stopped as soon as these develop. The use of female sex hormones will not prevent virilization in females.

In pre-pubertal boys – enlargement of the penis, frequent erections, acne, skin pigmentation, hairiness and stunting of growth.

In pre-pubertal girls – enlargement of the clitoris, increase in pubic hair, loss of periods and stunting of growth.

In post-pubertal males – they may knock out sperm production, cause the testes to shrink and cause impotence (failure to attain or maintain an erection), changes in libido, chronic erections (priapism), bladder disorders, male-type baldness, enlargement of the breasts.

Damage to the liver

Anabolic steroids may, rarely, damage the liver, producing jaundice.

Risks of cancer

Long-term use of anabolic steroids may, rarely, cause blood-filled cysts in the liver and spleen; these have been associated with liver failure and bleeding into the abdomen. Withdrawal of the drug usually results in complete disappearance of the cysts. Benign and malignant cancers of the liver have been reported; these cancers have a good blood supply and may burst, causing life-threatening bleeding into the abdomen.

There is also a very rare risk of cancer of the prostate and kidneys.

Risks in elderly people

Anabolic steroids may increase the risk of developing enlargement of the prostate gland and cancer of the prostate.

Table 73.1 Anabolic steroid preparations

Preparation	*Drug*	*Dosage form*
Anapolon 50	oxymetholone	Tablets
Deca-Durabolin	nandrolone	Depot injections
Durabolin	nandrolone	Depot injections
Stromba	stanozolol	Tablets

Warnings on the use of anabolic steroids

Anabolic steroids should not be used in people who are allergic to any one of them, or in anyone who has a disorder of liver function. They should not be used in patients who suffer from cancer of the prostate, cancer of the breast in males or in some females or in patients with severe kidney disorders or porphyria. Liver damage and jaundice may occur at relatively low doses with certain anabolic steroids (e.g. oxymetholone). In women with breast cancer, anabolic steroids may cause a rise in blood calcium level by stimulating the 'dissolving' of bone (osteoporosis). Fluid retention caused by anabolic steroids may trigger heart failure, kidney failure or liver failure in people suffering from existing disease of their heart, kidneys or liver. Anabolic steroids should be used with caution in anyone suffering from heart failure, impaired kidney function, high blood pressure, diabetes, epilepsy, migraine or enlarged prostate gland.

Anabolic steroids should be stopped immediately:

- In women – if they develop hoarseness of their voice, acne, more hair on their faces or changes with their periods
- In men – if they develop acne and or worsening of acne, and/or if they develop frequent and persistent erections of the penis
- In anyone – if they develop nausea, vomiting, changes in skin colour or ankle swelling

Liver function tests should be carried out before and at regular intervals during treatment of individuals taking anabolic steroids.

In pre-pubertal boys and girls, X-rays of the long bones should be carried out to determine whether the ends of the long bones have stopped growing.

Blood fat levels should be measured before and at regular intervals during treatment; if they are raised, treatment should not be started or it should be stopped.

74

Drugs and sex

Definitions

Impotence means the inability to perform the sexual act owing to some failure of the reflex mechanisms involved. As women can perform the sexual act without these reflexes being activated by sexual arousal and without reaching orgasm the term 'impotence' is principally applied to males. It implies a failure to attain or maintain an erection.

Orgasm is the climax of excitement in the sexual act. In males it occurs at the same time as ejaculation.

Ejaculation is the emission of seminal fluid (semen) and represents orgasm in males.

Premature ejaculation is the emission of seminal fluid at the beginning of the sexual act.

Our interest in sex, our sexual drive (*libido*) and our ability to carry out the sexual act to its climax are influenced by many factors, particularly by our emotions. It is often therefore very difficult to unravel why an individual should lose sexual drive, find it difficult to be 'turned-on', fail to get an orgasm, fail to get an erection or fail to ejaculate.

Against such a complex background you would think that sexual problems produced by drugs would be fairly easy to recognize and to treat. Surely it should not be too difficult to show that a particular drug caused a particular sexual problem – if the problem started when you were taking the drug and cleared up after you stopped the drug, you should have a good idea that it was that particular drug that caused your sexual problem. You would think that sexual problems created by drugs would be well documented. This is not the case, however, and we know very little about which drugs produce which sexual problems. This lack of information really reflects our inhibited attitude to sexual problems and our inability to discuss them, even with doctors. Unfortunately, many doctors know virtually nothing about how to diagnose and treat sexual problems and therefore seldom question their patients about such matters. Yet against this background of ignorance, each year millions of tablets and capsules are prescribed by doctors that could cause sexual problems in many patients.

It is obvious therefore that what we do know about the damaging effects of drugs on our sex lives is only the tip of the iceberg. There must be thousands of people whose sex lives are being damaged by drugs prescribed by doctors and/or bought from pharmacists, drug stores or from herbalists.

Sexual problems caused by drugs

Many drugs prescribed by doctors or bought over the counter can interfere with our interest in sex and our sexual activities (see later). Different people react differently to drugs, and as a result of taking a drug, some of us may just not feel like sex or can't be 'turned-on'. Some may be 'turned-on' but not be able to get an erection or reach a climax; and if some men get an erection they may be unable to maintain it long enough to have sexual intercourse. Other men get an erection but ejaculate too early, often before they have even 'started' and some may fail to ejaculate any semen (i.e. have an orgasm).

You will notice that most of these problems refer to men; this is because we know almost nothing about sexual problems created by drugs in women. The reasons for this are complex and are tied up in our cultural and social attitudes to sexual activities as they apply to both men and women. It is beyond the scope of this book for me to discuss these problems further except to say that if a man fails to get an erection it is fairly obvious, to say the least, and makes sexual intercourse impossible. Whereas, if a woman fails to have an orgasm it is less 'visually' obvious and does not interfere with the 'physical' performance of the sexual act.

Failure to attain or maintain an erection obviously challenges a male's self-image. This is probably why we hear more about men's problems than women's problems – because men may complain more.

Most reported drug-related sexual problems in women are either an increase or a decrease in libido. We know little about the effects of drugs on women's sexual pleasure and ability to have orgasms; but sexual arousal and pleasure from sexual activities, including orgasm, are determined by many cultural, social and emotional factors that influence our sexual beliefs, attitudes and expectations. These may therefore prevent women from complaining to doctors (particularly male doctors) about such matters, so we really do not have any idea how many women suffer from damage to their sex lives because of some drug treatment that they are taking.

Against this background of our lack of knowledge about the damaging effects of drugs on our sex lives the message is clear: if you are on regular daily treatment with a drug or drugs and experience any change in your sex life, *always* check whether it could be your treatment that is causing the problem.

A few examples of drugs that may damage your sex life

The following is just a very brief guide to some of the drugs that may affect your sex life, but, as stated above, if you develop any change in your sex life, always ask 'is it due to any drug I am taking?' – and this includes alcohol!

Anticholinergic drugs

Anticholinergic drugs (Chapter 2) can block the response to stimulation of the nerves that are closely involved in sexual arousal and in the sexual act. These drugs may have a damaging effect on your sex life. In men they may interfere with attaining and maintaining an erection, and may cause a failure to ejaculate.

NOTE Anticholinergic drugs may be present in medicines used to treat blocked and runny nose (cold symptoms), coughs, hayfever, asthma, indigestion, the painful colic of diarrhoea, kidney pain (renal colic), painful periods, certain heart disorders, certain eye disorders and parkinsonism.

Drugs used to treat raised blood pressure (hypertension)

Apart from those individuals with severe raised blood pressure, many people who are taking drug treatment for their hypertension may have no symptoms from the disease. What symptoms they do experience are more often caused by their drug treatment, and some of these symptoms may be sexual. Drugs used to treat hypertension probably cause more sexual problems than any other group of drugs, yet someone who is prescribed these drugs usually has to stay on them for life.

Diuretics (water tablets)

A major group of drugs used to treat hypertension are the diuretics. They are also used to treat heart failure. In some people diuretic drugs may produce failure to attain or maintain an erection and difficulty in ejaculating.

Anti-anxiety drugs (tranquillizers), sedatives and sleeping drugs

Any anti-anxiety drug or sleeping drug may reduce libido in some patients and it is important to consider this. Equally, by reducing anxiety and tension they may increase libido. However, long-term use may so affect your mood as to reduce your interest in sex.

Anti-anxiety drugs are often referred to as 'tranquillizers' or 'sedatives'.

Anti-depressant drugs

Monoamine-oxidase inhibitors may affect ability to attain or maintain an erection and cause a failure to ejaculate. In some people they may increase libido.

Tricyclic and other cyclic anti-depressant drugs may affect libido and cause problems with attaining or maintaining an erection in some individuals.

Lithium may cause problems with attaining or maintaining an erection in some people.

Anti-psychotic drugs

These drugs are used to relieve symptoms in people suffering from serious mental disorders such as schizophrenia. In some patients these drugs may cause problems with attaining or maintaining an erection and also failure to ejaculate. They may also reduce libido.

Oral contraceptives

Despite the fact that millions of women have taken oral contraceptives over the past three decades there is surprisingly little information about the effects of oral contraceptives on sexual desires and performance. The pill may increase libido in some women but not in others, and this effect has been related to freedom from the risk of pregnancy in the former and depression of mood in the latter.

Warnings *In this section are included very few examples of drugs that may damage your sex life. However, different people react differently to any one drug, and these harmful effects on sex lives may occur in some individuals and not in* *others. Therefore, the risks are not a reason for not taking a particular drug, but they are a reason for considering the possibility if you develop some change in your sex life and you are taking a drug or drugs regularly.*

Always check with your doctor or pharmacist if you suspect that a drug you are taking is affecting your sex life.

Drugs used in the treatment of sexual problems

A large proportion of married couples have some difficulty with their sex lives. However, 'difficulty' as felt by the individual partner or the couple may be interpreted differently by different people. Without getting too involved, it goes back to what I was saying earlier about the many complex factors that determine our attitudes towards sex and towards our sexual expectations. These are all bound up by our inhibitions and feelings of guilt and our beliefs that to talk about details of the sexual act and what pleases or displeases us is somehow 'dirty' or 'taboo'.

The common sexual problems in marriage include lack of interest in sex, failure to be aroused, and/or failure to get an orgasm in women and failure to attain or maintain an erection or premature ejaculation in men.

Unfortunately, most doctors are not trained to advise on sexual problems. They may share our ignorance and suffer from our inhibitions and guilts, and it is easy to understand why some doctors may find it difficult to discuss intimate sexual problems with their patients. Also, because there is usually no specific drug that they can prescribe to treat sexual problems, one of their main responses (the issuing of a prescription) to a patient's problem is removed from them. Therefore they feel 'impotent' to do anything!

Male sex hormones

Male sex hormones are discussed in Chapter 72. They influence libido in both men and women. This is because libido in women is determined by the amounts of natural male sex hormone they produce in their bodies. This is not affected by removal of the ovaries, so women who have had both their ovaries removed may experience little change if any in their libido. It is, however, affected by the removal of their adrenal glands or their pituitary gland (the master gland). This is because, under stimulation from the pituitary gland, the adrenal glands normally produce both male and female sex hormones in both men and women. It follows, therefore, that drugs that stop the activity of the adrenal glands (e.g. the corticosteroids) may reduce the production of sex hormones sufficiently to affect libido.

If male sex hormones are given to women, their libido increases but they will also grow a beard and develop a deep voice, a large clitoris and male-type baldness and acne. This is hardly a price to pay for an increase in libido. In men there is little indication, if any, for using male sex hormones to improve libido and sexual performance. In a man whose libido has totally gone, and who does not even get an erection or masturbate, it may occasionally be worth testing his male hormone production. It may help to give such an individual a small daily dose of testosterone if these tests show that he is not producing male hormones.

Drugs such as clomiphene and bromocriptine, which are used to increase testosterone production in men whose testes are not functioning properly, have no effect on libido or sexual performance in men who have no disorder of their testicles.

Other drugs

Levodopa used to treat parkinsonism has produced some startling effects in a few such individuals suffering from parkinsonism. In patients previously withdrawn and quiet because of the effects of their disorder, the drug may cause them to become over-excited and active (hypomanic); this may include excessive sexual arousal and inappropriate sexual behaviour – so much so that some patients can expose themselves and try to seduce members of staff. This applies to both men and women. Some men may develop frequent erections and start masturbating regularly for the first time in years. These effects are probably due to the fact that levodopa corrects a deficiency of the special nerve transmitter, dopamine, in the brain and elsewhere. In people who do not suffer from parkinsonism, the drug has no effect on sexual activities.

Amphetamines and amphetamine-related slimming drugs These drugs increase libido and sexual activity in both men and women. They may prolong erection time. A large dose injected into a vein may produce a marked sexual arousal. However, high doses and regular use have the opposite effects and decrease both interest in sex and the ability to carry out the act.

Vitamin E Although vitamin E is often called the 'sex vitamin' there is no evidence that it improves libido and sexual performance in humans.

Papaverine dilates blood vessels and, if injected directly into the penis, will produce an erection in men who fail to get an erection because of some nerve disorder (e.g. a spinal injury, multiple sclerosis) that stops the blood vessels in the penis filling with blood and making the penis erect (organic impotence). This treatment may also be useful in men who have a disorder of the blood vessels supplying the penis that causes an obstruction to the flow of blood into the penis on sexual arousal.

The dose required to get an erection varies from person to person and with the cause. Men with nerve damage require smaller doses than men with damage to the blood vessels. Persistent erections lasting for a few hours may occur in a few men but these are not painful.

Papaverine has little or no place in the treatment of most cases of impotence because they are not usually due to an organic cause. Apart from proving to the individual that the 'mechanisms' to produce an erection are still intact, it is difficult to see what possible benefit it may have in emotional impotence.

Drugs used to decrease sexual activity

Female sex hormones – oestrogens

In both males and females libido is related to the production of male sex hormones; therefore research into drugs that could suppress libido has centred around drugs that counter the effects of male sex hormones (androgens). They are usually grouped as *anti-androgens* (anti-male sex hormones), and of course the female sex hormones, oestrogens, may be used as anti-androgens because of their effects on male sexual organs. Also, oestrogens cause a decrease in production of those hormones produced by the pituitary gland that stimulate the testes to produce the male sex hormone testosterone. However, although oestrogens decrease the sex drive in men the risks outweigh any possible benefits.

'Chemical castration' – anti-androgens

Certain progestogens have been found to have anti-male hormone effects (anti-androgen effects); one of these drugs, *cyproterone* (Androcur), is prescribed to men who have committed serious sexual offences against women and/or children. It has also been used to treat men who suffer from compulsive masturbation, indecent exposure, sado-masochism and hetero- and homo-paedophilia.

Cyproterone produces shrinking of the testes. It blocks the effects of male sex hormones and causes male sex drive to virtually disappear within about 2 weeks. The effects wear off in about 2 weeks after stopping the drug. It is also of use in treating cancer of the prostate gland that relies on male sex hormones for its growth.

Harmful effects Fatigue and lassitude are common for the first few months of treatment. The breasts may enlarge and occasionally they may produce milk and breast nodules may develop. It may cause weight gain, abnormalities of liver function, block sperm production, and, rarely, osteoporosis. Rarely it may cause acne, patchy body hair, increased growth of scalp hair, lightening of hair colour and female type of pubic hair growth.

Warnings *It should not be used in individuals with liver disease, malignant cancers (other than for cancer of the prostrate for which cyproterone may be used), wasting disorders or severe depression. It should not be used in youths under the age of 18 years because it may stop bone growth and sexual development. It should be used with caution in individuals with diabetes or adrenal insufficiency. Blood glucose, adrenal function and liver function should be monitored. It may impair ability to drive and operate machinery and it is not effective in chronic alcoholism.*

Anti-psychotic drugs

These drugs are used to treat schizophrenia and other serious mental illnesses and are discussed in detail in Chapter 41. In addition to relieving some of the distressing mental symptoms, they also damp down sexual drive and interest. In general, this is regarded as an undesirable harmful effect and yet they have been used in the past and may still be used in some psychiatric hospitals to damp down the sexual drive of patients who show too much interest in sex and/or who masturbate frequently. To achieve this effect, high regular doses have to be used which turns the patients into 'zombies'. Hopefully, this practice is decreasing; it is like putting the patient's brain in a 'chemical prison' where all emotions are denied.

Anti-depressant drugs

The harmful effects produced by some anti-depressant drugs include reduced libido and delay or failure to ejaculate. Because of these harmful effects they have sometimes been used to treat 'over-sexed' men and men who suffer from premature ejaculation. In men who are depressed, the lifting of mood which these drugs produce may well cause an improvement in libido and a reduction in premature ejaculations. However, in men who are not depressed their other harmful effects outweigh the benefits.

Aphrodisiacs

An aphrodisiac is any drug that stimulates sexual desire and performance; but no such drug exists. Aphrodisiacs work because people believe they work; the response is all in the mind. In other words, any dummy tablet, potion or concoction will work provided the person who takes it believes that it will work. Greek, Roman, Indian, Arabic and Oriental literature contains many descriptions of the sexual achievements of people who have taken various aphrodisiacs. Some of them – for example, Spanish fly (crushed beetles containing cantharidine) – may cause severe inflammation of the bowel with ulceration and death; others, such as rhino horn, threaten the very existence of a whole species of animal – the rhinoceros; yet none of them has any beneficial effect upon sexual activity other than in the mind.

Any improvement in sexual desire or activities produced by an aphrodisiac is what is called a *placebo effect.* (The word placebo comes from a Latin verb meaning 'to please'.) Doctors usually use the term placebo to describe a dummy tablet and they define a placebo effect as any effect produced by a dummy preparation. But of course the placebo effect has broader implications than just swallowing a dummy pill and experiencing some beneficial effect. It refers to the effects we feel and experience because we believe in something. It is closely wrapped up in our culture, values, beliefs and expectations. And if you think about it, it covers all kinds of remedies such as herbs, tonics, health foods and all kinds of practices through various alternative medical treatments to orthodox medicine.

75

Skin diseases

Skin applications

Skin applications used in medical treatment contain drugs that may produce benefits but may also produce harmful effects. They should therefore be used in the smallest concentrations, in the smallest amounts, over the smallest area of skin for the shortest duration of time possible. You should be as cautious when using skin applications as you would be about taking tablets by mouth. You would not dream of taking a handful of tablets at one go if you were only supposed to take one, nor should you apply a handful of cream when the instructions say 'apply sparingly'. Just think – a handful of cream is like a handful of tablets!

Bases in skin applications

The choice of the main base for creams and ointments and other skin applications is very important. It is often referred to as the 'vehicle' because it acts as the vehicle for carrying the active drug. The base, or vehicle, can affect the moisture of the skin and the ability of the active drug to penetrate the surface of the skin; it is this ability of the active drug to penetrate the skin that determines how effective treatment will be.

Additives in skin applications

There are numerous additives in skin applications. These may act as inert carriers for the active drug and others may soften the application, improve its texture, ensure its consistency over time and also repel water. Substances that produce these effects are usually paraffins, waxes, oils and silicones.

Certain additives are used to ensure the proper mixing of ingredients such as oily substances and watery substances. This is called emulsification and the additives are called emulsifiers. They are also used to make ingredients soluble and to help the cream to spread. Other additives are included to keep the skin application stable by stopping those chemical reactions that will spoil its consistency and effectiveness. These are called stabilizers. In addition, skin applications may contain soaps and detergents, preservatives, colouring agents and fragrances.

Types of skin applications

According to the base used, there are numerous skin applications available – creams, ointments, lotions, dusting powders, sprays and pastes. They are used for treating skin disorders in different stages of severity and in different areas of the body.

Lotions are semi-liquid preparations used to treat acute skin conditions where the skin is unbroken. Watery lotions act by evaporation and cool the skin. When used, they should be applied frequently. The addition of alcohol to a skin lotion increases its cooling effects. They are useful for applying in a thin layer over a large surface or on hairy areas of the skin. When the skin is broken, a drying agent (an astringent; see later) may be included in order to help seal the weeping surface of the skin.

Shake lotions (e.g. calamine lotion) are used for dry skin disorders (e.g. sunburn). They cool by evaporation and deposit a fine powder on the surface.

Dusting powders (e.g. talc) are useful for treating skin disorders that affect skin folds – under the arms, in the groin or under the breasts.

Creams either mix with water and are easily washed off or they are oily and not easily washed off. They are less greasy and easier to apply than ointments. They have an emollient effect (see later).

Barrier creams protect the skin against water and irritants, and they may contain talc and water repellents such as silicone.

Ointments are greasy and give more covering than creams, which helps to keep the skin moist. Ointments are more suitable for chronic, dry, scaly rashes (e.g. eczema). Most ointments contain mineral oil or wax and are insoluble in water.

Pastes are stiff preparations containing powdered solids such as starch or zinc oxide. They protect the skin and absorb unwanted moisture. They are useful for treating clearly defined, dry, scaly patches such as psoriasis.

Collodions are preparations that, when applied to damaged areas of skin such as small wounds or ulcers, dry to form a protective film. They are sometimes used to keep a drug in contact with the skin (as in the treatment of warts, discussed later in this chapter).

Soothing skin applications

Emollients

Any substance that sooths the surface of the skin is called an emollient. They are usually fats and oils that are soothing when applied to the skin. They are chiefly used as a base to which other active drugs (e.g. antibiotics) are added. They work in two principal ways:

- By forming an oil film over the surface of the skin, which prevents water from evaporating from the surface cells
- By retaining water in the cells on the surface of the skin

Oily emollients

Greasy emollient skin applications that prevent loss of water from the outer layer of the skin usually contain vegetable oils, animal fats, paraffin and related chemicals, and/or waxes.

The vegetable oils are usually cotton-seed oil, corn oil, peanut oil, almond oil and cocoa-bean oil. Animal fats are wool fats from the wool of sheep. These are of two types – wool fat (anhydrous lanolin) and hydrous wool fat (known just as lanolin) which is wool fat mixed with 20–30 per cent of water. Lanolin may produce skin allergies in some people. It is not used as often as it once was, and yet the message is still given that there is something magical about preparations that contain lanolin. It may also contain traces of toxic chemicals from sheep dips.

Paraffin-related preparations include mineral oil (liquid paraffin), white petroleum and yellow petroleum (e.g. Vaseline white and yellow petroleum jellies). Waxes are principally obtained from beeswax (yellow wax). White wax is bleached beeswax.

Spermaceti is a waxy substance from the sperm whale which is used to raise the melting point of ointments to stop them melting too easily when applied to warm skin, particularly in hot climates (they are therefore called cold creams). Because of the need to save the lives of sperm whales it has been replaced by jojoba oil in many countries. Jojoba oil comes from the beans of the jojoba bush, a native of northern Mexico and southern California.

Urea-containing emollients

Urea is a principal ingredient of emollients that help the cells in the skin to retain water. It is the end product of the breakdown of proteins in the body, and occurs in blood and body fluids and in the urine. It absorbs water from the atmosphere.

Choice of emollient preparation

There are many emollient preparations on the market and no particular one can be recommended over all the others. It is a matter of personal choice. Simple and cheap preparations are often as effective as very expensive preparations. The beneficial effects of emollients are short lived and they must be applied frequently.

Protective skin applications

A *demulcent* is a substance that coats and protects the surface of the skin. Demulcents are usually gums from stems, roots and branches of various plants; for example, gum arabic, gum tragacanth, liquorice root, agar and sodium alginate (from algae). Synthetic drugs such as methylcellulose are also used. Glycerin is a common constituent of skin applications, and mixed with starch it forms a jelly base called starch glycerite. Glycerin should be used only in low concentrations because it can be irritant. Propylene glycol is related to glycerin, and is used in lotions and ointments because it mixes with water (hydrophilic) and also dissolves in oils. Many other glycols are used to make water-soluble bases for ointments.

Protectives are applications used to cover the skin in order to protect it from contact with an irritating agent. They are insoluble and inactive, and cover the skin physically rather than having any chemical effect. They include *dusting powders*, which are used to protect the skin in certain areas (e.g. skin folds) and on the surfaces of ulcers and wounds. They are smooth and prevent friction, and some absorb moisture from the surface of the area to which they are applied. Those that do this help to decrease friction and prevent irritation (e.g. ones containing zinc oxide or starch). On open wounds they make a crust. Those that contain starch have to have an antiseptic added to stop the starch fermenting. Dusting powders often contain talc (which is mainly magnesium silicate), and of course talc is widely available as talcum powders.

Collodion forms a 'skin' and was used to close off small wounds, but it is now considered better to let the air get to a wound. Gauzes impregnated with petroleum jelly are useful as protective dressings to wounds although the tendency now is to use dry non-stick dressings.

Barrier creams are used to protect the skin against irritants that dissolve in water. They usually contain dimethicone (silicone) or a related silicone. These stick to the skin and repel water. They are available as ointments and sprays as well as creams. They provide protection against the irritating effects of soap, water, skin-cleansing agents and breakdown products from urine. They should not be used on inflamed or damaged skin or near the eyes because they may produce irritation. Barrier preparations may contain an astringent such as zinc oxide and/or an antiseptic such as cetrimide or cetylpyridinium. They may produce allergic skin reactions in some people.

Choice of protective

No one barrier preparation can be recommended over all the others, and they are probably no more effective than a simple cheap application such as zinc and castor oil ointment.

Corticosteroid skin applications

Corticosteroids (often referred to just as steroids) are discussed in detail in Chapter 62. The ones used to treat skin disorders have been selected because they have a dramatic effect in reducing inflammation and allergic reactions. When applied to the skin surface, corticosteroids are absorbed into the underlying tissues of the skin where they block the action of chemicals that cause inflammation. They relieve redness, soreness, swelling and irritation of the skin. However, they do not cure the disorder, but only suppress the reaction. Therefore, if the underlying skin disorder is not self-limiting or if the agent that caused the skin rash is not removed (e.g. contact dermatitis to make-up) the rash will flare up again when the corticosteroid preparation is stopped. It may even be worse than before – what is called a rebound effect. Sometimes abruptly stopping a corticosteroid preparation may produce a general reddening of the affected area of skin called 'rebound erythroderma'. This may be prevented by reducing gradually the strength and/or amount of the application applied over a period of several days.

Corticosteroid skin applications are used to treat disorders such as exzema, dermatitis and psoriasis. They are of no value in treating nettle rash (urticaria) or acne rosacea. They should not be used on damaged skin or ulcers. Lotions are useful for large areas, ointments for dry scaly areas and creams for acute weepy areas. Urea (see earlier, under 'Emollients') added to a corticosteroid preparation increases the effectiveness of the corticosteroid by improving the depth that it penetrates into the skin.

Harmful effects of corticosteroid skin applications

Prolonged use of a corticosteroid application may produce wasting of the deep layer of the skin. This wasting may occur especially on the face, flexures (bend of the knees and elbows) and on moist parts of the skin. It is particularly likely to occur when a corticosteroid is used under plastic dressings. The wasting produces a thinning of the skin with local flattened, depressed, stripy-looking areas that may take years to go away.

Corticosteroid skin applications may produce burning, itching, dryness and irritation at the site of application and irreversible 'stretch marks' (like those seen on the abdomen after pregnancy). Fine blood vessels under the surface of the skin may become prominent (telangiectasia) and may easily be damaged, resulting in 'bruising' under the skin.

Increased growth of hair on the skin, acne, white patches due to mild transient loss of pigment (which shows up on dark-coloured skin) and sometimes a dermatitis around the mouth in young women may also occur following the regular use of corticosteroid skin applications.

Warnings on the use of corticosteroid skin applications

Because corticosteroids reduce the body's response to infection and reduce inflammation an infection of the skin may spread without the normal warning signs such as redness, swelling and pain. This risk is very evident when corticosteroids are applied to the skin under a plastic dressing. Whilst such dressings appear to increase the effectiveness of the corticosteroid, they may also be associated with boils and thrush infections and may allow infections of the skin to spread. Corticosteroids may delay the healing of ulcers (particularly leg ulcers).

Harmful effects on the skin may appear within 1–2 weeks of starting treatment. Strong preparations should be used only at the start of treatment and then switched to mild preparations after a week or two. A corticosteroid application may cause an allergic skin rash, and this should always be considered if a rash does not respond to treatment or appears to get worse.

A proportion of corticosteroid drug applied to the skin may enter the blood circulation and produce general harmful effects. This is particularly likely to happen in babies, infants and children (who may also lick the ointment off the skin) and in adults who regularly use large amounts of a strong preparation over large areas of skin. Absorption is greatest from raw surfaces and is increased by occlusive dressings (see above).

NOTE napkins and plastic pants can act like an occlusive dressing. The skin of the face, genitals and skin folds absorbs more corticosteroid than do other areas.

Combining a corticosteroid with anti-infective drugs

Some skin disorders may get infected and become soggy with pus (e.g. infected eczema). In these infected skin disorders an application containing a corticosteroid and an anti-infective drug (e.g. an antibiotic) may be effective. Such a combination is also useful on skin rashes in areas where infection is likely to occur; for example, in the groins or around the anus. However, do not forget that there is a slight risk that an anti-infective drug may produce an allergic reaction that the corticosteroid may mask. Remember this point if a skin rash seems to be getting worse despite the fact that initially it improved with such a preparation.

Dangers of using corticosteroids on infected skin

The wrong use of corticosteroid skin applications or corticosteroids combined with an anti-infective drug in infective skin disorders may produce severe harmful effects. For example, if used to treat impetigo (a bacterial infection of the skin), a small localized patch may be turned into a serious widespread skin infection; a simple fungus infection (e.g. athlete's foot) may spread over a large area; and herpes simplex (cold sores) may spread to produce nasty redness, sores and ulcers over the face.

Hydrocortisone preparations that can be purchased from a pharmacist

Preparations of hydrocortisone that can be purchased from a pharmacist without a doctor's prescription must include concentrations of hydrocortisone of 1 per cent or less. They must not be sold for use in children under 10 years of age or in pregnancy without medical advice.

They must only be sold by the pharmacist to treat irritant dermatitis, contact allergic dermatitis or insect bites. They should *not* be used on the eyes, face, anus, genitals, broken skin, cold sores, acne or athlete's foot.

Available preparations include:

Hc 45 cream (hydrocortisone 1.0%)
Lanacort cream and ointment (hydrocortisone 1.0%)
Zenoxone cream (hydrocortisone 1.0%)

Table 75.1 Corticosteroid skin preparations

Preparation	*Drug*	*Dosage form*	*Strength*
Adcortyl	triamcinolone	Cream, ointment	0.1%
Betnovate	betamethasone	Cream, ointment, lotion, scalp application	0.1%
Betnovate RD	betamethasone	Cream, ointment	0.025%
Dermovate	clobetasol	Cream, ointment, scalp application	0.05%
Dioderm	hydrocortisone	Cream	0.1%
Diprosone	betamethasone	Cream, ointment, lotion (Diprosone Duopack: Diprosone cream plus Diprobase emollient)	0.05%
Efcortelan	hydrocortisone	Cream, ointment	0.5%, 1.0%, 2.5%
Eumovate	clobetasone	Cream, ointment	0.05%
Haelan	flurandrenolone	Cream, ointment	0.0125%
Haelan Tape	flurandrenalone	Adhesive film	4 micrograms/cm²
Halciderm	halcinonide	Cream	0.1%
hydrocortisone	hydrocortisone	Cream	0.5%, 1.0%, 2.5%
		Ointment	0.5%, 1.0%
		Lotion	1.0%
Hydrocortistab	hydrocortisone	Cream, ointment	1.0%
Hydrocortisyl	hydrocortisone	Cream, ointment	1.0%
Ledercort	triamcinolone	Cream, ointment	0.1%
Locoid	hydrocortisone-17-butyrate	Cream, lipocream, ointment, scalp lotion	0.1%
Metosyn	fluocinonide	Cream, ointment, scalp lotion	0.05%
Mildison Lipocream	hydrocortisone, 70% oil base	Cream	1.0%
Modrasone	alclometasone	Cream, ointment	0.05%
Nerisone	diflucortolone	Cream, oily cream, ointment	0.1%
Nerisone Forte	diflucortolone	Oily cream, ointment	0.3%
Preferid	budesonide	Cream, ointment	0.025%
Propaderm	beclomethasone	Cream, ointment	0.025%
Stiedex	desoxymethasone	Oily cream	0.25%
Stiedex LP	desoxymethasone	Oily cream	0.05%
Synalar	fluocinolone	Cream, ointment	0.025%

Table 75.1 Corticosteroid skin preparations (*cont.*)

Preparation	*Drug*	*Dosage form*	*Strength*
Synalar 1 in 4 Dilution	fluocinolone	Cream, ointment	0.00625%
Synalar 1 in 10 Dilution	fluocinolone	Cream	0.0025%
Synalar Gel	fluocinolone	Gel	0.025%
Topilar	fluclorolone	Cream, ointment	0.025%
Ultradil	fluocortolone	Cream, ointment	0.1%
Ultralanum Plain	fluocortolone	Cream, ointment	0.25% (pivolate) and 0.25% (hexanoate)

Differences in potency between corticosteroids

Some corticosteroids are more powerful than others and you should bear this in mind.

Mildly powerful corticosteroids include:

alclometasone
*fluocinolone
hydrocortisone (but note that hydrocortisone butyrate is a very powerful form of hydrocortisone and preparations containing urea become moderately powerful because it increases the penetration of the hydrocortisone into the skin)
methylprednisolone

Moderately powerful corticosteroids include:

clobetasone
desoxymethasone
*fluocinolone
fluocortolone
flurandrenolone

Powerful corticosteroids include:

beclomethasone
betamethasone
budesonide
*desoxymethasone
*diflucortolone
fluclorolone
fluocinolone
fluocinonide
hydrocortisone-17-butyrate
triamcinolone

* NOTE that the strength of the application is also important. The higher the concentration, the more powerful the preparation.

Very powerful corticosteroids include:

clobetasol
*diflucortolone
halcinonide

Table 75.2 Combined corticosteroid skin preparations

Preparation	*Drug*	*Dosage form*
Alphaderm	hydrocortisone (1%) urea	Cream
Alphosyl HC	hydrocortisone (0.5%), coal tar, allantoin	Cream
Calmurid HC	hydrocortisone (1%), urea, lactic acid	Cream
Carbo-Cort	hydrocortisone (0.25%), coal tar solution	Cream
Cobadex	hydrocortisone (0.5%, 1%), dimethicone	Cream
Diprosalic	betamethasone (0.05%), salicylic acid	Ointment, scalp lotion (in alcoholic solution)
Epifoam	hydrocortisone (1%), pramoxine (local anaesthetic)	Foam in aerosol
Eurax-Hydrocortisone	hydrocortisone (0.25%), crotamiton	Cream
Hydrocal	hydrocortisone (1.0%), calamine	Cream
Sential	hydrocortisone (0.5%), urea, sodium chloride	Cream
Stiedex Lotion	desoxymethasone (0.25%), salicylic acid	Lotion
Tarcortin	hydrocortisone (0.5%), coal tar extract	Cream

Allergic reactions to corticosteroid preparations

Some corticosteroid skin applications may contain additives which may cause allergic reactions; for example, butylated hydroxyanisole, chlorocresol, ethylenediamine, fragrances, lanolin, parabens, propylene glycol and sorbic acid. If your rash gets worse (e.g. more red) after applying a corticosteroid preparation, check its additive contents with your pharmacist or doctor – you may have to change to another preparation.

Table 75.3 Combined corticosteroid and anti-infective skin preparations

Preparation	*Drug*	*Drug group*	*Dosage form*
Adcortyl with Graneodin	triamcinolone (0.1%)	Corticosteroid	Cream, ointment
	neomycin	Anti-bacterial	
	gramicidin	Anti-bacterial	
Aureocort	triamcinolone (0.1%)	Corticosteroid	Cream, ointment
	chlortetracycline	Anti-bacterial	
Barquinol HC	hydrocortisone (0.5%)	Corticosteroid	Cream
	clioquinol	Antiseptic	
Betnovate-C	betamethasone (0.1%)	Corticosteroid	Cream, ointment
	clioquinol	Antiseptic	
Betnovate-N	betamethasone (0.1%)	Corticosteroid	Cream, ointment
	neomycin	Anti-bacterial	
Canesten-HC	hydrocortisone (1%)	Corticosteroid	Cream
	clotrimazole	Anti-fungal	
Daktacort	hydrocortisone (1%)	Corticosteroid	Cream, ointment
	miconazole	Anti-fungal	
Dermovate-NN	clobetasol (0.05%)	Corticosteroid	Cream, ointment
	neomycin	Anti-bacterial	
	nystatin	Anti-fungal	
Econacort	hydrocortisone (1%)	Corticosteroid	Cream
	econazole	Anti-fungal	
Framycort	hydrocortisone (0.5%)	Corticosteroid	Ointment
	framycetin	Anti-bacterial	
Fucibet	betamethasone (0.1%)	Corticosteroid	Cream
	fusidic acid	Anti-bacterial	
Fucidin H	hydrocortisone (1%)	Corticosteroid	Ointment, cream, gel
	sodium fusidate	Anti-bacterial	
Genticin HC	hydrocortisone (1%)	Corticosteroid	Cream, ointment
	gentamicin	Anti-bacterial	
Gregoderm	hydrocortisone (1%)	Corticosteroid	Ointment
	neomycin	Anti-bacterial	
	nystatin	Anti-fungal	
	polymixin B	Anti-bacterial	
Haelan-C	flurandrenolone (0.0125%)	Corticosteroid	Cream, ointment
	clioquinol	Antiseptic	

Table 75.3 Combined corticosteroid and anti-infective skin preparations (*cont.*)

Preparation	*Drug*	*Drug group*	*Dosage form*
Locoid C	hydrocortisone (0.1%)	Corticosteroid	Cream, ointment
	chlorquinaldol	Antiseptic	
Lotriderm	betamethasone (0.05%)	Corticosteroid	Cream
	clotrimazole	Anti-fungal	
Neo-Medrone	methylprednisolone (0.25%)	Corticosteroid	Cream
	neomycin	Anti-bacterial	
Nystadermal	triamcinolone (0.1%)	Corticosteroid	Cream
	nystatin	Anti-fungal	
Nystaform-HC	hydrocortisone (0.5%)	Corticosteroid	Cream, ointment (hydrocortisone 1%)
	chlorhexidine	Antiseptic	
	nystatin	Anti-fungal	
Pevaryl TC	triamcinolone (0.1%)	Corticosteroid	Cream
	econazole	Anti-fungal	
Propaderm-A	beclomethasone (0.025%)	Corticosteroid	Ointment
	chlortetracycline	Anti-bacterial	
Quinocort	hydrocortisone (1%)	Corticosteroid	Cream
	hydroxyquinoline	Antiseptic	
Stiedex LPN	desoxymethasone (0.05%)	Corticosteroid	Oily cream
	neomycin	Anti-bacterial	
Synalar C	fluocinolone (0.025%)	Corticosteroid	Cream, ointment
	clioquinol	Antiseptic	
Synalar N	fluocinolone (0.025%)	Corticosteroid	Cream, ointment
	neomycin	Anti-bacterial	
Terra-Cortril	hydrocortisone (1%)	Corticosteroid	Ointment, spray (hydrocortisone 0.17%)
	oxytetracycline	Anti-bacterial	
Terra-Cortril Nystatin	hydrocortisone (1%)	Corticosteroid	Cream
	oxytetracycline	Anti-bacterial	
	nystatin	Anti-fungal	
Timodine	hydrocortisone (0.5%)	Corticosteroid	Cream
	benzalkonium	Antiseptic	
	nystatin	Anti-fungal	
	dimethicone	barrier	

Table 75.3 Combined corticosteroid and anti-infective skin preparations (*cont.*)

Preparation	*Drug*	*Drug group*	*Dosage form*
Tri-Adcortyl	triamcinolone (0.1%)	Corticosteroid	Cream, ointment
	neomycin	Anti-bacterial	
	nystatin	Anti-fungal	
	gramicidin	Anti-bacterial	
Tri-Cicatrin	hydrocortisone (1%)	Corticosteroid	Ointment
	neomycin	Anti-bacterial	
	bacitracin	Anti-bacterial	
	nystatin	Anti-fungal	
Trimovate	clobetasone (0.05%)	Corticosteroid	Cream, ointment
	oxytetracycline	Anti-bacterial	
	nystatin	Anti-fungal	
Vioform-Hydrocortisone	hydrocortisone (1%)	Corticosteroid	Cream, ointment
	clioquinol	Antiseptic	

Local anaesthetic skin applications

Skin applications containing a local anaesthetic should seldom be used. This is because they may irritate the skin and produce allergic skin rashes, particularly if they are applied to large areas of the skin or if they are used regularly. Preparations usually include amylocaine, benzocaine, cinchocaine, lignocaine or prilocaine. See Chapter 28.

Drugs that destroy or dissolve tissue

Caustics are chemicals that destroy tissue by corrosion or burning. Some commonly used caustics include acetic acid, phenol, podophyllum, trichloroacetic acid, silver nitrate and potassium hydroxide. They are used to treat warts and corns. Silver nitrate solution should no longer be used because it may be absorbed from open wounds, to produce vomiting, diarrhoea and convulsions. Long-term use may cause silver to be deposited in the skin, producing a slate-blue colour. It may also be deposited in the eyes and teeth. This condition is known as *argyria.*

An eschar is the dry scab that forms when an area of skin has been burned, this is why caustics are sometimes referred to as *escharotics*.

Cauterization is local burning of tissue by the application of heat; for example, electric cautery used by surgeons to close off the ends of small blood vessels to stop them bleeding.

Table 75.4 Anti-bacterial skin preparations

Preparation	*Drug*	*Dosage form*
Achromycin	tetracycline	Ointment
Anaflex	polynoxylin (anti-bacterial/ anti-fungal)	Cream, paste, dusting powder, aerosol spray
Aureomycin	chlortetracycline	Cream, ointment
Bactroban	mupirocin	Ointment
Cidomycin	gentamicin	Cream, ointment
Colomycin	colistin	Sterile powder; for making into topical preparations, usually solution, powder or ointment
Flamazine	silver sulphadiazine	Cream
Framygen	framycetin	Cream
Fucidin	fusidic acid	Cream, gel, ointment, Caviject gel in single-dose applicator
Genticin	gentamicin	Cream, ointment
neomycin	neomycin	Cream, ointment
Sofra-Tulle	framycetin	Impregnated dressing
Ster-Zac Bath Concentrate	triclosan	Solution
Combination products		
Cicatrin	neomycin, bacitracin zinc	Cream, dusting powder, powder spray (Cicatrin Aerosol)
Graneodin	neomycin, gramicidin	Ointment
Polybactrin	neomycin, polymyxin B, bacitracin zinc	Powder in aerosol
Polyfax	polymyxin B, bacitracin zinc	Ointment
Soframycin	framycetin, gramicidin	Cream, ointment
Tribiotic	neomycin, bacitracin zinc, polymyxin B	Spray application (aerosol)

A *keratolytic* is a drug that 'dissolves' keratin, the protein in the cells of the hard outer layer of the skin (the epidermis). It loosens the cells and causes them to swell and go soft so that they can be cut off easily. Keratolytics are used to treat warts and corns. The most commonly used are benzoic acid, salicylic acid, acetic acid and resorcinol. Benzoic, salicylic and malic acids are ingredients of Aserbine solution, which is used to clean the slough off ulcers and wounds.

Astringent (drying) skin applications

Astringents are drugs that dry up the skin and can cause it to tighten up. They 'damage' the walls of cells in the surface layer of the skin (the epidermis). This makes water less able to pass into the cells and causes them to dry up and shrink. They are included in many skin applications. They harden the skin, dry up soggy areas of skin and can stop bleeding from minor abrasions.

Astringents in various dilutions are used for all manner of disorders – in throat lozenges, mouth washes, eye drops, ear drops and to shrink piles. In higher concentrations they are used as caustics (see earlier). The greatest use of astringents is in anti-perspirant sprays and applications (see later). The main ones are salts of aluminium.

Infections of the skin

The skin acts as a first line of defence against infection but it can become infected itself if it is damaged through injury, insect bites or because of inflammation caused by some skin condition such as eczema. It may be infected by bacteria, fungi or viruses. To treat these infections we use anti-bacterial, anti-fungal and anti-viral drugs. The skin may also become infected with parasites, and the treatment of these disorders is discussed in Chapter 59.

Anti-bacterial skin applications

Bacterial infections of the skin are usually referred to as *pyodermas* because pus is usually present. They may be primary, occurring in the absence of any skin disorder, or they may be secondary, occurring in the presence of some underlying skin disorder such as eczema.

There is an increased risk of infection if the natural protective barrier of the skin is harmed due to excessive exposure to water, excessive sweating or bathing, or damage to the skin from sunburn or using detergents.

Bacterial infections of the skin can usually be prevented by cleansing the area of damaged skin and, if necessary, applying an antiseptic preparation. When an infection has developed causing redness, swelling and pus formation, it may be necessary to use an antibiotic or other anti-bacterial preparation.

Anti-bacterial skin applications should *not* be used to treat skin conditions where there is no bacterial infection (e.g. weeping eczema), to treat fungal infections which may be mistaken for bacterial infections (e.g.

ringworm) or to treat virus infections (e.g. herpes) which are not sensitive to anti-bacterial drugs.

Anti-bacterial skin applications may be used *wrongly* to treat bacterial infections of the skin when an anti-bacterial drug by mouth would be more effective; for example, in treating an infection under the surface of skin (cellulitis). They may also be wrongly used to treat scabby skin conditions that would be better treated with a mild antiseptic (see later).

Harmful effects of antibiotics

Any skin application containing an antibiotic may irritate the skin and/or cause an allergic reaction. Irritation may be caused by the base of the preparation, and an allergic reaction producing redness and swelling may be caused by the antibiotic and/or by some additive in the preparation.

Reducing the risks

Antibiotics used in skin applications are usually the ones that are not used internally by mouth or injection. They are also the ones that are poorly absorbed through the skin and therefore they concentrate on the skin surface. Nevertheless, some of these drugs, if applied to large areas of the skin, may be absorbed into the bloodstream and cause harmful effects. For example, neomycin may be sufficiently absorbed into the bloodstream to cause damage to hearing, particularly in children and elderly people.

Anti-bacterial drugs that are used in skin applications but which are also used internally include chlortetracycline, fusidic acid, gentamicin and tetracycline.

An additional and serious hazard of any over-use of an anti-bacterial drug to treat skin disorders is the emergence of bacteria resistant to that drug. This problem is discussed in detail in Chapter 48.

Improving safety

If an anti-bacterial drug is necessary, then, like any other drug applied to the skin, the minimum amount of an application should be applied for the shortest length of time possible, and, if the disorder gets worse, treatment should be immediately stopped.

Resistant organisms are more common in hospitals because of the over-use of anti-bacterial drugs. Therefore, in hospitals, it is advisable to take a swab of any skin infection and send it to the laboratory for culture and tests for anti-bacterial sensitivity before treatment is started.

Table 75.5 Anti-fungal skin preparations

Preparation	*Drug*	*Dosage form*
Canesten	clotrimazole	Cream, solution, spray, dusting powder
Daktarin	miconazole	Cream, spray powder, dusting powder, twin pack (cream and dusting powder)
Ecostatin	econazole	Cream, lotion, spray, powder
Exelderm	sulconazole	Cream
Fungilin	amphotericin	Ointment
Nizoral	ketoconazole	Cream
Nystan	nystatin	Cream, ointment, gel
Pevaryl	econazole	Cream, lotion, spray powder (aerosol)
Pimafucin	natamycin	Cream
Trosyl	tioconazole	Nail solution
Combination products		
benzoic acid ointment, compound	benzoic acid, salicylic acid	Ointment
Monphytol	methyl undecenoate, propyl undecenoate, methyl salicylate, propyl salicylate, salicylic acid, chlorbutol	Paint
Multilind	nystatin, zinc oxide	Ointment
Mycota	zinc undecenoate, undecenoic acid. Spray: chlorphen and undecenoic acid	Cream, dusting powder, spray application in pressurized aerosol
Nystaform	nystatin, chlorhexidine	Cream, ointment
Phytex	tannic acid, boric acid, salicylic acid, methyl salicylate, acetic acid	Paint
Phytocil	phenoxypropanol, chlorophenoxyethanol, salicylic acid, menthol	Cream
Phytocil Powder	phenoxypropanol, chlorophenoxyethanol, zinc undecenoate	Dusting powder
Quinoped	benzoyl peroxide, potassium hydroxyquinoline sulphate	Cream
Timoped	tolnaftate, triclosan	Cream
Tinaderm-M	tolnaftate, nystatin	Cream
Tineafax	tolnaftate, zinc naphthenate	Ointment

Anti-fungal skin applications

Anti-fungal drugs have produced a dramatic improvement in the treatment of fungal skin disorders. Before the availability of very effective anti-fungal drugs the problem was always the lack of effective treatments; now the problem may be a lack of effective diagnoses.

Fungal infections of the skin may be misdiagnosed and mistreated; for example, the use of anti-bacterial and/or corticosteroid applications to treat an unrecognized fungal skin disorder may cause the fungus infection to become very much worse.

The diagnosis of a fungus infection is made more accurate by taking a scraping from the affected area of skin and examining it under the microscope. This will show the characteristic fungal threads (mycelia).

Anti-fungal drugs used in skin applications are listed in Table 75.5. For a discussion of the treatment of fungal and yeast infections, see Chapter 56.

Anti-viral skin applications

The use of anti-viral drugs to treat cold sores (herpes simplex), sexually transmitted genital herpes and shingles (herpes zoster) is discussed in Chapter 57.

Antihistamine skin applications

Antihistamines are discussed in detail in Chapter 10.

There are several skin applications available that contain an antihistamine but their use is very limited because they are not very effective and because they can actually cause allergic skin rashes. They may be of use for treating small areas such as an insect bite or a nettle rash but they are probably no more effective than just dabbing on calamine lotion or a simple cream. The regular use of an antihistamine preparation should be avoided; so should application to a large area of skin (e.g. for sunburn) because of the risk of producing an allergic rash. They should not be used in eczema. Diphenhydramine (in Caladryl cream and lotion) and promethazine may cause the skin to become sensitive to sunlight.

Antihistamine skin preparations include Anthical cream (mepyramine with zinc oxide), Anthisan cream (mepyramine), Caladryl cream and lotion (diphenhydramine with calamine and camphor), RBC cream (antazoline with calamine, camphor and cetrimide).

Antiseptics and disinfectants

An *antiseptic* is a chemical that prevents or limits infection in tissues by destroying or preventing the growth of micro-organisms. To be used as an antiseptic the chemical has to be sufficiently non-toxic to be applied to the skin or other surfaces of the body and yet toxic enough to kill infecting micro-organisms.

A *disinfectant* is a chemical that destroys micro-organisms (but not usually spores). The term is used to describe chemicals that are used to treat objects (e.g. for cleaning toilets, sterilizing surgical instruments) but it may also be used to describe chemicals used to treat the skin and other surfaces.

A *germicide* is a substance that destroys micro-organisms. The term is used by some manufacturers to describe antiseptics (e.g. germicidal soap, germicidal shampoo).

Some disinfectants are used as antiseptics in diluted strengths but often they are too irritant to use on the body. Some antiseptics are not strong enough to use as disinfectants.

Antiseptics and disinfectants belong to various groups of chemicals but their effects are the same – they kill and/or prevent the growth of micro-organisms. They include the following.

Alcohols (e.g. ethanol [ethyl alcohol] and isopropyl alcohol) are active against bacteria but not very active against fungi and viruses. In diluted forms they are useful for rapidly cleaning the skin but they should not be used on damaged skin. Repeated use may cause dryness and irritation. Methylated spirits in the form of surgical spirits may be used to clean the skin before an injection.

Caution should be used in applying alcohol preparations to the skin before surgery; patients have suffered severe burns when diathermy has been used following the cleaning of the skin with an alcohol.

Aldehydes are useful disinfectants but they are too irritant to use as antiseptics on the skin. They include formaldehyde (Emoform) and glutaraldehyde (ASEP, Cidex, Glutarol).

Detergents used as antiseptics include complex ammonia compounds such as benzalkonium, cetrimide, cetylpyridinium and domiphen. They are active against a wide range of bacteria and also against certain fungi and viruses. Their detergent action is useful for cleaning the skin and dirty wounds. They are made inactive by soaps, by proteins in pus and blood and by absorption on to cotton dressings and some plasters. Some people may become allergic to them after prolonged and repeated applications to the skin. Contact with the eyes should be avoided.

Chlorhexidine is active against many bacteria and some fungi and viruses. It is used as an antiseptic. It may, rarely, cause an allergic skin rash, and strong solutions may irritate the eyes. Chlorhexidine dental gel and mouth wash may discolour the tongue and teeth, and may initially cause stinging of the tongue and a transient loss of taste. Strong mouth washes may cause soreness of the mouth and occasionally swelling of the parotid salivary glands in the cheeks. Chlorhexidine is taken up by contact lenses and may cause irritation of the eye. It is made inactive by soaps and cork, and may cause a brown stain on fabrics if they are bleached with hypochlorite; a perborate bleach should be used instead. Its activity may also be reduced by pus and blood. Chlorhexidine gel should not be used with dentifrices.

Chlorine and chlorine-releasing chemicals are active against many bacteria, some bacterial spores and some viruses. They are used principally as disinfectants and to purify water. They include sodium hypochlorite (Chlorasol, Milton), chloramine, chlorinated lime (e.g. Dakin's solution), halazone and oxychlorosene.

Dyes are active against some bacteria, fungi and yeasts. There are two types of dyes used as antiseptics: acridine derivatives and brilliant dyes. *Acridine derivatives* include acriflavine, aminacrine and proflavine. They are slow acting and may occasionally cause allergic reactions. They have gone out of fashion. *Brilliant dyes* include brilliant green, crystal violet, magenta and malachite green. Except for crystal violet these are out of fashion. Crystal violet, although it has been associated with causing cancer in laboratory animals, is still sometimes used on intact skin to mark out the skin before surgery.

Mercurial compounds are active against bacteria and fungi. They include thiomersal, hydrargaphen, mercurochrome and nitromersol. Mercurial compounds are inactivated by pus and blood. The risks of using mercurial compounds as antiseptics generally outweigh their benefits and they have largely been replaced by safer antiseptics. Regular, long-term use of mercury compounds applied to the skin may cause nerve damage, kidney damage and dermatitis, stomach upsets, loose teeth and a blue line on the gums, and, rarely, allergic reactions.

Phenols and chlorinated phenols are active against bacteria and some are active against fungi. They include cresol, phenol, thymol, tar acids, chlorocresol, chloroxylenol, hexachlorophane and triclosan.

Cresol is used as a general disinfectant mixed with soap solution (Lysol).

Phenol (carbolic acid, TCP Liquid Antiseptic) is used as a disinfectant, and weak solutions are used as an antiseptic. It should not be applied to large wounds because sufficient may be absorbed to cause toxic effects on the brain and circulation. It is inactivated by pus and blood and other organic matter.

Thymol (compound thymol glycerin) is a more powerful disinfectant than phenol but it is easily inactivated by pus and blood and other organic matter, is not very soluble and irritates the skin. It is added in very small quantities to mouth-washes and gargles as a deodorant. Its harmful effects are similar to those produced by phenol.

Tar acids are phenol-like substances obtained from distillation of coal tar or petroleum fractions. They are used as disinfectants, but are too irritant to the skin to use as antiseptics.

Cholorocresol (Wright's Vaporizing Fluid) is a chlorinated phenol; it is a strong disinfectant that is more toxic than phenol.

Chloroxylenol (Dettol) is a chlorinated phenol. It is used as a disinfectant and is active against some bacteria (e.g. streptococci) but not against bacterial spores. It is also used as an antiseptic in diluted solutions. Its activity may be reduced by blood and pus and other organic matter, and, very rarely, it may cause an allergic reaction.

Hexachlorophane is a chlorinated phenol. It is active against some bacteria. It is used in low dilutions as an antiseptic mainly in soaps and creams. Ordinary soap and alcohol can rapidly reduce its antiseptic effects. Repeated use may sensitize the skin to sunlight and it may, rarely, cause allergic reactions. Newborn babies washed regularly with a hexachlorophane preparation (e.g. 3% emulsion) may, very rarely, absorb sufficient of the drug to cause harmful effects on the brain. The drug is absorbed through the skin and, in a pregnant mother, easily crosses into the baby. It is advisible, therefore, to restrict the use of this antiseptic in pregnancy, particularly during the first 3 months of pregnancy. It should not be applied internally (e.g. mouth, vagina, rectum) or to large areas of skin or under occlusive dressings. Its effectiveness is reduced by pus, blood and other organic matter.

Triclosan is a chlorinated phenol active against some bacteria. It is used as an antiseptic mainly in soaps, scrubs and deodorants. It may, rarely, cause a contact dermatitis.

Iodine preparations are used as disinfectants and antiseptics. Iodine is active against bacteria, fungi, spores, protozoa and viruses. Iodine preparations include cadexomer iodine, iodoform and povidone-iodine.

Cadexomer iodine is available as a powder of micro-beads containing iodine; the beads absorb fluid and release iodine. It may be used to treat infected leg ulcers and bed sores. It may cause redness and stinging, and some iodine may be absorbed, to cause harmful effects (see later).

Iodine insuflation, ointment, solution and paints may be used as antiseptics.

Iodoform (compound iodoform paint, in iodoform paste) slowly releases iodine when applied to the skin. It acts as a mild antiseptic.

Povidone-iodine is a complex of iodine with povidone, which is a polymer. It is used as an antiseptic principally to clean wounds and prepare the skin for surgery. Its activity is reduced by alkalis. It is soluble in water and alcohol. It is less irritant than iodine. Its application to large areas of raw skin or severe burns may result in the absorpton of sufficient iodine to cause toxic effects.

Harmful effects and warnings on the use of iodine compounds Iodine and iodine preparations applied to the skin may occasionally cause allergic reactions, which include nettle rash, patchy swellings of the skin, minute bleeding into the skin (purpura), fever, painful joints and swollen glands. Prolonged applications may cause iodism (see under treatment of underactive thyroid gland, Chapter 63).

Hydrogen peroxide is used as an antiseptic and deodorant. It releases oxygen and is used to clean wounds and ulcers. A solution of hydrogen peroxide is also useful for releasing dressings that are stuck to wounds. It is used as a mouth-wash and in ear drops for removing wax. Strong solutions may irritate and 'burn' the skin or mouth. Regular use of mouth-washes may affect the surface of the tongue.

Sunscreen and anti-sunburn skin applications

The beneficial effects of sunlight have long been recognized but it is only in the past 50 years that sunbathing in order to produce a tan has become fashionable; and it is only in more recent years that the harmful effects of too much sunlight on the skin have become well documented.

Ultraviolet radiation

Sunburn and suntan are caused by ultraviolet rays from the sun. This ultraviolet radiation is commonly referred to as ultraviolet light, but the light part of the radiation refers only to those rays that you can see. It should preferably be referred to as radiation. The spectrum of ultraviolet (UV) radiation is divided into three bands – UV-A, UV-B and UV-C.

UV-A (320–400 nm) is long-wave radiation that stimulates tanning but produces only mild redness. It is also the range in which most drugs that cause 'sunlight sensitivity' produce their harmful effects.

UV-B (290–320 nm) is the range that produces sunburn. It also causes tanning and vitamin D production. It is this range that is thought to produce cancer of the skin.

UV-C (200–290 nm) radiation from the sun does not reach the earth but artificial ultraviolet sources emit it. It does not cause tanning but causes redness.

Dangers of sunlight

Excessive exposure to the sun's rays without appropriate protection is harmful; it causes burning and ageing of the skin, cancer of the skin (see later) and cataracts.

The skin of white people is more susceptible to damage by the sun's rays than the skin of black people. Over-exposure to the sun's rays in white people causes the skin to age prematurely and become dry, thin and wrinkled.

Sunburn and suntan

Sunburn and suntan are caused by ultraviolet rays (UVR). The shorter ultraviolet rays cause burning and the longer rays cause tanning (see above). Tanning provides protection against ultraviolet rays and it results from the migration of the brown skin pigment, melanin, from cells in the base layer of the skin up into cells in the surface of the skin. Protection against ultraviolet rays is provided by both the melanin content of the skin and the capacity of the skin to produce new melanin – in other words, the tanning capacity of the skin. Tanning provides some protection against sunburn but the main protection against being burnt comes from a thickening of the surface layer of the skin.

Warning *Sunburn and the long-term harmful effects of the sun's rays on the skin are directly related to the total dose of UVR received by the skin. This is determined by the intensity, duration and frequency of exposure to the sun's rays.*

Exposure to the sun and skin cancer

The most common cancer of the skin related to exposure to the sun is a cancer of the basal layer of the skin (a *basal cell* epithelioma). It affects white people and, very rarely, black and orientals. It starts as a small raised nodule on the skin of the nose or face. It has pearl-like edges and it may ulcerate and erode into underlying tissues, when it is sometimes called a *rodent ulcer*. It must be removed surgically.

Another skin cancer that occurs on areas of skin exposed to the sun is a *squamous cell carcinoma*. This arises from the surface cells of the skin that have been damaged by the sun's rays. It appears as a nodule with an inflamed and hard base. It must be removed surgically.

A *melanoma* is a cancer of the pigment-producing cells of the skin. They start like a mole but they are dangerous because they invade the surrounding skin and spread around the body. They account for two-thirds of deaths from skin cancer and they occur at a relatively early age (35–40 years). The incidence of melanoma is increasing, and there is a definite relationship to exposure to the sun's rays. People at risk of developing a melanoma are white and have fair complexions and light-coloured eyes, and sunburn easily.

The incidence of melanoma between the sexes is equal, but women tend to develop melanoma on the exposed parts of their bodies (e.g. the legs) more than men who have a higher incidence on the trunk. The incidence increases the nearer you get to the equator, and appears to be rising among people who take holidays in hot sunny climates, particularly among those with red or fair hair and blue eyes who freckle easily and sunburn easily and tan with difficulty.

Warning *If a mole bleeds or if there is any change in texture, colour or size, seek medical advice immediately.*

Sunscreen preparations

Sunscreen preparations have an important function in so far as they can protect the structure and function of the skin from damaging rays. They are chemicals in the form of clear or milky solutions, gels, creams or ointments that reduce (filter out) the harmful rays. They work by absorbing, reflecting or scattering these rays.

The selection of a sunscreen preparation should depend upon two main factors – your liability to sunburn and your ability to tan.

Sunscreens for application to the skin are either chemical sunscreens or physical sunscreens.

Chemical sunscreens contain one or more chemicals that absorb ultraviolet light and thus filter out the harmful rays. They are usually colourless and should obviously not irritate or stain the skin. Frequently used products include para-aminobenzoates such as para-aminobenzoic acid (PABA), benzophenones such as mexenone, cinnamates such as cinoxate; and salicylates such as homosalate.

Physical sunscreens or *sunshades* contain particles that reflect and scatter the harmful rays. They include powders of titanium dioxide, talc, zinc oxide, kaolin, calcium carbonate, magnesium oxide, ferric chloride and ichthammol. The powders have to be dusted on to the skin or applied in water- or oil-based creams or ointments. They are usually unacceptably messy but they may be essential for people who are ultra-sensitive to the sun's rays. Physical sunscreens tend to melt in the heat of the sun.

Preparations that increase tanning

In recent years preparations containing methoxypsoralen (bergaptene) or bergamot oil (which contains methoxypsoralen) have been heavily promoted. The application of these formulations actually stimulates tanning, which may provide improved protection, but they may produce 'sunlight sensitivity' rashes and over-pigmentation of the skin. They are advertised for use during sunbathing and as applications to be applied in advance of sunbathing – as pre-sun applications. Their association with an increased risk of skin cancer has not been proved.

Effectiveness of sunscreen preparations

Two factors are used to compare the effectiveness of sunscreen applications – MED (minimal erythema dose) and SPF (sun protective factor).

Minimal erythema dose

The minimal erythema dose (MED) is the least exposure dose of ultraviolet radiation (of specified wavelength) that will produce redness (erythema) of the skin through an application of a sunscreen preparation. It indicates the amount of radiation that is getting through to the skin and also the sensitivity of the skin (the ease with which it goes red). For example, two MEDs may produce redness whereas ten MEDs may produce sunburn with blisters. The MED for blacks is very much higher (over thirty times) than that for whites.

Sun protection factor

The sun protection factor (SPF) is a measure of the effectiveness of a sunscreen preparation against the sun's rays. It is the ratio of the least amount of the sun's rays required to produce redness of the skin through a sunscreen preparation to the amount required to produce redness without any sunscreen application. It is the MED for protected skin divided by the MED for unprotected skin. The higher the SPF, the more effective is the application at preventing sunburn. For example, an SPF of 4 should allow people to remain four times longer in the sun without burning than they would normally be able to, and one of 8 would allow them to stay eight times longer in the sun without burning, and so on.

*SPF categories of sunscreen products**	*SPF*
Minimal sun protection	2–4
Moderate sun protection	4–6
Extra sun protection	6–8
Maximal sun protection	8–15
Ultra-sun protection	15 and over

* Preparations should state protection against both UVB and UVA.

Factors that influence the SPF

Many factors can influence the effectiveness of a sunscreen preparation; for example, your skin type (whether you are fair or dark skinned, whether you burn easily or not), your age (children with 'new' skin burn more easily than adults with 'old' skin), whether you sweat a lot or not, and which area of the skin you expose to the sun (topless women bathers will realize that the skin on the breasts, which is not normally exposed to the sun, will burn more easily than the skin on the arms or legs which is usually exposed to the sun). The 'strength' of the sun's rays will affect the effectiveness of a sunscreen preparation (the sun's rays are much stronger in summer than winter) and also the weather (cloudy or not) and the amount of reflection of the sun's rays in the area where you are sunbathing. The source of radiation will have an effect (e.g. the sun or a lamp) and the age and type of the artificial UV radiation you use will have an effect.

The concentration of a sunscreen application, the base (vehicle) used in the preparation, the thickness of the application, the effects of water on the application (e.g. after swimming), and the effects of temperature, humidity, wind and sweating on the application will all have an effect. In addition, the testing procedure is very important because the effectiveness of a sunscreen preparation out of doors may not be related to its performance indoors under laboratory conditions.

Categories of sunscreen preparations

Sunscreen preparations can be divided into three categories:

1. Sunscreen preparations that keep out about 95 per cent of burning rays – these may be called *anti-sunburn* preparations.
2. Sunscreen preparations that let through some of the tanning rays but keep out at least 85 per cent of burning rays – these may be called *suntan* preparations. You go red with these preparations but you do not burn. You will also tan.
3. Sunscreen preparations that block out all ultraviolet radiation. These reduce the risk of sunburn and tanning to a minimum – they may be called *sun blockers*. They are very visible and no transparent preparation is available. A good example is zinc oxide, which is often applied to the nose and ears by lifeguards.

NOTE Most sunscreen preparations on the market contain a mixture of the first two but remember that it is only the concentration of the active agent that makes the difference. Differing effectiveness may be achieved by the amount that you apply at any one time and the frequency with which you apply the preparation.

Some active agents may actually make the skin sensitive to the sun's rays by causing an allergic reaction (allergic photodermatitis); for example, aminobenzoic acid (see later) and padimate A.

Suntan products

'Suntan' products differ from 'anti-sunburn' products because they contain lower concentrations of sunscreen drugs; they therefore let more rays through. Some (e.g. aminobenzoic acid) may block off the burning rays but let tanning rays through. However, it is important to remember that suntan products do not 'promote' a tan, they help you to stop getting burned, and because of this you may be able to stay longer in the sun.

Warnings *Some suntan products do* **not** *contain sunscreen agents. They usually contain oils (e.g. cocoa butter oil). Some contain substances that stain the skin brown but which offer no protection; for example, iodine and tannic acid (responsible for the brown colour of tea).*

Tanning without the sun

Applications that are supposed to tan you without you having to sunbathe contain dyes such as dihydroxyacetone (DHA). This reacts with protein in the skin to make a yellow–brown colour. It stains the palms of the hands, can be washed off and fades off in several weeks. It offers *no* protection against the rays of the sun.

A preparation that contains the dye dihydroxyacetone (DHA) combined with another dye, lawsone, has some sunscreening effects. Lawsone is obtained from the dried leaves of henna, which is used for dyeing the hair.

Tanning preparations that can be taken by mouth

These contain substances such as canthaxanthin and/or beta-carotene.

Canthaxanthin is a synthetic dye used in the food and pharmaceutical industries to colour foods and medicines orangey-brown. This dye, when taken by mouth, enters the fat cells in the skin and dyes them orangey-brown. It dyes the skin everywhere, including palms of the hands and soles of the feet. Because of the different thickness of skin between people it produces different effects in different people. It also colours the motions brick-red.

Beta-carotene is a precursor of vitamin A and is responsible for the yellow–orange colour of certain fruits and vegetables (e.g. carrots). It is used as a dye in the food industry. When taken by mouth the dye colours the fat in the skin and produces similar effects to canthaxanthin (see above).

Warning *The doses of canthaxanthin and beta-carotene used to dye the skin are far in excess of the doses allowed as colouring agents in the food and pharmaceutical industries, and the medium- and long-term dangers of such doses are not known.*

Selecting a sunscreen preparation

Use a preparation made by a reputable firm but note that the most expensive preparations are not necessarily the best. Go by your history of how easily you burn and how easily you tan, and choose a preparation with an appropriate SPF. For example, if you are fair skinned and burn easily, start with a preparation with an SPF of 10 or more; if you are dark skinned, tan easily and rarely burn, start with an SPF of 6. As the skin tans you may need a preparation with a lower SPF. If you are sensitive to the sun's rays, have cancer of the skin or ageing of the skin, use a prepration with an SPF of 15 or more.

If you will sweat a lot or intend going in the water, be guided by additional points on whether the preparation is *sweat-resistant* (protects for up to 30 minutes of heavy continuous sweating), *water-resistant* (still protects you despite continuous exposure to water for up to 40 minutes) or *waterproof* (protects for up to 80 minutes in water).

Apply any sunscreen half an hour before going into the sun; if it contains aminobenzoic acid, apply it 2 hours before. Do not use any sunscreen preparation on children under the age of 6 months; keep them in the shade. In children aged 6 months to 2 years, always use an SPF of 4 or more.

The higher the SPF, the longer you can stay in the sun and the longer it will take for you to tan. You may need to use a preparation with a high SPF (8+) at the beginning of the summer and one with a lower SPF (e.g. 2–4) at the end of the summer.

Some sunscreen preparations may stain clothing, pucker vinyl fabric and stain fibreglass. Many people use too much or too little – apply equivalent to half a teaspoonful on neck and face, half a teaspoonful to each arm and shoulder, half a teaspoonful to the front of the body and half a teaspoonful to the back, and half a teaspoonful on each leg and foot. Apply after swimming or excessive sweating and about every 2 hours while in the sun.

If you get cold sores, *always* protect your lips with a preparation of SPF 15 or more.

Suntan preparations that dye the skin offer *no* protection against burning.

Use a sunscreen preparation that protects both against UV-A *and* against UV-B – read the instructions on the label very carefully before buying a preparation.

Avoid direct exposure between 10 a.m. and 2 p.m. (particularly at the beginning of the season). The nearer the equator you are, the greater the risk, even if the sky is cloudy.

Protect against reflection – wear sunglasses and a sunscreen on the face when skiing in the snow on a sunny day and wear a sunscreen on the face on a cloudy day. Remember that sand and water also reflect the burning rays of the sun and increase the risk of your getting sunburned.

Avoid contact with eyes and do not use a preparation if it irritates the skin or causes a rash.

Warning *When the body is covered in a sunscreen application the temperature control system of the skin may be affected and you may over-heat; therefore do not do hard physical exercise on a hot day when you are covered in a sunscreen preparation.*

Several chemicals in sunscreen preparations may cause contact dermatitis following application to the skin and some may make the skin allergic to the sun's rays. If you develop a rash, stop using that particular preparation.

People who develop a 'sunlight sensitivity' (see below) to sulphonamides, thiazide diuretics, the local anaesthetics procaine and benzocaine or to certain hair dyes may develop an allergic dermatitis to the sun's rays if they use sunscreen preparations that contain para-aminobenzoic acid (PABA) or its derivatives.

Sunscreen preparations form a physical barrier that protects the skin from harmful rays; they do not alter the skin or make it more resistant to the sun's rays. Therefore, sunscreen preparations should be applied frequently during exposure to the sun.

No sunscreen preparation completely protects the skin from harmful rays, so people who are fair skinned and burn easily should *never* expose themselves to the direct rays of the sun, even if they are using a sunscreen preparation.

People sensitive to the sun's rays

People suffering from sensitivity to the sun's rays often require a combination of two sunscreen preparations, the first application in an alcoholic solution which evaporates and then a second application of a cream on top.

The effectiveness of most drugs that can be taken by mouth for the protection of 'sunlight-sensitive' people has never been proven. The anti-malarial drugs (e.g. chloroquine) have been used for many years to provide protection but they are of limited use. There is no convincing evidence from adequate and well controlled studies of the effectiveness of beta-carotene (see earlier).

Drug-induced sensitivity to the sun's rays (photosensitivity)

In an individual who suffers from sensitivity to the sun's rays the skin is excessively sensitive to the sun's rays and goes red and burns very easily. Drugs are a common cause of sensitivity to the sun's rays. For example, tetracycline and sulphonamide anti-bacterial drugs, the anti-fungal drug griseofulvin, phenothiazine anti-psychotics, oral anti-diabetic drugs, thiazide diuretics, nalidixic acid used to treat urinary infections, oral contraceptive drugs, gold, diphenhydramine (an antihistamine) and, rarely, saccharin may cause sensitivity to the sun's rays.

Applications to the skin may also sensitize it to the sun's rays; for example, tar (the basis of tar and ultraviolet ray treatment for psoriasis) and hexachlorophane (an antiseptic present in numerous skin applications and toiletries). Various deodorants may also sensitize the skin to the sun's rays, and so too may sunscreen applications that contain aminobenzoic acid.

Warning *Remember if you burn more quickly than usual for you then always think – is it a drug I am taking or a skin application I am using? Check with your pharmacist whether it produces sensitivity to the sun's rays, and either stop the drug immediately or contact the doctor who prescribed the treatment.*

Sunlight allergy

Some people are actually allergic to the sun's rays and may develop severe dermatitis on exposed parts of their skin. Certain disorders may cause allergy to the sun's rays; for example, porphyria (a disorder of metabolism). If you develop a rash on the exposed parts of your skin, always seek medical advice (see page 1026).

Treatment of sunburn

The most common treatments for sunburn are calamine lotion and zinc lotion. Do not use applications containing an antihistamine because they may produce an allergic skin rash and usually in sunburn there is a fairly large area of skin to be treated. Corticosteroid skin applications (e.g. hydrocortisone) are very effective but should be used with caution.

Drug treatment of some common skin diseases

Acne

Acne is a general term used to describe inflammation of the oil-producing glands that surround hair roots. These glands – *sebaceous glands* – produce the skin's natural oil (or sebum) which acts as a water repellent.

Acne vulgaris (usually referred to just as acne) is the common form of acne, which usually starts at puberty. At this age, the sebaceous glands become active under the influence of male sex hormones (androgens), which are produced by the testes in males and by the adrenal glands in both males and females. The level of production of these hormones increases up to about the age of 25 years, after which it levels out. People who get acne do not have higher levels of male sex hormones than people who do not develop acne, and it may be that their sebaceous glands are more sensitive to stimulation by male sex hormone.

Acne (vulgaris) affects the sebaceous glands in the skin of the face, neck, middle of the chest and back. These are areas where the glands are most active. Although acne is related to the production of male hormones, it occurs only slightly more commonly in males than females. We do not know why some people get acne and others do not nor why some just get mild acne and others get severe acne.

In acne, the outlets from sebaceous glands get blocked by skin cells and debris, and this forms what are called blackheads (or comedones). The glands then swell up and become infected and inflamed, to produce the red pimples (papules) and yellow pimples (pustules) of acne (zits). If the outlet is blocked completely the glands may swell right up to form a cyst; some individuals may get an overgrowth of scar tissue (called keloid) which produces irregular lumps and bumps in the affected area.

Some drugs may cause acne

Corticosteroid drugs may make the grease glands more sensitive and trigger acne in some people. Acne may also be caused by bromides, ethionamide, haloperidol, halothane, iodides, isoniazid, lithium, phenytoin, trimethadione and male sex hormones.

Because we do not know why some individuals get acne and others do not, there are all kinds of ideas about what causes it. There is no convincing evidence that factors in the diet – for example, chocolates, fats or sugars – aggravate acne.

Acne may get worse if you are tense and anxious, and of course it may get better if you are less tense about your condition because you think or hope that the treatment you are using will help to improve it. Acne may get worse just before a period and this may be due to fluid retention caused by female sex hormones. The fluid retention may cause swelling of the outlets from the glands, causing them to become blocked. Sweating may produce similar effects. Oral contraceptive preparations that contain a high concentration of oestrogen may make acne worse.

Contact of the skin with oil may cause acne to develop; for example, working with engineering oils or the regular application to the face of cosmetics that contain oils.

People who live in sunny climates suffer less from acne than people who live in cloudy climates. This is why sun-ray treatment has been used, but its beneficial effects are unpredictable.

Treatment of acne

There is no specific treatment for acne and it is often best to use what suits you or try different treatments, but do not be persuaded to use expensive preparations when the simplest and cheapest may be the best.

When deciding on the treatment of acne it helps to divide it into superficial acne and deep acne, according to its severity.

Superficial acne is characterized by comedones – which may be open (blackheads) or closed (whiteheads) – inflamed pimples (papules) and small superficial cysts and swellings containing pus (pustules). In *deep* acne papules and pus-filled cysts also develop deep in the skin.

Healing without scars is common in superficial acne but scarring often occurs in deep acne.

Superficial acne usually responds to topical application whereas deep acne usually requires drugs by mouth in addition to topical applications.

Skin applications

Cleansing preparations The important part of treatment of acne is to keep the skin free from grease by cleaning the skin regularly. The application of a hot, wet, face cloth to the face followed by washing with ordinary soap and water may be all that is needed. If this does not work, a detergent solution such as cetrimide should be used. The affected area should be washed with the solution twice daily, avoiding too much rubbing. Cosmetics and other applications that contain fats or oils should not be used. Also, oily hair dressings should be avoided and the hair should be shampooed regularly.

Drying and peeling preparations In addition to keeping the skin clean and free from excess grease, it may be necessary to apply preparations that dry and peel the skin and stop blackheads from forming. Products that contain sulphur or salicylic acid are used for this purpose. Preparations containing resorcinol should not be used because of the risk of absorption into the blood stream and its effects in knocking out the production of thyroid hormones by the thyroid gland.

The most frequently used chemical is benzoyl peroxide, which is present in many preparations. It not only dries and peels the skin, it also has antiseptic properties.

Vitamin A derivatives A vitamin A derivative called tretinoin (Retin-A), applied as a cream, gel or lotion, may be useful in some individuals with moderately severe acne but it may produce redness and peeling for several days. Too frequent use may cause dermatitis, so it may help to use the application once daily before going to bed and to use a benzoyl peroxide application in the mornings. Tretinoin should not be applied to the eyes, up the nose or on the creases of the mouth. The acne may appear to be worse at first, and it may take up to 4 weeks before any improvement occurs.

Abrasive preparations Abrasives may be used to help peeling and cleansing of the skin, and some individuals may occasionally find these of benefit. They include Brasivol and Ionax.

Anti-bacterial preparations A *tetracycline* antibiotic (e.g. Topicycline) applied to the skin may help to reduce bacterial infection in the sebaceous glands and may possibly produce some anti-inflammatory effects. A tetracycline antibiotic application may be worth trying in mild acne, but it may produce an allergic rash in susceptible individuals and it may cause bacteria on the skin to become resistant to tetracyclines. Other antibiotics included in acne applications include clindamycin (Dalacin T solution) and erythromycin (Stiemycin solution in Zineryt with zinc acetate).

For the use of anti-bacterial drugs by mouth, see later.

Antiseptic preparations Hydroxyquinoline kills bacteria and fungi, and is included in some acne preparations. It may produce irritation and redness.

Benzoyl peroxide, which is used as a peeling agent (see earlier), also has antiseptic properties. It is a popular constituent of acne applications. It may cause an initial stinging effect and, rarely, an allergic reaction. It may bleach hair and clothes.

Sulphur, which is used to produce peeling, also possesses some antiseptic effects.

Warning *Greasy creams or ointments and corticosteroid applications may make acne worse.*

Drugs taken by mouth to treat acne

Antibiotics Bacteria that normally live in the oil-producing (sebaceous) glands may produce irritant substances from the oil which cause inflammation. Antibiotics (e.g. tetracyclines) that dissolve in fat can kill these bacteria and help to reduce the inflammation. Therefore, if the acne is moderate or severe or does not respond to local applications, it is worth adding an anti-bacterial drug by mouth such as a tetracycline (e.g.

doxycycline, minocycline or oxytetracycline) or co-trimoxazole or erythromycin. The anti-bacterial drug must be taken daily; maximum improvement usually occurs within 3–4 months but sometimes treatment has to be continued for a longer period. This is powerful treatment and any benefit must be balanced against the risks of taking an anti-bacterial drug daily for such a long period of time.

Warnings *Tetracycline antibiotics should not be used in pregnancy, so women taking a tetracycline daily by mouth for the treatment of their acne should not be pregnant and should avoid getting pregnant while on treatment.*

Long-term use of antibiotics applied to the skin and/or taken by mouth may cause a superinfection of the skin around the nose and central part of the face, causing redness and pustules. Treatment of this superinfection is often difficult, and should be based on trying to identify the infecting micro-organism, testing its sensitivity to antibiotics and using the appropriate antibiotic.

Hormones Male sex hormones are associated with the development of acne, and female sex hormones (oestrogens) may therefore reduce some of their effects. Obviously oestrogens cannot be used in males, and, because of the risks of oestrogens (see page 891), they should not be used alone in females. A combination of an oestrogen with a progestogen reduces the risks, so a combined oral contraceptive may help acne in some women, but note that contraceptive pills with a high proportion of oestrogen may make acne worse.

Cyproterone is an anti-male sex hormone and, combined with an oestrogen (ethyniloestradiol), it may be beneficial in women who suffer from severe acne that has not responded to other treatments. The combination product is marketed under the name of Dianette. It also helps to reduce male-type hair growth (e.g. on the face) in women and can act as an oral contraceptive.

Isotretinoin This is a vitamin A derivative that is effective in some people with severe and nodular acne, and may prevent scarring. It reduces oil production and helps to unblock hair follicles, alters bacterial growth in the sebaceous glands and produces peeling of the superficial layer of the skin. It is best used in individuals who have failed to respond to antibiotics by mouth and/or who have severe deep acne.

It may produce serious harmful effects (see Table 75.6), so any possible benefits need to be weighed against the risks. It should be used only when other treatments have failed and only under specialist supervision.

Zinc There is no convincing evidence from adequate and well controlled studies that zinc sulphate by mouth has any beneficial effect.

Table 75.6 Drugs used by mouth to treat acne – harmful effects and warnings

Antibiotics

tetracyclines
See Chapter 51. Long-term use may, rarely, cause headache and visual disturbances.

erythromycin
See Chapter 53.

co-trimoxazole
See Chapter 54.

Hormones

Dianette
Contains cyproterone (an anti-androgen) and ethinyloestradiol (an oestrogen).

Harmful effects include nausea, vomiting, headaches, tension in the breasts, changes in body weight, changes in libido, mental depression and a pigmented rash on the face (chloasma).

Changes in periods include reduction in flow, missed periods (pregnancy must be excluded; see procedure under the pill, Chapter 67).

Bleeding between periods may be limited to 'spotting' or may be like a period (break-through bleeding). If persistent, a full medical examination should be carried out, including internal examination and a cervical smear.

Effect on the thyroid gland The amount of iodine bound to proteins in the blood increases and this may interfere with tests of thyroid function.

Effects on the blood chemistry Dianette may change the ratios of proteins in the blood and increase the level of copper, iron and alkaline phosphatase.

Warnings When Dianette is also used as a contraceptive, all the instructions that apply to the use of the combined contraceptive pill should be followed (see Chapter 67). Alternative mechanical contraceptive protection (e.g. a condom) should be used during the first 14 days of treatment. If a menstrual period has not begun by the end of the course, pregnancy must be excluded before continuing with the next month's course of treatment (see Chapter 67). Dianette should not be used in women with thrombosis or a history of thrombosis, sickle-cell anaemia, raised blood fat levels, acute or chronic liver disease, a history of itching and/or jaundice in pregnancy, breast cancer, cancer of the womb, undiagnosed vaginal bleeding, or in women with otosclerosis whose hearing deteriorated during pregnancy. For other warnings on the use of Dianette, see the combined contraceptive pill (Chapter 67).

Dianette should be stopped immediately:

- If you develop migraine and have never previously suffered from migraine
- If migraine attacks become more frequent and/or severe
- If unusual and/or severe headaches occur
- If you develop any disturbance of vision or a suspicion of a thrombosis
- If you develop jaundice
- Six weeks before a surgical operation and during the time confined to bed because of an illness or accident
- If you develop a moderate to severe rise in blood pressure
- If you become pregnant

All users should have a complete medical examination, including examination of the breasts, internal examination, blood pressure and cervical smear *before* starting treatment with Dianette. The drug should be used with caution in women with severe depression, varicose veins, diabetes, raised blood pressure, epilepsy, otosclerosis, multiple sclerosis, porphyria, heart disease, disease of the circulation, kidney disease, chloasma, fibroids or asthma, and in contact lens wearers. All these individuals should be carefully monitored, and if there are any signs of worsening of the diseases the drug should be stopped. The risk of chloasma (pigmentation on the face), which often does not clear up completely after the drug has been stopped, is reduced by avoiding excessive exposure to the sun's rays.

Risks in pregnancy Dianette should not be used in pregnancy or in anyone thinking of becoming pregnant.

Table 75.6 Drugs used by mouth to treat acne – harmful effects and warnings (*cont.*)

Risks in breast feeding It should not be used in breast-feeding mothers.

isotretinoin (Roaccutane)
Harmful effects include dryness of the skin with scaling, thinning, redness (especially of the face) and itching; dryness of the nose with nose bleeds; dry eyes and conjunctivitis; opacities of the cornea; thinning of the hair; nausea, malaise, drowsiness and sweating. The skin may be easily damaged and blisters may occur. Raised blood pressure in the brain may occur when isotretinoin is used with antibiotics. It may cause hearing difficulties, mood changes, irregular periods, painful muscles, painful joints and reduced ability to do vigorous exercise, changes in liver function tests, and raised blood fat and glucose levels. Changes in the growing ends of bones may occur, causing premature stopping of bone growth.

Warnings Isotretinoin should be used only to treat severe acne or acne that is complicated by cysts and which has failed to improve on all other types of treatment. It should not be used in anyone with impaired kidney or liver function. Tests of liver function and blood fat levels should be carried out before treatment, after 1 month and then at regular intervals during treatment. Repeated courses of treatment are not recommended. Users should not donate blood either during treatment or for 1 month after stopping treatment.

Risks in pregnancy This drug causes abnormalities in unborn babies, so do not use it in pregnancy. In any woman of child-bearing age, pregnancy should be excluded before starting treatment; any woman on treatment must avoid sexual intercourse or practise contraception (but not the pill) for 1 month before treatment, during treatment and for at least 1 month after the drug is stopped.

Warning Pregnancy occurring during treatment or within 4 weeks of stopping treatment carries a serious risk that the baby will have been damaged.

Risks in breast feeding Do not use in breast-feeding mothers.

Acne rosacea

Acne rosacea is a chronic flushing of the forehead, nose, cheeks and chin, with red pimples (acne papules) and yellow pimples (acne pustules). It is more common in people with fair complexions and it usually comes on in middle age. More women than men suffer from acne rosacea, and it is usually made worse by sunlight. The nose may be affected and become enlarged (rhinophyma).

No cause is known, and treatment consists of trying to avoid those things that make the face flush – hot drinks (particularly tea), sitting in front of a hot fire, hot spicy food and alcohol. Regular daily use for a month or two of an antibiotic by mouth such as oxytetracycline may control the acne pimples in some people, particularly if it is combined with local treatments discussed earlier under the treatment of acne vulgaris.

Corticosteroid applications should not be used to treat acne rosacea because they make it worse and may cause a severe flare-up if treatment is stopped, which is then very difficult to treat.

Athlete's foot (tinea pedis)

See discussion on the treatment of fungal infections in Chapter 56.

Athlete's foot is ringworm of the feet. It is common among people who bath together (e.g. boys in boarding schools, miners). It affects the skin between the toes and is usually worse on one foot. The hands may be infected through scratching the feet. If the feet are often warm and moist the infection may spread over the foot. The skin becomes soft and soggy (macerated) and little blisters may develop. This may lead to a secondary infection with bacteria, resulting in blisters containing pus.

Treatment

Scrapings from the infected area should be examined under the microscope in order to confirm the diagnosis of a fungus infection before treatment is started. An effective treatment is a local application of an anti-fungal preparation; for example, clotrimazole (Canesten), sulconazole (Exelderm), miconazole (Daktarin) or econazole (Ecostatin) ointment. If one of these does not work and the infection is severe, griseofulvin tablets by mouth should be added to the treatment and taken for 6–8 weeks. Compound benzoic acid ointment (Whitfield's ointment) is fairly effective but messy, and other preparations are less effective. A combination containing an anti-fungal drug and a weak corticosteroid may be used in the first few days of treatment if the area is severely inflamed (see Table 75.3).

Baldness

Male-type baldness

One of the most common causes of hair loss is male-type baldness in which there is a characteristic loss of hair from the temples and crown. Initially, the loss of hair is replaced by fine downy hair but eventually this stops growing and the loss of hair becomes permanent. Some hormonal change may probably be one of the main causes of male-type baldness, and although it mostly affects men it may sometimes affect women – when it produces a diffuse thinning of the hair.

In recent years much publicity has been given to the use of the drug minoxidil to treat male-type baldness in men. Minoxidil is used to treat raised blood pressure, and one of its harmful effects when taken by mouth is to produce hair growth even in bald men. As a result of this observation a 2% application of minoxidil (Regaine) is marketed for the treatment of male-type baldness in both men and women. Minoxidil appears to act by increasing the blood supply to the skin of the scalp. It also increases the length of hair follicles and reduces the number of white blood cells around them.

Harmful effects of minoxidil applications include local itching, dermatitis, dryness of the skin and allergic reactions. Some of the active drug may be absorbed into the blood stream and cause low blood pressure and palpitations, chest pain, fluid retention (e.g. ankle swelling), shortness of breath, headache and dizziness. It should not be applied to broken skin.

During the first 4 months of treatment there is very little hair growth and it takes up to 12 months to see any benefit. If there is no real improvement after 12 months the treatment should be stopped. In general, fewer than half the men treated will develop a cosmetically acceptable growth of hair. Best results are obtained on a small patch of balding on the crown which has been present for only a few years. Only about one-third of women achieve a moderate regrowth, one-third minor regrowth and one-third no regrowth at all.

An important limitation of minoxidil applications is that if they are stopped, the growth of hair stops and the baldness becomes as extensive as if it had never been treated. The new growth of hair will be shed within 2–3 months of stopping treatment.

Comment The benefits of an acceptable growth of hair need balancing against the risks of having to apply the application regularly over many years and the lack of knowledge about any long-term harmful effects.

Alopecia areata

Alpoecia areata is a sudden loss of hair occurring in clear-cut round areas. It is not associated with any skin disease or general disease, and there is no scarring of the bald patch of skin. Any area of skin may be involved but most often the scalp and beard are affected. There are broken stumps of hairs at the edge of the bald patch if it is spreading but they are absent if it is not spreading. Rarely, this type of alopecia may affect the whole scalp or the whole body.

We do not know what causes alopecia areata and there is no cure. Therefore, do not waste your money on purchasing special preparations, attending hair clinics or seeing private specialists. Recovery is poor if the alopecia is extensive and/or begins in childhood. New patches of alopecia occurring in adults often clear up in 2–3 months but they may recur.

An injection of a corticosteroid such as triamcinolone directly into a small patch of alopecia may cause a tuft of hair to grow but this may soon fall out and there is little point in such treatment.

Other causes of alopecia without scarring of the skin include constant tension of the hair as produced by tight rollers or brushing the hair back and using tight grips. Also some mentally disturbed individuals may twist and pull their hair out in patches; this is referred to as trichotillomania.

Alopecia with scarring of the bald patch of skin may occur with infections of the scalp; for example, a bacterial infection such as a boil, a fungal infection such as ringworm or a virus infection such as shingles. The treatment is to treat the underlying infection. Some chronic skin conditions may cause alopecia with scarring; for example, lupus erythematosus. Burns, injury and radiation treatment may also cause scarring alopecia.

Temporary thinning of the hair

Loss of hairs from the scalp is natural because each hair goes through its own cycle of a very long period of growth (anagen phase), followed by a resting period (telogen phase) when it may fall out. Normally about 10 per cent of hairs are in a resting phase and therefore loss of hair is usually nothing to worry about.

Temporary thinning of the hair may follow a serious illness or childbirth, but it is *temporary* and there is no evidence that any specific treatment is of benefit.

Diffuse loss of hair may also occur in individuals suffering from disorders of the thyroid or pituitary glands, or from diabetes. Some drugs may cause loss of hair; for example, heparin, cyclosporin and anti-cancer drugs. Loss of hair may occur in some skin disorders of the scalp (e.g. eczema and psoriasis).

Although it is popularly believed that taking vitamins and minerals is beneficial in preventing or treating loss of hair, there is no convincing evidence of any relationship between diet and hair loss.

Bedsores (decubitus ulcer, pressure sores, trophic ulcer)

Bedsores are pressure sores that occur when an immobile patient has been left in the same position for too long. They occur on the bony points of the bottom, lower back, heels and elbows, and they can affect not only the skin but also deep tissues such as muscle and bone.

Loss of the feelings of pain and pressure and thinness of the fat and muscle between the skin and bones predispose to bedsores. Wasting, malnutrition, anaemia and infection increase the risks, as do paralysis and poor circulation. Pressure on an area of skin for more than a few hours in an immobilized person may block the local circulation sufficiently to cause its death. Infrequent turning of the individual, friction and irritation from wrinkled bedding and clothing will contribute to the damage, and moisture from sweating, urine and faeces will make the skin soft and fragile.

Once they have developed, bedsores are very difficult to treat, and the answer lies in trying to prevent them. This includes frequent turning (at least every 2 hours) and special mattresses. People in wheel-chairs should have pressure-relieving pillows and be able to shift their position every 15 minutes. Protective sheepskin or synthetic sheepskin pads should be placed under pressure areas, and padded rings used to surround bony points.

The skin should be inspected every day, *using adequate light*, in order to identify early signs of danger from pressure such as patches of redness and/or hardness of the underlying skin.

Cleanness and dryness help to protect the skin, and bed-clothing should be clean and unwrinkled. Over-sedation should be avoided and physiotherapy should be carried out when possible. The application of talc will reduce friction and absorb sweat, and an oily cream rubbed into the pressure areas at regular intervals will help to protect the skin, particularly in patients who are incontinent. Barrier creams that contain silicones are frequently used to protect the skin on pressure areas from getting too wet and irritated, although there is no evidence that they are any more effective than an oily cream such as zinc and castor oil cream.

As for treating pressure sores, you name it, it has been tried. This tells us that there is no specific treatment. If there were, we would all use it. The important part of treatment is to treat the whole person. In addition to appropriate general and specific treatments for the main disorders, the patient should receive a nutritious diet with added vitamins and minerals. Particular attention should be paid to diagnosing and treating any other underlying disorder that could hinder the healing of bedsores; for example, anaemia, diabetes or a urinary tract infection. The bedsores should be treated with applications that may help to heal them and at least not make them worse. Simple applications are often better than more heroic methods. There is no convincing evidence that zinc salts by mouth help to heal ulcers more quickly than any other treatments.

Any areas of skin that show early signs of damage should be left exposed, free from pressure and kept dry. Gentle massage will help to improve the circulation. Unfortunately, the size of apparant damage of the skin surface may not indicate the degree of damage to underlying tissues, which can be extensive.

Once the skin has broken down and ulcerated, treatment is difficult because the ulcer fills with pus and dead tissue. If this is cleaned out, it will help healing. This should be done by cutting out some of the debris and applying a preparation that helps to get rid of the slough (e.g. cadexomer, Iodosorb; see below) and cleansing using hydrogen peroxide (e.g. Hioxyl). Deep ulcers including muscle and bone will need surgical cleaning and skin grafting.

Preparations used to clean ulcers (U)

Cleaning the slough from ulcers and drying them up may help to relieve local infection and encourage healing. Available preparations include the following. No one preparation can be recommended over all the others.

Aserbine cream and solution contains desloughing agents – malic acid, benzoic acid, salicylic acid and propylene glycol.

Betadine ointment contains the antiseptic povidone-iodine.

Chlorasol solution, for cleansing ulcers, contains sodium hypochlorite.

Debrisan powder and paste absorb exudates; they contain a polymer, dextranomer.

Flamazine cream contains the anti-bacterial antiseptic silver sulphadiazine.

Hioxyl cream contains hydrogen peroxide, an antiseptic cleaner.

Iodosorb powder and ointment dry up exudate and act as an anti-bacterial antiseptic. Iodosorb contains a polymer cadexomer combined with iodine in micro-beads. The beads absorb the fluid to form a gel which releases the iodine.

Varidase powder contains protein-dissolving enzymes (streptokinase and streptodornase) that dissolve the slough and help to clean the ulcer.

Boils

A hair follicle is a minute tube in the skin containing a hair root. A *boil*, or a furuncle, is a localized infection of a hair follicle. The infection causes a hot, red, painful swelling with pus and dead tissue in its centre. A *carbuncle* is a cluster of boils with the infection spreading under the skin; it may be associated with fever and flu-like symptoms.

The important part of treatment of boils is to prevent the infection spreading; therefore *do not* squeeze a boil, apply a plaster, or damage the surrounding skin by applying a hot poultice. An antibiotic ointment (e.g. chlortetracycline) or an antiseptic solution such as chlorhexidine will help to stop the spread of infection if applied on and around the boil. If it is a large boil or carbuncle or if the boil is up the nose or on the centre of the face, it may be necessary also to take an antibiotic by mouth; for example, a penicillinase-resistant penicillin such as cloxacillin (see Chapter 49).

In people with recurrent boils anywhere on the body, their urine should be tested for sugar to make sure they do not have diabetes, and an anti-bacterial ointment should be applied up the nose every night for 2 weeks to knock out the source of infection, which is usually a staphylococcus that lives up the nose in 40–60 per cent of people and may infect the skin. Naseptin cream, which contains chlorhexidine (an antiseptic) and neomycin (an antibiotic), or Bactroban nasal ointment, which contains the antibiotic mupirocin, are effective for this purpose. Unfortunately, the bacteria may recolonize the nose once treatment has stopped.

Chilblains

Chilblains are caused by cooling of the hands and feet and/or the whole of the body in susceptible individuals. They affect mainly toes and fingers, and are caused by constriction of the small arteries in the fingers and toes on exposure to cold, followed by dilatation of the arteries that results in swelling of the skin with itching and burning.

The best treatment for chilblains is prevention – central heating, warm clothes and physical exercise.

In cold weather, protection against getting the hands and feet cold and wet is important; therefore, socks and gloves should be worn and kept as dry as possible. Insulated boots or shoes will be beneficial, and it is also important to keep the rest of the body warm because chilling of the body can affect the circulation in the hands and feet. Head covering is very important because body heat can be lost from the head.

Drugs used to improve the circulation should not be used, and any ointment that produces redness and burning because it irritates the skin or dilates the arteries may do more harm than good. High doses of calcium or vitamin D have not been shown to be of value. No drug treatment can be recommended, whether by mouth or applied locally to the chilblains. Try to prevent them, but if you develop chilblains just apply a simple greasy ointment (e.g. Vaseline petroleum jelly) to protect the skin.

Corns (callosities, calluses)

A *corn* is a painful pea-sizd swelling of the skin due to an over-growth of the surface cells caused by pressure and friction. They are found principally on the toes over bony areas. The term *callus* also refers to a small defined swelling of the skin due to an over-growth of the surface cells caused by pressure and friction, but they may occur on the hands and feet or any part of the body where there is localized pressure and friction.

Prevention is the best treatment for corns and calluses. Avoid localized pressure and friction on any part of the skin; for example, to prevent corns, wear soft, well fitting shoes.

Treatment of corns and calluses involves softening with a keratolytic such as salicylic acid and rubbing with a nail file or pumice stone and paring the lesion down with a razor blade.

Dandruff

Dandruff is the term that is usually applied to ordinary scaling of the skin of the scalp. It is not a disease; it is part of a normal process of shedding cells from the surface of the skin. However, cells shed from the body cannot be seen, whereas in the hair they can and therefore they are of cosmetic interest. People with dandruff seem to shed surface cells on their scalp more quickly than people without dandruff, and the cells that are shed clump together and are visible. We do not know why some people suffer more from dandruff than others. There is no evidence that it can spread from person to person and there is no convincing evidence that it is caused by a bacterial or fungus infection. Excessive dandruff may be associated with skin disorders such as eczema or psoriasis and with a condition called seborrhoeic dermatitis (or seborrhoeic eczema) – see later.

Treatment There is no cure for dandruff, only control. Any detergent shampoo is of use in treating ordinary dandruff. If used at least two or three times a week, a detergent shampoo will keep the hair clean of dandruff but of course a detergent shampoo will not prevent the production of scales by the scalp.

The scalp should be well massaged, the shampoo left in contact with the scalp for several minutes and then thoroughly washed off. Any shampoo left on the scalp may cause the dandruff to stick together and be even more visible.

Detergent antiseptics are sometimes used in shampoos (e.g. benzalkonium and cetrimide) although the antiseptic effects have never been shown to be beneficial over and above the detergent effects.

Drug additives in shampoos Shampoos that contain drugs to treat dandruff are often referred to as *medicated shampoos.* Certain drug additives are included in shampoos because they may reduce the production of cells from the skin of the scalp, dissolve the particles of dandruff or break them up into smaller pieces, relieve itching and/or act as an antiseptic.

Reducing the production of dandruff

Selenium sulphide (Selsun) and pyrithione zinc (Head and Shoulders) reduce the rate of growth of cells on the scalp and this may help to reduce dandruff formation. Because their effectiveness depends upon the time that they are in contact with the scalp, these shampoos should remain in contact with the scalp for a total of 4–6 minutes before being washed off. However, this length of time for contact with the scalp must be balanced against the fact that prolonged contact increases the risks of the individual developing harmful effects.

Selenium sulphide should be rinsed from the hair thoroughly; otherwise it may discolour it. Frequent use produces an odour and an oily scalp. It may 'burn' the skin under the finger nails and irritate the eyes. The hands and nails should be thoroughly washed after use. It should not be used within 48 hours of applying hair colouring or permanent wave preparations. Selenium sulphide is *dangerous if swallowed.*

Zinc pyrithione also kills bacteria and fungi, and, although it is insoluble and not absorbed through the skin, it should not be used on damaged skin. It may, rarely, cause contact dermatitis.

Breaking up dandruff particles

Preparations that break up and loosen dandruff particles contain keratolytics, which dissolve the cement that holds the cells together. They include sulphur, salicyclic acid and allantoin; they all rely on a reasonable amount of contact time with the skin and yet with shampoos the contact time is usually minimal. However, ointments and pastes are not acceptable because they are messy; therefore preparations in water or alcohol are used. They may be moderately effective in controlling dandruff but they can irritate the skin and the eyes. Resorcinol should not be used because it may be absorbed from broken skin and affect the thyroid gland.

Warning *Products that break up dandruff particles also act on keratin in the hair, which may damage the hair.*

Tar products

Tar products break up the dandruff but they smell and they may stain the skin and hair. They also make the skin sensitive to sunlight. They are useful for treating psoriasis of the scalp.

Anti-itching preparations

These include menthol, eucalyptol, phenol, resorcinol, pine tar and methylsalicylate. They may irritate the skin and eyes, and be harmful if they are swallowed. The temporary relief from itching which they may produce has no real part to play in the treatment of dandruff.

Warning *Corticosteroid applications (e.g. hydrocortisone) should not be used to treat itching associated with ordinary dandruff.*

Anti-infective preparations

The antiseptics cresol, thymol and phenol are included in some shampoos. They may irritate the scalp and are of very doubtful benefit because there appears to be no relationship between infection and dandruff.

Eczema and dermatitis

The terms dermatitis and eczema mean the same thing – a superficial non-infective inflammation of the skin which may be acute, moderately acute (sub-acute) or long lasting (chronic). When acute, the skin is red, swollen, blistered, weeping, crusted, scaling and often itching. Scratching and rubbing may cause bleeding and scarring. When it is chronic the skin may be dry, thickened, scaling, itching and scarred.

Skin specialists in the USA use the term dermatitis for all types of dermatitis. In the UK, however, they use the term eczema to describe dermatitis caused by a sensitivity to some factor from inside of the body (e.g. allergic dermatitis caused by food allergy), and the term *contact dermatitis* to describe dermatitis caused by contact with some factor outside of the body (e.g. dermatitis due to a cosmetic).

Atopic eczema (atopic dermatitis)

This is chronic eczema that usually occurs in individuals with a family history of allergic disorders (e.g. eczema, hayfever, asthma). *Atopy* means an inherited tendency to develop eczema, asthma and/or hayfever in response to certain substances taken into the body by mouth or breathed in. The cause is unknown but it is considered to be an abnormal allergic response.

Atopic eczema starts in infancy and usually clears in childhood but can continue into adolescence and adult life. Itching is a major problem, particularly in the night, and scratching can cause bleeding and scarring. It typically appears as redness and scarring in the folds of the arms and legs and on the eyelids, neck and wrists. Atopic eczema may become infected and cause further problems. Stress, high environmental temperatures, changes in humidity, certain types of clothing (e.g. wool), various ointments and creams, and certain foods may make atopic eczema worse.

Other eczemas

Nummular eczema appears as coin-shaped patches of eczema on the front of the arms and legs and trunk. Its cause is unknown. It occurs most commonly in middle-aged people under emotional stress. It is subject to flare-ups and quiet periods, and is worse if the skin is dry and in winter months. The coin-shaped patches start with itching followed by the development of minute blisters (vesicles) and small pimples (papules).

Lichen simplex (localized scratch dermatitis, neuro-dermatitis) is a chronic superficial patch of eczema in a localized area caused by rubbing and scratching. Women are affected more than men and it is probably psychological. The patches are well demarcated, scarred and often pigmented. A common site is on the back of the neck, but they may also occur on the legs, arms and ankles. The patches itch, which results in scratching and damage to the skin.

Varicose eczema (stress dermatitis) is a localized patch of eczema around the ankles which is associated with varicose veins. It is often red, scaly and may be discoloured brown.

Contact dermatitis

This is an acute or chronic inflammation of the skin, often in well demarcated patches, caused by substances in contact with the skin. It may be caused by a direct irritant (irritant dermatitis) or by an allergic reaction (allergic dermatitis).

Irritant and allergic contact dermatitis look very similar but an allergic reaction may be more red and there may be more small blisters (vesicles) and swelling of the skin.

Irritant contact dermatitis Contact with irritants may damage normal healthy skin and also cause an existing dermatitis to flare up.

Weak irritants such as soap and water may take several days of continuous contact to trigger dermatitis, whereas strong irritants such as acids, powerful detergents and phenol antiseptics may cause damage to the skin within minutes.

Allergic contact dermatitis is caused by a delayed allergic reaction to some substance. The skin first becomes sensitized by contact with the substance, which triggers a delayed allergic response. This may not appear for days, months or even years, despite the fact that the individual's skin may have been in direct contact with the substance daily (e.g. make-up or ointment for their eczema).

Substances that may cause allergic contact dermatitis include:

- Ingredients in creams, ointments, pastes, toiletries, etc. applied to the skin for the treatment of skin diseases (e.g. local anaesthetics, antibiotics, antiseptics) and additives in topical preparations such as preservatives, stabilizers, bases, fragrances
- Industrial solvent cleansers
- Flowers and plants (e.g. primrose, poison ivy and poison oak)
- Chemicals used in the manufacture of clothing, gloves, shoes
- Metal compounds, such as nickel (in rings, jewellery, watches and buttons), chrome and mercury
- Dyes used in clothing, hair dyes, etc.
- Cosmetics

Patch testing may be used to identify a substance that is suspected of causing allergic contact dermatitis. Strips of adhesive containing patches of substances that commonly cause allergy are available and they are placed on an area of skin for 48 hours. The optimum concentrations of most substances for patch testing have now been worked out; this is important because too strong a concentration may cause direct irritation and be mistaken for an allergic reaction, and too weak a concentration may produce no reaction. The results are compared with patch tests of inert substances (controls).

Preventing contact dermatitis If possible the offending substance should be identified and contact avoided; otherwise any treatment will be ineffective. People made sensitive to the sun's rays should avoid exposure to sunlight.

Treatment of acute eczema and acute dermatitis

If the lesions are acute and wet, wet soaks containing an astringent such as aluminium acetate may help. If there is a risk of infection, an antiseptic soak such as potassium permanganate may be beneficial.

To relieve the inflammation and itching, a powerful corticosteroid cream should be used for the first few days and then switched to a milder preparation. Only hydrocortisone cream should be used on the face because the others may cause harmful effects on the skin (see earlier).

If the condition is severe and extensive, it may be necessary to add a corticosteroid by mouth for a few days.

If infection is present a combined corticosteroid/antibiotic cream should be used (see Table 75.3). If the infection is severe it may be necessary to use an antibiotic by mouth after a swab has been taken to identify the infecting micro-organism and the appropriate antibiotic to use.

Treatment of dry, scaly eczema and dermatitis

Over a period of time the irritated skin becomes thick and scaly and itchy, resulting in much scratching. Dry, scaly patches are best treated with a soothing skin application (e.g. an emollient).

A mainstay of treatment, particularly in atopic eczema, is the use of a corticosteroid ointment.

When the skin is very thick and scaly, it may help to use a substance that peels the skin, such as salicylic acid, coal tar or ichthammol.

Salicylic acid helps to make the skin smooth but it may cause an allergic contact rash in some people; if applied to large areas of skin, it may be absorbed into the blood stream, to cause symptoms like those produced by an overdose of aspirin (salicylism).

Coal tar relieves itching and helps to make the skin smooth but is messy to apply and it smells. For arms and legs it is best applied as coal tar bandages, which also help to prevent individuals from scratching themselves. Coal tar baths may help if the eczema is extensive. Combining coal tar with hydrocortisone (a corticosteroid) may be beneficial in some individuals suffering from chronic eczema. There is no evidence that combining coal tar with zinc oxide or salicylic acid is any more beneficial than coal tar on its own.

Ichthammol is milder than coal tar and may be used in less severe cases. A useful treatment for skin creases (flexures) of the elbows and knees is to apply zinc paste and ichthammol bandages.

If itching and scratching are a problem, zinc oxide or calamine lotion may help, but generally it is best to cover the area with coal tar bandages (see above). If itching is severe at night, an antihistamine by mouth may help, particularly if it is one that produces drowsiness e.g. trimeprazine (Vallergan).

Some general principles for treating atopic eczema

Diet Avoid anything that appears to make the condition worse. The main culprits are cows' milk, eggs, cheese, fish, chicken and wheat. Food colourings and/or preservatives may also aggravate eczema.

Bathing helps to soothe the skin and relieve itching but the water should not be too hot. A soothing ointment should be applied to the skin first and it may help to add a moisturizer or oil to the bath water.

Drying It is important to dry the skin by gentle patting rather than rubbing, which may damage the skin.

Clothing Use cotton clothing next to the skin because wool may irritate and synthetic fibres may stop it from 'breathing', causing it to become hot and itchy. It may help to wear cotton mittens and cotton socks in bed at night.

Bedding Use cotton or poly-cotton pillow cases and sheets, and change them regularly because skin flakes and dried ointments may cause itching. Use pillows and mattresses with synthetic fillings, and use a plastic under-sheet covered by a cotton one. Do not use rubber under-sheets.

The house should be kept as clean as possible with regular vacuuming and dusting with a damp cloth. The temperature should not be too hot and the atmosphere should be kept moist.

Nails Keep finger nails clean and short, with no sharp points.

Breast feeding may protect babies with a family history of eczema, asthma, and/or hayfever from developing eczema and this should continue for at least 3–6 months. Supplementation with cows' milk should be avoided but weaning on to cereals, vegetables and fruit may be started at 3 months.

We do not fully know how beneficial it is for breast-feeding mothers to avoid foods known to make eczema worse – for example, eggs, cheese, cows' milk – but if they do, they will need to take extra calcium because these are calcium-rich foods.

Bottle-fed babies may be fed on soya feeds or pre-digested milk (e.g. Pregestimil) that has had the milk protein (casein) broken down, but we do not know about their long-term benefits.

Warning *Because a baby may become sensitized to food proteins within the first few months of its life, it is probably best to avoid cows' milk until after 12 months of age and not to use eggs until 2 years of age.*

Oil of evening primrose Evening primrose oil is discussed in Chapter 45. The active fatty acid (gamolenic acid) of evening primrose oil is available in capsules (Epogam) to treat atopic eczema. It may relieve symptoms and produce an improvement in some children. It may cause nausea, diarrhoea and headache.

Dermatitis of the hands

If you have dermatitis of the hands, avoid direct contact with biological powders or detergents when washing or washing dishes. Wear cotton gloves inside plastic gloves. To wash yourself, use pure soap that contains no perfume, colours or chemicals. Try to avoid direct contact of the hands with shampoos, polishes, solvents (turpentine), hair creams, hair dyes and detergents. Avoid peeling fruits and vegetables, especially oranges, grapefruits, lemons, with unprotected hands. Avoid direct contact with anything that may make the rash worse.

Dermatitis caused by the sun's rays

In some individuals, dermatitis may occur on parts of their skin exposed to the sun's rays. The dermatitis may be one of two types – phototoxic or photoallergic.

Phototoxic dermatitis is like an exaggerated sunburn. It is caused by chemicals in contact with the skin, making it sensitive to the sun's rays. These chemicals are present in some perfumes, coal tar preparations and certain oils. Treatment involves avoiding contact with the sensitizing chemical and avoiding direct exposure to the sun's rays until the dermatitis has healed.

Photoallergic dermatitis is an allergic reaction to the sun's rays caused by the skin being made sensitive by the application of some chemicals; for example, after-shave lotions, sunscreen preparations, topically applied sulphonamide anti-bacterial preparations, antihistamine applications and local anaesthetic applications. Treatment involves stopping the use of the applications and avoiding exposure to the sun's rays until the dermatitis has healed.

NOTE Drugs taken internally may cause either phototoxic dermatitis or photoallergic dermatitis (see 'Allergic drug rashes', later).

Seborrhoeic dermatitis

The term 'seborrhoeic dermatitis' is misleading because the disorder has nothing to do with the production of oil by the sebaceous glands (see under 'Acne'). It is an inflammatory, scaling skin disease affecting principally the scalp and face but also other areas of the body.

There are two distinct types of seborrhoeic dermatitis – the adult type and the infantile type.

The adult type is more common in men and in people who suffer from dandruff. The dermatitis affects the scalp and central part of the face and it may also affect the ears (otitis externa), eyebrows and eyelids. It may also affect the middle of the chest and back, the armpits, groins and underneath the breasts. The affected areas are red and scaly, and yellow crusts develop. Dandruff may be severe and the scalp may itch.

Treatment depends upon the area affected and the severity. It traditionally involved the use of applications containing sulphur, salicylic acid and/or coal tar. Topical corticosteroids produce a rapid improvement but the disorder returns when treatment is stopped.

The skin of sufferers from seborrhoeic dermatitis contains high levels of fatty acids which become infected by a fungus (*pityrosporum*) producing inflammation. Treatment with an anti-fungal drug (e.g. ketoconazole: Nizoral) can be effective. An alternative is lithium succinate which has both anti-inflammatory and anti-fungal properties. It is combined with zinc sulphate in Efalith ointment. It should not be used in children and applied with caution in people with psoriasis. Contact with the eyes and mouth should be avoided.

The infantile type of seborrhoeic dermatitis affects young infants, causing scaling of the scalp and red patches on the body and folds of the arms. It usually requires no treatment and clears up on its own in a few weeks. Rarely, it may be necessary to apply hydrocortisone cream but this should be used with great caution.

Sometimes infants develop a thick yellow crust on the scalp (cradle cap) and they may also develop nappy rash. If cradle cap is severe, it may be worth rubbing olive oil on to the scalp and shampooing with a baby shampoo each day. For the treatment of nappy rash, see later.

Impetigo

Impetigo is an infection of the skin caused by certain bacteria (staphylococci) that normally live up the nose in about 40 per cent of us. The bacteria may spread from the nose of adults to cause skin infection in newborn babies, and they may spread among young children. The infection spreads from the nose to small cuts or abrasions on the skin of one child and then by close contact with other children. It usually affects exposed areas of skin – face, hands and knees – and forms sores with honey-coloured crusts. The affected areas may go red and get worse if they become secondarily infected with streptococci. Impetigo may also develop as small blisters; it is then labelled bullous impetigo.

The infecting bacteria that cause impetigo are usually resistant to penicillin, and so chlortetracycline ointment is the treatment of choice. This usually works quickly and very effectively. If the impetigo is severe and the patient has a temperature, indicating some 'blood poisoning', flucloxacillin should also be given by mouth. Before applying antibiotic ointment, the crusts should be soaked off with liquid paraffin or povidone-iodine or sodium hypochlorite. It is very important that the children with impetigo be kept away from school until the sores have completely healed up; they should also have their own towels.

Insect stings and bites

Stinging insects inject venom by a piercing organ (a sting) which is attached to the rear end of females but not to males. It acts as the female's depositor of eggs (ovipositor). Bee stings are barbed, so when a bee pulls away after stinging you it disembowels itself and dies. Wasp and ant stings are not barbed and they live to sting again. When stinging you, bees and wasps use their feet to cling on, whereas ants use their mouth.

Biting insects include mosquitoes, fleas and lice. They bite the skin and suck blood.

Reactions to insect stings

The injected venom causes a local reaction at the site of injection, which produces pain, redness, swelling and itching. A sting of the tongue or mouth may produce severe swelling which may interfere with breathing. In addition, people may become allergic to the venom. The first sting sensitizes them and any subsequent sting may produce a severe allergic reaction. Within minutes of the sting, the individual may develop redness and itching at the site of injection, and go on to develop a more generalized allergic reaction such as nettle rash (urticaria) and swelling of the face and lips. Some individuals may develop a severe allergic reaction (anaphylactoid shock) in which they start to wheeze, their blood pressure falls; they may collapse and their throat may swell up and start to suffocate them. They may also develop nausea, vomiting and diarrhoea. If not treated immediately, they may die. For a discussion of acute allergic reactions and their treatment, see Chapter 10.

Reactions to insect bites

Insect bites may produce local redness, swelling and itching at the site of the bite. If the bite is in the mouth or tongue it may produce severe swelling that may interfere with breathing.

Heat spots

Young children may develop what are commonly called 'heat spots', which are often put down to a change in water or diet. In actual fact these small red spots are usually due to insect bites in children who have become allergic to them because of previous such bites. Skin specialists call it papular urticaria (urticaria is another name for nettle rash). In addition to the small red spots there are often tiny blisters.

This condition is produced by dog and cat fleas, and the important part of treatment is to treat the dog and cat with an insecticide and also any rugs or chairs that the animal sits in. If the itching is severe, calamine lotion containing 1% phenol may help.

Other insects may also produce 'heat spots' – for example midges, sand fleas and fleas from birds. Some people (especially young girls) may develop large blisters round their ankles after walking in the grass on a summer's evening. Insect repellents such as dimethyl phthallate may help.

Treatment of insect bites and stings

The area should be cleansed and a cooling lotion applied (e.g. calamine lotion). Bee stings should be removed by scraping with a finger nail or knife before cleaning. If the reaction is fairly severe, an antihistamine should be taken by mouth. An application containing hydrocortisone may be very effective at relieving the itching and soreness.

Most over-the-counter preparations used to relieve the symptoms of an insect bite or sting contain one or more of the following – a *counter-irritant* such as camphor or menthol; a *local anaesthetic* such as benzocaine; an *antihistamine*; a *skin protectant* such as zinc oxide or calamine; or an *antiseptic* such as phenol or cresol. These may help but some may irritate the skin.

Insect repellents

Insect repellents do not kill insects, but keep them away. They give off a vapour that puts the insects off. Although many thousands of compounds have been tested as insect repellents, only a few are effective and safe enough to use on the skin. The best all-round repellent is diethyltoluamide. Others include dimethyl phthalate and butopyronoxyl. Mixtures often work better against a wide range of insects. They may irritate the skin and should be used with caution around the eye because they may cause a burning sensation.

People who are allergic to insect stings should use an insect repellent and carry a supply of an antihistamine drug with them at all times in summer and autumn. If they are stung, they should take an antihistamine tablet immediately; if an acute mild allergic reaction occurs, they should take an inhalation of an adrenaline-like drug from an inhaler (see Chapter 10) to abort an attack. Individuals who are at risk of developing such an allergy should carry an inhaler with them (e.g. Medihaler-Epi). If the attack is moderate or severe, adrenaline should be given by injection. For the treatment of allergic emergencies, see Chapter 10.

Itching skin (pruritus)

Itching is an irritation of the skin that produces the urge to scratch. It is also known as pruritus. It probably occurs because of the release of chemicals in the skin, triggered by inflammation, allergy, certain diseases (see later) or contact with an irritant substance. Although scratching provides temporary relief, it may damage the skin and produce inflammation and even bleeding. This may make the condition worse and set up a vicious circle of scratching and itching, which may continue long after the original cause of the itching has been removed.

Different people react differently to itching: some scratch like mad and others hardly at all. Children with eczema may scratch with their nails so much that they draw blood. The intensity of itching may vary in individuals; it may be worse in bed at night, it may be less if they are concentrating and worse if they are bored. Generalized itching is often worse in bed.

Local itching of the skin may be due to parasitic infections such as scabies, to infestation with body lice, to eczema, psoriasis, nettle rash (urticaria), fungus infections (e.g. athlete's foot) or chickenpox. General diseases may also cause itching of the skin; for example, diabetes, obstructive jaundice, certain types of cancer (e.g. Hodgkin's disease) and kidney diseases. An allergic reaction to a drug may produce itching, and some women develop itching skin during pregnancy.

Itching in the elderly (senile pruritus) appears to be related to advancing age although no actual cause has been found. It may be due to a dry skin and poor circulation. The great risk is that an individual may think that he or she has an infestation and applies all sorts of substances to the skin which may trigger dermatitis.

Itching around the anus and itching of the vagina are discussed later.

Anti-itching skin applications

Irritation of the skin causes a release of chemicals that dilate the blood vessels and cause fluid to accumulate under the skin. This response produces itching and inflammation. Applications used to relieve itching include the following.

Cooling lotions such as calamine lotion are frequently used to relieve mild itching caused by sunburn, nettle rash or insect bites. They relieve itching and irritation by cooling the skin and producing counter-irritation (see page 460) which helps to block out the sensation of itching.

Emollient creams (soothing creams) may help to relieve itching caused by a dry skin.

Antiseptic skin applications used to relieve itching usually include phenol, benzyl alcohol, balsam of Peru or chlorbutol. They do not act as antiseptics but as irritants, and that is their problem – they may irritate the skin. They produce counter-irritation and help to block out the sensation of itching. Phenol (1%) in calamine lotion may be used to stop the generalized itching caused by lice, provided other specific treatment is carried out (see later). It may also be used to treat senile pruritus (see earlier).

Local anaesthetic skin applications usually contain cinchocaine, benzocaine or amylocaine. They numb the nerve endings to the skin and may help to reduce the sensation of itching. They may be of benefit for treating very small localized patches of itching such as an insect bite but in general they are not recommended because they may irritate the skin and may cause allergic rashes.

Antihistamine creams and lotions usually contain mepyramine, diphenhydramine, promethazine or antazoline. They block the effects of histamine and may be useful for treating small areas such as insect bites but they are not recommended for larger areas because they may produce allergic skin rashes and there are doubts about how effective they really are.

Menthol and camphor applied to the skin produce a cooling effect but they may irritate the skin and should not be used.

Crotamiton (e.g. Eurax) produces a redness and warmth of the skin and relieves itching. It may be useful in some individuals but should not be applied to inflamed skin because it will make it worse. However, there is little evidence that it works any more effectively than calamine lotion, which is probably as effective as most other applications, particularly if 1% phenol is added.

Corticosteroids. If itching is associated with inflammation, a corticosteroid application (e.g. hydrocortisone) is the most effective application to use; for example, for treating itching caused by eczema.

Warning *Itching caused by an underlying disease (see earlier) cannot be helped* *by skin applications. When possible the underlying disease must be treated, but it may help to take an anti-itching drug by mouth.*

Drugs taken by mouth to relieve itching

There are two main groups of drugs that are taken by mouth to relieve itching. These are the *antihistamines* and the *phenothiazines* (anti-psychotic drugs). One of the most commonly used is the antihistamine trimeprazine (Vallergan).

Itching rashes produced by allergy to drugs or other substances should be treated with an antihistamine by mouth. The severe itching that accompanies obstructive jaundice may be relieved by the male sex hormone testosterone. It has also been tried in senile pruritus but without much success. Cholestyramine (Questran) may help the itching in liver and gall bladder disease because it reduces the blood level of bile salts, which is high in these disorders and may be a cause of the itching.

Comment

It is very important that someone who has a generalized itch should be examined very carefully and any underlying disorder diagnosed and treated if possible. In general, anti-itching drugs by mouth are not all that effective in relieving itching; nevertheless, they should be tried because chronic itching may produce tension and depression and interfere with sleep.

To relieve the symptoms of itching different treatments should be tried until some benefit is achieved – in other words, treatment should be tailored to the individual's needs. For example, calamine lotion with 1% phenol may help an elderly person with a generalized itch and an antihistamine at night may help a child with eczema.

When itching is severe, it can present a real problem – which is why some unexpected treatments have been reported. For example, cimetidine may help the itching of Hodgkin's disease, and aspirin may help the pain, redness and itching of the skin which may occasionally occur in people with cancer of the breast.

Itching anus (pruritus ani)

Pruritus ani is soreness and itching around the anus and genital area. It may be triggered by some local problem in the anus such as a tear (fissure) or by piles, and made worse by applying various ointments that irritate this sensitive area – for example, preparations containing a local anaesthetic. It may follow a course of antibiotics by mouth which may cause thrush around the anus. Threadworm in children may produce pruritus ani and ringworm from athlete's foot fungus may cause it in adults. In addition, there is often a psychological factor so that the itching is worse when the individual is tense or anxious.

Where there is no evidence of infection (e.g. thrush) and no other obvious cause for the itching, a corticosteroid ointment (e.g. hydrocortisone) will provide relief but it should only be used for as short a period of time as possible. You should avoid using any application that contains an antiseptic or a local anaesthetic because they will only irritate the skin and make it worse. Too much washing with soap also irritates the surface and makes the itching worse. Bland soothing applications containing a mild astringent may help (e.g. bismuth oxide or zinc oxide).

Itching vagina (pruritus vulvae)

Pregnancy, diabetes and vaginal discharge may cause itching of the vagina. Antibiotics by mouth may cause a thrush infection of the vagina and produce itching. Deodorant sprays, vaginal wipes and contraceptive creams may produce vaginal irritation, as may contact with rubber (e.g. with condoms or caps).

In treating pruritus vulvae any underlying disorder of the vagina or vulva should be dealt with; for example, any vaginal discharge should be treated, as should any underlying disease that could cause the irritation (e.g. diabetes). If there is a thrush infection an anti-fungal cream should be used, and an oestrogen cream will help vaginal irritation in post-menopausal women. When there is no evidence of an infection or other obvious cause of the itching, relief may usually be obtained by applying a corticosteroid cream (e.g. hydrocortisone).

Lice

Head lice (pediculosis capitis)

Head lice spread by direct person-to-person contact and by contact with infected combs and hats. It is a common infestation among school children. Infestation may occasionally cause itching but usually all that can be seen are eggs (nits) on the hair shafts. The eggs mature in about 3–4 days and then the lice can most often be found at the back of the head and behind the ears.

Treatment Effective treatments include applying lotions or shampoos containing benzyl benzoate, carbaryl, malathion, permethrin or phenothrin. The instructions provided by the manufacturer should be carefully followed. Lindane is no longer used because there are now strains of treated lice that are resistant to it.

Warning *Head lice may become resistant to any of these products and it is advisable that health authorities introduce a policy to rotate their use in order to attempt to reduce the risk of resistance developing to any one of them.*

Body lice (pediculosis corporis)

These lice are spread from person to person by direct contact or by contact with clothing. Lice and eggs can be found in the clothing. The person with body lice itches, and scratches. Such people should be bathed and given clean clothing. Calamine lotion with 1% phenol will reduce the itching. An emulsion of benzyl benzoate or lindane should be applied to the affected areas of the body, left on for 24 hours and then washed off. This treatment should be repeated two or three times.

Crabs (pediculosis pubis)

This infestation affects the pubic hairs and causes severe itching in the groins. In adults it is spread by close sexual contact. The underclothes should be washed and the infected person should take a bath and then apply a *carbaryl, lindane* or *malathion* lotion to the affected area. The lotion should be left on for 1–12 hours and then washed off. This treatment may have to be repeated daily for 3 days.

NOTE It may also be necessary to treat beards or moustaches if these have become infested.

Treating infected clothing

Most parasites that infect the skin may also contaminate clothing and bedding of an affected person. Therefore, following treatment of the body to remove the parasites, it is important to get rid of the lice and eggs from clothing and bedding. Those that can be washed should be washed in hot water and dried in a hot drier. Items that cannot be washed in water should be placed in plastic bags that should be tied and left for a sufficient length of time to ensure that the parasites have died – they cannot survive more than a few days without their human host. The time for such

Table 75.7 Preparations used to treat head lice and body lice

Preparation	*Drug*	*Dosage form*
Ascabiol	benzyl benzoate	Emulsion
benzyl benzoate	benzyl benzoate	Application, shampoo
Carylderm	carbaryl	Lotion, shampoo
Clinicide	carbaryl	Liquid
Derbac-M	malathion	Liquid
Derbac Shampoo	carbaryl	Shampoo
Full Marks	phenothrin	Shampoo
Lyclear	permethrin	Conditioner
Prioderm	malathion	Lotion, cream shampoo
Quellada Application PC	lindane	Shampoo
Suleo-C	carbaryl	Lotion, shampoo
Suleo-M	malathion	Lotion

Warning *Applications used to treat lice infestation may produce irritation and stinging of the skin. This may be very painful if the application comes in contact with eyes, mouth or other moist membranes (e.g. vagina). Applications should be kept away from the eyes. Clinic workers who apply the applications should wear rubber gloves.*

isolation of clothing is 2 days for scabies, 10 days for head and pubic lice (crabs) and 30 days for body lice.

Nappy rash

The term 'nappy rash' can mean anything from slight redness in the nappy area to a severe dermatitis with sores. Prevention is better than cure. Use disposable nappies, avoid tight-fitting plastic pants and regularly apply zinc and castor oil cream. If you use ordinary nappies regularly soak them in a detergent antiseptic (e.g. 2% cetrimide). Expose the baby's bottom to the air for a short time each day. Change the nappy the moment it is wet or soiled, and clean the skin with oil or petroleum jelly (Vaseline) instead of soap or water if it is very sore.

If the rash is mild, a detergent antiseptic ointment may help (e.g. one that contains benzalkonium); if it is severe, try a corticosteroid but only a mild corticosteroid should be used (e.g. hydrocortisone). Remember that nappies and plastic pants can increase the absorption of the corticosteroid into the bloodstream, so use such treatment for only the shortest duration of time and in the smallest effective amounts possible.

If *infection* is suspected, it is often beneficial to apply a corticosteroid with an antibiotic for a few days (see Table 75.3). If there is evidence of thrush (little white patches), an anti-fungal drug should be used instead of an anti-bacterial drug. Once it is cleared, be absolutely meticulous about trying to prevent it coming back.

Warning *Some preparations applied to the bottoms of babies in the hope of preventing nappy rash may actually cause a rash; for example, preparations that contain antiseptics, tars, phenol, sulphur and salicylic acid. Hard soaps may also irritate the skin, and bleach or detergents left on nappies that have not been adequately rinsed may irritate the skin and cause a rash.*

Psoriasis

The skin is continually being renewed and, as dead cells are shed from the surface, new cells underneath take their place. This process maintains the normal surface of the skin (the epidermis). However, in psoriasis the process is disturbed and in certain areas of the skin new cells are produced at an excessive rate while the shedding of old cells remains normal and cannot keep pace with the number of new skin cells pushing out on to the surface. As a result, these new cells pile up to produce patches of thickened skin covered in silvery scales. The patches heal over without producing a scar.

The spread and extent of these patches of psoriasis vary between acute attacks and chronic attacks, and are affected by the age of the patient. Patches of psoriasis may vary in size from a fraction of a centimetre to large areas affecting the skin of the whole of the trunk. Psoriasis may affect the finger nails, scalp, skin folds, elbows, knees, palms, soles, the back and the buttocks. The eyebrows and the skin around the anus and genitals and the navel may occasionally be affected. It may also be associated with arthritis affecting a few or many joints (psoriatic arthropathy).

We do not know what is the underlying cause of psoriasis. It usually starts between the age of 10 and 40 years and recurs throughout the affected individual's life.

Psoriasis runs in families. The onset is usually gradual but an acute attack of tonsillitis may bring on an acute attack of psoriasis in a susceptible child. In adults, hot weather and sunshine improve the condition and lack of sunshine makes it worse. Stress has been identified as a factor that may bring on an attack. It is much more common in white people than non-white people and affects men and women equally. The fact that it may be worse at puberty and at the menopause and better during pregnancy suggests an hormonal link. It is now well recognized that certain drugs may aggravate psoriasis – for example, chloroquine used to treat malaria and rheumatoid arthritis, chlorpropamide used to treat diabetes, lithium used to treat depression and the withdrawal of corticosteroid drugs used to treat psoriasis (see later).

Treatment of psoriasis

There is no cure for psoriasis but treatment can provide effective control by reducing the size of the patches and reducing inflammation. Treatment varies according to the severity and extent of the psoriasis and the areas affected.

Acute psoriasis that comes on in childhood (acute guttate psoriasis) usually clears up on its own in 2–3 months, and sometimes treatment may actually make it worse. All that is needed is a simple emollient cream.

Treatment of mild to moderate psoriasis

For mild psoriasis, a soothing ointment (emollient) may be all that is necessary. If it is moderately severe, it may be worth trying a tar product at night and an emollient in the day-time. An application of dithranol for half an hour in the day-time may be added to the treatment. In addition, a corticosteroid application may be used. Exposure to the sun's rays may help but sunburn should be avoided because psoriasis may develop at the site of any damage to the skin.

Skin applications work better if the thickened scales are removed first. This is often best achieved by having a daily bath containing an oil emulsion and then rubbing off the scales using a bland cream.

Preparations used to treat mild to moderate psoriasis

Tar products Tar products are antiseptic, they relieve itching and they help to peel the skin (keratolytics). They are useful for treating chronic patches of psoriasis. Tar may increase the release of chemicals involved in producing inflammation (prostaglandins). Tar products are available as creams, ointments, pastes, lotions, bath oils, shampoos, soaps and gels.

Harmful effects produced by tar products include boils, staining of the skin, sensitization of the skin to the sun's rays and irritation of the skin, producing dermatitis. Tar products are smelly and often messy to apply. They may increase the tendency to sunburn for up to 24 hours after application, and other drugs that produce sensitivity to the sun's rays may make this worse (e.g. tetracyclines, phenothiazines, sulphonamides). Tar products should preferably not be used around the anus and genitals because there is an association between contact with tar in these areas and cancer of the skin, although such cancers have not been reported in patients suffering from psoriasis and treated with tar products.

Dithranol should be used with caution because it may irritate the surrounding skin. A ring of petroleum jelly (Vaseline) should therefore be applied around the patch of psoriasis before applying the dithranol. It may stain the skin and clothing black. It works just as well if it is left on for about 20–30 minutes and then washed off than if it is left on all night. Low concentrations of dithranol should be used to start with and then the concentration gradually increased. Fair-skinned people are more sensitive to dithranol than dark-skinned people. Dithranol is messy and it is better to use a brand preparation such as Dithrocream or Psoradrate.

Both *tar* and *dithranol* should be avoided on the face because they may irritate the skin. They should also be avoided in skin folds because they may cause boils to develop. In these areas an emollient should be used. An alternative is to apply a corticosteroid cream, but only to the patches (see later).

Skin softeners Applications that soften the skin and help it to peel, work by loosening keratin, a protein in the outer layer of the skin (keratolytics). They may be useful for getting rid of thick scales of psoriasis, and are useful as additional treatment to coal tar and dithranol in mild to moderate psoriasis (see above) and for use on areas of skin sensitive to tar and dithranol (e.g. the face and skin folds). They include *sulphur*, *salicylic acid*, *allantoin* and *resorcinol*. However, they are irritant and should not be applied over large areas because they may be absorbed, to produce harmful effects (see earlier).

Corticosteroid applications may be very beneficial, particularly the more potent ones. However, they may lose their effectiveness if used every day for more than 2–3 weeks. It may therefore help to alternate treatment every 1 or 2 weeks between a corticosteroid and an emollient.

Harmful effects of corticosteroid applications on the skin are discussed earlier. They may be absorbed into the bloodstream to produce harmful effects (see Chapter 62). This is particularly likely to happen if they are applied under adhesive or plastic dressings, to large areas of the body, or if highly concentrated and/or potent forms are used, and/or if large amounts are applied at regular intervals.

The strength and number of applications of a corticosteroid should be gradually reduced as the treated patches of psoriasis improve. Hydrocortisone is the only corticosteroid that should be applied to the face. Thick patches of psoriasis that are resistant to applications may be injected under the skin with a solution of a corticosteroid such as triamcinolone. Such treatment should not be repeated within about 3 weeks in order to avoid wasting of the skin.

Warnings *Psoriasis may get very much worse if corticosteroid applications are stopped suddenly. This flare-up may be complicated by pustules (little pimples* *containing pus) and may prove very difficult to treat. Therefore, applications must be stopped gradually over several days by using smaller and smaller amounts and/or by slowly reducing the strength of corticosteroid application that is used.*

Anti-itching products Bland emollient creams are the applications of choice to stop itching. Local anaesthetics and antihistamine preparations should *not* be used because they may produce irritation and allergy.

Treatment of severe and/or chronic psoriasis

The treatment of severe and/or chronic psoriasis goes in fashions and 'old-fashioned' treatments are now back in favour – for example, local applications of coal tar, dithranol and skin softeners (e.g. salicylic acid). These are usually applied after a bath and after rubbing off the scales.

Ultraviolet B radiation is the basis of the good old-fashioned treatment called Ingram's method. It consists of a warm bath containing a tar solution, a dose of ultraviolet radiation B(UVB) to produce redness and then the application of tar or dithranol paste to the patches of psoriasis. The tar and dithranol make the patches of psoriasis sensitive to the ultraviolet radiation. Repeated every day this treatment is effective and most cases clear up well in about 3–6 weeks.

PUVA treatment Methoxsalen and other psoralen drugs act on DNA in cells to slow down their rate of division. The drugs are activated by exposure of the skin to ultraviolet A radiation (UVA). Methoxsalen is used in PUVA treatment (psoralens and ultraviolet A radiation), of large chronic patches of psoriasis.

The methoxsalen is applied to the affected areas as a suspension or given by mouth and followed by ultraviolet irradiation 2 hours later. This is timed to coincide with peak concentrations of the drug in the bloodstream. Treatments with gradually increasing doses of UVA are repeated two or three times a week until the psoriasis has cleared up. This usually averages about twenty treatments. The rash may not return for several months but, if necessary, the skin can be kept clear with one PUVA treatment every 1–3 weeks.

PUVA treatment should be used with caution in anyone taking any other drug that sensitizes the skin to ultraviolet radiation. *Immediate harmful effects* include nausea, itching and painful reddening of normal areas of skin and, occasionally, blistering. Patients should avoid exposure to sunshine for several days after treatment. *Long-term harmful effects* of repeated treatments may include a small risk of ageing of the skin, and possibly a rare risk of developing skin cancer (particularly in fair-skinned people with a history of having had treatment for skin cancer or of having had radiation treatment in the past) and cataracts. PUVA treatment should therefore be used with caution in younger people.

Methotrexate is a drug used to treat cancer. It stops cells dividing and, because of this action, it has been found to be useful in some patients suffering from severe chronic psoriasis; however, because of the risks, it should be used only under hospital supervision to treat psoriasis that has not responded to any other treatment. Other drugs of this type that have been tried include hydroxyurea.

Local applications of methotrexate have so far proved useless. For the treatment of psoriasis associated with arthritis, see Chapter 30, under 'Rheumatoid arthritis'.

Etretinate (Tigason) Although vitamin A is involved in skin development and function, it has proved of no use in treating psoriasis. However, etretinate (Tigason), which is related to vitamin A, reduces scaling and improves psoriasis when given by mouth. It slows down the rapid rate of cell division in skin cells and reduces the production of keratin – the hard protein that forms the outer layer of the skin. Unfortunately, serious risks may easily outweigh any benefits. Women of child-bearing age should avoid sexual intercourse or take contraceptive precautions during treatment and for 1 year after treatment because the drug may damage unborn babies. Pregnancy should be excluded before starting this drug. Etretinate is combined with PUVA treatment in a regimen sometimes referred to as Re-PUVA. This may be effective when all other treatments have failed.

Corticosteroids by mouth When the corticosteroids were introduced, skin specialists were quick to use them to treat psoriasis. Given by mouth they had a dramatic effect in clearing up psoriasis, but it was the old story. They were used with great enthusiasm until it was realized that if you try to reduce the dose or stop them, the psoriasis flares up and is worse than it was before treatment was started. What is more, these flare-ups proved very difficult to treat. It is now accepted that there is no place for corticosteroids by mouth or injection in the treatment of psoriasis.

Psoriasis of the hands and feet

This is difficult to treat but may be helped by the application of a corticosteroid cream and wearing plastic gloves on the hands or plastic bags on the feet at night.

Psoriasis of the scalp

Scalp psoriasis with itching may respond to a corticosteroid scalp lotion (e.g. betamethasone). If the areas on the scalp are not very thickened, dithranol ointment or a tar-based shampoo (e.g. Polytar) may help. If the patches are very thick, it may be necessary to add an ointment containing salicylic acid or sulphur in order to soften them. Dithranol can be helpful on the scalp but it may turn blond and red hair purple.

Warnings *The trouble with psoriasis is that, although you can clear it up quite effectively with the treatments discussed above, it nearly always returns; this is what makes it difficult for patients because in the end they get fed up with all the effort involved in going to hospital departments and applying ointments and dressings. Unfortunately, apart from using an ultraviolet lamp at home there is nothing that will lengthen the quiet periods of the disease, and once it flares up the only choice is to go through the whole ritual of treatment again.*

Table 75.8 Drugs used to treat psoriasis – harmful effects

allantoin
No reported harmful effects

coal tar
May cause irritation and an acne-like rash of the skin. It may also make the skin sensitive to ultraviolet radiation and stain the skin, hair and fabric

corticosteroids
See earlier in this chapter

dithranol
May cause a burning sensation when applied to the skin. Some people may be allergic to it and therefore it should be tried on a small area of the skin first in order to check for sensitivity. It stains the skin reddish-brown and it may also stain hair and fabric. It should not be used in a concentration greater than 0.1% and it should not be applied more than once daily. It should not be used in people with kidney disease

ichthammol
Contains ammonium salts and sulphur. It may cause irritation of the skin and produce allergic reactions in some individuals

resorcinol
May irritate the skin. Absorption through damaged skin or prolonged regular use may stop the thyroid gland from producing thyroid hormones, leading to under-activity of the gland

salicylic acid
May cause excessive drying and irritation of the skin in some people. If applied to large areas of skin, it may produce symptoms like an overdose of aspirin (see Chapter 27)

sulphur
No harmful effects reported

etretinate (Tigason)
Harmful effects Most harmful effects are related to dose and clear up if the dose is reduced or the drug is stopped. There is a narrow margin between the dose that produces benefits and the dose that produces harmful effects, so treatment should always be tailored to the individual's response and the dose carefully adjusted. The following harmful effects have been reported and should be considered whenever the drug is used by mouth: dryness of the mouth, eyes and nose; dryness of the skin with scaling, thinning and redness (especially on the face); itching, skinning of the palms and soles, fragility of the skin; loss of hair, especially 4–8 weeks after starting

Table 75.8 Drugs used to treat psoriasis – harmful effects (*cont.*)

treatment (clears up when drug is stopped); nausea, sweating, drowsiness, painful muscles, painful joints and reduced tolerance to exercise. Rarely, liver damage with jaundice may occur, and raised blood fat levels have been reported (this is related to dose and may be controlled by diet including reduced alcohol intake).

Warnings Etretinate should not be used in anyone with liver or kidney disease. Long-term use may produce bone changes, so this should be avoided in children. If bone joint or muscle pains develop, tests should be carried out (e.g. X-rays) to check on any bone changes and, if present, the drug should be stopped. Tests of liver function and blood fat levels should be carried out before treatment starts, after 1 month of treatment and then every 3 months. Patients should be told of the risks of hair loss and be warned not to take more vitamin A than is recommended in a normal diet. Patients should not be blood donors during treatment and for 1 year after treatment. Maximum benefit occurs after 2–4 weeks. Treatment should not continue for more than 6–9 months and there should be a rest period of 3–4 months before repeating treatment.

Scabies

Scabies is due to an invasion of the outer layer of the skin (the epidermis) by a mite called *Sarcoptes scabiei.* The infection is spread from person to person by close skin contact such as holding hands or sleeping together. Successful infection is caused by a fertilized female burrowing into the skin, where she lives for the rest of her life. As she burrows along the skin she lays her eggs every day for several weeks. The eggs hatch in a few days and the larvae leave the burrows and shelter in hair roots where they develop into adult mites. They then mate and set the whole cycle going again, which takes about 2 weeks.

The mites burrow in the skin particularly on the hands and feet, and after about a month an itchy rash develops at the infected sites because the individual has become sensitive (allergic) to the mites. The rash characteristically affects the wrists, ankles, fingers, buttocks, abdomen and genitals. It does not occur above the neck in adults. With any future infestation itching will start almost straight away because the individual has become allergic. Infected individuals may scratch so much that they damage the skin and dermatitis may develop – which may also become infested. Massive infestation may occur in individuals who are immune deficient (e.g. AIDS).

Treatment

It is absolutely essential to treat every member of the household who may have skin-to-skin contact, whether they are itching or not. It is also important to treat sexual partners. An individual may have no symptoms but be able to spread the disease for up to 8 weeks after becoming infected.

After washing well, an application of a monosulfiram solution (e.g. Tetmosol) should be applied all over the body from the neck downwards, preferably with a paint brush and by some other member of the household. (Washing well is now recommended in preference to a hot bath because the bath may increase the absorption of the drug into the bloodstream and possibly increase the risk of harmful effects.) This should be repeated next morning. Benzyl benzoate (Ascabiol) and lindane (Quellada) are just as effective as monosulfiram. Another drug that may be used is malathion (Derbac-M, Prioderm), but it may not be as effective as the others. Lotions and solutions are easier to apply than creams and ointments.

Monosulfiram (Tetmosol) soap may be used daily instead of ordinary soap as long as the infection lasts. Crotamiton (Eurax) lotion or cream may help to reduce the itching which may continue for up to 3 months after successful treatment of the infection.

Harmful effects of anti-scabies drugs

Benzyl benzoate (Ascabiol) is irritating and difficult to apply because it is in an emulsion wax base. Applications for infants should be diluted.

Crotamiton (Eurax) is useful for relieving the itching that is associated with scabies but it should be used *after* treatment with a more effective drug. It may produce redness of the skin and a sensation of warmth. It should not be used if there is dermatitis, and it should not be applied near the eyes.

Lindane (Quellada) may produce irritation of the skin. Because of the risk of absorption through the skin to produce nerve damage, it should be used with caution in children, and only in weak concentrations.

Malathion (Derbac-M, Prioderm) may produce skin irritation and allergic reactions.

Monosulfiram (Tetmosol) Adults treated with monosulfiram should avoid drinking alcohol. This is because monosulfiram is related to *disulfiram* (Antabuse), which is used to treat alcoholism. If taken by mouth, disulfiram produces no reactions unless alcohol is taken and then the individual develops flushing of the face, throbbing headache, a rapid pulse, irritation in the throat, giddiness, nausea, vomiting, chest pain and confusion. This is known as a disulfiram reaction (or Antabuse reaction), and a similar reaction may occur in a person using monosulfiram who also drinks alcohol.

Sweating and and body odour

The *eccrine sweat glands* are distributed all over the skin surface but particularly on the palms, soles, face and armpits. They produce sweat, which consists of water, various salts and some waste products, and play an important role in maintaining the body's temperature. A rise in body temperature produces sweating on the face and upper trunk; the water in the sweat evaporates and helps to cool the body.

Sweating on the palms, soles, face and armpits can be triggered by an emotional stimulation (e.g. fear). Sweating of the face may also be produced by eating hot, spicy foods. On average, we produce about 1 litre of sweat per day. Sweat is normally odourless but some foods and drugs can give it an odour.

Apocrine glands, which develop at puberty, open near hair roots and are concentrated in the armpits, around the nipples and around the genitals and anus. They produce an odourless secretion that bacteria break down into odorous substances – body odour (BO). Secretions from apocrine glands contain substances whose 'smell' may attract the opposite sex.

Sweating

Sweating that causes wetness is due to water being produced by the eccrine sweat glands faster than it evaporates – and obviously in areas like the armpits it does not evaporate very quickly. A blockage of sweat glands may cause the sweat to leak under the skin surface, causing irritation. This is called prickly heat, and is common in tropical countries.

Body odour

Body odour (BO) is caused principally by bacteria breaking down the secretions of the apocrine sweat glands. They produce waste products that smell, and hairy sites (like under the arms) act as reservoirs for these waste products.

Wetness due to excessive sweating from eccrine sweat glands and body odour (BO) from the secretions of apocrine glands are therefore two different processes.

Antiperspirants

Antiperspirants are substances that reduce the amount of sweat produced by the eccrine sweat glands. Most antiperspirants contain salts of aluminium and/or zinc which dry the skin and shrink the pores, closing off the openings of the sweat glands. In other words, they probably act as astringents (see earlier) although we really do not know how they work.

The antiperspirant market is worth millions of pounds. Antiperspirants are available in every size, shape and colour of container, as pads, sprays, roll-ons and creams, and with every possible smell. Some may stain fabric, others are acidic and may irritate the skin, and some may produce allergic skin rashes (e.g. those that contain aluminium salts).

Deodorants

Deodorants contain substances that change odour without reducing the production of sweat. Therefore deodorants are not antiperspirants, but many antiperspirants contain deodorants and some antiperspirants may be effective deodorants.

Deodorants usually contain perfumes to cover up body odour and/or antiseptics or anti-bacterial drugs to knock out the bacteria that produce the smelly waste products.

Antiseptics such as hexachlorophane and benzalkonium are frequently used in deodorant preparations. Hexachlorophane may produce allergic skin rashes, and benzalkonium and related complex ammonium compounds are inactivated by washing with soap and may irritate the skin. Some deodorants contain antibiotics that may be harmful because the individual may become allergic to the antibiotic and, furthermore, the bacteria may develop a resistance to the antibiotic – which will limit its future use for some more important medical problem.

In addition to obvious problems that may be caused as a result of applying an antiseptic or an antibiotic to large areas of the skin every day, some people may also become allergic to the perfume used in deodorants.

Sweaty feet

Over-sweating of the soles is a common complaint and produces a bad odour due to the bacteria breaking down the sweat. The sweating may be so severe that the skin on the soles becomes white and soggy. A 10% solution of glutaraldehyde dabbed on the feet or 3% formalin foot soaks are usually effective. Rubber-soled shoes should be avoided, and cotton socks may help. Wearing open sandals in summer may also help.

Feminine deodorant preparations

Mucus from the vagina and grease and secretions from the glands in the skin around the vagina and anus are broken down by bacteria, and the waste products produced can cause an odour. Other causes of odour include semen in the vagina, old blood, any infection in the vagina, copper intra-uterine devices (IUDs) and occasionally portions of tampons that have been left inside the vagina and forgotten.

The healthy vagina cleanses itself by means of its secretions and the area around the vagina and anus can be kept clean by regular washing with soap and water, so there is seldom any need to use feminine deodorant preparations. These may take the form of mist or powder sprays or pre-moistened towelettes (wipes) for application to the outside area around the vagina. They may contain substances that may irritate the vagina. If sprays are used too close to the vagina, the chemical may enter the urethra and produce irritation (see cystitis, Chapter 33).

Chemicals may enter the bloodstream much more easily from the surface of the vagina than from the skin; therefore any applications should be used with utmost caution, particularly during pregnancy when the chemical may enter the mother's bloodstream and pass through into the baby.

Warts

There are many types of viruses that cause warts. Warts may appear at any age but are more common in children. They may be single or multiple. They may disappear without treatment in months or years, and they may recur at the same site or at different sites. Patients who are immune deficient due to drugs or disease (e.g. AIDS) may suffer from an extensive attack of warts.

The common types of warts often affect the hands and feet. The latter are often referred to as plantar warts or verrucae.

Most wart applications contain a caustic or keratolytic, which removes the keratin layer and destroys the underlying layer of the skin. Commonly used ones include acetic acid, lactic acid, salicylic acid, nitric acid and formaldehyde. Most of these preparations will irritate the surrounding skin, and, because warts clear up on their own, it is not necessary to subject little children to such treatments.

Simple remedies are best for handwarts, e.g. salicylic acid collodion. A sticking plaster should be put over the warts after the application has dried.

Stronger preparations containing formaldehyde (Veracur) or glutaraldehyde (Novaruca, Glutarol, Verucasep) or bromine complexes (benzalkonium chloride–bromine; Callusolve) may work on some plantar warts in some people but their effectiveness is difficult to predict. Preparations containing formaldehyde or glutaraldehyde may irritate the skin and cause allergic rashes; they also have an unpleasant smell. Formalin solution (3%) used as a foot soak may help multiple plantar warts; or a tape impregnated with 40% salicylic acid may be helpful, if it is kept in place for several days at a time. Skin specialists may burn some warts with liquid nitrogen or they may surgically remove large and ugly warts.

Posalfilin, which contains podophyllum resin 20% and salicylic acid is also suitable for treating plantar warts (verrucae). The application should be applied directly on to the wart or warts, and contact with the surrounding skin should be avoided because it may irritate. A sticking plaster should then be applied over the treated wart and left in place until the next treatment is due – which is usually once or twice daily. Dead skin should be removed with a pumice stone before the next application.

Podophyllotoxin is the active ingredient of podophyllum obtained from American mandrake. It kills cells and is present in Condyline and Warticon solutions. It is used to treat warts around the anus and genitals. It should not be allowed to touch the surrounding skin, and a soft paraffin dressing should be applied over the application for protection. *Harmful effects* include irritation and pain at the site of application. If absorbed into the bloodstream, it may cause damage to nerves. Because of this only a few warts should be treated at any one time. It should *not* be used in pregnancy.

Allergic drug rashes

You may become allergic to a drug at any time whether you have taken it for only a day or two or for several years. Some patients may have an immediate and severe allergy to the very first dose of a drug if they have taken that drug before and become allergic to it. Allergic reactions are the commonest cause of skin rashes produced by drugs.

Allergic reaction may be one of four types:

1. A sudden drug reaction (anaphylactic reaction) in which there is an excessive release of histamine and related chemicals, causing wheezing, swelling of the throat so the individual cannot breathe and a sudden fall in blood pressure causing collapse. Such a reaction may follow an injection of penicillin in a patient who has had penicillin before and become allergic to it. This highlights the danger of using penicillin and other antibiotics in skin applications when the same antibiotic may have to be used subsequently by injection or by mouth.
2. A drug reaction where the drug affects the platelets in the blood and the small blood vessels, producing a skin reaction called *purpura* – small pin-point bleedings into the skin.

3. A drug reaction where the individual develops serium sickness – fever, swollen glands, painful joints and nettle rash or a measles-like rash.
4. A delayed allergic skin rash after a drug has been applied to the skin, producing a rash like eczema. Following the development of this allergy the allergic rash may recur if the drug is re-applied to the skin, given by injection or taken by mouth. It may also be produced by other drugs that are chemically similar (i.e. there is cross-allergy). For example, if an application of drug A has caused an allergic eczema-like rash on the part of the skin to which it was applied, then if a chemically related drug (drug B) is taken (even by mouth), the eczema can flare up in *exactly the same* part of the skin to which drug A had been applied.

Examples of skin rashes produced by drugs

Red, measles-like rashes

amitriptyline (an anti-depressant drug)
oral anti-diabetic drugs
diuretic drugs (used to treat raised blood pressure and heart failure)
gold salts (used to treat rheumatoid arthritis)
penicillins and cephalosporins (antibiotics)
phenylbutazone (used to treat rheumatoid arthritis)
sulphonamide drugs (anti-bacterial drugs)

Nettle rash (urticaria)

aspirin NOTE Cross allergy with other anti-rheumatic drugs and with orange dye (tartrazine) in orange squash, foodstuffs and some medicines
enzymes (e.g. streptokinase used to treat coronary thrombosis)
penicillins and cephalosporins (antibiotics)
X-ray contrast media

Blistering rashes

penicillamine (used to treat rheumatoid arthritis)

Red Blotches (erythema multiforme)

barbiturates (sleeping drugs, sedatives and anti-epileptics)
penicillins (antibiotics)
phenylbutazone (used to treat rheumatoid arthritis)

sulphonamides (anti-bacterial drugs)

Skinning, with death of patches of skin (toxic epidermal necrolysis)

barbiturates (sleeping drugs and sedatives, anti-epileptics)
phenytoin (used to treat epilepsy)
phenylbutazone (used to treat rheumatoid arthritis)
sulphonamides (anti-bacterial drugs)

Pin-point bleeding into the skin (purpura)

indomethacin (used to treat rheumatoid arthritis)
phenylbutazone (used to treat rheumatoid arthritis)
quinine (used to treat malaria and night cramps)
sulphonamides (anti-bacterial drugs)
thiazide diuretics (used to treat raised blood pressure and heart failure)

Fixed drug rashes

Fixed drug rashes are so called because they always occur at the same site. They start within 1–2 hours of taking the drug and fade away when the drug is stopped. They form a red disc-like rash which may have a blister in the middle. They may occur anywhere on the skin and even in the mouth.

barbiturates (sleeping drugs and sedatives and anti-epileptics)
chlordiazepoxide (anti-anxiety drug)
metronidazole (anti-bacterial drug)
phenacetin (banned pain reliever)
phenolphthalein (laxative)
phenylbutazone (used to treat rheumatoid arthritis)
sulphonamides (anti-bacterial drugs)

Acne

Acne has been discussed earlier. It may be caused by the following drugs:

bromides (previously used as sedatives)
corticosteroids
ethambutol (used to treat tuberculosis)
ethionamide (used to treat leprosy)
phenytoin (used to treat epilepsy)
iodides (used to treat thyroid disease, as antiseptics, in some cough medicines and as contrast media for X-rays)
isoniazid (used to treat tuberculosis)

male sex hormones
phenobarbitone (used to treat epilepsy)

Lichenoid rashes

These are small raised areas that can look like eczema and psoriasis.

chloroquine (used to treat malaria and rheumatoid arthritis)
mepacrine (used to treat malaria)
methyldopa (used to treat raised blood pressure)
para-amino salicylic acid (used to treat tuberculosis)
quinidine (used to treat disorders of heart rhythm)
quinine (used to treat malaria and night cramps)

Sensitivity of the skin to the sun's rays

There is sunburn on exposed parts according to the dose used.

chlorothiazide (a diuretic used to treat raised blood pressure and heart failure)
chlorpromazine (used to treat serious mental illness)
sulphonamides (anti-bacterial drugs)
tetracyclines (anti-bacterial drugs)

Allergic skin reactions to the sun's rays

all antibiotics
chlorpromazine (used to treat serious mental illness, and nausea and vomiting)
sulphonamides (anti-bacterial drugs)
sulphonylureas (oral anti-diabetic drugs)

Dermatitis with peeling of the skin (exfoliative dermatitis)

carbamazepine (used to treat epilepsy)
gold salts (used to treat rheumatoid arthritis)
phenindione (used to stop blood from clotting)
phenylbutazone (used to treat rheumatoid arthritis)
streptomycin (anti-bacterial drug, used to treat tuberculosis)

Eczema

This usually follows taking a drug by mouth or injection after the patient has been made allergic to that particular drug by a previous application to the skin.

antibiotics
antihistamines
methyldopa (used to treat raised blood pressure)
para-amino compounds (e.g. para aminobenzoic acid in sunscreen preparations)

Treatment of allergic drug rashes depends upon the severity of the rash. Stopping the drug immediately and taking an antihistamine drug by mouth is usually all that is needed. However, if the drug is excreted slowly from the body because of impaired liver or kidney function (e.g. in old age), the toxic levels of the drug may persist in the bloodstream and cause the drug rash to get progressively worse, in which case it is best for a corticosteroid to be given by mouth for a few days until the rash improves.

Warning on drug allergies

Allergy to a drug is for life, so it is important that people allergic to a drug should carry a warning card with them at all times in case of a medical or surgical emergency or accident.

Cancer

Definitions

Cancer is a general term used to describe a wide variety of diseases caused by abnormal new growth of tissue.

Neoplasia means an abnormal new growth of tissue and is used as a euphemism for cancer.

Neoplasm means any new formation of tissue and is used as a euphemism for cancer.

Malignant implies a danger to life.

Benign implies no danger to life.

Tumour means a swelling.

Cancer

After coronary heart disease, cancer is the second commonest cause of death in the Western world. The most common sites for cancer are the lungs, large bowel and breast. In children aged 3–13 years, cancer of the blood (leukaemia) is the commonest cause of death.

The cause of many cancers remains unknown but we do know, for example, that there is a direct relationship between cigarette smoking and cancer of the lungs, sunlight and skin cancer, a sexually transmitted factor and cancer of the cervix, and radiation and leukaemia.

Benign and malignant cancers

Benign cancers contain large numbers of dividing cells but they remain orderly within the tissue of their origin.

In *malignant* cancer the dividing cells are not orderly, they grow rapidly and are disordered in their growth and multiplication, so under the microscope it can be seen that the cells are at different stages of division and often do not resemble the cells of the tissue from which they have grown. Furthermore, with malignant cancer the cells in the primary growth may invade surrounding tissues and they may also leave the tissue of origin and spread through the blood stream and the lymph to other tissues. This process of breaking loose from the primary growth and spreading round the body is called metastasis, and the groups of cancer cells that spread and start growing elsewhere are called metastases or secondaries. For example, cells from malignant cancer of the lung may spread to settle in bone.

Classification of cancers

Cancers are classified into three major groups. *Carcinomas* arise from cells on surface linings; for example, on the skin or on linings of internal organs such as the lining of the stomach or bronchial tubes. *Sarcomas* arise from cells in supportive and other tissues (e.g. muscle, bone); and *leukaemias* and *lymphomas* arise from bone marrow tissue that forms white blood cells and from lymph tissue, respectively.

Cancers developing in the various tissues of the body have different types of cells and some are more malignant than others; this is why it is very important to take a biopsy and examine the cancer cells under the microscope. The information obtained from this examination will influence the types of treatment to be given – surgery and/or radiotherapy and/or drugs – and the extent and nature of these treatments.

Signs of cancer

The signs produced by a cancer will depend upon its location in the body, its size and whether it is benign or malignant. Signs therefore vary – for example, from a painless swelling caused by a cancer in muscle to blood in the motions from an ulcerating cancer of the colon.

Treatment of cancer

The treatment of cancer will depend on many factors such as its type, its location, whether it is benign and localized and can be removed surgically or whether it is malignant and has spread to adjacent and/or other tissues in the body. Treatment often involves a mixture of surgery, radiotherapy and drugs, and the main decision on treatment is whether to go for a 'cure' or to go for maximum relief of symptoms (palliative treatment). Obviously, someone with a localized cancer has a greater chance of survival than one in whom the cancer has spread (metastasized). The age, general condition and physical response of the individual will also influence the outcome, as can the emotional response of that person to the cancer and to the knowledge that he or she has a cancer. These are all important factors and involve decisions by the patient as well as by the doctor. Therefore, in the effective treatment of cancer there is a need for good communication and co-operation between doctors and patients. Patients need to know what they are suffering from, what treatment options are open to them and what the predicted outcome would be with and without surgery and/or radiotherapy and/or drugs.

Assessing the nature and extent of a cancer

At a technical level cancer specialists talk about 'staging', which means assessing the extent and nature of the cancer over time. The internationally recognized staging system is known as the TNM classification. T defines the extent of the cancer, N defines the extent of spread into local lymph glands (nodes) that drain the area in which the cancer is growing, and M defines the presence or absence of metastases (i.e. spread to other tissues and organs in the body). Numbers are then added to indicate further development according to agreed criteria; for example, M0 means no metastases whereas M1 means metastases present. This clinical staging is supported by the results of examinations under the microscope of sections of the cancer taken by biopsy. In addition, other techniques add to the doctor's assessment; for example, the results of a scan. Finally, what is called the patient's performance status is assessed. This assessment determines the level of functional impairment the cancer is producing. It involves assessment of any local impairment (e.g. breathlessness due to a cancer of the bronchial tube) and a general assessment of the patient's fitness and ability to perform everyday activities of life.

A further and very important part of caring is to assess the patient's response to treatment. This clearly may vary from a complete response (the disappearance of the cancer and the absence of any new cancer developing) to no response.

Drug treatment of cancer

For some historical reason doctors talk about chemotherapy of cancer instead of drug treatment. This is confusing because the term was originally used to describe the drug treatment of infectious diseases, and you will still hear some doctors referring to sulphonamides as chemotherapeutic agents. This is not necessary and we should talk about the drug treatment of cancer and the drug treatment of infectious diseases. Because drugs used to treat cancer are toxic to dividing cells, they are also referred to as cytotoxic drugs.

Principles of drug treatment of cancer

It is important not to make too many general statements about cancer and its treatment. This is because there are many different cancers and many different causes of cancer. They affect different people differently and they affect many different tissues in the body. Cancers also respond differently to different treatments and different patients respond differently to the effects of treatment. This means that cancer treatment must always be tailored to an individual's needs, which may well change over time as the patient responds or fails to respond to treatment. The treatment of cancer is a good example of the importance of treating the whole patient – his or her physical, social, emotional and spiritual needs.

How do anti-cancer drugs work?

All cells in the body go through regular cycles of growth and multiplication, some much faster than others. This growth and multiplication of cells is directly linked to different stages in the production and separation of chromosomes for the transmission of characteristics of the particular cell undergoing division – for example, a skin cell becomes a skin cell and not a kidney cell. Chromosomes are thread-like structures found in the nucleus of every cell; they contain genes that are formed by a chain of proteins known as DNA (deoxyribonucleic acid). This chain of proteins (DNA) carries special codes (genetic codes) for the newly developing cells which ensures that the cells develop exactly like their 'parent' cells. DNA is helped in this by another chain of proteins called RNA (ribonucleic acid) which acts as a messenger for the coding. This means that new skin cells will not only look like skin cells but they will also function as skin cells, just like their 'parent' cells, and this functioning will be quite different from cells in other tissues. It also means that these cells will be able to divide and 'transmit' their coding to new cells.

Since the observation in the First World War that mustard gas destroyed dividing cells, thousands of substances have been tested for their anti-cancer effects; today we have at least thirty effective anti-cancer drugs available. Anti-cancer drugs interfere with the growth of cells and their multiplication. Different drugs act at different stages in these processes. This gives the advantage that drugs with different actions can be combined to produce a more toxic effect on cancer cells than each drug used separately.

Anti-cancer drugs work more effectively on rapidly dividing cells, which is why, as well as destroying cancer cells that are rapidly dividing, they also destroy normal cells that divide rapidly; for example, cells in the bone marrow, hair root cells, and cells lining the mouth, stomach and intestine. This means that, in addition to their effects on cancer cells, they may also damage the bone marrow and knock out red blood cell production, resulting in anaemia; white cell production, resulting in susceptibility to infections; and platelet production, resulting in bleeding. They can also damage the cells of hair roots and cause loss of hair (alopecia); and the cells in the lining of the stomach and intestine, producing nausea, vomiting and diarrhoea.

Early diagnosis is important

Small cancers tend to be more sensitive to anti-cancer drugs than large ones because their cells usually divide more rapidly and their blood supply is better, which means the drugs can get into the cancer more effectively. This stresses the importance of early diagnosis and early treatment, which may include surgery and/or radiotherapy with drug treatment.

Benefits and risks

The gap between the beneficial effects of anti-cancer drugs in killing cancer cells and their harmful effects in damaging normal cells is, unfortunately, very narrow. Therefore, patients need very careful monitoring – regular physical examinations, including blood and urine tests. In addition, because of the risk to normal cells, only a certain maximum dose of an anti-cancer drug can be used at any one time, which means that not all of the cancer cells will be killed. This is why it is necessary to give repeated doses of anti-cancer drugs at intervals over several months to several years.

There must be gaps between courses of anti-cancer drugs in order to allow any damaged normal cells in the body to fully recover before the next course of anti-cancer drug is given. Therefore, in order to preserve normal cell function in the body, particularly in the bone marrow, anti-cancer drugs are usually given with a gap of at least 3 weeks between each course of treatment. This gives time for the bone marrow cells to return to normal function before the next dose.

Combination treatment can be very successful

As stated earlier, different anti-cancer drugs work at different stages in cell growth and division. Therefore, by using two, three or even four different anti-cancer drugs together to damage cell growth and division at different stages of division, a more effective result can be achieved. This combination approach requires detailed knowledge of the patient, the cancer and the available drugs, and in capable hands it has produced remarkable results in people suffering from cancers such as Hodgkin's disease, leukaemia, cancer of the breast, ovary, lung and testes, and several childhood cancers. These days we can talk about curing some cancers with drug treatment.

The principles involved in combined anti-cancer drug treatment are that each drug must have been shown to be effective on its own against the particular type of cancer being treated and that drugs which act in the same way should not be combined. Also, the doses of each drug used should be less than if it were being used on its own.

NOTE Certain cancers may respond to treatment with a single drug which is safer than using a combination of drugs. On the other hand, not every cancer is sensitive to anti-cancer drug treatment, and using drugs in such instances will only subject the individual to the risks of unnecessary harmful effects.

Examples of combination treatments are:

- MOPP treatment – a combination of mustine, Oncovin (vincristine), procarbazine and prednisolone
- MVPP treatment – a combination of mustine, vinblastine, procarbazine and prednisolone
- ABVD treatment – a combination of Adriamycin (doxorubicin), bleomycin, vinblastine and dacarbazine

Harmful effects of anti-cancer drugs

A number of anti-cancer drugs will cause death of local tissue if allowed to leak from the site of injection, so they must be injected with great care.

Whenever an anti-cancer drug is given in a dose sufficient to kill cells in a patient's cancer, it also kills normal cells in other tissues of the body, particularly those that divide rapidly (see earlier). This is the main problem with anti-cancer drugs and it often limits their effective use.

Harmful effects include the following.

Damage to the lining of the mouth, stomach and intestine

Anti-cancer drugs may produce ulceration of the mouth, nausea, vomiting and diarrhoea. Nausea and vomiting may be particularly severe and put people off treatment. The worst drugs for producing nausea and vomiting are cisplatin, mustine, dacarbazine, cyclophosphamide and doxorubicin. Thrush infections of the mouth and intestine may occur.

Drugs used to treat nausea and vomiting caused by anti-cancer drugs are discussed in Chapter 14. It may be helpful to start these anti-vomiting drugs before the anti-cancer drug treatment starts and to continue them for 24 hours afterwards. For anti-cancer drugs that produce severe vomiting it may also help to give dexamethasone (a corticosteroid) by mouth before and 6 hours after treatment and/or a benzodiazepine such as lorazepam by mouth before and 6 hours after. If the vomiting is severe, both these drugs may be given by injection into a vein. Lorazepam makes people drowsy and reduces their memory for what was happening to them. Lorazepam injections should not be used in patients with chronic chest disorders, and should be used with caution in the elderly.

NOTE Most of the drugs used to relieve nausea and vomiting may make you drowsy and affect your ability to drive.

Baldness

Anti-cancer drugs damage cells in hair roots and the hair falls out. Attempts to prevent this on the scalp have not been too successful, and it is important for patients to know that their hair will re-grow normally once the drug treatment is stopped. The degree of baldness will vary between different drugs and between different individuals.

Damage to blood-forming tissues in the bone marrow

All anti-cancer drugs except vincristine and bleomycin damage blood-forming cells in the bone marrow, with the result that they may knock out red blood cell production, causing anaemia; white cell production, causing a reduced resistance to infections; and platelet cells involved in blood clotting, producing a risk of bleeding. This damage usually shows itself after about 7–10 days but may be delayed with drugs such as carmustine, lomustine and melphalan. Regular blood counts should be carried out before, during and after treatment. If, between courses of treatment, the bone marrow does not show signs of full recovery the next course of treatment should be delayed or the doses reduced. In patients with a low white cell count, any fever or sore throat should be treated immediately with a course of antibiotics by injection, once tests have been carried out to try to identify the infecting micro-organism and its sensitivity to antibiotics.

Damage to sex organs

Anti-cancer drugs may affect the ovaries in women, causing loss of periods or irregular periods. They may produce sterility in both men and women. The majority of children treated before puberty with anti-cancer drugs do not become sterile. After puberty, anti-cancer drugs may damage female eggs (ova) and male sperm. Therefore, both male and female patients should avoid sexual intercourse or practise contraception during the period that they are receiving anti-cancer drugs and for 6 months after the treatment has stopped. If fertility does not return within 2 years it is unlikely to. Young males should consider sperm banking before treatment starts.

Risk of gout

Gout is discussed in Chapter 32. Because anti-cancer drugs kill cancer cells, there may be a rapid increase in the release of proteins (purines) from the damaged cells. The breakdown of these large amounts of cell proteins by the liver will cause a rise in the levels of uric acid in the blood, and this rise may trigger gout and cause kidney damage in susceptible individuals.

Risk of producing another cancer

There is a very rare risk with certain anti-cancer drugs used to treat certain types of cancer that cancer of the blood may develop many years after treatment of the cancer. For example, leukaemia may follow the treatment of cancer of the ovary with an alkylating anti-cancer drug (see below).

Specific harmful effects

Some anti-cancer drugs may occasionally produce specific damage to certain organs. For example, doxorubicin may damage the heart, cisplatin may damage the kidneys and bleomycin may produce scarring of the lungs.

Different types of anti-cancer drugs

Alkylating agents

These damage DNA (the genetic coding on genes). In addition to the general harmful effects discussed earlier, these drugs may damage sperm production in males, causing infertility early in treatment which is usually permanent. In females there is less risk of infertility but the drugs may damage the ovaries and cause early menopause. They may damage white cell production and, rarely, cause acute leukaemia in patients who have had continuous and prolonged treatment for conditions such as cancer of the ovary, particularly when used along with radiation treatment.

Alkylating agents include:

busulphan (Myleran)
carmustine (BiCNU)
chlorambucil (Leukeran)
cyclophosphamide* (Endoxana)
estramustine (Estracyt)
ethoglucid (Epodyl)
ifosfamide* (Mitoxana)
lomustine (CCNU)
melphalan (Alkeran)
mitobronitol (Myelobromol)
mustine
thiotepa (Thiotepa)
treosulfan (Treosulfan)

Anti-metabolites

These chemicals are taken into the nucleus of new cells where they combine with chemicals (enzymes) to prevent division of the cells.

Anti-metabolites are available that stop the effect of any one of three enzymes that use folic acid, purine or pyrimidine as building blocks. They are therefore known as folic acid antagonists, purine antagonists and pyrimidine antagonists. They are used to treat leukaemias and various

* Cyclophosphamide and ifosfamide damage the lining of the bladder and urinary tract. This is caused by a breakdown product of the drug (acrolein). Mesna (Uromitexan) reacts with this product and makes it inactive. Mesna is therefore given with cyclophosphamide and ifosfamide.

cancers (e.g. breast and colon), and have produced dramatic and long-lasting cures in the treatment of choriocarcinoma (a cancer that develops from the tissues of an unborn baby inside the uterus). Pyrimidine antagonists may damage the nails and the lining of the mouth, and cause loss of hair. Folic acid antagonists may interfere with the body's immune response to infection and foreign tissues (e.g. kidney transplants).

Anti-metabolites used to treat cancer include:

cytarabine (Alexan, Cytosar)
fluorouracil (Efudix, Fluoro-uracil)
mercaptopurine (Puri-Nethol)
methotrexate* (Maxtrex)
thioguanine (Lanvis)

Cytotoxic antibiotics (U)

These interfere with the ability of DNA to duplicate itself into dividing cells (replication). They can mimic the damaging effects of radiation on cells and so they should not be given as well as radiotherapy because of the serious risk to normal cells.

Cytotoxic antibiotics are used to treat leukaemias, various cancers (e.g. breast) and certain cancers in childhood. They include:

actinomycin D (Cosmegen Lyovac)
bleomycin
doxorubicin (Doxorubicin Rapid Dissolution)
epirubicin (Pharmorubicin)
mitomycin (Mitomycin C Kyowa)
plicamycin (mithramycin, Mithracin)

Vinca alkaloids

These are chemicals extracted from periwinkle (*Vinca rosea*) that stop cell division. In addition to the harmful effects described earlier, they may

* Folinic acid (Calcium Leucovorin, Refolinon) tablets or injections are used to compensate for the blocking of folic acid produced by methotrexate. This helps the cells of the bone marrow and other cells (e.g. in the lining of the mouth, stomach and intestine) to recover more quickly. Folinic acid should be given about 8–24 hours after the start of methotrexate treatment.

cause nerve damage in the arms and legs, producing numbness and pins and needles, and weakness and damage to the nerves of the intestine, producing a bloated abdomen with constipation. The nerves slowly recover once treatment is stopped. They are used to treat leukaemia and various cancers (e.g. of the breast and lungs). They include:

etoposide (Vepesid)
vinblastine (Velbe)
vincristine (Oncovin)
vindesine (Eldisine)

Cytotoxic immunosuppressants

Some anti-cancer drugs (cytotoxic drugs) are used to suppress the immune response in patients suffering from autoimmune disease or to prevent rejection of a transplanted organ (e.g. a kidney). They include *azathioprine* (Azamune, Berkaprine, Immunoprin, Imuran) and, occasionally, *chlorambucil* (Leukeran) or *cyclophosphamide* (Endoxana). These drugs are not specific in their actions and they may damage blood-forming cells in the bone marrow, with the result that they may knock out red cell production, causing anaemia, white cell production, causing a reduced resistance to infection, and platelet cells involved in blood clotting, producing a risk of bleeding. Repeated blood counts are necessary in patients receiving these drugs. Because these drugs interfere with the immune response (i.e. they cause immune deficiency) the patient is prone to develop infections by bacteria, fungi or viruses. Azathioprine is metabolized in the body to mercaptopurine (see earlier), and doses should be reduced if treatment with allopurinol (to reduce the blood uric acid level) is also given. Azathioprine may also damage the liver.

An important drug used to suppress immunity is cyclosporin (Sandimmun). It inhibits the multiplication of T-lymphocytes and is discussed in Chapter 9.

Other anti-cancer drugs

These are listed below, with some of their specific harmful effects which may occur *in addition* to those discussed earlier.

Amsacrine (Amsidine) is similar to doxorubicin. It may cause a fall in blood potassium levels, producing serious disorders of heart rhythm.

Carboplatin (Paraplatin) is related to cisplatin; it is less harmful to the kidneys, hearing and nerves but more harmful to the bone marrow. It produces less nausea and vomiting. A course of treatment should not be repeated within 4 weeks.

Cisplatin (Neoplatin, Platinex) is a platinum drug with an alkylating action. It may damage the kidneys, hearing and nerves, and cause a fall in blood magnesium levels.

Dacarbazine (DTIC-Dome) It is not known how this drug works. It produces severe nausea and vomiting. It may infrequently cause flu-like symptoms after large single doses about 7 days after treatment. These symptoms last 7–21 days and may recur with subsequent treatments. Rarely, it may cause liver damage.

Hydroxyurea (Hydrea) probably works by interfering with the synthesis of DNA. Very rarely, it may cause disorientation, hallucinations and convulsions, kidney damage and impaired liver function.

Mitozantrone (Novantrone) It is not fully understood how this works. It may, rarely, damage the heart and colour the urine blue–green for 24 hours after a dose. Very rarely, it may cause a transient blueness of the whites of the eyes.

Interferons used to treat cancer

Preparations of interferons include Intron A, Roferon-A and Wellferon.

In 1957 it was discovered that cells infected with a virus produce a substance that protects other cells from infection with that virus. These substances (highly active glycoproteins) are known as interferons. They act on the surface of cells, causing the cell to produce proteins that protect the cell against damage fom viruses.

Interferons act specifically on cells from a specific animal; for example, mouse interferon is inactive in human cells. There are three major types of human interferon and they are standardized by their ability to reduce the replication of viruses in tissue culture – 1 unit of interferon is roughly the amount that reduces virus replications in tissue culture by half. The three sources of interferon are human white blood cells, fibroblasts and lymphocytes.

Interferon has been tried in the prevention of certain virus infections: for example, herpes simplex (cold sores), influenza, viral infections of the eyes and herpes zoster (shingles). Some of the results are encouraging but there is need for much more research.

In the treatment of cancer, interferon has been shown to be of benefit in some experimental tumours in mice but we need more well controlled studies of the effects of interferon in human cancer. Interferons possess actions which obviously could have a beneficial effect. They stop replication of DNA and RNA tumour viruses; they have been shown to inhibit growth of cancer cells; they increase the activity of protective white cells (phagocytosis) and increase the effects of killer-cells – both activities leading to destruction of cancer cells; they also affect the immune system by inhibiting (and increasing in some cases) antibody production, and therefore may be able to reduce the number of cancer-protecting antibodies that are known to block the body's natural immune response to cancers. However, the usefulness of interferons in treating cancer remains unestablished.

Sex hormones and antagonists used to treat cancer

Certain cancers of the breast and prostate may require sex hormones for their continued growth, and the use of drugs that act against them, reduce their production or block their effects may produce beneficial effects.

Breast cancers dependent on oestrogens (female sex hormones)

Some breast cancers and their secondary deposits require oestrogen for their continued growth, and a drug such as tamoxifen (Emblon, Noltam, Nolvadex, Tamofen) which blocks oestrogen receptors in the body can produce very beneficial effects in some women. It offers an effective alternative to removal of the ovaries in pre-menopausal women and is a very effective treatment in post-menopausal women who suffer from oestrogen-dependent cancer of the breast.

A progestogen may be added to the treatment in pre-menopausal women who have had their ovaries removed, and in post-menopausal women.

Despite removal of the ovaries or the use of a drug such as tamoxifen (which blocks the effects of oestrogens), some oestrogen is still made in the body from male sex hormones produced by the adrenal glands. Removal of the adrenal glands was used in the past to prevent this extra production of oestrogen in women with oestrogen-dependent breast cancer but this treatment has now been replaced by the use of aminoglutethimide (Orimeten) which successfully blocks the conversion of male sex hormones to oestrogens in the tissues of the body. However, because it also blocks the production of corticosteroids by the adrenal glands, it is necessary to give additional treatment with a corticosteroid.

Prostate cancer dependent on androgens (male sex hormones) (U)

Cancer of the prostate gland relies on male hormones for its growth. Treatment of the primary cancer and any secondaries may be helped by removal of the testes, which produce most of the male sex hormone (testosterone) in the body.

An alternative to castration is to use a drug that stimulates the pituitary gland to increase its production of the hormone gonadotrophin, which then over-stimulates the testes to produce the male sex hormone testosterone. This causes the concentration of testosterone in the blood to rise to a peak which then switches off the production of gonadotrophin by the pituitary. The result is that the testes stop producing testosterone. Two such drugs are available: *buserelin* (Suprefact) and *goserelin* (Zoladex). These are hormones that stimulate the pituitary gland to secrete gonadotrophin.

After castration or the use of buserelin or goserelin, aminoglutethimide may be used to knock out any production of male sex hormone by the adrenal glands, and corticosteroids will need to be given as a supplement.

Other treatments of cancer of the prostate gland include the use of an oestrogen (female sex hormone) to counter the effects of the male sex hormone in the body. These include ethinyloestradiol, fosfestrol (Honvan), stilboestrol and polyestradiol (Estradurin) which is long acting.

Thyroid cancers dependent on thyroid stimulation

Some cancers of the thyroid gland rely on thyroid-stimulating hormone produced by the pituitary gland. The production of this hormone is determined by the level of thyroid hormone (thyroxine) in the blood stream. If this is high the production is reduced, and vice versa. Therefore one treatment of thyroid cancer involves testing to see whether it is sensitive to thyroid-stimulating hormone. If it is, the patient is given thyroid hormone, which depresses the production of the thyroid-stimulating hormone by the pituitary gland.

Table 76.1 Hormones and antagonists used to treat cancer – harmful effects and warnings

Oestrogens (stilboestrol; fosfestrol: Honvan; ethinyloestradiol; polyestradiol: Estradurin)
See Chapter 66

Progestogens (gestronol: Depostat; medroxyprogesterone: Depo-Provera, Farlutal, Provera; megestrol: Megace; norethisterone: Primolut N, Utovlan, SH420)
See Chapter 66

Androgens and anabolic steroids (drostanolone: Masteril; nandrolone: Deca-Durabolin, Durabolin)
See Chapters 72 and 73

aminoglutethimide (Orimeten)
Harmful effects Transient dizziness, sleepiness, lethargy, unsteadiness, nausea, vomiting and diarrhoea may occur at start of treatment and usually clear up after 6–8 weeks. They are related to the dose used. Drug rash with fever may occur after 7–14 days and usually clears up after 7–10 days despite continuing with treatment; if it does not clear up, the dose should be reduced or stopped temporarily and the dose of corticosteroid increased. Blood disorders and reduced thyroid function may occur.

Warnings In some people, aminoglutethimide may suppress the production of aldosterone and cause a fall in blood sodium and a rise in blood potassium, and a fall in blood pressure resulting in dizziness. If this happens the patient should be given mineralo-corticosteroid replacement treatment (e.g. fludrocortisone daily or on alternate days). The individual's blood count and blood chemistry should be checked at regular intervals while on treatment. The response of the patient to stress may be impaired. The drug may increase the breakdown of oral anti-coagulant drugs, anti-diabetic drugs and synthetic corticosteroids.

buserelin (Suprefact)
Harmful effects include hot flushes, reduced libido, transient irritation of the nose following nasal application and allergic reactions.

Warnings Buserelin should not be used in people who are allergic to it or to benzyl alcohol. Testosterone levels in the blood should be monitored and the dose adjusted accordingly. Improvement will not occur until 'chemical castration' has been achieved. The patient may get worse at the start of treatment. This flare-up can be prevented by adding an anti-androgen (e.g. cyproterone) for the first 3 weeks of treatment.

cyproterone acetate (Cyprostat)
Harmful effects include fatigue, tiredness, changes in body weight (up or down), enlargement of the breasts with milk production and occasionally nodules in the breasts, dryness of the skin and patchy loss of hair, anaemia, reduction of adrenal function in children, changes in blood sugar levels which may affect control of diabetes, worsening of mental depression, recurrence of thrombosis in patients with a history of thrombophlebitis, reduced sperm count and reduced amount of fluid in ejaculation, infertility and some shrinking of the testes; abnormal sperm may produce abnormalities in any babies that are conceived. It may affect liver function, and long-term use may cause anaemia.

Warnings Cyproterone should be used with caution in individuals with liver disease. Tests of liver function and blood counts should be carried out before and at regular intervals during treatment. It should not be used in anyone with severe mental depression, and used with utmost caution in patients who have had a previous thrombosis with embolism.

goserelin (Zoladex)
Harmful effecs include hot flushes, swelling and tenderness of the breasts, skin rashes and decreased libido.

Warnings Goserelin should be used with caution in patients with blockage of the outlets from the kidneys (ureters) or with

Table 76.1 Hormones and antagonists used to treat cancer – harmful effects and warnings (*cont.*)

compression of the spinal cord. The initial disorder may get worse at the start of treatment; this flare-up can be prevented by adding an anti-androgen (e.g. cyproterone) for the first 3 weeks of treatment.

tamoxifen (Noltam, Nolvadex, Tamofen)
Harmful effects are generally mild; they include hot flushes, nausea, a fall in white blood cells and a fall in platelets. Occasionally, it may cause skin rash, vaginal bleeding, itching of the vagina, stomach and bowel upsets, dizziness, light-headedness and fluid retention (e.g. ankle swelling). Thrombosis of a deep vein may occur very rarely with high doses, which may also cause blurred vision due to damage to the retina and/or cornea, especially if high doses are continued for a long period of time. Patients with secondary cancer in bone may experience more pain, sometimes associated with a rise in blood calcium levels.

Warnings Before treatment for breast cancer or infertility pre-menopausal women should be carefully examined in order to ensure that they are not pregnant. Some pre-menopausal women treated for breast cancer may lose their periods and in these women there is a risk of swelling of the ovaries due to cysts. This is reversible and occurs at a dose of 40 mg twice daily.

77

How to use drug treatments effectively and safely

At least two out of every five people do not take a prescribed drug as directed; they miss out one or more doses each day, or one or more days' treatment each week; some may not even get their prescription dispensed from a pharmacy and some may stop a course of treatment before it is completed. They may not take a drug as directed because they forget, their symptoms clear up, they do not believe in the treatment, or for many other reasons.

Failure to take a course of drugs as directed is referred to as *non-compliance* and it is a principal cause of failed treatments. Non-compliance may not matter with some short-term treatments such as cold remedies but it is important with others; for example, it is absolutely necessary to take and complete a short-term course of antibiotics for an infection – provided of course that the antibiotic was prescribed to treat a bacterial infection and not a virus infection which does not need antibiotic treatment. Similarly with long-term treatments, non-compliance may not matter; for example, in the treatment of rheumatic disorders with non-steroidal anti-inflammatory drugs (NSAIDs). These drugs relieve pain and swelling in the affected joints but they do not affect the progress of the underlying disorder. However, with some long-term treatments, failure to take just one dose could be dangerous; for example, insulin treatment in diabetes.

There is evidence that patients who have good relationships with their doctors and who understand their treatments are more likely to take their drug treatments as directed. Therefore, if it is important for you to take a drug treatment as directed, your doctor could help by explaining to you the nature of your disorder and why you have to take the treatment, the expected benefits or possible risks of the treatment and the consequences if no treatment is given. It will also help if the doctor prescribes drug treatments only when necessary and tries to avoid too many drug treatments at the same time (often referred to as poly-pharmacy). The latter occurs more often with elderly patients.

Several different drug treatments at the same time will involve you in having to remember to take different drugs – often at different times of the day, which may be very confusing. Furthermore, similar shaped tablets or similar coloured tablets (e.g. green or blue) may add to the confusion, particularly if your eyesight is impaired. Your doctor may therefore provide further help by considering the shape and colour of tablets and capsules and by prescribing as simple a treatment schedule as possible. For example, you may find it easier to remember to take one long-acting preparation daily than one ordinary tablet three times a day. It may also help you if the times for taking the drug fit in with your daily routine; for example, at meal-times.

How to use drug treatments effectively and safely

Before being prescribed a drug by a doctor

- Tell your doctor of any other drugs you are taking, whether prescribed or bought over the counter from a pharmacy, drug store, herbalist, health food shop or any other outlet
- Tell your doctor if you are pregnant (or trying to get pregnant) or are breast feeding
- Tell your doctor if you suffer from any allergies and particularly if you have suffered from an allergic reaction to a drug in the past
- Tell your doctor about any disorder you may be suffering from, particularly kidney or liver disease, which may affect your response to drug treatment (see page 1079)

Before being dispensed a prescription drug and/or before purchasing a drug over the counter

- Inform your pharmacist of any other drug you are taking, whether prescribed or bought over-the-counter from a pharmacy, drug store, herbalist, health food shop or any other outlet
- Inform your pharmacist if you are pregnant (or trying to get pregnant) or are breast feeding
- If you have difficulty opening child-resistant containers, ask the pharmacist to put your drug into an easy-to-open container

Before taking a drug

You should know why you have to take the drug

You should know what is wrong with you and what are the expected benefits and possible risks of drug treatment compared with no treatment.

You should know the names of the drug(s) you are taking

It would help if all patients on regular daily treatment carried a drug treatment card with them at all times.

Make sure that you always receive the same brand preparation of a drug as you had previously.

You should know what times to take the drug

You should be absolutely clear about whether a drug should be taken at intervals in the day-time (e.g. three times daily) or at equal intervals throughout the day and night (e.g. three times in 24 hours – i.e. every 8 hours). The latter timing is very important with certain drugs; for example, antibiotics. In order to avoid waking in the night you should also know whether you can double the bed-time dose and then take the next dose the first thing in the morning.

You should be absolutely clear about the meaning of 'take as before', 'take when necessary', 'take as required'; and you should know the maximum daily dose above which you should not go – check with your pharmacist.

You should know how to take the drug

All drugs to be taken by mouth should be swallowed with a non-alcoholic drink at meal-times, because, if nothing else, it may help you to remember to take your drug as directed.

Any drug that may damage the lining of the stomach and produce pain, indigestion, ulceration and/or bleeding (e.g. aspirin, anti-rheumatic drugs) should be taken *with* food or *just after* food.

Drugs that should *not* be taken with meals because their absorption from the stomach into the bloodstream may be affected include isoniazid, rifampicin, tetracycline antibiotics (except doxycycline and minocycline), narrow-spectrum antibiotics (e.g. penicillin V) and some oral anti-diabetic drugs. They should be taken between meals.

Drugs that may interact with each other in the stomach should be taken 2 hours apart; for example, tetracycline antibiotics and antacids.

Ask your pharmacist for a special instruction leaflet on how to take the following preparations:

- Liquids by mouth
- Tablets to dissolve in the mouth or under the tongue
- Applications to be applied to the eyes, ears or nose
- Inhalers (sprays, aerosols, nebulizers, etc.)
- Skin applications

- Rectal suppositories and applications
- Vaginal pessaries and applications

Warnings ***Enteric-coated*** *tablets have a special coating that protects the drug from acid in the stomach and the drug is not released until it enters the intestine. This is important with drugs whose effect may be reduced by acid. These enteric-coated tablets should not be sucked or chewed, but swallowed whole with a non-alcoholic drink. Any alkali may damage the acid-resistant coating, so they should not be taken with indigestion mixtures or with milk.*

Sustained-release *(prolonged-release) tablets or capsules are prepared so that their effects last over a prolonged period of time, which reduces the number of doses that have to be taken each day. They should not be sucked, crushed or chewed, but swallowed whole with a cupful of non-alcoholic fluid.*

NOTE *They may contain enough drug for two or three standard doses and so they could be harmful if they were chewed and released all their drug in one go.*

Tablets to be dissolved *in the mouth or under the tongue should not be swallowed or chewed.*

Chewable tablets *should be chewed into little pieces and swallowed with a cupful of non-alcoholic fluid. Chewable tablets that are acidic may cause dental decay (e.g. chewable vitamin C tablets).*

To avoid damaging the oesophagus *(gullet) you should always sit straight up (or, better still, stand up) to swallow any tablet or capsule that may irritate the lining, and you should take them with a full cup of a non-alcoholic fluid no later than half an hour before you go to bed.*

You should not take certain drugs with milk *(e.g. tetracycline antibiotics) because the calcium in the milk may form a compound (chelate) with the drug that will prevent it from being absorbed from the stomach into the bloodstream. Take them 2 hours apart.*

Some acidic fruit juices *(e.g. grapefruit juice, orange juice) may interfere with the absorption of certain antibiotics (e.g. penicillin G). Take them 1 hour apart.*

You should know whether you can drink alcohol whilst taking a drug

Read Chapter 87.

You should know whether you can drive a motor vehicle

Read Chapter 88.

NOTE If you are advised that a drug may affect your driving, this may also mean that you should not engage in hazardous work or hazardous sports, operate moving machinery, fly an aeroplane or carry out any activity that may put your life or the life of others at risk. Always take advice from your doctor and/or pharmacist.

You should know when and how to stop taking a drug

You should know whether you have to complete a course of treatment as directed (e.g. antibiotics) or whether you can stop the drug when you feel better (e.g. pain relievers).

Do not stop a course of antibiotics just because your symptoms have cleared up; complete the whole course in order to prevent a flare-up of the bacterial infection and/or the emergence of resistant bacteria.

With many daily treatments that continue for more than a few weeks or months you should stop the treatment *slowly* by reducing the daily dose gradually over several days to several weeks.

It may be *dangerous* to stop certain drugs suddenly; for example, corticosteroids and beta blockers. Drugs that can produce addiction (such as sleeping drugs and anti-anxiety drugs) should also be stopped slowly.

Stopping a drug suddenly may also cause a severe flare-up of your disorder or cause it to recur, sometimes worse than it was before treatment was started.

If you develop any new symptoms while taking a drug, check with your pharmacist or doctor whether the symptoms could be due to the drug(s) you are taking and seek advice on whether you should continue to take the drug as directed, reduce the dosage and stop the drug slowly over several days or stop the drug immediately.

Read Chapter 78 on harmful drug effects and what to do if you develop them. For example, if you develop symptoms of allergy (e.g. nettle rash and wheezing), you should immediately stop the drug and contact your doctor. However, most harmful drug effects are related to the dose and may easily be stopped or reduced if the strength of each dose is reduced and/or if the number of doses each day is reduced by extending the times between each dose.

You should know what to do if you miss a dose

This may be of little consequence with drugs that are prescribed to reduce a symptom (e.g. pain, nausea), but with certain diseases, to miss a single dose may be very serious; for example, insulin treatment of diabetes.

You must know whether you can take a missed dose as soon as you remember and how close to the next dose you can take it, or whether you can miss it out and double the next dose. The latter may be possible with a drug that has a wide margin of safety between its effective dose and the dose that will produce harmful effects (e.g. penicillins), but with drugs that have a narrow margin of safety (e.g. anti-cancer drugs) it could be dangerous to double a dose and produce an excessive rise in the concentration of the drug in the blood.

With oral contraceptives it is important that you should know exactly what to do if you miss a dose.

You should know what to do if you are taking more than one course of treatment

You should know what to do with regard to each drug treatment, and you should know whether you can take the different drugs together at one time or whether you should take them separately; for example, you should take a tetracycline antibiotic and an antacid at least 2 hours apart.

You should know the risks if two drugs interact with each other (see drug–drug interactions, Chapter 89) or if a drug could interact with chemicals in certain foods.

NOTE the risk of chemicals in certain foods interacting with MAOI antidepressant drugs (see Chapter 39).

NOTE that alcohol may interact with a large number of drugs and have its effects increased (see Chapter 87).

NOTE that calcium in milk, yoghurt and cheese can bind to tetracycline antibiotics to form a compound (a chelate) that is insoluble and prevents the tetracycline from being absorbed into the bloodstream; this will reduce its effectiveness.

You should know whether you should be on a special diet

Sometimes it is important to eat or to avoid certain foods if you are taking a certain drug. For example, it may help to eat foods high in potassium if you are taking loop or thiazide diuretics (water tablets) regularly every day because these drugs increase the loss of potassium in the urine. A diet low in purines may help some patients being treated for gout, and of course diabetic patients should avoid excessive use of refined sugars.

Always check with your doctor or pharmacist whether it is necessary to change your diet if you are on long-term drug treatment.

You should not continue obtaining repeat prescriptions without having medical check-ups at regular intervals

You should try to avoid the habit of regularly obtaining repeat prescriptions without seeing your doctor. This may be convenient for you but it denies your doctor the opportunity to examine you to assess your progress and to decide whether you are benefiting from the treatment or whether you are developing any harmful effects. It will help him or her to decide whether to stop, reduce or change your treatment.

With certain drugs it may be necessary for you to have regular blood tests, tests on your heart, liver function tests, breathing tests and/or kidney function tests. Depending on your treatment, you may also need special check-ups on your eyes, ears or skin. To go on picking up repeat prescriptions without having these examinations could result in serious problems.

You should know not to exceed the stated dose of a drug, and the consequences if you do

To exceed the stated dose of a drug may not necessarily increase its beneficial effects but it may increase its harmful effects. This is particularly true of drugs that have a narrow margin of safety between the effective dose and the dose that produces harmful effects.

Some drugs may produce tolerance in which you find yourself having to increase the dose of a drug in order to achieve the same level of effect that was produced initially – this may have particularly dangerous consequences with drugs that may produce addiction (e.g. sleeping drugs or anti-anxiety drugs).

Some drugs are not broken down and excreted quickly, and they or their active breakdown products may stay in the body for many hours, days or even weeks; if an increased daily dose is taken this will add to the amount of drug already in the body, pushing it up to a toxic level. The harmful effects produced by this toxic level of drug in the body may not always appear straight away but may develop slowly over several days. This is particularly dangerous with any drug that affects the brain because drowsiness, intoxication and confusion may gradually develop which, in elderly people, may be put down to their age or, even worse, to senile dementia.

NOTE Drugs given in 'standard' doses may accumulate in the body, to reach toxic levels if their rate of breakdown is slowed down by impaired liver function or their rate of excretion by the kidneys is slowed down due to impaired kidney function. This is why drugs should be used with caution in patients with impaired kidney or liver function and in elderly people whose kidney or liver function may be impaired because of their age; they will require reduced dosages.

You should know when and how to dispose of drugs

Do not hoard drugs. You should dispose of unwanted drugs or expired drugs (see later) by flushing them down the toilet or, preferably, returning them to your pharmacist.

You should know how to store drugs

Keep all drugs in their original containers with their labels intact.

Keep the lid or cap on tightly in order to prevent the drug preparation from deteriorating.

Do not store drugs in a bathroom cabinet – it is too warm and moist. They should be kept in a cool, dry place away from direct sunlight, and well out of the reach of children.

NOTE Some drugs have to be kept in a refrigerator (see warning label).

You should know the expiry date of your drug preparation

Expiry dates are estimates of the ageing of a drug preparation. Exposure to air, moisture, heat or sunlight may cause:

- A deterioration of the drug which may result in a reduced amount of active drug in the preparation
- A chemical change, which may make the drug or some constituent of the drug preparation more toxic
- A change in the rate at which a drug preparation dissolves, to release the active drug once it has entered the stomach

In general, tablets and capsules are more stable than liquid preparations to be taken by mouth or solutions for injection.

You should know what to do if you are taking a drug by mouth and you develop vomiting and/or diarrhoea

Vomiting and/or diarrhoea may reduce the amount of drug that you absorb into the bloodstream. This reduced absorption may make your treatment less effective, for example; find out what to do if you are taking an oral contraceptive and you develop vomiting and/or diarrhoea.

You should know that certain drugs may affect the results of laboratory blood tests

Some drugs can interfere with results of laboratory tests, giving either a false negative or a false positive reading. Before being sent for a blood test you must tell your doctor of any drugs you are taking, whether prescribed or bought over the counter from a pharmacy, drug store, herbalist, health food shop or other outlet.

You should know that you can become allergic to various additives in drug preparations

Drug preparations contain many additives, including colouring agents to which certain people may become allergic. *Tartrazine* is a colouring agent used to give food and drug preparations a yellowish colour (but it may also be included in turquoise, green and maroon colours). A small number of individuals are allergic to tartrazine and when exposed to it they may develop nettle rash; patchy swelling of the skin, lips and mouth (angioedema); runny nose and wheezing.

Allergy to tartrazine is more often seen in people who are allergic to aspirin and it should be noted that anyone who is allergic to aspirin may also be allergic to other non-steroidal anti-inflammatory drugs (NSAIDs) used to treat rheumatic disorders.

Other additives include:

- *Diluents* (e.g. lactose, starch, dextrose) to add bulk in order to make a capsule or tablet larger
- *Disintegrants* (e.g. starch) to speed up the rate at which a drug dissolves in the stomach
- *Special coatings* to improve its taste and colour and to protect it from the light, moisture and air (see also 'enteric coatings' earlier)
- *Preservatives*

Some special warnings

Mouth and gum preparations

After applying a drug preparation to the gums or inside the mouth, spit any excess out – if you swallow it, the drug may be absorbed into your bloodstream and produce harmful effects.

NOTE Babies and infants cannot spit, so it is safer not to use preparations to be applied to the mouth or gums of babies and infants (e.g. teething preparations).

Nose drops

Nose drops may run down the back of the throat and down the cheeks on to the lips and be licked off. This may lead to excessive absorption of the drug into the bloodstream and harmful effects.

Ear drops

Ear drops that are too cold or too warm may produce vertigo. You should warm the container in the palms of the hands for a few minutes.

Eye drops

Eye drops may run down the nose and down the cheeks on to the lips and be licked off. This may lead to excessive absorption into the bloodstream and produce harmful effects; this may be particularly dangerous in infants and young children.

Children

Keep all drugs out of reach of children.

Before giving a drug to a child always check the dose on the label.

Do not give children under the age of 12 years any preparation that contains aspirin.

Do not give any drug to a child under the age of 5 years without seeking advice from your doctor or pharmacist.

Some harmful drug effects and what to do if you develop them

Harmful drug effects can affect any tissue or organ in the body. In this chapter I list some examples of the organs and tissues that may be affected, and under each example are listed some of the drugs that may produce these effects. I also provide some simple advice on what to do if you develop symptoms that could be caused by the drug or drugs you are taking.

Remember that most people do not experience harmful effects from drugs and that most harmful effects are mild and usually related to the dose. Reducing the dose will nearly always clear up the trouble. These harmful effects are basically an exaggeration of the drug's effects, and they can very easily be *predicted* and *prevented* by treatment being tailored to your own needs and responses, particularly if you may be vulnerable to harmful drug effects; for example, if you are elderly.

With regard to *unexpected* harmful effects, we learn about these over time. We have a good source of information about unexpected harmful effects from established drugs and we are learning all the time about unexpected reactions from new drugs. (Note the importance of reporting any new symptom if you are receiving drug treatment.)

With established drugs we know what can happen in some people and we know that these unexpected reactions are rare but can be serious. We also know which types of patients are more likely to develop these reactions, and so we should also be able to predict and prevent many so-called 'unexpected' harmful effects.

Spotting the early signs

A part of being able to prevent unexpected (and often serious) harmful effects is being able to recognize the very earliest signs and symptoms that something is going wrong. It is therefore very important that you seek advice straight away for any 'new' symptoms that develop while you are taking a drug. For example, a sore throat may be the very earliest sign that your white blood cell production in the bone marrow is being affected by a drug and prompt action (stopping the drug, a full blood count and appropriate treatment) could stop this serious harmful effect before it has gone too far.

Warning *Always consult your doctor to check whether any new symptom that you develop is being caused by the drug or drugs that you are taking, or if the symptoms for which you are being treated get worse. If you are taking a drug preparation that has only recently been introduced on to the market, report any new symptom or medical event (e.g. a fall resulting in a fractured wrist) to your doctor who should report it straight away to a centre that monitors harmful drug effects. This centre will then be able to spot whether a new drug is beginning to cause problems and to issue warnings to doctors.*

The importance of warnings on drug use

There is no doubt that there could be a significant reduction in the extent and severity of harmful effects to drugs if we noted and acted upon the warnings on their use. I have listed the important warnings under the various drug groups and individual drugs, and you should make yourself familiar with these warnings for the particular drug or drugs you are taking. Also note that one drug may interact with another, to produce harmful effects, so do not take drugs unnecessarily and always check with your pharmacist whether it is safe to take any drug with another – an obvious example and a potentially dangerous one is the use of alcohol with any drug that depresses the activity of the brain. Likewise you should always check whether it is safe to drink alcohol or engage in hazardous occupation or sport if you are taking a drug or drugs.

Tell your doctor

Before being prescribed any drug, advise the doctor of your age (drugs are more harmful if you are elderly), whether you are pregnant or breast feeding, whether you suffer from allergies, whether you have previously had an allergic reaction to a drug, whether you have a genetic disorder, liver or kidney disease, heart trouble or a circulatory disorder, whether you have chest trouble, gout, diabetes or any disease other than the one the treatment is for.

Ask your pharmacist

Ask your pharmacist about any potential drug interactions and whether you can drink alcohol with the drug you have been prescribed or have just purchased. Also ask if you can drive a motor vehicle or engage in a hazardous occupation or sport (e.g. working up ladders, mountain climbing).

In addition, ask your pharmacist for a leaflet that explains how to use the drug preparation effectively and safely. This is particularly important with drug applications to be applied to the eyes, nose or ears, to be inhaled or applied up the anus or vagina.

NOTE Many elderly people are at a disadvantage because their prescriptions are picked up by relatives or friends or, if they are in a home, by the warden or a member of staff. An additional problem is that many prescriptions to elderly people are repeats and may carry vague instructions such as 'take as before'. Elderly people are also likely to be on complicated schedules which involve taking several different drugs at different times of the day.

If you are elderly or if you look after an elderly person, consult with the prescribing doctor to check whether the treatment could be made more simple in terms of the number of doses and the times for taking them. Also consult your pharmacist about preparing clear labels on how and when to take the drugs and a clear indication what each drug is for.

Some common harmful drug effects

Allergic reactions

Allergy is discussed in Chapter 10. Whether you develop an allergic reaction to a drug depends principally on the drug and upon your own predisposition to develop allergic reactions.

The chemical make-up of a drug preparation will affect its potential for causing allergic reactions in some people, as will the way you take it (e.g. applied to the skin, eyes or nose, or taken by mouth or by injection). Your own predisposition to develop an allergic reaction to a drug depends upon many factors; for example, you are more prone to develop an allergic reaction to a drug if you suffer from eczema, asthma or hayfever, and especially if you have previously suffered from an allergic reaction to any other drug. Other factors may include your age, sex and nutrition.

Allergic reactions most frequently cause skin rashes, and different drugs cause different types of skin rash (Chapter 75). Fever is a common allergic reaction, as is swelling of patches of the skin, lips and mouth (angio-oedema). Serum sickness is caused by some drugs, particularly antibiotics and antisera. The main symptoms are fever, nettle rash, painful joints, swollen glands, wheezing and patchy swellings of the skin. Severe allergic reactions are referred to as *anaphylactic* reactions and they are discussed in Chapter 10. They may cause nettle rash, swelling of the throat, wheezing and collapse due to a sudden fall in blood pressure. Allergic reactions may also cause blood disorders, liver damage, damage to the walls of blood vessels, asthma and kidney damage.

Advice *At the first sign of a skin rash, wheezing, fever or any other 'new' symptom, consult your doctor to see whether you should stop the drug immediately. Be especially cautious if you have ever suffered from a previous allergic reaction to a drug, particularly if you have asthma. Drugs from the same group may be particularly dangerous – for example, if you are allergic to one penicillin you may be allergic to other penicillins and to cephalosporins. If you are allergic to aspirin or to the orange dye tartrazine in foods and drink, you may be allergic to non-steroidal anti-inflammatory drugs (NSAIDs) used to treat rheumatoid arthritis and rheumatic disorders (Chapter 30).*

Bleeding

High doses of anti-coagulants (anti-blood-clotting drugs) may cause bleeding. The early signs may be bruising, nose bleeds, bleeding gums and blood in the urine.

Advice *If you are taking anti-coagulant drugs always carry a warning card with you and consult your doctor immediately if you develop bruising or bleeding. You will need a blood clotting test and the dose of your drug changed and/or an antidote. Always check whether you have taken any other drug that may increase the effects of the anti-coagulant you are taking (see Chapter 89).*

NOTE Any drug that damages the bone marrow may knock out blood platelets, which will cause bruising, little red spots on the skin (petechiae) and bleeding (e.g. nose bleeds, bleeding gums) – see 'Blood disorders', later.

Blood cholesterol and fat levels

Combined oral contraceptives ('the pill') may cause a rise in blood cholesterol and fats in some women.

Advice *If you have a raised level of cholesterol and/or fat in the blood, you* *should be most cautious about using the pill, particularly those containing a high dose of oestrogen.*

Blood disorders

Some drugs may, rarely, damage the bone marrow and interfere with the production of red blood cells, white blood cells and/or platelets. The production of all three groups of cells may be damaged or a drug may just damage one group (e.g. the red blood cells, causing anaemia). Drugs may also damage red blood cells in the circulation and cause them to burst (haemolysis), producing what is called haemolytic anaemia. They may also damage the oxygen-carrying red pigment (haemoglobin) in red blood cells.

When a drug damages the bone marrow and knocks out the production of all cells, it is called *aplastic anaemia*. This causes anaemia because of a lack of red blood cells, a lowered resistance to infection because of a lack of white blood cells, and a tendency to bleed and bruise easily (purpura) due to a lack of platelets. Some drugs may cause aplastic anaemia and, although it is *very rare*, it is important to be aware of the risk. The blood disorder may come on suddenly or slowly over several weeks or months.

Drugs that may, very rarely, damage the bone marrow and cause blood disorders include some anti-bacterial drugs (e.g. chloramphenicol, sulphonamides), anti-epileptic drugs (e.g. carbamazepine, primidone), antihistamines (e.g. chlorpheniramine), anti-malarial drugs (e.g. chloroquine, pyrimethamine), anti-arrhythmic drugs (e.g. procainamide, quinidine), anti-cancer drugs, diuretics (e.g. acetazolamide, chlorothiazide), anti-anxiety drugs (e.g. meprobamate), anti-psychotic drugs (phenothiazines), anti-diabetic drugs (sulphonylureas; e.g. chlorpropamide, tolbutamide).

Advice *With drugs known to cause aplastic anaemia, regular blood tests to check for damage to blood cell production are useful but it is also important to look for early symptoms. If you start to look pale, feel weak and tired, dizzy, develop palpitations and become breathless on exertion, your red cell production may be affected; if you develop a sore throat, fever or chills, your white cell production may be affected; and if you develop little red spots on your skin (petechiae), bruise easily and/or develop nose bleeds, bleeding gums, heavy menstrual periods or blood in your motions, your platelet production may be affected. At the* ***earliest*** *indication of any trouble, consult your doctor immediately to check whether the drug you are taking might cause the problems. If it could, the drug should be stopped immediately and a full blood test carried out.*

Very rarely, a drug may specifically damage red cell production, causing anaemia. This is referred to as *red cell aplasia* and it may possibly be caused by gold used to treat rheumatoid arthritis or by azathioprine (an immuno-suppressant drug).

Advice *If you develop paleness, tiredness, dizziness, palpitations, breathlessness on exertion or any new symptom, consult your doctor to check whether a drug you are taking could be causing the symptoms. If it could, the drug should be stopped straight away and a full blood test carried out.*

Specific damage to white blood cells is more common but is very rare considering the millions of drugs used every day. It is called *agranulocytosis* and appears to be caused by direct allergic damage to white blood cells in the circulation and by damage to white cell production in the bone marrow. Examples of drugs that may, very rarely, produce allergic damage to circulating white blood cells include sulphonamides, sulphonylurea anti-diabetic drugs, some anti-psychotic drugs, some anti-thyroid drugs, phenylbutazone, and quinidine used to treat disorders of heart rhythm. Anti-psychotic drugs (e.g. phenothiazines) may, very rarely, knock out white blood cell production by the bone marrow. This risk is increased in elderly patients and when high doses of the drugs are used over long periods of time.

Advice *If you develop a sudden fever, chills and/or a sore throat, consult your doctor immediately to see whether the drug you are taking could cause the problems. If it could, the drug should be stopped straight away and a full blood test carried out.*

Occasionally, a drug may specifically knock out platelet production in the bone marrow, causing a fall in blood platelets (*thrombocytopenia*) causing purpura – widespread red spots on the skin (petechiae), bruising, nose bleeds, bleeding gums, blood in the motions and heavy menstrual periods. Any drug that causes aplastic anaemia (see earlier) may cause thrombocytopenic purpura by damaging the bone marrow. Some drugs may, very rarely, produce allergic damage to platelets in the blood circulation; for example, the diuretic drug acetazolamide used to treat glaucoma, the diuretic drug hydrochlorothiazide used to treat heart failure and raised blood pressure, methyldopa also used to treat raised blood pressure, the anti-bacterial drug rifampicin, sulphonamide drugs and several others. This type of allergy can last for years.

Advice *If you develop pin-sized red spots in the skin, bruise easily, develop nose bleeds, bleeding gums, blood in your motions or heavy menstrual periods, consult your doctor immediately to check whether the drug you are taking could cause the symptoms. You will need a full blood test and bleeding tests.*

Destruction of red blood cells in the circulation (haemolytic anaemia)

This may be a direct 'allergic' type of reaction between the drug and red blood cells, or the drug may damage the function of the red blood cells. The latter is more likely to occur in people with a genetic abnormality of their red blood cells (see glucose-6-phosphate dehydrogenase deficiency, in Chapter 47).

A warning of the 'allergic' type of reaction causing haemolytic anaemia is given in a special test of the blood called Coombe's test. Several drugs may, rarely, cause a positive Coombe's test or frank haemolytic anaemia; they include cephalothin and methyldopa.

Glucose-6-phosphate dehydrogenase (G6PD) deficiency is discussed in Chapters 47 and 85. The main drugs causing damage to the red blood cells in individuals with such a deficiency are anti-malarial drugs such as quinine and pyrimethamine; pain relievers such as aspirin; and anti-bacterial drugs such as the sulphonamides, nitrofurantoin and chloramphenicol. Vitamins C and K may also cause problems.

Advice *If you develop paleness, tiredness, dizziness, breathlessness on exertion, palpitations, yellowness of the skin or eyes or any new symptom, contact your doctor to check whether the symptoms are caused by the drug you are taking and whether you need an immediate full blood test.*

Folic acid deficiency anaemia

Folic acid is a vitamin that is essential for red blood cell production in the bone marrow. Several drugs may interfere with the supply of folic acid to the bone marrow or block its use by the cells in the bone marrow.

Drugs that block its use (folic acid antagonists) include methotrexate, used to treat leukaemia and arthritis associated with psoriasis; pyrimethamine, used to treat malaria; the anti-bacterial drug trimethoprim, which is in co-trimoxazole; and triamterene, a diuretic drug.

Anti-epileptic drugs such as phenytoin, phenobarbitone and primidone may affect the absorption of folic acid from the intestine, its transport in the blood and its use by cells. Impaired absorption of folic acid from the intestine may be caused by sulphasalazine, used to treat ulcerative colitis; and oral contraceptives may possibly interfere with the absorption of folic acid from the intestine.

Advice *Any drug that may cause folic acid deficiency anaemia should be used with caution in someone who suffers from a disorder that may also produce folic acid deficiency; for example, pregnancy, cirrhosis of the liver or a disorder of the intestine that may impair absorption of folic acid (e.g. ulcerative colitis, Crohn's disease). If you develop any symptoms suggestive of anaemia (paleness, weakness* *and tiredness, dizziness, palpitations or breathlessness on exertion), consult your doctor to check whether any drug you are taking could be causing the symptoms. You may need a full blood test.*

Vitamin B_{12} deficiency causing anaemia (see Chapter 47) may be produced by certain drugs that interfere with its absorption into the blood stream from the intestine – for example, the antibiotic neomycin; biguanide anti-diabetic drugs; colchicine, used to treat gout; and possibly oral contraceptives in some women.

Advice *If you find yourself becoming pale, tired and weak, dizzy, develop palpitations and become breathless on exertion, consult your doctor to check whether any drug that you are taking may be causing the symptoms. You may need a full blood test.*

Blood pressure rise

Drugs that produce adrenaline-like effects on the body (sympathomimetic drugs) – for example in nasal decongestants, cold remedies, slimming drugs and anti-asthma drugs – may cause a rise in blood pressure, which may be dangerous in patients with heart disease (e.g. angina). They may also interact with certain drugs used to treat heart failure and angina, and they may interact with MAOI anti-depressants, to cause a severe rise in blood pressure (see dangers of this in Chapter 39).

Advice *If you suffer from heart disease (e.g. angina) or raised blood pressure, avoid – or use with utmost caution –any drug that may produce adrenaline-like effects on the body (see the discussion of sympathomimetic drugs in Chapter 2). If you are taking an MAOI anti-depressant, carry a warning card with you at all times (see Chapter 39).*

Blood pressure fall

A drug may cause a fall in blood pressure: if it depresses the function of the heart (see under Heart) and causes a reduced output of blood from the heart; if it dilates veins, causing blood to pool in the veins and therefore reducing the amount of blood returning to the heart; and if it dilates the arteries, producing a reduction in the resistance to the flow of blood (peripheral resistance) – see control of blood pressure in Chapter 21. Some drugs may produce a combination of these effects.

Drugs that cause a fall in blood pressure by causing dilatation of arteries and/or veins include those used to treat raised blood pressure, angina and heart failure. The blood pressure may fall suddenly in a severe allergic reaction and under a general anaesthetic. Sleeping drugs, sedatives, anti-anxiety drugs, anti-psychotic drugs and anti-depressant drugs may cause a fall in blood pressure.

The symptoms of a sudden fall in blood include dizziness, light-headedness, faintness and fainting.

Standing upright after lying or sitting down normally causes a sharp fall in the return of blood to the heart. This effect is immediately compensated for by reflex actions that correct the output from the heart and adjust the blood pressure. If these reflex actions do not occur, the blood pressure drops and the individual may feel faint and fall to the gound on standing up after lying or sitting down. This effect is called *postural hypotension* or *orthostatic hypertension* (low blood pressure on changing posture). Several drugs may cause postural hypotension by interfering with those reflex actions that normally respond immediately to the fall in the return of blood to the heart on standing up. They include vasodilator drugs used to treat angina and heart failure, and some drugs used to treat raised blood pressure.

Advice *If you find yourself feeling dizzy, light-headed or faint when you stand up after sitting or lying down, consult your doctor to check whether the symptoms are due to the drugs you are taking. See also harmful effects that may cause faint feelings (later).*

Blood sugar levels

A *raised blood sugar* (blood glucose) causing diabetes can occasionally be triggered by corticosteroids, thiazide diuretics and, rarely, by loop diuretics, diazoxide, oestrogens and oral contraceptives. The diabetes appears to develop in people who are susceptible because of some genetic factor (e.g. some near blood relative with diabetes) or in people with latent diabetes who develop a high blood sugar if they have an infection or undergo stress, become pregnant or are overweight.

Advice *If you have a close blood-relative who suffers from diabetes, or if you have produced sugar in your urine in the past (e.g. in pregnancy) then be most cautious about using any drug that may send up your blood sugar and watch out for early signs (see below). If you suffer from diabetes then you may need to use a different drug or increase the dose of your insulin or anti-diabetic drug by mouth.*

If you become thirsty, pass large volumes of urine, feel tired, lack energy, lose weight or develop any new symptoms consult your doctor to check whether the drug you are taking could cause the problems and ask for a urine test and blood test for sugar.

A *low blood glucose* (hypoglycaemia) may be caused by drugs used to treat diabetes (see Chapter 65).

Some drugs increase the blood-glucose-lowering effects of insulin, and drugs used by mouth to treat diabetes. Some beta blockers increase the effects of insulin and they may also mask the symptoms of hypoglycaemia. Clofibrate used to lower blood fat levels can cause a low blood glucose in diabetics taking sulphonylurea anti-diabetic drugs by mouth.

NOTE Alcohol may cause a serious fall in the blood glucose level in some under-nourished people and in diabetic patients on insulin or anti-diabetic drugs by mouth, particularly if they are underweight.

Advice *If you are a diabetic on insulin injections or anti-diabetic drugs by mouth, check with your doctor as to the possible risk of any interactions with alcohol and other drugs which may lower your blood sugar and trigger a hypoglycaemic attack.*

Bones

Osteoporosis is a reduction in the volume of bone, which makes them fragile and prone to fracture (see discussion in Chapter 68). The long-term regular daily use of corticosteroids may cause osteoporosis and fractures; so may the long-term use of the anti-blood-clotting drug heparin.

Interference with vitamin D in the body, causing *bone softening* (*rickets* in children and *osteomalacia* in adults) may occur in patients on long-term treatment with anti-epileptic drugs. The bones may become soft in people who take antacids containing aluminium hydroxide regularly every day for years on end. The aluminium hydroxide reduces the absorption of phosphates from the intestine into the blood stream, and this affects the laying down of calcium phosphate in bones. Bone softening may also be caused by the regular long-term use of laxatives, which may result in an excessive loss of calcium in the stools. Also, laxatives that contain liquid paraffin may interfere with the absorption of vitamin D, which will also cause bone softening.

Advice *If you develop bone pains or tenderness on pressure, muscle weakness (e.g. difficulty walking up stairs), or a fracture following a fall or any other new symptom, consult your doctor to check whether any drug you are taking may have contributed to the problem. You will need tests of your blood chemistry and X-rays of some of your bones.*

NOTE An infant with rickets may be restless, fretful, pale and have flabby muscles. Sweating of the head is common and the abdomen may be distended.

Breasts

Several drugs – for example, the diuretic drug spironolactone, digoxin used to treat heart failure, the male sex hormone testosterone, the anti-fungal drug griseofulvin and the female sex hormone stilboestrol – may occasionally cause the breasts to become enlarged in both males and females. (This is referred to as *gynaecomastia.*) Oestrogens (e.g. in the pill) may also cause the breasts to enlarge.

Several drugs may, rarely, cause milk to come from the breasts in males and females. This is called *galactorrhoea.* Examples include some anti-psychotic drugs (e.g. chlorpromazine, prochlorperazine, trifluoperazine, perphenazine, promazine and haloperidol); the benzodiazepine anti-anxiety drug chlordiazepoxide; the anti-blood-pressure drugs methyldopa and reserpine; the tricyclic anti-depressant drugs imipramine and amitriptyline; the amphetamine drug dexamphetamine; female sex hormones (oestrogens) and oral contraceptives.

Most of the drugs that cause milk production may also cause loss of menstrual periods in women, loss of libido in men, and enlargement of the breasts in both men and women, although it is more obvious in men than in women.

Advice *If you develop any breast enlargement or discomfort of the breasts or start to produce milk, consult your doctor to check whether any drug you are taking may cause the problem. If it does, consider stopping the drug. The problem will clear up in a few weeks after the drug has been stopped.*

Breathing

Some drugs dry up the bronchial tubes and make it *hard to cough up phlegm* e.g. anticholinergic drugs, antihistamine drugs, and tricyclic and cyclic anti-depressants.

Advice *If you suffer from asthma, chronic bronchitis or other chronic chest disorders, these drugs may make it hard for you to cough up phlegm; therefore, be cautious about using them.*

Several drugs may cause *wheezing,* and if you suffer from asthma or chronic bronchitis this may produce serious problems. For example, beta blockers should not be used by patients with asthma.

Advice *If you develop wheezing or your wheezing gets worse, consult your doctor as to whether any drug you are taking could cause the wheezing and, if so, whether you should change to another drug.* NOTE *Beta blockers should not be stopped suddenly (see Chapter 20).*

Acute and sometimes severe wheezing may occur in patients who develop an *allergic reaction to a drug.* Read about the dangers of aspirin and related drugs used to treat rheumatic disorders (Chapter 30), antibiotics (Chapter 48) and antisera (Chapter 11). See also the treatment of acute allergic emergencies (Chapter 10).

Advice *Stop any drug immediately at the first sign of an allergic reaction – itching, skin rash, swelling of the lips, wheezing, faintness; see under Allergic reactions (earlier).*

The infusion of excessive amounts of fluids into a vein may cause 'fluid on the lung' (*pulmonary oedema*).

High doses of morphine and related drugs (Chapter 27) may depress breathing and may be dangerous in patients with chronic chest trouble, as may sleeping drugs and tranquillizers.

Advice *If you suffer from asthma, chronic bronchitis or other chest trouble and your breathing gets worse, consult your doctor to check whether any drug you are taking could make your condition worse.*

Whether you have chest trouble or not and develop any new chest symptoms such as a cough, wheezing, breathlessness or pain in the chest, you should consult your doctor to check whether any drug you are taking may be causing the symptoms.

Cancer

The trouble with proving whether or not a drug causes cancer is that it may take up to 20 years from exposure to a cancer-producing agent to the actual development of a cancer. In addition, other factors in the environment may contribute to the risks; for example radiation in the atmosphere, exposure to industrial chemicals and food additives.

The long-term use of oral contraceptives and the possible but very rare risk of developing cancer of the breast, womb or liver requires further research, as does the risk of using hormone replacement therapy. There is a very rare risk of cancer of the vagina in teenage girls whose mothers took the female sex hormone stilboestrol in the first 3 months of their pregnancy.

Some anti-cancer drugs may, very rarely, cause leukaemia 1–5 years after treatment of a cancer. Ultraviolet irradiation used to treat psoriasis may, rarely, cause skin cancer. However, most claims that particular drugs cause cancer remain unsubstantiated.

Circulation to the arms and legs

Some drugs affect the circulation by causing the arteries to constrict (vasoconstriction), which reduces the blood supply to the tissues. This may produce coldness of the fingers and toes. Very rarely, it may be so severe that it produces pains in the legs on walking, and gangrene of the tips of the fingers and/or toes. The regular long-term use of ergotamine to prevent migraine may, rarely, cause this serious harmful effect (see Chapter 29).

Advice *Consult your doctor at the earliest sign of any circulatory trouble, such as coldness, blueness or tingling in the fingers or toes. Also check with your doctor whether any drug you are taking may be causing the problem (note that cigarette smoking affects the circulation).*

Constipation

Some drugs may cause constipation and this can be a particular problem in elderly people, pregnant women and patients debilitated by a serious illness.

Drugs that commonly cause constipation (see Chapter 17) include narcotic pain relievers (e.g. codeine and morphine), anti-cholinergic drugs, some anti-psychotic drugs (e.g. chlorpromazine) and some tricyclic and cyclic anti-depressant drugs. Indigestion remedies containing aluminium or calcium salts can constipate, as may iron salts.

Advice *If you develop constipation, check with your doctor as to whether it could be caused by any drug you are taking. It may be necessary to stop or change your treatment. If you are severely ill and in pain and need to take morphine or a related drug regularly every day, it may be necessary to give you a laxative as well.*

Diarrhoea

The regular use of laxatives may cause problems, particularly in older people (see Chapter 17).

Drugs that may occasionally cause diarrhoea include anti-bacterial drugs, especially those with a broad spectrum of action. The diarrhoea may be caused by a direct irritant effect on the intestine (e.g. sulphonamides, tetracyclines and, possibly, ampicillin) or it may be caused by disturbing the normal balance of bacteria and fungi in the intestine. This causes what is called a superinfection of the intestine (see Chapter 53) which may be serious because the micro-organism that causes this additional infection is often resistant to the antibiotic being used. Some antibiotics (e.g. clindamycin and lincomycin) may occasionally produce a very serious type of colitis called pseudomembranous colitis (see Chapter 48).

Other drugs that may cause diarrhoea include indigestion remedies containing magnesium salts, some anti-blood-pressure drugs e.g. bethanidine, debrisoquine and methyldopa, and some beta blockers. An overdose of digoxin or a related drug used to treat heart failure may cause diarrhoea; so may iron preparations, the anti-fungal drug flucytosine, and chenodeoxycholic acid used to treat gall stones. Colchicine used to treat acute gout may cause vomiting and diarrhoea. Very rarely, morphine-related drugs may cause diarrhoea rather than constipation, in which case the drug must be stopped.

Advice *If you develop diarrhoea, consult your doctor to check whether any drug you are taking may be causing it.* NOTE *Never self-treat diarrhoea caused by a drug, particularly diarrhoea caused by antibiotics.*

Ears

Some drugs may damage the ears and affect hearing and/or produce noises in the ears and/or dizziness. Particularly dangerous are the aminoglycoside antibiotics (e.g. gentamicin, kanamycin, neomycin, polymyxin, streptomycin). The damage to hearing and balance may occur if any of these drugs is applied locally to an ear that has a perforated ear drum, to wounds, as bladder wash-outs, or taken by mouth or injection. Other potentially harmful drugs inlude the diuretics ethacrynic acid and frusemide. Aspirin and quinine and chloroquine used to treat malaria may cause dizziness and noise in the ears if used in high doses.

Warning *The use of an aminoglycoside antibiotic with the diuretics ethacrynic acid or frusemide increases the risk of damage to hearing and balance.*

The *risk of deafness* from drug treatment is related to the concentration of the drug in the middle ear, which is related to the dose and frequency of dosing, how the drug is given (e.g. applied to the ears, by mouth or by injection) and the rate at which the body gets rid of the drug. The last is important and any defect in the breakdown of a drug by the liver and/or its excretion by the kidneys will cause the concentration of the drug in the blood to reach toxic levels.

Unborn babies are particularly vulnerable to drugs that can cause deafness, taken by their mothers. The greatest damage is done in the first 3 months of pregnancy while the hearing mechanisms are developing.

Advice *If you develop any deterioration in your hearing, hear noises or ringing in your ears and/or develop dizziness or vertigo, check with your doctor immediately as to whether any drug you are taking may damage your hearing or balance.*

Any drug that is known to damage the ears should be used only when absolutely necessary and in the smallest effective dose for the shortest duration of time possible. If you have to take such a drug, you should have your hearing and balance tested before and at regular intervals during treatment. *If you have kidney disease, the dose should be reduced and tests of kidney function should be carried out at regular intervals. These warnings also apply to elderly people, who are particularly vulnerable because their kidney function may be impaired. If you have a hearing difficulty or a disorder of balance or if you are blind, you should be treated most cautiously with any of these drugs.*

Eyes

Drugs may occasionally affect the conjunctiva, cornea, pupil, lens and retina of the eyes, damage the main nerve to the eyes (the optic nerve), cause swelling of the head of the nerve at the back of the eye (papilloedema), affect colour vision, produce other visual disturbances and affect the movement of the eyes (causing symptoms such as double vision).

Advice *If you develop any eye symptoms at all, no matter how trivial, check with your doctor as to whether any drugs you are taking may cause the problem. Also see an ophthalmic optician (optometrist) for a full eye examination. If there is any possibility that a drug is causing the trouble, it should be stopped.*

Colour vision

Some drugs may, very occasionally, affect colour vision; for example, sulphonamides, streptomycin, methaqualone (a sleeping drug), barbiturates, digoxin and related drugs used to treat heart failure, some diuretic drugs (e.g. chlorothiazide and frusemide), monoamine oxidase inhibitor (MAOI) anti-depressants and nalidixic acid used to treat urinary infections.

Conjunctivitis

Allergic reactions to drugs may cause conjunctivitis; for example, aspirin and some anti-rheumatic drugs. Damage to the conjunctivae may occur due to an allergic-type reaction (Stevens–Johnson syndrome) caused very rarely by sulphonamides (especially in children) and other drugs.

Carbamazepine (an anti-epileptic drug) and allopurinol (used to treat gout) may, very rarely, damage the mucous lining of the conjunctivae, mouth and vagina.

Advice *If you develop any irritation, redness or soreness of the eyes, check with your doctor as to whether any drug you are taking could cause the problem.*

Cornea

The cornea is the window of the eye and its transparency can be damaged by drugs causing opacities, which may interfere with vision. Very rarely, the anti-psychotic drug chlorpromazine and the anti-malarial drugs chloroquine and hydroxychloroquine, used in high doses to treat rheumatoid arthritis, may cause opacities of the cornea. Indomethacin used to treat rheumatoid arthritis may, very rarely, cause corneal opacities and also damage the retina of the eyes. Gold used to treat rheumatoid arthritis may also, very rarely, cause corneal opacities. Regular use of very high doses of vitamin D can cause calcium to be deposited in the cornea, to produce opacities and interfere with vision.

Some drugs (e.g. oral contraceptives) may cause the cornea to swell so that people are unable to wear their contact lenses.

Advice *At the earliest sign of any new problem with your vision, consult your doctor to check whether any drug you are taking may cause the problem; also see an ophthalmic optician (optometrist) for a complete eye check-up.*

If you wear contact lenses and develop difficulty in wearing them or they become discoloured, consult your ophthalmic optician (optometrist) for a check-up.

Dry eyes

Anti-cholinergic drugs (Chapter 2) may cause dry eyes; so may certain drugs used to treat raised blood pressure (e.g. ganglion blockers, Chapter 21). Some beta blockers may occasionally cause dryness of the eyes. The anti-viral drug idoxuridine may occasionally reduce tear production when applied to the eyes and some anti-psychotic drugs may, rarely, cause a reduced tear production in some people.

Advice *At the earliest sign that your eyes are becoming irritated and/or dry consult your doctor to check whether any drug you are taking may be causing the problem.*

Lens

The lens of the eye is transparent, and may occasionally be damaged by drugs, causing opacities (cataracts). Chlorpromazine and some other antipsychotic drugs may cause opacities of the lens of the eyes, and so may the long-term use of corticosteroids.

Advice *At the earliest sign of any new impairment of your vision, consult your doctor to check whether any drug you are taking might cause the problem. Also consult your ophthalmic optician (optometrist) for a full eye examination.*

Optic nerve

Damage to the main nerve to the eye (the optic nerve), producing impaired vision, may, very rarely, be caused by drugs; for example, ethambutol, isoniazid and streptomycin used to treat tuberculosis, sulphonamides, chlorpropamide used to treat diabetes, and penicillamine used to treat rheumatoid arthritis.

Advice *At the earliest sign of any new impairment of your vision, consult your doctor to check whether any drug you are taking may cause the problem. Also consult your ophthalmic optician (optometrist) for a full eye examination.*

Visual hallucinations (seeing things that are not there) may, very occasionally, be caused by drugs; for example, aspirin and related drugs, the anti-epileptic drug primidone, the pain reliever pentazocine, the antidiabetic drug chlorpropamide, the diuretic drug frusemide and the beta blocker propranolol. Atropine, hyoscine and cyclopentolate eye drops may occasionally cause visual hallucinations and nightmares in children (see Chapter 35), and of course LSD produces vivid and sometimes terrifying visual hallucinations.

Advice *If you start seeing things that are not there in reality, consult your doctor immediately to check whether any drug you are taking may cause the problem.*

Pupils

Drugs that constrict or dilate the pupils can affect vision. Those that dilate the pupils may trigger an attack of glaucoma in susceptible individuals (see Chapter 35).

Constriction of the pupils may be caused by certain drugs (e.g. carbachol, neostigmine and related drugs). Morphine, chloral hydrate and antipsychotic drugs may make the pupils small and interfere with focusing.

Dilatation of the pupils may be caused by several drugs; for example, anti-cholinergic drugs (Chapter 2), antihistamines, some drugs used to treat raised blood pressure (e.g. ganglion blockers; Chapter 21), monoamine oxidase inhibitor (MAOI) anti-depressants, tricyclic and cyclic antidepressants, amphetamines ('speed') and LSD.

Advice *At the earliest sign of any new impairment of your vision, consult your doctor to check whether any drug you are taking may cause the problem. Also consult your ophthalmic optician (optometrist) for a full eye examination.*

Retina

Some drugs may, rarely, damage the pigmentaton of the retina at the back of the eyes and interfere with vision; for example, chloroquine and related anti-malarial drugs used in high doses to treat rheumatoid arthritis, antipsychotic drugs, and digoxin and related drugs used to treat heart failure.

Swelling (oedema) of the retina may, very rarely, be caused by oral contraceptives, and high concentrations of oxygen given to premature babies may damage the retina. Quinine used to treat malaria and also used to treat night cramps may, very rarely, damage the retina.

Advice *At the earliest sign of any new impairment of your vision, consult your doctor to check whether any drug you are taking may cause the problem. Also consult your ophthalmic optician (optometrist) for a full eye examination.*

Eyelids

Acute allergic reactions to drugs may cause the eyelids to swell up. This may occur whether the drug is taken by mouth or applied to the eyelids (e.g. antibiotic ointment applied to treat a stye). Eye make-up may also cause a local allergic reaction with swelling of the eyelids. Primidone used to treat epilepsy may occasionally cause the eyelids to swell up, and excessive doses of vitamin A may cause swelling of the eyelids with loss of eyebrows and eyelashes.

Drooping upper eyelids may, very rarely, be caused by beta blockers, and drugs that produce adrenaline-like effects on the body (sympathomimetic drugs, Chapter 2) may cause the upper lids to retract and make you look as if you are staring.

Advice *If you develop swelling of the eyelids or any changes to the eyelids, consult your doctor to check whether it could be related to any drug you are taking – whether by mouth or applied to the eyelids.*

Faint feelings

Any drug that dilates the blood vessels (vasodilator) may cause a sudden and severe drop in blood pressure, causing you to develop light-headedness, dizziness and faintness. You may collapse (faint), and this can be harmful because you may fall and injure yourself. Glyceryl trinitrate and other drugs used to treat angina may cause this problem. The fainting is often preceded by a throbbing headache, flushing of the face and rapid beating of the heart.

Advice *It may help to take these drugs while you are sitting down rather than standing up; also, their harmful effects are likely to wear off over a few days of treatment. A fall in blood pressure on standing up after sitting or lying down may occur with some anti-blood-pressure drugs.*

If you feel light-headed or faint after taking a drug, sit or lie down immediately until the faintness goes off. The attacks usually become less frequent and severe over time, but if they do not, contact your doctor about changing your treatment. Elderly people are particularly prone to develop faintness and dizziness with vasodilator drugs used to treat angina and heart failure, anti-blood-pressure drugs and diuretics (water tablets). They may fall and injure themselves. They must check with their doctor.

Fever

Very rarely, some drugs may cause a fever – usually in the first few days of treatment; examples include the antibiotic rifampicin, procainamide used to treat disorders of heart rhythm, the anti-blood-pressure drugs hydralazine and methyldopa, penicillamine used to treat rheumatoid arthritis and vaccines. The fever may be due to an 'allergic-type' response or an inflammatory response.

Advice *If you develop a fever following the start of drug treatment, consult your doctor to check whether the fever could possibly be caused by the drug you are taking or whether it is due to some other cause.*

Malignant hyperpyrexia syndrome (malignant hyperthermia)

A few patients may be very sensitive to certain drugs and they may develop a sudden and serious rise in temperature, rigidity of the muscles and severe acidity of the blood. Early warning signs are stiffness of the jaw, rapid beating of the heart and mottling of the skin. This is a very rare reaction which is due to a genetic 'fault' in such individuals that makes them very vulnerable to inhalational anaesthetics (e.g. ether, halothane) when given with a muscle relaxant (e.g. suxamethonium). The condition is serious and life threatening.

Advice *If you have a close relative who has died under an anaesthetic, advise your doctor because you may be at risk.*

Growth

The long-term daily use of corticosteroids in children causes stunted growth. Male sex hormones given to pre-pubertal children will also cause stunting of growth by causing the long bones to stop growing. Drugs that cause under-activity of the thyroid gland may also cause failure to grow. Tetracycline antibiotics slow down bone growth and affect the growth of the teeth.

Advice *You should be aware of the dangers of any long-term drug treatment in children, which should be used only when the expected benefits will outweigh the obvious risks involved. Tetracycline drugs should not be used in children under 12 years of age, in pregnant women or by breast-feeding mothers.*

Headaches

Drugs that cause blood vessels to dilate (e.g. glyceryl trinitrate and related drugs used to treat angina) may cause a throbbing headache. Monoamine oxidase anti-depressants may cause severe and dangerous headache when taken with certain foods or drugs (see Chapter 39); withdrawal of some drugs after regular daily use may cause headaches – for example ergotamine used to treat migraine, amphetamines ('speed'), caffeine (in tea, coffee, cocoa and colas) and benzodiazepine anti-anxiety drugs.

Corticosteroids (whether taken by mouth or applied to the skin) may, very rarely, cause headaches, particularly if they are stopped suddenly.

Advice *If you develop headache when taking any drug, consult your doctor to check whether the drug could be causing the headache and to ask whether to* *stop the drug. Anti-migraine drugs containing ergotamine may cause headache.*

If you get a headache when you do not have your regular daily amounts of coffee, tea or colas, it is a warning that you may be overdosing with coffee, tea or cola on the other days of the week.

Heart

Drugs used to treat heart disease are responsible for most harmful effects on the heart caused by drugs. They are well recognized and can be predicted and easily prevented because they are related to the dose used. A reduction in dose will reduce the harmful effects.

Common harmful effects of drugs on the heart include slowing of the pulse rate, increase of the pulse rate, palpitations, and a fall in blood pressure producing light-headedness, faintness and dizziness. The fall in blood pressure may occur with some drugs especially on standing up after sitting or lying down. Other harmful effects include disorders of heart rhythm and depression of the function of the heart.

Drugs that may produce disorders of heart rhythm or rate include digoxin and related drugs, drugs used to treat disorders of heart rhythm, drugs that produce adrenaline-like effects in the body (sympathomimetic drugs, Chapter 2), beta blockers, levodopa used to treat parkinsonism, tricyclic and cyclic anti-depressants, and clonidine used to treat raised blood pressure and migraine.

Drugs that may depress the function of the heart include beta blockers, quinidine and procainamide used to treat disorders of heart rhythm and digoxin and related drugs used to treat heart failure and disorders of heart rhythm.

Advice *If you develop slow or fast beating of your heart, palpitations, light-headedness, faintness or any new symptom, consult your doctor to check whether any drug you are taking could cause the problem.*

Hypothermia

A fall in body temperature may be caused by drugs, particularly the ones that affect consciousness; for example, sleeping drugs, sedatives, anti-anxiety drugs and anti-psychotic drugs.

Advice *Elderly people are particularly vulnerable to hypothermia, so these drugs should be used with great caution; if possible, they should not be used at all,* *particularly in elderly people living alone without adequate heating.*

The intravenous use of blood and fluids straight from a refrigerator may cause hypothermia which may be dangerous in babies and elderly people. All intravenous products should be brought slowly up to at least room temperature before being given.

Infections

Some drugs may reduce our resistance to infections; others may alter the environment in which micro-organisms live (e.g. on the skin or in the intestine) and cause a disturbance in the natural balance between, for example, bacteria and fungi. This is why people taking antibiotics may develop thrush of the mouth or anus, or why they may develop an over-growth of a virulent micro-organism that causes colitis (see Chapter 48).

Our resistance to infection is reduced by corticosteroids and signs of inflammation are reduced by their anti-inflammatory effects. The danger is that patients may not have the signs caused by inflammation (e.g. swelling and pain) and yet the underlying infection may be getting worse. Anti-inflammatory drugs (NSAIDs) used to treat rheumatic and other disorders may also relieve the signs of inflammation caused by an underlying infection without having any effect on the underlying disease that is causing the inflammation.

Anti-cancer drugs may damage cells in the bone marrow which produce white blood cells. This causes a fall in the number of white blood cells in the blood and a reduction in our ability to fight an infection. Immuno-suppressive drugs reduce our natural resistance to infection. They are used to prevent rejection of transplanted organs. Anti-bacterial drugs may kill some micro-organisms and allow others to multiply and cause an additional infection (a superinfection). Any drug that dries up the eyes, nose, mouth, breathing tubes or skin may also lower the resistance to infection in these areas and predispose to infection.

Advice *Before starting taking any drug that reduces the body's resistance or response to infection, it is important that you should have a full medical check-up to make sure that you do not have some underlying infection (e.g. tuberculosis of the lungs). It is also important that you have regular medical check-ups during treatment, and that you report to your doctor immediately if you develop a sore throat, fever or chills, or any new symptoms.*

If you are taking antibiotics and develop any 'new' symptom, consult your doctor to check whether it is due to the antibiotic. Do not self-treat symptoms; for example, it is dangerous to take an anti-diarrhoea remedy for diarrhoea caused by an antibiotic. The treatment is to stop the antibiotic immediately and consult your doctor. The same warnings apply to the use of anti-fungal drugs and anti-viral drugs, and drugs used to treat parasites and worms.

Joints

Painful and swollen joints, skin rashes and swollen glands may occur in acute allergic reactions, and anticoagulants may cause bleeding into a joint. Injections of corticosteroids into joints may damage the injected joint.

Advice *If you develop any new aches and pains in your joints, consult your doctor to check whether any drug you are taking may cause the problem.*

Kidneys *(see Chapter 84)*

Certain drugs may occasionally damage the kidneys, producing various degrees of kidney failure that may be acute and sudden or come on slowly over many years of regular daily use. Drugs may damage the kidney tissues directly or damage the blood vessels in the kidneys. Kidney failure may also be caused by thrombosis inside the blood vessels of the kidneys.

Advice *Any drug should be used with caution if you have impaired kidney function because of the risk of defective excretion and a toxic rise in the level of the drug in the blood. Equally, any drug known to produce kidney damage should be used with utmost caution, and tests of kidney function should be carried out before and at regular intervals during treatment. If there is any suggestion that kidney function is becoming impaired, the drug should be stopped immediately.*

There are always special risks in the elderly, who may have impaired kidney function without the doctor knowing. This is why it is important to carry out tests of kidney function in elderly people before using any drug that may damage the kidneys or any drug that is excreted unchanged by the kidneys.

If you develop any new symptom such as feeling unwell, loss of appetite, nausea and/or vomiting, lack of energy and/or changes in the volume of urine you pass, ankle swelling or feeling drowsy and fuddled, contact your doctor straight away to check whether any drug you are taking may affect your kidney function. You will need urine tests and tests of your kidney function.

Liver *(see Chapter 83)*

Some drugs may occasionally damage the liver. This damage may or may not be related to the dose and/or duration of treatment. It may be mild or severe and threaten life. It may suddenly develop or slowly come on over the years (like liver damage caused by alcohol). Clearly, any drug known to damage the liver should be used with utmost caution if you have impaired liver function. Also, tests of liver function should always be carried out before and at regular intervals during treatment when any such drug is used. At the earliest sign of impaired function of the liver the drug should be stopped.

Advice *Unfortunately, routine liver function tests carried out at regular intervals during treatment are not a very effective method of monitoring for harmful effects to the liver and you should report to your doctor immediately for liver function tests if you develop symptoms such as feeling unwell, lack of energy, loss of appetite, nausea, vomiting, diarrhoea, chills, headache, yellowness of the skin and eyes, pale stools and/or dark urine. (The last may occur particularly with drugs that interfere with the excretion of bile from the liver.)*

Most drugs are broken down in the liver, and certain drugs may affect the chemical processes involved in this breakdown and speed up or slow down the breakdown of other drugs. This will affect their blood levels and, therefore, their beneficial effects (see Chapter 89).

Advice *If you are taking more than one drug and develop any new symptoms or your previous symptoms get worse, consult your doctor to check whether the drugs you are taking are interacting and causing the problem.*

Menstrual periods

Oral contraceptives may cause loss of periods and other problems. In some women the loss of periods may continue long after the oral contraceptive has stopped. You should be cautious about using the pill if you have irregular periods, and you should be aware of the risk of loss of periods. Several other drugs may cause loss of periods, usually associated with the production of milk from the breasts – see earlier, under Breasts.

Advice *If as a girl you were late starting your periods and/or your periods were previously irregular, you may be more prone to develop a loss of periods on the pill than women who started their periods early or at a 'normal' age and whose periods were previously regular.*

If you develop any changes to your periods, always consult your doctor to check whether any drug you are taking may be causing the problem.

Mental symptoms

Any drug that affects the brain may produce mental symptoms. These include drowsiness, depression, insomnia, nightmares, anxiety, tension, irritability, restlessness and feelings of extreme well-being (euphoria). Mental symptoms may be mild or severe and may be caused by sleeping drugs, sedatives, anti-anxiety drugs, anti-depressant drugs, anti-psychotic drugs, stimulants (amphetamines) and morphine-related drugs. These kinds of mental symptoms may also be caused by drugs such as levodopa to treat parkinsonism, anti-cholinergic drugs, digoxin and related drugs used to treat heart failure, corticosteroids and some anti-tuberculous drugs (e.g. isoniazid). Several other drugs may cause drowsiness; for example, antihistamines used to treat allergies and methyldopa used to treat raised blood pressure.

Advice *If you feel drowsy, depressed, cannot sleep, have nightmares, feel tense, irritable or anxious, feel restless, develop any change in mood or any other symptom that is 'new' to you, consult your doctor about whether your drug treatment is causing the problem and whether you should reduce the dose or stop treatment. Remember that many of these symptoms may be made worse by drinking alcohol and that you should not drive a motor vehicle if the drug affects you in this way, because it may impair your ability to drive. Always check harmful effects and warnings on each drug you are taking.*

Some drugs may cause *confusion*, which may present as inability to think or by muddled thinking, clouding of the mind, disorientation in space and time (the individual may not know where he or she is or what day it is), quiet or noisy behaviour, inability to concentrate, loss of memory, forgetfulness and mood changes. The mood changes may vary from anxiety and aggression to depression, fear and withdrawal. Delirium or serious schizophrenia-like symptoms may, very rarely, develop.

These symptoms may be caused by many drugs; for example, digoxin and related drugs used to treat heart failure, anticholinergics, antihistamines, sleeping drugs, anti-anxiety drugs, corticosteroids, anti-tuberculous drugs (e.g. isoniazid), levodopa and bromocriptine used to treat parkinsonism, penicillins, and cimetidine used to treat peptic ulcers.

Advice *If you become the slightest bit confused, it is very important that you consult your doctor to check whether you are taking any drug that may cause the confusion. Do not forget that elderly people are particularly vulnerable to the confusing effects of certain drugs and may be misdiagnosed and mistreated as 'senile'. Elderly people are a particular problem if they live alone and become forgetful and muddled. Doctors and nurses should always consider whether a patient's drug treatment is causing any physical or mental symptoms.*

Depression may occasionally be a problem with several groups of drugs; for example, reserpine and methyldopa used to treat raised blood pressure, corticosteroids, levodopa used to treat parkinsonism, depot injections of anti-psychotic drugs, wear-off effects of amphetamines, fenfluramine for slimming, and in some women the oral contraceptive may possibly cause depression but whether it is the oestrogen or the progestogen in the pill is not clear.

Advice *If you develop any symptoms of depression you should consult your doctor to check whether it is due to a drug you are taking.*

Occasionally, some drugs may cause *excitement* and a marked lift in mood along with restlessness and over-activity. They may cause serious mental symptoms and the individual may become manic.

Some drugs may produce a *schizophrenia-like illness*, which can be very serious. Some individuals may become paranoid and feel persecuted and have hallucinations. Amphetamines (speed) are particularly dangerous in this respect.

Advice *If you become excitable and over-active or develop any new mental symptoms or your previous mental symptoms get worse, you should check with your doctor as to whether your drug treatment could possibly be the cause.*

Hallucinations, particularly seeing things that are not 'real', but also sometimes hearing, feeling and smelling things that are not 'real' may, rarely, occur with some drugs; for example, levodopa used to treat parkinsonism. Amantadine, also used to treat parkinsonism, may cause hallucinations when taken with anti-cholinergic drugs.

Advice *If you develop any 'new' sensation, whether you see it, hear it, feel it or smell it, you should consult your doctor to check whether any drug you are taking could be causing the problem.*

Mouth

Some drugs may cause a *dry mouth*; for example, anti-cholinergics, tricyclic and cyclic anti-depressants and antihistamines.

Advice *With anti-depressant drugs the dry mouth and other effects usually wear off in a few weeks and it is important to continue treatment. With other drugs the only treatment is to stop the drug if the dry mouth becomes a problem.*

Warning *Avoid eating too many sweets to relieve a dry mouth because a dry mouth increases the risk of developing dental decay, which is made more likely by the sugar in the sweets.*

Some drugs cause an *increased production of saliva* – for example, pilocarpine used to treat glaucoma and neostigmine used to treat myasthenia gravis – but this seldom causes problems.

The *sense of taste* may be reduced by some drugs; for example, penicillamine usd to treat rheumatoid arthritis and the anti-fungal drug griseofulvin.

Some drugs may cause a *metallic taste* in the mouth; for example, metformin used to treat diabetes and the anti-bacterial drug metronidazole.

Some drugs may cause the *breath to smell*; for example, isosorbide dinitrate used to treat angina.

Advice *If you develop loss of taste, a metallic taste in the mouth or bad breath, consult your doctor to check whether any drug you are taking may be causing this problem.*

Allergic reactions to drugs can affect the mouth, producing sudden swelling of the lips and lining of the mouth, and be associated with nettle rash and wheezing (see acute allergic reactions, Chapter 10). Local anaesthetic injections used by dentists may trigger a local allergic reaction.

Advice *If you develop any swelling of the lips or mouth, stop the drug immediately and consult your doctor.*

Allergic-type reactions to drugs may also produce *inflammation and ulcers of the mouth* (stomatitis). The reaction may recur in one particular part of the mouth every time a certain drug is taken. This sort of recurrent reaction is called a 'fixed drug eruption' and it may occasionally occur with, for example, phenolphthalein in laxatives and sulphonamides.

Gold used to treat rheumatoid arthritis may, rarely, produce widespread ulceration of the mouth. Antibiotics may, occasionally, cause vitamin deficiency and produce a sore mouth and tongue and also cause thrush. Several anti-cancer drugs may cause a sore mouth (e.g. cyclophosphamide, chlorambucil and bleomycin). Aspirin preparations and potassium preparations may cause a sore mouth and ulcers if they are sucked or chewed.

Advice *If you develop soreness of the mouth, with or without ulcers, consult your doctor to check whether any drug you are taking may be causing the problem.*

NOTE Some people may develop an allergic reaction to an ingredient in toothpaste. If you develop a sore mouth which you think may be caused by a particular brand of toothpaste, stop using it and change to another brand preparation.

Whitish spots in the mouth (lichenoid eruptions) may be caused by an allergic reaction to a drug.

Advice *Consult your doctor if you develop whitish spots in the mouth to check whether they may be caused by a drug you are taking.*

Some drugs may cause *swelling of the gums and overgrowth* of the gums; for example, the anti-epileptic drug phenytoin.

Advice *If you develop swelling of the gums, consult your doctor to check whether any drug you are taking may have caused the problem.*

NOTE Regular daily effective cleaning of the teeth can help to prevent or reduce gum disorders. Therefore, in children or mentally handicapped people taking phenytoin it is important to make sure that they clean their teeth regularly and effectively every day.

Some drugs may cause *systemic lupus erythematosus* (see later), which produces soreness and ulceration of the mouth and affects the skin and various tissues and organs throughout the body.

Advice *If you develp a skin rash with a sore mouth or any new symptom and you are taking a drug that may cause systemic lupus erythematosus, consult your doctor immediately.*

Some drugs may cause *Stevens–Johnson syndrome,* which may vary from a mild skin rash with soreness of the mouth to a severe skin rash and severe ulceration and blisters in the mouth. It may be associated with ulcers in the urethra and vagina and on the eyes.

Advice *At the very first sign of a skin rash associated with soreness in the mouth, genitals or eyes you should consult your doctor immediately.*

Some drugs may *discolour* the lining of the mouth and gums either by direct contact or via the blood stream after being absorbed from the stomach. Heavy metals (e.g. lead, zinc, copper, bismuth) may discolour the gums, and anti-psychotic drugs may, rarely, produce a blue–grey colour of the gums.

Advice *If you develop any discoloration of your gums or lining of your mouth, consult your doctor to check whether it is due to any drugs you are taking.*

Sucking antibiotic preparations (e.g. penicillin) may cause you to develop a *black hairy tongue*; De-Nol, used to treat indigestion and peptic ulcers (see Chapter 15), may cause a *black tongue.*

Advice *If you develop any discoloration of your tongue, consult your doctor to check whether it is due to any drugs you are taking.*

Antibiotics and corticosteroids may trigger a *thrush infection* of the mouth.

Advice *If you develop white patches in your mouth or on your tongue, consult your doctor. You may need to take an anti-thrush drug.*

Drugs that cause an *immune deficiency* may trigger infections of the mouth that may be bacterial, fungal or viral (e.g. cold sores). These may be very serious.

Advice *If you are taking an immunosuppressive drug or corticosteroids and develop an infection in your mouth, consult your doctor straight away.*

Some drugs can cause abnormal *movements of the tongue and lips* (see anti-psychotic drugs, Chapter 41); others may *damage the nerves* supplying the mouth, causing pins and needles and numbness in the mouth and lips.

Advice *If you develop any involuntary movement of your tongue or lips or if you develop any numbness or pins and needles around the lips or mouth, consult your doctor to check whether the symptoms are caused by the drug(s) you are taking.*

NOTE Drugs that damage bone marrow and interfere with red and white blood cell and platelet production may cause soreness, ulceration and bleeding of the gums – see under Blood disorders. Also, anti-coagulant drugs may cause bleeding of the gums if the dose is not carefully controlled or if they are taken with drugs that increase their effects.

Muscles

Some drugs may cause *painful muscles* (myalgia); for example, drugs that alter the blood chemistry (such as diuretics), guanethidine used to treat raised blood pressure and suxamethonium used as a muscle relaxant.

Advice *If you develop painful muscles, cramps and/or twitching of a muscle or* *muscles, consult your doctor to check whether the symptoms are caused by any drug you are taking.*

Weakness of the muscles (myopathy) may be caused by certain drugs; for example, corticosteroids may occasionally affect the muscles of the upper legs and make it difficult to stand up from a sitting position and difficult to walk up stairs. Corticosteroids may, rarely, affect the muscles around the shoulders and make it difficult to raise the arms. Carbenoxolone used to treat peptic ulcer may produce muscular weakness associated with a low blood potassium level. Other types of muscle weakness may, rarely, be caused by, for example, bezafibrate and clofibrate used to lower blood fat levels and by penicillamine used to treat rheumatoid arthritis.

Advice *If you develop any weakness in a muscle or muscles, consult your doctor to check whether the problem is caused by any drug which you are taking.*

Nerves

Some drugs may cause *damage to nerves*, producing pins and needles, numbness and burning in the hands and feet, arms and legs, and face, and some may cause weakness of the arms and legs. Examples of drugs that may occasionally or rarely affect nerves and produce symptoms include some anti-depressant drugs, some beta blockers (e.g. propranolol), some anti-diabetic drugs (e.g. chlorpropamide, tolbutamide), some drugs used to treat migraine (e.g. ergotamine), some anti-tuberculous drugs (e.g. isoniazid, streptomycin) and some anti-bacterial drugs (e.g. colistin, nitrofurantoin).

Advice *If you develop numbness, burning, pins and needles or weakness in your hands and feet, arms and legs or face, consult your doctor to check whether any drug you are taking may be damaging your nerves and causing the symptoms.*

Nose

Harmful drug effects on the nose are caused most frequently by using nasal drops and sprays to relieve congestion. These preparations usually contain a sympathomimetic drug, which at first dries up the nose and clears the air passages but when the effects wear off may cause a rebound swelling of the lining of the nose.

Some anti-blood-pressure drugs (e.g. methyldopa, reserpine) may cause a blocked nose.

Advice *If you develop a blocked nose or catarrh, consult your doctor to check whether any drug you are taking may be causing the problem.*

Nose bleeds may occur in patients taking anticoagulant drugs, and a *loss of the sense of smell* may occur very rarely in patients taking aminoglycoside antibiotics.

Advice *If you are taking anti-coagulant drugs, always carry a warning card with you. If you develop a nose bleed, consult your doctor. You will need a blood test to check your blood clotting. Also check whether you have been taking any other drug that may increase the effects of the anti-coagulant you are taking (see Chapter 89).*

If you lose your sense of smell consult your doctor to check whether any drug you are taking may be causing the problem.

Parkinsonism and other disorders of movement

The worst culprits for causing disorders of movement are the anti-psychotic drugs, which may produce involuntary movements from simple restlessness to serious disorders such as parkinsonism and tardive dyskinesia (see Chapter 41).

Advice *If you develop any abnormal movement* ***(no matter how slight)*** *of your tongue, eyes, face, neck, arms or legs, consult your doctor to check whether any drug you are taking could be causing the problem.*

Passing urine

Sleeping drugs, sedatives, antihistamines, anti-cholinergics, anti-depressants, morphine-related pain relievers and certain anti-blood-pressure drugs may interfere with the ability to pass urine. In elderly men with enlarged prostate glands this may cause problems that lead to an inability to pass urine, causing retention of urine.

Advice *If you have any difficulty in passing urine, always advise the doctor before he or she prescribes a drug for you and always check with a pharmacist before you buy a drug over-the-counter. If you develop any difficulty passing urine, consult your doctor straight away to check whether any drug you are taking may be causing the problem.*

Some drugs predispose to the development of *kidney stones*, and others may cause crystals to develop in the urine (e.g. sulphonamides).

Advice *If you suffer from kidney trouble or gout always advise the doctor before he or she prescribes a drug for you. If you develop any pain in your kidneys or pain on passing urine, consult your doctor straight away to check whether any drug you are taking may be causing the problem.*

Phaeochromocytoma

Phaeochromocytomas produce excessive quantities of noradrenaline and adrenaline. Some drugs may stimulate the release of noradrenaline and adrenaline; for example, several general anaesthetics (e.g. cyclopropane, trichloroethylene, halothane) and anti-blood-pressure drugs (e.g. methyldopa, gaunethidine, bethanidine, debrisoquine).

Advice *If you suffer from a phaeochromocytoma, doctors should not prescribe any of these drugs to you and you should not purchase any over-the-counter drug without checking with a pharmacist.*

Salivary glands

Some drugs (e.g. phenylbutazone) may, rarely, cause the salivary glands in the cheeks and neck to swell up. Iodine may occasionally cause the glands to swell up like mumps (iodine mumps) and certain drugs may produce pain in the cheeks (e.g. gaunethidine and bethanidine used to treat raised blood pressure).

Advice *If you develop swollen glands and/or pain in the face or neck, consult your doctor to see whether the symptoms are caused by any drug you are taking.*

Seizures

Some drugs may cause seizures (e.g. 'fits') in apparently 'normal' people and can trigger seizures in people suffering from epilepsy. Drugs that may, very rarely, cause seizures include anti-psychotic drugs, tricyclic antidepressants, the anti-tubercular drugs cycloserine and isoniazid, and high intravenous doses of penicillins, insulin and lignocaine.

Advice *If you develop a seizure, consult your doctor who should consider whether it was due to a drug you are taking and, if necessary, stop or change your treatment.*

Sex

The effects of drugs on sex are discussed in Chapter 74.

Advice *If your sex life changes in any way, always ask yourself – is it due to any drug I am taking? Drugs may cause changes in sexual desire (libido), which may increase, decrease or disappear; they may make it more difficult for you to be 'turned-on', they may cause you to fail to attain or maintain an erection, or to ejaculate if you are a man or to have an orgasm if you are a woman. See Chapter 74 about lack of information about the effects of drugs on sexual activities.*

Sexual characteristics

Male sex hormones and anabolic steroids may produce masculinity in females. These changes include hairiness, deep voice, enlarged clitoris and increased libido.

NOTE that, except occasionally in the treatment of certain cancers, these drugs should not be used in women.

Skin

Several skin disorders caused by drugs are listed in Chapter 75.

Advice *If you develop any sort of skin rash while on drug treatment, consult your doctor to check whether your drug treatment is causing the problem. With drugs known to produce serious allergic reactions, stop the drug immediately at the first sign of a rash and consult your doctor.*

Sensitivity to the sun's rays

Damage to skin (sunburn) caused by the sun's rays may develop within a few hours of taking a drug that makes the skin sensitive to the sun's rays and it usually clears up quickly if the drug is stopped. This is called a *phototoxic* reaction. A drug may also make the skin allergic to the sun's rays (*photo-allergy*). This develops more slowly and takes longer to recover – it is often like eczema. However, both reactions are often mixed together.

Advice *If you find yourself burning more easily than usual from the sun's rays (or artificial ultra-violet rays) and/or if you develop a rash on exposed areas of* *skin, do not expose yourself to the sun's rays or artificial ultra-violet rays until you have consulted your doctor as to whether your drug treatment is causing the problem.*

Always ask yourself – is my skin rash or sunburn due to any drug I am taking, and check with your doctor.

Stomach and intestine

Stomach

Loss of appetite, nausea and vomiting are very common everyday symptoms; they are also commonly caused by drugs. Some people appear to be more sensitive to some drugs than others but some drugs are more prone than others to produce these symptoms; for example, digoxin and related drugs used to treat heart failure, morphine and related pain-relieving drugs, oestrogens, theophylline used to treat asthma, and levodopa used to treat parkinsonism. Some drugs (e.g. iron salts) may directly irritate the lining of the stomach and cause nausea and vomiting.

Advice *If your stomach upsets appear to be caused by a drug preparation irritating your stomach, it will help if you take the drug with a non-alcoholic drink with or after food, and not on an empty stomach.*

NOTE *Many stomach upsets caused by drugs are related to the dose and it will help to reduce the dose. Consult your doctor.*

If symptoms are caused by a drug's effects on the vomiting centre in the brain (e.g. morphine and related drugs), it may be necessary to take an anti-vomiting drug at the same time (see Chapter 14). Consult your doctor.

Stomach ulcers and bleeding

Aspirin and non-steroidal anti-inflammatory drugs interfere with the natural protective lining of the stomach and may produce indigestion, ulceration and bleeding from the stomach and intestine in some people.

Advice *You should not take any of these drugs if you have a peptic ulcer (e.g. stomach ulcer, duodenal ulcer, oesophageal ulcer) or a history of peptic ulcers. You should always take these drugs with a non-alcoholic drink with or after food and not on an empty stomach. You should stop them immediately and consult your doctor if you develop indigestion or pain in the stomach and/or if your stools look black like tar (this means that there is blood present in the stools from a bleeding ulcer higher up the intestine or in the stomach), and/or if you develop* *any symptoms of anaemia – paleness, tiredness, weakness, palpitations, dizziness and breathlessness on exertion.*

Heartburn can be made worse by anti-cholinergic drugs in people who suffer from a hiatus hernia or acid reflux (see Chapter 15).

Indigestion may be caused or made worse by alcohol, coffee, theophylline used to treat asthma, and reserpine used to treat raised blood pressure.

Advice *If you develop indigestion or heartburn, consult your doctor to check whether the problem may be caused by any drug you are taking.*

Ulcers of the oesophagus (gullet)

Potassium tablets may cause ulcers of the oesophagus, especially if there is already some disorder of the oesophagus or if the tablets are swallowed without a drink. Emepronium (an anticholinergic drug), previously used to treat incontinence of urine in elderly people, may cause ulcers of the oesophagus.

Advice *When swallowing any tablet or capsule, always stand up or sit up straight and take it with a good drink of non-alcoholic fluid. Consult your doctor if you develop any pain or discomfort in the centre of your chest, to check whether it could be due to any drug you are taking.*

Ulcers of the intestine

Ulcers of the intestine may be caused by specially coated tablets (enteric-coated tablets) that are designed to break down in the intestine rather than in the stomach; for example, potassium chloride tablets.

Advice *If you develop any abdominal pain or other new symptoms, consult your doctor to check whether any drugs you are taking could cause the problem.*

Inflammation of the pancreas (pancreatitis) producing nausea, vomiting and severe abdominal pain may, very rarely, be caused by drugs (e.g. sulphonamides). However, alcohol is one of the main culprits.

Advice *Report immediately to your doctor if you develop vomiting with severe abdominal pain and show him the drugs you have been taking whether prescribed or bought over-the-counter from a chemist or herbalist.*

Absorption of drugs from the stomach and intestine

Some drugs may interfere with the absorption of other drugs from the stomach and intestine; for example, indigestion remedies interfere with the absorption of tetracycline antibiotics. Such drugs should be taken at least 2 hours apart. They may also interfere with the absorption of vitamins such as vitamin B_{12} and folic acid, producing anaemia.

Advice *Never take more than one drug at the same time without checking that this is safe to do. One drug may interact with another, to produce harmful effects, or the effectiveness of one drug may be reduced or increased by the other (see Chapter 89).*

Stress response

High doses and regular daily use of corticosteroids will cause the adrenal glands to shrink, and this will damage your response to stress produced by an infection or injury (e.g. surgery). They also affect the response of the pituitary gland. Read about this danger in Chapter 62, on corticosteroids.

Advice *Discuss your need to take corticosteroids with your doctor, and always carry a steroid warning card with you at all times.*

NOTE Although there is much less risk with inhalations of corticosteroids and with the application of corticosteroids to the skin, there may still be a risk that sufficient corticosteroid is absorbed into the blood stream to produce harmful effects; therefore these preparations should always be used cautiously, particularly in children.

Advice *Make yourself familiar with the various harmful effects that corticosteroids may produce and, at the slightest sign of any problems, consult your doctor. Note the necessity to use the smallest effective dose possible.*

Systemic lupus erythematosus

Systemic lupus erythematosus is a very rare disorder in which the body produces antibodies that damage various tissues and organs in the body – it may damage the skin, lining of the mouth, blood vessels, joints, kidneys, blood, brain and nervous system, lungs, heart and spleen and produce mental symptoms. Examples of drugs that, very rarely, may cause lupus erythematosus include anti-epileptic drugs (ethosuximide, phenytoin, primidone, troxidone), anti-blood-pressure drugs (e.g. hydralazine), anti-tuberculous drugs (e.g. isoniazid), anti-thyroid drugs (e.g. propylthiouracil), beta blockers (e.g. practolol), anti-psychotic drugs (e.g. chlorpromazine) and anti-rheumatic drugs (e.g. penicillamine).

Advice *If you develop a skin rash with a sore mouth or any 'new' symptoms, consult your doctor immediately to check whether any drug you are taking could cause the problem.*

Teeth

Tetracycline antibiotics interfere with the development of teeth and stain them yellow; they should not be used in children under 12 years of age, in the last 6 months of pregnancy or while breast feeding. Liquid iron medicines stain the teeth black and should be taken through a straw. Some anti-cancer drugs make the teeth sensitive to pain.

Testes

Some anti-cancer drugs may damage the testes and produce infertility (see Chapter 76).

Thrombosis

Oral contraceptives may, very rarely, cause thrombosis. This risk is discussed in detail in Chapter 67.

Thyroid gland

Regular use of iodine-containing medicines (e.g. cough medicines) may produce a goitre and cause an under-active thyroid gland (see Chapter 63).

Advice *You should not take iodine-containing medicines regularly every day for more than a few days. The symptoms of under-active thyroid gland (Chapter 63) include gain in weight, feeling cold, tiredness, vague aches and pains, forgetfulness, changes in menstrual periods and dry skin. If you develop any of these symptoms, consult your doctor to check whether they may be caused by any drug you are taking.*

NOTE Aminoglutethimide, oral anti-diabetic drugs (sulphonylureas) and lithium used to treat depression may also cause under-activity of the thyroid gland.

Several drugs may interfere with *tests of thyroid function* (e.g. oral contraceptives).

Advice *If you are to be sent for a thyroid test, your doctor should always check what drugs you are taking and stop any that may interfere with the results of the test.*

79

Pregnancy and the risks of drug treatments

Definitions

Embryo refers to the developing baby from conception up to the eighth week of development inside its mother's womb.

Fetus refers to the developing baby from the eighth week up to birth.

Pregnancy may be divided into three periods, each of 3 months. These are referred to as *trimesters* and we talk about the first, second and third trimesters.

Abnormalities in a baby at birth are referred to as *congenital malformations* – they may be external (e.g. affecting an arm or a leg), internal (e.g. affecting the heart) or microscopic (e.g. affecting the cells of the brain). They are irreversible and cannot be corrected by the subsequent growth and development of the baby. A malformation may be hereditary (passed on from parent to child) or it may be caused by some external factor (e.g. a drug).

A factor that is associated with congenital malformations is referred to as a *dysmorphogen* (deformity producing). If it produces extensive physical abnormalities, it is referred to as a *teratogen* (monster producing) and is said to be *teratogenic.*

Risks of drug treatments in the first 3 months of pregnancy (the first trimester)

The most critical period for an unborn baby is during its first 3 months of life and yet for the first 2 months the mother may not even know she is pregnant. From the third to the eleventh week the cells in the baby multiply and develop into an almost fully formed baby. During this period (3–11 weeks) a baby is more sensitive to harmful effects in its environment than at any other time in its life. Before this period the embryo either dies or the damaged cells are replaced; after this stage major abnormalities cannot be produced because organs have developed.

Any damage occurring between the third and eleventh weeks will be *irreversible* and result in an abnormality at birth. Agents that can damage the baby include X-rays, virus infections (e.g. german measles), chemicals, poisons and drugs.

The extent and nature of any damage to the baby will be determined by the stage of development (e.g. whether its arms or legs have developed), by its 'genetic' susceptibility to damage and by the physical state of the mother. With regard to the last factor there is an increased risk of damage to the baby if the mother's nutritional state is poor, if she is an alcoholic or a drug addict or if she suffers from a chronic disease such as diabetes, raised blood pressure or toxaemia of pregnancy.

Thalidomide is an example of a drug that can damage a baby during its early stages of development and result in physical abnormalities at birth. However, there is no direct relationship between the chemical structure of a drug, its actions and effects on the body in adults and its specific damaging effects on an unborn baby. For example, drugs chemically related to thalidomide do not produce congenital abnormalities. It is therefore very difficult to predict which drug may cause damage to an unborn baby, except of course with some anti-cancer drugs which damage all cells as well as cancer cells.

Studies of the damaging effects of drugs in pregnant animals may provide a warning of a drug's potential damaging effects on human babies but the trouble is that different animals react differently to different drugs. Animal studies may therefore suggest caution on the future use of a specific drug in pregnancy but in general we have to rely on information collected from pregnant women over the years. The collection and interpretation of such information comes under the description of epidemiology (the study of the distribution and causes of diseases in a defined population). We may therefore talk about the epidemiology of congenital malformations – the study of the distribution and causes of malformations in newborn babies.

Epidemiological studies of the safety of a drug in pregnancy are difficult because they require that an adequate number of pregnant women have taken the drug and they should be designed in such a way that factors other than the drug can be discounted. Also, it is equally important to study, over the *same* period of time, an adequate number of pregnant mothers who did not take the drug during pregnancy. This latter, or control, group of mothers has to be used in order to assess whether babies born to mothers who took a specific drug actually developed more abnormalities than the babies of mothers who did not take that drug during pregnancy.

There are many other difficulties in proving whether a particular drug taken during pregnancy caused a particular abnormality in a newborn baby, and it is even more difficult to prove that a drug taken during pregnancy caused abnormalities that develop later in life; for example, microscopic damage to the tissues of the kidneys, heart and brain in an embryo that may result in abnormal functioning of these organs later in life.

A major problem in studying whether a specific drug caused a specific effect is the time lapse between taking a drug in the first few weeks of pregnancy and the subsequent delivery of the baby some 8–9 months later. There is also the problem that the mother may have been exposed to other drugs, either prescribed or bought over-the-counter; to alcohol; to caffeine in tea, coffee and colas; to cigarette smoke; and to various chemical and radiation hazards in the environment. It is therefore important to bear in mind the difficulties in trying to prove a direct cause and effect relationship between the use of a drug in pregnancy and a subsequent deformity in a baby.

Because of these many difficulties, there is no convincing evidence from adequate and well controlled studies of the safety of many drugs in the first 3 months of pregnancy; it is therefore wise to be cautious about using any drug during this critical period when the embryo is developing into an almost fully formed baby.

NOTE Despite all these problems and warnings, drugs appear to account for only about 1–5 per cent of the 20,000 or so babies born with an abnormality each year in the UK.

Risks of drug treatments in the middle 3 months (second trimester) and last 3 months (third trimester) of pregnancy

After the first 3 months of life there is little further development of organs to be completed and the baby spends the rest of pregnancy growing and developing the functions of its various organs. However, the brain and nervous system continue to develop right through pregnancy and in the first few months of life, and these can be damaged at any stage, producing impaired mental development and/or future behavioural disorders.

Because the blood circulation of the mother is linked directly to the baby's circulation through the placenta, any drug she takes may enter the baby's bloodstream, to affect the baby. This may occur any time during the second and third trimesters and during labour.

Drug treatment that may produce harmful effects on the pregnant mother

Any drug treatment is always a balance of benefits and risks for the individual being treated, whether pregnant or not. However, in addition, pregnant mothers are more vulnerable to certain drugs because they are pregnant. For example, the risk of liver damage from erythromycin estolate is greater in pregnant women and large dose of tetracyclines intravenously may produce liver damage.

Several drugs that may be used in pregnant women may affect the womb and cause a delay in labour. These include calcium channel blockers, diazoxide and the intravenous use of sympathomimetic drugs given to treat asthma. Aspirin and non-steroidal anti-inflammatory drugs (NSAIDs) can delay and prolong labour by blocking prostaglandins which cause the womb to contract.

Table 79.1 Drugs that should not be used, or used with caution, in pregnancy

Drug	*Harmful effects*
ACE inhibitors	Do not use in pregnancy. They may affect the blood pressure and kidney function of the baby before and after it is born. They may also produce defects of the skull in the baby
alcohol	Regular daily use during first 3 months may damage the baby (it is teratogenic). Regular daily use during the last 6 months may retard growth of the baby, and regular daily use in the last 3 months may cause addiction in the baby so that a newborn baby of an alcoholic mother may develop withdrawal symptoms
aminoglycoside antibiotics	Use during the last 6 months may damage the nerves of hearing and balance in the baby. Deafness may occur with streptomycin and kanamycin; smaller risk with gentamicin and tobramycin
amiodarone	Releases iodine after absorption into the body. If used in last 6 months, it could possibly cause goitre and under-active thyroid gland in the baby
anabolic steroids	May cause masculinization of female babies if used at any stage during pregnancy
anaesthetics (general)	May depress breathing in the unborn baby if used towards the end of pregnancy and in the newborn baby if used during labour
anaesthetics (local)	If large doses are used at delivery, may depress breathing and cause floppy limbs and slow heart rate in the newborn baby. *Prilocaine* and *procaine* may cause methaemoglobinaema (an abnormal haemoglobin in red blood cells, making them unable to carry oxygen)
androgens (male sex hormones)	May cause masculinization of female babies if used at any stage during pregnancy

Table 79.1 Drugs that should not be used, or used with caution, in pregnancy (*cont.*)

Drug	*Harmful effects*
anti-anxiety drugs	*Benzodiazepines* If large doses are used during labour, may depress the newborn baby's breathing and cause floppy limbs and drowsiness. Regular daily use in the last weeks of pregnancy may cause drowsiness and floppy limbs for a few days and possibly withdrawal symptoms in the baby
	All anti-anxiety drugs may produce drowsiness and depress breathing in the newborn baby if used at the end of pregnancy and/or during labour
anti-asthma drugs	Large doses of *salbutamol, terbutaline* and related selective beta-stimulant drugs injected into a vein to treat an acute attack of asthma may cause a delay in the onset of labour if used at the end of pregnancy
	Theophylline may cause irritability and difficulty with breathing in newborn babies if used in the last 3 months of pregnancy
anti-coagulant drugs by mouth	May damage the baby if used during first 3 months (they are teratogenic). In the last 6 months they may produce bleeding in the unborn baby, and if used near delivery they may cause bleeding in the newborn baby. See use of anti-coagulant drugs in pregnancy (Chapter 26)
anti-cancer drugs	Anti-cancer drugs damage all cells, so there is a risk of damage to the cells of the unborn baby if they are used in pregnancy. Alkylating agents and folic acid blockers (folate antagonists) cause a high risk; other anti-cancer drugs cause a lower risk
anti-depressants: tricyclic and related drugs	Regular daily use during last 3 months of pregnancy may occasionally produce rapid heart rate, irritability, spasm of muscles and convulsions in newborn babies
MAOIs	Do not use in pregnancy unless absolutely essential
anti-diabetic drugs (oral)	*Metformin* should not be used during pregnancy. *Sulphonylureas* should, preferably, not be used. If used at the end of pregnancy, they may cause hypoglycaemia (low blood glucose) in the newborn baby. Insulin should be used instead (see Chapter 55). If for some special reason sulphonylureas are used, they should be stopped 3 days before delivery. If used at the end of pregnancy, *tolbutamide* may increase the risk of kernicterus in jaundiced babies, especially if they are premature. It displaces the bile pigment, bilirubin, from being bound to proteins in the blood
anti-epileptics	See discussion in Chapter 37. If used in first 3 months there is a risk of damaging the baby. Regular daily use of *phenobarbitone* and other barbiturates in the last 3 months may produce withdrawal effects in the newborn baby. *Phenytoin* and *phenobarbitone* interfere with vitamin K clotting factors and may cause bleeding in newborn babies. Vitamin K should be given to the mother before delivery and to the baby after delivery. *Sodium valproate* may damage the baby's nervous system if used in the first 3 months, and if used in the last 3 months of pregnancy may cause bleeding and liver damage in the newborn baby

Table 79.1 Drugs that should not be used, or used with caution, in pregnancy (*cont.*)

Drug	*Harmful effects*
antihistamines	No evidence of harm but use with caution during pregnancy, particularly during first 3 months. Manufacturers recommend that the following antihistamines should not be used in pregnancy: Clarityn (loratadine), Congesteze (azatadine with pseudoephedrine), Hismanal (astemizole) and Primalan (mequitazine)
anti-inflammatory drugs (NSAIDs)	Regular daily use at the end of pregnancy may cause breathing difficulties in the newborn baby due to a raised blood pressure in the lungs, caused by closing off of a bypass vessel (ductus arteriosus) before delivery rather than after delivery. This is due to their effects on prostaglandins. May also cause delayed onset of labour and prolonged labour. Should not be used in the last 3 months of pregnancy
anti-malarials	There are rare risks of using anti-malarial drugs in pregnancy but benefits outweigh these risks. However, do not use them for other purposes during pregnancy (e.g. chloroquine or hydrochloroquine to treat rheumatoid arthritis or quinine to treat night cramps). Regular use in last 3 months of *chloroquine* may damage the retina of the baby's eyes. *Primaquine* may damage the newborn baby's red blood cells, causing haemolytic anaemia, and methaemoglobinaemia (an abnormal haemoglobin in red blood cells, making them unable to carry oxygen). *Maloprim* contains *dapsone*, which also produces these harmful effects. Folic acid supplement should be given to the mother. *Fansidar* contains *sulfadoxine*, a sulphonamide that may produce similar harmful effects. It may also increase the risk of kernicterus in newborn babies that are premature or jaundiced. *Maloprim* and *Fansidar* also contain *pyrimethamine*, which may damage the baby if used in the first 3 months of pregnancy. *Quinine* may damage the baby if used in high doses during the first 3 months of pregnancy. Pregnant women taking *proguanil* should be given folic acid supplements. Do not use *mefloquine* in pregnancy. Animal studies show it to be toxic to fetuses
anti-psychotics	Regular daily use in the last 3 months may produce movement disorders in the newborn baby
anti-thyroid drugs	The dose should be reduced towards the end of pregnancy because there is a risk of producing goitre and under-active thyroid glands in newborn babies (may also be produced by the use of iodine in the last 6 weeks). *Carbimazole*, if used regularly in last 6 months, may cause a patch of baldness on the scalp in newborn babies (aplasia cutis). *Radioactive iodine* may knock out the baby's thyroid gland permanently
aspirin	If aspirin is used regularly at the end of pregnancy, it may cause bleeding in the newborn baby, delay and prolong labour, and increase bleeding from the mother during childbirth. Do not use

Table 79.1 Drugs that should not be used, or used with caution, in pregnancy (*cont.*)

Drug	*Harmful effects*
	in last week. Because it blocks prostaglandins, high doses may affect breathing in the newborn baby (see under anti-inflammatory drugs) and, because it displaces the bile pigment bilirubin from blood proteins, it may increase the risk of kernicterus in premature and/or jaundiced babies. For other possible harmful effects, see anti-inflammatory drugs. Do not use in last week of pregnancy
azathioprine	May, very rarely, damage the baby if used in first 3 months
Aztreonam	Manufacturer advises that it should not be used in pregnancy
barbiturates	Regular daily use in last 3 months may produce withdrawal effects in the newborn baby. They may depress the newborn baby's breathing if used at the end of pregnancy or during labour
beta blockers	If used at the end of pregnancy may produce a low blood glucose (hypoglycaemia) in the newborn baby. They may slow down the heart rate of the baby before it is born and after it has been born, particularly if the mother has severe raised blood pressure which may impair the flow of blood through the placenta
bethanidine	Should not be used to treat raised blood pressure in pregnancy. If used in last 3 months, it may cause a reduced blood flow through the placenta to the baby. May cause fall in blood pressure on standing up after sitting or lying down (postural hypotension) in the mother
captopril	Should not be used at all during pregnancy because it may affect the blood pressure and kidney function of the baby before and after it is born. It may also produce defects of the skull in the baby
carbenoxolone	Do not use in the last 3 months of pregnancy. Causes retention of sodium and fluids in the mother.
chenodeoxycholic acid	If used at any time during pregnancy there is a possibility that it could affect the baby's metabolism
chloramphenicol	If used in high doses at the end of pregnancy, it may cause the 'grey syndrome' in newborn babies. This consists of vomiting, distension of the abdomen, an ashen-grey colour, poor breathing and a low temperature. The baby may become blue and shocked and die in a few days
ciprofloxacin	Should not be used in pregnancy. It may damage the joints of fetuses in pregnant animals
cisapride	Manufacturer advises that it should not be used in pregnancy
clofibrate	Should not be used in pregnancy because there is a possibility that it could interfere with growth and development because of its anti-cholesterol effect
contraceptives, oral	Should not be used in first 3 months; rare risk of damage to the baby
corticosteroids	Regular daily use of high doses (e.g. greater than 10 mg of prednisolone daily or the equivalent for the other corticosteroids)

Table 79.1 Drugs that should not be used, or used with caution, in pregnancy (*cont.*)

Drug	*Harmful effects*
	during the last 6 months may knock out the adrenal glands in the unborn and in the newborn baby
co-trimoxazole (contains trimethoprim and sulphamethoxazole)	Should not be used in pregnancy. Use of trimethoprim in first 3 months of pregnancy may damage the baby. It produces anti-folic acid effects. For harmful effects of sulphamethoxazole, see entry on sulphonamides
cyclosporin	May interfere with the growth of the unborn baby
danazol	If used at any stage during pregnancy, it may cause masculinization of a female baby due to its weak male hormone effects
dapsone	Regular use at the end of pregnancy may damage the newborn baby's red blood cells, causing haemolytic anaemia. It may also cause methaemoglobinaemia (an abnormal haemoglobin in red blood cells, making them unable to carry oxygen). The mother should be given supplements of folic acid during treatment
debrisoquine	Should not be used to treat raised blood pressure in pregnancy. If used in last 3 months, it may cause a reduced blood flow through the placenta to the baby. May cause fall in blood pressure on standing up after sitting or lying down (postural hypotension) in the mother
Dianette	If used at any stage during pregnancy, it may cause feminization of male babies due to the anti-male hormone effects of cyproterone which it contains. Should not be used
diazoxide	Prolonged regular daily use in last 6 months may cause loss of hair and disorders of blood glucose levels in the newborn baby. If used during labour, it may stop the womb from contracting
diethylpropion	Should not be used; it may damage the unborn baby
dihydroergotamine	Do not use in pregnancy. It may cause the womb to contract
diltiazem	Should be used with caution because it may produce abnormalities of fetuses in pregnant animals. If used near or during labour, it may stop the womb from contracting and inhibit labour
distigmine	Should not be used in pregnancy because it may cause the womb to contract
disulfiram (Antabuse)	Use in first 3 months may damage the baby due to toxic break-down products of alcohol products when it is taken with alcohol
diuretics	Should not be used to treat blood pressure in pregnancy because they reduce the volume of body fluids in the mother, which may cause a reduced blood flow through the placenta to the baby. The use of *thiazide diuretics* at the end of pregnancy may damage the bone marrow of the newborn baby, causing a reduction in platelets (thrombocytopenia) and resulting in bleeding and bruising

Table 79.1 Drugs that should not be used, or used with caution, in pregnancy (*cont*)

Drug	*Harmful effects*
enalapril	Should not be used at all during pregnancy because it may affect the blood pressure and kidney function of the baby before and after it is born. Also damages fetuses when given to pregnant animals
enoxacin	Should not be used in pregnancy. May damage joints of fetuses in pregnant animals
ergotamine	Should not be used in pregnancy because it may cause the womb to contract
etretinate	Should not be used in pregnancy because there is a high risk of it damaging the baby. Avoid sexual intercourse or use effective contraception 1 month before and during treatment, and for 2 years after treatment is stopped
fenofibrate	Should not be used in pregnancy. Damages fetuses in pregnant animals
flecainide	Damages fetuses in pregnant animals; therefore should be used with caution in first 3 months
fluconazole	Should not be used in pregnancy. High doses may damage fetuses in pregnant animals
flucytosine	If used in first 3 months, it may damage the baby
ganciclovir	Should not be used in first half of pregnancy. May damage the unborn baby
gold salts	*Auranofin* damages fetuses in pregnant animals. Should not be used in pregnancy. *Gold injections* (aurothiomalate) – should not be used in pregnancy Women of child-bearing potential should avoid sexual intercourse or use effective contraception during and for 3 months after treatment with gold salts
griseofulvin	Should not be used in pregnancy; damages fetuses in pregnant animals
guanethidine	Should not be used to treat raised blood pressure in pregnancy. If used in last 3 months, may cause a reduced blood flow through the placenta to the baby. May cause fall in blood pressure on standing up after sitting or lying down (postural hypotension) in the mother
heparin	Prolonged use may cause osteoporosis
hydralazine	Should not be used in first half of pregnancy. May damage fetuses in pregnant animals
iodine and iodides	Regular daily use in last 6 months may produce a goitre or under-active thyroid gland in newborn babies. Note that some cough medicines contain iodides. *Radioactive iodine* should not be used in pregnancy because it may knock out the baby's thyroid gland permanently
isotretinoin	Should not be used in pregnancy because there is a high risk of damage to the baby. Sexual intercourse should be avoided or effective contraception used for 1 month before, during and for 1 month after treatment

Table 79.1 Drugs that should not be used, or used with caution, in pregnancy (*cont.*)

Drug	*Harmful effects*
isradipine	If used at the end of pregnancy it may prolong labour
itraconazole	Should not be used in pregnancy. May damage fetuses in pregnant animals. In women of child-bearing potential, sexual intercourse should be avoided or effective contraception used during and for 1 month after treatment
ketoconazole	Should not be used in pregnancy. Damages fetuses in pregnant animals
lisinopril	Should not be used in pregnancy. See entry under captopril
lithium	If used in first 3 months, there is a low risk that it may damage the baby. Regular daily use in the last 6 months may cause goitre in the newborn baby and also lithium toxicity – floppy limbs and blueness. The dose in pregnancy has to be increased but should be carefully controlled by carrying out repeated estimates of the concentration of lithium in the mother's blood
mebendazole	Should not be used in pregnancy. Damages fetuses in pregnant animals
menadiol sodium phosphate (vitamin K)	Use at the end of pregnancy may damage blood cells and cause haemolytic anaemia in the newborn baby. It may also increase the risk of a jaundiced baby developing kernicterus
metaraminol	Should not be used in pregnancy because it can reduce the blood supply to the baby through the placenta
metronidazole	High-dose treatment should not be used in pregnancy
metyrapone	Should not be used in pregnancy. May damage production of steroids by the placenta
minoxidil	May produce excessive growth of hair in newborn baby if used in last 3 months of pregnancy
misoprostol	Should not be used in pregnancy. May make the womb contract
nalidixic acid	Causes damage to joints in fetuses of pregnant animals – use with caution throughout pregnancy
narcotic pain relievers (opioid analgesics)	If used at the end of pregnancy and/or during labour, may depress breathing in the newborn baby. Withdrawal effects in the newborn baby may occur if mother was addicted. May stop stomach from emptying in the mother, with a risk that she may vomit during labour and inhale the vomit
neostigmine	If used in high doses at the end of pregnancy, may produce muscle weakness in the newborn baby
nifedipine	Should not be used in pregnancy. Damages fetuses in pregnant animals. May inhibit labour because it stops the womb from contracting
nitrofurantoin	If used at the end of pregnancy, may damage red blood cells in the newborn baby and cause haemolytic anaemia
non-steroidal anti-inflammatory drugs (NSAIDs)	See anti-inflammatory drugs

Table 79.1 Drugs that should not be used, or used with caution, in pregnancy (*cont.*)

Drug	*Harmful effects*
noradrenaline	Should not be used in pregnancy – may reduce the blood supply to the baby through the placenta
octreotide	Should not be used in pregnancy; may damage growth of unborn baby
oestrogens	Should not be used in pregnancy. If used in first 3 months, may cause abnormalities in the newborn baby. *Diethylstilboestrol* – high doses in first 3 months of pregnancy may cause cancer of the vagina in female offspring some 15–20 years later
omeprazole	Should not be used in pregnancy. Damages fetuses in pregnant animals
penicillamine	Should not be used in pregnancy; may damage the baby
phenobarbitone	See entry on anti-epileptic drugs. Regular daily use of phenobarbitone towards the end of pregnancy may affect the production of blood-clotting factors that require vitamin K. This may cause bleeding in the newborn baby. Vitamin K_1 should be given to the mother before delivery and to the baby at birth
phenytoin	See entry on anti-epileptic drugs. Regular daily use of phenytoin towards the end of pregnancy may affect the production of blood-clotting factors that require vitamin K. This may cause bleeding in the newborn baby. Vitamin K_1 should be given to the mother before delivery and to the baby at birth
piperazine	Should not be used in pregnancy except on medical advice
podophyllum resin	Should not be used in pregnancy. May be absorbed from the skin, to cause abnormalities and/or death of the unborn baby
povidone-iodine	Should not be used in last 6 months of pregnancy because enough iodine may be absorbed from a local application to damage the unborn baby's thyroid gland
progestogens	Use of high doses in first 3 months may damage the baby. Should be used with caution
pyridostigmine	The use of large doses at the end of pregnancy may cause muscle weakness in newborn babies
quinapril	See under ACE inhibitors
quinine	Use of high dose in first 3 months may damage the baby. Benefits outweigh risks in treating malaria but *not* in treating night cramps (see under anti-malarial drugs)
quinolones	Should not be used in pregnancy. May damage the joints of fetuses in pregnant animals
reserpine	Regular daily use at the end of pregnancy may cause slowing of the heart rate, drowsiness and a stuffy nose in newborn babies
rifampicin	Should be used with caution in pregnancy. High doses may damage fetuses in pregnant animals. If used at the end of pregnancy there is an increased risk of the newborn baby developing bleeding due to a low prothrombin level in the blood

Table 79.1 Drugs that should not be used, or used with caution, in pregnancy (*cont.*)

Drug	*Harmful effects*
simvastatin	Should not be used in pregnancy. It may damage fetuses in pregnant animals. Women of child-bearing potential should avoid sexual intercourse or use a mechanical means of contraception during treatment, not the pill
sleeping drugs	If used at the end of pregnancy or during labour they may depress breathing in the newborn baby. (For risks of *barbiturates*, see entry 'barbiturates'; for risks of *benzodiazepines*, see under entry on anti-anxiety drugs.) *Thalidomide* damages the baby if used in the first 3 months of pregnancy
spironolactone	Breakdown products may produce cancer in rats, therefore use with caution
streptokinase	Should not be used in pregnancy because of potential risk of bleeding in the unborn baby and the risk of premature separation of the afterbirth in the first 18 weeks of pregnancy. May cause bleeding in the mother if used after labour
sulphasalazine	Sulphasalazine (Salazopyrin) is used to treat ulcerative colitis and Crohn's disease. It is broken down in the intestine into an aspirin-related drug (see entry 'aspirin') and a sulphonamide drug (see entry 'sulphonamides'). Could possibly cause haemolytic anaemia in newborn babies. Folic acid supplements should be given to the mother
sulphonamides	Should not be used in the last 3 months of pregnancy; may cause damage to red blood cells in newborn babies, causing haemolytic anaemia. There is also an increased risk of kernicterus in jaundiced babies and a risk of methaemoglobinaemia (an abnormal haemoglobin in red blood cells which makes them unable to carry oxygen)
tetracyclines	Tetracycline antibiotics are deposited in the teeth of the developing baby. They will produce discoloration of the milk teeth if used from the 14th week, and of the permanent teeth if used in last 3 months. Large doses intravenously may damage the mother's liver
thiabendazole	Should not be used in pregnancy. Damages fetuses in pregnant animals
tinidazole	Should not be used in first 3 months of pregnancy. May damage the baby
tocainide	May cause damage to fetuses in pregnant animals; therefore use with caution in first 3 months
trilostane	Should not be used in pregnancy because it interferes with the production of sex hormones by the placenta
trimethoprim	Should not be used in pregnancy. Use in first 3 months may damage the baby. It blocks the use of folic acid. Note entry on *co-trimoxazole*

Table 79.1 Drugs that should not be used, or used with caution, in pregnancy (*cont.*)

Drug	*Harmful effects*
tribavirin	Should not be used in pregnancy or in women of child-bearing potential
urokinase	Should not be used in pregnancy because of the potential risk of bleeding in the unborn baby and the risk of premature separation of the afterbirth in the first 18 weeks of pregnancy. Should not be used in mothers after labour because of risk of haemorrhage
vaccines (live)	Viruses from live vaccines enter the baby in the mother's womb and there is a potential risk of damage to the baby if used in first 3 months
verapamil	If used towards the end of pregnancy, it may inhibit labour
vidarabine	Damages fetuses in pregnant animals; therefore it should be used with caution in first 3 months
vigabatrin	Do not use in pregnancy. Animal studies show it to be toxic to fetuses
vitamins	Excessive doses of *vitamin A* and liver which contains high amounts of Vitamin A in first 3 months may damage the baby. *Vitamin K* products (but not vitamin K_1) may cause bleeding in the newborn baby if given at the end of pregnancy. Also displaces the bile pigment bilirubin from blood proteins and therefore increases the risk of kernicterus in jaundiced babies, especially if they are premature
xamoterol	Should not be used in pregnancy. May damage fetuses in pregnant animals
X-rays	If used in pregnancy there is an increased risk of leukaemia developing in childhood

80

Breast feeding and the risks of drug treatments

Most drugs taken by a breast-feeding mother will be excreted in her breast milk, and whilst the concentration will vary according to which drug she takes it will usually be in such a low amount as not to affect the baby. However, newborn babies, particularly if they are premature, may not be able to excrete even a small amount of a drug and therefore, if the drug is taken regularly every day by the mother, the drug may accumulate in the baby and produce toxic effects.

In general, only about 1 per cent of a drug taken by a breast-feeding mother appears in her breast milk; however, some drugs may actually appear in larger concentrations than in the mother's blood because they are concentrated in breast milk (e.g. iodine, which is present in some cough medicines and could affect the baby's thyroid gland).

Drugs that easily dissolve in fat will enter breast milk more readily than will drugs that are not very soluble in fat. Also, if the concentration of a drug in the mother's blood is higher than normal because she is unable to excrete the drug efficiently as a result of some kidney disorder, the concentration of that drug in her breast milk will also be higher than normal. This means that such mothers should take drugs with utmost caution and only under strict medical supervision.

There is a lack of information from adequate and well controlled studies on the safety of most drugs in breast-feeding mothers, whether they are prescribed or bought over-the-counter from a pharmacist, drug store, herbalist, health food shop or other outlets. Therefore, if you are breast feeding, it is wise only to take a drug regularly every day if the expected benefits to you outweigh any possible risk to the baby. In other words, use drugs with caution, not in high doses and preferably only when necessary. These warnings also apply to the use of alcohol, caffeine in tea, coffee and colas, and smoking.

Table 80.1 Drugs that enter breast milk and may affect the baby

Drug groups	*Possible harmful effect on the infant*
alcohol	Large amounts of alcohol may affect the baby
amiodarone	High concentrations in milk could release iodine (see 'iodine' under 'thyroid drugs')
anti-anxiety drugs	Large doses of *barbiturates* may produce drowsiness. Do not use if possible *Benzodiazepines* may produce drowsiness, lethargy, failure to thrive and weight loss. Do not use in repeated doses *Meprobamate* and related anti-anxiety drugs: concentrate in breast milk and may produce drowsiness. Do not use. NOTE Meprobamate is combined with aspirin and ethoheptazine in Equagesic
anti-bacterials	*Chloramphenicol* may damage the bone marrow, producing blood disorders. Do not use, or stop breast feeding *Tetracyclines* Risk of harmful effects on the teeth may be avoided because calcium in the breast milk may reduce absorption into the baby's blood stream. However, better not to use if possible *Sulphonamides* Risk of damage to the red blood cells (haemolytic anaemia) in G6PD-deficient babies and kernicterus in jaundiced newborn, particularly with long-acting sulphonamides. Similar risks apply to the use of *co-trimoxazole* because it contains a sulphonamide, sulphamethoxazole *Metronidazole* Large amount in the milk, do not breast feed for 24 hours after large single doses. May produce a bitter taste in the milk and put the baby off sucking *Nalidixic acid* May cause damage to red blood cells (haemolytic anaemia) – use with caution *Nitrofurantoin* may produce damage to red blood cells (haemolytic anaemia) in G6PD-deficient babies
anti-cancer drugs	Do not breast feed
anti-coagulants	Risk of bleeding with oral anti-coagulants. Do not use *phenindione* With *warfarin* and *nicoumalone* give vitamin K *Heparin* is not excreted in breast milk
anti-depressants	Accumulation of breakdown products of *doxepin* in the baby may cause drowsiness and affect breathing *Lithium* enters breast milk and may produce lethargy and floppy limbs if the concentration in the mother's milk is high because the level of the drug in her blood has not been well controlled. If the baby loses fluid because of diarrhoea the risks will be greater. Unless strict monitoring of the blood level of lithium in the mother is possible, it is safer not to breast feed
anti-diabetics	*Sulphonylureas* may possibly produce a fall in blood glucose
anti-epileptics	*Ethosuximide* may make the baby over-excitable and cause poor sucking. *Phenobarbitone* and *primidone* may produce drowsiness. *Phenobarbitone* and *phenytoin* may cause methaemoglobinaemina (an abnormal haemoglobin in red blood cells, making them unable to carry oxygen)

Table 80.1 Drugs that enter breast milk and may affect the baby (*cont.*)

Drug groups	*Possible harmful effect on the infant*
anti-malarials	Benefits of treatment of malaria outweigh the risks. NOTE *Fansidar* contains *sulphadoxine* and *Maloprim* contains *dapsone*, both of which may, rarely, damage the red blood cells and produce haemolytic anaemia, especially in G6PD-deficient babies. They may also cause kernicterus in jaundiced babies
anti-psychotics	Animal studies suggest possibility of harmful effects on developing nervous system; therefore, if taking any of these drugs, probably better not to breast feed *Chlorpromazine* may produce drowsiness *Sulpiride* is present in large amounts in breast milk; therefore do not use
anti-viral drugs	*Idoxuridine* may make the milk taste unpleasant and put the baby off sucking Do not use *ganciclovir* because of risk of harmful effects
aspirin	Do not use aspirin because of possible risk of Reye's syndrome (see Chapter 27). Regular daily use may affect platelet production and cause bleeding and bruising if the newborn baby's store of vitamin K is low
asthma drugs	*Theophylline* may produce irritability; sustained-release preparations may be safer *Ephedrine* may produce irritability and disturbed sleep (note its use in some cough remedies)
atropine	May produce anti-cholinergic harmful effects (see Chapter 2)
beta blockers	Should be used with caution. May possibly cause a slowing of the heart and a low blood glucose
bromocriptine	Suppresses milk production
caffeine (e.g. in tea, coffee, cola drinks)	Regular intake of large amounts can affect the baby, making it restless. Newborn babies cannot break caffeine down in the liver until they are about 3–6 months old. They have to excrete it unchanged in their urine
calcitonin	Do not use if you are breast feeding – it stops milk production in animals
carbimazole	Do not use. May affect the baby's thyroid gland
carisoprodol	Concentrated in breast milk; therefore do not use if you are breast feeding
ciprofloxacin	Do not use if breast feeding. High concentrations in breast milk of animals
clemastine	May produce drowsiness and irritability
colchicine	Should be used with caution because of its potential harmful effects on cells
cold and cough remedies	*Ephedrine* and *pseudoephedrine* may produce irritability and disturbed sleep *Aspirin* – see 'aspirin' *Bromides* may cause drowsiness and skin rash

Table 80.1 Drugs that enter breast milk and may affect the baby (*cont.*)

Drug groups	*Possible harmful effect on the infant*
	Iodine Concentrated in breast milk, may cause goitre or underactive thyroid gland. Stop breast feeding. Do not use cough medicines that contain iodine *Theophylline* – see under 'asthma drugs' *Anti-cholinergic* drugs – risk of anti-cholinergic harmful effects (see Chapter 2)
corticosteroids	Regular daily use of high doses (10 mg of prednisolone or equivalent) could possibly reduce the functioning of the adrenal glands. Baby must be medically examined at regular intervals
cyproterone	Use with caution. May have anti-male sex hormone effects on the baby
danazol	Should not be used. May possibly cause male hormone effects on the baby
dapsone	Use with caution. Slight risk of damage to baby's red blood cells (haemolytic anaemia)
diuretics	*Spironolactone* should not be used because of reported risk of cancer in rodents Large doses of *thiazide* diuretics may suppress milk production
enoxacin	Should not be used. High concentrations in breast milk of animals
ergotamine	May produce vomiting, diarrhoea, convulsions and poor circulation. Repeated doses may dry up the milk. Do not use
etretinate	Should not be used because of potential harmful effects
female sex hormones	*Oestrogens* High doses suppress milk production *Progestogens* High doses suppress milk production
gold salts	Should not be used. They are excreted in breast milk and there is a possible risk of harmful effects (e.g. skin rash)
indomethacin	Is present in high amounts in breast milk; convulsions have been reported. Do not use
iodine	See thyroid drugs
isoniazid	Mother and baby should be given pyridoxine (vitamin B_6) to prevent risk of nerve damage
isotretinoin	Should not be used because of risk of harmful effects
laxatives	Large doses of stimulant laxatives (e.g. cascara, danthron, senna) may cause diarrhoea *Phenolphthalein* should not be used. It may cause diarrhoea and skin rash
male sex hormones	Should not be used. May cause masculinization of female babies and precocious sexual development of male babies. High doses suppress milk production
mesalazine	May cause diarrhoea
narcotic pain relievers	Regular daily use of high doses can produce addiction in the baby *Methadone* in an addicted mother may produce withdrawal symptoms in the baby. May breast feed if on maintenance therapy

Table 80.1 Drugs that enter breast milk and may affect the baby (*cont.*)

Drug groups	*Possible harmful effect on the infant*
	Morphine 'Normal' doses may not be harmful. In an addicted mother, may produce withdrawal symptoms in the baby – do not breast feed *Diamorphine* Addicted mothers should not breast feed their babies
nifedipine	Do not use
octreotide	Should not be used because of risk of harmful effects
oestrogens	High doses stop milk production (see under oral contraceptives)
oral contraceptives	*Combined oestrogen/progestogen preparations* may reduce milk flow if mother is having difficulty or if the dose of oestrogen is above 50 micrograms *Progestogen-only* contraceptives do not affect milk flow once it has started and may be used when breast feeding
povidone-iodine	May be absorbed from the vagina and the iodine concentrated in the breast milk, to produce harmful effects on the thyroid gland (see 'thyroid drugs')
progestogens	High doses stop milk production (see under oral contraceptives)
sleeping drugs	Large doses of *barbiturates* may produce drowsiness. Do not use if possible *Benzodiazepines* may produce drowsiness, lethargy, failure to thrive and weight loss. Do not use in repeated doses *Chloral hydrate* and related sleeping drugs (e.g. chloral betaine, triclofos) may produce drowsiness
smoking	Smoking more than 20 cigarettes a day may reduce milk production and cause jitteriness in the baby
sulphasalazine	May very rarely cause bloody diarrhoea. May possibly damage red blood cells, producing haemolytic anaemia in G6PD-deficient babies
thyroid drugs	*Thyroxine* and *liothyronine* may affect laboratory tests for under-active thyroid gland *Anti-thyroid* drugs may block the production of thyroid hormones by the thyroid gland, particularly in newborn babies. Babies must be carefully monitored for signs of under-activity of their thyroid glands *Iodine* concentrated in breast milk; may cause goitre or under-active thyroid gland. Stop breast feeding *Radioactive iodine* may knock out the thyroid gland permanently. Do not breast feed. With diagnostic doses, do not breast feed for 24 hours
vitamins	Prolonged use of high doses of *vitamin A* may possibly produce harmful effects High doses of *vitamin D* may produce a raised blood calcium level
Thiamine	Severely thiamine-deficient mothers should not breast feed because of toxic products in their milk

81

Babies, infants and children, and the risks of drug treatments

When it comes to giving drugs to babies, infants and young children, it is important to remember that they are not 'little adults'. Many of their organs and tissues are not fully developed. In particular, their liver and kidneys may not be developed enough to break down certain drugs and to excrete them, which may cause toxic levels of the drug in the blood stream and the appearance of harmful effects.

Babies, infants and young children may easily become over-sensitive to the effects of drugs, because their bodies are rapidly affected by loss of fluids (e.g. due to diarrhoea and/or vomiting or to fever), or to changes in the acidity of the blood which may occur in sick children. A drug given to a child who is suffering from dehydration, who has a fever or whose acidity of the blood is increased may develop an exaggerated response to that drug; therefore, any drug should be given with utmost caution in these conditions.

The doses of drugs used to treat many minor illnesses in babies, infants and young children are scaled-down versions of adult dosages and scientifically calculated doses are not available. These doses have usually been developed over time and in general they are satisfactory. However, they are not satisfactory when treating more serious illnesses, particularly with drugs that have a narrow margin of safety between an effective dose and a harmful dose. With these drugs a safe dose may be calculated from the child's weight or surface area, and such doses may be appropriate with some drugs but not with others; this is why in some countries (e.g. the USA) certain drugs with narrow margins of safety are not allowed to be used to treat babies, infants and young children. These restrictions may well help to protect some children but they may also deny others the benefits of a potentially useful drug.

Against such a background, it makes sense not to use drugs in premature babies and babies up to the age of 1 month unless it is absolutely necessary, and to use drugs with utmost caution in older babies, infants and young children. Most commonly occurring illnesses in otherwise healthy babies, infants and young children are mild and self-limiting and do not need treating; some more serious ones can be prevented – for example, german measles, mumps, measles, polio, whooping cough and tetanus (see Chapter 11).

When drug treatment is used in babies, infants and young children, the dosage schedule should be as simple as possible (e.g. twice daily instead of four times daily) and the drug preparation should be as palatable as possible.

NOTE Certain commonly used drugs should not be used in children; for example, aspirin and tetracycline antibiotics.

Sugar

Many medicines contain sugar, which may be harmful to children's teeth – particularly if the medicine has to be taken regularly every day. It is therefore important when possible to use *sugar-free medicines*, whether tablets, capsules, liquids or diluting solutions. Consult your pharmacist.

A medicine should never be added to a baby's milk; it may react with the milk, which will interfere with its absorption from the baby's intestine and the baby may not get the full recommended dose.

Colouring agents and other additives

A few children may be sensitive to certain colouring agents (e.g. tartrazine) or some other additive in a medicine. If you suspect that your child is sensitive to an additive in a medicine, whether liquid, tablets or capsules, check with your pharmacist. Some manufacturers are now excluding from their preparations those additives that may cause problems. (The same advice applies to adults.)

82

Elderly people and the risks of drug treatments

Most doctors talk about elderly people as being aged 65 years or over; this is not because we want to label all people over 65 years as elderly, but when talking about drug treatment it does help to remind us to be cautious in someone who is turned 65 years. In this book I also use the term 'old elderly' to refer to patients over 75 years of age. Again, this is not meant to be derogatory; it is to remind us that these people, when ill, are particularly vulnerable to the effects of drugs.

If you are 65 years of age or over, you are more likely to be suffering from more disorders and to be taking more drugs regularly every day than are younger people. You are also more likely to suffer from the harmful effects of drugs. This risk may be slight if you are aged from 65 to 75 years, but if you are over 75 years of age the risks increase.

As we reach 'old' age our bodies undergo changes that may affect how we deal with drugs. We undergo changes in our total body fat, lean body mass and total body water; in the blood flow to various organs and tissues (e.g. to the brain); changes in the protein content of the blood, which may affect the transport of drugs; changes in the functioning of the kidneys and liver; changes in our ability to control our temperature (note the risk of hypothermia in elderly people); and changes in our ability to control our blood pressure with changes of posture; for example, we may become light-headed and faint if we stand up quickly from sitting or lying down. As we get older we also may become more sensitive to the effects of certain drugs (e.g. sleeping drugs).

Harmful effects from drugs will be more likely if our kidneys become less efficient at excreting drugs. If this happens, 'normal' doses of drugs used in younger people may produce harmful effects because the blood level of the active drug may rise to toxic levels due to reduced excretion by the kidneys. Harmful effects may also occur if our liver becomes less efficient at breaking drugs down.

Because of the various effects of ageing, elderly people may be more prone to develop:

- Drowsiness, hangover and confusion from sleeping drugs, anti-anxiety drugs and anti-psychotic drugs

- Dizziness, light-headedness, fainting and falls from anti-blood-pressure drugs
- Dizziness and weakness caused by disturbances of the blood chemistry from water tablets (diuretics) and laxatives
- Difficulties with passing urine from various drugs, including anti-depressants, anti-cholinergic drugs, antihistamines and drugs used to treat parkinsonism
- Constipation from narcotic pain relievers
- Eye problems from anti-cholinergic drugs and many other drugs
- More severe stomach ulceration and bleeding from anti-rheumatic drugs
- More bone marrow damage, producing anaemia and other blood disorders from using anti-bacterial drugs such as the sulphonamides and co-trimoxazole

In addition, because elderly people may be taking several drugs each day, they run an increased risk of developing harmful effects from one drug interacting with another (see Chapter 89).

Warnings on the use of drug treatments in the elderly

The observation that different people react differently to the same drug applies particularly to elderly people, and so we must avoid generalizations on drug use in the elderly. The treatment of elderly people should always be tailored to their individual needs. In addition, an elderly person's response to treatment should be carefully monitored over time, which means that elderly people on drug treatments should be seen and examined regularly by their doctors with the overall aim of producing the maximum benefits for minimum risks. This may be achieved by continuing drug treatment *only* when it is necessary and by using the minimum effective daily dosages for the shortest duration of time possible.

Relatives, friends, neighbours or carers who collect repeat prescriptions for elderly people month after month without their being seen and examined by their doctor do not do these elderly people a great favour. It would be far better if they were seen and examined by their doctors at regular intervals – at least once every 2–3 months.

Harmful effects from drugs are likely to be more frequent and/or severe in elderly people than in younger people; therefore all drugs should be used with caution by elderly people. You should check the harmful effects and warnings specific to any drug that you are taking and you should note specifically when you should take a reduced dosage and when you should have tests of your kidney function and other tests. Also you should not expect drug treatment for all your symptoms; no drug treatment may be much better and safer.

In elderly people the harmful effects of some drugs may be more frequent or severe. The following list includes some examples. (See also drug use in mild kidney failure Chapter 84)

Table 82.1 Examples of harmful effects of drug treatments in the elderly

Drug groups	*Harmful effects*
Anti-anxiety drugs (benzodiazepines)	Increased risk of harmful effects – drowsiness, ataxia, confusion. Small doses should be used
anti-asthma drugs	*Theophylline* Increased risk of harmful effects, especially nausea and confusion, due to raised blood levels. Small doses should be used to start treatment and then increased by very small amounts *Ephedrine* may cause retention of urine, especially in elderly men with enlarged prostate glands
anti-bacterial drugs	*Tetracyclines* Increased risk of harmful effects due to reduced excretion by kidneys. Also may cause rise in waste products in the blood (e.g. urea). Should be used with caution *Aminoglycosides* Reduced excretion by kidneys; therefore increased risk of harmful effects, especially deafness. Smaller dose should be used, and blood levels monitored *Co-trimoxazole* Increased risk of blood disorders. Should be used with caution *Nitrofurantoin* Increased risk of nausea and nerve damage because of reduced excretion. Should not be used if possible
anti-blood-pressure drugs	Increased risk of a drop in blood pressure on standing up after sitting or lying down (postural hypotension). This may cause light-headedness, dizziness and faintness, and elderly people may fall. Also, an excessive drop in blood pressure may trigger a stroke. Starting doses should be small, and any increase in dose should be small. Treatment should be built up gradually, and a rapid and excessive drop in blood pressure should be avoided Anti-blood-pressure drugs that cause severe postural hypotension should not be used; for example, *bethanidine, debrisoquine, guanethidine* The excretion of some ACE inhibitors such as *captopril* and *enalapril* may be reduced; therefore their doses should be reduced, particularly the starting doses
anti-coagulant drugs	Increased risk of bleeding. Smaller doses should be used of all anti-coagulant drugs and do not use *heparin* in full doses over a prolonged period of time
anti-depressants	*Tricyclic anti-depressants* Increased risk of harmful effects due to reduced excretion and raised blood levels – especially anti-cholinergic effects (such as blurred vision, dry mouth, constipation, difficulty in passing urine and confusion); may cause more problems for elderly people than younger people. A drop in blood pressure may occur on

Table 82.1 Examples of harmful effects of drug treatments in the elderly (*cont.*)

Drug	*Harmful effects*
	standing up after sitting or lying down (postural hypotension). This may cause light-headedness, dizziness and faintness and elderly people may fall. Smaller doses should be used Risk of damage to bone marrow by *mianserin* may be increased, causing a fall in white blood cells. Should be used with caution and in smaller doses The excretion of *trazodone* may be reduced, causing a rise in blood level and an increased risk of harmful effects (e.g. sedation). Smaller doses should be used *Lithium* Reduced excretion and increased risk of harmful effects. Smaller dose should be used. Increase in the volume of urine produced by lithium may cause dehydration and incontinence
anti-diabetic drugs	Increased risk of prolonged low blood glucose (hypoglycaemia) with *sulphonylureas* *Chlorpropamide* should not be used because it is long acting. Short-acting ones such as *tolbutamide* should be used
anti-inflammatory drugs (non-steroidal: NSAIDs)	Harmful effects of NSAIDs may affect elderly people more severely than younger people; for example, bleeding from the stomach and intestine and fluid retention
anti-parkinsonism drugs	Increased risk of harmful effects from *levodopa* and *bromocriptine*, especially confusion, serious mental symptoms, behaviour disorders and blood pressure changes. A drop in blood pressure may occur on standing up after sitting or lying down (postural hypotension). This may cause light-headedness, dizziness and faintness and elderly people may fall. Smaller doses should be used The risks of *amantadine* causing confusion and hallucinations are increased. Smaller dose should be used *Anti-cholinergic drugs* may cause confusion, difficulty passing urine, constipation and other harmful effects that are not well tolerated. Use smaller dose There is an increased risk of *selegiline* causing harmful effects (e.g. confusion and agitation) – smaller dose should be used
anti-peptic-ulcer drugs	*Carbenoxolone* Fluid retention increases the blood volume and increases the risk of developing a raised blood pressure, oedema (e.g. ankle swelling) and heart failure. The drug also causes a low potassium level which may be harmful, especially in patients who are taking digoxin or a related drug. Do not use in high doses or for prolonged periods of time *Cimetidine and ranitidine* Excretion by the kidneys is reduced, causing a rise in blood level and increased risk of harmful effects (e.g. confusion). Dose should be reduced
anti-psychotic drugs	Increased risk of harmful effects – parkinsonism and other movement disorders, anti-cholinergic effects (difficulty passing urine, constipation). A drop in blood pressure may occur on standing up after sitting or lying down (postural hypotension). This may cause light-headedness, dizziness, and faintness and elderly people may

Table 82.1 Examples of harmful effects of drug treatments in the elderly (*cont.*)

Drug	*Harmful effects*
	fall. Other blood pressure changes and temperature changes may also occur. Should not be used, or used with caution in smaller doses
beta blockers	Harmful effects on heart may be more frequent. Breakdown of *propranolol* in liver may be reduced and blood level may rise, producing increased risk of harmful effects Increased blood levels may occur with beta blockers that are excreted by the kidney, producing harmful effects; for example, *atenolol, nadolol, pindolol* and *sotalol*. The doses should be reduced. Smaller doses should be used at start of treatment
corticosteroids	Increased risk of osteoporosis, especially in women
digoxin	Excretion by the kidneys is reduced, causing a rise in blood level and an increased risk of harmful effects. The dose should be reduced. Treatment should be reviewed at regular intervals
diuretics	*Thiazide diuretics* and *loop diuretics*. Risk of producing dehydration and a low blood sodium level. A drop in blood pressure may occur on standing up after sitting or lying down (postural hypotension). This may cause light-headedness, dizziness and faintness and elderly people may fall. Increased volume of urine may cause incontinence or retention of urine. Risk of low blood potassium especially in elderly people on a poor diet. Smaller doses should be used. Effect of loop diuretics may be reduced and higher doses may be needed *Potassium-sparing diuretics* Increased risk of a raised blood potassium *Combinations of a thiazide diuretic with a potassium-sparing diuretic* Risk of low blood sodium. Should not be used, or used only in small doses
metoclopramide	Increased risk of movement disorders (e.g. parkinsonism). Should not be used regularly over prolonged periods of time
narcotic pain relievers	Increased risk of harmful effects from *dextropropoxyphene, methadone, pethidine* and *pentazocine*, due to raised blood levels
sleeping drugs	Increased risk of harmful effects on the brain which may be prolonged; for example, drowsiness in the day-time, ataxia, falls, confusion and restlessness. Do not use regularly every night if possible *Barbiturate* sleeping drugs should not be used. Only small doses of short-acting *benzodiazepines* should be used The elimination of *chlormethiazole* from the body may be impaired, and cause a raised blood level and an increased risk of harmful effects. Smaller doses should be used
thyroid drugs	Smaller doses should be used because of risk of triggering angina

83

Liver disease and the risks of drug treatments

Functions of the liver

The liver receives blood from the general circulation via a main artery called the hepatic artery, and blood returning from the intestine, spleen, pancreas and gall bladder via the portal vein. Blood from the liver is returned to the general circulation via the hepatic vein. Within the liver are microscopic canals that link up to form bile ducts. These drain bile into the gall bladder where it is concentrated (see later).

Liver cells carry out a whole range of activities, which include:

- The maintenance of blood glucose levels by storing or releasing glucose into the bloodstream
- The production of proteins from amino acids derived from proteins in the food
- The production of anti-blood-clotting proteins
- The production of many factors involved in the body's resistance to infection and injury
- The production of special proteins for the blood that act as 'shuttle' proteins to transport various substances (e.g. iron)
- The breakdown of fats and fatty acids, and formation of lipids. In the liver these are attached to proteins to form lipoproteins, which are released into the blood to supply muscles and other tissues with a source of energy or to be stored in fat deposits. In addition, cholesterol is also converted into bile acids (see later) which are passed into the bile and then the intestine where they help with the digestion of fats in food

Bile

Bile contains a red pigment called bilirubin. It is produced in the liver, spleen and bone marrow from breakdown of the red pigment, haemoglobin, in red blood cells. It is produced from the iron compound, haem, after removal of the iron which is recycled. This red pigment enters the bloodstream, becomes attached to certain proteins (albumins) and is transported to the liver. The liver cells secrete it into the bile after it has been combined with another chemical (glucuronic acid). This process is called conjugation, and the conjugated bilirubin passes through the bile and into the intestine where bacteria in the bowel convert it to a substance that colours the motions brown.

Bile also contains bile acids, which are made from cholesterol. They pass out into the duodenum where they break down fats in the food. Most of them are reabsorbed back into the bloodstream, returned to the liver and re-excreted into the bile.

The recycling of bile acids from the intestine to the liver and back to the intestine enables the bile acids to be used over and over again, which is useful because it allows a lot of bile acid to enter the intestine from a relatively small supply. New bile acids are made only to replace those lost in the faeces.

Bile acids are responsible for the absorption of fat and fat-soluble vitamins (A, D, E, K) from the food. A deficiency of bile acids can occur in liver disease, obstruction to the flow of bile (e.g. by a gall stone) and in certain disorders of the intestine.

Vitamins and minerals

The liver holds large stores of vitamins A, D and B_{12} which can last for months. It also has small stores of vitamin K and folates (folic acid) which are soon used up if there is a deficiency in the food. Vitamin K is used to form blood-clotting factors. The liver also stores iron.

Hormones

Several hormones are principally broken down in the liver; these include insulin, glucagon, growth hormone, corticosteroids, oestrogens and parathyroid hormones. The liver is also a main site of action for some hormones.

Drug breakdown (drug metabolism)

Most drugs are broken down by enzymes in the liver to inactive compounds which are soluble in water so that they can be excreted in the urine and in the bile. However, some drugs are converted into active compounds and it is better therefore to talk about drug metabolism rather than drug breakdown.

Certain drugs may increase or decrease the metabolism of other drugs in the liver. This may decrease or increase the concentration of the affected drugs in the bloodstream, causing problems in treatment. This is an example of what is known as a drug interacton (see Chapter 89).

Immune response

The liver plays a part in the body's defence system. It destroys worn out red cells, removes bacteria from the blood and plays a part in preventing proteins from food getting into the general circulation and producing an allergic reaction.

Jaundice

Jaundice is a term applied to a yellow colour of the skin, eyes and other tissues that results from an increase in the bile pigment bilirubin (see earlier), in the blood and other body fluids. All internal tissues and fluids are coloured yellow except the brain because bilirubin cannot pass through the normally protective barrier between the blood and the brain. However, this can happen in newly born babies and this is why certain types of jaundice in newborn babies may be harmful to the brain (see Chapter 26).

Disorders that cause jaundice may be put into three groups, as follows.

Jaundice due to destruction of red blood cells This occurs in haemolytic anaemia (see Chapter 47) where there is excessive destruction of red blood cells, producing large amounts of pigment in the blood. Except in newborn babies, the liver can cope very well with large amounts of bilirubin in the blood and jaundice is only mild in haemolytic anaemia.

Jaundice due to liver damage If the liver cells are damaged, bilirubin is not transported into the bile and its concentration in the blood increases. Also, the damaged liver cells may block the bile canals and cause bilirubin to enter the bloodstream. The common causes of acute liver disease are viruses (viral hepatitis), drugs and alcohol. The jaundice may be mild to severe.

Jaundice due to a block in the bile system This is called cholestatic jaundice, and is due to a blockage in the flow of bile anywhere between the duodenum and the liver cells. An impacted gall stone, cancer of the gall duct or narrowing due to scarring from previous surgery may block the large gall duct. Drugs and alcohol are important causes of damage to liver cells and of damage and blockage to the small bile ducts in the liver. The jaundice is severe and yellowish-green. Some individuals develop severe itching (pruritus), loss of appetite and a metallic taste in the mouth.

Chronic liver disease

There are two main forms of chronic liver disease – chronic hepatitis and cirrhosis. There are many causes of these disorders, which include alcohol and drugs.

Chronic hepatitis is a patchy death of liver cells associated with signs of chronic inflammation.

Cirrhosis is a widespread death of liver cells followed by scarring (fibrosis) and distortion of the liver produced by shrinking in some parts and overgrowth in others.

Alcohol directly damages the liver cells after years of exposure (5–15 years) to large daily doses. It produces cirrhosis of the liver.

Drugs can cause both chronic hepatitis and cirrhosis. The long-term use of methotrexate to treat cancer and methyldopa to treat raised blood pressure have, very rarely, been associated with these disorders, and so have phenylbutazone and sulphonamides.

Liver failure

Rarely, the liver can go into acute failure, causing jaundice and damage to the brain (encephalopathy) producing restlessness, drowsiness, confusion, disorientation, yawning, slurred speech, convulsions and unconsciousness. The damaging effects on brain function are thought to be due to a rise in the blood levels of ammonia and nitrogenous compounds, which can interfere with the transmission of nerve impulses. Acute viral hepatitis is the commonest cause and drugs are the next. Aspirin may cause severe liver failure in children and adolescents (see Chapter 27).

Treatment

Treatment of acute liver failure involves the withdrawal of all foods that contain nitrogen (e.g. proteins) and an attempt to reduce the production of nitrogen substances by bacteria in the bowel by giving an antibiotic, neomycin, to kill the bacteria. Neomycin is used because it is poorly absorbed into the bloodstream. In addition, a lactulose laxative is given. This also has the advantage that it increases the acidity in the bowel, which limits the absorption of ammonia into the bloodstream and promotes the use of nitrogen by bacteria that normally live in the bowel. Restlessness is controlled by injecting a small dose of diazepam (Valium) into a vein. Swelling of the brain (cerebral oedema), which is a frequent cause of death, is treated by infusing a diuretic, mannitol, rapidly into a vein.

Fluid retention

Sodium and water retention may occur in chronic liver disease, leading to retention of excessive fluid in the tissues (oedema), thus producing swelling (e.g. ankle swelling) and an abnormal accumulation of fluid in the abdominal cavity. This latter is called ascites and produces swelling of the abdomen. The volume of the blood becomes reduced and this affects the kidneys, which triggers the release of the hormone aldosterone (see Chapter 22) by the adrenal glands that in turn causes retention of sodium and loss of potassium.

Treatment

Treatment involves a low-salt diet and the use of a diuretic which blocks the effects of aldosterone (see Chapter 22). The diuretic acts against the effects of aldosterone and produces an increase of sodium in the urine and, therefore, water. It also causes retention of potassium.

Viral hepatitis

Hepatitis means inflammation of the liver, and virus infections are an important cause. Several specific hepatitis viruses can be recognized by laboratory tests. Other viruses include Epstein-Barr virus (glandular fever virus), herpes viruses, yellow fever virus, Lassa fever virus, but these are not generally included in the term viral hepatitis.

Acute hepatitis A (infective jaundice)

This disease is caused by the highly infectious type A virus and is usually spread by human faeces entering the body via the mouth; for example, infected persons who handle food can spread the disease by having faeces on their fingers due to lack of good hygiene when they have been to the lavatory. Little children can also spread the disease in a similar way. It may also be spread by infected blood transfusions and among sexual partners, particularly homosexuals through oral–anal contact. Infected persons excrete the virus in their faeces for about 2 weeks before and 1 week after the illness. The time between picking up the infection and the appearance of symptoms (the incubation period) is about 1 month.

For about 2 weeks infected individuals feel ill, develop headaches, chills, loss of appetite, nausea, vomiting and diarrhoea. They then become jaundiced (yellow), the urine becomes dark and the faeces pale. Slowly the symptoms clear up over 3–6 weeks. Milder cases do not become jaundiced. Most people recover fully although a few may relapse. Many may feel under the weather for several months after an attack.

Treatment

There is no specific treatment for hepatitis A, and good hygiene is the best form of prevention. Contacts can be protected by an injection of an immunoglobulin (see Chapter 11). This provides protection for 3 months and is useful for people travelling in areas where there is much of it about and hygiene is poor.

Acute hepatitis B (serum hepatitis)

Unlike type A, this virus has not been grown in a laboratory although it can be detected in the blood of infected persons. Blood and blood products are the main source of the type B virus. Infection may come from a transfusion with infected blood or from blood products. The latter account for the high incidence of hepatitis B among haemophiliac patients. Intravenous drug addicts spread hepatitis B by sharing dirty needles contaminated with infected blood. Tattooing and acupuncture may also spread this disease if contaminated needles are re-used.

Proteins from the virus have been detected in saliva, urine, semen and vaginal secretions; in addition to infection via blood and blood products, the virus can spread from one person to another by close sexual contact. This occurs largely among homosexual men. However, most of the world's hepatitis B carriers are found in the Far East, where the majority are infected from their mothers at birth.

Humans are the only source of hepatitis B and it takes about 3 months from the time of first infection to the appearance of positive blood tests for antibodies. Therefore a negative test in a contact does not necessarily exclude the possibility of disease. The disease is usually more severe than that described under hepatitis A, and skin rashes and arthritis are common complications. *Hepatitis D* appears to require hepatitis B to be effective; it causes acute and chronic liver damage.

Risk from carriers

A major risk of hepatitis B is that people who have no evidence of having had the disease may carry the virus. They have positive antibody tests for the virus and they can carry the virus for years. Some of these individuals eventually develop chronic liver disease (e.g. cirrhosis) and there is a rare but increased risk of their developing cancer of the liver.

The risk from carriers of hepatitis B is that they can spread the disease by sexual contact and by contact with their blood and other body fluids (e.g. saliva and urine), so special precautions should be taken by medical, nursing and dental staff when these patients are undergoing treatment.

People whose resistance to infection is lowered due to immune deficiency are susceptible to the condition. This may be because of disease (e.g. AIDS and certain cancers of lymph glands and lymph tissues), because of drugs that suppress their immune response (e.g. drugs given to prevent rejection of transplanted organs) or because they are undergoing long-term kidney dialysis.

Treatment

The best treatment for hepatitis B is prevention – screening blood donors, using sterile and preferably disposable needles etc., and using a condom and taking other sensible precautions during sexual intercourse. A hepatitis B vaccine is available for people at high risk of getting the disease (see Chapter 11), and for those who become infected accidentally (e.g. medical laboratory workers) an immunoglobulin (antibody) preparation is available (see Chapter 11). Infection acquired in adulthood may respond to treatment with interferon-alfa.

Hepatitis C, D and E

Once type A and B viruses were recognized, it was soon realized that other 'agents' could transfer infective hepatitis and trigger a defence response in the body (antibody formation). These were referred to as non-A and non-B hepatitis. A virus transmitted via blood and blood products, and also from a pregnant mother to her baby, has been identified as *hepatitis C* virus (HCV) and antibodies have been isolated. It appears to be a cause of chronic hepatitis following blood transfusions and rarely it can cause liver cancer. *Hepatitis E* has been identified as causing hepatitis non-A and non-B transmitted by the faeces (see earlier under hepatitis A). It can infect people immune to hepatitis A and can be very serious in pregnant women. For *Hepatitis D* see under *Acute hepatitis B*.

Treatment

Immunoglobulin (see Chapter 11), used to provide short-term protection against hepatitis A, may also protect against non-A, non-B hepatitis.

Harmful effects of drugs on the liver

Drugs that produce jaundice without liver damage

Drugs can increase the blood level of bilirubin and produce jaundice by damaging red blood cells (haemolytic anaemia, see Chapter 47). The jaundice is mild and is present without any damage to the liver.

Certain drugs, such as the sulphonamides and aspirin and related drugs, can displace bilirubin from attachment to protein in the blood; this causes 'free' bilirubin to circulate in the blood. This may produce very serious consequences if these drugs are taken in late pregnancy. The 'free' bilirubin passes from the mother into the baby's blood and then into its brain and spinal cord where it damages the nervous tissue. This disorder is known as *kernicterus* and, if severe, it appears on the second or third day of life with convulsions, drowsiness and risk of death. Less severe kernicterus may cause athetosis (slow involuntary movements, particularly of the arms and legs), spasticity (rigid spasm of muscles) and mental defects later in life.

Drugs that produce jaundice by interfering with the functions of the liver

Certain male sex hormones and body-building steroids can interfere with the excretion of bile pigment by the liver. They produce a chemical block that results in a deep jaundice similar to that produced when a gall stone blocks the flow of bile through the bile ducts into the intestine. Female sex hormones (oestrogens, including those used in the 'pill') can produce similar effects. Women who develop jaundice while on the pill also run the risk of getting jaundice during pregnancy. With these drugs the risk of getting jaundice is related to the dose of drug used – the higher the dose, the greater the risk.

Allergic drug reactions that produce jaundice

The anti-psychotic drug chlorpromazine, which is also used to prevent vomiting, can produce a similar kind of jaundice. This reaction is not related to the dose of chlorpromazine but appears to be an 'allergic' type of reaction in someone who is sensitive to the drug (about 0.5 per cent of people). The jaundice develops within the first 4 weeks of treatment and is associated with fever, nausea, vomiting and generalized itching. There may be some damage to liver cells. The jaundice and liver damage clear up within a few weeks or months after the drug is stopped.

Generalized allergic reactions may occasionally involve the liver producing jaundice; for example, allergic reaction to sulphonamides, penicillin, imipramine, phenytoin and para-aminosalicylic acid (PAS). These reactions may also be associated with some damage to the cells of the liver.

Drugs that damage the cells of the liver

Some drugs may damage liver cells directly and others may produce damage that looks like viral hepatitis. The similarity between the acute hepatitis produced by these drugs and that produced by viral hepatitis has sometimes caused problems when trying to decide whether the hepatitis was drug-related or not. This hepatitis-like drug reaction is not related to the dose of the drug used, though the risk may be increased by repeated use of the drug. It may occur up to 3 weeks after stopping the drug, and about one in five patients dies.

In addition to acute hepatitis, drugs may cause chronic hepatitis and cirrhosis (see earlier).

Warnings ***Alcohol*** *is a drug that may produce both acute liver damage (alcoholic hepatitis) and long-standing liver damage (cirrhosis).*

Aspirin *may cause liver damage in children, and should not be used in anyone under the age of 12 years.*

Liver disease and the use of drugs

The benefits and risks of taking a drug may change in a person with severe liver disease. Therefore, in these individuals drug treatments should be used as little as possible, and if they have to be used then the smallest possible dose of the drug for the shortest duration of time should be used.

Response to drugs by patients with liver disease

There are several ways in which the benefits and risks of drugs can be affected in patients with impaired liver function due to liver disease. These include the following.

Impaired liver function due to liver disease may slow the breakdown of a drug and result in a drug reaching a higher concentration in the blood, to produce toxic effects. Where a drug (e.g. rifampicin and fusidic acid) is excreted through the bile, any impairment of liver function and/or obstruction to the flow of bile through the bile system will result in a higher concentration of the drug in the blood to produce toxic reactions.

Proteins in the blood are an important method of transportation and storage of drugs, but if liver function is impaired there may be a fall in the production of these proteins by the liver, which results in a reduced amount of drug attached to the proteins and a higher level of 'free' drug in the bloodstream. It is this level of 'free' drug that determines a drug's beneficial and harmful effects. The anti-epileptic drug phenytoin is an example of a drug that may produce harmful effects if there is a fall in blood proteins; so is the corticosteroid drug prednisolone.

Impaired liver function may increase the harmful effects of certain drugs; for example, the liver is involved in the manufacture of blood-clotting factors and any impairment of liver function may reduce blood clotting and increase the risks of bleeding in people taking anti-coagulant drugs by mouth.

Drugs that can worsen the complications of liver disease

In patients with severe liver disease who run the risk of developing liver failure (see earlier) any drug that depresses the function of the brain should either be avoided or used with caution because they may cause the individual to go into a coma. They include sedatives, sleeping drugs, anti-anxiety drugs and morphine-related pain relievers. Diuretics (water tablets) may trigger a coma because they will increase the loss of potassium in the urine. Also, any drug that causes constipation may increase the absorption of ammonia compounds from the bowel and increase the risk of coma.

In patients with severe liver disease who have developed fluid retention (see earlier), diuretics should be used with utmost caution because of the serious risk of producing a low blood potassium level which may trigger coma. Drugs that contain a lot of sodium (e.g. some indigestion mixtures and some penicillin salts) should be used with caution, and so should drugs that cause sodium and water to be retained from the urine (e.g. carbenoxolone, corticosteroids and phenylbutazone). In addition to diuretics, any drug that causes potassium loss in the urine (e.g. carbenoxolone, corticosteroids) should be used with caution.

Some drugs are inactive until converted into an active form by the liver; for example, cortisone is converted to hydrocortisone, and prednisone to prednisolone by the liver. It therefore makes sense to use prednisolone or hydrocortisone and not prednisone or cortisone in someone with impaired liver function.

Use of drugs that may damage the liver

Some drugs are known to damage the liver and it is possible to *predict* that there will be a risk of liver damage if these drugs are used. Therefore such drugs should *not* be used in people with evidence of impaired liver function because liver damage may occur even if they are used in small doses.

The damage that some other drugs produce on the liver may be *unpredictable* and occur only in certain individuals and not in others. These reactions cannot be predicted because they are peculiar to the individual being treated – they are *idiosyncratic.* But, analysis of reports on such events makes it possible to identify those drugs that may produce such idiosyncratic reactions and they should be used with caution. However, there is no evidence that people with impaired liver function are more prone to develop such idiosyncratic liver damage than are people with normal liver function. Nevertheless, when patients with liver disease are being treated it is safer to avoid using *any drug* that is known to produce liver damage whether idiosyncratic or not. This is because if a drug damages the liver and produces jaundice in a patient with liver disease, it may not be possible to determine whether the jaundice was caused by the drug or by a worsening of the disease, which could have serious implications for treatment.

If it is necessary (i.e. life saving) to treat a patient with impaired liver function with a drug that is known to cause liver damage, tests of liver function should be carried out before and at regular intervals during treatment, and the drug should be stopped if there is any evidence of worsening of liver function. Unfortunately these tests are not that useful and it is important for patients to seek *immediate medical advice* on whether to stop such a drug if they develop symptoms suggestive of new liver damage such as lethargy, nausea, jaundice (yellowness of the eyes and/or skin), feeling unwell, dark urine, pale stools or any *new* symptom.

Use of drug treatments in patients with impaired liver function

As already discussed, the liver plays an important role in the breakdown of drugs in the body, and this activity may be affected by any disease or damage to the liver that impairs its function. Nevertheless, the cells of the liver have a remarkable ability to carry on functioning effectively despite being damaged; therefore, when discussing the risks of drug treatments in liver disease, patients are classified according to whether the disease has caused a mild or moderate impairment of liver function or a severe impairment.

Mild to moderate impairment of liver function

If a disease has produced only a mild or moderate impairment of liver function, drugs may be used but they should be used with caution – particularly those drugs that have a narrow margin of safety between the concentration in the blood that produces beneficial effects and the concentration that produces harmful effects. Smaller doses should be used in order to prevent toxic levels accumulating in the blood, and frequent measurements of the level of the drug in the blood should be carried out if possible.

Severe impairment of liver function

Severe impairment of liver function causes jaundice; affects the brain, producing tremor, dementia and coma; and produces fluid retention (ankle swelling) and excess fluid in the abdomen, causing it to swell (ascites). Kidney function may also become impaired in an individual suffering from liver disease and result in reduced excretion of drugs in the urine. In patients with this degree of liver impairment, drugs should not be used unless the benefits will outweigh the risks, and no drug that is known to produce liver damage should be used.

In patients with a severe impairment of liver function, many drugs may further impair brain function and trigger dementia and coma (hepatic encephalopathy). This is particularly likely to occur with sleeping drugs, sedatives and narcotic pain relievers.

Brain function in people with severe impairment of liver function may also be affected if the blood potassium falls or if the concentration of ammonia-type products rises. This means that any drug that may cause a fall in blood potassium (e.g. water tablets: diuretics) should not be used; nor should any drug that causes constipation because this would give bacteria in the intestine time to break food down into ammonium compounds which are then absorbed into the bloodstream to trigger coma in a patient with a severe impairment of liver function.

Fluid retention and the fluid in the abdomen (ascites) in patients with severely impaired liver function may be made much worse by any drug that causes further fluid retention in the body; for example, many non-steroidal anti-inflammatory drugs (NSAIDs) used to treat rheumatoid arthritis and related disorders, corticosteroids, and carbenoxolone used to treat peptic ulcers.

In severe impairment of liver function the amount of protein in the blood is reduced and this may affect the transport of drugs in the blood. If this happens, the amount of free drug in the blood may rise to toxic levels. This may occur with the anti-epileptic drug phenytoin and with the corticosteroid drug prednisone. In addition, some drugs are excreted in the bile (e.g. rifampicin and fusidic acid), and in liver disease the bile ducts may be blocked, causing these drugs to accumulate in the body and produce harmful effects.

The blood supply to the liver

Drugs taken by mouth that are rapidly broken down in the liver the first time they pass through it may reach toxic levels in the blood if they bypass the liver. This may happen if blood that normally goes straight to the liver from the intestine is shunted out into the general circulation without entering the main functioning parts of the liver. This can occur in cirrhosis of the liver. In these disorders drugs such as propranolol or chlormethiazole, which are broken down very rapidly on their first passage through the liver, will soon reach toxic levels in the main bloodstream and produce harmful effects. The oral doses of such drugs should be reduced.

Table 83.1 A guide to drugs that should not be used, or used with caution, in liver disease

Drug	*Advice*
amiodipine	Should be used with caution. Reduce dose
anabolic steroids	Should not be used. Risk of liver damage and jaundice which is related to dose
androgens (male sex hormones)	Should not be used. Risk of fluid retention, liver damage and jaundice which is related to dose
antacids	Do not use *antacids* that contain *aluminium* or *calcium*, which may constipate (see risk of constipation in liver failure, earlier). Also, do not use antacids that contain high amounts of sodium in patients who have fluid retention due to liver failure; for example, *magnesium trisilicate* mixture and *Gaviscon*
anti-anxiety, sedative and sleeping drugs	Increased risk of coma. Should not be used, or use a small dose of lorazepam or oxazepam. Dose of chlormethiazole by mouth should be reduced
anti-coagulant drugs (by mouth)	Should not be used, especially if prothrombin time is prolonged due to impaired liver function
anti-depressants	*MAOI anti-depressants* or *iprindole* (a tricyclic anti-depressant) should not be used. They may cause liver damage in certain individuals (idiosyncratic reactions). Other *tricyclic anti-depressants* may be used but their sedative effects may be increased
antihistamines	Should not be used; may trigger coma
anti-inflammatory pain relievers (non-steroidal: NSAIDs)	Should be used with caution. Increased risk of bleeding from the stomach and intestine, and increased risk of fluid retention
anti-psychotics	Should not be used. Can trigger coma. *Phenothiazines*, especially *chlorpromazine*, may also cause liver damage

Table 83.1 A guide to drugs that should not be used, or used with caution, in liver disease (*cont.*)

Drug	*Advice*
aspirin	Should not be used. Increased risk of bleeding from the stomach and intestine
azathioprine	Should be used with caution. Its effectiveness may be reduced because of impaired metabolism to active products, and its harmful effects may be increased because of an increased concentration of the unchanged drug in the bloodstream
bacampicillin	Use with caution in severe impairment because toxic breakdown products may accumulate and further damage the liver
benorylate	Should not be used; contains aspirin – see entry for aspirin
bezafibrate	Should not be used in severe impairment. Increased risk of harmful effects
carbenoxolone	Should not be used in severe impairment. It produces fluid retention and a low blood potassium, which may trigger coma
chenodeoxycholic acid	Should not be used in chronic liver disease. Increased risk of harmful effects on the liver. Of no benefit if patient's gall bladder does not function normally
chloramphenicol	Should not be used. Increased risk of bone marrow damage, causing blood disorders
chlormethiazole	Should be used with caution; reduce dose. Increased risk of coma
chlorpropamide	Should not be used. Increased risk of low blood glucose (hypoglycaemia) and also a risk of liver damage, producing jaundice
cholestyramine	Should be used with caution. Reduces the absorption of fat-soluble vitamins (A, D, E, K). A deficiency of vitamin K may lead to a further reduction in prothrombin, resulting in bleeding
cimetidine	Dose should be reduced. Increased risk of confusion
cisapride	Halve dose initially. Increased risk of harmful effects
clindamycin	Should be used with caution; reduce dose. Increased risk of confusion
clofibrate	Should not be used in severe impairment. Increased risk of harmful effects
clomiphene	Should not be used in severe impairment. Increased risk of harmful effects
contraceptives (oral)	See 'oral contraceptives'
corticosteroids	Should be used with caution. Cortisone and prednisone are converted to the active corticosteroids hydrocortisone and prednisolone by the liver. Therefore, if there is evidence of impaired liver function, use hydrocortisone or prednisolone instead of cortisone or prednisone
cough mixtures	Cough mixtures that contain morphine-related narcotics (e.g. codeine and pholcodine) should not be used in severe impairment

Table 83.1 A guide to drugs that should not be used, or used with caution, in liver disease (*cont.*)

Drug	*Advice*
cyclofenil	Should not be used in severe impairment. Increased risk of harmful effects
cyproterone	Should not be used. Increased risk of dose-related harmful effects
dantrolene	Should not be used. May cause severe liver damage
dehydrocholic acid	Should not be used in liver disease that interferes with the excretion of bile
diuretics	*Thiazide diuretics* and *loop diuretics* may cause a low blood potassium and trigger coma. They may also produce an increased risk of a raised blood magnesium level in patients with alcoholic cirrhosis. *Potassium-sparing diuretics* are of benefit and may be more beneficial than giving potassium supplements in order to prevent coma
doxorubicin	Should be used with caution. Dose should be reduced according to concentration of bilirubin in the blood
epirubicin	Should be used with caution. Reduce dose according to concentration of bilirubin in the blood
ergotamine	Should not be used in severe impairment. Increased risk of harmful effects
erythromycin	Should be used with caution. May cause liver damage in certain people (idiosyncratic). *Erythromycin estolate* should not be used because it may cause liver damage with jaundice
etretinate	Should not be used. May worsen impairment of liver function
female sex hormones	Oestrogens or progestogens should not be used. Increased risk of harmful effects
flecainide	Should not be used in severe impairment, or used with utmost caution by reducing the daily dosage. Its breakdown is reduced in severe impairment
fluoxetine	Dose should be reduced in severe impairment. Increased risk of harmful effects
fluvoxamine	Reduce dose in severe impairment. Increased risk of harmful effects
fusidic acid	Should not be used, or use with utmost caution by reducing the daily dosage. Its excretion through the bile may be reduced in liver disease and also the risk of liver damage is increased
gemfibrozil	Should not be used in severe impairment. Increased risk of harmful effects
gold salts	Should not be used in severe impairment. Risk of damage to the liver
idarubicin	Reduce dose according to blood level of bilirubin
iprindole	Should not be used. Increased risk of liver damage in certain individuals (idiosyncratic reactions). See 'Anti-depressant drugs' entry
isoniazid	Should not be used. Increased risk of liver damage in certain individuals (idiosyncratic reactions)

Table 83.1 A guide to drugs that should not be used, or used with caution, in liver disease (*cont.*)

Drug	*Advice*
isotretinoin	Should not be used. May worsen impairment of liver function
isradipine	Reduce dose. Increased risk of harmful effects
itraconazole	Should not be used; related to ketoconazole (below)
ketoconazole	Should not be used if possible. May accumulate and cause damage to liver cells, producing a hepatitis reaction
labetalol	Dose by mouth should be reduced; impaired liver function may cause increased blood levels
lignocaine	Should not be used in severe impairment, or use with utmost caution by reducing the dose. Increased risk of harmful effects because breakdown is reduced in severe impairment
lincomycin	Should not be used if possible. Increased risk of harmful effects
Lomotil	Lomotil contains *diphenoxylate*, which is related to morphine. Should not be used in severe impairment because of increased risk of coma
magnesium sulphate	Should not be used to treat liver coma if there is a risk of kidney failure developing
metformin	Should not be used. Increased risk of lactic acidosis
methotrexate	May produce liver damage that is dose related. In patients with impaired liver function it should not be used to treat disorders that are not life threatening (e.g. psoriasis)
methyldopa	Should not be used. Risk of damage to the liver
metoprolol	Should be used with caution. Dose by mouth should be reduced. Increased risk of harmful effects
metronidazole	Should be used with caution. In severe impairment, dose should be reduced. Increased risk of harmful effects
mexiletine	Should not be used in severe impairment, or used with utmost caution by reducing the daily dose. Breakdown is reduced in severe impairment, producing increased risk of harmful effects
monoamine oxidase inhibitors	Should not be used. May cause liver damage in certain individuals (idiosyncratic reactions)
nalidixic acid	Should be used with caution; partially metabolized in liver
narcotic pain relievers (opioid analgesics)	Should not be used. May trigger coma. Higher blood levels may occur when given by mouth
nicardipine	Should be used with caution. Dose should be reduced. Increased risk of harmful effects
nifedipine	Should be used with caution. Dose should be reduced because excretion may be impaired, increasing risk of harmful effects
niridazole	Should be used with caution because the risk of harmful effects on the brain and nervous system is increased in patients with cirrhosis

Table 83.1 A guide to drugs that should not be used, or used with caution, in liver disease (*cont.*)

Drug	*Advice*
	of the liver and in liver disorders where the blood from the intestines bypasses the liver and is shunted out into the main circulation
nitroprusside (sodium)	Should not be used in severe impairment. Increased risk of harmful effects
oestrogens	Do not use – see oral contraceptives
omeprazole	Reduce dose in severe liver disease to not more than 20 mg daily. Increased risk of harmful effects
oral contraceptives	Should not be used in women with active liver disease or in women with a history of jaundice or itching in the last 2 months of pregnancy
oxprenolol	Should be used with caution. Dose by mouth should be reduced. Increased risk of harmful effects
paracetamol	Large doses should not be used because the overdose required to produce liver damage may be smaller in patients with liver disease
phenobarbitone	Should be used with caution. May trigger coma in severe impairment
phenothiazines	Should not be used. They may trigger coma and cause liver damage, especially chlorpromazine
phenytoin	Breakdown is reduced in severe impairment; therefore the dose should be reduced to prevent risk of harmful effects
plicamycin	Should not be used if possible. Increased risk of harmful effects
prednisolone	See 'corticosteroids' entry
prednisone	See 'corticosteroids' entry
primidone	Should be used with caution. May trigger coma in severe impairment
procainamide	Do not use, or reduce dose. Increased risk of harmful effects
progestogens	Should not be used. Increased risk of harmful effects
propafenone	Dose should be reduced. Increased risk of harmful effects
propranolol	Should be used with caution. Dose by mouth should be reduced. Increased risk of harmful effects because breakdown may be reduced in severe impairment and by the drug bypassing the liver and being shunted into the main circulation
pyrazinamide	Should not be used. Increased risk of liver damage in certain individuals (idiosyncratic reactions)
ranitidine	Should be used with caution. Dose should be reduced. Increased risk of confusion
rifampicin	Should not be used, or dose should be reduced in patients with severe impairment. Risk of liver damage is increased because of reduced excretion in the bile, leading to increased blood levels
simvastatin	Dose should be reduced. Risk of liver damage

Table 83.1 A guide to drugs that should not be used, or used with caution, in liver disease (*cont.*)

Drug	*Advice*
sleeping drugs	Increased risk of coma. See entry 'anti-anxiety, sedative and sleeping drugs'
sodium valproate	Should not be used if possible. Occasional risk of liver damage and liver failure, especially in first 6 months of treatment
suxamethonium	The production of pseudocholinesterase, which breaks down suxamethonium, may be reduced in severe liver disease; therefore should be used with utmost caution in severe liver disease because it may cause patients to stop breathing for prolonged periods
talampicillin	Should be used with caution in severe impairment because toxic breakdown products may accumulate and damage the liver
tetracyclines	Large intravenous doses should not be used because of risk of damage to the liver. Increased risk of worsening of kidney function in severe liver impairment
theophylline	Should be used with caution in serious impairment because of increased risks of harmful effects. Dose should be reduced
thiopentone	Should be used with caution in severe impairment. Dose should be reduced to start off anaesthesia
tocainide	Should not be used in severe impairment, or used with utmost caution by reducing the dose. Breakdown is reduced in severe impairment, increasing the risk of harmful effects
tolbutamide	Should not be used. Increased risk of low blood glucose (hypoglycaemia). May produce liver damage with jaundice
tricyclic anti-depressants	See entry 'anti-depressants'
ursodeoxycholic acid	Should not be used in chronic liver disease. Of no benefit if patient's gall bladder does not function normally
verapamil	Should be used with caution. Dose should be reduced. Excretion is impaired and blood levels increase with doses by mouth or intravenously; therefore increased risk of harmful effects
warfarin	Should not be used, especially if prothrombin time is prolonged because of impaired liver function
zidovudine	May accumulate due to reduced breakdown; therefore increased risk of harmful effects
zopiclone	Reduce dose. Increased risk of harmful effects

Kidney disease and the risks of drug treatments

We have two kidneys, one on each side of the spine just below the diaphragm.

Functions of the kidneys

In health, the volume and constituents of the body fluids are kept within very narrow limits by complex mechanisms. The kidneys play the main role in maintaining these limits. They control the body's water and salts, and they maintain the acidity of the blood at a constant level. They retain substances in the blood that the body needs in order to function effectively (e.g. glucose, proteins, amino acids, bicarbonate and phosphate) and they excrete waste products (e.g. urea).

Tests of kidney function

Most of the problems produced by kidney disease affect the whole body. They include disturbances in the chemical composition of body fluids, raised blood pressure, anaemia and bone disease. Therefore, when the function of the kidneys is being tested the patient requires a general physical examination as well as tests of the chemistry of the blood and tests for anaemia. In addition, there are specific tests of the urine and of kidney function (see later). The rate at which the kidneys filter urine is measured (renal clearance), and the acidity and specific gravity of the urine are also measured. In addition, special X-rays of the kidney may be necessary and examination of the bladder and urinary tract using special viewers (cystoscopes).

Disease of the kidneys

The term 'glomerulonephritis' is used to describe an inflammatory disease that affects the glomeruli in both kidneys. The glomeruli are microscopic tufts of small blood vessels (capillaries) which lie within small round microscopic bodies or corpuscles at the beginning of the urine-collecting ducts (nephrons) of the kidneys. It is through the capillaries in the glomeruli that blood is filtered into the nephrons to produce urine.

There are three main types of glomerulonephritis – proliferative (widespread), minimal lesion and membranous. These are terms based principally upon microscope examination of the diseased kidneys.

The *proliferative* type follows some infection (e.g. streptococcal tonsillitis) and the damage is produced as a result of an immune reaction in which antibody complexes block the capillaries in the glomeruli. The acute form occurs more commonly in childhood and adolescence but may develop at any age. Most children recover but only about 50 per cent of adults do so. Those who do not, progress to develop a raised blood pressure (hypertension) and chronic kidney failure (see later). In a few individuals the acute attack may advance rapidly to produce raised blood pressure, reduced output of urine, convulsions and death from heart failure or kidney failure. A small group of patients may go on to develop nephrotic syndrome, a condition in which there is excessive excretion of proteins in the urine and a reduced level of proteins in the blood, which causes excessive amounts of fluid to be retained in the tissues (oedema).

The *minimal lesion* type affects principally children and young adults whilst the *membranous* type affects people over 30 years of age. They both come on slowly over months and years, and gradually they develop nephrotic syndrome – the amount of protein in the urine increases, the blood protein level falls and excessive fluid is retained in their tissues (oedema). The swollen tissues are widespread throughout the body, particularly under the skin. The face may look white and puffy, and fluid may accumulate in the lungs. Gradually the individual develops a low resistance to infection, muscle wasting and softening of the bones. The blood fat levels (cholesterol) are increased, the blood proteins markedly reduced and there is retention of sodium and water by the failing kidneys and loss of potassium.

A *chronic* form of glomerulonephritis may develop slowly over years without any history of kidney disease or it may follow an attack of the proliferative type (see earlier). As the kidney failure progresses, the water and salt balance of the body fluids becomes severely disturbed, the acidity of the blood increases and waste products accumulate in the blood (e.g. urea). This results in a state known as uraemia, which is the end stage of kidney disease (see later). These individuals pass large volumes of urine, anaemia, itching, weakness, nausea, vomiting or diarrhoea, raised blood pressure, headaches, nerve damage, loss of vision, breathlessness, disorders of brain function, and bone pains due to bone softening. Without treatment they deteriorate, develop muscular twitching, fits and drowsiness, and go into a coma and die.

There is no drug treatment that cures chronic glomerulonephritis. Treatment involves a special diet, correcting the body's salts and fluids, treating anaemia and any infection, and relieving the symptoms of nausea, vomiting, hiccoughing and bone pains.

Kidney dialysis

In people with chronic glomerulonephritis, kidney dialysis preserves life and should be started before symptoms of uraemia become too incapacitating and before they have to give up work. An alternative treatment is *peritoneal dialysis.* A dialysing fluid is introduced into the abdomen, left for about 6 hours and then drawn off again. It takes with it the toxic products that the kidneys cannot excrete. The process is repeated four times in every 24 hours and patients can get on with their work because they wear a plastic bag round the waist to collect the fluid.

Kidney transplant

Provided the tissues match well, a kidney transplant into a patient with chronic kidney failure can have a dramatic effect on life expectancy. Individuals who receive a kidney from a living relative do better than those who receive a kidney from a 'dead' patient. Nevertheless, the survival rates after transplantation are impressive. Much of this is due to effective drug treatment that prevents rejection of the transplanted organ by the use of cyclosporin or other immuno-suppressive drugs and the use of corticosteroids.

Kidney failure

Uraemia is the term used to describe the signs and symptoms produced by kidney failure (renal failure). These are due to retention of nitrogen waste products in the blood (e.g. urea), to disturbances in the salt and water balance in the body and to changes in the acidity of the blood.

Kidney failure may be triggered by drugs (see later) or diseases that damage the kidneys, by any disorder that reduces the blood supply to the kidneys or by any disorder that obstructs the flow of urine from the kidney.

Examples of diseases that damage the kidneys are glomerulonephritis (see earlier), severe hypertension (raised blood pressure), diabetes, gout and virus infections. Drugs that damage the kidneys are discussed next.

Drugs that may cause kidney damage

Drugs may damage the kidneys directly or they may interfere with the function of the kidneys.

Direct damage is a chemical effect and it is not difficult to understand how this can happen. The kidneys take about one-quarter of the blood pumped out by the heart at rest. Because drugs are carried round the body in the blood, at any one time large amounts of a drug are not only passing through the kidneys but are also reaching very high concentrations as the blood is filtered to form urine. This means that the kidney cells are exposed to these very high concentrations of the drug. In addition, drugs also pass into the urine and so the cells are exposed to a double risk – from high concentrations of the drug in the blood and from high concentrations in the urine.

Certain drugs may produce *indirect damage* in the kidneys. For example, some drugs used to prevent gout cause increased excretion of uric acid in the urine; this excess uric acid may precipitate out to form crystals, which damage the tubules. Some sulphonamide drugs may also precipitate in the urine to form crystals which produce local damage. Overdosage with vitamin D may cause excessive calcium to be excreted in the urine, which may produce kidney damage, and over-use of diuretics (water tablets) may damage the kidney by producing excessive loss of sodium and potassium. Drugs used to prevent the blood from clotting (anti-coagulants) may produce bleeding into the kidneys if the dose is not carefully controlled.

Allergic reactions to drugs may cause damage to the kidneys. These reactions may produce several different types of injury to the kidneys and may be caused by a whole range of drugs, from gold used to treat rheumatoid arthritis to the penicillins used to treat infection.

Kidney disease increases the risks of using certain drugs

Problems with the excretion of drugs

In people whose kidneys are not functioning effectively because of disease (see earlier), the harmful effects of drugs that are normally excreted wholly or largely by the kidneys may increase. This is because the defective excretion of the drug in the urine will lead to an accumulation of the drug in the blood and, as the concentration in the blood increases, the risk of toxic effects from the drug also increases. This may be more dangerous with some drugs than others. With certain drugs there is a narrow range between the concentration of the drug in the blood that produces beneficial effects and the concentration that produces harmful effects. With these drugs, any impaired excretion of the drug in the urine will soon push the concentration of the drug in the blood up into toxic levels (e.g. gentamicin). The problem is not as dangerous with those drugs in which there is a wide range between the concentrations in the blood required to produce beneficial effects and those that produce harmful effects (e.g. penicillin).

Problems with the transport of drugs in the blood

A drug is carried around the blood in two forms. It may be *free* in solution – to exert its effects until it is metabolized in the liver and then excreted in the urine. It may also travel around in the blood attached or *bound* to protein molecules (usually albumin). When it 'piggy-backs' in this way it is not active and is not metabolized or excreted. There is always a steady balance between the amount of free drug in the blood and that bound to proteins. Any fall in the level of free drug will cause a release of the drug from the proteins to maintain the balance.

As much as 99 per cent of a drug may be bound to proteins and so anything that reduces this amount produces a very high rise in free drug in the blood. Therefore, it helps to regard the binding of a drug to proteins in the blood as not only a transport system but also as an effective storage system for the drug from which free drug can be drawn.

Kidney disease (see earlier) may cause a significant reduction in the concentration of proteins in the blood and also affect the binding capacity of the proteins. This means that with certain drugs the amount of free drug in the blood will soon reach toxic levels unless the dose is reduced accordingly.

Problems with drugs that cause kidney damage

Any drug that is known to cause kidney damage (see earlier) may obviously make any kidney disease worse. Some drugs cause an increase in waste products in the blood and may put an extra burden on the kidneys. A good example of this is the tetracycline antibiotics. They affect protein production in the body and, if given to elderly patients whose kidney function may be finely balanced, they can tip them over into kidney failure. The kidneys just cannot cope with the extra protein waste products being produced (e.g. urea). These increase in the blood and start to produce drowsiness and other symptoms of early uraemia (see earlier). Obviously, this also happens to patients whose kidney function is impaired by disease.

Drug treatments in patients with kidney disease

As already discussed, several diseases of the kidneys may impair their function and interfere with the filtration of drugs from the blood into the urine and/or the active secretion of drugs into the urine. Because the kidneys are the principal route of excretion of most drugs from the body, *any* impairment of kidney function will cause problems with drugs that are excreted by the kidneys either as the active drug or in a partly broken down form. Failure to excrete a drug effectively will cause the level of the drug in the blood to rise to toxic levels and produce harmful effects, particularly those drugs that have a narrow margin of safety between the concentration of the drug in the blood that produces benefits and the concentration in the blood that produces harmful effects. Also, the sensitivity of some patients to some drugs is increased if their kidney function is impaired.

Many problems that are caused by drugs in people with impaired kidney function could have been predicted and prevented. They could have been predicted by carrying out tests to determine the degree of impaired kidney function and they could be prevented by using smaller doses or by using drugs known *not* to cause problems in patients with impaired kidney function.

Assessment of kidney function

Glomerular filtration rate

The efficiency of the kidneys is measured by their ability to clear certain substances from the blood into the urine. These substances must pass freely through the kidney filtering systems and must not be absorbed or excreted into the urine by the kidneys. In other words, the quantity excreted in the urine must be identical with the quantity that passed through the kidneys' filters (glomeruli). The clearance of such a substance from the blood into the urine therefore gives an indication of the rate at which the filters are filtering the blood – this is calculated by multiplying the concentration in the urine by the volume of urine passed per minute and dividing by the concentration in the blood. The result is called the glomerular filtration rate (GFR). In an average adult the GFR is about 120 ml/minute.

An injection of the polysaccharide inulin may be used to measure glomerular filtration rate but usually in clinical practice the clearance by the kidneys of creatinine is used by collecting a 24-hour sample of urine and a single blood sample. Creatinine is a breakdown product of muscle metabolism and the amount excreted daily in the urine is constant for each individual, regardless of diet but depending entirely on the blood flow through the kidneys.

A defective creatinine clearance (excretion) gives a warning that certain drugs will also fail to be excreted effectively and the dose will have to be reduced proportionately. However, it is important to point out that creatinine clearance is a fairly crude measure of kidney function. Kidney function has to fall to about 25 per cent of normal capacity before the creatinine in the blood increases. Therefore, any rise in creatinine level in the blood is a strong warning to use any drug that is excreted by the kidneys with utmost caution.

Concentration of creatinine in the blood

An alternative to measuring creatinine clearance is to use the concentration of creatinine in the blood as a rough guide to kidney function. However, this is a *very* rough guide unless it is corrected for the age, weight and sex of the patient. Charts (nomograms) are available that allow the blood creatinine level to be corrected for these factors.

Impairment of kidney function

Impairment of kidney function is usually divided into three groups:

	GFR (millilitres/minute)	*Blood creatinine level* (micromoles/litre)
mild impairment	20–50	150–300
moderate impairment	10–20	300–700
severe impairment	Less than 10	Greater than 700

Impaired kidney function with advancing age

Kidney function declines with age and, because many elderly people have a reduced muscle mass, the amount of creatinine they produce will also be reduced. Therefore the level of creatinine in their blood will not give a true indication of the degree of impaired kidney function from which they may be suffering. *It is therefore safer for all elderly people to be treated as if they have a mild degree of impairment of their kidney function.*

Reducing the dosage of drugs in people with impaired kidney function

In anyone with impaired kidney function it is important to reduce the dose of some drugs. The extent of any reduction in the dose of such a drug will depend upon whether the drug is excreted in the urine unchanged or whether it is partly broken down in the liver first; the extent of impaired functioning of the kidneys; the potential of the drug for producing harmful effects; and the margin of safety between the concentration of the drug in the blood that produces beneficial effects and the concentration that produces harmful effects.

The over-all daily dosage of a drug may be lowered by reducing the size of each dose or by increasing the interval of time between doses (e.g. 8-hourly instead of 6-hourly).

Table 84.1 If kidney function is impaired the following drugs should be used with caution

Drug	*Action*
Mild impairment or if individual is elderly	
acetohexamide	Should be used with caution. May cause prolonged fall in blood glucose (hypoglycaemia)
acyclovir	Dose should be reduced. Possible transient rise in waste products in the blood (e.g. urea)
aminoglycosides	Dose should be reduced and blood levels monitored. Increased risk of kidney damage, deafness and paralysis of muscles due to neuro-muscular block
amphotericin	Should be used intravenously only if no alternative. Increased risk of kidney damage
anti-inflammatory pain relievers (non-steroidal: NSAIDs)	Should not be used if possible. Increased risk of fluid retention and worsening of kidney function
baclofen	Smaller doses should be used. Excreted by kidneys. Increased risk of muscle weakness and sedation
bezafibrate	Dose should be reduced. Risk of worsening of kidney function
capreomycin	Dose should be reduced. Increased risk of nerve damage, deafness, and paralysis of muscles due to neuromuscular block
captopril	Should not be used if possible. If used, dose should be reduced and effects monitored carefully. Excreted by kidneys. Increased risk of raised blood potassium and worsening of kidney function
cephalosporins	Dose should be reduced. Increased risk of harmful effects with cefoxitin, ceftazidime, ceftizoxime, cefuroxime, cefamandole, cephazolin and cephadrine
chloroquine	Maximum daily dose should be reduced to 75 mg. Increased risk of harmful effects with prolonged use because the drug accumulates in the body

Table 84.1 If kidney function is impaired the following drugs should be used with caution (*cont.*)

Drug	*Action*
clofibrate	Dose should be reduced. Increased risk of muscle weakness and worsening of kidney function
colistin	Dose should be reduced. Increased risk of nerve and kidney damage, and paralysis of muscles due to neuromuscular block
digoxin	Dose should be reduced (250 mcg daily). Increased risk of disorders of heart rhythm, nausea, confusion and visual disturbances
disodium etidronate	Maximum daily dose should be reduced to 5 mg/kg daily. Increased risk of harmful effects
disopyramide	Dose should be reduced according to degree of impairment. Increased risk of depression of the heart and disorders of heart rhythm; and also anticholinergic effects – dry mouth, blurred vision, constipation and difficulty passing urine
doxorubicin	Dose should be reduced. Increased risk of harmful effects
enalapril	Dose should be reduced. Increased risk of raised blood potassium and worsening of kidney function. Avoid use if possible
fenofibrate	Dose should be reduced. Increased risk of harmful effects
flecainide	Dose should be reduced. Increased risk of harmful effects
fluconazole	Dose should be reduced. Increased risk of harmful effects
flucytosine	Dose should be reduced. Increased risk of blood disorders due to damage to the bone marrow. Also increased risk of liver damage
ganciclovir	Dose should be reduced. Increased risk of harmful effects
hydroxychloroquine	Dose should be reduced (maximum 75 mg daily). Increased risk of harmful effects with prolonged use because the drug accumulates in the body
latamoxef	Dose should be reduced. Increased risk of harmful effects
lisinopril	Dose should be reduced – see 'captopril'
lithium	Dose should be reduced and blood levels monitored. Increased risk of nausea and vomiting and of harmful effects on brain and nervous system
methotrexate	Dose should be reduced. Accumulates in the body to produce risk of kidney damage
milrinone	Dose should be reduced and response monitored
nizatidine	Dose should be reduced (150 mg daily). Increased risk of harmful effects
penicillamine	Do not use, or reduce dose. Increased risk of kidney damage
pentamidine	Dose should be reduced. Increased risk of harmful effects
perindopril	Dose should be reduced – see captopril
potassium-sparing diuretics	Blood potassium levels should be monitored. High risk of raised blood potassium
procainamide	Do not use, or reduce dose. Increased risk of nerve damage

Table 84.1 If kidney function is impaired the following drugs should be used with caution (*cont.*)

Drug	*Action*
propylthiouracil	Dose should be reduced. Increased risk of harmful effects
quinapril	Dose should be reduced at start of treatment. See 'captopril'
teicoplanin	Dose should be reduced after 4 days
tocainide	Dose should be reduced. Increased risk of harmful effects
vancomycin	Intravenous injections should be used with caution. Increased risk of loss of hearing and kidney damage
zidovudine	Dose should be reduced. Excreted by kidneys. Increased risk of harmful effects
The following drugs should be added to the list if kidney impairment is *moderate*	
alcuronium	Dose should be reduced. May cause prolonged paralysis with large or repeated doses
allopurinol	Maximum daily dose should be reduced to 200 mg daily. Increased risk of harmful effects and rashes
alteplase	Use with caution. Excreted by the kidneys
amiodarone	Accumulation of iodine from metabolism of drug may affect the functioning of the thyroid gland
atenolol	Dose should be reduced. Increased risk of harmful effects. Excreted unchanged in the urine
Augmentin (co-amoxiclav)	Dose should be reduced. Increased risk of harmful effects. Contains amoxicillin and clavulanic acid
azlocillin	Dose should be reduced. Increased risk of harmful effects
aztreonam	Dose should be reduced. Increased risk of harmful effects
beta blockers	Slowing of the heart rate and fall in blood pressure may occur with atenolol, pindolol and sotalol. They may reduce blood flow to the kidneys and worsen the impairment of function
bezafibrate	Dose should be reduced. Increased risk of muscle weakness and worsening of kidney function
bleomycin	Dose should be reduced. Increased risk of harmful effects
bumetanide	May need higher doses
carbenicillin	Dose should be reduced. Increased risk of damage to the nerves and bleeding. Note carbenicillin has a high content of sodium
cefadroxil	Dose should be reduced. Increased risk of harmful effects
cefsulodin	Dose should be reduced. Increased risk of harmful effects
cetirizine	Dose should be reduced. Increased risk of harmful effects
chloroquine	Dose should be reduced. Mild to moderate – max. 75 mg daily. Moderate – max. 50 mg daily. Increased risk of harmful effects with prolonged use
cimetidine	Dose should be reduced. Increased risk of confusion, and temporary worsening of kidney function may occur

Table 84.1 If kidney function is impaired the following drugs should be used with caution (*cont.*)

Drug	*Action*
ciprofloxacin	Half dose should be used. Increased risk of harmful effects
cisapride	Should start with half dose and progress should be monitored
clofibrate	Dose should be reduced. Increased risk of muscle weakness and worsening of kidney function
cyclophosphamide	Dose should be reduced. Increased risk of harmful effects
digoxin	Dose should be reduced (125–250 mcg daily). Increased risk of harmful effects due to disturbances of salt and water balance
disopyramide	Dose should be reduced. Increased risk of harmful effects
enoxacin	Initial dose should be reduced and effects monitored carefully. Excreted by kidneys. Increased risk of raised blood potassium and worsening of kidney function
famotidine	Dose should be reduced. Increased risk of harmful effects
fenofibrate	Dose should be reduced. Increased risk of harmful effects
fluoxetine	Should start with smaller doses and response should be monitored
fluvoxamine	Should start with smaller doses and response should be monitored
frusemide	May need higher doses. Deafness may follow rapid intravenous injection
hydroxychloroquine	Mild to moderate – max. 75 mg daily. Moderate – max. 50 mg daily. Increased risk of harmful effects with prolonged use
ifosfamide	Dose should be reduced. Increased risk of harmful effects
magnesium salts (in antacids and health salts)	Should not be used, or used in reduced dose. Note that magnesium carbonate mixture and magnesium trisilicate mixture are also high in sodium
melphalan	Dose should be reduced. Increased risk of harmful effects
mercaptopurine	Dose should be reduced. Increased risk of harmful effects
methotrexate	Should not be used. May accumulate in the body and produce kidney damage
nadolol	Increased risk of harmful effects. Excreted unchanged by the kidney; therefore dose should be reduced
narcotic pain relievers	Increased risk of harmful effects on the brain. Small doses should be used. Codeine, dihydrocodeine or morphine should not be used
nicardipine	Should start with small doses, and progress should be monitored. Increased risk of harmful effects
nifedipine	Should start with small doses, and progress should be monitored. May cause reversible worsening of kidney function
nitroprusside	See 'sodium nitroprusside' in Table 84.2
nizatidine	Dose should be reduced (150 mg on alternate days). Increased risk of harmful effects
pancuronium	Dose should be reduced. May cause prolonged paralysis with large and repeated doses

Table 84.1 If kidney function is impaired the following drugs should be used with caution (*cont.*)

Drug	*Action*
pindolol	Dose should be reduced. Excreted unchanged by the kidneys; therefore increased risk of harmful effects
piperacillin	Dose should be reduced. Increased risk of harmful effects
procarbazine	Dose should be reduced. Increased risk of harmful effects
sotalol	Dose should be reduced. Excreted unchanged by the kidneys; therefore increased risk of harmful effects
sulpiride	Should not be used, or dose reduced because of increased risk of harmful effects
temoxicillin	Dose should be reduced. Increased risk of harmful effects
thioguanine	Dose should be reduced. Increased risk of harmful effects
ticarcillin	Dose should be reduced. High in sodium
Timentin	Dose should be reduced. Contains clavulanic acid and ticarcillin. Increased risk of harmful effects
tubocurarine	Dose should be reduced. May cause prolonged paralysis with high or repeated doses
vigabatrin	Do not use by injection if possible. Increased risk of hearing and kidney damage
xamoterol	Dose should be reduced. Excreted by kidneys. Increased risk of harmful effects
The following drugs should be added to the list if kidney impairment is *severe*	
acebutolol	Should start with small doses. Increased risk of harmful effects from the accumulation in the body of active breakdown products
allopurinol	Maximum daily dose should be reduced to 100 mg. Increased risk of harmful effects and rashes
amoxycillin	Dose should be reduced. Increased risk of skin rashes
ampicillin	Dose should be reduced. Increased risk of skin rashes
amylobarbitone	Dose should be reduced. Increased risk of drowsiness
anti-anxiety drugs	Should start with small dose. Increased risk of harmful effects on the brain
anti-psychotic drugs	Should start with small doses. Increased risk of harmful effects on the brain (e.g. movement disorder)
azathioprine	Dose should be reduced. Increased risk of blood disorders due to damage to bone marrow
bacampicillin	Dose should be reduced. Increased risk of rashes
benzylpenicillin (penicillin G)	Maximum daily dose should be reduced to 6 g. Nerve damage may occur with high doses – may cause convulsions
beta blockers	Should start with small doses. Increased risk of slowing of the heart rate and fall in blood pressure with metoprolol and propranolol. They may also reduce the blood flow to the kidneys and worsen kidney function

Table 84.1 If kidney function is impaired the following drugs should be used with caution (*cont.*)

Drug	*Action*
cefotaxime	Smaller doses should be used. Increased risk of harmful effects
cephalexin	Maximum daily dose should be reduced to 500 mg. Increased risk of harmful effects
chloramphenicol	Should not be used unless no alternative. Dose and response should be monitored carefully. Risk of dose-related damage to bone marrow, producing serious blood disorders
cimetidine	Dose should be reduced. Increased risk of confusion
colchicine	Should not be used, or dose should be reduced if no alternative
co-trimoxazole	Maximum daily dose should be reduced to 960 mg. Increased risk of blood disorders and skin rashes. May cause worsening of kidney function
diazoxide	Dose should be reduced to 75–150 mg intravenously. Risk of increased fall in blood pressure if given intravenously
digitoxin	Maximum daily dose should be reduced to 100 micrograms. Increased risk of harmful effects due to disturbances of salt and water balance
digoxin	Dose should be reduced (less than 125 mcg daily). Increased risk of harmful effects due to disturbances of salt and water balance
disopyramide	Dose should be reduced. Increased risk of harmful effects
domperidone	Dose should be reduced by 30–50 per cent. Increased risk of harmful effects on the brain (e.g. movement disorders)
gemfibrozil	Starting dose should be reduced. Increased risk of harmful effects
gliclazide	Should start with small doses. Increased risk of low blood glucose (hypoglycaemia)
glipizide	Should start with small doses. Increased risk of low blood glucose (hypoglycaemia)
gliquidone	Dose should be reduced. Increased risk of low blood glucose level (hypoglycaemia)
hydralazine	Should start with small doses. Increased blood pressure-lowering effects. Also, possible increased risk of systemic lupus erythematosus
insulin	May need reduced dose of insulin. Impaired response to low blood glucose level (hypoglycaemia) may occur
isoniazid	Maximum daily dose should be reduced to 200 mg. Increased risk of nerve damage, especially in people who break the drug down slowly
methyldopa	Should start with small dose. Increased risk of low blood pressure and sedation
metoclopramide	Should not be used, or used in small doses. Increased risk of movement disorder

Table 84.1 If kidney function is impaired the following drugs should be used with caution (*cont.*)

Drug	*Action*
metoprolol	Should start with small doses. High blood levels after taking the drug by mouth may reduce blood supply to kidneys and further impair kidney function
mezlocillin	Dose should be reduced. Possible risk of nerve damage with high doses
pamidronate sodium	Doses should divided throughout the day
phenobarbitone	Should not be used in large doses. Increased risk of drowsiness
piperazine	Dose should be reduced. Increased risk of nerve damage
pivampicillin	Increased risk of skin rashes
prazosin	Should start with small doses. Increased risk of blood pressure-lowering effects and fall in blood pressure on standing up after sitting or lying down (postural hypotension). Also, increased risk of harmful effects on the nervous system
primidone	Should not be used in large doses. Increased risk of sedation
proguanil	Should not be used, or use reduced doses. Increased risk of blood disorders
propranolol	Should start with small doses. High blood levels after the drug is taken by mouth may reduce blood supply to kidneys and affect kidney function. Increased risk of harmful effects
ranitidine	Should be used in half normal dose. Increased risk of harmful effects (e.g. confusion)
sleeping drugs	Should not be used, or start with small doses. Increased risk of harmful effects
sulphasalazine	Increased risk of rashes and blood disorders; also, risk of crystals forming in the urine and producing further kidney damage. Must drink plenty of fluids
sulphonamides	Increased risk of rashes and blood disorders; also, risk of crystals forming in the urine and producing further kidney damage. Must drink plenty of fluids
tolazamide	Dose may need reducing. Increased risk of low blood glucose (hypoglycaemia)
tolbutamide	Dose may need reducing. Increased risk of low blood glucose (hypoglycaemia)
trimethoprim	Dose should be reduced. Possible risk of a worsening in kidney function

Table 84.2 Dependent upon the degree of kidney impairment the following drugs should not be used

Drug	*Action*
acetazolomide	Should not be used in severe impairment. May cause increased acidity of the blood (metabolic acidosis)
acetohexamide	Should not be used in severe impairment
acrivastine	Should not be used in moderate or severe impairment. Excreted by kidneys. Increased risk of harmful effects
amantadine	Should not be used in mild, moderate or severe impairment. Excreted by kidneys. Increased risk of harmful effects (e.g. agitation, confusion, hallucinations)
anti-inflammatory pain relievers (non-steroidal: NSAIDs)	Should not be used in severe impairment nor, if possible, in moderate or mild impairment. May cause increase in fluid retention and worsening of kidney function
aspirin	Should not be used in severe impairment nor, if possible, in moderate or mild impairment. May cause increase in fluid retention and worsening of kidney function. Increased risk of bleeding from the stomach and intestine
azapropazone	Should not be used in moderate or severe impairment. Excreted by the kidneys. Increased risk of harmful effects
bethanidine	Should not be used in moderate or severe impairment. May cause severe fall in blood pressure on standing up after sitting or lying down (postural hypotension), and reduced blood flow to the kidney which may worsen impairment of function
bezafibrate	Should not be used in severe impairment. May cause worsening of kidney function
carbenoxolone	Should not be used in severe impairment. Increased risk from fluid retention
cephalothin	Should not be used in mild, moderate or severe impairment. Risk of kidney damage
chloroquine	Should not be used for prolonged treatment in severe impairment. Increased risk of harmful effects
chlorpropamide	Should not be used in mild, moderate or severe impairment. Risk of prolonged fall in blood glucose (hypoglycaemia)
cinoxacin	Should not be used in moderate or severe impairment. Increased risk of harmful effects (e.g. nausea and rashes)
cisplatin	Should not be used in mild, moderate or severe impairment if possible. Risk of damage to the kidneys
clofibrate	Should not be used in severe impairment. Risk of muscle weakness and worsening of kidney function
codeine	Should not be used in moderate or severe impairment. Risk of increased or prolonged effects. See entry 'narcotic pain relievers'

Table 84.2 Dependent upon the degree of kidney impairment the following drugs should not be used (*cont.*)

Drug	*Action*
Colven	Should not be used in severe impairment. Contains high amounts of sodium
cyloserine	Should not be used in mild, moderate or severe impairment. Increased risk of harmful effects.
debrisoquine	Should not be used in moderate or severe impairment. Risk of severe fall in blood pressure on standing up after sitting or lying down (postural hypotension), and reduced blood flow to the kidney which may worsen kidney function
De-Nol and De-Noltab	Should not be used in severe impairment. Increased risk of harmful effects from bismuth
dextropropoxyphene	Should not be used in severe impairment. Increased risk of harmful effects on the brain and nervous system
diflunisal	Should not be used in severe impairment. Excreted by kidneys. See entry 'anti-inflammatory pain relievers'
dihydrocodeine	Should not be used in moderate or severe impairment. Increased risk of harmful effects on the brain and nervous system
disodium etidronate	Should not be used in severe impairment. Excreted by kidneys. Increased risk of harmful effects
ergotamine	Should not be used in moderate or severe impairment. May cause nausea, vomiting and risk of constriction of arteries that supply the kidneys, causing a worsening of kidney function
ethacrynic acid	Should not be used in severe impairment. Risk of deafness following intravenous injection
ethambutol	Should not be used in mild, moderate or severe impairment. Risk of damage to the main nerves of the eyes (optic nerves)
etidronate disodium	See disodium etidronate
etretinate	Should not be used in mild, moderate or severe impairment. Increased risk of harmful effects
fluoxetine	Should not be used in severe impairment
Fybogel	Should not be used in severe impairment. Contains high amounts of potassium
gallamine	Should not be used in moderate or severe impairment. May cause prolonged paralysis
Gaviscon	Should not be used in severe impairment. Contains high amounts of sodium
glibenclamide	Should not be used in severe impairment. Risk of a prolonged fall in blood glucose (hypoglycaemia)
gold salts	Should not be used in mild, moderate or severe impairment. Risk of damage to the kidneys

Table 84.2 Dependent upon the degree of kidney impairment the following drugs should not be used (*cont.*)

Drug	*Action*
guanethidine	Should not be used in moderate or severe impairment. Increased risk of fall in blood pressure on standing after sitting or lying down (postural hypotension). May reduce the blood flow to the kidneys and worsen the impairment of function
hexamine	Not effective if there is any mild, moderate or severe impairment of kidney function
hydroxychloroquine	Should not be used for prolonged treatment in severe kidney failure. Increased risk of harmful effects
inosine pranobex	Should not be used in mild, moderate or severe impairment. Broken down to uric acid
isotretinoin	Should not be used in mild, moderate or severe impairment. Increased risk of harmful effects
lincomycin	Should not be used in moderate or severe impairment (use clindamycin instead)
lithium	Should not be used in moderate or severe impairment. Increased risk of harmful effects
magnesium salts (e.g. in indigestion mixtures and laxatives)	Should not be used in severe impairment because of the risk of magnesium accumulating in the body to produce toxic effects. Should not be used, or used in reduced dose, in moderate impairment. Magnesium carbonate and magnesium trisilicate also contain a high amount of sodium
mesalazine	Should not be used in severe impairment. Increased risk of harmful effects
metformin	Should not be used in mild, moderate or severe impairment. Increased risk of lactic acidosis
methocarbamol	Should not be used in mild, moderate or severe impairment. May cause an increased blood urea and increased acidity of the blood (acidosis)
methotrexate	Should not be used in moderate or severe impairment. May accumulate to produce kidney damage
morphine	Should not be used in moderate or severe impairment. May produce increased and prolonged effects
nalidixic acid	Should not be used in moderate or severe impairment. Increased risk of vomiting, rashes and sensitivity of the skin to sunlight
narcotic pain relievers (opioid analgesics)	Increased risk of harmful effects on the brain. Codeine, dihydrocodeine or morphine should not be used in moderate or severe impairment, nor dextropropoxyphene or pethidine in severe impairment
neomycin	Should not be used in mild, moderate or severe impairment. Risk of deafness and kidney damage

Table 84.2 Dependent upon the degree of kidney impairment the following drugs should not be used (*cont.*)

Drug	*Action*
nitrofurantoin	Should not be used in mild, moderate or severe impairment. Risk of nerve damage
nitroprusside	See 'sodium nitroprusside'
picamycin	If possible should not be used in mild, moderate or severe impairment. Increased risk of harmful effects
potassium salts	Should not be used routinely in moderate or severe impairment. Increased risk of a rise in blood potassium levels
potassium-sparing diuretics	Should not be used in moderate or severe impairment. Increased risk of a rise in blood potassium levels
probenecid	Should not be used in moderate or severe impairment. Ineffective and increased risk of harmful effects
salt substitutes	Should not be used regularly in moderate or severe impairment. Risk of raised blood potassium levels
Sandocal	Should not be used in severe impairment. High content of potassium
sodium bicarbonate	Should not be used in severe impairment. Increased risk of harmful effects
sodium nitroprusside	Thiocyanide accumulates in the body; therefore prolonged use should be avoided in moderate or severe impairment
sodium salts	Should not be used in severe impairment. Increased risk of harmful effects
Solpadeine	Should not be used in severe impairment. Contains high amounts of sodium
sulindac	Should not be used in moderate or severe impairment. Excreted by kidneys; risk of fluid retention and worsening of impairment of kidney function
sulphadiazine	Should not be used in severe impairment. High risk of crystals forming in the urine and causing kidney damage
sulphinpyrazone	Will be ineffective in moderate or severe impairment. Do not use
talampicillin	Should not be used in severe impairment. Risk that toxic breakdown products will accumulate in the body
tetracyclines (except doxycycline and minocycline)	Should not be used in mild, moderate or severe impairment because of risk of accumulation of protein breakdown products in the blood (e.g. urea) and worsening of kidney function. Use doxycycline or minocycline if necessary
thiazide diuretics (except metolazone)	Ineffective in moderate or severe impairment. Metolazone effective, but may produce excessive amounts of urine
tolmetin	Do not use in severe impairment. Increased risk of harmful effects

Risks from drugs in impaired kidney function

Because of their various effects on the body certain drugs may be harmful in patients with impaired kidney function. These include:

- Drug preparations that are *high in sodium content* – e.g. carbenicillin, Colven, Gaviscon, magnesium trisilicate, Resonium A, Sandocal, sodium salts and Solpadeine Forte
- Drug preparations that are *high in potassium* – e.g. Fybogel, potassium-sparing diuretics, potassium citrate, potassium supplements, salt substitutes, Sandocal
- Drug preparations that produce *fluid retention* in the body – e.g. oestrogens, corticosteroids, carbenoxolone, non-steroidal anti-inflammatory drugs (NSAIDs)
- Drug preparations that may cause a *rise in protein waste products* in the blood (e.g. urea) – corticosteroids, corticotrophin (ACTH), tetracyclines
- Drug preparations that may *affect blood glucose levels* – e.g. insulin and oral anti-diabetic drugs; they may cause a prolonged fall in blood glucose level (hypoglycaemia); note that there is a risk of lactic acidosis from metformin
- Drug preparations that *depress the function of the brain* – e.g. sleeping drugs, anti-anxiety drugs and anti-psychotic drugs.
- Drug preparations that *contain vitamin A*; the blood level of vitamin A is raised in patients with long-standing kidney failure, and extra vitamin A will lead to excess of vitamin A in the body
- Drug preparations that are known to *damage the kidney*

Impaired kidney function may make the following drugs less effective or ineffective

- *Diuretics* (water tablets) – because they rely on efficient kidney function
- *Anti-blood-pressure drugs* – because the blood volume may increase in kidney failure due to the retention of salt and water in the body. This effect will counter the blood pressure-lowering effects
- *Drugs that increase the excretion of uric acid by the kidneys in the treatment of gout* – because these drugs rely on efficient kidney functioning to be effective
- *Drugs used to treat infections of the urinary tract* – because they rely on reaching a higher concentration in the urine than in the blood; if kidney failure is present, their concentration in the blood may rise to toxic levels because of impaired excretion in the urine. Nalidixic acid and nitrofurantoin should be avoided, and sulphonamides and trimethoprim and co-trimoxazole should be used in reduced dosage.

85

Inherited abnormalities and the risks of drug treatments

Allergy Some patients develop allergic reactions to drugs and others do not. This indicates that an individual's genetic make-up may predispose them to developing allergic reaction.

Bleeding disorders Patients with haemophilia are sensitive to aspirin, which prolongs the bleeding time.

Flushing Some people develop flushing of the face when they take certain drugs with alcohol.

Glaucoma Some people inherit an abnormality of the eyes which makes them prone to develop glaucoma when given certain drugs (see Chapter 35).

Glucose-6-phosphate-dehydrogenase (G6PD) deficiency (see Chapter 47) is an inherited abnormality of red blood cells affecting people from certain races which makes them prone to develop blood disorders in response to certain drugs.

Hereditary methaemoglobinaemia is a disorder that reduces the red pigment in red blood cells and reduces their oxygen-carrying capacity. This causes blueness (cyanosis). Affected individuals are much more likely to develop damage to their red blood cells from nitrates (e.g. used to treat angina) and those drugs that may also cause problems in G6PD deficiency.

Malignant hyperpyrexia This is a sudden unexplained rise in temperature, which may be fatal in certain patients undergoing general anaesthesia who have also been given the muscle relaxant suxamethonium. The patient develops rigidity of the muscles, over-breathing, increased acidity of the blood and a raised blood potassium; 60–70 per cent of patients die.

Porphyria is a biochemical abnormality in which porphyrins (pigments found in animals and plants) are not broken down properly and accumulate in the body, to cause a raised level of porphyrins in the blood and urine. It may be inherited or it may be acquired.

Acute idiopathic porphyria is inherited and is characterized by attacks of abdominal pain; damage to nerves, producing weakness, numbness and pins and needles in the arms and legs; and serious mental symptoms.

Acquired porphyria results from liver damage caused by alcohol or drugs (e.g. barbiturates, sulphonamides, griseofulvin, some anti-epileptic drugs, chlorpropamide, tolbutamide). These drugs may trigger an acute attack of porphyria, causing a sensitivity rash to sunlight associated with blisters, scarring and fragility of the skin, hairiness and defective wound healing.

Acute intermittent porphyria (hepatic porphyria) may be triggered by drugs (e.g. sulphonamides, barbiturates, oestrogens) in susceptible people. It causes abdominal pain, dark urine, nerve damage and mental symptoms.

Race

There are several examples of racial characteristics being associated with an increased risk of harmful effects from drugs; for example, glucose-6-phosphate-dehydrogenase deficiency in blacks, the ability to break down certain drugs only very slowly in Mediterranean Jews, and a relationship between an individual's blood group and an increased risk of harmful effects from certain drugs.

Stomas and the risks of drug treatments

The term 'stoma' is used to describe an opening that leads from the stomach or intestine out on to the surface of the abdomen. Such an opening is usually the result of surgery in which part of the intestine is removed or the intestine is cut through and the part that is still connected to the stomach is brought to the surface through an opening in the abdominal wall. The contents of the intestine pass through this opening and have to be collected in special bags. If the small intestine is brought to the surface it is called an *ileostomy*, and if the large intestine is brought to the surface it is called a *colostomy*.

Different problems with drug treatments will occur for patients according to which type of ostomy they have; for example, in people with an ileostomy the contents of the intestine are liquid and may cause skin irritation and loss of fluid and salts. In those with a colostomy from the descending colon the contents may be firm and constipation can be a problem.

Special problems always surround the opening, which may become irritated and sore, and there are appliances, cements and skin-protective preparations available to reduce these problems.

Problems of drug use in people with stoma

Special coated preparations

In someone with an ileostomy the transit time for the contents to move from the stomach to the opening may be decreased. This means that special coated tablets designed to resist the acid of the stomach until they are in the intestine (enteric coated) and tablets or capsules designed specifically to release their active drug slowly into the intestine (sustained-release preparations), may pass quickly through the intestine without having time to be broken down and the drug absorbed properly into the bloodstream. This will result in a reduced dose of the drug entering the body. None of these preparations should therefore be used to treat people with ileostomies. Liquid peparations or preparations chewed and crushed before swallowing are best.

Antacids (indigestion mixtures)

Antacids containing magnesium salts may cause diarrhoea and be a problem in people with an ileostomy, and individuals with a colostomy may develop constipation if they take an antacid containing aluminium.

Antibiotics

Antibiotics may alter the balance of bacteria and fungi that grow in the intestine and cause fungal infection around the stoma. Antibiotics may also cause diarrhoea and therefore loss of water and salts. Extra fluids should be taken while on antibiotic treatment.

Treating diarrhoea

Codeine, loperamide or diphenoxylate may be used to stop diarrhoea, but see comments on their use (Chapter 16). A bulking agent (see Chapter 16) may be of use but working out the appropriate dose to relieve the diarrhoea may be difficult and is often a matter of trial and error.

Digoxin

Patients with an ileostomy may lose fluids and electrolytes, particularly potassium; this may cause a fall in blood potassium levels. Such a fall will increase the toxicity of digoxin and therefore anyone with an ileostomy who has to take digoxin should be given supplements of potassium in liquid form.

Diuretic drugs (water tablets)

These drugs cause loss of water, sodium and potassium in the urine. This may add to the water and electrolyte loss that occurs in people with ileostomies. They may become dehydrated and develop a low blood potassium level. Individuals who need to take a diuretic (e.g. for heart failure) should be given supplements of potassium in a liquid preparation.

Iron preparations

Iron preparations may cause loose and dark motions and irritate the stoma. It may therefore be necessary to use iron injections. Obviously, sustained-release preparations of iron should not be used (see earlier).

Treating constipation

Enemas and wash-outs should not be used by people with ileostomies because they may cause excessive loss of fluids, leading to dehydration.

Someone with a colostomy may become constipated, and the best treatment is to increase the fluid intake and to use a bulk laxative (e.g. bran). A faecal softener may also be used, but not regularly. Stimulant laxatives should preferably be avoided because the stoma may become blocked in constipation and the laxative may produce irritation and perforation of the wall of the intestine above the blockage.

NOTE Special preparations for clearing the intestine before X-ray examination should not be used in anyone with an ileostomy because they may cause severe dehydration.

Pain relievers

Morphine and related pain relievers may cause constipation, and in anyone with a colostomy this may be troublesome. Commonly used morphine-related drugs include codeine, dextropropoxyphene and dihydrocodeine. These are often present in combined pain relieving preparations.

Aspirin and drugs used to treat rheumatic disorders may irritate the stomach and intestine and cause ulcers and bleeding; they are best avoided in people with ileostomies. Paracetamol is the safest mild pain reliever to use.

Potassium salts

Individuals with stomas who have to take supplementary potassium salts should take the liquid form and not sustained-release preparations (see above).

87

Risks of drug treatments in people who drink alcohol

Many drugs prescribed by doctors or purchased over-the-counter from pharmacies may increase the effects of alcohol (see below). It is safer never to drink alcohol when taking any of these drugs. Note the warnings on alcohol and driving and on drugs and driving.

Warning *Always check with your pharmacist whether any drug that you are prescribed or purchase may increase the effects of alcohol.*

Drugs that may increase the effects of alcohol

sleeping drugs
anti-anxiety drugs
anti-depressant drugs
anti-psychotic drugs
antihistamines (see Chapter 10)
narcotic pain relievers

NOTE There is an increased risk of death if one of these drugs is taken in overdose with alcohol.

Alcohol may increase the harmful effects of certain drugs

Alcohol causes arteries to dilate and this makes you flushed. This reaction may cause the blood pressure to fall on standing up after sitting or lying down, which may cause you to become light-headed and faint. This is called postural hypotension (fall in blood pressure on change of posture). This reaction may also be caused by several groups of drugs that dilate arteries, and when alcohol is taken along with these drugs the reaction may be severe.

Drugs that produce postural hypotension which may be made worse by alcohol include:

- *Drugs used to treat raised blood pressure* – e.g. ACE inhibitors, adrenergic neurone blockers, hydralazine, prazosin and labetalol
- *Drugs used to improve the circulation* – e.g. thymoxamine
- *Drugs used to treat angina* – nitrate vasodilators, calcium channel blockers

Other drug reactions with alcohol

The risk of bleeding from ulceration of the stomach may be increased if alcohol is taken with *aspirin.*

The risk of liver damage from an overdose of *paracetamol* is increased in alcoholics who may have liver damage.

Certain chemicals in alcoholic drinks (e.g. tyramine) may produce severe headache, a severe rise in blood pressure and a risk of brain haemorrhage in patients who are taking an *MAOI anti-depressant* or who have taken one in the previous two weeks.

The breakdown of alcohol is blocked by *cimetidine,* causing a rise in the blood level of alcohol and increasing the risks of intoxication.

Disulfiram reaction (Antabuse reaction)

Disulfiram (Antabuse) is used to treat alcohol abuse because it produces severe reactions to alcohol if you are taking the drug. This is supposed to put the individual off drinking alcohol. Taking alcohol, even in very small amounts, after taking disulfiram, produces flushing of the face, red eyes, a feeling of heat, throbbing headache, rapid beating of the heart and giddiness; in addition, there may be nausea, vomiting, sweating, deep breathing, chest pain, blurred vision, confusion and a fall in blood pressure. The effects come on quickly and last about $\frac{1}{2}$ to 1 hour but may go on for several hours.

The intensity and duration of the disulfiram reaction vary greatly between individuals and even very small amounts of alcohol in some individuals may produce alarming effects.

Other drugs that may produce a disulfiram (Antabuse) reaction

Drugs that may produce an 'Antabuse reaction' with alcohol include cefamandole, latamoxef, metronidazole, monosulfiram, procarbazine and tinidazole.

Table 87.1 Disulfiram (Antabuse) – harmful effects and warnings

Harmful effects At the start of treatment, disulfiram may cause an unpleasant taste in the mouth, nausea, vomiting, body odour, bad breath and reduced libido. Rarely, it may cause allergic dermatitis, damage to the nerves producing numbness and pins and needles in the arms and legs, and, very rarely, liver damage and serious mental symptoms. Very rare but serious harmful effects following alcohol may include collapse, disorders of heart rhythm, heart failure, unconsciousness, convulsions and death. It may cause confusion and mood changes when taken with metronidazole, isoniazid or paraldehyde. The intensity of the disulfiram reaction may be increased by chlorpromazine and amitriptyline, and decreased by diazepam.	*Warnings* Care should be taken when drinking alcohol. Severe reactions may occur and deaths have been reported following the drinking of large volumes of alcohol. Many liquid medicines and tonics contain sufficient alcohol to trigger a disulfiram reaction. Disulfiram should be used to treat a 'drink problem' only under strict medical supervision, and the manufacturer's guidelines should be carefully followed. It should not be used during a drinking episode. It should not be used in people with heart failure, coronary heart disease, pregnancy, severe mental illness (e.g. schizophrenia, depression) or drug addiction. It should be used with caution in anyone with impaired kidney or liver function, chronic heart trouble, diabetes or epilepsy.

Risks of drug treatments in people who drive

Many drugs affect the brain and may reduce the physical and mental skills, judgement and co-ordination that are required to drive any vehicle safely. Alcohol is the most commonly used drug that can impair driving ability, and its harmful effects can be quickly increased by a wide range of drugs prescribed by doctors and available for purchase from pharmacists.

Any drug that affects vision or balance or produces dizziness or vertigo, light-headedness, faintness, drowsiness, nervousness, tenseness, anxiety or mood changes may affect your ability to drive.

Warnings *Do not take any drug without checking with your pharmacist as to whether the drug can affect your driving ability.*

Do not drink even a small amount of alcohol and drive when you are taking a drug that may affect your driving ability.

The warnings on the dangers of alcohol and drugs on driving also apply to individuals who operate moving machinery, drive any machinery, carry out any hazardous occupation or pilot aircraft or perform any task which requires skill and judgement and which, if impaired, could endanger their life or the lives of others.

Drugs that may affect driving ability

Sleeping drugs, anti-anxiety drugs, anti-psychotic drugs, anti-depressant drugs, antihistamines and narcotic pain relievers produce sedation and may interfere with your ability to drive a motor vehicle. These harmful effects on driving ability are increased by alcohol.

Anti-epileptic drugs such as carbamazepine, phenytoin, phenobarbitone and primidone may produce drowsiness and interfere with your ability to drive in the first few weeks of treatment (see Chapter 37 on the use of anti-epileptic drugs and driving). Their harmful effects on driving will be increased in alcohol.

Anti-blood-pressure drugs cause a fall in blood pressure which may produce light-headedness and faintness. Do not drive at the start of treatment nor until you know that it is safe to do so. Also be cautious if the dose of anti-blood-pressure drug is increased or if another anti-blood-pressure drug is added to your treatment.

Beta blockers used to treat angina, raised blood pressure, anxiety, migraine and over-active thyroid gland may produce drowsiness and fatigue and impair your ability to drive motor vehicles. Do not drive until you know that it is safe to do so.

Insulin and oral anti-diabetic drugs used to treat diabetes may cause a fall in blood glucose levels (hypoglycaemia) and interfere with your ability to drive motor vehicles.

Eye drops that dilate the pupils may affect vision and interfere with your ability to drive a motor vehicle. Do not drive until the effects have worn off.

Anaesthetics used by dentists and for minor surgery may affect your ability to drive. Do not drive for 24–48 hours, depending upon the anaesthetic used, the duration of the anaesthetic and how you respond to anaesthetics.

Muscle relaxants used, for example, to treat muscle spasm (e.g. baclofen and dantrolene) may produce drowsiness and muscle weakness and increase the effects of alcohol. Do not drive until you know that it is safe to do so.

The anti-inflammatory drugs *indomethacin* and *phenylbutazone,* used to treat rheumatic disorders, may affect your ability to drive. Do not drive until you know that it is safe to do so.

Several drugs may produce *drowsiness* and interfere with your ability to drive; these include *hyoscine, cyproheptadine, ketotifen, pizotifen, procarbazine, thiabendazole.*

For warnings on individual drugs see appropriate tables on harmful effects and warnings.

89

Risks of one drug reacting with another drug (drug–drug interaction)

When two or more drugs are given together the effects produced may be greater or smaller than the total effects (the sum of the effects) produced when each drug is given separately. Some drugs may therefore *decrease* the effectiveness of certain other drugs and some drugs may *increase* the effects of certain other drugs and therefore increase the risks of harmful effects. The effect that one drug may have on the actions and effects of another drug is called a *drug interaction*, and many drugs may interact.

Drug interactions may be *beneficial*; for example, when two drugs produce an extra desired effect because the beneficial effects produced by one of the drugs add to the beneficial effects produced by the other drug, provided of course that the harmful effects produced by each drug are different and are not additive. On the other hand, some drug interactions may be *harmful* and undesired (see later).

The consequences of many drug interactions are largely unknown because of a lack of information on the extent and nature of drug interactions occurring in patients; yet multiple drug treatments are often used, particularly in elderly people.

Although we have some information from animal studies on the potential for some drugs to interact with others, it is usually not possible to measure the extent and nature of many drug interactions in humans, particularly in patients being treated for one or more disorders. As a consequence, drug interactions that reduce the effectiveness of a drug may easily go unrecognized and harmful effects created because of a drug interaction may also go unrecognized. However, it is important to note that probably only a small number of potential drug interactions recognized in research laboratories are important when treating people and that different individuals react differently to interactions. Not everyone treated with drugs known to interact will actually develop signs of that interaction (e.g. reduced or increased effects, or harmful effects). These differences between individuals may be related to constitutional (genetic) factors; for example, those people who have a genetic 'defect' which causes them to break a drug down more slowly in their liver than other individuals may experience more harmful effects if that drug is given with another drug that interacts to slow down its break-down even further – the blood level of the drug will soon rise to toxic levels. Also, certain people may be more vulnerable to the effects of drug interactions than other people; for example, old elderly people, seriously ill people, people with impaired functioning of their kidneys or liver, or people who have a reduced protein level in the blood which will affect the amount of free (active) drug in the blood.

Sites of drug interactions

A drug may interact with another drug in the syringe or infusion bag; in the stomach and intestine; in the blood stream; in the tissues; at the site of action; in the liver; in the kidneys; and in the urine.

In the syringe or infusion bag

If two drugs are left to mix together in a syringe or infusion bag, one drug may inactivate the other or cause it to precipitate from the solution. If this happens the drugs are said to be *incompatible*, and pharmacists make reference to lists of drug incompatibilities before deciding to mix drugs together. These interactions may occur without a visible change in the solution, and interactions may occur not only between the active drugs but also between the various chemicals that are used in a drug preparation (e.g. preservatives).

In the stomach and intestine

When two or more drugs are taken together by mouth, one drug may alter the rate or completeness of absorption of the other drug into the blood stream. Any drug that alters the acidity of fluids in the stomach and intestine or slows down or speeds up movements of the stomach and/or intestine may interfere with the absorption of another drug.

Drugs may bind to other drugs in the stomach and intestine to form an unabsorbable chemical (chelate), which will lessen the effect of the drug because some of it will not be absorbed. One drug may compete with another drug for absorption through the wall of the stomach or intestine, and the long-term use of some drugs may interfere with the absorption of nutrients from food, leading to malnutrition.

By killing bacteria in the intestine, anti-bacterial drugs may interfere with the absorption of drugs that rely on bacteria in the intestine to break them down or to synthesize them before absorption.

In the bloodstream

Many drugs and metabolites of drugs travel round in the bloodstream attached to proteins (this is referred to as *protein binding*). In this 'bound' form they act as a 'safe' store of drugs because it is only when a drug is free in the bloodstream that it can produce its beneficial and harmful effects. There is a careful balance between the amount of free 'active' drug in the bloodstream and the amount of 'inactive' drug bound to blood proteins. This balance may be disturbed if another drug enters the bloodstream and starts to take over the proteins and displaces the other drug, making it become 'free'. This results in a higher concentration of the 'free' drug in the bloodstream, which may reach toxic levels and produce harmful effects – depending of course on how efficiently the drug is broken down in the liver and excreted by the kidneys. This rise in 'free' drug in the bloodstream may be dangerous with drugs that have a narrow margin of safety between the concentration that produces beneficial effects and the concentration that produces harmful effects.

The *displacement* of one drug by another drug from the blood proteins (plasma proteins) will depend on how much affinity one drug has over the other for binding to proteins and upon their particular sites of attachment on the proteins. It will also depend upon the concentration of the displacing drug in the blood, which will have to be higher than the concentration required just to fill up all its own binding sites on the plasma proteins.

In the tissues

In addition to acting at their sites of action (receptor sites), some drugs may also bind themselves to certain tissues (e.g. muscle tissue). Like drugs bound to plasma proteins, drugs bound to tissues form an 'inactive' store, and there is a balance between the concentration of free drug in the bloodstream and the concentration of the drug bound in the tissues. Any drug that reduces the binding of another drug to its particular tissue will cause an increase in the concentration of the free (active) drug in the bloodstream, which may reach toxic levels and produce harmful effects.

At the site of action

Interactions that affect the actions and effects of drugs (their *pharmacodynamic effects*) are probably the most common type of drug interaction.

Pharmacodynamic interactions occur when two drugs act on the *same* target site in the body. They may work *together* to produce the following types of interactions:

- *Addition* – when the effects of two drugs that have the same actions are added together
- *Potentiation* – when one drug increases (makes more powerful) the action of another drug

Alternatively, drugs may interact to oppose each other's actions and produce what is referred to as *antagonism.* This may occur if the drugs work at the same site in the body but produce entirely opposite effects – physiological or non-competitive antagonism. However, the two drugs may act on the same receptors at their sites of action and therefore they will compete with each other, so one drug will block the effects of the other – competitive antagonism.

In the liver

Increased rate of drug metabolism in the liver

Many drugs that are soluble in fat stimulate enzymes in liver cells to metabolize other drugs more rapidly. The long-term use of these drugs will not only result in an increase in the rate of their own metabolism but will also increase the rate of metabolism of certain other drugs. This process is referred to as *enzyme induction* and, depending upon the particular drug and the dose used, the induction will develop over days or weeks and persist for days or weeks after the drug causing the induction has been stopped.

If the metabolism of a drug in the liver results in the breakdown of that drug to *inactive* breakdown products, the results of induction by another drug will be to increase its breakdown and reduce its effectiveness. Alternatively, if the products of metabolism of a drug are more active than the parent drug, a drug that produces induction of that drug in the liver will cause an increase in the effects and harmful effects of that drug by speeding up the release of *active* products (metabolites) from the liver into the bloodstream.

Decreased rate of drug breakdown in the liver

Drugs that block enzymes involved in drug metabolism in the liver may reduce the rate of breakdown of certain drugs, causing their blood level to rise and resulting in an increased risk of harmful effects. This process is referred to as *enzyme inhibition.*

Different drugs may block different enzymes in the liver, to produce different effects on different drugs. In terms of benefits to risks, the consequence of a slowing up in the breakdown of a drug in the liver by another drug will depend upon the margin of safety between the concentration of the drug in the blood stream that produces beneficial effects and the concentration that produces harmful effects. This means that the risk is greater with drugs that possess a narrow margin of safety compared with drugs with a wide margin of safety.

Changes in blood flow to the liver

The rate of metabolism of a drug in the liver is affected by the blood flow to the liver. Any drug that reduces the blood flow to the liver because it reduces the output of blood from the heart may *decrease* the breakdown of certain drugs in the liver, resulting in an increase in their effects and an increased risk of harmful effects. Conversely, those drugs that cause an increase in output of blood from the heart and an increase in the flow of blood to the liver may *increase* the breakdown of certain other drugs in the liver, with a consequent lessening of their effectiveness.

Some drugs are excreted by the liver into the bile and certain drugs may interact, to affect this excretion, resulting in an increased concentration of the affected drug in the blood.

A few drugs are broken down in the intestine (e.g. by bacteria) to their active forms and then absorbed into the blood stream to be taken to the liver. However, some of the 'parent' drug may also be absorbed into the bloodstream and taken to the liver where it is excreted into the bile and then re-enters the intestine to be broken down into its active forms. This process is referred to as *enterohepatic circulation* (intestine/liver circulation), and it can be slowed down by drugs that bind to the parent drug and prevent it from being recirculated.

Alternatively, an antibiotic may knock out the bacteria in the intestine that break a parent drug down into its active form (metabolite). This will reduce the availability of the 'active' drug for absorption into the blood stream and reduce the 'parent' drug's effectiveness.

In the kidneys

Many drugs may compete with each other for excretion by the kidneys – this may result in decreased excretion of one drug by another, causing a rise in the blood concentration of the affected drug and an increased risk of harmful effects.

In the urine

Drugs that increase or decrease the acidity of the urine may increase or decrease the excretion of certain drugs in the urine.

Table 89.1 Drug interactions

Drug	*Interactions*
ACE inhibitors	
alcohol	Increased lowering of blood pressure if taken together
anaesthetics	Increased lowering of blood pressure if taken together
anti-anxiety drugs	Increased lowering of blood pressure if taken together
anti-blood-pressure drugs (other)	Increased lowering of blood pressure if taken together
anti-depressants	Increased lowering of blood pressure if taken together
beta blockers	Increased lowering of blood pressure if taken together
calcium channel blockers	Increased lowering of blood pressure if taken together
carbenoxolone	Carbenoxolone counteracts blood pressure-lowering effect of ACE inhibitors
corticosteroids	Corticosteroids counteract blood pressure-lowering effects of ACE inhibitors
cyclosporin	Increased risk of a rise in blood potassium if taken together
diuretics	When taken with an ACE inhibitor, all diuretics produce an increased lowering of blood pressure, which can be severe. Potassium-sparing diuretics produce an increased risk of a rise in blood potassium and kidney failure if taken with an ACE inhibitor
levodopa	Increased lowering of blood pressure if taken together
lithium	Enalapril and possibly other ACE inhibitors reduce the excretion of lithium and increase its blood level
nitrate vasodilators	Increased lowering of blood pressure if taken together
NSAIDs	NSAIDs counteract blood pressure-lowering effects of ACE inhibitors. Increased risk of kidney failure if taken together. Also, risk of a rise in blood potassium levels with indomethacin and possibly other NSAIDs
oestrogens	Counteract blood pressure-lowering effects of ACE inhibitors
oral contraceptives	Counteract blood pressure-lowering effects of ACE inhibitors
phenothiazine anti-psychotic drugs	A severe fall in blood pressure on standing up after sitting or lying down (postural hypotension) may occur when chlorpromazine is taken with an ACE inhibitor. This may possibly occur with other phenothiazine anti-psychotic drugs
potassium salts	Increased risk of a rise in blood potassium if taken together
probenecid	Probenecid reduces excretion of captopril
acetazolamide (for other interactions, see under 'diuretics')	
anti-arrhythmics	Acetazolamide may make the urine alkaline and reduce the excretion of flecainide, mexiletine and quinidine. Occasionally this may cause a rise in blood levels

Table 89.1 Drug interactions (*cont.*)

Drug	*Interactions*
aspirin	Aspirin reduces excretion of acetazolamide and increases risk of harmful effects
digoxin and related drugs	Acetazolamide lowers blood potassium and may increase the risk of harmful effects from digoxin and related drugs
lithium	Acetazolamide increases excretion of lithium
loop and thiazide diuretics	Increased blood potassium-lowering effects if taken together
acyclovir	
probenecid	Probenecid reduces excretion of acyclovir and increases its blood level
zidovudine	Extreme lethargy may occur when zidovudine is given with intravenous acyclovir
adrenergic neurone blockers	
alcohol	Increased lowering of blood pressure if taken together
anaesthetics	Increased lowering of blood pressure if taken together
anti-anxiety drugs	Increased lowering of blood pressure if taken together
anti-blood pressure drugs (other)	Increased lowering of blood pressure if taken together
beta blockers	Increased lowering of blood pressure if taken together
calcium channel blockers	Increased lowering of blood pressure if taken together
carbenoxolone	Carbenoxolone counteracts blood pressure-lowering effects of adrenergic neurone blockers
corticosteroids	Corticosteroids counteract blood pressure-lowering effects of adrenergic neurone blockers
diuretics	Increased lowering of blood pressure if taken together
levodopa	Increased lowering of blood pressure if taken together
nitrate vasodilators	Increased lowering of blood pressure if taken together
NSAIDs	NSAIDs counteract blood pressure-lowering effects of adrenergic neurone blockers
oestrogens	Oestrogens counteract blood pressure-lowering effects of adrenergic neurone blockers
oral contraceptives	Oral contraceptives counteract blood pressure-lowering effects of adrenergic neurone blockers
phenothiazine anti-psychotics	Increased lowering of blood pressure if taken together
pizotifen	Pizotifen counteracts blood pressure-lowering effects of adrenergic neurone blockers
sleeping drugs	Increased lowering of blood pressure if taken together

Table 89.1 Drug interactions (*cont.*)

Drug	*Interactions*
sympathomimetics	Some sympathomimetics, used for slimming and in cough and cold remedies, may counteract blood pressure-lowering effects of adrenergic neurone blockers
tricyclic anti-depressants	Tricyclic anti-depressants counteract blood pressure-lowering effects of adrenergic neurone blockers
alcohol	
anti-anxiety drugs	Increased sedation if taken together
anti-bacterials	Alcohol produces disulfiram-like reaction with cefamandole, latamoxef, metronidazole, nimorazole and tinidazole
anti-blood pressure drugs	Increased lowering of blood pressure if taken together
anti-coagulants	Alcohol increases effects of warfarin and nicoumalone, and increases risk of bleeding
anti-depressants	Alcohol increases sedative effects of tricyclic anti-depressants. Tyramine in some alcoholic and non-alcohol drinks may trigger a serious rise in blood pressure when taken with an MAOI or within 2 weeks of taking an MAOI (see Chapter 39)
anti-diabetics	Increased lowering of blood glucose if taken together. Alcohol may cause flushing in susceptible individuals when taken with chlorpropamide. Increased risk of lactic acidosis if alcohol is taken with metformin
antihistamines	Increased sedation if taken together
anti-psychotics	Increased sedation if taken together
monosulfiram	Alcohol may trigger a disulfiram-like reaction if taken with monosulfiram
procarbazine	Alcohol may trigger a disulfiram-like reaction if taken with procarbazine
sleeping drugs	Increased sedation if taken together
allopurinol	
anti-coagulants	Allopurinol increases effects of nicoumalone and warfarin. Increased risk of bleeding
azathioprine	Allopurinol increases effects of azathioprine. Increased risk of harmful effects
cyclophosphamide	Allopurinol increases effects of cyclophosphamide. Increased risk of harmful effects
mercaptopurine	Allopurinol increases effects of mercaptopurine. Increased risk of harmful effects
alpha blockers	
alcohol	Increased lowering of blood pressure if taken together. Alcohol increases sedative effects of indoramin

Table 89.1 Drug interactions (*cont.*)

Drug	*Interactions*
anaesthetics	Increased lowering of blood pressure if taken together
anti-anxiety drugs	Increased lowering of blood pressure if taken together
anti-blood pressure drugs (other)	Increased lowering of blood pressure if taken together
anti-depressants	Increased lowering of blood pressure if taken together
anti-psychotics	Increased lowering of blood pressure if taken together
beta blockers	Beta blockers increase risk of a severe fall in blood pressure with the first dose of the alpha blockers doxazosin, prazosin and terazosin
calcium channel blockers	Increased lowering of blood pressure if taken together
carbenoxolone	Carbenoxolone counteracts blood pressure-lowering effects of alpha blockers
corticosteroids	Corticosteroids counteract blood pressure-lowering effects of alpha blockers
diuretics	Diuretics increase the risk of a severe fall in blood pressure with the first dose of the alpha blockers doxazosin, prazosin and terazosin
levodopa	Increased lowering of blood pressure if taken together
nitrate vasodilators	Increased lowering of blood pressure if taken together
NSAIDs	NSAIDs counteract blood pressure-lowering effects of alpha blockers
oestrogens	Oestrogens counteract blood pressure-lowering effects of alpha blockers
oral contraceptives	Oral contraceptives counteract blood pressure-lowering effects of alpha blockers
sleeping drugs	Increased lowering of blood pressure if taken together
amantadine	
anti-blood-pressure drugs	Do not use methyldopa, metirosine or reserpine with amantadine because their harmful effects include movement disorders
anti-cholinergic drugs	Amantadine may increase the harmful effects of anticholinergic drugs
anti-psychotics	Do not use anti-psychotics with amantadine because their harmful effects include movement disorders
domperidone	Do not use domperidone with amantadine because its harmful effects include movement disorders
metoclopramide	Do not use metoclopramide with amantadine because its harmful effects include movement disorders
tetrabenazine	Do not use tetrabenazine with amantadine because its harmful effects include movement disorders

Table 89.1 Drug interactions (*cont.*)

Drug	*Interactions*
aminoglutethimide	
anti-coagulants	Aminoglutethimide increases breakdown and reduces effects of nicoumalone and warfarin
dexamethasone	Aminoglutethimide increases breakdown and reduces effects of dexamethasone
digitoxin	Aminoglutethimide increases breakdown and reduces effects of digitoxin
theophylline	Aminoglutithamide increases breakdown and reduces effects of theophylline
aminoglycosides	
amphotericin	Increased risk of kidney damage if taken together
cephalosporins	Increased risk of kidney damage if taken together, especially with cephalothin
cisplatin	Increased risk of kidney damage and possibly loss of hearing if taken together
cyclosporin	Increased risk of kidney damage if taken together
loop diuretics	Increased risk of loss of hearing if taken together
muscle relaxants	Aminoglycosides increase the effects of non-depolarizing muscle relaxants (e.g. tubocurarine)
neostigmine	Aminoglycosides counteract effects of neostigmine
pyridostigmine	Aminoglycosides counteract effects of pyridostigmine
vancomycin	Increased risk of loss of hearing and kidney damage if taken together
amiodarone	
anti-arrhythmics	Amiodarone adds to the effects of disopyramide, flecainide, procainamide and quinidine, producing increased risks of disorders of heart rhythm affecting the ventricles and depression of the heart
anti-coagulants	Amiodarone blocks breakdown of nicoumalone and warfarin. Increased risk of bleeding
phenytoin	Amiodarone blocks breakdown of phenytoin and increases its blood level
beta blockers	When taken together there is an increased risk of slowing of the heart rate, heart block (A/V) and depression of the heart
calcium-channel blockers	When amiodarone is taken with diltiazem or verapamil there is an increased risk of slowing the heart rate, heart block (A/V) and depression of the heart
cimetidine	Cimetidine increases the blood level of amiodarone
digoxin	Amiodarone causes an increase in blood level of digoxin (the maintenance dose should be halved)

Table 89.1 Drug interactions (*cont.*)

Drug	*Interactions*
diuretics	Acetazolamide, loop diuretics and thiazides may cause a fall in blood potassium level and increase the risk of harmful effects of amiodarone
amphotericin	
aminoglycosides	Increased risk of kidney damage if taken together
cephalothin	Increased risk of kidney damage if taken together
cyclosporin	Increased risk of kidney damage if taken together
anabolic steroids	
anti-coagulants	Anabolic steroids increase effects of nicoumalone, phenindione and warfarin. Increased risk of bleeding
anaesthetics (general)	
adrenaline	Risk of disorders of heart rhythm if adrenaline given with volatile anaesthetics such as cyclopropane or halothane
anti-anxiety drugs	Increased sedative effects if taken together
anti-blood-pressure drugs	Increased lowering of blood pressure if taken together
anti-psychotics	Increased lowering of blood pressure if taken together
beta blockers	Increased lowering of blood pressure if taken together
levodopa	Risk of disorders of heart rhythm if levodopa is given with volatile anaesthetics such as cyclopropane or halothane
noradrenaline	Risk of disorders of heart rhythm if noradrenaline is given with volatile anaesthetics such as cyclopropane or halothane
sleeping drugs	Increased sedative effects if taken together
verapamil	Increased lowering of blood pressure and slowing of heart rate if taken together
antacids	
anti-arrhythmics	Antacids make urine alkaline and reduce excretion of flecainide, mexiletine and quinidine. May occasionally increase blood levels
anti-bacterials	Antacids reduce absorption of ciprofloxacin, ofloxacin, pivampicillin, rifampicin and tetracyclines (except doxycycline and minocycline) from the intestine. This may reduce their effectiveness
anti-fungals	Antacids reduce absorption of itraconazole and ketoconazole from the intestine and may reduce their effectiveness
anti-malarials	Antacids reduce absorption of chloroquine and hydroxychloroquine (also used to treat rheumatoid arthritis) from the intestine, and may reduce their effectiveness

Table 89.1 Drug interactions (*cont.*)

Drug	*Interactions*
anti-psychotics	Antacids reduce absorption of phenothiazines from the intestine and may reduce their effectiveness
aspirin	Antacids make the urine alkaline and increase the excretion of aspirin in the urine, making it less effective
diflunisal	Antacids reduce absorption of diflunisal from the intestine and may make it less effective
dipyradimole	Do not take with antacids
lithium	Sodium bicarbonate increases excretion of lithium by the kidneys and lowers its blood level
oral iron	Magnesium trisilicate reduces absorption of iron salts from the intestine and may reduce their effectiveness
penicillamine	Antacids reduce absorption of penicillamine from the intestine and may reduce its effectiveness
sucralfate	Antacids neutralize the acid in the stomach whereas sucralfate requires acid to work effectively – do not take together
anti-anxiety drugs see entries under 'benzodiazepines'	
anti-arrhythmics	
	Any combination of two or more anti-arrhythmic drugs will produce increased effects on the heart. See entry under each drug
anti-cholinergics	
amantadine	Increased anti-cholinergic effects if taken together
anti-arrhythmics	Increased anti-cholinergic effects if anti-cholinergics given with disopyramide Atropine delays absorption of mexiletine from the intestine
anti-depressants	Increased anti-cholinergic effects if taken together
antihistamines	Increased anti-cholinergic effects if taken together
anti-psychotics	Increased anti-cholinergic effects if taken together, and anti-cholinergics may reduce blood levels of phenothiazines
cisapride	Anti-cholinergics counteract effects of cisapride on the stomach and intestine
domperidone	Anti-cholinergic drugs used to treat intestinal colic may block the effects of domperidone on the stomach and intestine
ketoconazole	Anti-cholinergics reduce absorption of ketoconazole from the intestine and may reduce its effectiveness
metoclopramide	Anti-cholinergic drugs used to treat intestinal colic may counteract the effects of metoclopramide on the stomach and intestine
nitrate vasodilators	Dryness of mouth caused by anti-cholinergics may make it difficult to dissolve nitrate tablets under the tongue and may reduce their effectiveness

Table 89.1 Drug interactions (*cont.*)

Drug	*Interactions*
anti-depressants (tricyclics)	
adrenaline	Risk of blood pressure and disorders of heart rhythm if taken together
alcohol	Increased sedation if taken together
anti-anxiety drugs	Increased sedation if taken together
anti-blood-pressure drugs	Increased lowering of blood pressure if taken together Tricyclic anti-depressants may counteract blood pressure-lowering effects of adrenergic neurone blockers Tricyclic anti-depressants may counteract blood pressure-lowering effects of clonidine and increase risk of a rebound rise in blood pressure when clonidine is stopped
anti-cholinergics	Increased anti-cholinergic effects if taken together
anti-epileptics	Tricyclic anti-depressants counteract anti-epileptic effects. Increased risk of seizures. Anti-epileptics increase breakdown, reduce blood level and may reduce effectiveness of tricyclic anti-depressants
antihistamines	Increased anti-cholinergic effects if taken together
anti-psychotics	Phenothiazines may increase anticholinergic effects of tricyclic anti-depressants
cimetidine	Cimetidine blocks breakdown and increases blood levels of amitriptyline, desipramine, doxepin, imipramine, nortriptyline, and probably other tricyclic anti-depressants
disulfiram	Disulfiram blocks breakdown of tricyclic anti-depressants and increases blood levels Amitriptyline increases risk of disulfiram producing a reaction when disulfiram is taken with alcohol
fluoxetine	Fluoxetine increases blood levels of some tricyclic anti-depressants
MAOIs	See Chapter 39. Avoid MAOIs 2 weeks before, during and 5 weeks after treatment. Increased risk of harmful effects with lithium
nitrate vasodilators	Tricyclic anti-depressants dry the mouth and make it difficult to dissolve a nitrate tablet under the tongue, thus making it less effective
noradrenaline	Risk of raised blood pressure if taken together
oral contraceptives	Oral contraceptives counteract beneficial anti-depressant effects of tricyclics but increase the risk of harmful effects by increasing the blood level of the anti-depressant
sleeping drugs	Increased sedation if taken together
anti-diabetics	
alcohol	Alcohol increases blood glucose-lowering effects of anti-diabetic drugs. Alcohol may cause flushing of face in susceptible individuals when taken with chlorpropamide. Alcohol produces an increased risk of lactic acidosis with metformin

Table 89.1 Drug interactions (*cont.*)

Drug	*Interactions*
anti-bacterials	Chloramphenicol, co-trimoxazole and sulphonamides increase effects of sulphonylureas Rifampicin increases breakdown and reduces effects of sulphonylureas
azapropazone	Azapropazone increases effects of sulphonylureas
beta blockers	Beta blockers increase blood glucose-lowering effects of anti-diabetic drugs but may mask some of the warning signs of hypoglycaemia (e.g. tremor, sweating)
cimetidine	Cimetidine blocks excretion of metformin by the kidneys and increases its blood level
clofibrate and related drugs	Clofibrates may improve effects of anti-diabetics by producing additive effects
corticosteroids	Corticosteroids counteract blood glucose-lowering effects of anti-diabetic drugs
diazoxide	Diazoxide counteracts blood glucose-lowering effects of anti-diabetics
diuretics	Loop and thiazide diuretics counteract blood glucose-lowering effects of anti-diabetic drugs Chlorpropamide increases risk of a fall in blood sodium levels with combined thiazide and potassium-sparing diuretic treatment
lithium	Lithium may affect blood glucose levels, and dose of insulin or oral anti-diabetic drugs may need changing
MAOI anti-depressants	MAOIs increase blood glucose-lowering effects of anti-diabetic drugs
miconazole	Miconazole increases effects of sulphonylureas
nifedipine	Nifedipine may reduce effectiveness of anti-diabetic drugs
octreotide	Octreotide affects blood glucose levels, and dose of insulin or oral anti-diabetic drugs may need changing
oral contraceptives	Oral contraceptives counteract blood glucose-lowering effects of anti-diabetic drugs
phenylbutazone	Phenylbutazone increases effects of sulphonylureas
sulphinpyrazone	Sulphinpyrazone increases effects of sulphonylureas
antihistamines	
alcohol	Increased sedation if taken together
anti-anxiety drugs	Increased sedation if taken together
anti-cholinergics	Increased anti-cholinergic effects if taken together
anti-depressants (tricyclics)	Increased anti-cholinergic effects if taken together
betahistine	Betahistine counteracts effects of antihistamines
sleeping drugs	Increased sedation if taken together

Table 89.1 Drug interactions (*cont.*)

Drug	*Interactions*
anti-psychotic drugs	
ACE inhibitors	Increased lowering of blood pressure if taken together. Risk of severe fall in blood pressure on standing up after sitting or lying down (postural hypotension) when chlorpromazine is given with an ACE inhibitor. May possibly occur with other anti-psychotics
alcohol	Increased sedation if taken together
anaesthetics (general)	Increased lowering of blood pressure if taken together
antacids	Antacids reduce absorption of phenothiazines from intestine and may reduce their effectiveness
anti-anxiety drugs	Increased sedation if taken together
anti-blood-pressure drugs	Increased lowering of blood pressure if taken together. Methyldopa, metirosine and reserpine increase the risk of movement disorders from anti-psychotic drugs
anti-cholinergics	Increased anti-cholinergic effects if taken together, and anti-cholinergics may reduce blood levels of phenothiazines
anti-epileptics	Anti-psychotic drugs counteract effects of anti-epileptics. Increased risk of seizures
bromocriptine	Anti-psychotic drugs counteract prolactin-lowering effects of bromocriptine
calcium channel blockers	Increased lowering of blood pressure if taken together
carbamazepine	Carbamazepine increases breakdown of haloperidol and reduces its blood level
desferrioxamine	Manufacturer recommends that desferrioxamine should not be given with prochlorperazine
indomethacin	Indomethacin interacts with haloperidol to produce severe drowsiness
lithium	Increased risk of movement disorders and nerve damage if phenothiazines or haloperidol are taken with lithium
MAOIs	Oxypertine interacts with MAOIs to cause stimulation of the brain and a rise in blood pressure (see Chapter 39)
metoclopramide	Increased risk of movement disorders if taken together
propranolol	Propranolol increases blood level of chlorpromazine
rifampicin	Rifampicin increases breakdown of haloperidol and reduces blood level
tetrabenazine	Increased risk of movement disorders if taken together
tricyclic anti-depressants	Increased anti-cholinergic effects if taken together (particularly phenothiazines)

Table 89.1 Drug interactions (*cont.*)

Drug	*Interactions*
aspirin	
acetazolamide	Aspirin reduces excretion of acetazolamide in urine and may increase its harmful effects
antacids	Antacids may make urine alkaline and increase excretion of aspirin in urine, making it less effective
anti-coagulants	Aspirin increases risk of bleeding due to its effects on platelets when taken with anti-coagulants
anti-epileptics	Aspirin increases effects of phenytoin and sodium valproate
anti-gout drugs	Aspirin reduces effects of probenecid and sulphinpyrazone
domperidone	By its effect on movements of the stomach and intestine, domperidone helps to increase the absorption of aspirin and to improve its effectiveness.
methotrexate	Aspirin delays excretion of methotrexate and increases risk of harmful effects
metoclopramide	By its effect on movements of the stomach and intestine, metoclopramide helps to increase the absorption of aspirin and to improve its effectiveness
spironolactone	Aspirin counteracts the diuretic effect of spironolactone
azathioprine	
allopurinol	Allopurinol increases the effects of azathioprine and increases the risk of harmful effects
aztreonam	
anti-coagulants	Aztreonam increases the effects of nicoumalone and warfarin. Increased risk of bleeding
barbiturates	
anti-arrhythmics	Barbiturates increase breakdown of disopyramide and quinidine, and reduce blood levels
anti-bacterials	Barbiturates increase breakdown of chloramphenicol, doxycycline and metronidazole
anti-coagulants	Barbiturates increase breakdown of nicoumalone and warfarin, and may reduce effects
anti-depressants (tricyclics)	Tricyclic anti-depressants counteract anti-epileptic effects of barbiturates. Increased risk of seizures. Barbiturates increase breakdown and reduce blood levels of tricyclics
anti-epileptics	Use of the barbiturates phenobarbitone or primidone with any other anti-epileptic drug may increase risk of harmful effects from these drugs (e.g. increased drowsiness), without more effective control of seizures. The blood levels of other anti-epileptic drugs may be changed which may make it difficult to determine the most effective dose

Table 89.1 Drug interactions (*cont.*)

Drug	*Interactions*
anti-psychotics	Anti-psychotic drugs counteract anti-epileptic effects of barbiturates. Increased risk of seizures
corticosteroids	Barbiturates increase breakdown of corticosteroids and may reduce their effects
cyclosporin	Barbiturates increase breakdown of cyclosporin and may reduce its effects
digitoxin	Barbiturates increase breakdown of digitoxin and reduce its effects
griseofulvin	Phenobarbitone increases breakdown of griseofulvin and reduces its effects
isradipine	Barbiturates reduce effects of isradipine
oral contraceptives	Barbiturates increase breakdown of oral contraceptives and may reduce their effectiveness
theophylline	Barbiturates increase breakdown of theophylline and may reduce its effectiveness
thyroxine	Barbiturates increase breakdown of thyroxine and may reduce its effectiveness
benzodiazepines	
alcohol	Increased sedation if taken together
anaesthetics (general)	Increased sedation if taken together
anti-blood pressure drugs	Benzodiazepines increase blood pressure-lowering effects of anti-blood pressure drugs
anti-depressants	Increased sedation if taken together
antihistamines	Increased sedation if taken together
anti-psychotics	Increased sedation if taken together
cimetidine	Cimetidine blocks breakdown of benzodiazepines, and increases their blood levels
clonazepam	Benzodiazepines increase breakdown of clonazepam (used to treat epilepsy) and may reduce its effectiveness
disulfiram	Disulfiram blocks breakdown of chlordiazepoxide and diazepam, causing increased sedation
erythromycin	Erythromycin blocks breakdown of triazolam and increases its blood level
levodopa	Benzodiazepines occasionally counteract the effects of levodopa
narcotic pain relievers	Increased sedation if taken together
beta blockers	
alcohol	Increased blood pressure-lowering effects if taken together
alpha blockers (selective)	Beta blockers increase the risk of a fall in blood pressure with the first dose of a selective alpha blocker

Table 89.1 Drug interactions (*cont.*)

Drug	*Interactions*
anaesthetics	Increased blood pressure-lowering effects if taken together
anti-anxiety drugs	Increased lowering of blood pressure if taken together
anti-arrhythmics	Increased risk of effects on the heart (e.g. slowing of heart rate) if taken together Increased risk of slowing of heart rate if amiodarone is taken with a beta blocker
anti-blood-pressure drugs	Other anti-blood-pressure drugs increase the lowering of blood pressure produced by beta blockers
anti-diabetic drugs	Beta blockers increase blood glucose-lowering effects of anti-diabetic drugs and may mask some of the warning signs of hypoglycaemia (e.g. tremor, sweating)
calcium channel blockers	With beta blockers there is an increased risk of slowing of heart rate with diltiazem; an occasional increased risk of a severe fall in blood pressure and heart failure with nifedipine; and an occasional increased risk of a severe fall in blood pressure, heart failure and, rarely, stopping of the heart (asystole) with verapamil
carbenoxolone	Carbenoxolone counteracts blood pressure-lowering effects of beta blockers
chlorpromazine	Concentration of chlorpromazine in the blood is increased by propranolol
cimetidine	Cimetidine increases blood levels of labetalol and propranolol
clonidine	Beta blockers increase risk of a rebound rise in blood pressure on stopping clonidine
corticosteroids	Corticosteroids counteract blood pressure-lowering effects of beta blockers
digoxin and related drugs	Increased risk of slowing of heart rate if taken together
diuretics	Increased lowering of blood pressure if taken together. Fall in blood potassium caused by loop and thiazide diuretics may increase risk from sotalol producing disorders of heart rhythm (ventricular arrhythmia)
ergotamine	Increased risk of cold fingers and toes (peripheral vasoconstriction) if taken together
fluvoxamine	Fluvoxamine increases blood level of propranolol
muscle relaxants (neuromuscular blocking drugs)	Propranolol (in large doses) increases effects of neuromuscular blocking drugs
neostigmine	Propranolol counteracts effects of neostigmine
NSAIDs	NSAIDs counteract blood pressure-lowering effects of beta blockers
pyridostigmine	Propranolol counteracts effects of pyridostigmine
reserpine	Increased risk of slowing of the heart rate if reserpine is taken with beta blockers

Table 89.1 Drug interactions (*cont.*)

Drug	*Interactions*
rifampicin	Rifampicin increases breakdown of propranolol and reduces its blood level
sleeping drugs	Increased lowering of blood pressure if taken together
sympathomimetics	Adrenaline and noradrenaline may produce a serious rise in blood pressure, especially with non-selective beta blockers Sympathomimetics in cough and cold medicines and slimming drugs may also trigger severe rise in blood pressure if taken with beta blockers
thyroxine	Thyroxine increases breakdown of propranolol and reduces its effect
xamoterol	Beta blockers counteract effects of xamoterol and xamoterol reduces effects of beta blockers
betahistine	
antihistamines	Antihistamines counteract the effects of betahistine
bromocriptine	
anti-psychotic drugs	Anti-psychotic drugs counteract the effects of bromocriptine in lowering blood levels of prolactin and in parkinsonism
domperidone	Domperidone counteracts the effects of bromocriptine in lowering blood levels of prolactin (milk-producing hormone)
metoclopramide	Metoclopramide counteracts the effects of bromocriptine in lowering blood levels of prolactin (milk-producing hormone)
buspirone	
MAOIs	Do not use together (see Chapter 39)
calcium salts	
digoxin and related drugs	Large intravenous doses of calcium can trigger disorders of heart rhythm in people taking digoxin or a related drug
tetracyclines	Calcium salts reduce absorption of tetracyclines from the intestine and may reduce their effectiveness
thiazide diuretics	Increased risk of a rise in blood calcium levels if taken together
calcium channel blockers	
anaesthetics	Verapamil increases blood pressure-lowering effects of general anaesthetics. Also risk of slowing of heart rate
anti-arrhythmics	Diltiazem and verapamil increase risk of harmful effects on the heart produced by amiodarone. Verapamil may increase blood level of quinidine and cause severe fall in blood pressure
anti-blood-pressure drugs	Increased lowering of blood pressure if given together
anti-diabetics	Nifedipine may occasionally affect blood glucose control of anti-diabetic drugs

Table 89.1 Drug interactions (*cont.*)

Drug	*Interactions*
anti-epileptics	Diltiazem and verapamil increase effects of carbamazepine. Effects of isradipine and probably nicardipine and nifedipine are reduced by carbamazepine, phenobarbitone, phenytoin and primidone
anti-psychotics	Increased lowering of blood pressure if taken together
beta blockers	Beta blockers may interact to produce an increased risk of slowing of heart rate with diltiazem; occasional increased risk of severe fall in blood pressure and heart failure with nifedipine and verapamil and, rarely, stopping of heart (asystole) with verapamil
cimetidine	Cimetidine blocks breakdown of some calcium channel blockers and increases their blood levels
cyclosporin	Diltiazem, nicardipine and verapamil increase blood levels of cyclosporin
digoxin	Calcium channel blockers may increase effects of digoxin. Verapamil increases risk of slowing of the heart from digoxin
lithium	Diltiazem and verapamil may increase nerve damage caused by lithium without increasing its blood level
muscle relaxants (non-depolarizing)	Verapamil increases effects of non-depolarizing muscle relaxants (e.g. tubocurarine)
rifampicin	Rifampicin increases breakdown of verapamil and possibly isradipine and reduces their blood levels
theophylline	Diltiazem and verapamil increase effects of theophylline
carbamazepine	
anti-bacterials	Carbamazepine increases breakdown of doxycycline and reduces its effects Erythromycin and isoniazid increase blood levels of carbamazepine
anti-coagulants	Carbamazepine increases breakdown of nicoumalone and warfarin and reduces their effects
anti-depressants	Anti-depressants counteract anti-epileptic effects of carbamazepine. Increased risk of seizures. Viloxazine increases blood level of carbamazepine Anti-epileptics increase breakdown of tricyclic anti-depressants, and decrease their blood levels. Do not use with MAOIs
anti-epileptics	Interactions between anti-epileptic drugs may increase effects and harmful effects (e.g. sedation) without improved control of seizures and cause changes in blood levels which may make it difficult to work out effective doses
anti-psychotics	Anti-psychotic drugs counteract effects of anti-epileptic drugs. Increased risk of seizures Carbamazepine increases breakdown of haloperidol and reduces its blood level
calcium channel blockers	Diltiazem and verapamil increase effects of carbamazepine Carbamazepine reduces effects of isradipine

Table 89.1 Drug interactions (*cont.*)

Drug	*Interactions*
cimetidine	Cimetidine blocks breakdown of carbamazepine and increases its blood level
clonazepam	Carbamazepine increases breakdown of clonazepam and reduces its effects
corticosteroids	Carbamazepine increases breakdown of corticosteroids and reduces effects
cyclosporin	Carbamazepine increases breakdown of cyclosporin and reduces its blood level
danazol	Danazol blocks breakdown of carbamazepine and increases its effects
dextropropoxyphene	Dextropropoxyphene increases effects of carbamazepine
digitoxin	Carbamazepine increases breakdown of digitoxin and reduces its effects
lithium	Carbamazepine may increase risk of nerve damage from lithium without causing an increase in the blood level of lithium
oral contraceptives	Carbamazepine increases breakdown of oral contraceptives and reduces their contraceptive effectiveness
theophylline	Carbamazepine increases breakdown of theophylline and reduces its effects
thyroxine	Carbamazepine increases breakdown of thyroxine and reduces its effects
carbenoxolone	
anti-blood-pressure drugs	Carbenoxolone counteracts blood pressure-lowering effects of anti-blood-pressure drugs
corticosteroids	Increased risk of a fall in blood potassium level if taken together
digoxin and related drugs	Carbenoxolone may cause a fall in blood potassium levels and increase harmful effects from digoxin and related drugs
Diuretics	Carbenoxolone counteracts diuretic effects of diuretics. Carbenoxolone increases risk of a fall in blood potassium levels from acetazolamide and from thiazide and loop diuretics Amiloride and spironolactone may block ulcer-healing effects of carbenoxolone
cardiac glycosides see digoxin and related drugs	
cephalosporins	
alcohol	A disulfiram-like reaction may occur if alcohol is taken with cefamandole and latamoxef
aminoglycosides	Cephalothin increases risk of kidney damage from aminoglycosides
amphotericin	Cephalothin increases risk of kidney damage from amphotericin

Table 89.1 Drug interactions (*cont.*)

Drug	*Interactions*
anti-coagulants	Cefamandole and latamoxef increase effects of nicoumalone and warfarin. Increased risk of bleeding
loop diuretics	Loop diuretics increase risk of kidney damage from cephalothin
probenecid	Probenecid reduces excretion of cephalosporins in the urine and increases their blood levels
vancomycin	Increased risk of kidney damage if cephalothin is taken with vancomycin
chloramphenicol	
anti-coagulants	Chloramphenicol increases anti-coagulant effects of nicoumalone and warfarin. Increased risk of bleeding
anti-diabetics	Chloramphenicol increases effects of sulphonylureas
phenobarbitone	Phenobarbitone increases breakdown of chloramphenicol and reduces its blood level
phenytoin	Chloramphenicol increases blood level of phenytoin and increases risk of harmful effects
rifampicin	Rifampicin increases breakdown of chloramphenicol and reduces its blood level
chlormethiazole for general interactions, see benzodiazepines	
chloroquine and hydroxychloroquine	
antacids	Antacids reduce absorption of chloroquine and hydroxychloroquine from the intestine and may reduce their effectiveness
cimetidine	Cimetidine blocks breakdown of chloroquine and increases blood level
neostigmine	Chloroquine and hydroxychloroquine counteract effects of neostigmine
pyridostigmine	Chloroquine and hydroxychloroquine counteract effects of pyridostigmine
cholestyramine	
anti-coagulants	Cholestyramine may increase effects of nicoumalone, phenindione and warfarin. Increased risk of bleeding
digoxin and related drugs	Cholestyramine reduces absorption of digoxin and related drugs from the intestine and may reduce their effectiveness
paracetamol	Cholestyramine reduces absorption of paracetamol from the intestine and may reduce its effectiveness
phenylbutazone	Cholestyramine reduces absorption of phenylbutazone from the intestine and may reduce its effectiveness
thiazide diuretics	Cholestyramine reduces absorption of thiazide diuretics from the intestine and may reduce their effectiveness

Table 89.1 Drug interactions (*cont.*)

Drug	*Interactions*
thyroxine	Cholestyramine reduces absorption of thyroxine from the intestine and may reduce its effectiveness
vancomycin	Cholestyramine counteracts the effects of vancomycin by mouth
cholinergics	
anti-bacterials	Aminoglycosides, clindamycin, lincomycin and polymyxins counteract effects of neostigmine and pyridostigmine
chloroquine	Chloroquine counteracts effects of neostigmine and pyridostigmine
lithium	Lithium counteracts effects of neostigmine and pyridostigmine
propranolol	Propranolol counteracts effects of neostigmine and pyridostigmine
quinidine	Quinidine counteracts effects of neostigmine and pyridostigmine
suxamethonium	Demacarium, ecothiopate (in eye drops), neostigmine and pyridostigmine increase the effects of suxamethonium
tubocurarine and related drugs	Demacarium and ecothiopate eye drops, neostigmine and pyridostigmine counteract effects of non-depolarizing muscle relaxants such as tubocurarine
cimetidine	
anti-arrhythmics	Cimetidine increases blood levels of flecainide, lignocaine, procainamide, propafenone and quinidine
anti-coagulants	Cimetidine blocks breakdown and increases effects of nicoumalone and warfarin. Increased risk of bleeding
anti-epileptics	Cimetidine blocks breakdown of carbamazepine and phenytoin and increases their blood levels
anti-fungals	Cimetidine reduces absorption of itraconazole and ketoconazole from the intestine and may reduce their effectiveness
benzodiazepines	Cimetidine blocks breakdown of benzodiazepines and increases their blood levels
beta blockers	Cimetidine blocks breakdown of labetalol and propranolol, and increases their blood levels
calcium channel blockers	Cimetidine blocks breakdown of some calcium channel blockers and increases their blood levels
chlormethiazole	Cimetidine blocks breakdown of chlormethiazole and increases its blood level
chloroquine	Cimetidine blocks breakdown of chloroquine and increases its blood level
fluorouracil	Cimetidine increases blood levels of fluorouracil
metformin	Cimetidine blocks excretion of metformin by the kidneys and increases its blood level
metronidazole	Cimetidine blocks breakdown and increases the blood level of metronidazole

Table 89.1 Drug interactions (*cont.*)

Drug	*Interactions*
narcotic pain relievers	Cimetidine blocks breakdown and increases the blood levels of narcotic pain relievers (particularly pethidine)
quinine	Cimetidine blocks breakdown of quinine and increases its blood level
rifampicin	Rifampicin increases breakdown of cimetidine and reduces its blood level
sucralfate	Cimetidine blocks acid production in the stomach but sucralfate requires acid to work effectively. Therefore do not take together to treat peptic ulcers
theophylline	Cimetidine blocks breakdown of theophylline and increases its blood level
tricyclic anti-depressants	Cimetidine blocks breakdown and increases the blood levels of amitriptyline, desipramine, doxepin, imipramine, and nortriptyline
ciprofloxacin	
antacids	Antacids reduce absorption of ciprofloxacin from the intestine and may reduce its effectiveness
iron	Oral iron reduces absorption of ciprofloxacin from the intestine and may reduce its effectiveness
theophylline	Ciprofloxacin increases the blood level of theophylline
cisapride	
anti-cholinergics	Anti-cholinergics counteract effects of cisapride on movements of the stomach and intestine
narcotic pain relievers	Narcotic pain relievers counteract effects of cisapride on movements of the stomach and intestine
cisplatin	
aminoglycosides	Increased risk of kidney damage and possibly loss of hearing if taken together
clindamycin	
muscle relaxants	Clindamycin increases effects of non-depolarizing muscle relaxants such as tubocurarine
neostigmine	Clindamycin counteracts effects of neostigmine
pyridostigmine	Clindamycin counteracts effects of pyridostigmine
clofibrate and related drugs	
anti-diabetics	Clofibrate and related drugs may improve blood glucose-lowering effects of anti-diabetic drugs
anti-coagulants	Clofibrate and related drugs increase effects of nicoumalone, phenindione and warfarin. Increased risk of bleeding

Table 89.1 Drug interactions (*cont.*)

Drug	*Interactions*
clonazepam see general interactions under 'benzodiazepines'	
anti-epileptic drugs (other)	Carbamazepine, phenobarbitone and phenytoin increase breakdown of clonazepam
clonidine	
alcohol	Increased lowering of blood pressure if taken together
anaesthetics	Increased lowering of blood pressure if taken together
anti-anxiety drugs	Increased lowering of blood pressure if taken together
anti-blood-pressure drugs (others)	Increased lowering of blood pressure if taken together
anti-depressants (tricyclics)	Tricyclic anti-depressants counteract blood pressure-lowering effects of clonidine and increase risk of a rebound rise in blood pressure which may occur when clonidine is stopped
anti-psychotics	Increased lowering of blood pressure if taken together
beta blockers	Beta blockers produce a risk of a rebound rise in blood pressure when clonidine is stopped
calcium channel blockers	Increased lowering of blood pressure if taken together
carbenoxolone	Carbenoxolone counteracts blood pressure-lowering effects of clonidine
corticosteroids	Corticosteroids counteract blood pressure-lowering effects of clonidine
diuretics	Increased lowering of blood pressure if taken together
levodopa	Increased lowering of blood pressure if taken together
oestrogens	Oestrogens counteract blood pressure-lowering effects of clonidine
oral contraceptives	Oral contraceptives counteract blood pressure-lowering effects of clonidine
sleeping drugs	Increased lowering of blood pressure if taken together
colestipol	
anti-coagulants	Colestipol may increase effects of nicoumalone, phenindione and warfarin. Increased risk of bleeding
digoxin and related drugs	Colestipol reduces absorption of digoxin and related drugs from the intestine and may reduce their effectiveness
paracetamol	Colestipol reduces absorption of paracetamol from the intestine and may reduce its effectiveness
phenylbutazone	Colestipol reduces absorption of phenylbutazone from the intestine and may reduce its effectiveness
thiazide diuretics	Colestipol reduces absorption of thiazide diuretics from the intestine and may reduce their effectiveness

Table 89.1 Drug interactions (*cont.*)

Drug	*Interactions*
thyroxine	Colestipol reduces absorption of thyroxine from the intestine and may reduce its effectiveness
vancomycin	Colestipol counteracts the effects of vancomycin by mouth
contraceptives (oral)	
anti-bacterials	Rifampicin increases breakdown of both combined and progestogen-only oral contraceptives, with a possibility that their contraceptive effects may be reduced Ampicillin, tetracycline and other broad-spectrum antibiotics may occasionally reduce contraceptive effects of combined oral contraceptives
anti-blood-pressure drugs	Combined oral contraceptives counteract the blood pressure-lowering effects of drugs used to treat raised blood pressure
anti-coagulants	Oral contraceptives counteract the anti-coagulant effects of nicoumalone, phenindione and warfarin, and reduce their effectiveness
anti-depressants	Oral contraceptives may counteract the anti-depressant effects of tricyclic anti-depressants. However, blood levels of tricyclics may be increased, causing an increased risk of harmful effects.
anti-diabetics	Oral contraceptives counteract the blood glucose-lowering effects of insulin and oral anti-diabetic drugs
anti-epileptics	Carbamazepine, phenobarbitone, phenytoin and primidone increase the breakdown of oral contraceptives and reduce their contraceptive effectiveness
barbiturates	Phenobarbitone and primidone increase the breakdown of oral contraceptives and reduce their contraceptive effectiveness
cyclosporin	Oral contraceptives increase the blood level of cyclosporin
diuretics	Combined oral contraceptives counteract the diuretic effects of diuretics
griseofulvin	Griseofulvin increases breakdown of oral contraceptives and reduces their contraceptive effectiveness
theophylline	Combined oral contraceptives delay the excretion of theophylline and increase its blood level
corticosteroids and corticotrophin	
aminoglutethimide	Aminoglutethimide increases breakdown of dexamethasone
anti-blood-pressure drugs	Corticosteroids and corticotrophin counteract blood pressure-lowering effects of anti-blood-pressure drugs
anti-diabetics	Corticosteroids and corticotrophin counteract blood glucose-lowering effects of insulin and oral anti-diabetics
anti-epileptics	Carbamazepine, phenobarbitone, phenytoin and primidone increase breakdown of corticosteroids and reduce their effects
barbiturates	Phenobarbitone and primidone increase breakdown of corticosteroids and may reduce their effects

Table 89.1 Drug interactions (*cont.*)

Drug	*Interactions*
carbenoxolone	Increased risk of a fall in blood potassium if taken together
diuretics	Corticosteroids and corticotrophin counteract the diuretic effects of diuretics Acetazolamide, loop diuretics and thiazides increase the risk of a low blood potassium from corticosteroids and corticotrophin
rifampicin	Rifampicin increases breakdown of corticosteroids and reduces their effects
sympathomimetics	Risk of a fall in blood potassium if high doses of corticosteroids are given with high doses of fenoterol, pirbuterol, reproterol, rimiterol, ritodrine, salbutamol, and terbutaline
co-trimazole see sulphonamides	
cyclophosphamide	
allopurinol	Allopurinol increases risk of harmful effects from cyclophosphamide
muscle relaxants (depolarizing)	Cyclophosphamide increases effects of suxamethonium
cyclosporin	
ACE inhibitors	Increased risk of rise in blood potassium if taken together
anti-bacterials	Aminoglycosides, ciprofloxacin and co-trimoxazole: increased risk of kidney damage if taken together Erythromycin: increases blood level of cyclosporin Rifampicin: reduces blood level of cyclosporin
anti-epileptics	Phenobarbitone, phenytoin and primidone increase breakdown and reduce blood level of cyclosporin
anti-fungals	Amphotericin increases risk of kidney damage from cyclosporin Ketoconazole and possibly fruconazole block breakdown and increase blood level of cyclosporin
barbiturates	Phenobarbitone and primidone increase breakdown and reduce blood level of cyclosporin
calcium channel blockers	Diltiazem, nicardipine and verapamil increase blood levels of cyclosporin
danazol	Danazol blocks breakdown of cyclosporin and increases its blood level
potassium salts	Increased risk of a rise in blood potassium if taken together
potassium-sparing diuretics	Increased risk of a rise in blood potassium if taken together
progestogens	Progestogens block breakdown and increase blood level of cyclosporin
danazol	
anti-coagulants	Danazol blocks breakdown of nicoumalone and warfarin and increases their effects. Increased risk of bleeding

Table 89.1 Drug interactions (*cont.*)

Drug	*Interactions*
carbamazepine	Danazol blocks breakdown of carbamazepine and increases its blood level
cyclosporin	Danazol blocks breakdown of cyclosporin and increases its blood level
dapsone	
probenecid	Probenecid reduces excretion of dapsone, increases its blood level and increases risk of harmful effects
desferrioxamine	
prochlorperazine	Do not use desferrioxamine with prochlorperazine
dextrothyroxine	
anti-coagulants	Dextrothyroxine increases effects of nicoumalone and warfarin. Increased risk of bleeding
diazoxide	
alcohol	Increased lowering of blood pressure if taken together
anaesthetics	Increased lowering of blood pressure if taken together
anti-anxiety drugs	Increased lowering of blood pressure if taken together
anti-blood-pressure drugs	Increased lowering of blood pressure if taken together
anti-depressants	Increased lowering of blood pressure if taken together
anti-diabetics	Diazoxide counteracts blood glucose-lowering effects of anti-diabetic drugs
anti-psychotics	Increased lowering of blood pressure if taken together
calcium channel blockers	Increased lowering of blood pressure if taken together
carbenoxolone	Carbenoxolone counteracts blood pressure-lowering effects of diazoxide
corticosteroids	Corticosteroids counteract blood pressure-lowering effects of diazoxide
diuretics	Increased lowering of blood pressure if taken together
levodopa	Increased lowering of blood pressure if taken together
nitrate vasodilators	Increased lowering of blood pressure if taken together
NSAIDs	NSAIDs counteract blood pressure lowering effects of diazoxide
oestrogens	Oestrogens counteract blood pressure-lowering effects of diazoxide
oral contraceptives	Oral contraceptives counteract blood pressure-lowering effects of diazoxide
sleeping drugs	Increased lowering of blood pressure if taken together

Table 89.1 Drug interactions (*cont.*)

Drug	*Interactions*
digoxin and related drugs	
aminoglutethimide	Aminoglutethimide increases breakdown of digitoxin and reduces its effects
anti-arrhythmics	Amiodarone, propafenone and quinidine may increase blood levels of digoxin (halve the maintenance dose)
barbiturates	Barbiturates increase breakdown of digitoxin and reduce its effects
beta blockers	Beta blockers increase harmful effects of digoxin and related drugs on the heart. Risk of slowing of heart rate
calcium channel blockers	Calcium channel blockers may increase effects of digoxin Verapamil increases risk of slowing of heart rate from digoxin and related drugs
calcium salts	Large intravenous doses of calcium may trigger disorders of heart rhythm in individuals on digoxin and related drugs
carbenoxolone	Carbenoxolone may cause a fall in blood potassium level and increase risk of harmful effects from digoxin and related drugs
cholestyramine	Cholestyramine may reduce absorption of digoxin and related drugs and may reduce their effectiveness
colestipol	Colestipol may reduce absorption of digoxin and related drugs and may reduce their effectiveness
diuretics	Acetazolamide, loop diuretics and thiazides may cause a fall in blood potassium and increase risk of harmful effects from digoxin and related drugs Spironolactone increases effects of digoxin
erythromycin	Erythromycin increases effects of digoxin
NSAIDs	NSAIDs may worsen heart failure, reduce the function of the kidneys and increase the blood level of digoxin and related drugs
quinine	Quinine raises the blood level of digoxin (halve maintenance dose)
rifampicin	Rifampicin increases breakdown of digitoxin and reduces its effects
suxamethonium	Suxamethonium increases risk of disorders of heart rhythm from digoxin and related drugs
dipyridamole	
antacids	Do not use dipyridamole with antacids
anti-coagulants	Dipyridamole increases effects of anti-coagulants due to its effects on the blood platelets
disopyramide	
Anti-arrhythmics (other)	Amiodarone interacts with disopyramide to increase the risk of ventricle disorders of the heart (ventricular arrhythmias) Disopyramide increases risks of harmful effects on the heart from any other anti-arrhythmic drug

Table 89.1 Drug interactions (*cont.*)

Drug	*Interactions*
anti-bacterials	Rifampicin reduces blood level of disopyramide and may reduce its effects Erythromycin increases blood level of disopyramide and increases risk of harmful effects
anti-cholinergics	Increased anti-cholinergic harmful effects if taken together
anti-epileptics	Phenobarbitone, phenytoin and primidone reduce blood level of disopyramide
barbiturates	Phenobarbitone and primidone reduce blood level of disopyramide
diuretics	Acetazolamide, loop diuretics and thiazide diuretics may cause a fall in blood potassium levels and increase the risk of harmful effects from disopyramide
nitrate vasodilators	Disopyramide may cause a dry mouth and make it difficult to dissolve nitrate tablets under the tongue. May reduce their effectiveness
disulfiram	
alcohol	A disulfiram reaction occurs if taken together
anti-coagulants	Disulfiram increases effects of nicoumalone and warfarin. Increased risk of bleeding
anti-depressants (tricyclics)	Disulfiram blocks breakdown of tricyclic anti-depressants and increases their blood levels Amitriptyline increases risk of disulfiram producing a reaction when taken with alcohol
benzodiazepines	Disulfiram blocks breakdown of chlordiazepoxide and diazepam, increases blood levels and increases risk of harmful effects (e.g. sedation)
phenytoin	Disulfiram blocks breakdown of phenytoin, increases its blood level and increases risk of harmful effects
diuretics	
ACE inhibitors	Diuretics increase effects of ACE inhibitors and may cause a serious drop in blood pressure. Also risk of a rise in blood potassium with potassium-sparing diuretics ACE inhibitors increase risk of a rise in blood potassium with potassium-sparing diuretics
alpha blockers	Diuretics produce an increased risk of a drop in blood pressure with first dose of selective alpha blockers
anti-arrhythmics	Loop and thiazide diuretics may cause a fall in blood potassium levels and increase the risk of harmful effects from amiodarone, disopyramide, flecainide and quinidine. The fall in blood potassium levels may also counteract the effects of lignocaine, mexiletine and tocainide Acetazolamide reduces excretion of quinidine and increases its blood level
anti-bacterials	Loop diuretics increase the risk of deafness from aminoglycosides, polymyxins and vancomycin. Loop diuretics increase the risk of kidney damage from cephalothin

Table 89.1 Drug interactions (*cont.*)

Drug	*Interactions*
anti-diabetics	Loop and thiazide diuretics counteract the blood glucose-lowering effects of anti-diabetic drugs. Chlorpropamide increases risk of a fall in blood sodium level from combined use of a thiazide and potassium-sparing diuretics
aspirin	Aspirin counteracts diuretic effect of spironolactone. Aspirin reduces excretion of acetazolamide and increases risk of harmful effects
calcium salts	Increased risk of a rise in blood calcium if thiazides and calcium salts are taken together
carbenoxolone	Increased risk of a fall in blood potassium when carbenoxolone is taken with acetazolamide or a loop or thiazide diuretic Carbenoxolone counteracts diuretic effects of diuretics Amiloride and spironolactone counteract ulcer-healing effects of carbenoxolone
cholestyramine	Cholestyramine reduces absorption of diuretics from the intestine and reduces their effectiveness
corticosteroids and corticotrophin	Increased risk of a fall in blood potassium if corticosteroids or corticotrophin are given with acetazolamide or a loop or thiazide diuretic Corticosteroids and corticotrophin counteract diuretic effect of diuretics
cyclosporin	Cyclosporin increases risk of a rise in blood potassium from potassium-sparing diuretics
digoxin and related drugs	Acetazolamide and loop and thiazide diuretics may cause a fall in blood potassium level and increase harmful effects of digoxin and related drugs Spironolactone increases effects of digoxin and related drugs
diuretics (others)	Increased risk of a fall in blood potassium if acetazolamide, loop diuretics or thiazides are given together A combination of metolazone and frusemide may produce a severe diuresis
indapamide	Increased risk of low blood potassium if indapamide is given with a loop or thiazide diuretic
lithium	Loop diuretics and thiazides reduce excretion of lithium, increase blood levels and increase risk of harmful effects. (Loop diuretics are safer than thiazides) Acetazolamide increases excretion of lithium
NSAIDs	Diuretics increase risk of kidney damage from NSAIDs NSAIDs counteract diuretic effects of diuretics, particularly indomethacin Indomethacin and possibly other NSAIDs increase the risk of a rise in blood potassium level from potassium-sparing diuretics
oestrogens	Oestrogens counteract diuretic effects of diuretics
oral contraceptives	Oral contraceptives counteract diuretic effects of diuretics
potassium salts	Potassium salts increase the risk of a rise in blood potassium levels from potassium-sparing diuretics

Table 89.1 Drug interactions (*cont.*)

Drug	*Interactions*
sotalol	Acetazolamide and loop and thiazide diuretics may cause a fall in blood potassium levels and increase the risks of sotalol producing disorders of heart rhythm (ventricular arrhythmia)
trilostane	Trilostane increases risk of a raised blood potassium level from potassium-sparing diuretics
domperidone	
anti-cholinergics	Anti-cholinergics counteract effects of domperidone on movements of the stomach and intestine
bromocriptine	Domperidone counteracts the prolactin-lowering effects of bromocriptine
narcotic pain relievers	Narcotic pain relievers counteract effects of domperidone on movements of the stomach and intestine
doxapram	
sympathomimetics	Risk of a rise in blood pressure if taken together
theophylline	Increased risk of stimulation of the brain and nervous system if taken together
enoxacin	
anti-coagulants	Enoxacin increases effects of nicoumalone and warfarin. Increased risk of bleeding
theophylline	Enoxacin increases blood level of theophylline
ergotamine	
beta blockers	Increased constriction of peripheral arteries, producing coldness of fingers and toes if taken together
erythromycin	Erythromycin increases risk of harmful effects (ergotism) from ergotamine
erythromycin	
alfentanil	Erythromycin increases blood level of alfentanil
anti-coagulants	Erythromycin increases effects of nicoumalone and warfarin. Increased risk of bleeding
carbamazepine	Erythromycin blocks breakdown of carbamazepine and increases its blood level
cyclosporin	Erythromycin blocks breakdown of cyclosporin and increases its blood level
digoxin	Erythromycin may increase effects of digoxin
disopyramide	Erythromycin increases blood level of disopyramide and increases risk of harmful effects
ergotamine	Erythromycin may increase risk of harmful effects (ergotism) from ergotamine

Table 89.1 Drug interactions (*cont.*)

Drug	*Interactions*
theophylline	Erythromycin blocks breakdown of theophylline and increases its blood level
triazolam	Erythromycin blocks breakdown of triazolam and increases its blood level
ethosuximide	
anti-depressants	Anti-depressants counteract effects of ethosuximide. Increased risk of seizures
anti-epileptics (other)	Interactions between anti-epileptic drugs may increase effects, increase sedation and affect blood levels making it difficult to monitor treatment
anti-psychotics	Anti-psychotics counteract effects of ethosuximide. Increased risk of seizures
isoniazid	Isoniazid increases blood level of ethosuximide and risk of harmful effects
etretinate	
methotrexate	Etretinate increases the blood level of methotrexate
flecainide	
antacids and kaolin	Antacids and kaolin make urine alkaline and reduce excretion of flecainide. Occasionally this may increase blood levels
anti-arrhythmics (other)	Amiodarone increases blood level of flecainide and increases risk of ventricular arrhythmias Flecainide increases risk of harmful effects on the heart from any other anti-arrhythmic drug
cimetidine	Cimetidine blocks breakdown of flecainide and increases its blood level
diuretics	Acetazolamide and loop and thiazide diuretics may cause a fall in blood potassium level and increase risks from flecainide Acetazolamide may occasionally reduce the excretion of flecainide, increase blood levels and increase effects
fluconazole	
anti-coagulants	Fluconazole increases effects of nicoumalone and warfarin. Increased risk of bleeding
cyclosporin	Fluconazole may possibly block breakdown and increase blood level of cyclosporin
phenytoin	Fluconazole increases effects of phenytoin
fluorouracil	
cimetidine	Cimetidine blocks breakdown of fluorouracil and increases its blood level

Table 89.1 Drug interactions (*cont.*)

Drug	*Interactions*
fluoxetine	
anti-depressants (other)	Fluoxetine increases blood levels of some tricyclics MAOIs should not be used for 2 weeks before, during and for 5 weeks after treatment with fluoxetine; it may cause agitation and nausea with tryptophan
flutamide	
warfarin	Flutamide may increase effects of warfarin
fluvoxamine	
anti-coagulants	Fluvoxamine may increase effects of nicoumalone and warfarin. Increased risk of bleeding
MAOI anti-depressants	Fluvoxamine increases effects of MAOIs on the brain and nervous system (see Chapter 39)
propranolol	Fluvoxamine increases blood level of propranolol
ganciclovir	
	Increased risk of damage to the bone marrow, producing blood disorders when taken with any other drug that may damage the bone marrow
zidovudine	Damage to bone marrow, producing serious blood disorders, may occur if taken together
glyceryl trinitrate and other nitrate vasodilators	
alcohol	Increased lowering of blood pressure if taken together
anaesthetics	Increased lowering of blood pressure if taken together
anti-anxiety drugs	Increased lowering of blood pressure if taken together
anti-blood-pressure drugs	Increased lowering of blood pressure if taken together
anti-cholinergics	Anti-cholinergics may reduce effectiveness of nitrate vasodilator preparations dissolved under the tongue because they may produce dryness of the mouth
anti-depressants	Increased lowering of blood pressure if taken together
anti-psychotics	Increased lowering of blood pressure if taken together
calcium channel blockers	Increased lowering of blood pressure if taken together
carbenoxolone	Carbenoxolone counteracts blood pressure-lowering effects of glyceryl trinitrate and other nitrate vasodilators
corticosteroids	Corticosteroids counteract blood pressure-lowering effects of glycerol trinitrate and other nitrate vasodilators
disopyramide	Disopyramide may reduce effectiveness of nitrate vasodilator preparations dissolved under the tongue because it may produce dryness of the mouth

Table 89.1 Drug interactions (*cont.*)

Drug	*Interactions*
diuretics	Increased lowering of blood pressure if taken together
levodopa	Increased lowering of blood pressure if taken together
oestrogens	Oestrogens counteract blood pressure-lowering effects of glyceryl trinitrate and other nitrate vasodilators
oral contraceptives	Oral contraceptives counteract blood pressure-lowering effects of glyceryl trinitrate and other nitrate vasodilators
sleeping drugs	Increased lowering of blood pressure if taken together
tricyclic anti-depressants	Tricyclic anti-depressants may reduce effectiveness of nitrate vasodilator preparations dissolved under the tongue because they may produce dryness of the mouth
griseofulvin	
anti-coagulants	Griseofulvin increases breakdown of nicoumalone and warfarin and reduces their effects
oral contraceptives	Griseofulvin increases breakdown of oral contraceptives and reduces their contraceptive effectiveness
phenobarbitone	Phenobarbitone increases breakdown of griseofulvin and reduces its effects
guar gum	
penicillin V	Guar gum reduces absorption of penicillin V from the intestine and may reduce its effectiveness
heparin	
anti-platelet drugs	Aspirin, dipyridamole and sulphinpyrazone increase effects of heparin and increase risk of bleeding
aspirin	Aspirin increases anti-coagulant effects of heparin and increases risk of bleeding
hydralazine	
alcohol	Increased lowering of blood pressure if taken together
anaesthetics	Increased lowering of blood pressure if taken together
anti-anxiety drugs	Increased lowering of blood pressure if taken together
anti-blood-pressure drugs	Increased lowering of blood pressure if taken together
anti-depressants	Increased lowering of blood pressure if taken together
anti-psychotics	Increased lowering of blood pressure if taken together
calcium channel blockers	Increased lowering of blood pressure if taken together
carbenoxolone	Carbenoxolone counteracts blood pressure-lowering effects of hydralazine

Table 89.1 Drug interactions (*cont.*)

Drug	*Interactions*
corticosteroids	Corticosteroids counteract blood pressure-lowering effects of hydralazine
diuretics	Increased lowering of blood pressure if taken together
levodopa	Increased lowering of blood pressure if taken together
nitrate vasodilators	Increased lowering of blood pressure if taken together
NSAIDs	NSAIDs counteract blood pressure-lowering effects of hydralazine
oestrogens	Oestrogens counteract blood pressure-lowering effects of hydralazine
oral contraceptives	Oral contraceptives counteract blood pressure-lowering effects of hydralazine
sleeping drugs	Increased lowering of blood pressure if taken together
influenza vaccine	
phenytoin	Influenza vaccine increases effects of phenytoin
interferons	
theophylline	Interferons block breakdown of theophylline and increase its effects
iron	
ciprofloxacin	Iron reduces the absorption of ciprofloxacin from the intestine and may reduce its effectiveness
levodopa	Iron may reduce the absorption of levodopa from the intestine and may reduce its effectiveness
magnesium trisilicate antacids	Magnesium trisilicate reduces absorption of iron from the intestine and may reduce its effectiveness
penicillamine	Iron reduces absorption of penicillamine from the intestine and may reduce its effectiveness
tetracyclines	Tetracyclines reduce absorption of iron from the intestine and may reduce its effectiveness (and vice versa)
trientine	Trientine reduces absorption of iron from the intestine and may reduce its effectiveness
zinc	Zinc reduces absorption of iron from the intestine and may reduce its effects (and vice versa)
isoniazid	
anti-epileptics	Isoniazid blocks the breakdown and increases the effects of carbamazepine, ethosuximide and phenytoin
itraconazole	
antacids	Antacids reduce the absorption of itraconazole from the intestine and may reduce its effectiveness
H_2-blockers	H_2-blockers reduce the absorption of itraconazole from the intestine and may reduce its effectiveness

Table 89.1 Drug interactions (*cont.*)

Drug	*Interactions*
rifampicin	Rifampicin increases breakdown of itraconazole and reduces its blood level
ketoconazole	
antacids	Antacids reduce the absorption of ketoconazole from the intestine and may reduce its effectiveness
anti-cholinergics	Anti-cholinergic drugs reduce the absorption of ketoconazole from the intestine and may reduce its effectiveness
anti-coagulants	Ketoconazole increases effects of nicoumalone and warfarin. Increased risk of bleeding
cyclosporin	Ketoconazole blocks breakdown of cyclosporin and increases its blood level
H_2-blockers	H_2-blockers reduce absorption of ketoconazole from the intestine and may reduce its effectiveness
phenytoin	Phenytoin reduces blood level of ketoconazole Ketoconazole increases effects of phenytoin
rifampicin	Rifampicin increases breakdown of ketoconazole and reduces its blood level
levodopa	
anaesthetics	Volatile anaesthetics (e.g. cyclopropane and halothane) increase risk of disorders of heart rhythm from levodopa
anti-blood-pressure drugs	Increased lowering of blood pressure if taken together
anti-psychotics	Anti-psychotics counteract effects of levodopa
benzodiazepines	Chlordiazepoxide, diazepam and lorazepam, and possibly other benzodiazepines, occasionally counteract effects of levodopa
iron	Iron may reduce the absorption of levodopa from the intestine and may reduce its effectiveness
MAOIs	Risk of hypertensive crisis if taken together (see Chapter 39)
metoclopramide	Metoclopramide increases blood level of levodopa
pyridoxine	Pyridoxine counteracts effects of levodopa unless a dopa-decarboxylase inhibitor is also given (see Chapter 36)
reserpine	Reserpine counteracts effects of levodopa
lignocaine	
acetazolamide	Low blood potassium caused by acetazolamide counteracts effects of lignocaine
anti-arrhythmics (other)	Increased risk of harmful effects on the heart if taken together
beta blockers	Increased risk of harmful effects on the heart if taken together. Propranolol increases risk of harmful effects from lignocaine

Table 89.1 Drug interactions (*cont.*)

Drug	*Interactions*
cimetidine	Cimetidine blocks breakdown of lignocaine and increases risk of harmful effects
diuretics	Low blood potassium caused by loop and thiazide diuretics counteracts effects of lignocaine
lincomycin	
kaolin	Kaolin reduces absorption of lincomycin from the intestine and may reduce its effectiveness
muscle relaxants	Lincomycin increases effects of non-depolarizing muscle relaxants (e.g. tubocurarine)
neostigmine	Lincomycin counteracts effects of neostigmine
pyridostigmine	Lincomycin counteracts effects of pyridostigmine
lithium	
ACE inhibitors	Enalapril and possibly other ACE inhibitors reduce excretion of lithium from the kidneys and increase its blood level
acetazolamide	Acetazolamide increases the excretion of lithium by the kidneys
anti-diabetics	Lithium may occasionally affect the effectiveness of insulin and oral anti-diabetic drugs
anti-epileptics	Carbamazepine and phenytoin may increase nerve damage from lithium without causing an increase in its blood level
anti-psychotics	Increased risk of movement disorders and possibly nerve damage when lithium is given with anti-psychotic drugs, particularly haloperidol
calcium channel blockers	Diltiazem and verapamil may increase nerve damage from lithium without causing any increase in its blood level
diuretics	Loop and thiazide diuretics reduce excretion of lithium in the urine, increase its blood level and increase the risk of harmful effects from lithium
fluoxetine	Fluoxetine increases the risk of harmful effects on the nervous system from lithium
fluvoxamine	Fluvoxamine increases the risk of harmful effects on the nervous system from lithium
methyldopa	Methyldopa may increase nerve damage from lithium without causing an increase in its blood level
metoclopramide	Increased risk of movement disorders if taken together. Metoclopramide increases risk of nerve damage from lithium
muscle relaxants	Lithium increases effects of muscle relaxants
neostigmine	Lithium counteracts effects of neostigmine
NSAIDs	NSAIDs reduce excretion of lithium by the kidneys and may possibly increase harmful effects

Table 89.1 Drug interactions (*cont.*)

Drug	*Interactions*
pyridostigmine	Lithium counteracts effects of pyridostigmine
sodium bicarbonate	Sodium bicarbonate increases excretion of lithium and reduces its blood level
theophylline	Theophylline reduces the excretion of lithium by the kidneys and reduces its blood level
magnesium salts	
muscle relaxants	Magnesium salts increase the effects of non-depolarizing muscle relaxants (e.g. tubocurarine)
MAOIs	
see Chapter 39	
mefloquine	
beta blockers	Increased risk of slowing of the heart if taken together
calcium channel blockers	Increased risk of slowing of the heart if taken together
digoxin	Increased risk of slowing of the heart if taken together
quinidine	Increased risk of harmful effects when quinidine is taken with mefloquine
quinine	Increased risk of harmful effects when mefloquine is taken with quinine
mepacrine	
primaquine	Mepacrine increases the blood level of primaquine and increases risk of harmful effects
mercaptopurine	
allopurinol	Allopurinol increases the effects and harmful effects of mercaptopurine
methotrexate	
co-trimoxazole	The anti-folic acid effects of methotrexate are increased by co-trimoxazole
etretinate	Etretinate increases blood levels of methotrexate
NSAIDs	Excretion of methotrexate by the kidneys is reduced and the risk of harmful effects increased by aspirin, azapropazone, diclofenac, indomethacin, ketoprofen, naproxen, phenylbutazone, and probably other NSAIDs
phenytoin	The anti-folic acid effects of methotrexate are increased by phenytoin
probenecid	Probenecid reduces excretion of methotrexate by the kidneys and increases the risk of harmful effects

Table 89.1 Drug interactions (*cont.*)

Drug	*Interactions*
pyrimethamine	The anti-folic acid effects of methotrexate are increased by pyrimethamine
trimethoprim	The anti-folic acid effects of methotrexate are increased by trimethoprim
methyldopa	
alcohol	Increased lowering of blood pressure if taken together
anaesthetics	Increased lowering of blood pressure if taken together
anti-anxiety drugs	Increased lowering of blood pressure if taken together
anti-blood-pressure drugs (others)	Increased lowering of blood pressure if taken together
anti-depressants	Increased lowering of blood pressure if taken together
anti-psychotics	Increased lowering of blood pressure if taken together. Methyldopa increases risk of movement disorders from anti-psychotic drugs
beta blockers	Increased lowering of blood pressure if taken together
calcium channel blockers	Increased lowering of blood pressure if taken together
carbenoxolone	Carbenoxolone counteracts blood pressure-lowering effects of methyldopa
corticosteroids	Corticosteroids counteract blood pressure-lowering effects of methyldopa
diuretics	Increased lowering of blood pressure if taken together
levodopa	Increased lowering of blood pressure if taken together
lithium	Methyldopa increases the risk of nerve damage from lithium without causing an increase in the blood level of lithium
nitrate vasodilators	Increased lowering of blood pressure if taken together
NSAIDs	NSAIDs counteract blood pressure-lowering effects of methyldopa
oestrogens	Oestrogens counteract blood pressure-lowering effects of methyldopa
oral contraceptives	Oral contraceptives counteract blood pressure-lowering effects of methyldopa
sleeping drugs	Increased lowering of blood pressure if taken together
metirosine	
anti-psychotics	Increased risk of movement disorders if taken together
levodopa	Metirosine counteracts effects of levodopa
metoclopramide	
anti-cholinergics	Anti-cholinergics counteract effects of metoclopramide on the stomach and intestine
anti-psychotics	Increased risk of movement disorders if taken together

Table 89.1 Drug interactions (*cont.*)

Drug	*Interactions*
aspirin	Metoclopramide increases absorption of aspirin from the intestine and increases its effectiveness
bromocriptine	Metoclopramide counteracts the prolactin-lowering effects of bromocriptine
levodopa	Metoclopramide increases blood level of levodopa
lithium	Increased risk of movement disorders and possibility of nerve damage if taken together
narcotic pain relievers	Narcotic pain relievers counteract effects of metoclopramide on the stomach and intestine
paracetamol	Metoclopramide increases absorption of paracetamol from the intestine and increases its effectiveness
reserpine	Increased risk of movement disorders if taken together
tetrabenazine	Increased risk of movement disorders if taken together
metronidazole	
alcohol	Alcohol may cause a disulfiram-like reaction if taken with metronidazole
anti-coagulants	Metronidazole increases effects of nicoumalone and warfarin. Increased risk of bleeding
cimetidine	Cimetidine blocks breakdown of metronidazole and increase its blood level
disulfiram	Severe mental symptoms (psychotic reaction) may occur if taken together
phenobarbitone	Phenobarbitone increases breakdown of metronidazole and reduces its blood level
phenytoin	Metronidazole blocks breakdown of phenytoin and increases its blood level
mexiletine	
antacids	Antacids make the urine alkaline, which reduces the excretion of mexiletine into the urine. This may occasionally increase blood levels and increase effects
anti-arrhythmics (other)	Increased risk of harmful effects on the heart if taken together
atropine	Atropine delays absorption of mexiletine from the intestine and may reduce its effectiveness
diuretics	Loop and thiazide diuretics counteract effects of mexiletine because they cause a fall in blood potassium levels Acetazolamide produces similar effects and may also reduce excretion of mexiletine in the urine and occasionally causes a rise in blood levels
narcotic pain relievers	Narcotic pain relievers delay absorption of mexiletine from the intestine

Table 89.1 Drug interactions (*cont.*)

Drug	*Interactions*
phenytoin	Phenytoin increases breakdown of mexiletine, and reduces its blood levels
rifampicin	Rifampicin increases breakdown of mexiletine and reduces its blood level
mianserin	
alcohol	Increased effects if taken together
anti-anxiety drugs	Increased effects if taken together
sleeping drugs	Increased effects if taken together
miconazole	
amphotericin	Amphotericin counteracts effects of miconazole
anti-coagulants	Miconazole increases effects of nicoumalone and warfarin. Increased risk of bleeding
anti-diabetics	Miconazole increases blood glucose-lowering effects of sulphonylurea oral anti-diabetics
phenytoin	Miconazole increases effects of phenytoin
monosulfiram	
alcohol	Disulfiram-like reaction if used together
muscle relaxants (depolarizing and non-depolarizing)	
antibiotics	Aminoglycosides, clindamycin, lincomycin and polymyxins increase effects of non-depolarizing muscle relaxants
anti-cancer drugs	Cyclophosphamide and thiotepa increase the effects of the depolarizing muscle relaxant suxamethonium
cholinergics	Demacarium, ecothiopate, neostigmine and pyridostigmine increase the effects of the depolarizing muscle relaxant suxamethonium but counteract the effects of non-depolarizing muscle relaxants
digoxin	The depolarizing muscle relaxant suxamethonium may interact with digoxin to cause disorders of heart rhythm
lithium	Lithium increases effects of muscle relaxants
magnesium salts	Intravenous magnesium increases effects of non-depolarizing muscle relaxants
propranolol	Propranolol increases effects of muscle relaxants
quinidine	Quinidine increases effects of muscle relaxants
verapamil	Verapamil increases effects of non-depolarizing muscle relaxants
nalidixic acid	
anti-coagulants	Nalidixic acid increases effects of nicoumalone and warfarin. Increased risk of bleeding

Table 89.1 Drug interactions (*cont.*)

Drug	*Interactions*
probenecid	Probenecid reduces excretion of nalidixic acid and increases risk of harmful effects
narcotic pain relievers	
anti-anxiety drugs	Increased sedation if taken together
anti-coagulants	Dextropropoxyphene may increase effects of nicoumalone and warfarin. Increased risk of bleeding
carbamazepine	Dextropropoxyphene increases effects of carbamazepine
cimetidine	Cimetidine blocks breakdown of pethidine and increases its blood level
cisapride	Narcotic pain relievers counteract effects of cisapride on stomach and intestine
domperidone	Narcotic pain relievers counteract effects of domperidone on stomach and intestine
erythromycin	Erythromycin increases blood level of alfentanil
MAOIs	Pethidine and possibly other narcotic pain relievers interact to affect the brain and blood pressure (see Chapter 39)
metoclopramide	Narcotic pain relievers counteract effects of metoclopramide on the stomach and intestine
mexiletine	Narcotic pain relievers delay absorption of mexiletine from the intestine
rifampicin	Rifampicin increases breakdown of methadone
sleeping drugs	Increased sedation if taken together
nefopam	
anti-cholinergics	Increased harmful effects if taken together
MAOIs	Manufacturer recommends that these drugs should not be used together
nitrofurantoin	
probenecid	Probenecid reduces excretion of nitrofurantoin in the urine and increases risk of harmful effects
NSAIDs (non-steroidal anti-inflammatory drugs)	
ACE inhibitors	NSAIDs counteract blood pressure-lowering effects of ACE inhibitors. Increased risk of a rise in blood potassium levels and kidney failure when indomethacin (and possibly other NSAIDs) is given with an ACE inhibitor
antacids	Antacids reduce the absorption of diflunisal from the intestine and may reduce its effectiveness
anti-blood-pressure drugs	NSAIDs counteract blood pressure-lowering effects of anti-blood-pressure drugs

Table 89.1 Drug interactions (*cont.*)

Drug	*Interactions*
anti-coagulants	Azapropazone and phenylbutazone increase the effects of warfarin. Increased risk of bleeding. This may also occur with diflunisal, flurbiprofen, mefenamic acid, piroxicam, sulindac and possibly with other NSAIDs
anti-diabetics	Azapropazone and phenylbutazone increase blood glucose-lowering effects of sulphonylurea oral diabetics
cholestyramine	Cholestyramine reduces absorption of phenylbutazone from the intestine and may reduce its effectiveness
digoxin	NSAIDs may make heart failure worse by causing fluid retention. They may impair kidney function and reduce the excretion of digoxin and increase its blood level
diuretics	Diuretics increase the risk of kidney damage from NSAIDs NSAIDs (particularly indomethacin) counteract the effects of diuretics Indomethacin and possibly other NSAIDs increase the risk of a rise in blood potassium from potassium-sparing diuretics Indomethacin may interact with triamterene, to impair kidney function
haloperidol	Indomethacin and haloperidol may interact to produce severe drowsiness
lithium	The excretion of lithium is reduced and the risk of harmful effects increased by diclofenac, ibuprofen, indomethacin, mefenamic acid, naproxen, phenylbutazone, piroxicam, and probably other NSAIDs
methotrexate	The excretion of methotrexate may be delayed and its harmful effects increased by azapropazone, indomethacin, ketoprofen, phenylbutazone and probably other NSAIDs
phenytoin	Azapropazone and phenylbutazone increase the effects of phenytoin
probenecid	Probenecid delays the excretion of indomethacin, ketoprofen and naproxen by the kidneys and increases their blood levels
thyroxine	Phenylbutazone may affect tests of the level of thyroxine in the blood, causing a false low value
octreotide	
anti-diabetics	Octreotide affects blood glucose levels, and the dose of insulin and oral diabetics may need reducing
omeprazole	
anti-coagulants	Omeprazole increases the effects of warfarin. Increased risk of bleeding
phenytoin	Omeprazole increases effects of phenytoin
oral contraceptives	see contraceptives (oral)

Table 89.1 Drug interactions (*cont.*)

Drug	*Interactions*
paracetamol	
cholestyramine	Cholestyramine reduces the absorption of paracetamol from the intestine and may reduce its effectiveness
metoclopramide	Metoclopramide speeds up absorption of paracetamol from the intestine and increases its effectiveness
penicillamine	
antacids	Antacids reduce absorption of penicillamine from the intestine and may reduce its effectiveness
iron	Iron reduces absorption of penicillamine from the intestine and may reduce its effectiveness
zinc	Zinc reduces absorption of penicillamine from the intestine and may reduce its effectiveness
penicillins	
antacids	Antacids reduce absorption of pivampicillin from the intestine and may reduce its effectiveness
contraceptives (oral)	Broad-spectrum penicillins (e.g. ampicillin) may possibly reduce the contraceptive effectiveness of combined oral contraceptives
guar gum	Guar gum reduces absorption of penicillin V from the intestine and may reduce its effectiveness
probenecid	Probenecid reduces the excretion of penicillins by the kidneys
phenindione	
anabolic steroids	Oxymetholone, stanozolol and other anabolic steroids increase the effects of phenindione. Increased risk of bleeding
aspirin	Aspirin increases the effects of phenindione. Increased risk of bleeding
cholestyramine	Cholestyramine increases or decreases the effects of phenindione
clofibrate group	The clofibrate group of drugs increase the effects of phenindione. Increased risk of bleeding
dipyridamole	Dipyridamole increases the effects of phenindione. Increased risk of bleeding
oral contraceptives	Oral contraceptives counteract anti-coagulant effects of phenindione
thyroxine	Thyroxine increases the effects of phenindione. Increased risk of bleeding
vitamin K	Vitamin K in some tube feeds may counteract the effects of phenindione

Table 89.1 Drug interactions (*cont.*)

Drug	*Interactions*
phenytoin	
anti-arrhythmics	Amiodarone increases the blood level of phenytoin Phenytoin reduces the blood level of disopyramide, mexiletine and quinidine
anti-bacterials	Chloramphenicol, isoniazid and metronidazole increase the blood level of phenytoin Co-trimoxazole increases the blood level and increases the anti-folic acid effects of phenytoin Rifampicin reduces the blood level of phenytoin Phenytoin reduces the blood level of doxycycline
anti-coagulants	Phenytoin increases breakdown of nicoumalone and warfarin, and may reduce their effects (*but* may also increase their effects)
anti-depressants	Anti-depressants counteract anti-epileptic effects of phenytoin. Increased risk of seizures Viloxazine increases the blood level of phenytoin Phenytoin reduces the blood levels of tricyclic anti-depressants
anti-epileptics	If phenytoin is taken with another anti-epileptic drug there is an increase in harmful effects without increased seizure control. There may also be changes in blood levels and difficulty with monitoring (see Chapter 37)
anti-fungals	Fluconazole, ketoconazole and miconazole increase the blood level of phenytoin Phenytoin reduces the blood level of ketoconazole and possibly of other anti-fungal drugs
anti-psychotics	Anti-psychotics counteract anti-epileptic effects of phenytoin. Increased risk of seizures
aspirin	Aspirin increases the blood level of phenytoin
azapropazone	Azapropazone increases the blood level of phenytoin
cimetidine	Cimetidine blocks breakdown of phenytoin and increases its blood level
corticosteroids	Phenytoin increases breakdown of corticosteroids and reduces their effects
cyclosporin	Phenytoin increases breakdown of cyclosporin and reduces its blood level
digitoxin	Phenytoin increases breakdown of digitoxin
disulfiram	Disulfiram increases the blood level of phenytoin
folic acid	Folic acid may occasionally reduce the blood level of phenytoin
influenza vaccine	Influenza vaccine increases the effects of phenytoin
isradipine	Phenytoin reduces the effects of isradipine
lithium	Phenytoin may increase nerve damage from lithium without increasing the blood level of lithium

Table 89.1 Drug interactions (*cont.*)

Drug	*Interactions*
Methotrexate	Methotrexate reduces absorption of phenytoin. Increased antifolic acid effect if taken together
omeprazole	Omeprazole increases the effects of phenytoin
oral contraceptives	Phenytoin increases breakdown of oral contraceptives and reduces their contraceptive effectiveness
phenylbutazone	Phenylbutazone increases the blood level of phenytoin
sucralfate	Sucralfate reduces the absorption of phenytoin from the intestine and may reduce its effectiveness
sulphinpyrazone	Sulphinpyrazone increases the blood level of phenytoin
theophylline	Phenytoin increases breakdown of theophylline and reduces its blood level
thyroxine	Phenytoin increases breakdown of thyroxine
pizotifen	
adrenergic neurone blockers	Pizotifen counteracts blood pressure-lowering effects of adrenergic neurone blockers
polymyxins	
muscle relaxants	Polymyxins increase effects of muscle relaxants (depolarizing and non-depolarizing)
potassium salts	
ACE inhibitors	Increased risk of a rise in blood potassium level if taken together
cyclosporin	Increased risk of a rise in blood potassium level if taken together
potassium-sparing diuretics	Increased risk of a rise in blood potassium level if taken together
primaquine	
mepacrine	Mepacrine increases blood level of primaquine and may increase risk of harmful effects
probenecid	
anti-bacterials	Probenecid reduces excretion and increases blood levels of cephalosporins, dapsone, nalidixic acid, nitrofurantoin and penicillins
anti-virals	Probenecid reduces excretion of acyclovir and zidovudine and increases their blood levels
aspirin	Aspirin counteracts the effects of probenecid
captopril	Probenecid reduces excretion of captopril
methotrexate	Probenecid reduces excretion of methotrexate and increases risk of harmful effects
NSAIDs	Probenecid delays excretion and increases blood levels of indomethacin, ketoprofen and naproxen

Table 89.1 Drug interactions (*cont.*)

Drug	*Interactions*
pyrazinamide	Pyrazinamide counteracts effects of probenecid
procainamide	
anti-arrhythmics (other)	Increased risk of harmful effects on heart if taken together Amiodarone increases the blood level of procainamide
cimetidine	Cimetidine blocks breakdown of procainamide and increases its blood level
procarbazine	
alcohol	Disulfiram-like reaction if taken together
progestogens	
cyclosporin	Progestogens block breakdown of cyclosporin and increase its blood level
propafenone	
anti-coagulants	Propafenone blocks breakdown and increases blood level of nicoumalone and warfarin. Increased risk of bleeding
cimetidine	Cimetidine increases blood level of propafenone
digoxin	Propafenone increases blood level of digoxin
quinidine	Quinidine increases blood level of propafenone
pyrazinamide	
probenecid	Pyrazinamide counteracts effects of probenecid
sulphinpyrazone	Pyrazinamide counteracts effects of sulphinpyrazone
pyrimethamine	
methotrexate	Increased anti-folic acid effects if taken together
quinidine	
acetazolamide	Acetazolamide may reduce excretion of quinidine and occasionally increase its blood level. It may also cause a fall in blood potassium and increase the risk of harmful effects from quinidine
antacids	Antacids make the urine alkaline, which may reduce excretion of quinidine. The blood level of quinidine may occasionally be increased
anti-arrhythmics (other)	Increased risk of harmful effects on the heart if taken together Amiodarone increases blood level of quinidine and increases risk of serious disorders of heart rhythm (ventricular arrhythmias)
anti-coagulants	Quinidine increases effects of nicoumalone and warfarin. Increased risk of bleeding
anti-epileptics	Phenobarbitone, phenytoin and primidone increase breakdown of quinidine and reduce its blood level

Table 89.1 Drug interactions (*cont.*)

Drug	*Interactions*
barbiturates	Barbiturates increase breakdown of quinidine and reduce its blood level
cimetidine	Cimetidine blocks breakdown of quinidine and increases its blood level
digoxin	Quinidine increases the blood level of digoxin; maintenance dose of digoxin should be halved
diuretics	Loop diuretics and thiazides may cause a fall in blood potassium level and increase risk of harmful effects from quinidine
muscle relaxants	Quinidine increases effects of muscle relaxants (polarizing and non-polarizing)
neostigmine	Quinidine counteracts effects of neostigmine
pyridostigmine	Quinidine counteracts effects of pyridostigmine
rifampicin	Rifampicin increases breakdown of quinidine and reduces its blood level
verapamil	Verapamil increases blood level of quinidine; possibility of a severe fall in blood pressure
quinine	
cimetidine	Cimetidine blocks breakdown of quinine and increases blood level
digoxin	Quinine increases blood level of digoxin; maintenance dose of digoxin should be halved
quinolones	
antacids	Antacids reduce absorption of ciprofloxacin and ofloxacin
anti-coagulants	Ciprofloxacin, enoxacin and nalidixic acid increase effects of nicoumalone and warfarin
cyclosporin	Quinolones increase the risk of kidney damage from cyclosporin
iron	Oral iron reduces absorption of ciprofloxacin
probenecid	Probenecid reduces excretion of nalidixic acid in the urine and increases the risk of harmful effects
theophylline	Ciprofloxacin and enoxacin increase the blood level of theophylline
sucralfate	Sucralfate reduces absorption of ciprofloxacin
zinc salts	Ciprofloxacin reduces absorption of zinc
reserpine and related drugs	
alcohol	Increased lowering of blood pressure if taken together
anaesthetics (general)	Increased lowering of blood pressure if taken together
anti-anxiety drugs	Increased lowering of blood pressure if taken together
anti-blood-pressure drugs (others)	Increased lowering of blood pressure if taken together

Table 89.1 Drug interactions (*cont.*)

Drug	*Interactions*
anti-psychotics	Increased risk of movement disorders if taken together
beta blockers	Increased slowing of heart rate if taken together
calcium channel blockers	Increased lowering of blood pressure if taken together
carbenoxolone	Carbenoxolone counteracts blood pressure-lowering effects of reserpine and related drugs
corticosteroids	Corticosteroids counteract blood pressure-lowering effects of reserpine and related drugs
diuretics	Increased lowering of blood pressure if taken together
levodopa	Increased lowering of blood pressure if taken together Reserpine and related drugs counteract effects of levodopa
MAOIs	Risk of stimulation of brain and rise in blood pressure if taken together (see Chapter 39)
metoclopramide	Increased risk of movement disorders if taken together
nitrate vasodilators	Increased lowering of blood pressure if taken together
NSAIDs	NSAIDs counteract blood pressure-lowering effect of reserpine and related drugs
oestrogens	Oestrogens counteract blood pressure-lowering effects of reserpine and related drugs
oral contraceptives	Combined oral contraceptives counteract blood pressure-lowering effects of reserpine and related drugs
sleeping drugs	Increased lowering of blood pressure if taken together
rifampicin	
antacids	antacids reduce absorption of rifampicin from the intestine and may reduce its effectiveness
anti-arrhythmics	Rifampicin increases breakdown and reduces blood levels of disopyramide, mexiletine and quinidine
anti-coagulants	Rifampicin increases breakdown and reduces effects of nicoumalone and warfarin
anti-diabetics	Rifampicin increases breakdown and may reduce effects of chlorpropamide, tolbutamide and possibly other sulphonylurea oral anti-diabetic drugs
anti-fungals	Rifampicin increases breakdown of itraconazole and ketoconazole, and reduces their blood levels
chloramphenicol	Rifampicin increases breakdown of chloramphenicol and reduces its blood level
cimetidine	Rifampicin increases breakdown of cimetidine and reduces its blood level
corticosteroids	Rifampicin increases breakdown and may reduce effects of corticosteroids

Table 89.1 Drug interactions (*cont.*)

Drug	*Interactions*
cyclosporin	Rifampicin increases breakdown and reduces the blood level of cyclosporin
digitoxin	Rifampicin increases breakdown of digitoxin and may reduce its effects
haloperidol	Rifampicin increases breakdown of haloperidol and reduces its blood level
isradipine	Rifampicin may possibly increase breakdown of isradipine and reduce its blood level
methadone	Rifampicin increases breakdown of methadone and may reduce its effects
oral contraceptives	Rifampicin increases breakdown of combined oral contraceptives and progestogen-only contraceptives and reduces their contraceptive effectiveness
phenytoin	Rifampicin increases breakdown and reduces blood level of phenytoin. Increased risk of seizures
propranolol	Rifampicin increases breakdown of propranolol and reduces its blood level
theophylline	Rifampicin increases breakdown of theophylline and reduces its blood level
thyroxine	Rifampicin increases breakdown of thyroxine and may reduce its effects
verapamil	Rifampicin increases breakdown of verapamil and reduces its blood level
simvastatin	
anti-coagulants	Simvastatin may increase the effects of nicoumalone and warfarin. Increased risk of bleeding
sodium valproate	
anti-depressants	Anti-depressants counteract the effects of sodium valproate. Increased risk of seizures
anti-epileptics (other)	If sodium valproate is taken with another anti-epileptic drug there is an increased risk of harmful effects without increased seizure control. There may also be changes in blood levels and difficulty with monitoring (see Chapter 37)
anti-psychotics	Anti-psychotics counteract the effects of sodium valproate. Increased risk of seizures
aspirin	Aspirin increases the effects of sodium valproate
sucralfate	
antacids	Antacids neutralize the acid in the stomach whereas sucralfate requires the acid to work effectively. Therefore do not take together

Table 89.1 Drug interactions (*cont.*)

Drug	*Interactions*
antibiotics	Sucralfate reduces absorption of tetracyclines and ciprofloxacin from the intestine and may reduce their effectiveness
peptic ulcer-healing drugs	Sucralfate requires acid in the stomach to work effectively, therefore do not take sucralfate with any drug that reduces acid production
phenytoin	Sucralfate reduces absorption of phenytoin from the intestine and may reduce its effectiveness
warfarin	Sucralfate reduces absorption of warfarin from the intestine and may reduce its effectiveness
sulphinpyrazone	
anti-coagulants	Sulphinpyrazone increases effects of nicoumalone and warfarin. Increased risk of bleeding
anti-diabetics	Sulphinpyrazone increases blood glucose-lowering effects of sulphonylurea oral anti-diabetic drugs
aspirin	Aspirin counteracts the excretion of uric acid by sulphinpyrazone
phenytoin	Sulphinpyrazone increases the blood level of phenytoin
pyrazinamide	Pyrazinamide counteracts effects of sulphinpyrazone
theophylline	Sulphinpyrazone reduces blood level of theophylline
sulphonamides and co-trimoxazole	
anaesthetics	Sulphonamides increase the effects of thiopentone
anti-coagulants	Sulphonamides increase the effects of nicoumalone and warfarin. Increased risk of bleeding
anti-diabetics	Sulphonamides increase the effects of sulphonylurea oral anti-diabetic drugs. Increased risk of low blood glucose (hypoglycaemia)
cyclosporin	Increased risk of kidney damage if taken together
methotrexate	Co-trimoxazole increases anti-folic acid effect of methotrexate and may increase risk of harmful effects
phenytoin	Co-trimoxazole increases anti-folic acid effects of phenytoin and increases its blood level
sympathomimetics	
adrenergic neurone blockers	Sympathomimetics in cough and cold remedies and in slimming drugs may counteract blood pressure-lowering effects of adrenergic neurone blockers
anaesthetics	Risk of disorders of heart rhythm if adrenaline or isoprenaline are given with volatile anaesthetics
beta blockers	Adrenaline and noradrenaline may cause a serious rise in blood pressure if taken with a beta blocker, particularly with non-selective beta blockers. This reaction may also occur with sympathomimetics included in cough and cold remedies and slimming drugs

Table 89.1 Drug interactions (*cont.*)

Drug	*Interactions*
corticosteroids	Increased risk of a low blood potassium level if corticosteroids are given with high doses of the adrenostimulant asthma drugs: fenoterol, pirbuterol, reproterol, rimiterol, ritodrine, salbutamol and terbutaline
doxapram	Risk of a rise in blood pressure if taken together
MAOIs	See Chapter 39
tricyclic anti-depressants	Adrenaline and noradrenaline may cause a rise in blood pressure and disorders of heart rhythm when given with tricyclics. Adrenaline in local anaesthetic preparations may not produce these harmful effects
tamoxifen	
anti-coagulants	Tamoxifen increases the effects of nicoumalone and warfarin. Increased risk of bleeding
tetrabenazine	
MAOIs	Risk of stimulation of brain and raised blood pressure if taken together (see Chapter 39)
tetracyclines	
antacids	Antacids reduce absorption of tetracyclines from the intestine and may reduce their effectiveness
anti-epileptics	Carbamazepine, phenobarbitone, phenytoin and primidone increase breakdown of doxycycline and reduce its blood level
barbiturates	Barbiturates increase breakdown of doxycycline and reduce its blood level
dairy products	Dairy products reduce absorption of tetracyclines (except doxycycline and minocycline) from the intestine and may reduce the effectiveness of tetracyclines
iron salts	Iron salts reduce the absorption of tetracyclines from the intestine and may reduce their effectiveness. Tetracyclines reduce the absorption of iron salts from the intestine and may reduce their effectiveness
oral contraceptives	Tetracyclines may reduce contraceptive effectiveness of oral contraceptives
quinapril	Quinapril tablets contain magnesium carbonate which reduces absorption of tetracyclines and reduces their effectiveness
sucralfate	Sucralfate reduces absorption of tetracyclines from the intestine and may reduce their effectiveness
zinc salts	Zinc salts reduce the absorption of tetracyclines from the intestine and may reduce their effectiveness

Table 89.1 Drug interactions (*cont.*)

Drug	*Interactions*
theophylline	
aminoglutethimide	Aminoglutethimide reduces the blood level of theophylline
anti-bacterials	Ciprofloxacin, enoxacin and erythromycin increase the blood level of theophylline Rifampicin reduces the blood level of theophylline
anti-epileptics	Carbamazepine, phenobarbitone, phenytoin and primidone reduce the blood level of theophylline
barbiturates	Barbiturates reduce the blood level of theophylline
calcium channel blockers	Diltiazem and verapamil increase the blood level of theophylline
cimetidine	Cimetidine increases the blood level of theophylline
interferons	Interferons increase the blood level of theophylline
lithium	Theophylline increases excretion of lithium and reduces its blood level
oral contraceptives	Combined oral contraceptives increase the blood level of theophylline
sulphinpyrazone	Sulphinpyrazone reduces the blood level of theophylline
sympathomimetics	Increased risk of a low blood potassium level if theophylline is given with high doses of the adrenostimulant asthma drugs: fenoterol, pributerol, reproterol, rimiterol, ritodrine, salbutamol and terbutaline
viloxazine	Viloxazine increases the blood level of theophylline
thiotepa	
suxamethonium	Thiotepa increases the effects of suxamethonium
thyroxine	
anti-coagulants	Thyroxine increases the effects of nicoumalone, phenindione and warfarin. Increased risk of bleeding
anti-epileptics	Carbamazepine, phenobarbitone, phenytoin and primidone increase breakdown of thyroxine and may reduce its effects
barbiturates	Barbiturates increase breakdown of thyroxine and may reduce its effects
cholestyramine	Cholestyramine reduces absorption of thyroxine from the intestine and may reduce its effectiveness
phenylbutazone	Phenylbutazone affects blood tests for thyroxine, giving a false low result
propranolol	Thyroxine increases breakdown of propranolol and may reduce its effects
rifampicin	Rifampicin increases breakdown of thyroxine and may reduce its effects

Table 89.1 Drug interactions (*cont.*)

Drug	*Interactions*
tocainide	
anti-arrhythmics (others)	Increased risk of harmful effects on the heart if taken together
diuretics	Loop diuretics and thiazides may cause a fall in blood potassium level which will counteract the effects of tocainide Acetazolamide may cause a fall in blood potassium level, which counteracts the effects of tocainide
trazodone	
alcohol	Increased sedation if taken together
anti-anxiety drugs	Increased sedation if taken together
sleeping drugs	Increased sedation if taken together
trientine	
iron salts	Trientine reduces absorption of iron salts from the intestine and may reduce their effectiveness
trilostane	
potassium-sparing diuretics	Increased risk of a rise in blood potassium level if taken together
trimethoprim	
methotrexate	Trimethoprim increases anti-folic acid effects of methotrexate
tryptophan	
MAOIs	Stimulation of the brain and confusion if taken together (see Chapter 39)
valproate see sodium valproate	
vancomycin	
anti-bacterials (others)	Increased risk of deafness if vancomycin is taken with an aminoglycoside Increased risk of kidney damage if vancomycin is taken with an aminoglycoside or a cephalosporin (particularly cephalothin)
cholestyramine	Cholestyramine counteracts effects of oral vancomycin
diuretics	Increased risk of deafness if vancomycin is taken with a loop diuretic
viloxazine	
anti-epileptics	Viloxazine increases the blood levels of carbamazepine and phenytoin
theophylline	Viloxazine increases the blood level of theophylline

Table 89.1 Drug interactions (*cont.*)

Drug	*Interactions*
vitamins	
anti-coagulants	Vitamin K (in some tube feeds) counteracts effects of oral anti-coagulants (e.g. nicoumalone, phenindione and warfarin)
levodopa	Pyridoxine counteracts effects of levodopa but not when it is combined with a dopa-decarboxylase inhibitor
phenytoin	Folic acid occasionally reduces the blood level of phenytoin
warfarin	
alcohol	Alcohol increases the effects of warfarin. Increased risk of bleeding
allopurinol	Allopurinol may increase the effects of warfarin. Increased risk of bleeding
aminoglutethimide	Aminoglutethimide reduces the effects of warfarin
anabolic steroids	Anabolic steroids (e.g. oxymetholone, stanozolol) increase the effects of warfarin. Increased risk of bleeding
anti-arrhythmics	Amiodarone, propafenone and quinidine may increase the effects of warfarin. Increased risk of bleeding
anti-bacterials	Aztreonam, cefamandole, chloramphenicol, ciprofloxacin, co-trimoxazole, erythromicin, latamoxef, metronidazole and sulphonamides increase the effects of warfarin. Increased risk of bleeding Rifampicin reduces the effects of warfarin Enoxacin, nalidixic acid, neomycin and tetracyclines may increase the effects of warfarin. Increased risk of bleeding
anti-epileptics	Carbamazepine, phenobarbitone, and primidone reduce the effects of warfarin Phenytoin may increase or decrease the effects of warfarin
anti-fungals	Fluconazole, ketoconazole and miconazole increase the effects of warfarin. Increased risk of bleeding Griseofulvin reduces the effects of warfarin
aspirin	Increased risk of bleeding when aspirin is given with warfarin due to aspirin's effects on platelets
barbiturates	Barbiturates reduce the effects of warfarin
chloral (hydrate and betaine)	Chloral may increase the effects of warfarin. Increased risk of bleeding
cholestyramine	Cholestyramine may increase or decrease the effects of warfarin
cimetidine	Cimetidine increases the effects of warfarin. Increased risk of bleeding
clofibrate group	Bezafibrate, clofibrate and gemfibrozil increase the effects of warfarin. Increased risk of bleeding
danazol	Danazol increases the effects of warfarin. Increased risk of bleeding
dextropropoxyphene	Dextropropoxyphene increases the effects of warfarin. Increased risk of bleeding

Table 89.1 Drug interactions (*cont.*)

Drug	*Interactions*
dipyridamole	Increased risk of bleeding due to the effects of dipyridamole on platelets
disulfiram	Disulfiram increases the effects of warfarin. Increased risk of bleeding
fluvoxamine	Fluvoxamine may increase the effects of warfarin. Increased risk of bleeding
NSAIDs	Effects of warfarin increased by azapropazone and phenylbutazone and occasionally by diflunisal, flurbiprofen, mefenamic acid, piroxicam, sulindac and other NSAIDs. Increased risk of bleeding
omeprazole	Omeprazole increases the effects of warfarin. Increased risk of bleeding
oral contraceptives	Oral contraceptives reduce the effects of warfarin
simvastatin	Simvastatin may increase the effects of warfarin. Increased risk of bleeding
sucralfate	Sucralfate reduces absorption of warfarin from the intestine and may reduce its effects
sulphinpyrazone	Sulphinpyrazone increases the effects of warfarin. Increased risk of bleeding
tamoxifen	Tamoxifen increases the effects of warfarin. Increased risk of bleeding
thyroxine and dextrothyroxine	Thyroxine and dextrothyroxine increase the effects of warfarin. Increased risk of bleeding
vitamin K	Vitamin K (present in some tube feeds) reduces the effects of warfarin
zidovudine	
	Increased risk of harmful effects when given with other drugs that may damage the kidneys or bone marrow
anti-virals (other)	Severe lethargy may occur when intravenous acyclovir is given to individuals taking zidovudine Severe damage to bone marrow, producing serious blood disorders, may occur when zidovudine and ganciclovir are given together
zinc	
anti-bacterials	Tetracyclines and ciprofloxacin reduce the absorption of zinc salts from the intestine and may reduce their effectiveness (and vice versa)
iron	Iron salts reduce absorption of zinc salts from the intestine and may reduce their effectiveness (and vice versa)
penicillamine	Zinc salts reduce the absorption of penicillamine and may reduce its effectiveness

Appendix 1

Generic prescription drugs and their brand names

NOTES
1. An asterisk (*) indicates that the preparation has other ingredients
2. (ext.) indicates that the preparation is for external use only

acebutolol
Secadrex*
Sectral
acetazolamide
Diamox
acetic acid
Aci-jel
Phytex* (ext.)
acetohexamide
Dimelor
acetomenaphthone
Ketovite*
acetylcysteine
Fabrol
Ilube*
Parvolex
acetylsalicylic acid – *see* **aspirin**
acipimox
Olbetam
aclarubicin
Aclacin
acrivastine
Semprex
acrosoxacin
Eradacin
actinomycin D
Cosmegen Lyovac
activated dimethicone – *see* **dimethicone (activated)**
acyclovir
Zovirax
adrenaline
Epifrin
Eppy
Ganda*
Isopto Epinal*
Marcain with adrenaline*
Medihaler-Epi
Simplene
Xylocaine*
alclometasone
Modrasone (ext.)
alcuronium
Alloferin
alfentanil hydrochloride
Rapifen
alginic acid
Algitec*
Gastrocote*
Gastron*
Gaviscon*
Pyrogastrone*
Topal*
allopurinol
Hamarin
Zyloric
allyloestrenol
Gestanin
almasilate
Malinal
aloxiprin
Palaprin forte
alprazolam
Xanax
alprostadil
Prostin VR
alteplase
Actilyse
aluminium hydroxide
Actonorm*
Diovol*
aluminium hydroxide gel
Aludrox
Aludrox SA*
Aluhyde*
Andursil*
APP*
Mucaine*
Polycrol*
Theodrox*
aluminium hydroxide gel, dried
Alu-cap
Asilone*
Caved-S*
Gastrocote*
Gastron*
Gaviscon*
Gelusil*
Kolanticon*
Maalox*
Mucogel*
Pyrogastrone*
Siloxyl*
Topal*
Unigest*
aluminium hydroxide/ magnesium carbonate co-dried gel
Algicon*
Aludrox (tablets)*
Andursil*
Polycrol*
Simeco*
aluminium oxide
Andursil*
Brasivol (ext.)
alverine citrate
Alvercol*

Spasmonal
amantadine hydrochloride
Mantadine
Symmetrel
ambutonium bromide
Aludrox SA*
amethocaine
Eludril spray*
Minims Amethocaine
Noxyflex*
amikacin
Amikin
amiloride
Amilco*
Frumil*
Hypertane*
Kalten*
Lasoride*
Midamor
Moducren*
Moduret 25*
Moduretic*
Navispare*
Normetic*
Vasetic*
aminoglutethimide
Orimeten
aminophylline
Pecram
Phyllocontin Continus
Theodrox*
aminosalicylic acid – *see* **mesalazine**
amiodarone
Cordarone X
amitriptyline
Lentizol
Limbitrol*
Triptafen*
Triptafen-M*
Tryptizol
amlodipine
Istin
amoxapine
Asendis
amoxycillin
Amoram
Amoxil
Augmentin*
Galenamox
amphotericin
Fungilin
Fungizone
ampicillin
Amfipen
Ampiclox*
Dicapen
Magnapen*
Penbritin
Vidopen
amsacrine
Amsidine
amylobarbitone
Amytal
Sodium Amytal
Tuinal*
ancrod
Arvin
anistreplase
Eminase
antazoline
Otrivine-Antistin*
RBC* (ext.)
Vasocon-A*
antidiuretic hormone
DDAVP*
Glypressin*
aprotinin
Trasylol
aspirin
Angettes
Aspav*
Aspellin* (ext.)
Caprin
Co-codaprin
Codis*
Doloxene Compound*
Equagesic*
Hypon*
Laboprin*
Migravess*
Nu-Seals aspirin
Platet
Robaxisal forte*
Solprin
astemizole
Hismanal
atenolol
Beta-adalat*
Kalten*
Tenif*
Tenoret 50*
Tenoretic*
Tenormin
atracurium besylate
Tracrium
atropine sulphate
Isopto Atropine*
Lomotil*
Minims Atropine
Opulets Atropine
auranofin
Ridaura
azapropazone
Rheumox
azatadine
Congesteze*
Optimine
azathioprine
Azamune
Berkaprine
Immunoprin
Imuran
azlocillin
Securopen
aztreonam
Azactam
bacampicillin
Ambaxin
bacitracin
Cicatrin* (ext.)
Polybactrin* (ext.)
Polybactrin Soluble GU*
Polyfax* (ext.)
Tri-Cicatrin* (ext.)
Tribiotic* (ext.)
baclofen
Lioresal
beclomethasone
Becloforte
Becodisks
Beconase
Becotide
Propaderm (ext.)
Propaderm-A* (ext.)
Ventide*
belladonna extract
Alophen*
Bellocarb*
Carbellon*
belladonna liquid extract
Aluhyde*
bendrofluazide
Aprinox
Centyl
Centyl-K*

Corgaretic*
Inderetic*
Inderex*
Neo-NaClex
Neo-NaClex-K*
Prestim*
benethamine penicillin G
Triplopen*
benorylate
Benoral
benoxinate – *see* **oxybuprocaine**
benperidol
Anquil
benserazide
Madopar*
benzathine penicillin G
Penidural
benzhexol
Artane
Bentex
Broflex
benzocaine
AAA Spray*
Intralgin* (ext.)
Medilave*
Merocaine*
Transvasin* (ext.)
Tyrozets*
benzoyl peroxide
Acetoxyl (ext.)
Acnegel (ext.)
Acnidazil* (ext.)
Benoxyl (ext.)
Benoxyl with sulphur* (ext.)
Benzagel (ext.)
Nericur (ext.)
Panoxyl (ext.)
Quinoderm* (ext.)
Quinoderm with hydrocortisone* (ext.)
Quinoped* (ext.)
benzthiazide
Dytide*
benztropine mesylate
Cogentin
benzydamine hydrochloride
Difflam (ext.)
Difflam Oral Rinse
benzyl benzoate
Anugesic-HC*
Anusol HC*
Ascabiol (ext.)
Sudocrem* (ext.)
benzylpenicillin – *see* **penicillin G**
bephenium hydroxynaphthoate
Alcopar
betahistine
Serc
betaine hydrochloride
Kloref*
Kloref-S*
betamethasone
Betnelan
Betnesol
Betnesol-N*
Betnovate (ext.)
Betnovate Rectal*
Betnovate-C* (ext.)
Betnovate-N* (ext.)
Bextasol
Diprosalic* (ext.)
Diprosone (ext.)
Fucibet* (ext.)
Lotriderm* (ext.)
Vista-Methasone
Vista-Methasone N*
betaxolol
Betoptic
Kerlone
bethanechol
Myotonine
bethanidine sulphate
Bendogen
Esbatal
bezafibrate
Bezalip
biperiden
Akineton
bisacodyl
Dulcolax
bismuth subnitrate
Caved-S*
Roter*
bisoprolol
Emcor
Monocor
bran
Fybranta*
Lejfibre
bretylium tosylate
Bretylate
brilliant green
Variclene* (ext.)
bromazepam
Lexotan
bromocriptine
Parlodel
brompheniramine
Dimotane prep's.
Dimotapp*
buclizine
Migraleve*
budesonide
Preferid (ext.)
Pulmicort
Rhinocort
bufexamac
Parfenac (ext.)
bumetanide
Burinex
Burinex K*
bupivacaine
Marcain
Marcain with adrenaline*
buprenorphine
Temgesic
buserelin
Suprefact
buspirone
Buspar
busulphan
Myleran
butethamate
CAM*
butobarbitone
Soneryl
butriptyline
Evadyne
cadexomer iodine
Iodosorb
caffeine
Cafadol*
Cafergot*
Doloxene Compound*
Glykola*
Hypon*
Labiton*
Migril*
Parahypon*
Pardale*
Propain*
Syndol*

Uniflu*
calcitonin – *see also* **salcatonin**
Calcitare
calcitriol
Rocaltrol
calcium (salts)
Calcimax*
Calcium Sandoz
Chocovite*
Miol* (ext.)
Nutracel*
Octovit*
Sandocal*
calcium carbonate
APP*
Cacit
Calcichew
Citrical
Gaviscon*
Nulacin*
Rabro*
Sandocal*
Titralac*
calcium gluconate
Chocovite*
calcium heparin
Calciparine
Minihep Calcium*
calcium leucovorin – *see* **folinic acid**
calcium sulphaloxate
Enteromide
canrenoate potassium
Spiroctan-M
capreomycin sulphate
Capastat
captopril
Acepril
Acezide*
Capoten
Capozide*
carbachol
Isopto Carbachol*
carbamazepine
Tegretol
carbaryl
Carylderm (ext.)
Clinicide (ext.)
Derbac Shampoo (ext.)
Suleo-C (ext.)
carbenicillin sodium
Pyopen
carbenoxolone sodium
Biogastrone
Bioplex
Bioral
Duogastrone
Pyrogastrone*
carbidopa
Sinemet*
carbimazole
Neo-Mercazole
carbocisteine
Mucodyne
carboplatin
Paraplatin
carboprost
Hemabate
carfecillin
Uticillin
carisoprodol
Carisoma
carmustine
Bicnu
carteolol
Cartrol
Teoptic
cefaclor
Distaclor
cefadroxil
Baxan
cefamandole
Kefadol
cefixime
Suprax
cefotaxime
Claforan
cefoxitin
Mefoxin
cefsulodin
Monaspor
ceftazidime
Fortum
ceftizoxime
Cefizox
cefuroxime
Zinacef
cefuroxime axetil
Zinnat
cellulose
Nilstim*
cephalexin
Ceporex
Keflex
cephalothin
Keflin
cephazolin
Kefzol
cephradine
Velosef
cetirizine
Zirtek
chenodeoxycholic acid
Chendol
Chenofalk
chloral betaine
Welldorm tablets
chloral hydrate
Noctec
Welldorm elixir
chlorambucil
Leukeran
chloramphenicol
Actinac* (ext.)
Chloromycetin
Chloromycetin hydrocortisone*
Kemicetine
Minims chloramphenicol
Opulets chloramphenicol
Sno Phenicol
Tanderil chloramphenicol*
chlorbutol
Cerumol*
Eludril Mouthwash*
Monphytol* (ext.)
chlordiazepoxide
Librium
Limbitrol*
Tropium
chlormethiazole
Heminevrin
chlormezanone
Lobak*
Trancopal
chloroquine
Avloclor
Nivaquine
chlorothiazide
Saluric
chlorpheniramine maleate
Haymine*
Piriton
chlorpromazine

Largactil
chlorpropamide
Diabinese
chlortetracycline
Aureocort* (ext.)
Aureomycin
Deteclo*
Propaderm-A* (ext.)
Trimovate* (ext.)
chlorthalidone
Hygroton
Hygroton K*
Kalspare*
Lopresoretic*
Tenoret 50*
Tenoretic*
cholestyramine
Questran
choline magnesium trisalicylate
Trilisate
choline salicylate
Audax
Teejel*
choline theophyllinate
Choledyl
cilastatin
Primaxin*
cimetidine
Algitec*
Dyspamet
Tagamet
cinchocaine
Nupercainal (ext.)
Proctosedyl*
Scheriproct*
Ultraproct*
Uniroid*
cinnarizine
Stugeron
cinoxacin
Cinobac
ciprofloxacin
Ciproxin
cisapride
Alimix
Prepulsid
clavulanic acid
Augmentin*
Timentin*
clemastine
Tavegil
clindamycin
Dalacin C
Dalacin T (ext.)
clioquinol
Barquinol HC* (ext.)
Betnovate-C* (ext.)
Haelan-C* (ext.)
Locorten-Vioform*
Oralcer*
Synalar C* (ext.)
Vioform-hydrocortisone* (ext.)
clobazam
Frisium
clobetasol
Dermovate (ext.)
Dermovate-NN* (ext.)
clobetasone butyrate
Eumovate
Eumovate-N*
Trimovate* (ext.)
clofazimine
Lamprene
clofibrate
Atromid-S
clomiphene
Clomid
Serophene
clomipramine
Anafranil
clomocycline
Megaclor
clonazepam
Rivotril
clonidine hydrochloride
Catapres
Dixarit
clopamide
Viskaldix*
clorazepate potassium
Tranxene
clotrimazole
Canesten
Canesten-HC*
Lotriderm* (ext.)
cloxacillin sodium
Ampiclox*
Orbenin
clozapine
Clozaril
co-amilofruse
Frumil*
Lasoride*
co-amilozide
Amilco*
Hypertane*
Moduret 25*
Moduretic*
Normetic*
co-amoxiclav
Augmentin*
co-beneldopa
Madopar*
co-careldopa
Sinemet*
co-codamol
Paracodol*
co-codaprin
Codis*
co-danthrusate
Normax*
co-dergocrine mesylate
Hydergine
co-dydramol
Paramol*
co-fluampicil
Magnapen
co-proxamol
Distalgesic*
Paxalgesic*
co-trimoxazole
Bactrim*
Chemotrim*
Comox*
Fectrim*
Laratrim*
Septrin*
codeine phosphate
Benylin*
Co-codamol*
Co-codaprin*
Codis*
Diarrest*
Dimotane Co*
Formulix*
Galcodine
Hypon*
Kaodene*
Migraleve*
Paracodol*
Parahypon*
Pardale*
Phensedyl*
Propain*
Solpadol*
Syndol*

Tercoda*
Terpoin*
Tylex*
Uniflu*
colestipol
Colestid
colistin
Colomycin
corticotrophin
Acthar
cortisone
Cortistab
Cortisyl
crotamiton
Eurax (ext.)
Eurax-hydrocortisone* (ext.)
cyanocobalamin
BC 500*
Cytacon
Cytamen
Ketovite Liquid*
Octovit*
Solivito N*
cyclandelate
Cyclobral
Cyclospasmol
cyclizine
Cyclimorph*
Diconal*
Migril*
Valoid
cyclofenil
Rehibin
cyclopenthiazide
Navidrex
Navidrex-K*
Navispare*
Trasidrex*
cyclopentolate
Minims cyclopentolate
Mydrilate
Opulets cyclopentolate
cyclophosphamide
Endoxana
cyclosporin
Sandimmun
cyproheptadine
Periactin
cyproterone acetate
Androcur
Cyprostat
Dianette*
cytarabine
Alexan
Cytosar
dacarbazine
DTIC-Dome
danazol
Danol
danthrolene sodium
Dantrium
danthron
Co-danthrusate*
Codalex*
Normalex*
dapsone + pyrimethamine
Maloprim*
debrisoquine sulphate
Declinax
demeclocycline
Deteclo*
Ledermycin
desferrioxamine
Desferal
desipramine
Pertofran
desmopressin
DDAVP*
Desmospray
desogestrel
Marvelon*
Mercilon*
desoxymethasone
Stiedex prep's (ext.)
Stiedex LP N* (ext.)
dexamethasone
Decadron
Dexa-Rhinaspray*
Maxidex*
Maxitrol*
Otomize*
Sofradex*
dexamphetamine
Dexedrine
dexfenfluramine
Adifax
dexpanthenol
Concavit*
Lipoflavonoid*
Lipotriad*
dextranomer
Debrisan (ext.)
dextromethorphan hydrobromide
Actifed*
Benylin*
Lotussin*
Sudafed*
dextromoramide
Palfium
dextropropoxyphene
Co-Proxamol*
Distalgesic*
Doloxene
Doloxene Compound*
Paxalgesic*
diazepam
Alupram
Atensine
Diazemuls
Stesolid
Tensium
Valium
diazoxide
Eudemine
dichlorphenamide
Daranide
diclofenac
Rhumalgan
Valenac
Volraman
Voltarol
Voltarol Emugel (ext.)
dicyclomine hydrochloride
Diarrest*
Kolanticon*
Merbentyl
dienoestrol
Ortho Dienoestrol
diethylcarbamazine
Banocide
diethylpropion hydrochloride
Apisate*
Tenuate Dospan
diflucortolone valerate
Nerisone (ext.)
diflunisal
Dolobid
digoxin
Lanoxin
dihydrocodeine
Co-dydramol*

DF 118
DHC Continus
Paramol*
dihydroergotamine
Dihydergot
diltiazem
Adizem
Angiozem
Britiazim
Tildiem
dimenhydrinate
Dramamine
dimethicone
Cobadex* (ext.)
Conotrane* (ext.)
Diovol*
Kolanticon*
Rikospray silicone* (ext.)
Siopel* (ext.)
Sprilon* (ext.)
Timodine* (ext.)
Translet barrier cream* (ext.)
Unigest*
dimethicone (activated)
Actonorm*
Altacite Plus*
Andursil*
Asilone*
Infacol
Maalox*
Piptalin*
Polycrol*
Siloxyl*
Simeco*
dimethindene maleate
Fenostil Retard
Vibrocil*
dimethyl sulphoxide
Herpid* (ext.)
Iduridin*
Rimso-50
Virudox* (ext.)
dinoprost
Prostin F2 alpha
dinoprostone
Prepidil
Prostin E2
diphenhydramine
Benylin*
Caladryl* (ext.)
Guanor*
Histalix*
Lotussin*
Propain*
Uniflu*
diphenoxylate
Lomotil*
diphenylpyraline
Eskornade*
Histryl
Lergoban
dipipanone
Diconal*
dipivefrin
Propine
dipyridamole
Persantin
Vasyrol
disopyramide
Dirythmin SA
Rythmodan
distigmine
Ubretid
disulfiram
Antabuse
dobutamine
Dobutrex
docosahexaenoic acid (DHA)
Maxepa*
docusate sodium
Co-danthrusate*
Dioctyl
Dioctyl ear drops*
Fletchers' Enemette
Molcer
Normax*
Waxsol
domiphen bromide
Bradosol
Bradosol Plus*
domperidone
Evoxin
Motilium
dopamine
Intropin
dopexamine
Dopacard
dothiepin
Prothiaden
doxapram
Dopram
doxazosin
Cardura
doxepin
Sinequan
doxycycline
Nordox
Vibramycin
doxylamine
Syndol*
droperidol
Droleptan
Thalamonal*
dydrogesterone
Duphaston
econazole nitrate
Econacort* (ext.)
Ecostatin
Gyno-Pevaryl
Pevaryl (ext.)
Pevaryl TC* (ext.)
eicosapentaenoic acid (EPA)
Maxepa*
enalapril
Innovace
enoxacin
Comprecin
enoximone
Perfan
ephedrine
CAM*
Davenol*
Franol*
Franol Plus*
Haymine*
Phensedyl*
epirubicin
Pharmorubicin
epoetin
Eprex
Recormon
epoprostenol
Flolan
ergometrine maleate
Syntometrine*
ergotamine tartrate
Cafergot*
Lingraine
Medihaler-ergotamine
Migril*
erythromycin
Erymax
Erythrocin
Erythromid

Erythroped
Ilosone
Stiemycin (ext.)
Zineryt* (ext.)
estramustine
Estracyt
ethacrynic acid
Edecrin
ethambutol
Myambutol
Mynah*
ethamsylate
Dicynene
ethinyloestradiol
BiNovum*
Brevinor*
Conova 30*
Dianette*
Eugynon 30*
Femodene*
Femodene ED*
Loestrin 20*
Loestrin 30*
Logynon*
Logynon ED*
Marvelon*
Mercilon*
Microgynon 30*
Minulet*
Neocon 1/35*
Norimin*
Ovran*
Ovran 30*
Ovranette*
Ovysmen*
Schering PC4*
Synphase*
Trinordiol*
TriNovum*
TriNovum ED*
ethoglucid
Epodyl
ethoheptazine citrate
Equagesic*
ethosuximide
Emeside
Zarontin
ethyl nicotinate
Transvasin* (ext.)
ethyl salicylate
Dubam* (ext.)
ethynodiol diacetate
Conova 30*
Femulen
etidronate
Didronel
etodolac
Lodine
etoposide
Vepesid
etretinate
Tigason
famotidine
Pepcid PM
felbinac
Traxam (ext.)
fenbufen
Lederfen
fenfluramine
Ponderax
Fenofibrate
Lipantil
fenoprofen calcium
Fenopron
Progesic
fenoterol
Berotec
Duovent*
fentanyl
Sublimaze
Thalamonal*
ferric ammonium citrate
Lexpec with iron*
Lexpec with iron-M*
ferric chloride
Glykola*
ferrous fumarate
BC 500 with iron*
Ferrocap
Ferrocap-F 350*
Fersaday
Fersamal
Folex-350*
Galfer
Galfer FA*
Givitol*
Meterfolic*
Pregaday*
ferrous gluconate
Ferfolic SV*
Fergon
ferrous glycine sulphate
Ferrocontin
Ferrocontin Folic*
Plesmet
ferrous succinate
Ferromyn
ferrous sulphate
Fefol*
Fefol-Vit*
Fefol Z*
Feospan
Ferrograd
Ferrograd C*
Ferrograd Folic*
Fesovit*
Fesovit Z*
Folicin*
Octovit*
Pregnavite forte F*
Slow-Fe
Slow-Fe Folic*
flavoxate
Uripas
flecainide acetate
Tambocor
fluclorolone
Topilar (ext.)
flucloxacillin sodium
Floxapen
Ladropen
Magnapen*
Stafoxil
Staphlipen
fluconazole
Diflucan
fludrocortisone acetate
Florinef
flumazenil
Anexate
flumethasone
Locorten-Vioform*
flunisolide
Syntaris
flunitrazepam
Rohypnol
fluocinolone
Synalar (ext.)
Synalar C* (ext.)
Synalar N* (ext.)
fluocinonide
Metosyn (ext.)
fluocortolone
Ultradil (ext.)
Ultralanum (ext.)
Ultraproct*
fluorometholone
FML
FML-Neo*

fluoxetine
Prozac
flupenthixol
Depixol
Fluanxol
fluphenazine
Modecate
Moditen
Motipress*
Motival*
flurandrenolone
Haelan (ext.)
Haelan-C* (ext.)
flurazepam
Dalmane
flurbiprofen
Froben
fluspirilene
Redeptin
flutamide
Drogenil
fluvoxamine
Faverin
folic acid
Fefol*
Fefol-Vit*
Fefol Z*
Ferfolic SV*
Ferrocap-F 350*
Ferrocontin Folic*
Ferrograd Folic*
Folex-350*
Folicin*
Galfer FA*
Givitol*
Ketovite*
Lexpec
Lexpec with iron*
Lexpec with iron-M*
Meterfolic*
Pregaday*
Pregnavite forte F*
Slow-Fe Folic*
Solivito N*
folinic acid
Refolinon
formaldehyde
Veracur (ext.)
foscarnet
Foscavir
fosfestrol
Honvan
framycetin sulphate
Framycort*
Framygen
Sofradex*
Soframycin
Soframycin* (ext.)
Sofra-Tulle (ext.)
frangula
Normacol Plus*
Rabro*
Roter*
frusemide
Diumide-K Continus*
Dryptal
Frumil*
Frusene*
Lasikal*
Lasilactone*
Lasipressin*
Lasix
Lasix + K*
Lasoride*
FSH – *see* urofollitrophin
fusafungine
Locabiotal
fusidic acid – *see* sodium fusidate
gallamine triethiodide
Flaxedil
gammaglobulin – *see* immunoglobulin
gamolenic acid
Epogam
ganciclovir
Cymevene
gemeprost
Cervagem
gemfibrozil
Lopid
gentamicin sulphate
Cidomycin
Garamycin
Genticin
Genticin HC* (ext.)
Gentisone HC*
Minims Gentamicin
gestodene
Femodene*
Femodene ED*
Minulet*
gestronol hexanoate
Depostat
glibenclamide
Daonil
Euglucon
Semi-daonil
gliclazide
Diamicron
glipizide
Glibenese
Minodiab
gliquidone
Glurenorm
glutaraldehyde
Glutarol (ext.)
Novaruca (ext.)
Verucasep (ext.)
glyceryl trinitrate
Coro-Nitro
Deponit
Nitrocine
Nitrocontin Continus
Nitrolingual
Nitronal
Percutol (ext.)
Suscard Buccal
Sustac
Transiderm-Nitro
Tridil
glycopyrronium bromide
Robinul
Robinul Neostigmine*
gonadorelin
Fertiral
HRF
gonadotrophin (human chorionic)
Gonadotrophon LH
Pregnyl
Profasi
gonadotrophin (human menopausal)
Humegon
goserelin
Zoladex
gramicidin
Adcortyl with Graneodin* (ext.)
Graneodin* (ext.)
Neosporin*
Sofradex*
Soframycin* (ext.)
Tri-Adcortyl* (ext.)
Tri-Adcortyl Otic*
griseofulvin
Fulcin

Grisovin
growth hormone – *see* **somatrem**
guaiphenesin
Actifed*
Bricanyl Expectorant*
Dimotane Expectorant*
Sudafed*
guanethidine monosulphate
Ganda*
Ismelin
guar gum
Guarem
Guarina
halcinonide
Halciderm (ext.)
haloperidol
Dozic
Fortunan
Haldol
Serenace
heparin calcium
Minihep Calcium*
Monoparin Ca
Uniparin Ca
heparin sodium
Hep-Flush (ext.)
Heplock (ext.)
Hepsal (ext.)
Minihep Sodium*
Monoparin
Multiparin
Unihep
Uniparin
hexachlorophane
Anacal*
Dermalex* (ext.)
Ster-Zac DC (ext.)
Ster-Zac Powder (ext.)
Torbetol* (ext.)
hexamine
Hiprex
hexetidine
Oraldene
homatropine
Minims Homatropine
homatropine methyl bromide
APP*
hydralazine
Apresoline
hydrochlorothiazide
Acezide*
Amilco*
Capozide*
Co-Betaloc*
Dyazide*
Esidrex
Hydromet*
Hydrosaluric
Hypertane*
Kalten*
Moducren*
Moduret 25*
Moduretic*
Normetic*
Secadrex*
Serpasil Esidrex*
Sotazide*
Tolerzide*
Triamco*
Vasetic*
hydrocortisone
Actinac* (ext.)
Alphaderm* (ext.)
Alphosyl HC* (ext.)
Anugesic-HC*
Anusol HC*
Barquinol HC* (ext.)
Calmurid HC* (ext.)
Canesten-HC*
Carbo-Cort* (ext.)
Chloromycetin Hydrocortisone*
Cobadex* (ext.)
Colifoam
Corlan
Daktacort* (ext.)
Dioderm (ext.)
Econacort* (ext.)
Efcortelan
Efcortesol
Epifoam*
Eurax-hydrocortisone* (ext.)
Framycort*
Fucidin H* (ext.)
Genticin HC* (ext.)
Gentisone HC*
Gregoderm* (ext.)
Hydrocal* (ext.)
Hydrocortistab
Hydrocortisyl (ext.)
Hydrocortone
Mildison Lipocream (ext.)
Neo-Cortef* (ext.)
Nystaform-HC* (ext.)
Otosporin*
Proctofoam HC*
Proctosedyl*
Quinocort* (ext.)
Quinoderm with hydrocortisone* (ext.)
Sential* (ext.)
Solu-Cortef
Tarcortin* (ext.)
Terra-Cortril* (ext.)
Terra-Cortril nystatin* (ext.)
Timodine* (ext.)
Tri-Cicatrin* (ext.)
Uniroid*
Vioform-hydrocortisone* (ext.)
Xyloproct*
hydrocortisone-17-butyrate
Locoid (ext.)
Locoid C* (ext.)
hydroflumethiazide
Aldactide*
Hydrenox
hydrogen peroxide
Hioxyl (ext.)
hydrotalcite
Altacite
Altacite Plus*
hydroxocobalamin
Cobalin-H
Lipoflavonoid*
Lipotriad*
Neo-Cytamen
hydroxyapatite
Ossopan
hydroxychloroquine sulphate
Plaquenil
hydroxyprogesterone hexanoate
Proluton
hydroxyurea
Hydrea
hydroxyzine
Atarax
hyoscine
Buscopan

Omnopon
scopolamine
Scopoderm
hypromellose
Ilube*
Isopto Alkaline
Isopto Atropine*
Isopto Carbachol*
Isopto Carpine*
Isopto Epinal*
Isopto Frin*
Isopto Plain
Maxidex*
Maxitrol*
Tears Naturale*
ibuprofen
Brufen
Fenbid Spansule
Junifen
Motrin
Proflex (ext.)
idarubicin
Zavedos
idoxuridine
Herpid* (ext.)
Idoxene
Iduridin*
Kerecid*
Virudox* (ext.)
ifosfamide
Mitoxana
imipenem
Primaxin*
imipramine hydrochloride
Tofranil
immunoglobulin
Endobulin
Gamimune-N
Gammabulin
Humotet
Kabiglobulin
Sandoglobulin
INAH (isonicotinic acid hydrazine) – *see* isoniazid
indapamide
Natrilix
indomethacin
Flexin Continus
Imbrilon
Indocid
Indocid PDA
Indolar SR
Indomod
indoramin
Baratol
Doralese
inosine pranobex
Imunovir
inositol nicotinate
Hexopal
insulins – *see* Chapter 65
interferon
Intron A
Roferon-A
Wellferon
iodine – *see* povidone-iodine
ipecacuanha
Alophen*
ipratropium bromide
Atrovent
Duovent*
Rinatec
iprindole
Prondol
iron dextran complex
Imferon
iron polysaccharide complex
Niferex
iron sodium edetate
Sytron
iron sorbitol/citric acid complex
Jectofer
isoaminile citrate
Isoaminile linctus
isocarboxazid
Marplan
isoconazole
Travogyn
isoetharine
Bronchilator*
Numotac
isometheptene
Midrid*
isoniazid
Mynah*
Rifater*
Rifinah*
Rimactazid*
isoprenaline
Duo-Autohaler*
Intal Compound*
Iso-Autohaler
Medihaler-Duo*
Medihaler-Iso
Saventrine
isosorbide dinitrate
Cedocard
Isoket
Isordil
Soni-slo
Sorbichew
Sorbid SA
Sorbitrate
Vascardin
isosorbide mononitrate
Elantan
Elantan LA
Imdur
Ismo
Isotrate
MCR-50
Monit
Mono-Cedocard
isotretinoin
Roaccutane
isoxsuprine
Duvadilan
ispaghula
Colven*
Fybogel
Isogel
Manevac*
Regulan
isradipine
Prescal
itraconazole
Sporanox
kanamycin
Kannasyn
ketoconazole
Nizoral
Nizoral (ext.)
Nizoral Shampoo (ext.)
ketoprofen
Alrheumat
Orudis
Oruvail
ketotifen
Zaditen
labetalol
Trandate
lactulose
Duphalac
laevulose
Emetrol*

Rehidrat*
lanatoside C
Cedilanid
levobunolol
Betagan
levodopa
Brocadopa
Larodopa
Madopar*
Sinemet*
levonorgestrel
Cyclo-Progynova*
Eugynon 30*
Logynon*
Logynon ED*
Microgynon 30*
Microval
Norgeston
Ovran*
Ovran 30*
Ovranette*
Trinordiol*
LH – *see* **gonadotrophin (chorionic)**
LHRH – *see* **buserelin, gonadorelin, goserelin**
lignocaine
Betnovate Rectal*
Bradosol Plus
Calgel* (ext.)
Depo-Medrone with Lidocaine*
EMLA* (ext.)
Instillagel* (ext.)
Minims Lignocaine and Fluorescein*
Xylocaine
Xylocard
Xyloproct*
lincomycin
Lincocin
lindane
Quellada (ext.)
liothyronine sodium
Tertroxin
liquorice deglycyrrhizinized
Caved-S*
Rabro*
lisinopril
Carace
Zestril
lithium (salts)
Camcolit
Efalith (ext.)
Liskonium
Litarex
Phasal
Priadel
lofepramine
Gamanil
lomustine
CCNU
loperamide
Imodium
loprazolam
Dormonoct
loratadine
Clarityn
lorazepam
Almazine
Ativan
loxapine
Loxapac
lymecycline
Tetralysal
lypressin
Syntopressin
lysuride
Revanil
magnesium alginate
Algicon*
Gaviscon Infant*
magnesium carbonate
Algicon*
APP*
Bellocarb*
Caved-S*
Nulacin*
Roter*
Topal*
magnesium citrate
Picolax*
magnesium hydroxide
Actonorm*
Aludrox SA*
Aludrox Tablets*
Andursil*
Carbellon*
Diovol*
Maalox*
Mucaine*
Mucogel*
Octovit*
Polycrol*
Simeco*
magnesium oxide
Asilone*
Kolanticon*
Nulacin*
Rabro*
Siloxyl*
magnesium trisilicate
Aluhyde*
APP*
Bellocarb*
Gastrocote*
Gastron*
Gaviscon*
Gelusil*
Nulacin*
Pyrogastrone*
malathion
Derbac-M (ext.)
Prioderm (ext.)
Suleo-M (ext.)
maprotiline hydrochloride
Ludiomil
mazindol
Teronac
mebendazole
Vermox
mebeverine
Colofac
Colven*
mebhydrolin
Fabahistin
mecillinam
Selexidin
medazepam
Nobrium
medroxyprogesterone
Depo-Provera
Farlutal
Provera
mefenamic acid
Dysman
Ponstan
mefloquine
Lariam
mefruside
Baycaron
megestrol
Megace
melphalan
Alkeran
menadiol sodium diphosphate
Synkavit

menotrophin
Pergonal
mepenzolate bromide
Cantil
mepivacaine
Estradurin*
meprobamate
Equagesic*
Equanil
meptazinol
Meptid
mequitazine
Primalan
mercaptopurine
Puri-Nethol
mesalazine
Asacol
Pentasa
mesna
Uromitexan
mesterolone
Pro-Viron
mestranol
Menophase*
Norinyl-1*
Ortho-Novin 1/50*
metaraminol
Aramine
metformin
Glucophage
methadone
Physeptone
methicillin sodium
Celbenin
methixene
Tremonil
methocarbamol
Robaxin
Robaxisal forte*
methoserpidine
Decaserpyl
methotrexate
Maxtrex
methotrimeprazine
Nozinan
methoxamine
Vasoxine
methyclothiazide
Enduron
methylcellulose
Celevac
Cologel
Nilstim*
methyl cysteine
Visclair
methyldopa
Aldomet
Dopamet
Hydromet*
methylphenobarbitone
Prominal
methylprednisolone
Depo-Medrone
Depo-Medrone with Lidocaine*
Medrone
Medrone acne lotion* (ext.)
Neo-Medrone cream* (ext.)
Solu-Medrone
methysergide maleate
Deseril
metipranolol
Glauline
Minims Metipranolol
metoclopramide
Gastrese LA
Gastrobid Continus
Gastroflux
Gastromax
Maxolon
Metox
Migravess*
Paramax*
Parmid
Primperan
metolazone
Metenix
metoprolol
Betaloc
Betaloc-SA
Co-Betaloc*
Lopresor
Lopresor SR
Lopresoretic*
Metoros
metronidazole
Elyzol
Flagyl
Flagyl Compak*
Metrolyl
Zadstat
metyrapone
Metopirone
mexenone
Uvistat* (ext.)
mexiletine
Mexitil
mezlocillin
Baypen
mianserin hydrochloride
Bolvidon
Norval
miconazole nitrate
Acnidazil* (ext.)
Daktacort* (ext.)
Daktarin
Gyno-Daktarin
Monistat
midazolam
Hypnovel
milrinone
Primacor
minocycline
Minocin
Minocin 50
minoxidil
Loniten
Regaine (ext.)
misoprostol
Cytotec
mitozantrone
Novantrone
monosulfiram
Tetmosol (ext.)
morphine
Cyclimorph*
MST Continus
Nepenthe
Oramorph
mupirocin
Bactroban (ext.)
Bactroban Nasal
nabilone
Cesamet
nabumetone
Relifex
nadolol
Corgard
Corgaretic*
naftidrofuryl
Praxilene
nalbuphine
Nubain
nalidixic acid
Mictral*
Negram
Uriben

naloxone
Narcan
naltrexone
Nalorex
nandrolone decanoate
Deca-Durabolin
Deca-Durabolin 100
nandrolone phenylpropionate
Durabolin
naphazoline
Vasocon-A*
naproxen
Naprosyn
Synflex
natamycin
Pimafucin
nedocromil
Tilade
nefopam hydrochloride
Acupan
neomycin
Adcortyl with Graneodin* (ext.)
Audicort*
Bretnesol-N*
Cicatrin* (ext.)
Dermovate-NN* (ext.)
Dexa-Rhinaspray*
Eumovate-N*
FML-Neo*
Graneodin* (ext.)
Gregoderm* (ext.)
Maxitrol*
Minims neomycin
Naseptin*
Neo-Cortef* (ext.)
Neo-Medrone cream* (ext.)
Neosporin*
Nivemycin*
Otomize
Otosporin*
Polybactrin* (ext.)
Polybactrin Soluble GU*
Predsol-N*
Stiedex LP N* (ext.)
Synalar N* (ext.)
Tri-Adcortyl* (ext.)
Tri-Adcortyl Otic*
Tri-Cicatrin* (ext.)
Tribiotic* (ext.)
Uniroid*
Vibrocil*
Vista-Methasone N*
neostigmine
Prostigmin
Robinul neostigmine*
netilmicin
Netillin
nicardipine
Cardene
niclosamide
Yomesan
nicofuranose
Bradilan
nicotinyl alcohol tartrate
Ronicol
nicoumalone
Sinthrome
nifedipine
Adalat
Adalat IC
Adalat Retard
Beta-Adalat*
Calcilat
Coracten
Tenif*
nimodipine
Nimotop
nimorazole
Naxogin 500
Nitrazepam
Mogadon
Nitrados
Remnos
Somnite
Unisomnia
nitrofurantoin
Furadantin
Macrodantin
nizatidine
Axid
noradrenaline
Levophed
norethisterone
BiNovum*
Brevinor*
Estrapak*
Loestrin 20*
Loestrin 30*
Menophase*
Menzol
Micronor
Neocon 1/35*
Noriday
Norimin*
Norinyl-1*
Noristerat
Ortho-Novin 1/50*
Ovysmen*
Primolut N
SH 420
Synphase*
TriNovum*
TriNovum ED*
Trisequens*
Utovlan
Norfloxacin
Utinor
norgestrel
Cyclo-progynova*
Neogest
Prempak-C*
Schering PC4*
nortriptyline hydrochloride
Allegron
Aventyl
Motipress*
Motival*
noxythiolin
Noxyflex*
Noxyflex S
nystatin
Dermovate-NN* (ext.)
Flagyl Compak*
Gregoderm* (ext.)
Multilind* (ext.)
Mysteclin*
Nystadermal* (ext.)
Nystaform* (ext.)
Nystaform-HC* (ext.)
Nystan
Nystavescent
Terra-Cortril nystatin* (ext.)
Timodine* (ext.)
Tinaderm-M* (ext.)
Tri-Adcortyl* (ext.)
Tri-Adcortyl Otic*
Tri-Cicatrin (ext.)
Trimovate* (ext.)
octreotide
Sandostatin

oestradiol
Cyclo-Progynova*
Estraderm (ext.)
Estrapak*
Hormonin*
Progynova
Trisequens*
oestriol
Hormonin*
Ortho-Gynest
Ovestin
Trisequens*
oestrogen
Premarin
Prempak-C*
oestrone
Hormonin*
ofloxacin
Tarvid
olsalazine
Dipentum
omeprazole
Losec
ondansetron
Zofran
orciprenaline
Alupent
orphenadrine
Biorphen
Disipal
Norflex
oxatomide
Tinset
oxazepam
Oxanid
oxerutin
Paroven
oxethazaine
Mucaine*
oxpentifylline
Trental
oxprenolol
Slow-Pren
Slow-Trasicor
Trasicor
Trasidrex*
oxybuprocaine
Minims Benoxinate
Opulets Benoxinate
oxymetazoline
Afrazine
oxymetholone
Anapolon 50

oxypertine
Integrin
oxyphenbutazone
Tanderil
Tanderil
Chloramphenicol*
oxytetracycline
Berkmycen
Imperacin
Terra-Cortril* (ext.)
Terra-Cortril
nystatin* (ext.)
Terramycin
Trimovate* (ext.)
oxytocin
Syntocinon
Syntometrine*
pamidronate
Aredia
pancuronium bromide
Pavulon
papaveretum
Aspav*
Omnopon
Omnopon
Scopolamine*
papaverine
APP*
paracetamol
Cafadol*
Calpol
Co-codamol*
Co-dydramol*
Co-proxamol*
Disprol paed.
Distalgesic*
Formulix*
Fortagesic*
Lobak*
Medised*
Midrid*
Migraleve*
Paldesic
Pameton*
Panadol
Panaleve
Paracodol*
Parahypon*
Parake*
Paramax*
Paramol*
Pardale*
Paxalgesic*

Propain*
Salzone
Solpadol*
Sudafed-co*
Syndol*
Tylex*
Uniflu*
pemoline
Volital
penbutolol
Lasipressin*
penicillamine
Distamine
Pendramine
penicillin G sodium
Bicillin*
Crystapen
Triplopen*
penicillin V potassium
Distaquaine V-K
Stabillin V-K
V-Cil-K
pentaerythritol tetranitrate
Cardiacap
Mycardol
pentazocine
Fortagesic*
Fortral
peppermint oil
Carbellon*
Colpermin
Mintec
Tercoda*
pepsin
Muripsin*
pericyazine
Neulactil
perindopril
Coversyl
permethrin
Lyclear (ext.)
perphenazine
Fentazin
Triptafen*
Triptafen-M*
pethidine hydrochloride
Pamergan P100*
phenazocine
Narphen
phenazopyridine
Uromide*
phenelzine

Nardil
phenethicillin potassium
Broxil
phenindamine
Thephorin
phenindione
Dindevan
pheniramine maleate
Daneral SA
phenolphthalein
Agarol*
Alophen*
Kest*
phenoperidine
Operidine
phenothrin
Full Marks (ext.)
phenoxybenzamine
Dibenyline
phenoxymethylpenicillin – *see* **penicillin V**
phentermine
Duromine
Ionamin
phentolamine
Rogitine
phenylbutazone
Butacote
phenylephrine
Betnovate Rectal*
Bronchilator*
Dimotapp*
Duo-Autohaler*
Isopto Frin*
Medihaler-Duo*
Minims phenylephrine
Uniflu*
Vibrocil*
phenylpropanolamine
Dimotapp*
Eskornade*
phenytoin
Epanutin
pholcodine
Copholco*
Copholcoids*
Davenol*
Galenphol
Pavacol-D
Pholcomed
phytomenadione
Konakion
pilocarpine
Isopto Carpine*
Minims Pilocarpine
Ocusert Pilo
Opulets Pilocarpine
Sno Pilo
pimozide
Orap
pindolol
Viskaldix*
Visken
pipenzolate methobromide
Piptal
Piptalin*
piperacillin
Pipril
piperazine
Antepar
Pripsen*
piperazine estrone sulphate
Harmogen
pipothiazine palmitate
Piportil Depot
pirbuterol
Exirel
pirenzepine
Gastrozepin
piretanide
Arelix
piroxicam
Feldene
Feldene Gel (ext.)
pivampicillin
Miraxid*
Pondocillin
Pondocillin Plus*
pivmecillinam
Miraxid*
Pondocillin Plus*
Selexid
pizotifen
Sanomigran
podophyllotoxin
Condyline (ext.)
Warticon (ext.)
podophyllum
Posalfilin* (ext.)
poldine methylsulphate
Nacton
poloxamer '188'
Codalax*
polymyxin B
Aerosporin
Gregoderm* (ext.)
Maxitrol*
Neosporin*
Otosporin*
Polybactrin* (ext.)
Polybactrin Soluble GU*
Polyfax* (ext.)
Polytrim*
Terra-Cortril* (ext.)
Tribiotic* (ext.)
Uniroid*
polynoxylin
Anaflex
polyoestradiol
Estradurin*
polystyrene sulphonate
Calcium Resonium
Resonium-A
polythiazide
Nephril
potassium bicarbonate
Algicon*
Dioralyte*
Effercitrate*
Kloref*
Kloref-S*
Phosphate-Sandoz*
Pyrogastrone*
Sando-K*
potassium chloride
Burinex K*
Centyl-K*
Diarrest*
Dioralyte*
Diumide-K Continus*
Electrolade*
Glandosane*
Gluco-Lyte*
GoLytely*
Hygroton K*
Kay-Cee-L
Klean-prep*
Kloref*
Kloref-S*
Lasikal*
Lasix + K*
Leo K
Navidrex-K*
Neo-NaClex-K*
Nu-K
Rehidrat*
Sando-K*

Slow-K
povidone-iodine
Betadine
Disadine D.P. (ext.)
Inadine
Videne (ext.)
pravastatin
Lipostat
prazosin
Hypovase
prednisolone
Anacal*
Deltacortril
Deltastab
Minims Prednisolone
Precortisyl
Predenema
Pred Forte
Predfoam
Prednesol
Predsol
Predsol-N*
Scheriproct*
Sintisone
prednisone
Decortisyl
prilocaine
Citanest
EMLA* (ext.)
primidone
Mysoline
probenecid
Benemid
probucol
Lurselle
procainamide hydrochloride
Procainamide Durules
Pronestyl
procaine penicillin G
Bicillin*
Triplopen*
procarbazine
Natulan
prochlorperazine maleate
Buccastem
Stemetil
Vertigon
procyclidine
Arpicolin
Kemadrin
progesterone
Cyclogest
Gestone
proguanil
Paludrine
prolintane
Villescon*
promazine
Sparine
promethazine hydrochloride
Avomine
Medised*
Pamergan P100*
Phenergan
Phensedyl*
Sominex
propafenone
Arythmol
propantheline bromide
Pro-Banthine
propranolol
Bedranol SR
Berkolol
Inderal
Inderal LA
Inderetic*
Inderex*
propyl undecenoate
Monphytol* (ext.)
protriptyline
Concordin
proxymetacaine
Ophthaine
pseudoephedrine
Actifed*
Benelyn*
Congesteze*
Dimotane Co*
Dimotane Expectorant*
Dimotane Plus*
Galpseud
Sudafed
Sudafed-co*
Sudafed Plus
pyrantel embonate
Combantrin
pyrazinamide
Rifater*
Zinamide
pyridostigmine bromide
Mestinon
pyrimethamine
Daraprim
Fansidar*
Maloprim*
quinalbarbitone sodium
Seconal Sodium
Tuinal*
quinapril
Accupro
quinidine bisulphate
Kiditard
Kinidin Durules
ramipril
Tritace
ranitidine
Zantac
razoxane
Razoxin
reproterol
Bronchodil
reserpine
Serpasil
Serpasil Esidrex*
resorcinol
Eskamel* (ext.)
rifampicin
Rifadin
Rifater*
Rifinah*
Rimactane
Rimactazid*
rimiterol
Pulmadil
ritodrine
Yutopar
salbutamol
Aerolin Autohaler
Salbulin
Salbuvent
Ventide*
Ventodisks
Ventolin
Volmax
salcatonin
Calsynar
Miacalcic
salsalate
Disalcid
selegiline
Eldepryl
selenium sulphide
Lenium (ext.)
Selsun (ext.)
silver sulphadiazine

Flamazine (ext.)
simethicone – *see* **dimethicone (activated)**
simvastatin
Zocor
sodium acid phosphate
Carbalax*
Fletchers' phosphate*
Phosphate-Sandoz*
sodium alginate
Algitec*
Gastrocote*
Gaviscon*
Pyrogastrone*
sodium aurothiomalate
Myocrisin
sodium bicarbonate
Carbalax*
Caved-S*
Dioralyte*
Electrolade*
Gastrocote*
Gastron*
Gaviscon*
Gluco-Lyte*
GoLytely*
Klean-prep*
Mictral*
Phosphate-Sandoz*
Pyrogastrone*
Rehidrat*
Roter*
sodium cellulose phosphate
Calcisorb
sodium chloride
Diarrest*
Dioralyte*
Electrolade*
Glandosane*
Gluco-Lyte*
GoLytely*
Klean-prep*
Minims Artificial Tears*
Minims Saline
Miol* (ext.)
Normasol (ext.)
Opulets Saline
Rehidrat*
Sential* (ext.)
Sential E* (ext.)
Slow Sodium
Topiclens (ext.)
Uriflex S
sodium citrate
Benylin*
Diarrest*
Guanor*
Micolette*
Micralax*
Mictral*
Relaxit*
Urisal
sodium clodronate
Loron
sodium cromoglycate
Intal
Intal compound*
Nalcrom
Opticrom
Rynacrom
Rynacrom Compound*
sodium fluoride
En-De-Kay
Fluor-a-day
Fluorigard
Zymafluor
sodium fusidate
Fucibet* (ext.)
Fucidin
Fucidin H* (ext.)
Fucidin Intertulle
Fucithalmic
sodium heparin
Minihep Sodium*
Pump-Hep
sodium hypochlorite
Chlorasol (ext.)
sodium lactate
Hydromol* (ext.)
sodium lauryl sulphate
Relaxit*
sodium lauryl sulphoacetate
Micolette*
sodium nitroprusside
Nipride
sodium perborate
Bocasan
sodium phosphate
Fletchers' phosphate*
sodium picosulphate
Laxoberal
Picolax*
sodium sulphate
GoLytely*
Klean-prep*
sodium valproate
Epilim
somatropin
Genotropin
Humatrope
Norditropin
Saizen
sotalol hydrochloride
Beta-Cardone
Sotacor
Sotazide*
Tolerzide*
spectinomycin
Trobicin
spironolactone
Aldactide*
Aldactone
Diatensec
Lasilactone*
Spiretic
Spiroctan
stanozolol
Stromba
sterculia
Alvercol
Normacol
Normacol Plus*
Prefil
stilboestrol
Tampovagan stilboestrol and lactic acid*
streptodornase
Varidase*
streptokinase
Kabikinase
Streptase
Varidase*
sucralfate
Antepsin
sulbactam
Dicapen
sulconazole nitrate
Exelderm (ext.)
sulfadoxine
Fansidar*
sulfametopyrazine
Kelfizine W
sulindac
Clinoril

sulphabenzamide
Sultrin*
sulphacarbamide
Uromide*
sulphacetamide
Albucid
Minims
Sulphacetamide
Sultrin*
sulphadimidine
Sulphamezathine
sulphamethoxazole
Bactrim*
Chemotrim*
Comox*
Fectrim*
Laratrim*
Septrin*
sulphasalazine
Salazopyrin
sulphathiazole
Sultrin*
sulphinpyrazone
Anturan
sulpiride
Dolmatil
Sulpitil
suxamethonium chloride
Anectine
Scoline
talampicillin
Talpen
tamoxifen
Noltam
Nolvadex
Tamofen
teicoplanin
Targocid
temazepam
Normison
temocillin
Temopen
tenoxicam
Mobiflex
terazosin
Hytrin
terbutaline
Bricanyl
Bricanyl Expectorant*
Bricanyl SA
Monovent
terfenadine
Triludan
terlipressin
Glypressin*
terodiline
Micturin
testosterone
Primoteston Depot
Restandol
Sustanon
Virormone
tetrabenazine
Nitoman
tetracosactrin
Synacthen
tetracycline
Achromycin
Deteclo*
Mysteclin*
Sustamycin
Tetrabid
Tetrachel
Topicycline (ext.)
theophylline
Biophylline
Franol*
Franol Plus*
Labophylline*
Lasma
Nuelin
Pro-Vent
Sabidal SR
Slo-Phyllin
Theo-Dur
Uniphyllin Continus
thiabendazole
Mintezol
thiethylperazine
Torecan
thioguanine
Lanvis
thiopentone sodium
Intraval
thioridazine
Melleril
thymoxamine
Minims Thymoxamine
Opilon
thyroxine sodium
Eltroxin
tiaprofenic acid
Surgam
ticarcillin
Ticar
Timentin*
timolol maleate
Betim
Blocadren
Moducren*
Prestim*
Timoptol
tinidazole
Fasigyn
tioconazole
Trosyl
tobramycin
Nebcin
Tobralex
tocainide
Tonocard
tocopheryl
Concavit*
Ephynal
Ketovite*
Multibionta*
Octovit*
Vita-E
Vita-E Ointment (ext.)
tolazamide
Tolanase
tolbutamide
Rastinon
tolmetin
Tolectin
tolnaftate
Timoped* (ext.)
Tinaderm-M* (ext.)
Tineafax Cream* (ext.)
Tineafax Powder (ext.)
tramazoline
Dexa-Rhinaspray*
tranexamic acid
Cyklokapron
tranylcypromine sulphate
Parnate
Parstelin*
trazodone
Molipaxin
tretinoin
Retin-A (ext.)
tripotassium dicitratobismuthate
De-Nol
De-Noltab

triamcinolone
Adcortyl
Adcortyl with Graneodin* (ext.)
Adcortyl in Orabase
Audicort*
Aureocort* (ext.)
Kenalog
Ledercort
Lederspan
Nystadermal* (ext.)
Pevaryl TC* (ext.)
Tri-Adcortyl* (ext.)
Tri-Adcortyl Otic*
triamterene
Dyazide*
Dytac
Dytide*
Frusene*
Kalspare*
Triamco*
triazolam
Halcion
tribavirin
Virazid
trifluoperazine
Parstelin*
Stelazine
trifluperidol
Triperidol
triglycerides, omega 3
Maxepa*
trimeprazine
Vallergan
trimetaphan
Arfonad
trimethoprim
Bactrim*
Chemotrim*
Comox*
Fectrim*
Ipral
Laratrim*
Monotrim
Polytrim*
Septrin*
Syraprim
Trimopan
trimipramine
Surmontil
triprolidine
Actidil
Actifed*
Pro-Actidil
Sudafed Plus*
trisodium edetate
Limclair
tropicamide
Minims tropicamide
Mydriacyl
tubocurarine chloride
Jexin
Tubarine
tyrothricin
Tyrozets*
urofollitropin
Metrodin
urokinase
Ukidan
ursodeoxycholic acid
Destolit
Ursofalk
vancomycin
Vancocin
vasopressin – *see* **antidiuretic hormone**
vecuronium bromide
Norcuron
verapamil
Cordilox
Securon
Univer
vigabatrin
Sabril
viloxazine
Vivalan
vinblastine
Velbe
vincristine
Oncovin
vindesine
Eldisine
viper venom – *see* **ancrod**
vitamin K – *see* **phytomenadione**
warfarin
Marevan
xamoterol
Corwin
xipamide
Diurexan
xylometazoline
Otrivine
Otrivine-Antistin*
Rynacrom Compound*
zidovudine
Retrovir
zinc sulphate
Efalith* (ext.)
Fefol Z*
Fesovit Z*
Octovit*
Ocusol*
Solvazinc
Z Span Spansule
zinc undecenoate
Phytocil* (ext.)
zuclopenthixol
Clopixol

Appendix 2 *UPDATE*

New preparations

Aclarubicin (Aclacin, powder in vial)
Is an anti-cancer drug used to treat acute non-lymphatic leukaemia in individuals who have failed to respond to first line treatment. It is an anthracycline and produces effects similar to those of doxorubicin (page, 1061).

Harmful effects include dose related damage to bone marrow, resulting in a fall in white cells and platelets in the blood. It may cause nausea, vomiting, diarrhoea, sore mouth and changes in liver function. Rarely, it may damage the heart, cause allergic reactions and alopecia. Infusions may cause phlebitis at the site of injection.

Warnings It should not be used in pregnancy, in breast feeding mothers or in individuals with severe bone-marrow impairment. It should be used with caution in people with impaired kidney, liver or heart function, or raised blood uric acid levels. Blood tests and tests of heart function should be carried out at regular intervals.

Acrivastine (Semprex capsules)
Is a non-sedative antihistamine, see page 94.
Harmful effects It may rarely produce drowsiness.

Warnings It should not be used in people with kidney failure. It should be used with caution in pregnancy and when breast feeding. It may increase the effects of alcohol and affect ability to drive (see harmful effects and warnings on the use of antihistamines, page 96). It should not be used in children under 12 years of age or in elderly people.

Cetirizine (Zirtek tablets)
Is a non-sedative antihistamine, see page 94.
Harmful effects include stomach and bowel upsets, dry mouth, dizziness, headache, drowsiness and agitation.

Warnings Do not use if breast feeding. It should be used with caution in people with impaired kidney function and in pregnancy. It may increase the effects of alcohol and affect ability to drive. Do not use in children under 12 years of age.

Carboprost (Hemebate solution in ampoules)
Is a prostaglandin used to treat haemorrhage after childbirth due to failure of

the womb to contact (atony) – see page 953. Carboprost is recommended when oxytocin combined with ergometrine has failed.

Harmful effects include nausea, vomiting, high temperature, flushing and wheezing. Occasionally it may cause a rise in blood pressure, breathlessness and fluid on the lungs (pulomary oedema).

Warnings It should be used with caution if the womb is scarred from previous injury or if there is acute infection around the uterus (acute pelvic inflammatory disease). It should be used with caution in women with anaemia, asthma, diabetes, epilepsy, glaucoma, jaundice, or impaired heart, liver or kidney function. Individuals with heart and/or chest disorders should be monitored carefully and given additional oxygen if necessary.

Enoxaparin (Clexane)

Is a low molecular weight heparin (LMWH) obtained by breaking down the natural heparin molecule (by partial depolymerization). These low weight molecules have a greater effect against the formation of a thrombus but produce less risk of bleeding than the parent molecule of heparin. Their effects also last much longer and they need only be given once daily. Enoxaparin is used to prevent embolism from thrombi in veins (see pages 382, 389), particularly those associated with surgery. It is also used to prevent clotting during kidney dialysis.

Harmful effects include a fall in blood platelets (thrombocytopenia) and disorders of liver function. For other potential harmful effects see **heparin** page 392.

Warnings It should not be used to treat individuals with acute bacterial endocarditis, serious bleeding disorders, acute peptic ulcers, or who have suffered a stroke due to bleeding into the brain or who have a low blood platelet count. It should not be given by intramuscular injection. It should be used with caution in people with impaired liver function or a history of peptic or intestinal ulceration, in pregnancy, in breast-feeding mothers and in individuals with uncontrolled high blood pressure.

Erythropoietin (Eprex injections: epoetin alfa; Recormon injections: epoetin beta

Is used to treat anaemia associated with chronic kidney failure in individuals on kidney dialysis. Erythropoietin (see pages 705, 715) is a hormone, principally formed by the kidneys, that regulates the production of red blood cells by the bone marrow, a process known as erythropoiesis. The kidneys trigger the production of erythropoietin if the oxygen level in the kidney tissues falls. Kidney disease resulting in a failure of the kidneys to produce erythropoietin will cause anaemia, which can now be successfully treated with epoetin alfa or beta.

Harmful effects include flu-like symptoms, skin rashes, raised blood pressure and thrombosis at the site of injection. Rarely it may cause seizures.

Warnings It should not be used in children. It should be used with caution in people with raised blood pressure, coronary artery disease, a history of epilepsy, and during pregnancy. Drug treatment of blood pressure may be neccessary and diet and dialysis treatment may need to be adjusted. Tests for anaemia, blood pressure and chemistry of the blood should be carried out at regular intervals. Anaemia due to other causes should be treated.

Flutamide (Drogenil tablets)

Is an anti-male-sex-hormone drug (anti-androgen). It is used to treat cancer of the prostate gland (see page 1065).

Harmful effects include swelling and tenderness of the breasts with milk production. It may also cause nausea, vomiting, diarrhoea, increased appetite, tiredness and insomnia.

Warnings It should not be used in individuals who are sensitive to flutamide. It should be used with caution in men with heart disease because it may cause retention of fluids in the body. Regular tests of liver function should be carried out.

Fosinopril (Staril tablets)

Is an ACE inhibitor (see page 296) used to treat raised blood pressure.

Harmful effects include dizziness, stomach and bowel upsets, coughing, chest pain, skin rash, muscle and joint pains and taste disturbances. Rarely it may cause angioedema (stop immediately).

Warnings Should not be used in pregnancy and when breast feeding. It should be used with caution in individuals with impaired liver or kidney function, congestive heart failure or raised blood pressure associated with impaired kidney function.

Gamolenic acid (gamma-linolenic acid, GLA, Eflamast capsules)

Is obtained from oil of evening primrose (see pages 676–7). It is used to treat painful breasts (mastalgia) which may be cyclical (e.g. with menstrual periods) or non-cyclical. The discomfort appears to be due to sensitivity to female sex hormones which may be caused by an abnormal ratio of saturated to unsaturated fatty acids in the breast tissue. The pain can be relieved by reducing the ratio of these fatty acids by taking gamolenic acid which provides a high source of unsaturated fatty acids (see page 676). It may take up to six months to produce any benefit.

Harmful effects include nausea, headache and indigestion.

Warnings It should be used with caution in women with a history of epilepsy or who are pregnant. Cancer of the breast should be excluded before treatment.

Gestrinone (Dimetriose capsules)

Is used to treat endometriosis (see page 924). It has both anti-oestrogenic and anti-progestogenic properties. It reduces the secretion of LH and FSH by the pituitary gland and therefore reduces the release of oestrogens and progesterone by the ovaries. It also blocks progesterone receptors in endometrial tissues (i.e. the lining of the womb and other endometrial deposits, see page 924) causing them to shrink. It also dries up the menstrual periods. It offers an alternative to danazol (see page 924) and needs to be taken only twice weekly instead of daily.

Harmful effects include fluid retention, weight gain, acne, stomach and bowel upsets, changes in appetite, hot flushes, cramps, nervousness, depression, changes in libido, and very rarely male-type hair growth and voice changes.

Warnings It should not be used in women with severe heart, kidney or liver disorders, or when breast feeding. It should not be used in women with diabetes or raised blood-fat levels. It should not be used in pregnancy or if there is a risk of the woman being pregnant. Women on treatment should avoid sexual intercourse or use a barrier contraceptive (e.g. condom, cap). It may interact with anti-epileptic drugs, oral contraceptives and rifampicin.

Humegon

Freeze-dried preparation in ampoules contains human menopausal gonadotrophin (HMG), human follicle stimulating hormone (FSH) and human luteinizing hormone (LH). It is used to treat male and female infertility (see pages 942–5) due to inadequate gonadotrophin stimulation of the testes and ovaries respectively. It is also used to stimulate egg production in fertilization programmes.

Harmful effects include allergic reactions, and overdose may cause hyperstimulation syndrome. This may be mild (mild swelling of the ovaries, abdominal distension and pain), moderate (moderate swelling of the ovaries with more severe abdominal distension and pain plus nausea, vomiting and occasionally diarrhoea) or severe (severe enlargement of the ovaries with pronounced abdominal distension and pain, fluid in the abdomen and chest cavities, decreased blood volume, reduced production of urine and disturbances of the blood chemistry).

Warnings It should not be used to treat individuals with tumours of the pituitary gland, testes or ovaries. It should be used with caution if there is any abnormality of the genital organs. There is an increased risk of miscarriage and multiple pregnancies if pregnancy occurs.

Idarubicin (Zavedos powder in vials)

Is an anti-cancer drug related to daunorubicin. It is a cytotoxic antibiotic (see page 1061).

Harmful effects include damage to the bone marrow producing blood disorders and, rarely, damage to the heart. It may cause nausea, vomiting, diarrhoea, sore mouth and oesophagus, fever, chills and skin rashes. It may affect liver function, cause reversible alopecia and discoloration of the urine. Very rarely, the individual may develop very severe infections.

Warnings It should not be used in individuals with severe impairment of liver or kidney function, uncontrolled infections or who are breast feeding. It should be used with caution in people with impaired bone-marrow function, heart disease or who have received similar drugs in high doses. Patients over 55 years will need special care during the period when the bone marrow is not working. Uric acid levels should be checked at intervals. Any infections should be treated before treatment starts. Leakage at the site of injection may cause thrombophlebitis.

Leuprorelin (Prostap SR powder in vial for injection)
Is used to treat serious cancer of the prostate gland (see page 1065). It is a gonadotrophin-releasing hormone analogue that stimulates the pituitary gland to release LH and FSH, which initially stimulates the testes to produce testosterone but subsequently causes the pituitary to switch off the production of LH and FSH causing the blood level of testosterone to fall so that within about three weeks an effect similar to castration is achieved (chemical castration, see page 959).

Harmful effects include decreased libido, impotence, hot flushes, sweating, ankle swelling, fatigue and nausea. It may cause pain at the injection site and initially, when blood testosterone levels are up, it may cause bone pain and difficulty passing urine.

Warnings To reduce the flare-up of symptoms at start of treatment an anti-male sex hormone drug (anti-androgen) should be given 3 days before starting treatment and continued for 2–3 weeks.

Loratadine (Clarityn tablets)
Is a non-sedative antihistamine, see page 94.
Harmful effects include nausea, headaches, fatigue.

Warnings Do not use in pregnancy or when breast feeding. It should not be used in children under 12 years of age. It is not recommended for use in elderly people.

Norfloxacin (Utinor tablets)
Is a quinolone antibiotic (see page 758) used to treat infections of the urinary tract.

Harmful effects include nausea, heartburn, abdominal cramps, diarrhoea, loss of appetite, headache, dizziness, anxiety, irritability, sleep disturbances and skin rashes.

Warnings It should not be used in pregnancy and breast-feeding mothers. It should be used with caution in individuals who have suffered from epilepsy or who have impaired kidney function.

Ondansetron (Zofran tablets)
Is used to treat nausea and vomiting caused by anti-cancer drugs and radiotherapy (see pages 180–81). It is a 5HT blocker (see page 31) which is able to control vomiting induced by stimulation of receptors in the small intestine and the chemoreceptor trigger zone (CTZ).

Harmful effects include headache, flushing and constipation. Rarely, it may cause allergic reactions and occasionally alter liver function.

Warnings It should not be used in breast-feeding mothers and it should be used with caution in pregnancy.

Oxitropium (Oxivent inhaler)
An anticholinergic drug administered by inhaler to treat asthma (see page 147).

Harmful effects include local irritation of the nose and throat, dry mouth and nausea. Rarely it may produce general anticholinergic effects (see page 18) such as blurred vision and difficulty passing urine.

Warnings It should not be used by individuals allergic to atropine or ipratropium and it should be used with caution in people with glaucoma or enlarged prostate gland. Contact with eyes should be avoided. It should not be used in pregnancy or when breast feeding. It should be stopped if wheezing, coughing or tightness in the chest develops.

Pravastatin (Lipostat tablets)
Is used to treat people with raised blood cholesterol levels which have not responded to other treatments (see pages 372–8). It blocks the effects of an enzyme involved in the production of cholesterol. This reduces the level of cholesterol in the blood, which stimulates an increase in LDL receptors that help to reduce the level of LDL in the blood (see page 367). It differs from similar drugs insofar as it is hydrophillic (attracted to water), which impedes its uptake by cells. This reduces its effects on cholesterol production by the cells and may reduce the risk of harmful effects e.g. on the brain. However, it is actively taken up by the cells in the liver.

Harmful effects include nausea, vomiting, diarrhoea, fatigue, headache, muscle pains, chest pains and skin rashes.

Warnings It should not be used in pregnancy and breast-feeding mothers or in individuals with active liver disease, or on raised blood cholesterol due to a high LDL level. It should be used with caution in people with a history of liver disease or heavy alcohol drinking.

Pregnyl (powder in ampoules)
Contains human chorionic gonadotrophin (HCG). It is used to 'treat infertility in males and females (see pages 942–5).

Harmful effects include salt and water retention in the body and skin rashes.

Warnings It should not be used in individuals suffering from cancers dependent upon male sex hormones for their growth. Because it causes salt and fluid retention it should be used with caution in individuals with raised blood pressure, impaired kidney or heart function, epilepsy or migraine.

Ramipril (Tritace capsules)
Is an ACE inhibitor used to treat mild to moderate hypertension (see page 296). It is a pro-drug, which means that it is inactive until it is activated in the liver to form ramiprilat which is a long acting ACE inhibitor.

Harmful effects include nausea, vomiting, abdominal pains, diarrhoea, headache, dizziness, fatigue and cough. Rarely it may cause a marked fall in blood pressure, faintness, allergic reactions, angioedema, and impaired kidney function.

Warnings It should not be used in individuals with a history of angioedema, in pregnancy or in breast-feeding mothers. It should not be used in people with aortic stenosis or obstruction to the outflow of blood from the heart. It should be used with utmost caution in individuals with congestive heart failure and impaired liver function. Kidney function should be checked before and at regular intervals during treatment, and the dose reduced according to the degree of impaired function. Diuretic drugs should be stopped 2 to 3 days before starting treatment with ramipril otherwise there is an increased risk of a marked fall in blood pressure.

Salmeterol (Serevent inhaler, diskhaler)
A selective (beta) adrenoreceptor stimulant used to treat asthma (see pages 147–9). It is also used for treating asthma at night, exercise-induced asthma and wheezing associated with bronchitis. It is formulated to remain at the site of action in order to produce long-lasting effects (12 hours) so that it need only be taken twice daily. In addition to its bronchodilator effects (see page 147) salmeterol helps to control the release of chemicals (e.g. histamine, prostaglandins) that produce inflammation.

Harmful effects Rarely, it may cause tremor, headaches and palpitations (for other potential harmful effects see page 149, 163–4).

Warnings It should be used with caution in pregnancy and breast-feeding mothers and with selective beta blockers.

Scherisorb (Hydrogel)
Is used to remove sloughs from ulcers (see page 1017) and wounds. It maintains a moist environment, rehydrates dead tissue and absorbs sloughs.

Sertraline (Lustral capsules)

Is used to treat depression (see page 589). It increases the amount of the stimulant nerve transmitter 5-hydroxytryptamine (5HT, serotonin) in the brain by blocking its re-uptake by nerve cells. Because it has less effect on other stimulant nerve transmitters in the nervous system it produces less drowsiness than the tricyclic antidepressants and produces fewer anticholinergic effects and effects in the heart. It may possibly be safer in overdose.

Harmful effects include dry mouth, nausea, diarrhoea, tremor, sweating, indigestion and delayed ejaculation.

Warnings It should not be used in individuals with impaired kidney or liver function and it should be used with caution in pregnancy, breast-feeding mothers and people with unstable epilepsy.

Sodium clodronate (Loron capsules and infusion)

Is used to keep blood calcium levels (see page 694) within normal ranges in individuals suffering from a high blood calcium caused by certain cancers (e.g. cancer of the breast, kidney, bronchus) in which calcium is dissolved from bone into the bloodstream and also reabsorbed by the kidneys out of the urine and back into the blood. Sodium clodronate decreases blood calcium levels by suppressing the dissolving of bone and increasing the excretion of calcium in the urine without affecting the laying down of calcium in the bone.

Harmful effects Oral treatment may cause nausea or mild diarrhoea which may benefit from dividing the daily dose and taking it twice daily instead of once daily. Rarely, allergic reactions may occur, infusions may cause protein in the urine, and the blood calcium may fall below normal levels.

Warnings It should not be used in individuals with moderate to severe impairment of kidney function, or by mouth in people with inflammatory intestinal disorders, in pregnancy or in breast-feeding mothers. Blood calcium and phosphates should be measured during infusions. Kidney-function tests should be carried out before and during treatment by mouth and infusion. Duration of treatment (300 mg per day over two hours) should not exceed ten days and by mouth (4 to 8 capsules daily, one hour before or after food) should not exceed six months.

Terbinafine (Lamisil tablets)

An antifungal drug taken by mouth to treat severe or extensive ringworm (see page 783).

Harmful effects include nausea, abdominal pain, allergic skin rashes.

Warnings It should be used with caution in individuals with impaired kidney function, severe liver disease, during pregnancy and in breast-feeding mothers.

Vigabatrin (Sabril tablets)

Is an anti-epileptic drug (see page 571).

Harmful effects include drowsiness, fatigue, dizziness, irritability and nervousness. It may affect the memory and vision and cause excitation and agitation in children. Frequency of seizures may increase in individuals suffering from myoclonic seizures.

Warnings It should not be used in pregnancy or when breast feeding. It should be used with caution in individuals with impaired kidney function and in elderly people. Regular medical check-ups should be carried out and the drug should be withdrawn slowly over 2 to 4 weeks.

Index

NOTE

Drugs that should not be used, or used with caution, during pregnancy are listed on pages 1119–28.

Drugs that enter the breast milk and may affect the baby are listed on pages 1130–33.

Drugs that should not be used, or used with caution, in people with impaired liver function are listed on pages 1153–8.

Drugs that should not be used, or used with caution, in people with impaired kidney function are listed on pages 1166–77.

Drug interactions are listed on pages 1193–1246.

AAA 427
Abortion 951
  abortion pill 954
  prostaglandins in 951
ABVD therapy 1057
Accupro 302, 331
Acebutolol
  in angina 279
  in disorders of heart rhythm 350
  in hypertension 304
Acepril 302, 331
ACE inhibitors
  in heart failure 326
  in hypertension 296
Acetazolamide 317
  harmful effects and warnings 536, 567
  in epilepsy 570, 571
  in glaucoma 534, 535, 539
Acetic acid
  in cough expectorants 49
  in vaginal applications 948
  in wart applications 1046
Acetohexamide 873
Acetylcholine 11
Acetylcholine esterase 12
Acetylcysteine 51
Acezide 306
Achromycin 65, 526, 752, 989
Achromycin V 752
Acid reflux *see* Heartburn
Acidification of urine 488, 493
Aci-jel 947, 948
Acipimox 378
Acne 734, 1006–12
  pyridoxine in 678
Acne rosacea 1012
Acquired Immune Deficiency Syndrone *see* AIDS
Acridine antiseptics 995
Acriflavine 995
Acrivastine 94
Acrocyanosis 360
Acrolein 1060
Acromegaly 820
Acrosoxacin 758, 763
Actal 197
ACTH 840–41
Acthar Gel 824
Actidil 95
Actifed
Actilyse 272, 277, 397
Actinomycin D 1061
Actonorm 197
  in heartburn 213
Acupan 409
Acu Pulse Band 179
Acyclovir 788
  harmful effects and warnings 793
  in chickenpox 791
  in cold sores 172
  in herpes infections of the eyes 521, 527
  in herpes simplex infections 790
  in shingles 791
Adalat 277, 302, 365
Adcortyl and Graneodin 986
Adcortyl in Orabase 171
Adcortyl injections 452
Adcortyl skin preparations 983
Addiction *see* Drug dependence
Addisonian crisis (acute adrenal failure) 830
ADH *see* Anti-diuretic hormone
Adifax 649
Adizem continus *see* Dilitiazem
Adrenal cortex 827
  hormones produced by 827

Adrenal crisis *see* Adrenal failure
Adrenal failure 830–31
  acute 831
Adrenal glands 827–31
  acute failure of (adrenal crisis) 831
  failure of 831
  overactivity of 828, 829
  underactivity of 830
Adrenal medulla 28, 827
  hormones produced by 28, 827
Adrenaline
  harmful effects and warnings in eyes 536
  in anaphylactic shock 103
  in asthma 165, 166
  in glaucoma 533, 534, 539
  in insect stings and bites 1030
  in local anaesthetics 425
  uses of 25
Adrenergic neurone blocking drugs
  actions 27
  in hypertension 294
Adrenocortical steroids 62
Adrenocorticotrophic hormone *see* Corticotrophin
Adrenoreceptor stimulants (beta-stimulants)
  harmful effects and warnings 163–4
  in asthma 147–9, 160
  in premature labour 953–4
  preparations 165–8
Adriamycin 1057
Aerolin 165
Aerosporin 763
Afrazine 70
Agar 649
Ageing
  vitamin B complex in 678
  vitamin C in 678
  vitamin D in 678
  vitamin supplements in 678
Agranulocytosis 1083
AIDS 506–20
  and vaccinations 141
  drug treatment of 514
Akineton 552
Albacon 787
Albucid 526
Alclometasone 983, 984
Alcohol
  and risk of drug treatments 1183–5
Alcoholism
  vitamin B complex in 678
Alcopar 815
Alcuronium 19
Aldactide 329, 331
Aldactone 328
Aldomet 302
Aldosterone 827
  drugs which block (antagonists) 319
  overproduction of (aldosteronism) 829
Aldosterone antagonists 319
Alexan 1061
Alexitol 197
Alfentanil 419
Algicon 197
  in heartburn 213
Alginates 196
Alginic acid 196
Algitec 213
Alkalinisation of urine 488, 493
Alkeran 1060
Alka-Seltzer 412
Alkylating drugs 1060
Allantoin
  in psoriasis 1038
Allegron 499, 599
Aller-eze 94, 95
Allergic emergencies *see* Anaphylactic shock
Allergies 88–107, 1178
Allergic rhinitis *see* Hayfever
Alloferin 19
Allopurinol 479, 483
  harmful effects and warnings 481
Allyloestrenol 897, 901
Almasilate 197
Almazine 623
Alopecia *see* Baldness
Alopecia areata 1014–15
Aloxiprin 442, 451
Alpha-adrenoceptor blocking drugs *see* Alpha blockers
Alpha/beta blockers
  in angina 267
  in hypertension 294
Alpha blockers
  in disorders of the circulation 353
  in hypertension 293
Alphaderm 985
Alphosyl, HC 984
Alprazolam 625
Alrheumat 451
Altacite 197
  in heartburn 213
Alteplase 272
  harmful effects and warnings 397
Alu-Cap 197
Aludrox 197
Aludrox SA 230
Aluhyde 197, 230
Aluline 483
Alum 171
Aluminium acetate 62, 65
Aluminium hydroxide 197
  in antacids 193
Aluminium hydroxide and belladonna 197, 230
Aluminium salts
  in antacids 193, 197, 198, 199
Alunex 95
Alupram 470, 623
Aluzine 328
Alverine
  in diarrhoea 218
  in spasm of the intestine 229
Alzheimer's disease
  aluminium in 678
  vitamins in 678
Amantadine
  harmful effects and warnings 549, 793
  in influenza 788, 792–3
  in parkinsonism 547, 552, 553
Ambaxin 742
Ambenonium 13
Ambutonium 229
Amethocaine 427, 523, 528
Amfipen 742
Amikacin 757
Amikin 757
Amilko 329, 331
Amiloride
  harmful effects and warnings 334
  in heart failure 328, 329
Aminacrine 995
Aminobenzoic acid 675
  in sunscreens 1000, 1002, 1005
Aminoglutethimide
  harmful effects and warnings 1066
  in breast cancer 1064
  in Cushing's syndrome 829
Aminoglycosides 754–7
  harmful effects and warnings 754–6
Aminophylline
  in asthma 150

in emergency treatment of asthma 163
preparations to treat asthma 165, 166
5-Aminosalicylic acid (5-ASA) 225
Amiodarone 349
harmful effects and warnings 346
Amitriptyline
in bedwetting 499
in depression 599, 600
in migraine 434
Amlodipine
harmful effects and warnings 269
in angina 269
in hypertension 304
Ammonium chloride
in cough expectorants 49
to acidify the urine 493
Amodiaquine 798, 801
Amoebic dysentry 804
Amoxapine 599
Amoxil 742
Amoxycillin 738, 742
in bronchitis 734
in dental abscess 734
preparations 742
Amoxycillin/clavulinic acid (co-amoxyclav) 744
in typhoid fever 734
Amphetamines 638
and libido 972
in slimming 648
Amphotericin 780, 787
harmful effects and warnings 785
in preparations used to treat thrush of the mouth 174
in skin preparations 992
in vaginal infections 949
Ampicillin 738, 742, 743
in bronchitis 734
in gonorrhoea 506
Ampicillin/sulbactam 745
Ampiclox 744
Amsacrine 1062
Amsidine 1062
Amylobarbitone 582
Amytal 582
Anabolic steroids 961–6
in osteoporosis 930
Anaemias 704–25
aplastic 1082
aplastic, anabolic steroids in 962
haemolytic 720, 1084
folic acid deficiency 718–20, 1084
in chronic disease 713
in red cell aplasia 1083
iron-deficiency 705–15
megaloblastic 716, 719
pernicious 717
vitamin B12 deficiency 615, 715–18, 1085
Anaesthetics, local 423–7
harmful effects and warnings 426
in eye disorders 523
in insect stings and bites 1029
in itching 1031
in mouth ulcers 171
in slimming 651
in throat lozenges and pastilles 43
in urethral pain 494
preparations 427
skin preparations 988
Anaflex 174, 989
Anafranil 599
Analgesics *see* Pain-relieving drugs
Anaphylactic shock 102
treatment of 103
Anapolon-50 966
Ancrod 384
harmful effects and warnings 392
Andrews Liver Salts 244
Androcur 959, 973, 975
Androgens *see* Male sex hormones
Andursil 197
in heartburn 213
Anectine 20
Aneurine *see* Vitamin B_1
Anflam 983
Angettes 277
Angilol 349, 438
Angina 253–80
vitamin E in 679
Angioedema 89, 962
Angioneurotic oedema *see* Angioedema
Angiotensin 282
Angiotensin-converting enzyme inhibitors *see* ACE inhibitors
Anistreplase 273
harmful effects and warnings 397
Anorectics *see* Slimming drugs
Anorexia nervosa
zinc in 679
Anquil 636
Antabuse 1184, 1185
Antacids 190
minerals in 197
preparations 197
Antazoline 70
Antepar 816
Antepsin 207
Anthical 993
Anthisan 993
Anthraquinones 234
Anthrax vaccine 110
Anti-androgens *see* Anti-male sex hormones
Anti-anxiety drugs 605–25
and sex 970
Anti-arrhythmic drugs 343–51
Anti-bacterials 726–34
in diarrhoea 219
in eye disorders 521
in urinary tract infections 486
skin applications 990
suggested uses of 734
Antibiotics *see* Antibacterials
Anti-blood-clotting drugs *see* Anti-coagulants
Antibodies 77
Anti-cancer drugs 1054–67
Anti-cholinergic drugs 14–18
harmful effects and warnings 18
and sex 969
in asthma 145, 161
in cold remedies 38
in cough medicines 51
in diarrhoea 218
in peptic ulcers 195, 196, 200
in spasm of the intestine 229
in vomiting 176
uses of 16
Anticholinesterases 12–13
Anti-coagulants 383–93
in heart attacks 275
preparations 394
Anti-convulsants *see* Anti-epileptics
Anti-D (Rhesus) immunoglobulin 140, 737
Anti-depressant drugs 585–603
and sex 970
in bedwetting 499
in incontinence of urine 497
in urinary frequency 495

Anti-depressant drugs – *cont.*
lithium 596
monoamine oxidase inhibitors (MAOIs) 593–6
preparations 599–601
to decrease sexual activity 974
tricyclics 586–90
Anti-diabetic drugs 869–72
and sunlight sensitivity 1006
Anti-diarrhoeal drugs 217–9
Anti-diuretic hormone *see* Vasopressin
Anti-emetics *see* Anti-vomiting drugs
Anti-epileptics 570, 571
Anti-fibrinolytic drugs 396
harmful effects and warnings 398
Anti-fungal drugs 780–87
in eye diseases 522
in mouth infections 170, 174
in vaginal thrush 947
skin preparations 993
Anti-herpes simplex immunoglobulin 140
Antihistamines 90–7
harmful effects and warnings 96–7
actions of 90
in allergic disorders 91
in allergic emergencies 103–4
in cold remedies 36
in cough medicines 50
in eye diseases 523
in hayfever 105
in insect stings and bites 1029
in itching 1031, 1032
in motion sickness 178
in nausea and vomiting caused by morphine related drugs 180
in vertigo 183
in vomiting 176
skin preparations 993
Anti-hypertensive drugs 289–313
and sex 969
Anti-inflammatory drugs *see* NSAIDs
Anti-insulins 863
Anti-itching drugs 1030–33
in dandruff 1020
in eye disorders, dangers of 523
in itching anus 1032
in itching skin 1030–32
in itching vagina 1033
in psoriasis 1039
Anti-malarials 798–803
Anti-male sex hormones 959–73
in cancer of the prostate 1065
to decrease sexual activity 973
Anti-metabolites 1060, 1061
Anti-migraine drugs 430–38
Antimony compounds
in oriental sore 806
Antineoplastic drugs *see* Anti-cancer drugs
Anti-oestrogens 896
in breast cancer 1064
Anti-perspirants 1044
Anti-platelet drugs 379
Antipressan 277, 302
Antipruritics, topical *see* Anti-itching drugs
Anti-psychotics 627–37
harmful effects 627
abnormal movements caused by 633
and sex 970
and sunlight sensitivity 1006
depot injections of 634
in anxiety 619
in controlling behaviour 634
in schizophrenia 631
preparations 636, 637
to decrease sexual activity 974
warnings on use 365
Anti-rabies immunoglobulin 140
Antiseptics 994–7
in dandruff 1021
in insect stings and bites 1029
in mouth ulcers 171
in sore throat 42, 43
in vaginal infections 948
Antisera 110
harmful effects and warnings 142
Anti-spasmodics 229–31
Anti-tetanus immunoglobulin 140
Anti-thrombotic drugs 275, 277
Anti-thyroid drugs 848–50
Anti-tuberculous drugs 772–8
Antitussives *see* Cough suppressants
Anti-varicella-zoster immunoglobulin 140
Anti-venom
against ancrod 392
Anti-viral drugs 788–95
in AIDS 515
in eye disorders 521
skin preparations 993
Anti-vomiting drugs 176–86
in cancer treatment 180–82
in migraine 431
Antoin 412
Anturan 483
Anus
fissure of 249
itching of, (pruritus ani) *see* Itching
Anxiety 604–25
Anxiolytics *see* Anti-anxiety drugs
Aphrodisiacs 975
Aphthous ulcers 170
zinc in 679
Apisate 653
APP 197
Appetite stimulants 657
Appetite suppressants *see* Slimming drugs
Apresoline 302, 331
Aprinox 302, 328
Aprotinin 396
harmful effects and warnings 398
APSAC *see* Anistreplase
Apsifen 408, 451
Apsin VK 742
Apsolol 277, 302, 349, 438
Apsolox 277, 302, 349
Arachis oil 237
Aramine 26, 335
Arelix 302
Arfonad 302
Argipressin is synthetic vasopressin, *see* Vasopressin
Aromatic essential oils
in vapour rubs and inhalants 39
Arpicolin 552
Arpimycin 763
Arret *see* Loperamide
Artane 552
Arteriosclerosis
vitamin A in 679
vitamin C in 679
vitamin E in 679

Arthritis 464
 calcium in 679
 copper in 679
 fish oils in 679
 vitamin B complex in 679
 vitamin C in 679
Artracin 450
Arvin 392
Arvin Antidote 385, 392
Arythmol 349
5-ASA 225
Asacol 228
Ascabiol 1035, 1043
Ascalix 816
Ascorbic acid *see* Vitamin C
Asendis 599
ASEP 994
Aserbine 1017
Asilone 197, 213
Askit 412
Aspav 412
Aspergillosis 784
Aspirin
 harmful effects and warnings 404, 406, 453
 effects on platelets 395
 in chronic back pain 466
 in colds 34
 in dysmenorrhoea 923
 in gout 476
 in heart attacks 274, 275
 in migraine 430, 437
 in pain relief 405
 in PMS 920
 in preventing strokes 391
 in rheumatoid arthritis 442, 451, 452
Aspirin, paracetamol and codeine tablets 412
Aspirin-paracetamol ester *see* Benorylate
Astemizole 94
Asthma 143–68
 harmful effects and warnings of drugs used to treat 163
 aerosol nebulizer solutions in 159
 emergency treatment of 163
 inhaled preparations in 158
 preparations used to treat 165
 vitamin B complex in 679
 vitamin C in 679
Astringents
 in eye disorders 524
 in mouth ulcers 171
 in skin preparations 990
Atarax 623
Ataxia
 definition 618
Atenolol
 in angina 277, 280
 in disorders of heart rhythm 350
 in hypertension 302, 305
 in migraine 434
Atensine 470, 624
Atherosclerosis 355, 366
 pyridoxine in 679
 vitamin C in 679
 vitamin E in 679
Atherosclerosis obliterans 356
Athlete's foot 782, 1013
Ativan 571, 624
Atopy 1021
Atracurium 19
Atrial fibrillation 339
 anti-coagulants in 391
 in heart failure 327
Atromid-S 378
Atropine
 effects of 14
 in diarrhoea 218
 in disorders of heart rhythm 349
 in spasm of the intestine 229
 to dilate the pupils 525, 529, 530
 uses of 16
Atrovent 165
Attapulgite, activated 219
Attention-deficit disorders (ADD) 641
Audax 65
Audicort 65
Augmentin 739, 744
Auranofin 444
 harmful effects and warnings 459
Aureocort 986
Aureomycin 526, 752, 989
Aurothiomalate *see* Gold
Autism
 vitamin B complex in 679
 vitamin C in 679
Autoimmune disease 80
Aventyl 599
Avloclor 445, 803
Avomine 185
Axid 207
Azactam *see* Aztreonam
Azamune 83, 228, 446, 1062
Azapropazone
 harmful effects and warnings 453, 482
 in gout 476, 478, 479, 483
 in rheumatoid arthritis 452
Azatadine 94
Azathioprine
 immunosuppression and 82, 1062
 in Crohn's disease 223
 in rheumatoid arthritis 446
 in ulcerative colitis 225
Azidothymidine (AZT) *see* Zidovudine
Azlocillin 739, 743
AZT *see* Zidovudine
Aztreonam 748

Babies, infants and children, risks of drug treatments 1134–5
Bacampicillin 738, 742
Back pain
 chronic, treatment of 465–7
 vitamin C in 679
Bacillus Calmette-Guerin vaccine
Bacitracin 526
Baclofen
 harmful effects and warnings 468
 in chronic back pain 467
 preparations 470
Bactrim 770
Bactroban 71, 989, 1018
Baldness 1013–15
 oil of evening primrose in 678
 vitamin B complex in 678
 vitamins in 678
Balsam of Peru 1031
Banocide 815
Baratol 302
Barbiturates
 harmful effects and warnings 578–9
 in anxiety 618
 in sleeping disorders 574, 578
Barquinol HC 986
Barrier creams 977
Bassorin 649
Baxan 749
Baycaron 302, 328
Bayolin 742
BCG vaccine 110–12
Becloforte 165

Beclomethasone
in nasal preparations 70
in skin preparations 983, 984
preparations used to treat asthma 165
Becodisks 165
Beconase 70
Becotide 165
Bedranol SR 277, 302
Bedsores 1015–17
vitamin C in 679
zinc in 679
Bedwetting 498–500
Belladonna
in peptic ulcers 195
in spasm of the intestine 229
uses of 16
Bellocarb 197, 230
Bendrofluazide
in heart failure 328, 329
in hypertension 302, 303
Benemid 483
Benethamine penicillin 735, 737
Benoral 443
Benorylate
harmful effects and warnings 408, 453
in chronic back pain 466
in pain 409
in rheumatoid arthritis 443
Benoxinate *see* Oxybuprocaine
Benperidol 636
Benserazide 546, 552
Bentex 552
Benylin 37
Benzalkonium 994
in dandruff 1019
in nappy rash 1035
Benzalkonium chloride-bromine 1046
Benzathine penicillin 735, 737, 743
Benzhexol 16, 551, 552
Benzocaine 427
and sunlight sensitivity 1005
in lozenges, compound 171
in mouth ulcers 171
in slimming 651
Benzodiazepines
harmful effects and warnings 618
addiction to 605
as muscle relaxants 467
dependence 605
in anxiety 605
in migraine 432
in sleeping disorders 574, 579
tolerance 605
withdrawal of 605
withdrawal symptoms 603
Benzoic acid ointment, compound 992
in athlete's foot 1015
Benzophenones 1000
Benzoyl peroxide 1008
Benzthiazide 329
Benztropine 16, 551, 552
Benzydamine 171
Benzyl alcohol 1031
Benzyl benzoate
in lice 1034, 1035
in scabies 1043
Benzylpenicillin *see* Penicillin G
Bephenium
harmful effects and warnings 815
in hookworm 811
Bergamot oil 1000
Bergaptene 1000
Berkaprine 446, 1062
Berkatens 277, 302, 349
Berkmycen 752
Berkolol 277, 302, 349, 438, 624
Berkozide 302, 328
Berotec 165
Beta-Adalat 280, 306
Beta-adrenoceptor blocking drugs *see* Beta blockers
Beta-adrenoreceptor stimulants *see* Adrenoreceptor stimulants
Beta blockers 260
harmful effects and warnings 265
following heart attack 276
in angina 263–4
in anxiety 619
in glaucoma 533, 534
in hypertension 293
in migraine 434
in overactive thyroid disease 849
Beta-Cardone 277, 349
Beta-carotene 1003
in sunlight sensitivity 1005
Betadine 948, 1017
Betagan 539
Betahistine 183, 186
Beta-lactam antibiotics 748
Beta-lactamases 735
Betaloc 277, 302, 349, 438
Betamethasone 841, 843, 845
in eye preparations 527
in nasal preparations 70, 71
in psoriasis of the scalp 1041
in skin preparations 983, 984
preparations used to treat asthma 165
Beta stimulants *see* Adrenoreceptor stimulants
Betaxolol
harmful effects and warnings in eyes 536
in glaucoma 533, 539
in hypertension 304
Bethanechol 12
harmful effects and warnings 501
in retention of urine 500
Bethanidine 302, 303
harmful effects and warnings 308
Betim 277, 302, 438
Betnelan 844
Betnesol 65, 70, 527, 844
Betnesol-N 65, 71, 527
Betnovate 983
Betnovate-C 986
Betnovate-N 986
Betnovate rectal ointment 427
Betoptic 539
Bextasol 165
Bezafibrate
harmful effects and warnings 376
on blood cholesterol and fats 373, 378
Bezalip 378
Bicillin 744
BiCNU 1060
Biguanides
preparations 873
use in diabetes 870–72
Bilarcil 816
Bile 1141–2
Biltricide 717
BiNovum 914
Bioflavoids 675
Biogastrone 207
Biophylline 165
Bioplex 171
Bioral Gel 171
Biorphen 552

Biotin 667
Biperiden 16, 551, 552
Bisacodyl 233, 243
Bismuth chelate 204
Bismuth salts 196
Bisoprolol
in angina 278, 279
in hypertension 303, 304
Bitters 657
Blackwater fever 797
Bleeding disorders 379, 380
Bleomycin 1069
Blepharitis 535
Blindness
vitamin A in 679
Blocadren 278, 302, 438
Blood fats 366–78
blood levels of 370
deposits in arteries, *see* Atherosclerosis
drugs used to lower 372–8
screening, blood levels of 375
Blood pressure, low *see* Hypotension
Blood pressure, raised *see* Hypertension
Blood transfusion reactions 721
Body odour 1044–6
magnesium in 679
para-aminobenzoic acid in 679
pyridoxine in 679
zinc in 679
Boils 1017–18
zinc in 679
Bolvidon 599
Bonjela 171
Boron 930
Botulism antitoxin 112
Bowel
prevention of infection after surgery on 734
Bradilan 365, 378
Bradosol 427
Brain
drugs used to improve blood supply to 362
Bran 235
Brasivol 1009
Breast feeding 1129
and eczema 1025
drugs that enter the breast milk and may affect the baby 1130–33
Bretylate 349
Bretylium 349
harmful effects and warnings 346
Brevinor 913
Bricanyl 165, 954
Brilliant green 995
Britiazim 278
Brocadopa 552
Broflex 552
Brolene 521, 526
Bromazepam 624
Bromocriptine
harmful effects and warnings 549, 945
and testicular function 972
in infertility 944
in over-secretion of growth hormone 822
in over-secretion of prolactin 822
in parkinsonism 548, 552
Brompheniramine 94
Bronchiectasis 144
Bronchilator 167
Bronchitis 144, 734
vitamin A in 680
vitamin C in 680
Bronchodil 165
Bronchodilators
in asthma 145–51
in cough medicines 50
Broxil 742
Brufen 408, 451, 923
Bruises
vitamin C in 680
Buccastem 185
Budesonide
in nasal preparations 70
in skin preparations 983, 984
preparations used to treat asthma 165
Buerger's disease 356
Bumetanide 328
Bupivacaine 427
Buprenorphine 418, 422
Burinex 328
Burinex K 330
Burns
vitamin C in 680
vitamin E in 680
Buscopan 230
Buserelin 1065
harmful effects and warnings 1066
Buspar 624
Buspirone
harmful effects and warnings 622
in anxiety 619, 624
Busulphan 1060
Butobarbitone 583
Butopyronoxyl 1029
Butriptyline 599

Cadexomer iodine *see* Iodosorb
Cafadol 413
Cafergot 437
Caffeine 641–3
in pain relievers 412
in preparations used to treat acute migraine 437
Caladryl 993
Calamine lotion 1030
Calamine with phenol 1029, 1031
Calcichew 695
Calciferol *see* Ergocalciferol
Calcimax 695
Calciparine 394
Calcitare 470
Calcitonin 859
in osteoporosis 930
Calcitonin (pork)
harmful effects and warnings 470
in Paget's disease 470
Calcium 692–4
and tetany 693
high blood levels 694
in osteoporosis 929
low blood levels 693
supplements 695
Calcium carbonate
as antacid 192, 193, 198, 199
in diarrhoea 219
in physical sunscreens 1000
Calcium-channel blockers 268
harmful effects and warnings 269, 270
in angina 268
in hypertension 296
in migraine 434
Calcium gluconate 695
Calcium lactate 695
Calcium leucovorin 1063
Calcium salts
as supplements 695
in antacids 192, 193, 198, 199
Calcium-Sandoz 695
Calcium supplements 695
Calcium with vitamin D 695
Calgel 427
Callosities *see* Corns
Calluses *see* Corns

Callusolve 1046
Calmurid HC 985
Calsynar 470
CAM 167
Camcolit 599
Camphor
  in cooling
    applications 461, 1031
  in vapour rubs and
    inhalants 39
Cancer 1052–67
  and exposure to the
    sun 999
  carotene in 680
  drug treatment of 1054–67
  laetrile in 680
  selenium in 701
  vitamin C in 680
  vitamin E in 680
Canesten 65, 948, 992, 1013
Canesten-HC 986
Canker sores *see* Aphthous
    ulcers
Canthaxanthin 1003
Canrenoate
  harmful effects and
    warnings 334
  in heart failure 329
Canthaxanthin 1003
Cantil 230
Capastat 778
Caplenal 483
Capoten 302, 331
Capozide 306
Capreomycin 775, 778
  harmful effects and
    warnings 775
Caprin 442, 451
Captopril
  harmful effects and
    warnings 309
  in heart failure 331
  in hypertension 302, 303
  in Raynaud's disease 359
Carace 303, 331
Carbachol 12
  harmful effects and
    warnings 501
  harmful effects and
    warnings in eyes 536
  in glaucoma 539
  in retention of urine 500
  to constrict pupils 530
Carbalax 243
Carbamazepine
  harmful effects and
    warnings 567
  in depression 598, 600
  in diabetes insipidus 823
  in epilepsy 570, 571
Carbaryl 1034, 1035
Carbellon 197, 230
Carbenicillin 739
Carbenoxolone
  harmful effects and
    warnings 205
  in mouth ulcers 171
  in peptic ulcers 203
  preparations 207
Carbidopa 546, 553
Carbimazole 848
  harmful effects and
    warnings 853
Carbocisteine 51
Carbo-Cort 985
Carbolic acid 996
Carbonic anhydrase
    inhibitors 317
Carboplatin 1062
Carboprost 953
Cardene 278, 303
Cardiac glycosides 323–5
Cardiacap 278
Carfecillin 492, 739
Carisoma 467, 470
Carisoprodol
  harmful effects and
    warnings 468
  in chronic back pain 467
  preparations 470
Carmellose 172
Carmustine 1060
Carteolol
  harmful effects and
    warnings in eyes 536
  in angina 278
  in glaucoma 533, 539
Cartrol 278
Carylderm 1035
Cascara 233
Castor oil 235
Catapres 303
Cataracts 541
  calcium in 680
  drugs that may cause
    cataracts 541
  vitamin B_1 in 680
  vitamin C in 680
  vitamin E in 680
Catarrh 74
Caved-S 207
CCNU 1060
Cedilanid 331
Cedocard 278, 331
Cefaclor 749
Cefadroxil 749
céfixime 749
Cefizox 749
Cefotaxime 749
Cefoxitin 749
Cefsulodin 749
Ceftazidime 749
Ceftizoxime 749
Cefuroxime 749
  in gonorrhoea 506
Celbenin 742
Celevac 228, 650
Cellucon 228, 650
Central alpha
    stimulants 292–3
Centyl 303, 328
Centyl K 306, 330
Cephalexin 749
Cephalosporins 734,
    746–9
  harmful effects of 747
  in gall bladder
    infections 734
  warnings on use 748
Cephalothin 749
Cephamandole 749
Cephazolin 749
Cephradine 749
Ceporex 749
Ceratonia 219
Cerumol 62
Cervagem 954
Cesamet 185
Cetirizine 94
Cetrimide 994
  in dandruff 1019
  in nappy rash 1035
Cetylpyridinium 994
Charcoal, activated 218
Chemical castration 959, 973
Chemotrim 770
Chendol 251, 252
Chenodeoxycholic acid 251,
    252
Chenofalk 251, 252
Chickenpox 791
  passive immunization 140
Chilblains 361
  calcium in 1018
  vitamin B complex in 680
  vitamin D in 680
Chloral betaine 583
  harmful effects and
    warnings 579
Chloral hydrate 582, 583
  harmful effects and
    warnings 579
Chlorambucil
  in cancer 1060
  immunosuppression
    and 83, 1062
  in rheumatoid
    arthritis 446
Chloramine 995
Chloramphenicol

harmful effects and
warnings 758–9
in conjuctivitis 535, 734
in eye infections 526
in otitis externa 65
in typhoid fever 734
preparations 763–4
Chlorasol 995, 1017
Chlorbutol
in itching 1031
in motion sickness 179
in mouth ulcers 171
Chlordiazepoxide 624, 625
Chlorhexidine 995
in boils 1018
in mouth ulcers 171
in nasal preparations 71
Chlorinated lime 995
Chlorinated phenols 995
Chlorine 995
Chlormethiazole
harmful effects and
warnings 579
in epileptic
emergencies 566, 571
in sleeping disorders 579,
582
Chlormezanone
harmful effects and
warnings 623
in anxiety 619, 625
in chronic back pain 467
in sleeping disorders 580
preparations 470
Chlorocresol 995, 996
Chloromycetin 526, 763
Chloromycetin
Hydrocortisone 527
Chloroquine
harmful effects and
warnings 458, 758,
801
in amoebic dysentry 804
in malaria 798, 799, 800,
801, 803
in rheumatoid
arthritis 445
in sunlight
sensitivity 1005
Chlorothiazide
in heart failure 329
in hypertension 304
Chloroxylenol 995, 996
Chlorpheniramine
in allergies 94
in anaphylactic shock 103
Chlorpromazine
antipsychotic use of 636
in nausea and
vomiting 185
in thyroid crisis 853
preparations 186
Chlorpropamide
in diabetes insipidus 824
in diabetes mellitus 873
Chlortetracycline 752
in boils 1017
in eye infections 526
in impetigo 734, 1027
in skin preparations 989
in trachoma 542
Chlorthalidone
in diabetes insipidus 824
in heart failure 328
in hypertension 303
Chocovite 695
Cholecalciferol 669
Choledyl 165
Cholelithiasis 250
Cholera vaccine 113
Cholesterol 366–78
blood levels of 370
deposits in arteries *see*
Atherosclerosis
drugs used to lower
372–8
screening, blood levels
of 375
Cholestyramine
harmful effects and
warnings 376
in Crohn's disease 223
in itching 1032
on blood cholesterol and
fats 373, 378
Choline 675
Choline magnesium
trisilicate 442, 453
Choline salicylate dental
gel 171
Choline theophyllinate 150,
165, 166
Cholinergic drugs 12
to constrict pupils 530,
531
Cholinesterase inhibitors *see*
Anticholinesterases
Chorionic gonadotrophin *see*
Gonadotrophin
Chromium 698
Chronic obstructive airways
disease 144
Cicatrin 989
Ciclacillin 738
Cidomycin 65, 526, 757, 989
Cidex 994
Cigarette smoking
and blood fats, 369
and Buerger's disease 356
and heart disease 255
and hypertension 289
and peptic ulcers 189
and Raynaud's disease 358
vitamin B complex in 680
vitamin C in 680
Cilastatin 748
Cimetidine
harmful effects and
warnings 205
preparations 207
Cinchocaine 427
Cinnarizine
disorders of the
circulation 354, 364,
365
in motion sickness 178
in vertigo 183
preparations 186
Cinobac 492, 763
Cinoxacin 490, 491, 759
harmful effects and
warnings 763
Ciprofloxacin 490, 759, 763
harmful effects and
warnings 759
in gonorrhoea 734
in urinary infections 490
preparations 763
Ciproxin 763
Circulation
disorders of 352–365
drugs used to treat 365
harmful effects and
warnings of drugs used
to treat 364
Cirrhosis of the liver
and alcohol 1144
and drugs 1144
Cisapride 212
Cisplatin 1063
Citanest 427
Claforan 749
Clarityn 95
Clemastine 94
Clavulanic acid 739
Clindamycin 759, 763
Clinicide 1035
Clinoril 451
Clioquinol 66, 220, 986
Clobazam
in anxiety 624
in epilepsy 571
Clobetasol 983, 985
Clobetasone
in eye disorders 522, 527
in skin preparations 983,
984
Clofibrate
harmful effects and
warnings 376

Clofibrate – *cont.*
in diabetes insipidus 823
on blood cholesterol and fats 373, 378
Clofibrate group of drugs
on blood cholesterol and fats 373, 378
Clomiphene 896
harmful effects and warnings 944
and testicular function 972
in infertility 943
Clomid 896, 943, 944
Clomipramine 599
Clomocycline 753
Clonazepam
in epilepsy 570
in epileptic emergencies 566
Clonidine
harmful effects and warnings 312
actions 27
in hypertension 293, 303
in migraine 435
Clopamide 308
Clopixol 636
Clorazepate 625
Clotrimazole 780
in athlete's foot 1015
in skin preparations 992
in vaginal infections 948
Cloxacillin 738, 743, 744
in boils 1017
Clozaril 636
Cluster headaches 429
Coal tar
harmful effects and warnings 1041
in eczema and dermatitis 1024
in psoriasis 1037, 1038, 1039
in seborrhoeic dermatitis 1027
in dandruff products 1020
Co-amilofruse 329
Co-amilozide 329
Co-amoxiclav 739, 744
Cobadex 985
Cobalt 698
Cobutalin 165
Co-beneldopa 546
Co-Betaloc 306
Cocaine 643
in eye disorders 523, 528
in local anaesthesia 427
in slimming 651
Cocaine and homatropine eye drops 528
Co-careldopa 546
Cocoa butter oil 1003
Co-codamol 413
Co-codaprin 412
Codanin 413
Co-danthramer 234
Co-danthrusate 234
Codeine
harmful effects and warnings 410
in chronic back pain 466
in combined preparations 411
in cough 47
in diarrhoea 217
in migraine 430, 437
in osteoarthritis 465
in pain 409, 418
Co-dergocrine 363, 364, 365
Codis 412
Co-dydramol 413
Co-fluampicil 738, 744
Co-flumactone 329
Cogentin 552
Cojene 412
Colchicine 476, 478, 480
Cold sores *see* Herpes simplex
Colds 32–44
harmful effects and warnings of drugs used to treat colds 43
vitamin A in 680
vitamin C in 41, 57, 680
Colestid 378
Colestipol 373, 376, 378
Colifoam 228
Colistin 760, 763
in skin preparations 989
Collodions 977, 979
Colofac 230
Colomycin 763, 989
Colostomy 1180
Colpermin 230
Colven 230
Combantrin 817
Comox 770
Competitive neuromuscular blocking drugs 19
Complement system 78
Comprecin 763
Concordin 599
Condyline 1047
Congesteze 37
Conjugated oestrogens 891, 896
Conjunctivitis 535, 734
Conn's syndrome 829
Conova-30 913
Constipation 232–44
drugs that may cause 241
use of laxatives 242
vitamin B_1 in 680
Contraceptives, oral 902–18
and sex 970
and sunlight sensitivity 1006
combined 902–13
in acne 1010
in dysmenorrhoea 923
in endometriosis 924
in menorrhagia 922
in PMS 920
morning-after 916–18
phasic 902, 914
post coital 916
progestogen-only 902, 915–16
pyridoxine (vitamin B_6) in 906
vitamin B_{12} in 680
vitamin C in 680, 912
vitamin E in 680
Convalescence
anabolic steroids in 962
vitamin C in 680
Convulsions 559. *See also* Epilepsy
in feverish children 566
in MMR immunization 127
Coolant sprays 468
Cooley's anaemia 725
Coombe's test 1084
and methyldopa 312
Coparvax 87
Co-phenotrope 221
Copper 699
Co-prenozide 308
Co-proxamol 413
Cordarone X 349
Cordilox 278, 303, 349
Corgard 278, 303, 349, 438
Corgaretic 306
Corlan 171
Coronary artery disease 253–80
chromium in 682
evening primrose oil in 682
potassium in 682
selenium in 682
vitamin B complex in 682
vitamin C in 682
vitamin E in 682
Coronary thrombosis 253
Coro-Nitro 278
Corneal ulcer *see* eye diseases
Corns 1018–19

Corticosteroids 833–45
harmful effects 834–9
benefits and risks 843
emergency use of 843
equivalent doses 843
in allergies 99–100
in anaphylaxis 103
in asthma 152, 162
in Crohn's disease 223
in eczema and dermatitis 1023
in eye disorders 522, 535
in hayfever 106, 107
in itching 1031
in mouth ulcers 171
in psoriasis 1038, 1040, 1041
in replacement treatment 841
in rheumatoid arthritis 443, 452
in seborrhoeic dermatitis 1027
in stress 842
in ulcerative colitis 224
preparations by mouth and injection 843
skin preparations 980–88
suppressive treatment 842
warnings on use of 839–40
Corticosteroid/anti-infective skin preparations 986–8
Corticotrophin (ACTH) 840–41
in gout 476
preparations 825
Cortisol 827
Cortisone 841, 844
Cortistab 844
Cortisyl 844
Corwin 326, 336
Corynebacterium parvum 87
Cosalgesic 413
Co-simalcite 197
Cosmegen Lyovac 1061
Cosuric 483
Co-trimoxazole 769–71
harmful effects and warnings 769–70
in acne 1010
in bronchitis 734
in gonorrhoea 506
in sinusitus 734
in typhoid fever 734
Coughs 45–53
Cough medicines
cough mixtures 52
expectorants 48
soothing 46
suppressants (narcotic) 47
suppressants (non-narcotic) 47
Coumarins 385
Counter irritants 460, 1029
Coversyl 303
Crabs *see* Lice
Cream of tartar 244
Creams 977
Creatinine 1165
Cresol 995, 996
Cretinism 855
Crohn's disease 222–4, 226–7, 228, 826
Cromoglycate *see* Sodium cromoglycate
Crotamiton 1031, 1043
Crystal violet 995
Crystapen 742
Cushing's disease 821, 828
Cushing's syndrome 821, 828
Cyanocobalamin 718
Cyclandelate
harmful effects and warnings 364
and mental function in elderly 363
in disorders of the circulation 354, 365
Cyclimorph 422
Cyclizine 178, 183, 186, 422, 437
Cyclobral 365
Cyclofenil 896, 943, 944
Cyclogest 901
Cyclopenthiazide
in heart failure 329
in hypertension 304
Cyclopentolate
in iridocyclitis 535
to dilate the pupils 525, 529, 530
uses of 16
Cyclophosphamide
immunosuppression and 84
in cancer 1060, 1062
in rheumatoid arthritis 446
Cyclo-Progynova 901, 941
Cyclopyrrolones 580
Cycloserine 775, 778
Cyclospasmol 365
Cyclosporin 85
Cyklokapron 396, 398, 922
Cymevene 788
Cyproheptadine 94, 435
Cyprostat 1066
Cyproterone 959, 973, 1066
Cystitis 485, 487, 489
Cytarabine 1061
Cytosar 1061
Cytotec 207
Cytotoxic antibiotics 1061
Cytotoxic drugs *see* Anti-cancer drugs
Cytotoxic immunosuppressants *see* Immunosuppressants

Dacarbazine 1063
Dactinomycin *see* Actinomycin D
Dakin's solution 995
Daktacort 986
Daktarin 174, 787, 992, 1013
Dalacin C 763
Dalacin T 1009
Dalmane 582
Danazol 224, 922
Dandruff 1019–21
Daneral-SA 95
Danol 922, 924
Danthron 233, 234
Dantrium 467, 470
Dantrolene 467, 468, 470
Daonil 873
Dapsone (in Maloprim) 799
Daranide 539
Daraprim 803
Dazoxiben 360
DDAVP 823, 825
Deafness
vitamin A in 680
Debrisan 1017
Debrisoquine 303
Decadron 452, 844
Deca-Durabolin 966
Decaserpyl 303
Declinax 303
Decongestants
in allergies 100, 105
in colds 34–6
in cough medicines 51
in eye applications 524
nasal applications 35, 44, 69–70
oral 35, 37, 43
Decortisyl 844
Decubitus ulcers *see* Bedsores
Deglycyrrhizinized liquorice *see* Liquorice, deglycyrrhizinized
Dehydrocholic acid 252
Deltacortril 228, 844
Deltastab 452, 844
Demeclocycline 752, 753

Demulcent cough medicines *see* Soothing cough medicines
Demulcent skin applications 979
De-Nol 204, 207
De-Noltab 204, 207
Dental abscess 734
Dental caries *see* Dental decay
Dental decay
  fluoride in 697
  pyridoxine in 680
  vitamin C in 680
Deodorants 1045, 1046
Deoxycortone 841
Depixol 636
Depocillin 742
Depolarizing neuromuscular blocking drugs 20–21
Depo-Medrone 107, 844
Depo-Medrone with Lidocaine 427, 452
Deponit 278
Depo-Provera 901, 916, 917, 924
Depostat 901
Depression 584–603
  pyridoxine in 681
Dequalinium 174
Derbac 1035, 1043
Derbac-M 1035, 1043
Dermatitis 1021–27
  vitamin A in 681
  vitamin B complex in 681
Dermovate 983
Dermovate-NN 986
Desensitization *see* Hyposensitization
Deseril 438
Desipramine 600
Desmopressin 823, 824, 825
  in bedwetting 499
Desmospray 823, 825
Desogestrel 913
Desoxymethasone 983, 984
Destolit 251, 252
Deteclo 752
Dettol 996
DeWitt's Analgesic Pills 413
Dexamethasone 452, 527, 841, 843, 844
Dexamphetamine 640
Dexa-Rhinaspray 70
Dexedrine 640
Dexfenfluramine 649
Dextranomer 1017
Dextromethorphan 47
Dextromoramide 418, 422
Dextropropoxyphene 409, 410, 411, 418, 466
DF-118 411, 422
DHC Continus 411
Dhobie's itch 782
Diabetes 861–86
  chromium in 681
  magnesium in 681
  pyridoxine in 681
  vitamin A in 681
  vitamin C in 681
  vitamin E in 681
  zinc in 681
Diabetes insipidus 823
  preparations used to treat 826
Diabetes mellitus *see* Diabetes
Diabinese 873
Diamicron 873
Diamorphine 47, 418, 422
Diamox 539, 571
Dianette 1010, 1011
Diarrhoea 214
Diatensec 328
Diazemuls 470, 571, 624
Diazepam
  as a muscle relaxant 467, 470
  in anxiety 623, 624, 625
  in chronic back pain 467
  in epileptic emergencies 566, 571
  in migraine 433
Diazoxide 314
Dibenyline 303
Dicapen 745
Dichlorphenamide 317
  harmful effects and warnings 537
  in glaucoma 534, 539
Diclofenac
  harmful effects and warnings 453
  in gout 476
  in rheumatoid arthritis 452
Diconal 422
Dicyclomine 14, 16
  in diarrhoea 218
  in peptic ulcers 196
  in spasm of the intestine 229
Dicynene 396, 398, 922
Didronel 470, 471, 931
Dienoestrol 891, 896
Diethylcarbamazine 814, 815
Diethylpropion 648, 652, 653
Diethylstilboestrol 891
Difflam cream 462
Difflam oral rinse and spray 171
Diflucan 174, 787, 948
Diflucortolone
  in skin preparations 983, 984, 985
Diflunisal 442, 451, 453
Digitoxin
  in heart failure 331
  in disorders of heart rhythm 349
Digoxin
  harmful effects and warnings 324, 332
  in disorders of heart rhythm 349, 350
  in heart failure 323, 331, 853
Dihydergot 437
Dihydroergotamine 432, 436, 437
Dihydrocodeine 410, 419, 422, 466
Dihydroxyacetone (DHA) 1003
Dijex 197
Diltiazem 278, 280
Diloxanide 804, 815
Dimelor 873
Dimenhydrinate 178, 185
Dimethicone
  in antacids 196
  in barrier skin applications 979
Dimethindene 94
Dimethyl phthalate 1029
Dimotane 37, 95
Dimotapp 37
Dindevan 394
Dinoprostone 951, 954
Dinoprost
  in abortion 951
  in labour 952, 954
Dioctyl 62
Dioctyl sodium sulphosuccinate *see* Docusate sodium
Dioderm 983
Dioralyte 217
Diovol 197
  in heartburn 213
Dipentum 228
Diphenhydramine 94
  and sensitivity to sunlight 993
Diphenoxylate 217, 223
Diphenylpyraline 94
Diphtheria vaccines 114
Dipipanone 419, 422

Dipivefrin
harmful effects and
warnings 537
in glaucoma 533, 539
Dipotassium clorazepate *see* Clorazepate
Diprosalic 985
Diprosone 983
Dipyridamole 395
Dirythmin SA 350
Disalcid 442, 451
Disease, resistance to
vitamin A in 684
vitamin B complex in 684
vitamin C in 684
Disinfectants 994–7
Disipal 552
Disodium cromoglycate *see* Sodium cromoglycate
Disodium etidronate
harmful effects and warnings 471
in osteoporosis 931
in Paget's disease 470, 471
Disopyramide 346, 350
Distaclor 749
Distalgesic 413
Distamine 445
Distaquaine V-K 742
Distigmine 13, 500, 501
Disulfirim 1184, 1185
Dithranol 1038, 1039
Dithrocream 1038
Diumide-K Continus 330
Diuretics
harmful effects and warnings 333
and sex 970
carbonic anhydrase inhibitors 317
combined diuretics 323
combined diuretic + potassium 322
in elderly 319
in glaucoma 534
in heart failure 316
in hypertension 290
in PMT 921
in slimming 649
incontinence and 495
loop 318
main risks of 321
osmotic 317
potassium sparing 319
thiazide 318
(thiazide) and sunlight sensitivity 1006
types of 317
with potassium supplements 291
Diurexan 303
Dixarit 438
Doan's Backache Pills 414
Dobutamine
harmful effects and warnings 335
in heart failure 326
uses of 25
Dobutrex 26, 326, 335
Docusate sodium 234, 237
Dolmatil 636
Dolobid 408, 442, 451
Doloxene Co 412
Domical 599
Domiphen 994
Domperidone 176
harmful effects and warnings 185–6
and anti-cancer drugs 180
and bromocriptine 180
and levodopa 180
in radiation treatment 181
preparations 185, 186
Dopacard 326
Dopa-decarboxylase inhibitors 546
Dopamet 303
Dopamine
harmful effects and warnings 335
in heart failure 326
uses of 25, 29
Dopamine blockers 30
in vomiting 177
Dopamine precursors 545
Dopamine stimulants 29, 545
Dopaminergic drugs 545
Dopexamine 326
Doralese 501
Dormonoct 582
Dothiepin 600
Doxazosin 303, 310
Doxepin 600
Doxorubicin 1061
Doxycycline 753
in acne 1010
Dozic 636
Dracontiasis 814
Dramamine 185
Driving
and drugs 1186–87
Droleptan 636
Droperidol 636
Drug dependence
to narcotic pain relievers 420
to sleeping drugs 578, 620–21
to benzodiazepines 609–14
to sedatives 620–21
Drug interactions
table of drug–drug interactions 1193–1242
types of 1188–92
Dry mouth 173
Dryptal 303, 328
DTIC-Dome 1063
Dulcolax 243
Duo-Autohaler 167
Duodenal ulcers *see* Peptic ulcers
Duogastrone 207
Duovent 167
Duphaston 901, 924
Durabolin 966
Duromine 653
Dusting powders 977, 979
Duvadilan 954
Dyazide 306, 331
Dydrogesterone 897, 901
in dysmenorrhoea 924
in PMS 920
Dynese 197
Dysmenorrhoea 922–4
calcium in 683
Dyspamet 207
Dyspepsia 187
Dysrhythmias *see* Heart rhythm and rate, disorders of
Dytac 328
Dytide 329, 331

Ear wax *see* Ears
Ears
disorders of 61–6
otitis externa 62, 65
otitis media 64, 65, 734
removal of wax 61, 62
Ebufac 408, 451
Econacort 986
Econazole 780
in athlete's foot 1013
in skin preparations 992
in vaginal infections 949
Econocil VK 742
Ecostatin 949, 992, 1013
Ecothiopate 530
Eczema 1021–5
oil of evening primrose in 681
vitamin A in 681
vitamin B complex in 681
zinc in 681
Edecrin 328
Edrophonium 13

Efalith 1027
Efcortelan cream 983
Efcortelan ointment 983
Efcortelan soluble 844
Efcortesol 844
Effercitrate 493
Efudix 1061
Ejaculation 967
premature 967
Elantan 278, 331
Elavil 599
Eldepryl 552
Elderly people
harmful effects of drug treatments 1138–40
risks of drug treatments 1136–40
Eldisine 1062
Electrolade 217
Electrolyte and water replacement
oral, in acute diarrhoea 216, 217
Eltroxin 858
Eludril aerosol spray 427
Elyzol 765
Emblon 896, 943, 1064
Emcor 278, 303
Emepronium 16
Emeside 571
Emetine 804, 815
Eminase 273, 277, 397
EMLA 427
Emoform 994
Emollients 978–9, 1031
Emphysema 144
Emulsifiers 976
Enalapril
harmful effects and warnings 309
in heart failure 331
in hypertension 304
Endometriosis 924–5
Endoxana 84, 446, 1060, 1062
Enduron 303, 328
Enemas 241, 243
Engerix B 120
Eno 244
Enoxacin 760
Enoximone 326, 335
Entamizole 815
Enteric coated tablets 1071
Enteromide 770
Enuresis *see* Bedwetting
Epanutin 350, 571
Ephedrine 25
in asthma 165, 167
in bedwetting 499
in eye drops 524
in incontinence of urine 497
in nasal decongestants 37, 70
Epifoam 985
Epifrin 539
Epilepsy 558–71
driving 565
in pregnancy 564
status epilepticus 566
Epilim 571
Epirubicin 1061
Epodyl 1060
Epogam 1025
Epoprostenol 395
Eppy 539
Epsom Salts 244
Equagesic 413
Equanil 624
Eradacin 763
Ergocalciferol 669, 860
Ergometrine 952, 953
Ergometrine/oxytocin (syntometrine) 952, 953, 954
Ergot related drugs
harmful effects and warnings 436–7
Ergotamine 432, 436, 437
Erycen 763
Erymax 763
Erythrocin 763
Erythromelalgia 361
Erythromid 763
Erythromycin 734, 760, 763, 764
in acne 1010
in bronchitis 734
in gonorrhoea 504
in sinusitis 734
in syphilis 734
in tonsillitis 733
in trachoma 542
Erythropoietin 705, 715
Erythroped 764
Esbatal 303
Esidrex 303, 328
Essential fatty acids 676
Esterified oestrogens 891
Estracyt 1060
Estraderm 896, 941
Estradurin 427, 1065
Estramustine 1060
Estrapak 901, 941
Estropipate *see* Piperazine oestrone sulphate
Etafedrine 95
Ethacrynic acid 328
Ethambutol 776, 778
Ethamsylate 397, 398
in menorrhagia 922
Ethanol (*see also* Alcohol)
as antiseptic 994
Ethinyloestradiol 891, 896
in cancer of the prostate 1065
in oral contraceptives 913, 914
Ethisterone 897
Ethosuximide 568, 570, 571
Ethyl alcohol *see* Ethanol
Ethynodiol 897
in combined oral contraceptives 913
in progestogen-only contraceptives 917
Etidronate disodium
harmful effects and warnings 471
in osteoporosis 931
in Paget's disease 470, 471
Etodolac 451, 454
Etoposide 1062
Etretinate 1040, 1042
Eudemine 303
Euglucon 873
Eugynon-30 913
Eumovate 527, 983
Eumovate-N 527
Eurax 1031, 1043
Eurax-Hydrocortisone 985
Evacort 983
Evadyne 599
Evening primrose oil 676–7
in eczema 1025
in PMS 921
Exelderm 992, 1013
Exirel 165
Exophthalmos 847
Expectorants *see* Cough medicines
Expurhin 37
Exterol 62
Eye applications, lubricant 524
Eyelids
inflammation of 535
Eye diseases 521–42
allergic reactions affecting 538
drugs that cause dry eyes 540
dryness of 540
ulcers of (corneal) 538
vitamin B_2 in 681

Fabahistin 95
Fabrol 51
Faecal impaction 240

Faecal softeners 237–8
Famotidine 205, 207, 208
Fansidar 799, 800, 803
harmful effects and warnings 802
Fasigyn 769, 949
Fatigue
magnesium in 681
potassium in 681
vitamin B complex in 681
vitamin C in 681
vitamin E in 681
Fats 366–78
blood levels of 370
deposits in arteries *see* Atherosclerosis
drugs used to lower 372–8
screening, blood levels of 375
Faverin 599
Favus 782
Fe-cap 714
Fectrim 771
Fefol 715
Felbinac 462
Feldene 451
Feldene gel and Sports gel 462
Femafen 408
Female sex hormones 887–901
at menstruation 887
at puberty 887
at the menopause 890
in pregnancy 889
Femerital 414
Femodene 913
Femodene ED 913
Femulen 917
Fenbid 408, 451
Fenbufen 451, 454
Fenfluramine 648, 652, 653
Fennings Adult Cooling Powders 414
Fenofibrate 373, 377, 378
Fenoprofen 451, 453, 454
Fenopron 408, 451
Fenostil Retard 95
Fenoterol 25, 165, 167
Fentanyl 419
Fentazin 185, 636
Ferfolic SV 715
Fergon 714
Ferric ammonium citrate 715
Ferric chloride 1000
Ferric salts 708
Ferrocap 714
Ferrocap-F 715
Ferrocontin Continus 714
Ferrocontin Folic Continus 715
Ferrograd 714
Ferrograd Folic 715
Ferromyn 714
Ferrous fumarate 709, 714, 715
Ferrous gluconate 709, 714, 715
Ferrous glycine sulphate 709, 714, 715
Ferrous salts 708
Ferrous succinate 709, 714
Ferrous sulphate 709, 714, 715
dried 709
Fersaday 714
Fersamal 714
Fertiral 824, 944, 945
Fever
aspirin in 33–4
ibuprofen in 33–4
paracetamol in 33–4
Feverfew 431
Fibrinolytic drugs 396
harmful effects and warnings 397
in heart attack 252
Filariasis 814
Fish oils
harmful effects and warnings 376
following heart attack 276
in osteoporosis 930
on blood cholesterol and fats 374, 378
Flagyl 765, 949
Flamazine 989, 1017
Flavoxate
harmful effects and warnings 497
in incontinence of urine 497
in urinary frequency 495
Flaxedil 20
Flecainide 347, 350
Fletchers' enemas 243
Fletchers' Enemette 243
Flexin Continus 451
Flolan 395
Florinef 844
Floxapen 743
Fluanxol 599
Fluclorolone 984
Flucloxacillin 734, 738, 743, 744, 1027
Fluconazole 174, 781, 785, 787, 948
Flucytosine 781, 785, 787
Fludrocortisone 841, 844
Flumazenil
Flunisolide 70
Flunitrazepam 583
Fluocinolone 984
Fluocinonide 983, 984
Fluocortolone 984
Fluoride 697, 930
Fluorometholone 522, 527
Fluorouracil 1061
Fluoxetine 589, 591, 600
Flupenthixol 599, 636
Fluphenazine 637
Flurandrenolone 983, 984
Flurazepam 582
Flurbiprofen 451, 454
Flushing
and alcohol 1178
Fluspirilene 637
Fluvoxamine 589, 591, 599
FML 527
FML-Neo 527
Folates *see* Folic acid
Folex-350 715
Folic acid 666, 718
anti-cancer drugs and 719
anti-epileptic drugs and 719
deficiency of 719
oral contraceptive drugs and 719
pregnancy and 710, 715, 719
Folinic acid 1063
Follicle stimulating hormone (FSH), 821, 943, 945
Formaldehyde 994
in warts 1046
Formalin
in plantar warts 1047
in sweaty feet 1045
Fortagesic 411
Fortral 410, 422
Fortum 749
Fortunan 636
Foscavir 788
Fosfestrol 1065
Framycetin 526, 757
in skin preparations 989
Framycort 65, 527, 986
Framygen 65, 526, 989
Franol 167
FreAmine 111
Frisium 571, 624
Froben 451
Frumil 329, 331
Frusemide
in heart failure 328, 329
in hypertension 303
Frusene 329, 331

FSH *see* Follicle stimulating hormone
Fucibet 986
Fucidic acid 758
Fucidin 764, 989
Fucidin H 986
Fulcin 787
Full Marks 1035
Fungal infections 779–87
Fungilin 174, 787, 949, 992
Fungizone 787
Furadantin 492
Furamide *see* Diloxanide
Furuncle *see* Boils
Fusafungine 71
Fusidic acid 989
Fybogel 228
Fybranta 228
Fynnon Calcium Aspirin 413

Galactorrhoea 1088
Galfer 714
Galfer FA 715
Gall bladder
  disorders of 250
  infections of 734
  prevention of infection after surgery on 734
Gall stones 250
  vitamin C in 681
Gallamine 19
Galpseud 37
Gamanil 599
Gamma benzene hexachloride *see* Lindane
Gamma globulins *see* Immonoglobulins
Gamma-linolenic acid (GLA) 676
Gamolenic acid *see* Gamma-linolenic acid
Ganciclovir 788, 794
Ganda 539
Ganglion-blocking drugs 18, 28
  in hypertension 295
Gangrene
  vitamin E in 681
Garamycin 65, 526
Gargles
  in mouth disorders 173
  in sore throats 43
Gastrese LA 186
Gastric ulcers *see* Peptic ulcers
Gastrils 197
Gastritis 188
Gastrobid Continus 186
Gastrocote 198, 213
Gastroflux 186
Gastromax 186
Gastron 198, 213
Gastrozepin 200, 207
Gaviscon 198, 213
Gelusil 198
Gemeprost 954
Gemfibrozil 373, 376, 378
General anaesthesia *see* Anaesthesia, general
Genotropin 824, 826
Gentamicin 757
  after surgery 734
  in eye infections 526, 734
  in gall bladder infections 734
  in otitis externa 66
  in skin preparations 989
Gentian violet *see* Crystal violet
Genticin 66, 526, 757, 989
Genticin HC 986
Gentisone HC 66
German measles
  active immunization 117–19
  passive immunization 119
Germicides 994
Gestanin 901
Gestodene 913
Gestone 901
Gestronol 901
GFR *see* Glomerular filtration rate 1165
Giardiasis 804
Gigantism 820
GLA *see* Gamma-linolenic acid
Glandosane 173
Glandular fever
  skin rash caused by broad spectrum penicillins 739
  vitamin B complex in 681
  vitamin C in 681
Glauber's Salt 244
Glaucoma 531–9, 1178
  harmful effects and warnings of drugs used to treat 536–8
  closed angle (narrow angle, acute, congestive) 532
  drugs that may trigger closed angle glaucoma 532
  drugs used to treat glaucoma 533–5
  open angle (chronic, simple) 531
  vitamin C in 681
Glauline 539
Glibenclamide 873
Glibenese 873
Gliclazide 873
Glipizide 873
Gliquidone 873
Glomerular filtration rate (GFR) 1165
Glucagon 863
Glucocorticoids 832
Gluco-lyte 217
Glucophage 873
Glucose-6-phosphate dehydrogenase (G6PD) deficiency 724, 1084, 1178
Glucose tolerance factor (GTF) 698
Glurenorm 873
Glutaraldehyde 994
  in sweaty feet 1045
  in warts 1046
Glutarol 994, 1046
Glycerin 979, 247
Glycerol
  suppositories 243
Glyceryl trinitrate
  in angina 256, 278, 279, 280
  in heart failure 332
  in Raynaud's disease 360
Glycopeptide antibiotics 758
Glycopyrronium 16
  in spasm of the intestines 229
Glypressin 824, 826
Goitre 856–7
  drugs that may cause 857
  nodular 847
  thyrotoxic nodular 847
Gold 444
  harmful effects and warnings 459
  and sunlight sensitivity 1006
Gonadorelin 824, 944, 945
Gonadotrophin 825
  harmful effects and warnings 944
  human chorionic (HCG) 825, 826, 943
  human menopausal (HMG) 944
  in infertility 944
Gonadotrophin-releasing hormone (LHRH) 821, 824
Gonadotraphon LH 825, 943, 944
Gonorrhoea 505, 734
Goserelin 1065, 1066
Gout 472–83
  drugs that may cause 474

drugs used to prevent attacks 478–80
drugs used to treat acute attacks 476–8
Gramicidin 526
Graneodin 526, 989
Grave's disease 847
Gregoderm 986
Griseofulvin 781
harmful effects and warnings 785
and sunlight sensitivity 1006
in athlete's foot 1013
preparations 787
Grisovin 787
Growth hormone (GH)
in acromegaly 820
in gigantism 820
under-secretion of 823
GTN 300 mcg 278
Guaiacol 49
Guanethidine 304, 309
harmful effects and warnings in eyes 309, 537
in glaucoma 533, 539
in hypertension 294, 304
Guar gum
in diabetes 884
in slimming 650
Guarem 650, 884
Guarina 884
Gynaecomastia 1088
Gynatren 949
Gyno-Daktarin 949
Gyno-Pevaryl 949
Gynol 11

H_2 blockers
in heartburn 212
in peptic ulcer 201–2, 208–9
H_2 receptor antagonists *see* H_2 blockers
Haelan 983
Haelan-C 986
Haemolytic disease of the newborn 722
Haemophilia 1178
Haemorrhoids 245–9
vitamin C in 682
Hair (*see also* Baldness)
thinning of 1015
Hair loss *see* Alopecia *and also* Baldness
Halazone 995
Halciderm 983
Halcinonide 983, 985
Halcion 582
Haldol 636
Half-Inderal 278, 438, 624
Haloperidol
anti-psychotic use of 636, 637
in nausea and vomiting 182
Hamamelis 247
Hamarin 483
Harmful drug effects and
allergic reactions 1080
bleeding 1081
blood cholesterol and fat levels 1081
blood disorders 1082–5
blood pressure 1085–6
blood sugar 1086–7
bones 1087
breasts 1088
breathing 1088
cancer 1089–90
circulation 1090
constipation 1090
diarrhoea 1090
ears (hearing and balance) 1091–2
eyes 1092–5
eyelids 1095–6
faintness 1096
fever 1096
growth 1097
headaches 1097
heart 1098
hypothermia 1098
infections 1099–1100
joints 1100
kidneys 1100
liver 1101
menstrual periods 1101
mental symptoms 1102
mouth 1103
muscles 1106
nerves 1107
nose 1107
parkinsonism and movement disorders 1108
passing urine 1108
phaeochromocytoma 1109
salivary glands 1109
seizures 1109
sex 1110
sexual characteristics 1110
skin 1110
stomach and intestine 1111
stress response 1113
systemic lupus erythematosus 1113–14
teeth 1114
testes 1114
thrombosis 1114
thyroid gland 1114–15
ulcers, intestine 1112
ulcers, oesophagus 1112
ulcers, stomach 1112
Harmogen 896, 941
Hayfever 104–7
vitamin B complex in 682
vitamin C in 682
vitamin E in 682
Haymine 37
HBIG *see* Hepatitis B, Immunoglobulin
H-B-Vax 120
Hc45 982
HCG *see* Gonadotrophin, human chorionic
Head and Shoulders shampoo 1019
Headaches
cluster 429
migraine 428–9
vascular 430
Health salts 243
Heart attack
treatment of 271–2
Heartburn 210–13
in pregnancy, treatment of 213
Heart failure 314–36
Heart rhythm and rate disorders 337, 351
Heart valve infections
prevention of in dental treatment 734
Heat spots 1028
Hemabate 953
Heminevrin 571, 582
Heparin 383–4, 392, 394
Heparinised saline 394
Hepatitis
acute viral 1145–7
chronic 1144
vitamin C in 682
Hepatitis A 1145–6
passive immunization 120
Hepatitis B 1146–7
active immunization 119
passive immunization 120
Hepatitis C 1147
Hepatitis D 1147
Hepatitis E 1147
Hepatitis non-A, non-B 1147
Hep-Flush 394
Hepsal 394
Herbal remedies
as tonics 658
in slimming 651

Heroin *see* Diamorphine
Herpes simplex virus
infections 789–90
vitamin C in 680
zinc in 680
Herpes zoster *see* Shingles
Herpid 788
Hexachlorophane 995, 996
Hexamine 490, 491, 492
Hexopal 365
HGH *see* Gonadotrophin, human chorionic
Hiatus hernia 210
Hioxyl 1017
Hiprex 492
Hismanal 95
Histamine 89
Histamine H_2-antagonists *see* H_2 blockers
Histamine H_1-antagonists *see* Antihistamines
Histoplasmosis 784
Histryl 95
HLA system 80
HNIG *see* Immunoglobulin, human normal
Homatropine 16, 525, 529
Honvan 1065
Hookworm 811
Hormone replacement therapy (HRT) 931–41
harmful effects of 940
benefits of 933–4
HRT preparations 941
in dryness and shrinking of the vagina 926, 946
risks of 934–40
to prevent osteoporosis 933–4
to relieve menopausal symptoms 926, 933
Hormonin 896, 941
HRF 824
HRT *see* Hormone replacement therapy
5 HT *see* 5-Hydroxytryptamine
5 HT blockers 31
in vomiting 177
5 HT stimulants 30
HTIG *see* Tetanus immunoglobulin (human)
Humatrope 824
Hydatid disease (echinococcus) 810–11
Hydergine 365
Hydralazine
harmful effects and warnings 314
in heart failure 326, 331
in hypertension 295, 302
Hydrargaphen 995
Hydrea 1063
Hydrenox 303, 328
Hydrocal 985
Hydrochlorothiazide
in heart failure 328
in hypertension 303
Hydrocortisone 844, 845
in eczema and dermatitis 1023
in emergency treatment of asthma 163
in eye disorders 527
in infantile seborrhoeic dermatitis 1027
in itching 1031
in mouth ulcers 171
in nappy rash 1035
in rheumatoid arthritis 452
in thyroid crisis 853
injections of in anaphylactic shock 103
skin applications 982–8
Hydrocortisone butyrate 983, 984
Hydrocortistab 452, 844, 983
Hydrocortisyl 983
Hydroflumethiazide 328
Hydrogen peroxide
as antiseptic 997
to remove ear wax 61, 62
in bedsores 1017
Hydromet 306
HydroSaluric 303, 328
Hydrotalcite 198
Hydroxocobalamin 717, 718
Hydroxyapatite 695
Hydroxychloroquine 445, 458
Hydroxyprogesterone 897, 901
Hydroxyquinoline 1009
5-Hydroxytryptamine 30
Hydroxyurea 1063
Hydroxyzine 619, 623
Hygroton 303, 328
Hygroton K 306, 330
Hyoscine
in diarrhoea 218
in motion sickness 177
in spasm of the intestine 229
preparations 186
to dilate the pupils 525, 529
uses of 16
Hyoscyamine 16
in spasm of intestine 229
Hyperactivity in children 641
vitamin B complex in 682
vitamin C in 682
vitamin E in 682
Hypercalcaemia 694
Hyperkalaemia 691
Hypermagnesaemia 692
Hypernatraemia 689
Hyperphosphataemia 695
Hypertane 306, 329, 331
Hypertension 281–314
drugs that may cause 283
in elderly 300
in pregnancy 301
Hyperthyroidism 847–54
Hypnotics *see* Sleeping drugs
Hypocalcaemia 693
Hypoglycaemia 879–80
prevention of 880
treatment of 880
Hypokalaemia 690
Hypomagnesaemia 691
Hypon 413
Hyponatraemia 687
Hypophosphataemia 694
Hypopituitarism 822
Hyposensitization 100–102
Hypotears 529
Hypotension
postural (orthostatic) 1086
Hypothalamic and anterior pituitary preparations 825
Hypothalamic hormones 821
Hypothyroidism 854–6
Hypovase 303, 331, 365, 501
Hypromellose
in artificial tears 524, 529
Hysterectomy
prevention of infection following 734
Hytrin 303

Ibular 408
Ibumetin 408
Ibuprofen
harmful effects and warnings 455
in dysmenorrhoea 923
in fever 33
in migraine 431
in pain relief 408
in PMS 920
in rheumatoid arthritis 451
Ichthammol

in eczema and dermatitis 1024
in physical sunscreens 1000
in psoriasis 1041
Idoxene 527, 789
Idoxuridine 788
harmful effects and warnings 794
in herpes infections of the eyes 521, 527, 790
in shingles 791
Iduridin 788
Ifosfamide 1060
Ileostomy 1180
Ilosone 764
Ilube 529
Imbrilon 451
Imferon 712
Imipenem 748
Imipenem/cilastatin 748
Imipramine
in bedwetting 499
in depression 599, 600
Immune deficiency disorders 85
Immune reactions 78
Immune system 75–87
drugs that stimulate 87
drugs that suppress 81–5
Immunity
active immunity 108–9
definition 75
passive immunity 109–10
Immunization vaccines 110–42
Immunizations 108–42
Immunoglobulins
anti-D 140, 723
hepatitis B 139
human 138
normal 138
rabies 140
tetanus 140
varicella/zoster 140
Immunoprin 446, 1062
Immunostimulants 87
Immunosuppressants 81–5
harmful effects and warnings 82
cytotoxic 1062
in rheumatoid arthritis 446
Immunotherapy *see* Hyposensitization
Imodium 221, 228
Imperacin 752
Impetigo 734, 1027–8
Impotence 967
drugs that may cause 969–70
papaverine in treatment of 973
vitamin A in 682
Imunovir 789, 949
Imuran 82, 228, 446, 1062
Inabrin 408
Indanediones 385
Indapamide 304
Inderal 278, 303, 350, 438, 624
Inderetic 306
Inderex 306
Indigestion 187–8
Indocid 451
Indolar SR 451
Indomethacin
harmful effects and warnings 455
in chronic back pain 466
in gout 476, 478
in rheumatoid arthritis 451
Indomod 451
Indoramin
harmful effects and warnings 311
in benign prostatic hypertrophy 501
in hypertension 302
Infertility 942–5
harmful effects and warnings of drugs used to treat 944–5
drugs used to treat 943
in males 945, 957
vitamin E in 681
Influenza 792–3
amantadine in 792
vaccines 120–21
Ingram's treatment 1039
Inhalations
aromatic 39
steam 40
Inherited abnormalities
risks of drug treatment in 1178–9
Innovace 304, 331
Inosine pranobex 789
harmful effects and warnings 794
in vaginal infections 949
Inositol 675
Inositol nicotinate 354, 364, 365
Insect repellants 1029
Insect stings and bites 1028–30
allergy to 1029
Instillagel 427, 494
Insulins 861–3
harmful effects of 877–8
biphasic-acting combined insulin preparations 885–6
changing preparations 880
pork and beef 874
preparations of 874–5
short, intermediate and long acting insulin preparations 884–5
Intal 166
Intal Compound 168
Integrin 636
Interactions *see* Drug–drug interactions
Interferons 1063
Intestinal colic 227–31
drugs used to treat 15, 229–31
Intestinal spasm *see* Intestinal colic
Intralgin 427
Intron A 1063
Intropin 26, 326, 335
Iodides
in cough expectorants 49
Iodine
harmful effects of 850, 854
as antiseptic 997
in thyroid crisis 853
in thyroid disease 846, 850
radioactive 850
Iodoform 997
Iodosorb 997, 1016, 1017
Ionamin 653
Ionax 1009
Ipecachuanha 49
Ipral 771
Ipratropium
in asthma 146, 165, 167
in emergency treatment of asthma 163
in vasomotor rhinitis 68, 70
Iprindole 600
Iridocyclitis 535
Iron 705
harmful effects and warnings of iron by mouth 710, 714
and folic acid preparations 715
in iron deficiency anaemia 707
in tonics 656
injections 711
preparations by mouth 708, 714

Iron – *cont.*
- slow-release
  - preparations 709
- vitamin C and 709

Iron dextran injection 712
Iron sorbitol injection 713
Ironorm 714
Irritable bowel syndrome 227, 229
Ismelin 304
Ismo 278, 331
Isoaminile 47
Iso-Autohaler 166
Isocarboxazid 599
Isoconazole 950
Isoetharine 25, 165, 167
Isogel 228
Isoket 278, 331
Isometheptene 25, 433, 437
Isoniazid 734, 776, 778
Isoprenaline
- harmful effects and warnings 335
- in asthma 147, 166, 167
- in heart failure 326
- uses of 25

Isopropyl alcohol 994
Isopto
- alkaline 529
- atropine 529
- carbachol 530, 539
- carpine 530, 538, 539
- epinal 539
- frin 529
- plain 529

Isordil 279, 331
Isosorbide dinitrate
- in angina 257, 278–80
- in heart failure 331

Isosorbide mononitrate
- in angina 250, 278, 279
- in heart failure 331

Isotrate 279, 332
Isotretinoin 1010, 1012
Isoxsuprine 25, 954
Ispaghula
- in constipation 235
- in diarrhoea 219
- in slimming 649

Isradipine 304
Istin 304
Itching
- anus (pruritus ani) 1032–33
- skin (pruritus) 1030–32
- vagina (pruritus vulvae) 1033

Itraconazole 781, 786, 787
- in vaginal infections 950

Jaundice 1143–4
- drugs that cause 1148–9

Jectofer 713
Jexin 20
Jojoba oil 978
Joy-rides 186
Juno Junipah 244

Kabikinase 273, 277, 397
Kala-azar 805
Kalspare 306, 329, 331
Kalten 307
Kanamycin 757
Kannasyn 757
Kaolin
- in diarrhoea 218
- in physical sunscreens 1000

Kay-Cee-L 331
Kefadol 749
Keflex 749
Keflin 749
Kefzol 749
Kelfizine W 771
Kemadrin 552
Kemicetine 764
Kenalog 452, 844
Keratolytics 989
- in dandruff 1020

Kerecid 527, 789
Kerlone 304
Kernicterus 723
Ketanserin 360
Ketazolam
- as muscle relaxant 469

Ketoconazole 781, 786, 787
- in seborrhoeic dermatitis 1027
- in skin preparations 992
- in vaginal infections 949

Ketoprofen 455, 451
Ketotifen 97, 99
- in asthma 157, 162, 167

Kiditard 350
Kidney colic *see* Renal colic
Kidney disease 1159–62
- and problems with drug treatments 1176–7
- assessment of kidney function 1164–5
- drugs that may cause 1162
- drugs that should not be used 1173–6
- drugs to be used with caution 1166–72
- impairment and age 1165
- impairment, degree of 1165
- use of drugs in 1162–77

Kidney stones, *see* Renal stones
Kinidin Durules 350
Kloref 331
Kolanticon 198, 231
Kolantyl 231
Konakion 397, 399, 672
Kwells 186

Labetalol 27
- in angina 267, 279, 280
- in hypertension 304, 305

Labophylline 168
Labosept 174
Labour
- drugs used to induce and augment 951–952
- premature 953

Labrocol 279, 304
Lachesine 16
- to dilate pupils 529

Lacri-Lube 529
Lactic acid
- in warts 1046

Lactobacillus vaccine 947–8, 949
Lactulose 236
Ladropen 743
Laetrile 676
Lanatoside C 331
Lanolin 978
Lanoxin 331, 350
Lanvis 1061
Laractone 328
Laraflex 408, 451
Laratrim 771
Largactil 636
Lariam 186, 803
Larodopa 552
Lasikal 330
Lasilactone 307, 329, 331
Lasipressin 307
Lasix 328
Lasix + K 330
Lasoride 329
Lasma 166
Lasoride 329
Laxatives
- bulk forming 235–6
- faecal softeners 237–8
- in slimming 649
- osmotic 236–7
- stimulant 233–5

Learning disabilities
- vitamin C in 682
- vitamin E in 682
- vitamin supplements in 682

Lecithins 676
Ledercort 844, 983

Lederfen 451
Ledermycin 753
Lederspan 452
Leishmaniasis 805
  oriental sore 806
  visceral (kala-azar) 805
Lenacort 982
Lentizol 599
Leo K 331
Lergoban 95
Leukeran 83, 446, 1060, 1062
Levamisole 446
  harmful effects and warnings 815
  in hookworm 811
  in rheumatoid arthritis 446
  in roundworm 808
Levobunolol 533, 537, 539
Levodopa
  harmful effects and warnings 546, 550
  and sexual behaviour 972
  in parkinsonism 545, 552
  pyridoxine and 547
  vitamin C and 683
Levonorgestrel
  in combined contraceptives 913, 914
  in progestogen-only contraceptives 917
Levophed 26, 336
Levorphanol 419
Lexotan 624
Lexpec with Iron 715
Lexpec with Iron-M 715
LH and FSH releasing hormone (LHRH) 821
LHRH 821
Libido 967, 1088
Librium 624
Librofem 408
Lice
  body (pediculosis corporis) 1034
  head (pediculosis capitis) 1033–4
  pubic (crabs, pediculosis pubis) 1034
Lidifen 408, 451
Lignocaine
  harmful effects and warnings 347
  in disorders of heart rhythm 350
  in eye drops 528
  in local anaesthesia 427
Limbitrol 600
Lincocin 764
Lincomycin 761, 764
Lincosamide antibiotics 758
Lindane
  in lice 1034, 1035
  in scabies 1043
Lingraine 437
Lioresal 467, 470
Liothyronine 856, 858
Lipantil 378
Lipid-lowering drugs 372–5, 378
Lipoproteins 366–78
  blood levels of 370
  deposits in arteries *see* Atherosclerosis
  drugs used to lower 372–8
  screening, blood levels of 375
Lipostat 378
Lipids *see* Blood fats
Liquid paraffin
  in constipation 237
  in emollients 978
Liquifilm Tears 529
Liquorice
  in cough expectorants 49
  in peptic ulcers 203–4
  deglycyrrhizinized 203, 205, 207
Lisinopril
  harmful effects and warnings 310
  in hypertension 303, 305
  in heart failure 331
Liskonium 599
Litarex 599
Lithium 597, 599, 600
Lithium succinate/zinc sulphate
  in seborrhoeic dermatitis 1027
Lithium salts *see* Lithium
Livedo reticularis 360
Liver disease 1143–58
  harmful effects of drugs on 1148–9
  and the use of drugs 1149–53
  chronic hepatitis 1144
  cirrhosis 1144
  drugs that should not be used or used with caution 1153–8
  liver failure 1144–5
  virus hepatitis 1145–7
Lobak 414, 467, 470
Locabiotal 71
Local anaesthetics *see* Anaesthetics, local
Locoid 983
Locoid C 987
Locorten-Vioform 66
Lodine 451
Loestrin-20 913
Loestrin-30 913
Lofepramine 599
Logynon 914
Logynon ED 914
Lomotil 221
Lomustine 1060
Loniten 304
Loop diuretics *see* Diuretics
Loperamide
  in Crohn's disease 223
  in diarrhoea 217
Lopid 378
Loprazolam 582, 583
Lopresor 279, 304, 350
Lopresor SR 279, 304
Lopresoretic 307
Loratadine 94
Lorazepam
  in anxiety 623, 624
  in epilepsy 571
Lormetazepam 583
Losec 202, 206, 207
Lotions 977
  shake lotions 977
Lotriderm 987
Low blood pressure *see* Hypotension
Loxapac 637
Loxapine 636, 637
Ludiomil 599
Lumbago
  calcium in 683
  thiamine in 683
Lupus erythematosus
  with hydralazine 295
Luteinizing hormone (LH) *see* LH
Lyclear 1035
Lymecycline 753
Lynoestrenol 897
Lypressin 823, 824, 825
Lysergic acid diethylamide *see* Lysergide
Lysol 996
Lysuride 548, 550, 552

Maalox 198, 213
Macrodantin 492
Macrolide antibiotics 758
Madopar 546, 552
Magaldrate 198
Magenta 995
Magnapen 745
Magnesia, cream of, *see* Magnesium hydroxide

Magnesium 691–2
  high blood levels 692
  in osteoporosis 930
  in PMS 921
  low blood levels 691
Magnesium/aluminium salts
  in antacids 194, 197, 198, 199
Magnesium carbonate 198
Magnesium hydroxide 198
  in antacids 193
  in constipation 244
Magnesium oxide 1000
Magnesium salts
  in antacids 193, 197, 198, 199
  in osmotic laxatives 237
Magnesium sulphate 244
Magnesium trisilicate 198
Magnesium trisilicate and belladonna mixture 198 231
Malachite green 995
Malaria 796–803
  harmful effects and warnings of drugs used to treat 800
  prevention 799
  treatment 798
Malarivon 445
Malathion
  in lice 1034, 1035
  in scabies 1043
Male sex hormones 955–60
  harmful effects 957–8
  and libido 971–2
  in menopause 957
  in women 891
  preparations 960
  warnings on use 958–9
Malignant hyperthermia *see* Malignant hyperpyrexia syndrome
Malignant hyperpyrexia syndrome
  and suxamethonium 21, 1097, 1178
Maloprim 799, 800, 802, 803
Manganese 700
Mannitol 317
Mansil 816
Mantadine 552
Mantoux test 774
MAOIs *see* Anti-depressant drugs
Maprotiline 588, 591, 599
Marcain 427
Marevan 394
Marplan 599
Marvelon 913
Marzine 186
Maxagesic 408
Maxepa 378
Maxidex 527
Maxitrol 528
Maxolon 186
Maxtrex 446, 1061
Mazindol 649, 652
MCR-50 279
Measles, mumps and rubella vaccine (MMR) 126–8
Measles vaccine 122–4
Mebendazole
  harmful effects 815
  in hookworm 811
  in hydatid disease 811
  in roundworm 808
  in threadworms 807
Mebeverine
  in diarrhoea 218
  in spasm of the intestine 229
Mebhydrolin (Fabahistin) 95
Mecillinam 739, 740, 743
Meclozine 186
Medazepam 624
Medicort 982
Medihaler-Duo 168
Medihaler-epi 166, 1029
Medihaler-Ergotamine 437
Medihaler-Iso 166
Medilave 427
Medised 414
Medomet 304
Medrone 844
Medroxyprogesterone 897, 901, 916, 917
  in endometriosis 924
Mefenamic acid 408
  harmful effects and warnings 456
  in dysmenorrhoea 923
  in menorrhagia 922
  in pain 408
  in PMS 920
  in rheumatoid arthritis 452
Mefloquine 799, 800, 802, 803
Mefoxin 749
Mefruside
  in heart failure 328
  in hypertension 302
Megaclor 753
Melleril 637
Melphalan 1060
Memory loss
  vitamin B complex in 683
Menadiol 397, 671
  harmful effects and warnings 399
  in vitamin K deficiency in adults 672
  risks in newborn 672
Mengivac (A + C) 125
Ménière's disease 183
Meningitis vaccine 124–5
Meningococcal vaccine *see* Meningitis vaccine
Menopause 925–6
  and hormone replacement therapy 926
  and osteoporosis 928
  vitamin B complex in 683
  vitamin E in 683
Menophase 901, 941
Menorrhagia 922
Menotrophin 825, 826, 945
Menstrual periods 887–9
  fluid retention in 684
  heavy 922
  painful *see* Dysmenorrhoea
  pyridoxine in 684
  vitamin C in 684
  vitamin E in 684
Mental illness 626
Menthol
  in cooling applications 1031
  in vapour rubs and inhalants 39
Menzol 901
Mepacrine 805, 815
Mepenzolate 16
  in diarrhoea 218
  in spasm of the intestine 229
Mepivacaine 427
Meprobamate 619, 623, 624
Meptazinol 419, 422
Meptid 422
Mequitazine 94
Merbentyl 231
Mercaptopurine 1061
Mercilon 913
Mercurial compounds 995
Mercurochrome 995
Merocaine 427
Mesalazine 225, 227, 228
Mesna 84, 1060
Mesterolone 960
Mestranol
  in oral contraceptives 913
Metamucil 228
Metaraminol 25, 335
Metenix 304, 329
Meterfolic 715
Metformin 870–72, 873
Methadone
  in cough 47
  in pain 419, 422

Methaemoglobinaemia
hereditary 1178
Methenamine *see* Hexamine
Methicillin 738, 742
Methixene 16
in parkinsonism 551, 553
Methocarbamol 467, 469, 470
Methoserpidine 303
Methotrexate 446
in cancer 1061
in psoriasis 1040
in rheumatoid arthritis 446
Methotrimeprazine 637
Methoxamine 25, 336
Methoxsalen 1039
Methoxypsoralen 1000
Methyclothiazide
in heart failure 328
in hypertension 303
Methylcellulose
in constipation 235
in diarrhoea 219
in skin applications 979
in slimming 649, 650
Methylcysteine 51
Methyldopa 27, 292, 302, 303, 304, 312
Methylphenobarbitone 571
Methylprednisolone 841, 844, 845
in exophthalmos 847
in hayfever 107
in rheumatoid arthritis 452
Methyltestosterone 960
Methyprylone 580
Methysergide 435, 436, 438
Metipranolol 533, 537, 539
Metoclopramide
harmful effects and warnings 185–6
and anti-cancer drugs 180
in anaesthesia 181
in heartburn 212
in migraine 182, 431, 437
in radiation treatment 181
preparations 186
Metolazone
in heart failure 329
in hypertension 304
Metopirone 824, 825, 828
Metoprolol
in angina 277, 279
in disorders of heart rhythm and rate 349, 350
in hypertension 302, 304
in migraine 434, 438
Metosyn 983
Metox 186
Metriphonate 813, 816
Metrodin 824, 826, 943, 945
Metrolyl 765, 949
Metronidazole 764–5
harmful effects and warnings 765
after hysterectomy 734
in amoebic dysentry 804
in Crohn's disease 223
in dental abscess 734
in dracontiasis 815
in giardiasis 805
in peptic ulcers 204
in vaginal infections 947, 949
in Vincent's infection 172
Metyrapone 824, 825, 828, 829
Mexiletine 347, 350
Mexitil 350
Mezlocillin 738, 742
Miacaleic 470
Mianserin 588, 592, 599
Micolette 243
Miconazole 782, 786, 787
harmful effects and warnings 786
in athlete's foot 1013
in skin preparations 992
in thrush of the mouth 174
in vaginal infections 949
Micralax 243
Microgynon-30 913
Micronor 917
Microval 917
Mictral 492
Micturin 494, 498
Midamor 329
Middle ear infection (Otitis media) *see* Ears, disorders of
Midrid 437
Migrafen 408
Migraine 428–38
magnesium in 683
vitamins in 683
Migraleve 414, 437
Migravess 413, 431, 437
Migril 437
Mildison 983
Milk-alkali syndrome 193
Milk of Magnesia 244
Milk producing hormone *see* Prolactin
Milrinone 326
Milton 995
Mineralocorticoids 827, 832
replacement treatment with 841
Minerals 686–703
Minihep 394
Minihep calcium 394
Min-I-Jet Adrenaline 26
Min-I-Jet Calcium Chloride
Min-I-Jet Isoprenaline 26
Minims
amethocaine 427, 528
artificial tears 529
atropine 529
benoxinate (oxybuprocaine) 427, 528
castor oil 529
chloramphenicol 526
cyclopentolate 529
gentamicin 526
homatropine 529
lignocaine and fluorescein 427, 528
metipranolol 539
neomycin 526
phenylephrine 530
pilocarpine 530, 538, 539
prednisolone 527
sulphacetamide 526
thymoxamine
tropicamide 530
Minocin 753
Minocycline 753
in acne 1010
Minodiab 873
Minoxidil
harmful effects and warnings 314
in baldness 1013–14
in hypertension 295
Mintec 231
Mintezol 817
Minulet 913
Miotics 530–531
Miraxid 745
Misoprostol 204, 205, 207
Mithracin 1061
Mithracyn *see* Plicamycin
Mithramycin *see* Plicamycin
Mitozantrone 1063
Mitobronitol 1060
Mitomycin 1061
Mitomycin C Kyowa 1061
Mitoxana 1060
MMR vaccine *see* Measles, mumps and rubella vaccine
Mobiflex 451
Modecate 637
Moditen 637
Moditen Enanthate 637

Modrasone 983
Moducren 307
Moduret 307, 329, 331
Moduretic 307, 330, 331
Mogadon 583
Molcer 62
Molipaxin 599
Molybdenum 700
Monaspor 749
Monistat 949
Monit 279
Mono Cedocard 279
Monoamine-oxidase inhibitors *see* Anti-depressant drugs
Monoamine-oxidase-B inhibitors 549
Monocor 279, 304
Monoparin 394
Monoparin Calcium 394
Monospor 749
Monosulfiram 1043
Monotrim 771
Monovent 166
MOPP therapy 1057
Morphine
  in cough 47
  in diarrhoea 217
  in pain 418, 422
Mosquito bites
  thiamine in 683
Motilium 186
Motion sickness 175–9
  harmful effects and warnings of drugs used to treat 184–5
  preparations 185–6
Motipress 600
Motival 600
Motrin 408, 451
Mouth
  disorders of 169–79
Mouth ulcers 170
  zinc in 679
Mouth washes 173
Mrs Cullen's Powders 413
MST Continus 422
Mucaine 199, 213
Mucodyne 52
Mucogel 199
Mucolytics
  inhalation 51
  oral 51
Multilind 992
Multiparin 394
Multivitamin preparations
  uses of 660–61
Mumps vaccine 125–6
Mupirocin 71, 989
Muscle cramps
  calcium in 683
  potassium in 683
  vitamin C in 683
  vitamin E in 683
Muscle relaxants (skeletal)
  harmful effects and warnings 468
  in chronic back pain 467
  in osteoarthritis 465
  used in anaesthesia *see* Neuromuscular blocking drugs
Mustine 1060
MVPP therapy 1057
Myambutol 778
Myasthenia gravis 13, 755
Mycota 992
Mydriacyl 530
Mydriatics 525
Mydrilate 530
Myelobromol 1060
Myleran 1060
Mynah 778
Myocardial infarction 253 *see also* Heart attack
Myocardial ischaemia 253
Myocardol 279
Myocrisin 444
Myoneural blocking drugs *see* Neuromuscular blocking drugs
Myotonine 500, 501
Mysoline 571
Mysteclin 753
Myxoedema 854, 856

Nabilone 181, 186
Nabumetone 452, 456
Nacton 231
Nadolol
  in angina 278
  in disorders of heart rhythm 349
  in hypertension 303
  in migraine 434, 438
Naftidrofuryl
  harmful effects and warnings 364
  and mental function in elderly 363
  in disorders of the circulation 354, 365
Nalbuphine 419, 422
Nalcrom 228
Nalidixic acid 490, 492, 761, 764
  harmful effects and warnings 491
  and sunlight sensitivity 1006
Naloxone 415
Nandrolone 966
  in aplastic anaemia 962
Naphazoline 25, 524
Nappy rash 1035–6
Naprosyn 408, 451, 923
Naproxen
  harmful effects and warnings 456
  in dysmenorrhea 923
  in gout 476, 478
  in pain relief 408
  in rheumatoid arthritis 451, 452
Narcotic antagonists *see* Opioid antagonists
Narcotic pain relievers *see* Pain relieving drugs
Nardil 599
Narphen 422
Nasal decongestants *see* Decongestants
Nasal polyps *see* Nose
Naseptin 71
Natamycin 782, 787
  harmful effects and warnings 786
  in skin preparations 992
  in vaginal infections 950
Natrilix 304
Natulan *see* Procarbazine
Nausea 175–86
  harmful effects and warnings of drugs used to treat 184–5
  drugs used to treat 185–6
  in pregnancy 179–80
Navidrex 304, 329
Navidrex-K 307, 330
Naxogin 500, 816, 949
Nebcin 757
Nedocromil 156, 162, 167
Nefopam 409
Negram 492
Nelson's syndrome 828
Neocon 1/35 913
Neo-Cortef 66, 528
Neogest 917
Neo-Medrone 987
Neo-Mercazole 848, 853
Neomycin 757
  in eye infections 526
  in nasal preparations 70–71
  in skin preparations 989
Neo-NaClex 304, 329
Neo-NaClex-K 307, 330
Neoplatin 1063
Neosporin 526
Neostigmine 13
  harmful effects and warnings 502

in retention of urine 501
Nepenthe 422
Nephril 304, 329
Nerisone 983
Netillin 757
Netilmicin 757
Nettle rash *see* Urticaria
Neulactil 367
Neuromuscular blocking drugs 18
Niacin 662, 665
Niacinamide *see* Niacin
Nicardipine
in angina 278
in hypertension 303
Nickel 700
Niclosamide 810, 816
Nicofuranose
harmful effects and warnings 364
in disorders of the circulation 354, 365
on blood cholesterol and fats 378
Nicotinamide *see* Niacin
Nicotinic acid (*see also* Niacin) 662
harmful effects and warnings 364
and blood cholesterol and fats 373, 378
and its derivatives 354
and the circulation 354, 355
Nicotinic acid amide *see* Niacin
Nicotinyl alcohol 354
Nicoumalone 385, 393, 394
Nifedipine
harmful effects and warnings 269
in angina 277
in hypertension 302
in migraine 434
in Raynaud's disease 359, 365
Niferex 714
Nilstim 650
Nimodipine 354
Nimorazole
harmful effects and warnings 816
in Vincent's infection 172
in vaginal infections 947, 949
Nimotop 365
Nipride 304, 332
Niridazole 815, 816
Nitrados 583
Nitrate vasodilators
in angina 256
in heart attack 271
in heart failure 323
in Raynaud's disease 359
Nitrates *see* Nitrate vasodilators
Nitrazepam 583
Nitric acid 1046
Nitrocine 279, 332
Nitrocontin Continus 279
Nitrofurantoin 490, 491, 492
Nitroglycerine 259
Nitrolingual 279
Nitromersol 995
Nitronal 332
Nitroprusside 304, 305
harmful effects and warnings 335
in heart failure 326, 332
in hypertension 295, 304, 305
Nivaquine 445, 803
Nivemycin 757
Nizatidine 206, 207, 208
Nizoral 787, 949, 992, 1027
Nobrium 624
Noctec 583
Noltam 896, 943, 1064, 1067
Nolvadex 896, 943, 1064, 1067
Non-depolarizing muscle relaxants *see* Competitive neuromuscular blocking drugs
Non-gonococcal urethritis 504, 734
Non-specific urethritis (NSU) 504
Non-steroidal anti-inflammatory drugs *see* NSAIDs
Noradrenaline 21, 25, 336
Norcuron 20
Norditropin 825, 826
Nordox 753
Norethisterone 897, 901
in combined contraceptives 913, 914, 916
in dysmenorrhoea 924
in progestogen-only contraceptives 917
Norflex 467, 470
Norgeston 917
Norgestrel
in progestogen-only contraceptives 917
Noriday 917
Norimin 913
Norinyl-l 913
Noristerat 916, 917
Normacol 228
Normal immunoglobulin *see* Immunoglobulins, normal
Normax 234
Normetic 307, 330, 331
Normison 583
Nortriptyline
in bedwetting 499
in depression 599
Norval 600
Noscapine 47
Nose, disorders of 67–71
allergic disorders *see* Hayfever
blockage of 67
infections of 69–70
polyps of 68–9
rhinitis medicamentosa 69
vasomotor rhinitis 67–8
Novantrone 1063
Novaprin 408
Novaruca 1046
Noxyflex 427, 492
Noxythiolin 492
Nozinan 367
NSAIDs (Non-steroidal anti-inflammatory drugs)
harmful effects and warnings 447, 453
in chronic back pain 466
in dysmenorrhoea 922–4
in gout 476
in migraine 431
in osteoarthritis 465
in pain 406, 408
in rheumatic rubs 462
in rheumatoid arthritis 440
Nubain 422
Nuelin 166
Nu-K 331
Nulacin 199, 213
Numotac 166
Nupercainal 427
Nurofen 408
Nurse Sykes Powders 413
Nu-Seals Aspirin 277, 442, 451
Nystadermal 987
Nystaform 992
Nystaform-HC 987
Nystan 174, 787, 949, 992
Nystatin 782, 786, 787
in skin preparations 992

Nystatin – *cont.*
in thrush of the mouth 174
in vaginal thrush 946–7, 949

Ocusert Pilo 531, 538, 539
Oesophagitis 210
Oestradiol 891, 896
Oestradiol implants 941
Oestriol 891, 896
Oestrogens 891–6
harmful effects and warnings 892–4
in breast feeding 894, 895
in HRT 932
in menopause 926
in menorrhagia 922
in pregnancy 894
in vaginal dryness and shrinking 926, 946
natural 891
preparations 896
semi-synthetic 891
synthetic 891
to decrease sexual activity 973
Oestrone 891, 896
Ofloxacin 761, 764
Ointments 977
Olbetam 378
Olsalazine 225, 227, 228
Omega-3 marine triglycerides *see* Fish oils
Omeprazole 202, 206, 207
Omnopon 422
Omnopon-Scopolamine 16
Oncovin 1062
Ondansetron 181
Ophthalmic preparations *see* Eye preparations
Opilon 365
Opioid antagonists 415
Opioid pain relievers *see* Pain relieving drugs
Opium 217
Opthaine eye drops 427, 528
Opticrom 107, 523, 528
Optimine 95
Opulets
atropine 530
benoxinate (oxybuprocaine) 427, 528
chloramphenicol 526
cyclopentolate 530
pilocarpine 531, 538, 539
Orabase 172
Orabet 873
Orahesive 172
Oral contraceptives *see* Contraceptives, oral
Oral hypoglycaemic drugs *see* Anti-diabetic drugs, oral
Oral rehydration preparations *see* Electrolyte and water replacement
Oramorph 422
Orap 367
Orbenin 743
Orciprenaline 25, 165
Orgasm 967
Oriental sore 806
Orimeten 1064, 1066
Orphenadrine
harmful effects and warnings 469
in chronic back pain 467
in parkinsonism 551, 552
preparations 470
uses of 16
Ortho Dienoestrol 896, 941
Ortho-Gynest 896, 941
Ortho-Novin 1/50 913
Orudis 451
Oruvail 451
Ossopan 695
Osteitis deformans *see* Paget's disease of bone
Osteoarthritis 464–5
Osteomalacia 670
caused by drugs 1087
Osteoporosis 927–31
caused by drugs 1087
prevention of 929–31
Otitis externa *see* Ears, disorders of
Otitis media *see* Ears, disorders of
Otosporin 66
Ovestin 896, 941
Ovran 913
Ovran-30 913
Ovranette 913
Ovysmen 913
Oxamniquine 813, 816
Oxanid 624
Oxatomide 94, 97, 99
Oxazepam 624
Oxethazaine 196
Oxpentifylline 354, 364, 365
Oxprenolol
in angina 277, 279, 280
in anxiety 624, 625
in disorders of heart rhythm 349, 350, 351
in hypertension 302, 304, 305
Oxybuprocaine 427, 523, 528
Oxychlorosene 995
Oxycodone 422
Oxymetazoline 25, 70
Oxymetholone 962, 966
Oxymycin 753
Oxypertine 636
Oxyphenbutazone eye ointment 523
Oxyphenisatin 234
Oxytetracycline 752, 753
in acne 1010
in acne rosacea 1012
in gonorrhoea 504
Oxytocin 819, 820
harmful effects and warnings 952
in labour 952, 954
to prevent bleeding after abortion or childbirth 952, 953, 954

PABA *see* Para-aminobenzoic acid
Pacifene 408
Padimate A 1002
Padimates 1000
Paget's disease of bone 469–71
Pain 400–422
Pain-relieving drugs 401–22
combined narcotic/non-narcotic 411–15
narcotic 415–22
non-narcotic 402-15
Palaprin Forte 442, 451
Painful periods *see* Dysmenorrhoea
Palfium 422
Paludrine 803
Pamergan 422
Panadeine 414
Pancuronium 19
Pantothenic acid 667
Papaveretum 419, 422
Papaverine
in impotence 972
Para-aminobenzoic acid (PABA)
and sunlight sensitivity 1005
in sunscreen applications 1000
Paracetamol
harmful effects and warnings 408
dangers of overdose 407
in chronic back pain 466
in colds 34
in fever 34, 127

in migraine 430, 437
in osteoarthritis 465
in pain 407
in thyroid crisis 853
Paracodol 414
Paradeine 414
Paraesthesia *see* Pins and Needles
Parahypon 414
Parake 414
Paraldehyde 566, 568, 571
Paralgin 414
Paralysis agitans *see* Parkinson's disease
Paramax 432, 437
Paramol 414
Paraplatin 1062
Parasympathomimetics 11–12
Parathyroid glands
disorders of 859–60
Parathyroid hormone (parathormone, PTH) 859
Pardale 414
Parkinsonism 543–57
Parkinson's disease 543–57
Parlodel 552, 944, 945
Parmid 186
Parnate 600
Parstelin 600
Passive immunization 109, 138–40
Pastes 977
Pavulon 20
Paxadon 186
Paxalgesic 414
Paxofen 408, 451
PCP 512
Peak flow meters 144
Peanut oil 237
Pecram 166
Pectin 218
Penbritin 743
Pendramine 445
Penicillamine 445, 450, 459–60
Penicillin G 734, 735, 737
Penicillin V 734, 735, 736, 737, 742, 743, 744
Penicillin VK *see* Penicillin V
Penicillinases 735
Penicillins 735–45
harmful effects of 740, 741
anti-pseudomonal 739
broad spectrum 738
mecillinams (amidino) 739
penicillinase-resistant 737
penicillinase-sensitive 737
warnings on use 741, 742
Penidural 743
Pentaerythritol tetranitrate 258, 278, 279
Pentasa 228
Pentazocine
in combined preparations 411
in pain 410, 419, 422
in chronic back pain 466
Pentostam 817
Pepcid PM 207
Peppermint oil
in diarrhoea 218
in spasm of the intestine 229
Peptic ulcers 187–210
vitamins in 685
Perbuterol 25
Percutol 279
Perfan 326, 336
Pergonal 825, 826, 943, 945
Periactin 95
Pericyazine 637
Perindopril 303, 310
Permethrin 1034, 1035
Perphenazine 185, 636
Persantin 395
Persomnia 414
Pertofran 600
Pertussis vaccine *see* Whooping cough vaccine
Pethidine 419, 422
Petroleum jelly
in chilblains 1018
in cold sores 172
in emollients 978
in nappy rash 1035
in protective skin applications 979
Pevaryl 949, 992
Pevaryl TC 987
Phaeochromocytoma 28, 1109
Pharmorubicin 1061
Phasal 600
Phascolamin 651
Phenazocine 420, 422
Phenazopyridine 494
Phenelzine 599
Phenergan 95, 179
Phenethicillin 737, 742
Phenformin 870
Phenindamine 94
Phenindione 385, 393, 394
Pheniramine 94
Phenobarbitone
in epilepsy 570, 571
in epileptic emergencies 566
Phenol 995, 996, 1031
Phenolphthalein 234
Phenoperidine 420
Phenothiazines (*see also* Anti-psychotics)
and anti-cancer drugs 181
and morphine 181
and sunlight sensitivity 1005
in anaesthesia 181
in itching 1032
in radiation treatment 181
in vertigo 183
in vomiting 177, 182
Phenothrin 1034, 1035
Phenoxybenzamine 293, 303, 311
Phentermine 648, 653
Phenoxymethylpenicillin *see* Penicillin V
Phensic 413
Phentolamine 304, 312
Phenylbutazone
in ankylosing spondylitis 467
Phenylephrine
harmful effects and warnings 336
in asthma preparations 167
in decongestant eye drops 524
in nasal decongestants 35, 36, 37
to dilate the pupils 526, 530
uses of 25
Phenylpropanolamine
in incontinence of urine 497
in nasal decongestants 35, 36, 37
in slimming 648
uses of 25
Phenytoin
harmful effects and warnings 347, 568
in disorders of heart rhythm and rate 350
in epilepsy 570, 571
in epileptic emergencies 566
Phenytoin sodium *see* Phenytoin
Pholcodine 47
Phosphates *see* Phosphorus

Phosphorus
(phosphates) 694–6
Photosensitivity 1005
Phyllocontin 166
Physeptone 422
Physostigmine 13, 530, 531, 538, 539
and pilocarpine 530, 531
Phytex 992
Phytocil 992
Phytomenadione
harmful effects and warnings 399
in newborn 397
in vitamin K deficiency 672
Piles *see* Haemorrhoids
Pilocarpine 12, 530, 531, 534, 538, 539
and physostigmine 530, 531
Pimafucin 787, 950, 992
Pimozide 637
Pindolol
in angina 280
in hypertension 305
Pins and needles (paraesthesia)
pyridoxine in 683
Pipenzolate 16, 229
Piperacillin 739, 743
Piperazine
harmful effects and warnings 816
in roundworm 808
in threadworms 807
Piperazine oestrone sulphate *see* Oestrone
Piportil Depot 367
Pipothiazine palmitate
antipsychotic use of 637
Pipril 743
Piptal 231
Piptalin 231
Pirbuterol 165
Pirenzepine 16
harmful effects and warnings 206
in peptic ulcers 200–201, 207
Piretanide 302
Piriton 95
Piroxicam
in gout 476
in rheumatoid arthritis 451
Pitressin 823, 825
Pituitary gland 819–26
Pivampicillin 738, 743
Pivmecillinam 740, 743, 745
Pizotifen 433, 438
Plaquenil 445
Platet 277
Platinex 1063
Plesmet 714
Plicamycin 1061
Pneumococcal vaccine 130–31
Pneumocystis carnii (PCP) 512
Pneumovax II 131
Podophyllin 1046, 1047
Podophyllotoxin 1047
Podophyllum resin *see* Podophyllin
Poldine
in peptic ulcers 196
in spasm of the intestine 229
uses of 17
Poliomyelitis vaccine 131–2
Polybactrin 989
Polycrol 199, 213
Polyestradiol 1065
Polyethylene glycol
in artificial tears 524, 529
Polyfax 526, 989
Polyglutamates (folates) 618
Polymyxin B 761, 763
in eye infections 526
Polymyxins 758
Polynoxylin
in skin preparations 989
in thrush of the mouth 174
Polyps, nasal *see* Nose, disorders of
Polysaccharide-iron complex 714
Polythiazide 304
Polytrim 526
Polyvinyl alcohol
in artificial tears 524, 529
Ponderax 653
Pondocillin 743
Ponstan 408, 452, 922, 923
Posalfilin 1047
Post coital intra-uterine device 918
Potassium 689–91
Potassium chloride 331
Potassium citrate 492, 493
Potassium permanganate 1023
Potassium sparing diuretics *see* Diuretics
Potassium supplements 331
Povidone-iodine 997
in impetigo 1027
in vaginal applications 948
Powerin 413
Pravastatin 374, 378
Praxilene 365
Praziquantel
harmful effects and warnings 817
in schistosomiasis 813
in tapeworm 810
Prazosin
harmful effects and warnings 311
in benign prostatic hypertrophy 501
in disorders of the circulation 355, 365
in heart failure 326, 331
in hypertension 303
Pre-medication before surgery
use of anticholinergic drugs in 17
Precortisyl 228, 845
Pred Forte 527
Predenema 228
Predfoam 228
Prednesol 228, 845
Prednisolone 841, 843, 844, 845
in asthma 154
in Crohn's disease 223, 228
in eye disorders 527
in rheumatoid arthritis 443, 452
in ulcerative colitis 225, 228
Prednisone 844
Predsol 66, 228, 527
Predsol-N 66, 528
Preferid 983
Prefil 650
Pregaday 715
Pregnancy 1116–18
drugs that should not be used or used with caution 1119–28
heartburn in 213
hormonal changes in 889–90
nausea and vomiting in 179–80
Pregnancy, toxaemia of 301
folic acid in 685
pyridoxine in 685
Primidone 569, 570, 571
Premarin 896, 941
Premenstrual Syndrome (PMS)
Prempak-C 901, 941

Prepidil 954
Prepulsid 212
Prescal 304
Pressure sores *see* Bedsores
Prestim 307
Priadel 600
Prickly heat
  vitamin C in 684
Prilocaine 427
Primacor 326
Primalan 95
Primaquine 798, 802, 803
Primaxin 748
Primolut Depot 901
Primolut N 901, 924
Primoteston Depot 960
Primperan 186
Prioderm 1035, 1043
Pripsen 816
Pro-Actidil 95
Pro-Banthine 231, 494, 497
Probenecid
  harmful effects and warnings 482
  in gout 478, 483
  with antiobiotics 504
Probucol 374, 377, 378
Procainamide 348, 350
Procaine 427
  and sunlight sensitivity 1005
  in gonorrhoea 505
  in syphilis 734
  procaine penicillin 737, 742
Procarbazine 1057
Prochlorperazine
  as anti-psychotic 637
  in vomiting during pregnancy 179
  preparations to relieve vomiting 185, 186
Proctosedyl 427
Procyclidine 17, 551, 552
Profasi 826, 941, 944
Proflavine 995
Proflex 408
Proflex cream 462
Progesic 408, 452
Progesterone 897–901
  in PMS 919
Progestogens 897–901
  harmful effects and warnings 898–9
  depot injections of 897
  in breast feeding 899
  in dysmenorrhoea 923–4
  in menorrhagia 922
  in miscarriages 899
  in pregnancy 899
  synthetic 897
Proguanil 800, 801, 803
Progynova 896, 941
Prolactin 822
Promazine 637
Promethazine
  harmful effects and warnings 581
  and sensitivity to sunlight 993
  in allergies 94
  in motion sickness 178, 179
  in sleeping disorders 581, 583
  in vomiting of pregnancy 180
  preparations 185, 186
Prominal 571
Prondol 600
Pronestyl 350
Propaderm 983
Propaderm-A 987
Propafenone 348, 349
Propain 414, 437
Propamidine 521, 526
Propantheline
  harmful effects and warnings 497
  in diarrhoea 218
  in peptic ulcers 196
  in spasm of the intestine 229
  in urinary frequency 494
Propine 533, 539
Propranolol
  in angina 277, 278, 279
  in anxiety 624
  in disorders of heart rhythm 349, 350
  in hypertension 302, 303, 304
  in migraine 434, 438
  in overactive thyroid disease 849
  in thyroid crisis 853
Propylene glycol
  in skin applications 979
Propylthiouracil 848, 854
Prostacyclin *see* Epoprostenol
Prostaglandins
  in abortion 951
  in inflammation 402, 440
  in labour 952
  in peptic ulcers 204
  in Raynaud's disease 359
Prostate
  benign hypertrophy of 501
  evening primrose oil in 684
  zinc in 684
Prostigmin 501, 502
Prostin E2 951, 954
Prostin F2 alpha 951, 952, 954
Protamine sulphate 384, 392, 394
Prothiaden 600
Protirelin *see* Thyrotrophin-releasing hormone
Proton pump blockers 202
Proton pump inhibitors *see* Proton pump blockers
Protriptyline 599
Pro-Vent 166
Provera 901
Pro-Viron 960
Proxymetacaine 427, 523, 528
Prozac 600
Pruritus *see* Itching
Pruritus ani *see* Itching
Pruritus vulvae *see* Itching
Pseudocholinesterase 20
Pseudoephedrine
  in incontinence of urine 497
  in nasal decongestants 35, 36, 37
Psoradrate 1038
Psoralens 1039
Psoriasis 1036–42
  harmful effects and warnings of drugs used to treat 1041–2
  zinc in 684
Psychoneurosis 626
Psychosis 626
Psyllium
  in constipation 235
  in diarrhoea 219
  in slimming 649
Pteroylglutamic acid *see* Folic acid
PTH *see* Parathyroid hormone
Pulmadil 166
Pulmicort 166
Pulmonary embolism 382
  anti-coagulants in 390
  streptokinase in 390
  urokinase in 390
Pump-Hep 394
Pupils
  drugs that constrict 530–31
  drugs that dilate 525, 529
Puri-Nethol 1061
PUVA treatment 1039–40
Pyopen 743
Pyralvex 171
Pyrantel

Pyrantel – *cont.*
harmful effects and warnings 817
in hookworm 811
in roundworm 808
in threadworms 807
Pyrazinamide 776, 778
Pyridostigmine 13
Pyridoxine 664
in depression 598
in nausea and vomiting of pregnancy 180
in PMS 921
Pyrimethamine 799, 803
Pyrithione zinc shampoo 1019, 1020
Pyrogastrone 199, 207, 213

Quellada 1035, 1047
Questran 228, 378, 1032
Quinalbarbitone 583
Quinapril
harmful effects and warnings 310
in heart failure 332
in hypertension 302
Quinidine 348, 350
Quinine 799, 803
Quinocort 987
Quinolones 758
4-Quinolones *see* Quinolones
Quinoped 992

Rabies
active immunization 133
passive immunization 133, 140
immunoglobulin 134, 140
Rabies vaccine 133–4
Rabro 199, 207
Ranitidine 206, 208
Rashes caused by drugs 1047–51
Rastinon 873
Rauwolfia alkaloids 294, 313
Raynaud's disease 357–60
Raynaud's phenomenon 358
Raynaud's syndrome 357–60
RBC cream 993
Redeptin 637
Redoxon 493
Refolinon 1061
Refrigerants 462
Regaine 1014
Regulan 228
Rehibin 896, 943, 944
Rehidrat 217
Rehydration
oral 217
Reiter's disease 504
Relaxit 243
Relcofen 408
Relifex 452
Remnos 583
Renal colic
use of anticholinergic drugs in 17
Renal stones
and gout 472
magnesium in 682
pyridoxine in 682
Renin 282
Renin–angiotensin mechanism 282, 827
Reproterol 25, 165
Re-PUVA treatment 1040
Reserpine 294, 304, 313
Resorcinol 1038
Restandol 960
Restless legs
vitamin C in 684
Retin-A 1009
Retrovir 515
Revanil 552
Reye's syndrome
aspirin and 405
Rhesus factor 722, 723
Rheumatic fever
prevention of 734
Rheumatic rubs 460, 461
Rheumatoid arthritis 439–60
Rheumox 452, 483
Rhinitis medicamentosa *see* Nose
Rhinocort 70
Rhumalgan 452
Ribavirin *see* Tribavirin
Riboflavine 663
Rickets 670
Ridaura 444
Rifadin 764, 778
Rifampicin 762
harmful effects and warnings 777
in meningitis contacts 127, 734
in tuberculosis 773, 778
preparations 764, 778
Rifinah 778
Rimactane 764, 778
Rimactazid 778
Rimiterol 25, 165
Rinatec 70
Ringworm 782
Ritodrine 25
in premature labour 954
Rivotril 571
Roaccutane 1012
Robaxin 467, 470
Robaxisal Forte 413, 467, 470
Rochelle Salts 244
Roferon-A 1063
Rogitine 304
Rohypnol 583
Ronicol 365
Rosoxacin *see* Acrosoxacin
Roter 199
Roundworm 808
Rubefacients 460
Rubella *see* German measles
Rubella, normal immunoglobulin *see* German measles immunoglobulin 139
Rubella vaccine *see* German measles vaccine
Rynacrom 70, 106
Rythmodan 350

Sabidal 166
Saccharin
and sunlight sensitivity 1006
Saizen 825
Salazopryrin 228, 444
Salbulin 166
Salbutamol 25
in anaphylactic shock 103
in asthma 165, 166, 167
in emergency treatment of asthma 163
in premature labour 954
Salbuvent 166
Salcatonin 470
Salicylic acid
harmful effects and warnings 1041
in corns 1019
in eczema and dermatitis 1024
in psoriasis 1038, 1039
in warts 1046, 1047
Salicilic acid collodion 1046
Salicylates 403
Saline, isotonic 688
Saliva, artificial 173
Salsalate 442, 451, 456
Saluric 304, 329
Sandimmun 85
Sandocal 695
Sando-K 331
Sanomigran 438
Saventrine 336
Saventrine IV 26
Scabies 1042–1043
Schering PC4 917

Scheriproct 427
Schistosomiasis
(Bilharziasis) 811–13
acute (Katayama
fever) 813
swimmer's itch 813
Schizophrenia 626–37
folic acid in 684
vitamin B complex in 684
vitamin B_{12} in 684
vitamin C in 684
Scoline 20
Scopoderm 178, 186
Scopolamine *see* Hyoscine
Sea-legs 186
Seborrhoeic
dermatitis 1026–7
biotin in 684
pyridoxine in 684
vitamin B complex in 684
Secadrex 308
Seclodin 408
Seconal Sodium 583
Sectral 279, 304, 350
Securon 279, 304, 350
Securopen 743
Sedatives
and sex 970
definition 605
general warnings on
use 620–22
in anxiety 605
Select-A-Jet Dopamine 26
Selegiline 548, 551, 552
Selenium 701
in cancer 701
in coronary artery
disease 701
Selenium sulphide 1019,
1020
Selexid 743
Selexidin 743
Selsun 1019
Semi-Daonil 873
Semi-membranous
colitis 733
Semprex 95
Senna 233
Sential 985
Septrin 771
Serc 186
Serenace 637
Serophene 896, 943, 944
Serotonin *see* 5-
Hydroxytryptamine
Serpasil 304
Serpasil-Esidrex 308
Sex
and drugs 967–75
Sex hormones 832
in cancer 1064, 1065
Sexual activity
drugs used to
decrease 973
Sexual problems
drugs used to treat
971–2
Sexually transmitted
diseases 503–20
Shampoos
medicated 1019
Shingles 790–92
passive immunization 140
vitamin B complex in 684
vitamin B_{12} in 684
vitamin C in 684
Sickle cell anaemia 74
Silicon 701
Siloxyl 199, 213
Silver nitrate 171
Silver sulphadiazine 989
Simeco 199, 213
Simplene 539
Simvastatin 374, 377, 378
Sinemet 546, 553
Sinequan 600
Sinthrome 394
Sintisone 228, 845
Sinusitis 72, 734
Skin
allergy to the sun's
rays 1006
cancer of, caused by
sunlight 999
sensitivity to the sun's
rays 1005
Skin, ageing of
vitamin E in 681
Skin, dry
vitamin A in, 681
vitamin E in 681
Skin diseases 976–1051
Skin preparations
additives in 976
anti-bacterial 990
anti-fungal 993
antihistamine 993
antiseptics and
disinfectants 994
anti-viral 993
astringent 990
bases in 976
caustics 988
corticosteroid 980–8
emollients 978
keratolytic 989
local anaesthetic 988
protective 979
soothing 978
types of 977
Sleep disorders 572–83
drugs that may cause 573
Sleeping drugs 573–83
and sex 970
general warnings on
use 620–22
Slimming 646–53
Slimming drugs 648–53
and libido 972
Slo-Phyllin 167
Slow-Fe 714
Slow-Fe folic 715
Slow-K 331
Slow-Pren 279, 305
Slow-Trasicor 305, 624
Smallpox vaccine 134
Smell, loss of sense of
vitamin A in 683
zinc in 683
Sno Phenicol 526
Sno Pilo 538, 539
Sno Tears 529
Sodium 686–9
Sodium acid phosphate 243
Sodium Amytal 583
Sodium aurothiomalate *see*
Gold
Sodium bicarbonate
as antacid 192–3, 199
ear drops 62
to make the urine
alkaline 493
Sodium
carboxymethylcellulose
see Carmellose sodium
Sodium chloride
solutions 689
Sodium citrate 493
Sodium cromoglycate
harmful effects and
warnings 99, 156
actions 98
eye applications in
hayfever 107, 527
in asthma 155, 161, 165
in hayfever 106, 107
in nasal preparations 70
in ulcerative colitis 225
Sodium fusidate 762, 764
Sodium hypochlorite 995
in impetigo 1027
Sodium ironedetate 714
Sodium nitroprusside *see*
Nitroprusside
Sodium picosulphate 234
Sodium polystyrene
sulphonate resin 691
Sodium salicylate 452, 457
Sodium salts
in osmotic laxatives 237

Sodium stibogluconate 805, 817
Sodium valproate *see* Valproate
Sofradex 66, 528
Soframycin 66, 526, 757, 989
Sofra-Tulle 989
Solis 470, 624
Solpadeine 414
Solprin 452
Solu-Cortef 845
Solu-Medrone 845
Somatropin 824, 826
Sominex 583
Somnite 583
Soneryl 583
Soni-Slo 280
Sorbichew 280
Sorbid SA 280
Sorbitrate 280
Sotacor 280, 305, 350
Sotalol
  in angina 277
  in disorders of heart rhythm 349, 350
  in hypertension 302, 305
Sotazide 308
Sparine 637
Spasmonal 231
Spastic colon *see* Irritable bowel syndrome
Spectinomycin 762, 764
  in gonorrhoea 506, 733
Spermaceti 978
Spherocytosis, hereditary 724
Spiretic 329
Spiroctan 329
Spiroctan-M 329
Spirolone 329
Spironolactone 328, 329
  harmful effects and warnings 334
Sporanox 787, 950
Stabilizers 976
Stabillin V-K 743
Stafoxil 744
Stanozolol
  in angioedema 962
  in Behçet's syndrome 962
  in Raynaud's disease 359
  preparations 966
Starch blockers 651
Stelazine 186, 637
Stemetil 186, 637
Sterculia
  in constipation 235
  in diarrhoea 219
  in slimming 649, 650
Steroids 832
Steroids, anabolic *see* Anabolic steroids
Ster-Zac
  bath concentrate 989
Stesolid 470, 571, 624
Stevens–Johnson syndrome 1105
Stiedex 983, 985
Stiedex LPN 987
Stiemycin 1009
Stilboestrol 891, 896
  in cancer of the prostate 1065
Stimulants 638
Stomach ulcers *see* Peptic ulcers
Stomas
  risks of drug treatments 1180–82
Stramonium 17
Streptase 273, 277, 397
Streptokinase
  harmful effects and warnings 397
  in heart attack 272
Streptomycin 777, 778
Stroke
  treatment of 390
Stromba 966
Stugeron 186, 365
Sublimaze 419
Sucralfate 203, 206, 207
Sudafed 37
Sulbactam 745
Sulconazole
  in athlete's foot 1013
  in skin preparations 992
Suleo-C 1035
Suleo-M 1035
Sulfadoxine (in Fansidar) 799
Sulfametopyrazine 771
Sulindac
  harmful effects and warnings 457
  in gout 476
  in rheumatoid arthritis 451
Sulphacetamide
  in eye infections 524, 526
Sulphadiazine 771
Sulphadimethoxine 542
Sulphadimidine 734, 771
Sulphadoxine 799
Sulphaguanidine 771
Sulphaloxate, calcium 770
Sulphamethoxazole 769
  trimethoprim with 769
Sulphamezathine 771
Sulphasalazine
  harmful effects and warnings 226
  in Crohn's disease 223
  in rheumatoid arthritis 444
  in ulcerative colitis 225
  preparations 228
Sulphaurea 771
Sulphinpyrazone 478, 482, 483
Sulphonamides 766–71
  harmful effects and warnings 766–8
  and sunlight sensitivity 1006
Sulpiride 636
Sulphur 702
  in acne 1009
  in psoriasis 1038
  in seborrhoeic dermatitis 1027
Sulphonylureas 869–70
  harmful effects and warnings 869–70
  preparations 873
Sulpitil 637
Sultrin 950
Sun blockers 1002
Sun protection factor (SPF) 1001
Sunburn 998
  anti-sunburn preparations 997–1002
  treatment of 1006
  vitamin C in 685
  vitamin E in 685
  zinc in 685
Sunlight
  dangers of 998–9
Sunlight allergy 1006
Sunlight sensitivity 1005, 1026
Sunscreens 997–1005
Suntan 998, 1000, 1003
  preparations 1002–3
Superinfection 732
Suppositories
  laxative 241, 243
Suprefact 1065
Suramin 817
Surem 583
Surgam 452
Surmontil 600
Suscard Buccal 280, 332
Suspren 408
Sustac 280
Sustamycin 753
Sustanon 960
Suxamethonium 20
Sweating 1044–5

of feet 1045
Swimmer's itch 813
Symmetrel 553, 788
Sympathomimetics 22, 24, 26
decongestants 35–6, 37
in asthma 147–9
in bed wetting 499
in heart disease 326
in incontinence of urine 496–7
in premature labour 953
Synacthen 825, 826, 841
Synalar 984
Synalar 1 in 10 984
Synalar 1 in 4 984
Synalar C 987
Synalar N 987
Synalar Gel 984
Syndol 414
Synflex 408, 452
Synkavit 397, 399, 671, 672
Synphase 914
Syntaris 70
Syntocinon 952, 954
Syntopressin 823, 825
Syraprim 771
Systemic lupus erythematosus 1113–14
Sytron 714
Syntometrine 952, 953, 954

Tagamet 207
Talampicillin 738, 744
Talc
dusting powder 979
in physical sunscreens 1000
Talpen 744
Tambocor 350
Tamofen 896, 943, 1064, 1067
Tamoxifen 896
harmful effects and warnings 1067
in breast cancer 1064
in infertility 943
in PMS 922
Tampovagan Stilboestrol and Lactic Acid 896, 941
Tanderil eye ointment 523
Tapeworms 809–11
Tar *see* Coal tar
Tarcortin 985
Tardive dyskinesia 633–6
Targocid 764
Tarivid 764
Tavegil 95
TCP 996
Tear substitutes *see* Tears, artificial
Tears, artificial 524, 540
Tears Naturale 529
Teejel 171
Tegretol 571, 600
Teicoplanin 762, 764
Temazepam 583
Temgesic 422
Temocillin 744
Temopen 744
Tenif 280, 308
Tenoret-50 308
Tenoretic 308
Tenormin 280, 305, 351
Tenoxicam 451, 457
Tensium 470, 625
Tenuate Dospan 653
Teoptic 539
Terazosin 303, 311
Terbutaline
in asthma 165, 166
in emergency treatment of asthma 163
in premature labour 954
uses of 25
Terfenadine 94
Terlipressin 824, 825, 826
Terodiline
harmful effects and warnings 498
in incontinence of urine 497
in urinary frequency 494
Teronac 653
Terra-Cortril 66, 987
Terra-Cortril Nystatus 987
Terramycin 753
Tertroxin 858
Testosterone 897, 955, 960
and libido 972
Tetanus
active immunization 134–5, 140
anti-tetanus immunoglobulin 135
passive immunization 135–6, 140
Tetanus toxoids 134
Tetanus vaccine 134–5
Tetany 693
Tetmosol 1043
Tetrabenazine 30
Tetrabid 753
Tetrachel 753
Tetrachloroethylene 811, 817
Tetracosactrin 825, 826, 841
Tetracycline 752, 753
eye ointment in trachoma 542
in aphthous ulcers 171
in bronchitis 734
in eye infections 526
in malaria 799, 800
in non-gonococcal infection 734
in skin preparations 989
in syphilis 734
Tetracyclines
harmful effects and warnings 750–52, 1011
in acne 734, 1010, 1011
in gonorrhoea 504
in Reiter's disease 505
in toxoplasmosis 807
Tetralysal 753
Thalamonal 419
Thalassaemia 725
Theodrox 168
Theo-Dur 167
Theophylline
harmful effects and warnings 164
in asthma 149–51, 161
preparations used to treat asthma 165, 166, 167
Thephorin 95
Thiabendazole 811, 817–18
Thiamine *see* Vitamin B_1
Thiazides *see* Diuretics
Thiethylperazine 179, 186
Thioguanine 1061
Thiomersal 995
Thioridazine 637
Thiotepa 1060
Threadworms 807
Throat lozenges 42
Throat pastilles 42
Thromboangiitis obliterans *see* Buerger's disease
Thrombocytopenic purpura 1082
Thrombolytics 396
in heart attacks 272
preparations 277
Thrombophlebitis 362
vitamin E in 685
Thrombosis 381–99
Thrombus dissolving drugs *see* Thrombolytics
Thrush
of the mouth 169, 174
of the skin 783
of the vagina 783, 947
Thymol 995, 996
Thymol glycerin, compound 996

Thymoxamine
in disorders of the circulation 355, 364, 365
to reverse dilatation of pupils 526
Thyroid drugs 856, 858
in slimming 651
Thyroid gland
disorders of 846–58
Thyroid hormones 846
Thyroid stimulating hormone (TSH) 846
in thyroid cancer 1065
Thyrotoxicosis 847
Thyrotrophin-releasing hormone 821, 846
Thyroxine 856
Tiaprofenic acid 452, 458
Ticarcillin 739, 744
Ticarcillin/clavulanic acid 745
Tigason 1040, 1041
Tilade 167
Tildiem 280
Timentin 739, 745
Timocort 982
Timodine 987
Timolol
in angina 278
in glaucoma 533, 538, 539
in hypertension 302
in migraine 434, 438
Timoped 992
Timoptol 539
Tin 702
Tinaderm-M 992
Tineafax 992
Tinidazole 764–5
in amoebic dysentry 804
in giardiasis 805
in vaginal infections 947, 948, 949
Tinset 95
Tioconazole 782, 786, 992
Titanium dioxide 1000
Tixylix
Titralac 695
Tobralex 526
Tobramycin 526, 757
Tocainide 348, 350
Tocopherols *see* Vitamin E
Tofranil 499, 600
Tolanase 873
Tolazamide 873
Tolbutamide 873
Tolectin 452
Tolerzide 308
Tolmetin 452, 458
Tolnaftate 992
Tonics 654–8
Tonocard 351
Tonsillitis 734
Topal 199, 213
Topicycline 1009
Topilar 984
Torecan 179, 186
Toxoplasmosis 806
Trace elements 686
Trachoma 541
Tracrium 19
Tramil 415
Trancopal 625
Trandate 280, 305
Tranexamic acid 396, 398
in menorrhagia 922
Tranquillizers 605–6
Transiderm-Nitro 280
Transvasin 427
Tranxene 625
Tranylcypromine 600
Trasicor 280, 305, 351, 625
Trasidrex 308
Trasylol 396, 398
Travel sickness *see* Motion sickness
Traveller's diarrhoea 220–22
Traveltabs 179
Travogyn 950
Traxam 462
Trazodone 589, 592, 599
Tremonil 553
Trental 365
Treosulfan 1060
Tretinoin 1009
TRH *see* Thyrotrophin-releasing hormone
Tri-Adcortyl 988
Tri-Adcortyl Otic 66
Triamcinolone 841, 844
in alopecia areata 1014
in rheumatoid arthritis 452
in skin preparations 983, 984
Triamco 330, 331
Triamterene 328, 334
Tribavirin 789, 794
Tribiotic 989
Tri-Cicatrin 988
Triclofos 581, 583
Triclosan 989, 995, 996
Tricyclic anti-depressants *see* Anti-depressant drugs, tricyclic
Tridil 332
Trifluoperazine
harmful effects and warnings 858
as an anti-psychotic 637
in nausea and vomiting 186
Trifluperidol 637
Triglycerides *see* Blood fats
Tri-iodothyronine
in Raynaud's disease 360
in underactive thyroid 856
Trilisate 452
Trilostane 829
Triludan 95
Trimeprazine 94
in eczema 1024
in itching 1034
Trimetaphan 302, 313
Trimethoprim 769, 770, 771
in bronchitis 734
in eye infections 526
Trimipramine 600
Trimopan 771
Trimovate 988
Trinordiol 914
TriNovum 914
TriNovum ED 914
Triogesic 37
Triominic 37
Triperidol 637
Triple vaccine 116
Triplopen 745
Triprolidine 94
Triptafen 600
Trisequens 941
Trisilate 442
Trobicin 764
Trophic ulcers *see* Bedsores
Tropicamide 17, 525, 530
Tropium 625
Trosyl 782, 992
Tryptizol 499, 600
Tryptophan 598
TSH *see* Thyroid stimulating hormone
Tubarine 20
Tuberculin PPD *see* Tuberculin skin test
Tuberculin skin test 774
Tuberculosis 772–8
BCG vaccination against 110–12
isoniazid in prevention 734
skin test 774
Tubocurarine 19
Tuinal 583
Tylex 415
Typhoid vaccine 136–7
Typhus vaccine 137
Typhoid fever 734
Tyrozets 427

Ubretid 500, 501
Ukidan 273, 277, 398
Ulcerative colitis 224–8, 826
Ultradil 984
Ultralanum Plain 984
Ultraproct 427
Ultraviolet radiation 997–8
Uniflu with Gregovite C 37
Unigesic 415
Unigest 199
Unihep 394
Uniparin 394
Uniparin Calcium 394
Uniphyllin 167
Uniroid 427
Unisomnia 583
Univer 280, 305
Urea 317, 978, 980
Uriben 492, 764
Urinary tract, disorders
 of 484–502
 bedwetting 498–500
 cystitis 485, 487, 489
 drugs that may cause
 retention 500
 frequency 494–5
 incontinence 495–8
 infection 484–92
 retention 500–502
 urgency 494–5
Urisal 493
Urispas 495, 497
Urofollitrophin 824, 826, 945
Urokinase 273, 398
Uromide 771
Uromitexan 84, 1060
Ursodeoxycholic acid 251, 252
Ursofalk 251, 252
Urticaria 78, 1048
Uticillin 492
Utovlan 901, 924

Vaccination 109
Vaccines 110–42
 harmful effects and
 warnings 140–41
Vagifem 941
Vaginal disorders 946–9
 bacterial infections 948
 dryness and shrinking 946
 itching of (pruritus
 vulvae) 1033
 preparations used to
 treat 948, 949
 thrush 946
 trichomonal infections 947
Valium 467, 470, 571, 625
Vallergan 95, 1024, 1032
Valoid 186
Valproate (sodium
 valproate) 569, 570, 571
Vanadium 702
Vancocin 764
Vancomycin 762, 764
Vansil 816
Vapour rubs 39
Varicella *see* Chickenpox
Varicose veins
 vitamin C in 685
 vitamin E in 685
Varidase 1017
Vascardin 280, 332
Vascular headaches 430
Vaseline *see* Petroleum jelly
Vasocon A 107, 528
Vasodilators
 in heart failure 325–6
 in hypertension 295
Vasomotor rhinitis *see* Nose
Vasopressin 819, 820
 harmful effects and
 warnings 823–4
 in diabetes insipidus 823, 825
 over-secretion of *see*
 Diabetes insipidus
Vasoxine 26, 336
V-Cil-K 744
Veganin 413
Velbe 1062
Velosef 749
Ventide 168
Ventodisks 167
Ventolin 167, 954
Vepesid 1062
Veracur 1046
Verapamil
 harmful effects and
 warnings 269–70
 in angina 277, 278, 279, 280
 in disorders of heart
 rhythm 349, 350, 351
 in hypertension 302, 303, 304, 305
 in migraine 434, 438
Vercuronium 19
Veripaque 243
Vermox 815
Vertigo 182–6
Vertigon 186
Verucae *see* Warts, plantar
Verucasep 1046
Vi-Siblin 228
Vibramycin 753
Vibrocil 70
Vidarabine 789
 harmful effects and
 warnings 794
 in chickenpox 789
 in herpes infections of the
 eyes 521
 in shingles 792
Vidopen 744
Viloxazine 589, 593, 600
Vinblastine 1062
Vinca alkaloids 1061
Vincent's gingivitis *see*
 Vincent's infection
Vincent's infection 172
Vincent's stomatitis *see*
 Vincent's infection
Vincristine 1062
Vindesine 1062
Vioform-Hydrocortisone 988
Viral infections 788–95
Virazid 789
Virormone 960
Virudox 788
Visclair 51
Viskaldix 308
Visken 280, 305
Vista-Methasone 66, 70, 527
Vista-Methasone N 66, 71, 528
Vitamin A 661
 and libido 972
Vitamin B group 662
Vitamin B (thiamine) 663
Vitamin B_2 *see* Riboflavine
Vitamin B_3 *see* Niacin
Vitamin B_5 *see* Pantothenic
 acid
Vitamin B_6 *see* Pyridoxine
Vitamin B_{12} 667
 anaemia due to deficiency
 of 715–18
Vitamin C 668–9
 in cancer 669
 in colds 41
 in cold sores 669
 in rectal polyps 669
 in wound healing 669
 to acidify the urine 493
 to lower blood
 cholesterol 669
 to stimulate the immune
 system 669
Vitamin D 669–71
 anti-epileptic drugs
 and 670
 in osteoporosis 930
Vitamin D_2 *see* Ergocalciferol
Vitamin D_3 *see* Cholecalciferol
Vitamin E 672
Vitamin H *see* Biotin
Vitamin K 397, 399, 671

Vitamin K – *cont.*
and anti-coagulants 672
Vitamin K_1 671, 672
Vitamin K_2 671
Vitamins 659–85
daily requirements of 674
in tonics 656
multivitamin
preparations 660
Vivalan 600
Volmax 167
Volraman 452
Voltarol 452
Voltarol Emulgel 462
Volumatic 159
Vomiting 175–86
in pregnancy 179–80

Warfarin 385, 393, 394
Warticon 1047
Warts 1046–7
plantar 1046, 1047
vitamin E in 685
Waxes 978
Waxsol 62
Welldorm 583
Wellferon 1063
Whitfield's ointment 1013
Whooping cough
vaccine 128–30
Wool fat 978
Wound healing
vitamin A in 685
vitamin C in 685
vitamin E in 685
zinc in 685
Wright's Vaporizing
Fluid 41, 996

Xamoterol 25, 326, 336
Xanax 625
Xanthines *see* Theophyl-line, 149
Xanthine-oxidase inhibitor *see* Allopurinol
Xipamide
in heart failure 328
in hypertension 303
Xylocaine 427, 494
Xylocard 351, 427
Xylometazoline 25, 36, 70
Xyloproct 427

Yeast 657
Yellow fever vaccine 137
Yomesan 816
Yutopar 954

Zaditen 167
Zadstat 765, 950
Zantac 208
Zarontin 571
Zefringe 415
Zenoxone 982
Zestril 304, 332
Zidovudine 789
harmful effects and
warnings 795
in AIDS 515
ZIG *see* Varicella-zoster
immunoglobulin
Zimovane 583
Zinacef 749
Zinamide 778
Zinc 702
in acne 1010
in osteoporosis 930
Zinc oxide
in dusting powders 979
Zinc pyrithione *see* Pyrithione
zinc shampoo
Zinc sulphate eye drops 524, 526
Zineryt 1009
Zinnat 749
Zirtek 95
Zocor 378
Zoladex 1065, 1066
Zopiclone 580, 583
Zovirax 172, 527, 788
Zuclopenthixol 636
Zyloric 483

FOR THE BEST IN PAPERBACKS, LOOK FOR THE 

In every corner of the world, on every subject under the sun, Penguin represents quality and variety – the very best in publishing today.

For complete information about books available from Penguin – including Puffins, Penguin Classics and Arkana – and how to order them, write to us at the appropriate address below. Please note that for copyright reasons the selection of books varies from country to country.

In the United Kingdom: Please write to *Dept E.P., Penguin Books Ltd, Harmondsworth, Middlesex, UB7 0DA.*

If you have any difficulty in obtaining a title, please send your order with the correct money, plus ten per cent for postage and packaging, to *PO Box No 11, West Drayton, Middlesex*

In the United States: Please write to *Dept BA, Penguin, 299 Murray Hill Parkway, East Rutherford, New Jersey 07073*

In Canada: Please write to *Penguin Books Canada Ltd, 2801 John Street, Markham, Ontario L3R 1B4*

In Australia: Please write to the *Marketing Department, Penguin Books Australia Ltd, P.O. Box 257, Ringwood, Victoria 3134*

In New Zealand: Please write to the *Marketing Department, Penguin Books (NZ) Ltd, Private Bag, Takapuna, Auckland 9*

In India: Please write to *Penguin Overseas Ltd, 706 Eros Apartments, 56 Nehru Place, New Delhi, 110019*

In the Netherlands: Please write to *Penguin Books Netherlands B.V., Postbus 195, NL–1380AD Weesp*

In West Germany: Please write to *Penguin Books Ltd, Friedrichstrasse 10–12, D–6000 Frankfurt/Main 1*

In Spain: Please write to *Alhambra Longman S.A., Fernandez de la Hoz 9, E–28010 Madrid*

In Italy: Please write to *Penguin Italia s.r.l., Via Como 4, I-20096 Pioltello (Milano)*

In France: Please write to *Penguin Books Ltd, 39 Rue de Montmorency, F-75003 Paris*

In Japan: Please write to *Longman Penguin Japan Co Ltd, Yamaguchi Building, 2–12–9 Kanda Jimbocho, Chiyoda-Ku, Tokyo 101*

PENGUIN HEALTH

Audrey Eyton's F-Plus Audrey Eyton

'Your short cut to the most sensational diet of the century' – *Daily Express*

Baby and Child Penelope Leach

A beautifully illustrated and comprehensive handbook on the first five years of life. 'It stands head and shoulders above anything else available at the moment' – Mary Kenny in the *Spectator*

Woman's Experience of Sex Sheila Kitzinger

Fully illustrated with photographs and line drawings, this book explores the riches of women's sexuality at every stage of life. 'A book which any mother could confidently pass on to her daughter – and her partner too' – *Sunday Times*

A Guide to Common Illnesses Dr Ruth Lever

The complete, up-to-date guide to common complaints and their treatment, from causes and symptoms to cures, explaining both orthodox and complementary approaches.

Living with Alzheimer's Disease and Similar Conditions
Dr Gordon Wilcock

This complete and compassionate self-help guide is designed for families and carers (professional or otherwise) faced with the 'living bereavement' of dementia. With clear information and personal case histories, Dr Wilcock explains the brain's ageing process and shows how to cope with the physical and behavioural problems resulting from dementia.

Living with Stress Cary L. Cooper, Rachel D. Cooper and Lynn H. Eaker

Stress leads to more stress, and the authors of this helpful book show why low levels of stress are desirable and how best we can achieve them in today's world. Looking at those most vulnerable, they demonstrate ways of breaking the vicious circle that can ruin lives.

PENGUIN HEALTH

Living with Asthma and Hay Fever John Donaldson

For the first time, there are now medicines that can prevent asthma attacks from taking place. Based on up-to-date research, this book shows how the majority of sufferers can beat asthma and hay fever and lead full and active lives.

Anorexia Nervosa R. L. Palmer

Lucid and sympathetic guidance for those who suffer from this disturbing illness, and for their families and professional helpers, given with a clarity and compassion that will make anorexia more understandable and consequently less frightening for everyone involved.

Medicines: A Guide for Everybody Peter Parish

This sixth edition of a comprehensive survey of all the medicines available over the counter or on prescription offers clear guidance for the ordinary reader as well as invaluable information for those involved in health care.

Pregnancy and Childbirth Sheila Kitzinger

A complete and up-to-date guide to physical and emotional preparation for pregnancy – a must for all prospective parents.

Miscarriage Ann Oakley, Ann McPherson and Helen Roberts

One million women worldwide become pregnant every day. At least half of these pregnancies end in miscarriage or stillbirth. But each miscarriage is the loss of a potential baby, and that loss can be painful to adjust to. Here is sympathetic support and up-to-date information on one of the commonest areas of women's reproductive experience.

The Parents' A to Z Penelope Leach

For anyone with children of 6 months, 6 years or 16 years, this guide to all the little problems involved in their health, growth and happiness will prove reassuring and helpful.

PENGUIN HEALTH

Fighting Food Marilyn Lawrence and Mira Dana

Fighting Food explains how society, the media and the family contribute to the suppression of women's needs which can result in a range of serious eating disorders. The authors also clarify the three main kinds – anorexia, bulimia and compulsive eating – demonstrating the links between them and discussing the best methods of treatment.

Medicine The Self-Help Guide
Professor Michael Orme and Dr Susanna Grahame-Jones

A new kind of home doctor – with an entirely new approach. With a unique emphasis on self-management, *Medicine* takes an *active* approach to drugs, showing how to maximize their benefits, speed up recovery and minimize dosages through self-help and non-drug alternatives.

Defeating Depression Tony Lake

Counselling, medication and the support of friends can all provide invaluable help in relieving depression. But if we are to combat it once and for all we must face up to perhaps painful truths about our past and take the first steps forward that can eventually transform our lives. This lucid and sensitive book shows us how.

Freedom and Choice in Childbirth Sheila Kitzinger

Undogmatic, honest and compassionate, Sheila Kitzinger's book raises searching questions about the kind of care offered to the pregnant woman – and will help her make decisions and communicate effectively about the kind of birth experience she desires.

Care of the Dying Richard Lamerton

It is never true that 'nothing more can be done' for the dying. This book shows us how to face death without pain, with humanity, with dignity and in peace.